Clinical Drug Therapy

Rationales for Nursing Practice

Fifth Edition

Clinical Drug Therapy

Rationales for Nursing Practice

Fifth Edition

Anne Collins Abrams, R.N., M.S.N.

Associate Professor
Department of Baccalaureate and Graduate Nursing
College of Allied Health and Nursing
Eastern Kentucky University
Richmond, Kentucky

Consultant
Tracey L. Goldsmith, Pharm.D.

Clinical Manager
Department of Pharmacy Services
Hermann Hospital
Houston, Texas

Lippincott
Philadelphia • New York

Acquisitions Editor: Margaret Zuccarini
Assistant Editor: Sara Lauber
Project Editor: Sandra Cherrey Scheinin
Production Manager: Helen Ewan
Production Coordinator: Nannette Winski
Design Coordinator: Kathy Kelley-Luedtke

Fifth Edition

9 8 7 6 5 4 3 2

Library of Congress Cataloging in Publications Data

Abrams, Anne Collins.
     Clinical drug therapy : rationales for nursing practice / Anne
Collins Abrams ; consultant, Tracey L. Goldsmith. — 5th ed.
        p.   cm.
     Includes bibliographical references and index.
     ISBN 0-397-55372-2
     1. Chemotherapy.   2. Drugs.   3. Nursing.   I. Goldsmith, Tracey L.
II. Title.
     [DNLM: 1. Drugs—nurses' instruction.   2. Drug Therapy—nurses'
instruction.   3. Nursing Process.   QV 55 A161c 1998]
RM262.A27   1998
615.5'8—dc21
DNLM/DLC
for Library of Congress   97-23562
                                                                                            CIP

Care has been taken to confirm the accuracy of the information presented and to describe generally accepted practices. However, the authors, editors, and publisher are not responsible for errors or omissions or for any consequences from application of the information in this book and make no warranty, express or implied, with respect to the contents of the publication.

The authors, editors, and publisher have exerted every effort to ensure that drug selection and dosage set forth in this text are in accordance with current recommendations and practice at the time of publication. However, in view of ongoing research, changes in government regulations, and the constant flow of information relating to drug therapy and drug reactions, the reader is urged to check the package insert for each drug for any change in indications and dosage and for added warnings and precautions. This is particularly important when the recommended agent is a new or infrequently employed drug.

Some drugs and medical devices presented in this publication have Food and Drug Administration (FDA) clearance for limited use in restricted research settings. It is the responsibility of the health care provider to ascertain the FDA status of each drug or device planned for use in their clinical practice.

Preface

Purpose

The basic precepts underlying the previous editions of *Clinical Drug Therapy* continued to guide the writing of this fifth edition. The overall purpose is to promote safe, effective, and rational drug therapy by:

- Providing essential information that accurately reflects current practices in drug therapy
- Facilitating the acquisition, comprehension, and application of knowledge related to drug therapy. Application requires knowledge about the drug and the client receiving it.
- Identifying knowledge and skills the nurse can use to smooth the interface between a drug and the client receiving it.

Goals and Responsibilities of Nursing Care Related to Drug Therapy

- Preventing the need for drug therapy, when possible, by promoting health and preventing conditions that require drug therapy
- Using appropriate and effective nonpharmacologic interventions instead of, or in conjunction with, drug therapy when indicated. When used with drug therapy, such interventions may promote lower drug dosage, less frequent administration, and fewer adverse effects.
- Enhancing therapeutic effects by administering drugs accurately and considering clients' individual characteristics that influence responses to drug therapy.
- Preventing or minimizing adverse drug effects by knowing the major adverse effects associated with particular drugs, identifying clients with characteristics that may increase risks of experiencing adverse effects, and actively monitoring for the occurrence of adverse effects. When adverse effects occur, early recognition allows interventions to

minimize their severity. Because all drugs may cause adverse effects, nurses must maintain a high index of suspicion that symptoms, especially new ones, may be drug-induced.

- Teaching clients and caregivers accurate administration of medications, nonpharmacologic treatments to use with or instead of pharmacologic treatments, and when to contact a health care provider.

Organizational Framework

The content of *Clinical Drug Therapy* is organized into 11 sections, primarily by therapeutic drug groups and their effects on particular body systems. This approach helps the student make logical connections between major drug groups and the conditions for which they are used. It also provides a foundation for learning about new drugs, most of which fit into known groups.

The first section contains the basic information required to learn, understand, and apply drug knowledge in patient care. These chapters include drug names, laws and standards, schedules of controlled substances, cellular physiology, cellular response to injury (Chapter 1); pharmacokinetics, the receptor theory of drug action, factors that influence drug effects on body tissues (Chapter 2); dosage forms and routes and methods of accurate drug administration (Chapter 3); and guidelines for using the nursing process in drug therapy and general principles of drug therapy (Chapter 4).

Most drug sections include a chapter that reviews the physiology of a body system and several chapters that discuss drug groups used to treat disorders of that body system. The seven physiology review chapters are designed to facilitate understanding of drug effects on a body system. These include the central nervous (CNS), the autonomic nervous (ANS); and the endocrine, immune, respiratory, cardiovascular, and digestive systems. The chapters within each section emphasize therapeutic classes of drugs and prototypical or commonly used individual drugs. Drug chapter content includes a description of a condition for which a drug group is used; a general description of a drug group, including mechanism(s) of action, indications for use, and contraindications; and monographs or tables of individual drugs, with recommended dosages and routes of administration.

Additional clinically relevant information is presented under the headings of Nursing Process, Principles of Therapy, and Nursing Actions. Nursing process content emphasizes the importance of the nursing process in drug therapy, including assessment of the client's condition in relation to the drug group, nursing diagnoses, expected outcomes in terms of client characteristics, interventions and teaching indicated, and evaluation of the client's progress toward expected outcomes. Client teaching is separated from other interventions to emphasize its importance. Principles of therapy include client-related and drug-related factors that influence choices of drugs, dosages, and routes of administration. Each drug chapter includes a nursing actions table that states specific nursing responsibilities within the following categories: *Administer accurately, Observe for therapeutic effects, Observe for adverse effects, Observe for drug interactions*, and *Teach clients*.

Three sections include nutritional products, drugs used to treat infections, and drugs used to treat neoplastic, ophthalmic, and dermatologic disorders.

Important Features Continued From Previous Editions

- **Readability**. Since the first edition of *Clinical Drug Therapy* was published in 1983, many students and faculty have commented about the book's clear presentation style.
- **Organizational framework**. This allows the book to be used effectively as both a textbook and as a reference. As a textbook, students can read chapters in their entirety to learn the characteristics of major drug classes, their prototypical drugs or commonly-used representatives, their uses and effects in prevention or treatment of disease processes, and their implications for nursing practice. As a reference book, students can readily review selected topics for clinical laboratory practice or clinical nursing courses. Specific features that facilitate such uses include a consistent format and frequent headings that allow the reader to identify topics at a glance.
- **Extensive index**. Listings of generic and trade names of drugs, nursing process, and other topics provide rapid access to desired information.
- **Emphasis on FDA-approved therapeutic drugs**. Drugs used to treat common disorders and which are likely to be encountered in clinical nursing practice are presented.
- **Principles of therapy**. This presents guidelines for individualizing drug therapy in specific populations, particularly in children and older adults.

General principles about drug usage in children and older adults are included in Chapter 4; specific principles related to drug groups are included in the chapters where those drug groups are discussed. This approach, rather than separate chapters on pediatric and geriatric pharmacology, was chosen because knowledge about a drug is required before that knowledge can be applied to a specific population with distinctive characteristics and needs in relation to drug therapy.

- **Nursing Action Tables**. These emphasize nursing process before, during, and after drug therapy. The inclusion of rationales for nursing actions provides a strong knowledge base and scientific foundation.
- **Client teaching focus**. This promotes active and knowledgeable client participation in drug therapy regimens.
- **Review and Application Exercises**. These encourage students to test themselves in chapter content.
- **Appendices**. Included in these are Canadian drug names, Canadian drug laws and standards, the International System of Units (SI units), and selected miscellaneous drugs.

New Content in the Fifth Edition

- **Updated drug information.** Approximately 120 new drugs have been added. Many of these are additions to well-known drug groups (*e.g.*, cephalosporin and fluoroquinolone antibacterials, angiotensin converting enzyme inhibitors). However, several drugs represent significant advances in the drug therapy of some disease processes and some new drug groups. For type II diabetes mellitus (Chapter 27), two alpha-glucosidase inhibitors, a newer biguanide, and a drug that increases sensitivity of body tissues to insulin (called an insulin enhancer or an insulin resistance reducing agent) create exciting possibilities for better glycemic control with less hypoglycemia. For hypertension (Chapter 55), angiotensin II receptor antagonists offer considerable promise. For asthma (Chapter 47), leukotriene inhibitors prevent or reduce inflammation, the main pathophysiologic component of the disease, rather than simply treating symptoms. For many people with human immunodeficiency virus (HIV) infection (Chapter 39), multidrug regimens that include protease inhibitors greatly improve quality and quantity of life.

Combinations of drugs are increasingly being used. With type II diabetes mellitus, insulin and oral agents and combinations of oral agents are being used with reported success. For hypertension, the newest combination fixed-dose products contain an angiotensin converting enzyme (ACE) inhibitor and a calcium channel blocker. For HIV infection, the most effective treatment is concurrent administration of two or three drugs that act against the causative retrovirus.

In addition, several discontinued (by manufacturers), obsolete, or rarely used drugs have been deleted.

- **Major revision of most chapters.** Chapter revisions reflect current practices in drug therapy, integrate new drugs, explain the major characteristics of new drug groups, and present content in a clear, meaningful and visually-interesting way. For example:
  - Chapter 5 contains more information about the CNS neurotransmitters and receptors that form neurotransmission systems. This material is especially pertinent to the study of antipsychotic (Chapter 9) and antidepressant (Chapter 10) drugs, because the drugs act to normalize abnormal neurotransmission systems.
  - Chapter 33 includes more information about antibiotic-resistant microorganisms.
  - Chapter 38 features more information about multidrug resistant tuberculosis (MDR-TB).
  - Chapter 39 reflects "state-of-the-art" treatment of common viral infections, including acquired immunodeficiency syndrome (AIDS).
  - Chapter 64 contains several "cytoprotective" drugs that prevent or reduce some serious adverse effects of cytotoxic antineoplastic drugs.
- **Reorganization of chapters.** The total number of chapters has been reduced from 70 to 67. Chapter 1 was divided into two chapters because of its length. The previous Chapter 7 (Sedative-Hypnotics) and Chapter 8 (Antianxiety Drugs) are now combined in Chapter 8. This change decreases the emphasis on barbiturates, which are important historically but infrequently used in current practice, and increases the emphasis on benzodiazepines, which are commonly used for numerous purposes.
  - The most extensive reorganization involves the antimicrobial chapters. Now, all of the beta-lactam antibiotics (penicillins, cephalosporins, carbapenems, and a monobactam) are included in Chapter 34 and the fluoroquinolones are included with the aminoglycosides in Chapter 35 to reflect their increasing use and clinical importance.

New Features

- **New illustrations** include protein binding (Chapter 2), insulin secretion and interaction with insulin receptors in normal glucose metabolism

(Chapter 27), and the development of re-entry cardiac arrhythmias (Chapter 52).
- **New tables,** include aminoglycosides and fluoroquinolones (Chapter 35), antiarrhythmic drugs (Chapter 52), and cytoprotective drugs (Chapter 64).
- **Home care heading,** in the Principles section, expands the areas of nursing responsibility to the home care setting.
- **Visually attractive icons** highlight a range of features:

 Home Care

 Teach Clients

 Review and Application Exercises

- **Chapter opener pedagogy** include a list of terms, learning objectives, and a chapter outline to focus the student's attention on important chapter content.

Ancillary Teaching–Learning Aids

Nursing students must develop skills in critical thinking, information processing, decision making, collaboration, and problem solving. How can a teacher assist the student to develop these skills in relation to drug therapy? The goal of the ancillary package is to assist both student and teacher in this development. The following beliefs, concepts, and principles guided preparation of the materials:

- **Learning** is an active process of becoming informed or gaining knowledge through study and experience. Learning requires thinking about the material to be learned and manipulating it in ways to make the material meaningful to oneself. Thinking is a cognitive skill characterized by formulating ideas in the mind and considering them in relation to previous knowledge and experience. Just like psychomotor skills, cognitive skills can be enhanced by practice. Specific techniques include silent review and thinking about information; writing notes about text or lecture material; paraphrasing, summarizing, or self-questioning, (mentally, verbally, or in writing); completing written worksheets, learning exercises and projects; and verbally questioning others or discussing the material with other students or faculty.
- **Teaching** is promoting learning. Specific techniques include providing information or knowledge; providing or assisting the student to find

sources of information; giving instructions; varying teaching strategies to accommodate different learning styles; providing opportunities to work independently and with others; providing examples that relate the material being studied to actual or anticipated "real-life" experiences; providing experience and practice in solving problems; and providing experience and practice in developing critical thinking skills.

- **Critical thinking** is thoughtful, reasoned judgment based on appropriate collection and analysis of data. Data collection is guided by a strong knowledge base and sufficient depth and breadth of information to adequately reflect a given situation. Analysis of data requires application of knowledge and use of appropriate resources when additional information is needed. Critical thinking requires evidence to support its conclusions; it is not based on assumptions, uninformed opinions, superficial memorization of facts, or routines and rituals.

The student manual aims to engage the student's interest and active participation by providing a variety of learning exercises and opportunities to practice cognitive skills. Worksheets related to each chapter of the text (*e.g.*, matching and completion exercises; crossword puzzles) promote initial learning and review of terms, concepts, principles, and characteristics and uses of major drug groups. The worksheets can be completed independently or assigned and removed for review by the instructor. Clinical scenarios or case studies promote appropriate data collection, critical analysis of both drug-related and client-related data, and application of the data in patient care.

The instructor's manual facilitates use of the text in designing and implementing courses of study, whether in separate pharmacology courses or in nursing courses with integrated pharmacology. To fulfill this purpose, classroom and clinical teaching strategies are stated for each chapter of the text. The test bank portion assists the instructor in evaluating students' knowledge of drug information and their ability to apply that information in client care. The multiple choice test items, stated for each chapter of the text, follow the format of NCLEX. From these materials, each instructor can choose those relevant to his or her circumstances.

Anne Collins Abrams, RN, MSN

Contents

Section I

Introduction to Drug Therapy

1 Introduction to Pharmacology

Objectives

After studying this chapter, the student will be able to:

1 Differentiate between pharmacology and drug therapy.

2 Differentiate between generic and trade names of drugs.

3 Define a prototypical drug.

4 Select authoritative sources of drug information.

5 Differentiate the main categories of controlled substances in relation to therapeutic use and potential for abuse.

6 Discuss the role of the Food and Drug Administration.

7 Describe characteristics of normal cells in relation to drug therapy.

8 Describe cellular responses to injury, including inflammation.

Key Terms

Biotechnology	**Prostaglandins**
Drug therapy	**Prototype**
Generic name	**Scheduled drugs**
Inflammatory mediators	**Systemic effects**
Leukotrienes	**Trade name**
Pharmacology	

Pharmacology is the study of drugs (chemicals) that alter functions of living organisms. Drug therapy involves the use of drugs to prevent, diagnose, or cure disease processes or to relieve signs and symptoms without curing the underlying disease. When prevention or cure is not a reasonable goal, relief of symptoms can greatly improve quality of life and ability to function in activities of daily living. Drugs given for therapeutic purposes are usually called medications.

Drugs may be given for local or systemic effects. Drugs that have local effects, such as dermatologic preparations and local anesthetics, act mainly at the site of application. Those that have systemic effects are absorbed into the bloodstream and circulated to various parts of the body. Most drugs are given for their systemic effects.

Sources of Drugs

Historically, drugs were mainly derived from plants (*e.g.*, morphine), animals (*e.g.*, insulin), and minerals (*e.g.*, iron). Now most drugs are synthetic chemical compounds manufactured in laboratories. Technologic advances have enabled production of synthetic versions of many drugs originally derived from plants and animals, as well as new drugs. Synthetic drugs are more standardized in chemical characteristics, more consistent in their effects, and less likely to produce allergic reactions. Semisynthetic drugs (*e.g.*, many antibiotics) are naturally occurring substances that have been chemically modified.

Biotechnology (also called recombinant deoxyribonucleic acid [DNA] technology and genetic engineering) is increasing in importance as a source of drugs. This technology includes methods for manipulating DNA and ribonucleic acid (RNA) and recombining genes into hybrid molecules that can be inserted into living organisms (*Escherichia coli* bacteria are often used) and repeatedly reproduced. Each hybrid molecule produces a genetically identical molecule, called a clone. Cloning makes it possible to identify the DNA sequence in a gene and produce the protein product encoded by a gene, including insulin and several other body proteins. Cloning also allows production of the relatively large amounts needed for therapeutic or research purposes.

Drug Nomenclature

Drugs are classified according to their effects on particular body systems, their therapeutic uses, and their chemical characteristics. For example, morphine can be classified as a central nervous system (CNS) depressant, a narcotic analgesic, and an opiate. Individual drugs that represent groups of drugs are called *prototypes*. Morphine is the prototype of narcotic analgesics and is the standard with which other narcotic analgesics are compared. Drug classifications and prototypes are extremely stable, and most new drugs can be assigned to a group and compared with an established prototype.

Individual drugs may have several different names, but the two most commonly used are the generic name and the trade name. The *generic name* (*e.g.*, amoxicillin) is related to the chemical or official name and is independent of the manufacturer. The generic name often indicates the drug group (*e.g.*, drugs with generic names ending in "-cillin" are penicillins). The *trade* or *brand name* is designated and patented by the manufacturer. For example, amoxicillin is manufactured by several pharmaceutical companies, each of which assigns a specific trade name, such as Amoxil or Polymox. (Trade names are capitalized; generic names are lower case.) Drugs may be prescribed and dispensed by generic or trade name.

Sources of Drug Information

There are many sources of drug data. Among the most useful are pharmacology textbooks, drug reference books, and journal articles. For the beginning student of pharmacology, a textbook is usually the best source of information because it describes groups of drugs in relation to therapeutic uses. Thus, the student can get an overview of the major drug classifications and their effects. Nursing students usually need textbooks and other references to gain necessary drug knowledge and apply that knowledge to the nursing care of clients.

Drug reference books are most helpful in relation to individual drugs. Two authoritative sources are the *American Hospital Formulary Service* and *Drug Facts and Comparisons*. The former is published by the American Society of Health-System Pharmacists and updated periodically. The latter is published by the Facts and Comparisons division of Lippincott-Raven Publishers and updated monthly (looseleaf edition) or annually (hardbound edition). A widely available but less authoritative source is the *Physicians' Desk Reference* (PDR). The PDR, published yearly, is a compilation of manufacturers' package inserts for selected drugs. In addition, several major publishers of nursing textbooks publish drug reference handbooks, and many pharmacologic, medical, and nursing journals contain information about drugs. Journal articles often present information about drug therapy for clients with specific disease processes and may thereby facilitate application of drug knowledge in clinical practice.

Federal Drug Laws and Standards

Current drug laws and standards have evolved over many years, often as an effort to protect consumers. Although state laws regulate some aspects of drug use and distribution, federal laws regulate most major aspects. The first federal law, the Pure Food and Drug Act of 1906, established official standards and requirements for accurate labeling of drug products. This law was amended in 1912 (Sherley Amendment) to prohibit fraudulent claims of efficacy and in 1914 (Harrison Narcotic Act) to restrict and regulate the importation, manufacture, sale, and use of opium, cocaine, marijuana, and other drugs that the act defined as narcotics.

The next major legal development was passage of the Food, Drug, and Cosmetic Act in 1938. This law was the first to require proof of safety before a new drug could be marketed. One amendment in 1945 required governmental certification of biologic products, such as insulin and antibiotics. A second amendment in 1952 (Durham-Humphrey Amendment) designated drugs that must be prescribed by a physician and dispensed by a pharmacist (prescription drugs). A third amendment in 1962 (Kefauver-Harris Amendment) required proof of effectiveness for drugs to remain commercially available and gave the federal government the authority to standardize drug names. Overall, this law and its amendments regulate the manufacture, distribution, advertising, and labeling of drugs in an attempt to ensure safety and effectiveness. It also confers official status on drugs listed in *The United States Pharmacopeia*. The names of these drugs may be followed by the letters *USP*. Official drugs must meet standards of purity and strength as determined by chemical analysis or animal response to specified doses (bioassay). The Food and Drug Administration (FDA) is charged with enforcing the law. In addition, the Public Health Service regulates vaccines and other biologic products, and the Federal Trade Commission can suppress misleading advertisements of nonprescription drugs.

In 1970, the Comprehensive Drug Abuse Prevention and Control Act was passed. Title II of this law, called the Controlled Substances Act, regulates distribution of narcotics and other drugs of abuse and categorizes these drugs according to therapeutic usefulness and potential for abuse. These categories are described in Box 1-1. In addition to federal laws, state laws also regulate the sale and distribution of controlled drugs.

Additional developments include the Drug Regulation Reform Act of 1978, which shortened the time required for developing and marketing new drugs, and the Orphan Drug Act of 1983, which provided incentives to manufacturers (decreased taxes and competition) for producing drugs to treat certain serious disorders affecting relatively few people.

BOX 1-1. CATEGORIES OF CONTROLLED SUBSTANCES

Schedule I
Drugs that are not approved for medical use and that have high abuse potentials are included in this category (heroin, lysergic acid diethylamide [LSD], peyote, mescaline, tetrahydrocannabinol, marijuana).

Schedule II
These drugs are used medically and have high abuse potentials; abuse may lead to psychological or physical dependence. Included in this group are narcotic analgesics (*e.g.*, codeine, hydromorphone, methadone, meperidine, morphine, oxycodone, oxymorphone), central nervous system (CNS) stimulants (*e.g.*, cocaine, dextroamphetamine, methamphetamine, phenmetrazine, methylphenidate), and barbiturate sedative-hypnotics (amobarbital, pentobarbital, secobarbital).

Schedule III
These drugs have less potential for abuse than those in Schedules I and II. Abuse may lead to psychological or physical dependence. Included are mixtures containing small amounts of controlled substances, such as codeine, barbiturates not listed in other schedules, an antidiarrheal (paregoric), and some CNS stimulants (benzphetamine, phendimetrazine). In addition, male sex hormones (androgens and anabolic steroids) became Schedule III controlled substances in 1991 because of their widespread overuse to enhance athletic prowess and bodybuilding.

Schedule IV
Drugs in this category have some potential for abuse. Included are benzodiazepine antianxiety agents (*e.g.*, chlordiazepoxide, diazepam, lorazepam), benzodiazepine hypnotics (*e.g.*, flurazepam, temazepam); other sedative-hypnotics (phenobarbital, chloral hydrate), and some prescription appetite suppressants (diethylpropion, fenfluramine, mazindol, phentermine).

Schedule V
These products contain moderate amounts of controlled substances. They may be dispensed by the pharmacist without a physician's prescription but with some restrictions regarding amount, recordkeeping, and other safeguards. Included are antidiarrheal drugs, such as diphenoxylate and atropine (Lomotil).

DRUG APPROVAL PROCESSES

The FDA is responsible for approving new drugs and certain other aspects of drug use. The FDA reviews research studies (usually conducted or sponsored by a pharmaceutical company) about proposed new drugs; the organization does not test the drugs.

Before passage of the Food, Drug, and Cosmetic Act and its amendments, many drugs were marketed without confirmation of safety or efficacy. Since 1962, however, newly developed drugs have been extensively tested before being marketed for general use. The drugs are carefully evaluated at each step. Testing usually proceeds if there is evidence of safety and effectiveness but may be stopped at any time for inadequate effectiveness or excessive toxicity. Many potential drugs are discarded and never marketed; a few drugs are marketed but later withdrawn, usually because of adverse effects that become evident only when the drug is used in a large, diverse population.

Testing and Clinical Trials

The testing process begins with animal studies to determine potential uses and effects. The next step involves FDA review of the data obtained in the animal studies. The drug then undergoes clinical trials in humans. Most clinical trials use a randomized, controlled experimental design that involves selection of subjects according to established criteria, random assignment of subjects to experimental groups, and administration of the test drug to one group and a control substance to another group.

In Phase I, a few doses are given to a few healthy volunteers to determine safe dosages, routes of administration, absorption, metabolism, excretion, and toxicity. In Phase II, a few doses are given to a few subjects with the disease or symptom for which the drug is being studied, and responses are compared with those of healthy subjects. In Phase III, the drug is given to a larger and more representative group of subjects with studies designed to reduce bias. In double-blind, placebo-controlled designs, half the patients receive the new drug and half receive a placebo, with neither patients nor researchers knowing who receives which formulation. In crossover studies, subjects serve as their own controls; each subject receives the experimental drug during half the study and a placebo during the other half. Other research methods include control studies, in which some patients receive a known drug rather than a placebo, and subject matching, in which patients are paired with others of similar characteristics. Phase III studies help to determine whether the potential benefits of the drug outweigh the risks.

In Phase IV, the FDA evaluates the data from the first three phases for drug safety and effectiveness, allows the drug to be marketed for general use, and requires manufacturers to continue monitoring the drug's effects. Some adverse drug effects may become evident during the postmarketing phase as the drug is more widely used, especially in women of childbearing age, children, and the elderly, because these groups are often excluded from earlier clinical trials.

FDA Approval

The FDA approves about 20 to 25 new drugs annually. In 1992, procedures were changed to accelerate the approval process, especially for drugs to treat acquired immunodeficiency syndrome (AIDS). Since then, new drugs are categorized according to their review priority and therapeutic potential. "1P" status indicates a new drug reviewed on a priority basis and with some therapeutic advantages over similar drugs already available; "1S" status indicates standard review and drugs with few, if any, therapeutic advantages (*i.e.,* the new drug is similar to one already available).

The FDA also approves transfer of drugs from prescription to nonprescription (over-the-counter or OTC) status. Several drugs have received such approval, including cimetidine (Tagamet), clotrimazole (Gyne-Lotrimin), diphenhydramine (Benadryl), ibuprofen (Advil and others), and miconazole (Monistat 7). For drugs taken orally, indications for use may be different, and recommended doses are usually lower for nonprescription products.

Cellular Physiology

Because all body functions and disease processes and most drug actions take place at the cellular level, cellular physiology will be reviewed here. Each body cell has the capacity to function and respond to injury. Although cells differ in various tissues according to location and function, they have common characteristics as well. For example, all cells normally can exchange materials with their immediate environment to obtain energy from nutrients, synthesize complex molecules, and duplicate themselves. They also can communicate with each other through various body chemicals, such as neurotransmitters and hormones.

Cells (Fig. 1-1) are composed of *protoplasm*, which, in turn, is composed of water, proteins, lipids, carbohydrates, and electrolytes (potassium, magnesium, phosphate, sulfate, and bicarbonate). Within the protoplasm are several structures. The *nucleus* directs cellular activities by determining the type and amount of proteins, enzymes, and other substances to be produced. The *cytoplasm* surrounds the nucleus and contains the working units of the cell. The *endoplasmic reticulum* (ER) contains ribosomes, which synthesize enzymes and

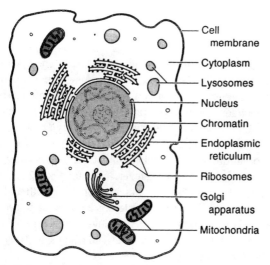

Figure 1-1
Schematic diagram of cell highlighting cytoplasmic organelles.

Labels in figure:
Cell membrane
Cytoplasm
Lysosomes
Nucleus
Chromatin
Endoplasmic reticulum
Ribosomes
Golgi apparatus
Mitochondria

other proteins. These include enzymes that synthesize glycogen, triglycerides, and steroids and those that detoxify drugs and other chemicals. Overall, the ER is important in the production of hormones by glandular cells and the production of plasma proteins and drug-metabolizing enzymes by liver cells.

The *Golgi complex* stores hormones and other substances produced by the ER. It also packages these substances into secretory granules, which then move out of the Golgi complex into cytoplasm and, following an appropriate stimulus, are released from the cell through the process of exocytosis (see below).

Mitochondria generate energy for cellular activities and require oxygen. *Lysosomes* are membrane-enclosed vesicles that contain enzymes capable of breaking down nutrients (proteins, carbohydrates, fats), foreign substances, and the cell itself. During phagocytosis, or when a cell becomes worn out or damaged, the membrane around the lysosome breaks, and the enzymes are released. Thus, lysosomal enzymes are important in the digestion of cellular debris and phagocytized antigens. However, lysosomal contents also are released into extracellular spaces, destroying surrounding cells. They may cause the tissue destruction that sometimes accompanies inflammatory reactions, including rheumatoid arthritis. In addition, the enzymes act on complement to produce component C5a and on kinins to produce bradykinin, both of which are inflammatory mediators (Box 1-2). Normally, the enzymes (proteases) are inactivated by enzyme inhibitors (antiproteases) in serum and synovial fluids, and excessive tissue destruction is prevented.

The *cell membrane* separates intracellular contents from the extracellular environment, provides receptors for hormones and other biologically active substances, participates in electrical events that occur in nerve and muscle cells, and helps regulate growth and proliferation.

Substances enter and leave the cell by several transport mechanisms. In addition to the basic mechanisms (*i.e.*, diffusion, osmosis, facilitated diffusion, and active transport), pinocytosis, phagocytosis, and exocytosis are important in inflammatory and immune processes. *Pinocytosis* involves the ingestion of small amounts of extracellular fluid and dissolved particles and is an important mechanism for the transport of proteins and electrolytes into cells. In this process, the cell membrane engulfs particles and forms a vesicle; the contents are eventually freed by lysosomal or other cytoplasmic enzymes. *Phagocytosis* resembles pinocytosis except that larger indentations occur in the cell membrane; these allow the cell to ingest large particles such as bacteria and cell debris. Microorganisms and particles become attached to phagocytic cells, where they are engulfed and killed or digested. *Exocytosis* is a mechanism for secreting intracellular substances into extracellular spaces. In this process, a fluid-filled sac fuses to the inner side of the cell membrane and opens to the external cell surface, where the contents are released into the extracellular fluid. Exocytosis allows the removal of cellular debris and the release of hormones and other substances synthesized inside the cell.

Cellular Injury and Response to Injury

Cellular injury may be caused by hypoxia, ischemia, microorganisms, chemicals, excessive heat or cold, radiation, and nutritional deficiencies or excesses. Chemicals, including therapeutic drugs, may injure the cell membrane and other cell structures, block enzymatic pathways, coagulate cell proteins (tissues), and disrupt the osmotic and ionic balance of the cell. Such injuries may result from the parent chemical or its metabolites. When cells are injured, the cell accumulates water, fats, and other normal components and excessive amounts or abnormal types of products synthesized within the cell. These reversible changes lead to edema and impaired cellular function. If the damage continues long enough or is not repaired, the changes become irreversible and result in cell death and tissue necrosis.

INFLAMMATORY AND IMMUNE RESPONSES

Cellular response to injury involves inflammation, a generalized reaction to any tissue damage. Inflammation is an attempt to remove the damaging agent and repair the damaged tissue. The hemodynamic aspect of inflammation includes vasodilation, which increases blood supply to the injured area, and increased capillary

BOX 1-2. CHEMICAL MEDIATORS OF INFLAMMATION AND IMMUNITY

Bradykinin is one of the inactive polypeptide kinins present in body fluids. Kinins become physiologically active in the presence of tissue injury. When tissue cells are damaged, white blood cells (WBCs) increase in the area and ingest damaged cells to remove them from the area. When the WBCs die, they release enzymes that activate kinins. The activated kinins increase and prolong the vasodilation and increased vascular permeability caused by histamine. They also cause pain by stimulating nerve endings for pain in the area. Thus, bradykinin may aggravate and prolong the erythema, heat, and pain of local inflammatory reactions. It also increases mucous gland secretion.

Complement is a group of plasma proteins essential to normal inflammatory and immunologic processes. More specifically, complement destroys cell membranes of body cells (*e.g.*, red blood cells, lymphocytes, platelets) and pathogenic microorganisms (*e.g.*, bacteria, viruses). The system is initiated by an antigen–antibody reaction or by tissue injury. Components of the system (called C1 through C9) are activated in a cascade type of reaction in which each component becomes a proteolytic enzyme that splits the next component in the series. Activation yields products with profound inflammatory effects. C3a and C5a, also called anaphylatoxins, act mainly by liberating histamine from mast cells and platelets, and their effects are therefore similar to those of histamine. C3a is the most abundant cleavage product, and it causes or increases smooth muscle contraction, vasodilation, vascular permeability, degranulation of mast cells and basophils, and secretion of lysosomal enzymes by leukocytes. C5a performs the same functions as C3a and also promotes movement of neutrophils and macrophages into the injured area (chemotaxis). In addition, it activates the lipoxygenase pathway of arachidonic acid metabolism (see leukotrienes, below) in neutrophils and macrophages, thereby inducing formation of even more substances that increase vascular permeability and chemotaxis. Thus, C5a is a powerful inflammatory agent.

In the immune response, the complement system breaks down antigen–antibody complexes, especially those in which the antigen is a microbial agent. It enables the body to produce inflammation and localize an infective agent. More specific reactions include increased vascular permeability, chemotaxis, and opsonization (altering a microbe or other antigen so it can be more readily phagocytized).

Cytokines are mediators released by lymphocytes and other body cells in response to antigens. Unlike antibodies, their characteristics are not determined by the antigen that stimulates their production. Cytokines may act on the same cells that produce them, on surrounding cells, or on distant cells (like hormones) if sufficient amounts reach the

bloodstream. Thus, these mediators act locally and systemically to produce inflammatory and immune responses, including increased vascular permeability and chemotaxis of macrophages, neutrophils, and basophils. Two major types of cytokines have been identified, interleukins (produced by leukocytes) and interferons (produced by T lymphocytes or fibroblasts). Interleukin-1 mediates several inflammatory responses, including fever, and interleukin-2 (also called T-cell growth factor) is required for the growth and function of T lymphocytes. Interferons are a group of cytokines that protect nearby cells from invasion by intracellular microorganisms, such as viruses and rickettsiae. They also limit the growth of some cancer cells.

Histamine is stored in most body tissue, mainly in mast cells and basophils. Mast cells are especially abundant in skin and connective tissue. Histamine is discharged from mast cells into the vascular system in response to certain stimuli (*e.g.*, antigen–antibody reaction, tissue injury, extreme cold, and some drugs). Once released, histamine is highly vasoactive, causing vasodilation (increasing blood flow to the area and producing hypotension) and increasing permeability of capillaries and venules (producing edema). Other effects include contracting smooth muscles in the bronchi (producing bronchoconstriction and respiratory distress), gastrointestinal (GI) tract, and uterus; stimulating salivary, gastric, bronchial, and intestinal secretions; stimulating sensory nerve endings to cause pain and itching; and stimulating movement of eosinophils into injured tissue. Histamine is the first chemical mediator released in the inflammatory response and immediate hypersensitivity reactions (anaphylaxis).

When histamine is released from mast cells and basophils, it diffuses rapidly from its area of release into other tissues. It then acts on target tissues through both histamine-1 (H_1) and histamine-2 (H_2) receptors. H_1 receptors are located mainly on smooth muscle cells in blood vessels and the respiratory and GI tracts. When histamine binds with these receptors, resulting events include contraction of smooth muscle, increased venular permeability, production of nasal mucus, stimulation of sensory nerves, pruritus, and vasodilation of capillaries in the skin. H_2 receptors are also located in the airways, GI tract, and other tissues. When histamine binds to these receptors, there is increased secretion of gastric acid by parietal cells in the stomach mucosal lining, increased mucous secretion and bronchodilation in the airways, contraction of esophageal muscles, tachycardia, inhibition of lymphocyte function, and degranulation of basophils (with additional release of histamine and other mediators) in the bloodstream. In allergic reactions, both types of receptors mediate hypotension (in anaphylaxis), skin flushing, and headache. The peak effects of histamine occur within 1 to 2 minutes of its release and may last as

BOX 1-2. (CONTINUED)

long as 10 minutes, after which it is inactivated by histaminase (produced by eosinophils), or N-methyltransferase.

Leukotrienes are a group of chemical mediators formed by the lipoxygenase pathway of arachidonic acid metabolism. Arachidonic acid is a fatty acid released from the phospholipids of cell membranes in response to tissue injury. Leukotrienes help regulate cellular responses to injury, including inflammation. Leukotrienes LTC4, LTD4, and LTE4 (formerly called slow-releasing substance of anaphylaxis or SRS-A because it is released slowly compared with histamine) cause sustained constriction of the bronchioles and are important mediators in bronchial asthma and immediate hypersensitivity reactions (anaphylaxis). The leukotrienes also may increase vascular permeability, extravasation of WBCs, and chemotaxis of neutrophils, basophils, eosinophils, and monocytes.

Prostaglandins are a group of chemical mediators formed by the cyclooxygenase pathway of arachidonic acid metabolism. Prostaglandins are found in virtually all body tissues and act locally in the area where they are produced to regulate many cellular functions before being rapidly inactivated. The specific type of prostaglandin produced and its effects depend on the tissue involved, the stimulus, the hormonal environment, and other factors. In the inflammatory process, prostaglandins cause or potentiate the vasodilation, vascular permeability, pain, and edema caused by other mediators (*e.g.*, bradykinin, histamine) in areas of tissue damage. They also regulate smooth muscle in blood vessels and the GI, respiratory, and reproductive systems; they protect GI mucosa from the erosive effects of gastric acid; they regulate the amount and distribution of renal blood flow; they control platelet function; and they maintain a patent ductus arteriosus in the fetus. More specifically, prostaglandin D_2 causes bronchoconstriction; E_2 causes vasodilation, bronchodilation, increased activity of GI smooth muscle, increased sensitivity to pain, and fever; F_2 causes bronchoconstriction, increased uterine contraction, and increased activity of GI smooth muscle; I_2 (prostacyclin) causes vasodilation and decreased platelet aggregation; and thromboxane A_2 causes vasoconstriction and increased platelet aggregation. Thus, prostaglandins may exert various and opposing effects in different body tissues.

Serotonin (5-hydroxytryptamine or 5-HT) is derived from the essential amino acid tryptophan and found in the brain (where it is an excitatory neurotransmitter), GI tract, and platelets. It is released by platelets activated by blood vessel injury. Its role in inflammatory and immune responses is not well understood. It reportedly causes vasoconstriction.

permeability, which allows fluid to leak into tissue spaces. The cellular aspect involves the movement of leukocytes (white blood cells [WBCs]) into the area of injury. WBCs are attracted to the injured area by bacteria, tissue debris, plasma protein fractions (complement), and other substances in a process called *chemotaxis*. Once they reach the area, they phagocytize causative agents and tissue debris.

Specific WBCs are granulocytes (neutrophils, eosinophils, and basophils) and nongranulocytes (monocytes and lymphocytes). Granulocytes often contain inflammatory mediators or digestive enzymes in their cytoplasm. *Neutrophils*, the body's main defense against pathogenic bacteria, are the major group of leukocytes in the bloodstream. Substances (*e.g.*, complement) released from infected or inflamed tissue cause them to migrate to the affected tissue. There, they localize the area of injury and phagocytize organisms or particles by releasing digestive enzymes and oxidative metabolites that kill engulfed pathogens or destroy other types of foreign particles. Neutrophils usually arrive within 90 minutes of injury, and their numbers increase greatly during the inflammatory process. They have a life span of about 10 hours and must be replaced frequently.

Eosinophils increase during allergic reactions and parasitic infections. In parasitic infections, they bind to and kill the parasites. In hypersensitivity reactions, they produce enzymes that inactivate histamine and leukotrienes (see Box 1-2) and may produce other enzymes that destroy antigen–antibody complexes. Despite these generally beneficial effects, eosinophils also may aggravate tissue damage by releasing cytotoxic substances. *Basophils* release histamine, a major chemical mediator in inflammatory and immediate hypersensitivity reactions.

Nongranulocytes arrive several hours after injury, and monocytes usually replace neutrophils as the predominant WBC within 48 hours. Monocytes are the largest WBCs, and their life span is much longer than that of the granulocytes. Monocytes can phagocytize larger sizes and amounts of foreign material than neutrophils. In addition to their activity in the bloodstream, monocytes can leave blood vessels and enter tissue spaces (then called fixed tissue macrophages), although they can again become mobile and re-enter the bloodstream in some circumstances. Tissue macrophages are widely distributed in connective tissue and other areas (*e.g.*, Kupffer's cells in the liver, alveolar macrophages in the lungs, others in the lymph nodes and spleen) and form the mononuclear macrophage system (formerly called the reticuloendothelial system).

Both mobile and fixed monocytes are important in inflammatory and immune processes as the phagocytic cells digest or encapsulate foreign material and cellular debris. *Lymphocytes* include B cells, which are involved in antibody formation (humoral immunity), and T cells, which are involved in both cell-mediated and humoral immunity. Both types of lymphocytes play major roles in the immune response.

Inflammatory (and immune) responses produce their effects indirectly, through complex and overlapping interactions among cytokines and other chemical mediators. Cytokines are substances produced by WBCs that induce WBC replication, phagocytosis, antibody production, fever, inflammation, and tissue repair (see Chap. 42). Chemical mediators are synthesized or released by mast cells, basophils, and other cells. Once activated, mediators may exert their effects on tissues locally or at distant target sites. They also may induce or enhance other mediators. Histamine and other important mediators are described in Box 1-2.

Characteristics of the Inflammatory Response

Local manifestations of inflammation include erythema, heat, edema, and pain. The erythema and heat result from vasodilation and increased blood supply, and edema results from leakage of blood plasma into the area. Pain is produced by the pressure of edema and secretions on nerve endings and by the chemical irritation of bradykinin, histamine, and other substances released by the damaged cells. Prostaglandins increase the pain and edema caused by other mediators. Systemic manifestations include leukocytosis, increased erythrocyte sedimentation rate, fever, headache, loss of appetite, lethargy, and weakness. Both local and systemic manifestations vary according to the cause and extent of tissue damage. Skeletal muscle may be broken down to provide the amino acids required for the synthesis of substances used to repair injured tissue, such as lymphokines, immunoglobulins, fibroblasts, and collagen.

Inflammation may be acute or chronic. Acute inflammation involves the hemodynamic and cellular responses to injury described previously. It is often precipitated by a self-limited stimulus, such as infection, which is rapidly controlled by host defenses. The inflamed area may heal completely, with the injured

tissue returning to normal or near-normal appearance and function; it may progress and develop a purulent exudate composed of WBCs, proteins, and tissue debris; or it may become chronic.

Chronic inflammation may result from recurrent or progressive episodes of acute inflammation or from a low-grade, smoldering type of tissue response to persistent irritants that cannot penetrate deeply or spread rapidly (*e.g.*, foreign bodies; some viruses and bacteria, such as tuberculosis bacilli; and injured or altered tissue around a tumor or healing fracture). It follows a less consistent pattern, lasts longer (often months or years), and involves fewer neutrophils and more monocytes and lymphocytes in the affected area. It also produces more scar tissue, deformities, and impaired function. Little information is available about the chemical mediators of chronic inflammation, but immunologic mechanisms are thought to play an important role.

REVIEW AND APPLICATION EXERCISES

1. What is the difference between local and systemic effects of drugs?

2. Can a client experience systemic effects of local drugs and local effects of systemic drugs? Why or why not?

3. Why is it helpful for nurses to know the generic names of commonly used medications?

4. Why must nurses understand cellular physiology in relation to drug therapy?

5. How do body cells respond to injury?

6. What roles do histamine and prostaglandins play in the inflammatory process?

SELECTED REFERENCES

Guyton, A.C. & Hall, J.E. (1996). *Textbook of medical physiology*, 9th ed. Philadelphia: W.B. Saunders.

Larocco, M. (1994). Inflammation and immunity. In C.M. Porth, *Pathophysiology: Concepts of altered health states*, 4th ed., pp. 243–264. Philadelphia: J.B. Lippincott.

Nies, A.S. & Spielberg, S.P. (1996). Principles of therapeutics. In J.G. Hardman, L.E. Limbird, P.B. Molinoff, & R.W. Ruddon (Eds.), *Goodman & Gilman's The pharmacological basis of therapeutics*, 9th ed., pp. 43–62. New York: McGraw-Hill.

2 Basic Concepts and Processes

Outline

Objectives

After studying this chapter, the student will be able to:

1 Describe the main mechanisms by which drugs cross biologic membranes and move through the body.

2 Define each process of pharmacokinetics.

3 Describe drug-related factors that influence each pharmacokinetic process.

4 Describe client-related factors that influence each pharmacokinetic process.

5 Discuss drug actions at the cellular level (pharmacodynamics).

6 Describe major characteristics of the receptor theory of drug action.

7 Differentiate between agonist drugs and antagonist drugs.

8 Identify signs and symptoms that may occur with adverse drug effects on major body systems.

Key Terms

Agonist	**Nephrotoxicity**
Agranulocytosis	**Passive diffusion**
Antagonist	**Pharmacodynamics**
Carcinogenicity	**Pharmacokinetics**
Displacement	**Protein binding**
Enzyme induction	**Receptor theory**
Enzyme inhibition	**of drug action**
Hepatotoxicity	**Teratogenicity**
Hypersensitivity	**Tolerance and cross-**
Leukopenia	**tolerance**

Drugs are chemicals that alter basic physiochemical processes in body cells. They can stimulate or inhibit normal cellular functions. To act on body cells, drugs given for systemic effects must reach adequate concentrations in blood and other tissue fluids surrounding the cells. Thus, they must enter the body and be circulated in the bloodstream. After they act on cells, they must be eliminated from the body, as are many other body chemicals. This chapter describes the concepts and processes essential to understanding drug effects.

Mechanisms of Drug Movement

The mechanisms of drug movement are passive diffusion, facilitated diffusion, and active transport.

Passive diffusion, the most common mechanism, involves movement of a drug from an area of higher concentration to one of lower concentration. For example, when an orally administered drug reaches the upper small intestine, its relatively high concentration promotes movement of its molecules into the bloodstream. The blood carries the molecules to other parts of the body; thus, drug concentration in the blood is low compared with that in the intestinal tract. When the drug molecules reach responsive cells, their greater concentration in the blood promotes movement of the drug into the fluids surrounding the cells or into the cells themselves. Passive diffusion continues until a state of equilibrium is reached between the amount of drug in the tissues and the amount in the blood.

Facilitated diffusion is a similar process, except that drug molecules combine with a carrier substance, such as an enzyme or other protein.

In *active transport*, drug molecules are moved from an area of lower concentration to one of higher concentration. This process requires a carrier substance and the release of cellular energy.

Drug movement, and therefore drug action, are affected by a drug's ability to cross cell membranes. For example, a drug given orally must pass through the cell membranes that line the intestinal tract, lymphatic vessels, and capillary walls to reach the bloodstream and circulate through the body. Cell membranes are complex structures composed of lipid and protein. Lipid-soluble drugs cross cell membranes by dissolving in the lipid layer; water-soluble drugs cross cell membranes through pores or channel openings. Lipid-soluble drugs can cross cell membranes more easily than water-soluble ones. Thus, most drugs are lipid-soluble.

Pharmacokinetics

Pharmacokinetics involves drug movement through the body (*i.e.*, "what the body does to the drug"). Specific processes are absorption, distribution, metabolism (biotransformation), and excretion.

ABSORPTION

Absorption is the process that occurs between the time a drug enters the body and the time it enters the bloodstream to be circulated. The rate and extent of absorption are affected by the dosage form of the drug, its route of administration, gastrointestinal function, and other variables. Dosage form is a major determinant of a drug's bioavailability (the amount of drug absorbed into the bloodstream).

Most oral drugs must be swallowed, dissolved in gastric fluid, and reach the small intestine before they are absorbed. Liquid medications are absorbed faster than tablets or capsules because they need not be dissolved. Increases in gastric emptying time and intestinal motility may lead to increased drug absorption by promoting contact with absorptive mucous membrane. However, they also may decrease absorption because some drugs are degraded in gastric fluids, and others may move through the intestinal tract too rapidly to be absorbed. For most drugs, the presence of food in the stomach slows the rate of absorption and may decrease the amount of drug absorbed.

Drugs injected into subcutaneous or intramuscular tissues are usually absorbed more rapidly than oral drugs because they move directly from the injection site to the bloodstream. Absorption is rapid from intramuscular sites because muscle tissue has an abundant blood supply. Because they are placed directly in the bloodstream, drugs injected intravenously bypass the barriers to absorption encountered by other drugs.

Other absorptive sites include the skin, mucous membranes, and lungs. Most drugs applied to the skin are given for local effects (*e.g.*, sunscreens). Systemic absorption is minimal from intact skin but may be considerable when the skin is inflamed or damaged. Also, a number of drugs have been specifically formulated for transdermal systemic absorption (*e.g.*, estrogen, nitroglycerin, scopolamine, clonidine). Some drugs applied to mucous membranes also are given for local effects. However, systemic absorption occurs from the mucosa of the oral cavity, nose, eye, vagina, and rectum. Drugs absorbed through mucous membranes pass directly into the bloodstream. The lungs have a large surface area for absorption of anesthetic gases and a few other drugs.

DISTRIBUTION

Distribution involves the transport of drug molecules within the body. Once a drug is injected or absorbed into the bloodstream, it is carried by the blood and tissue fluids to its sites of pharmacologic action, metabolism, and excretion. Drug molecules enter and leave the bloodstream through the capillaries. Distribution depends largely on the adequacy of blood circulation. Drugs are distributed rapidly to organs receiving a large blood supply, such as the heart, liver, and kidneys. Distribution to other internal organs, muscle, fat, and skin is usually slower.

An important factor in drug distribution is *protein binding* (Fig. 2-1). Most drugs form a complex with plasma proteins, mainly albumin, which act as carriers. Drug molecules bound to plasma proteins are pharmacologically inactive because the large size of the complex prevents their leaving the bloodstream through the small openings in capillary walls and reaching their sites of action, metabolism, and excretion. *Only the free or unbound portion of a drug acts on body cells.* As the free drug acts on cells, the decrease in plasma drug levels causes some of the bound drug to be released. Protein binding allows part of a drug dose to be stored and released as needed. This, in turn, maintains more even blood levels and reduces the risk of drug toxicity.

Protein binding also is the basis for some important drug–drug interactions. A drug with a strong attraction to protein-binding sites may displace a less tightly bound drug. The displaced drug then becomes pharmacologically active, and the overall effect is the same as taking a larger dose of the displaced drug.

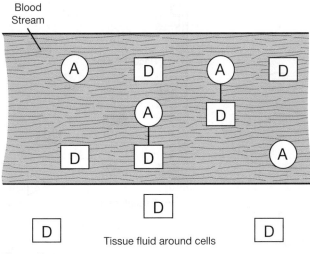

Figure 2-1
Plasma proteins, mainly albumin (A), act as carriers for drug molecules (D). Bound drug (A–D) stays in bloodstream and is pharmacologically inactive. Free drug (D) can leave the bloodstream and act on body cells.

Plasma protein binding is a method by which the body stores drugs. Some drugs also are stored in muscle, fat, or other body tissues and released gradually when plasma drug levels fall. Drugs that are highly bound to plasma proteins or stored extensively in other tissues have a long duration of action.

Drug distribution in the central nervous system (CNS) is unique. Although some drugs with high lipid solubility and other characteristics enter the brain and cerebrospinal fluid readily, many drugs do not because they cannot pass the blood-brain barrier. The blood-brain barrier is composed of capillaries with very tight walls that regulate diffusion of drug molecules from the bloodstream into brain tissue. Generally, this barrier acts as a selectively permeable membrane to protect the CNS. However, it also can make drug therapy of CNS disorders more difficult.

Drug distribution during pregnancy and lactation also is unique (see Chap. 67). During pregnancy, most drugs cross the placenta and may affect the fetus. During lactation, many drugs enter breast milk and may affect the nursing infant.

METABOLISM

Metabolism is the method by which drugs are inactivated or biotransformed by the body. Most often, an active drug is changed into one or more inactive metabolites, which are then excreted. Some active drugs yield metabolites that are also active and that continue to exert their effects on body cells until they are metabolized further or excreted. Other drugs (called prodrugs) are initially inactive and exert no pharmacologic effects until they are metabolized.

Most drugs are lipid-soluble, a characteristic that aids their movement across cell membranes. However, the kidneys, which are the primary excretory organs, can excrete only water-soluble substances. Therefore, one function of metabolism is to convert fat-soluble drugs into water-soluble metabolites.

Most drugs are metabolized by enzymes in the liver (called the microsomal, mixed-function oxidase, or the cytochrome P-450 enzyme system); red blood cells, plasma, kidneys, lungs, and gastrointestinal mucosa also contain drug-metabolizing enzymes. These enzymes, which are complex proteins in structure, catalyze the chemical reactions of oxidation, reduction, hydrolysis, and conjugation with endogenous substances, such as glucuronic acid or sulfate. With chronic administration, some drugs activate the hepatic enzymes, thereby accelerating drug metabolism. In a process called *enzyme induction*, the drugs stimulate liver cells to produce larger amounts of drug-metabolizing enzymes. Larger amounts of the enzymes then allow larger amounts of a drug to be metabolized during a given time. As a result, larger doses of the rapidly metabolized drug may be required to produce therapeutic effects.

Drugs that induce enzyme activity also may increase the rate of metabolism for endogenous steroidal hormones (*e.g.*, cortisol, estrogens, testosterone, and vitamin D). High-protein diets may aid production of drug-metabolizing enzymes. Metabolism also can be decreased or delayed in a process called *enzyme inhibition*, which most often occurs with concurrent administration of two or more drugs that compete for the same metabolizing enzymes. In this case, smaller doses of the slowly metabolized drug may be needed to avoid adverse reactions and toxicity from drug accumulation. The rate of drug metabolism also is reduced in infants because their hepatic enzyme system is immature; in people with impaired blood flow to the liver or severe hepatic or cardiovascular disease; and in people on low-protein diets.

When drugs are given orally, they are absorbed from the gastrointestinal tract and carried to the liver through the portal circulation. Some drugs are extensively metabolized in the liver, with only part of a drug dose reaching the systemic circulation for distribution to sites of action. This phenomenon is called the *first-pass effect*.

EXCRETION

Excretion refers to elimination of a drug from the body. Effective excretion requires adequate functioning of the circulatory system and of the organs of excretion (kidneys, bowel, lungs, and skin). Most drugs are excreted by the kidneys and eliminated unchanged or as metabolites in the urine. Some drugs or metabolites are excreted in bile, then eliminated in feces; others are excreted in bile, reabsorbed from the small intestine, returned to the liver (called *enterohepatic recirculation*), metabolized, and eventually excreted in urine. Some oral drugs are not absorbed and are excreted in the feces. The lungs mainly remove volatile substances, such as anesthetic gases. The skin has minimal excretory function. Factors impairing excretion, especially severe renal disease, lead to drug accumulation and potentially severe adverse reactions if dosage is not reduced.

SERUM HALF-LIFE

Serum half-life, also called *elimination half-time*, is the time required for the serum concentration of a drug to decrease by 50%. It is determined primarily by the drug's rates of metabolism and excretion. A drug with a short half-life requires more frequent administration than one with a long half-life.

When a drug is given at a stable dose, about four or five half-lives are required to achieve steady-state concentrations and develop equilibrium between tissue and serum concentrations. Because maximal therapeutic effects do not occur until equilibrium is established, some drugs are not fully effective for days or weeks. To maintain steady-state conditions, the amount of drug given must equal the amount eliminated from the body. When a drug dose is changed, an additional four to five half-lives are required to re-establish equilibrium; when a drug is discontinued, it is eliminated gradually over several half-lives.

Pharmacodynamics

Pharmacodynamics involves drug actions on target cells and the resulting alterations in cellular biochemical reactions and functions (*i.e.*, "what the drug does to the body").

RECEPTOR THEORY OF DRUG ACTION

Like the physiologic substances (*e.g.*, hormones and neurotransmitters) that normally regulate cell functions, most drugs exert their effects by chemically binding with receptors at the cellular level (Fig. 2-2). Receptors are mainly proteins located on the surfaces of cell membranes or within cells. Specific receptors include *enzymes* involved in essential metabolic or reg-

Figure 2-2
Cell membrane contains receptors for physiologic substances such as hormones (H) and neurotransmitters (NT). These substances stimulate or inhibit cellular function. Drug molecules (Da and Db) also interact with receptors to stimulate or inhibit cellular function.

ulatory processes (*e.g.*, dihydrofolate reductase, acetylcholinesterase), *proteins* involved in transport (*e.g.*, sodium, potassium adenosine triphosphatase) or structural processes (*e.g.*, tubulin), and *nucleic acids* (*e.g.*, DNA) involved in cellular protein synthesis, reproduction, and other metabolic activities.

When drug molecules bind with receptor molecules, the resulting drug–receptor complex initiates physiochemical reactions that stimulate or inhibit normal cellular functions. One type of reaction involves activation, inactivation, or other alterations of intracellular enzymes. Because almost all cellular functions are catalyzed by enzymes, drug-induced changes can markedly increase or decrease the rate of cellular metabolism. For example, an epinephrine–receptor complex increases the activity of the intracellular enzyme adenyl cyclase, which then causes the formation of cyclic adenosine monophosphate (cAMP). The cAMP, in turn, can initiate any one of many different intracellular actions, the exact effect depending on the type of cell.

A second type of reaction involves changes in the permeability of cell membranes to one or more ions. The receptor protein is a structural component of the cell membrane, and its binding to a drug molecule may open or close ion channels. In nerve cells, for example, sodium or calcium ion channels may open and allow movement of the ion or ions into the cell. This usually causes the cell membrane to depolarize and excite the cell. At other times, potassium channels may open and allow movement of potassium ions out of the cell. This action inhibits neuronal excitability and function. In muscle cells, movement of the ions into the cells may alter intracellular functions, such as the direct effect of calcium ions in stimulating muscle contraction.

A third reaction may modify the synthesis, release, or inactivation of the neurohormones (*e.g.*, acetylcholine, norepinephrine, serotonin) that regulate many physiologic processes.

Additional elements and characteristics of the receptor theory include:

1. The site and extent of drug action on body cells are determined primarily by specific characteristics of receptors and drugs. Receptors vary in type, location, number, and functional capacity. For example, many different types of receptors have been identified. Most types occur in most body tissues, such as receptors for epinephrine and norepinephrine (whether received from stimulation of the sympathetic nervous system or administration of drug formulations) and receptors for hormones, including growth hormone, thyroid hormone, and insulin. Some occur in fewer body tissues, such as receptors for opiates and ben-

zodiazepines in the brain and subgroups of receptors for epinephrine in the heart (beta$_1$-adrenergic receptors) and lungs (beta$_2$-adrenergic receptors). Receptor type and location influence drug action. The receptor is often described as a lock into which the drug molecule fits as a key, and only those drugs able to bond chemically to the receptors in a particular body tissue can exert pharmacologic effects on that tissue. Thus, all body cells do not respond to all drugs, even though virtually all cell receptors are exposed to any drug molecules circulating in the bloodstream.

The number of receptor sites available to interact with drug molecules also affects the extent of drug action. It is likely that a minimal number of receptors must be occupied by drug molecules to produce pharmacologic effects. Thus, if many receptors are available but only a few are occupied by drug molecules, few drug effects occur. In this instance, increasing the drug dosage increases the pharmacologic effects. Conversely, if only a few receptors are available for many drug molecules, receptors may be saturated. In this instance, if most or all receptor sites are occupied, increasing the drug dosage produces no additional pharmacologic effect.

Drugs vary even more widely than receptors. Because all drugs are chemical substances, chemical characteristics determine drug actions and pharmacologic effects. For example, a drug's chemical structure affects its ability to reach tissue fluids around a cell and bind with its cell receptors. Minor changes in drug structure may produce major changes in pharmacologic effects. Another major factor is the concentration of drug molecules that reach receptor sites in body tissues. Drug- and patient-related variables that affect drug actions are further described below.

2. When drug molecules chemically bind with cell receptors, pharmacologic effects are agonism or antagonism. *Agonists* are drugs that produce effects similar to those produced by naturally occurring hormones, neurotransmitters, and other substances. Agonists may accelerate or slow normal cellular processes, depending on the type of receptor activated. For example, epinephrine-like drugs act on the heart to increase the heart rate, and acetylcholine-like drugs act on the heart to slow the heart rate; both are agonists. *Antagonists* are drugs that inhibit cell function by occupying receptor sites. This prevents natural body substances or other drugs from occupying the receptor sites and activating cell functions. Once drug action occurs, drug molecules may detach from receptor molecules (*i.e.*, the chemical binding is reversible), return to the bloodstream, and circulate to the liver for metabolism and the kidneys for excretion.

3. Receptors are dynamic cellular components that can be synthesized by body cells and altered by endogenous substances and exogenous drugs. For example, prolonged stimulation of body cells with an excitatory agonist usually reduces the number or sensitivity of receptors. As a result, the cell becomes less responsive to the agonist (a process called receptor desensitization or down-regulation). Prolonged inhibition of normal cellular functions with an antagonist may increase receptor number or sensitivity. If the antagonist is suddenly reduced or stopped, the cell becomes excessively responsive to an agonist (a process called hyperreactivity, supersensitivity, or up-regulation). These changes in receptors may explain why some drugs must be tapered in dosage and discontinued gradually if withdrawal symptoms are to be avoided.

NONRECEPTOR DRUG ACTIONS

Relatively few drugs act by mechanisms other than combining with receptor sites on cells. These include:

1. Antacids, which act chemically to neutralize the hydrochloric acid produced by gastric parietal cells
2. Osmotic diuretics (*e.g.,* mannitol), which increase the osmolarity of plasma and pull water out of tissues into the bloodstream
3. Drugs that are structurally similar to nutrients required by body cells (*e.g.,* purines, pyrimidines) and that can be incorporated into cellular constituents, such as nucleic acids. This interferes with normal cell functioning. Several anticancer drugs act by this mechanism.
4. Metal chelating agents, which combine with toxic metals (*e.g.,* lead) to form a complex that can be more readily excreted.

Variables That Affect Drug Actions

Expected responses to drugs are largely based on those occurring when a particular drug is given to healthy adult males (18–65 years old) of average weight (150 lb [70 kg]). However, other groups of people (*e.g.,* women, children, the elderly, different ethnic or racial groups, and clients with diseases or symptoms for which the drugs are designed to treat) receive drugs and respond differently than healthy adult males. Therefore, some authorities propose that these other groups be included in clinical trials. In any client, however, responses may be altered by both drug- and client-related variables, some of which are described below.

DRUG-RELATED VARIABLES

Dosage

Although the terms *dose* and *dosage* are often used interchangeably, dose usually indicates the amount to be given at one time and dosage refers to the frequency, size, and number of doses. Dosage is a major determinant of drug actions and responses, both therapeutic and adverse. If the amount is too small or administered infrequently, no pharmacologic action occurs because the drug does not reach an adequate concentration at cellular receptor sites. If the amount is too large or administered too often, toxicity (poisoning) may occur. Because dosage includes the amount of the drug and the frequency of administration, overdosage may occur with a single large dose or with chronic ingestion of smaller amounts. Doses that produce signs and symptoms of toxicity are called *toxic doses.* Doses that cause death are called *lethal doses.*

Dosages recommended in drug literature are usually those that produce particular responses in 50% of the people tested. These dosages generally produce a mixture of therapeutic and adverse effects. The dosage of a particular drug depends on many characteristics of the drug (reason for use, potency, pharmacokinetics, route of administration, dosage form, and others) and of the recipient (age, weight, state of health, and function of cardiovascular, renal, and hepatic systems). Thus, the recommended dosages are intended only as guidelines for individualizing dosages.

Route of Administration

Routes of administration affect drug actions and responses largely by influencing absorption and distribution. For rapid drug action and response, the intravenous route is most effective because the drug is injected directly into the bloodstream. For many drugs, the intramuscular route also produces drug action within a few minutes because muscles have an abundant blood supply. The oral route generally produces slower drug action than parenteral routes. Absorption and action of topical drugs vary according to the drug formulation, whether the drug is applied to skin or mucous membranes, and other factors.

Drug–Diet Interactions

Food may alter the absorption of oral drugs. In many instances, food slows the absorption of oral drugs by slowing gastric emptying time and altering gastrointestinal secretions and motility. When tablets or capsules are taken with or soon after food, they dissolve more slowly; therefore, drug molecules are delivered to absorptive sites in the intestine more slowly. Food also may decrease absorption by combining with a drug to form an insoluble drug–food complex. In other instances, however, certain drugs or dosage forms demonstrate enhanced absorption with certain types of meals. For example, a fatty meal increases the absorption of some sustained-release forms of theophylline. Interactions that alter drug absorption can be minimized by spacing food and medications.

In addition, some foods contain substances that react with certain drugs. One such interaction occurs between tyramine-containing foods and monoamine oxidase (MAO) inhibitor drugs. Tyramine causes the release of norepinephrine, a potent vasoconstrictive agent, from the adrenal medulla and sympathetic neurons. Normally, norepinephrine is active for only a few milliseconds before it is inactivated by MAO. However, because MAO inhibitors prevent inactivation of norepinephrine, ingesting tyramine-containing foods with an MAO inhibitor may produce severe hypertension or intracranial hemorrhage. MAO inhibitors include the antidepressants isocarboxazid (Marplan) and phenelzine (Nardil) and the antineoplastic procarbazine (Matulane). Tyramine-rich foods to be avoided by clients taking MAO inhibitors include beer, wine, aged cheeses, yeast products, chicken livers, and pickled herring.

An interaction may occur between oral anticoagulants, such as warfarin (Coumadin), and foods containing vitamin K. Because vitamin K antagonizes the action of oral anticoagulants, large amounts of green leafy vegetables, such as spinach and other greens, may offset the anticoagulant effects and predispose the person to thromboembolic disorders.

A third interaction occurs between tetracycline, an antibiotic, and dairy products, such as milk and cheese. The drug combines with the calcium in milk products to form an insoluble, unabsorbable compound that is excreted in the feces.

Drug–Drug Interactions

The action of a particular drug may be increased or decreased by its interaction with another drug in the body. Most interactions occur whenever the interacting drugs are present in the body; some, especially those affecting the absorption of oral drugs, occur when the interacting drugs are given at or near the same time.

Interactions that can increase the therapeutic or adverse effects of drugs are as follows:

1. *Additive effects* occur when two drugs with similar pharmacologic actions are taken.
   Example: alcohol + sedative drug → increased sedation
2. *Synergism or potentiation* occurs when two drugs with different sites or mechanisms of action produce greater effects when taken together than either does when taken alone.

   Example: acetaminophen (non-narcotic analgesic) + codeine (narcotic analgesic) → increased analgesia
3. *Interference* by one drug with the metabolism or elimination of a second drug may result in intensified effects of the second drug.
   Example: cimetidine (Tagamet) inhibits drug-metabolizing enzymes in the liver and therefore interferes with the metabolism of many drugs (*e.g.*, benzodiazepine antianxiety and hypnotic drugs, calcium channel blockers, tricyclic antidepressants, some antiarrhythmics, beta-blockers and anticonvulsants, theophylline, and warfarin). When these drugs are given concurrently with cimetidine, they are more likely to cause adverse reactions and toxic effects. Cimetidine is a prescription drug for peptic ulcer disease and a nonprescription drug for heartburn.
4. *Displacement* of one drug from plasma protein-binding sites by a second drug increases the effects of the displaced drug. This increase occurs because the molecules of the displaced drug, freed from their bound form, become pharmacologically active.
   Example: aspirin (an anti-inflammatory/analgesic/antipyretic agent) + warfarin (an anticoagulant) → increased anticoagulant effect

Interactions in which drug effects are decreased are grouped under the term antagonism. Examples of such interactions are as follows:

1. In some situations, a drug that is a specific antidote is given to antagonize the toxic effects of another drug.
   Example: naloxone (a narcotic antagonist) + morphine (a narcotic analgesic) → relief of narcotic-induced respiratory depression. Naloxone molecules displace morphine molecules from their receptor sites on nerve cells so that the morphine molecules cannot continue to exert their depressant effects.
2. Decreased intestinal absorption of oral drugs occurs when drugs combine to produce nonabsorbable compounds.
   Example: aluminum or magnesium hydroxide (antacids) + oral tetracycline (an antibiotic) → binding of tetracycline to aluminum or magnesium, causing decreased absorption and decreased antibiotic effect of tetracycline
3. Activation of drug-metabolizing enzymes in the liver increases the metabolism rate of any drug metabolized primarily in the liver. Some anticonvulsants, antitubercular drugs, barbiturates, and antihistamines are known "enzyme inducers."

Example: phenobarbital (a barbiturate) + warfarin (an anticoagulant) → decreased effects of warfarin

4. Increased excretion occurs when urinary pH is changed and renal reabsorption is blocked.

Example: sodium bicarbonate + phenobarbital → increased excretion of phenobarbital. The sodium bicarbonate alkalinizes the urine, raising the number of barbiturate ions in the renal filtrate. The ionized particles cannot pass easily through renal tubular membranes. Therefore, less drug is reabsorbed into the blood and more is excreted by the kidneys.

CLIENT-RELATED VARIABLES

Age

The effects of age on drug action are most pronounced in neonates, infants, and older adults. In children, drug action depends largely on age and developmental stage. During pregnancy, drugs cross the placenta and may harm the fetus. Fetuses have no effective mechanisms for metabolizing or eliminating drugs because their liver and kidney functions are immature. Newborn infants (birth to 1 month) also handle drugs inefficiently. Drug distribution, metabolism, and excretion differ markedly in neonates, especially premature babies, because their organ systems are not fully developed. Older infants (1 month to 1 year) reach approximately adult levels of protein binding and kidney function, but liver function and the blood-brain barrier are still immature.

Children (1–12 years) experience a period of increased activity of drug-metabolizing enzymes so that some drugs are rapidly metabolized and eliminated. Although the onset and duration of this period are unclear, a few studies have been done with particular drugs. Theophylline, for example, is cleared much faster in a 7-year-old child than in a neonate or adult (18–65 years). After about 12 years of age, healthy children handle drugs similarly to healthy adults.

In older adults (65 years and older), physiologic changes may alter all pharmacokinetic processes. Changes in the gastrointestinal tract include decreased gastric acidity, decreased blood flow, and decreased motility. Despite these changes, however, there is relatively little difference in absorption. Changes in the cardiovascular system include decreased cardiac output and therefore slower distribution of drug molecules to their sites of action, metabolism, and excretion. In the liver, there is decreased blood flow and probably a decreased number of metabolizing enzymes. Thus, many drugs are metabolized more slowly, have a longer action, and are more likely to accumulate with chronic administration. In the kidneys, there is decreased blood flow, decreased glomerular filtration rate, and de-

creased tubular secretion of drugs. All of these changes tend to slow excretion and promote accumulation of drugs in the body. Impaired kidney and liver function greatly increase the risks of adverse drug effects. In addition, older adults are more likely to have acute and chronic illnesses that require multiple drugs or long-term drug therapy. Thus, possibilities for interactions among drugs and between drugs and diseased organs are greatly multiplied.

Body Weight

Body weight affects drug action mainly in relation to dose. The ratio between the amount of drug given and body weight influences drug distribution and concentration at sites of action. Generally, people heavier than average need larger doses, provided that their renal, hepatic, and cardiovascular functions are adequate. Recommended doses for many drugs are listed in terms of grams or milligrams per kilogram of body weight.

Genetic and Ethnic Characteristics

Drugs are given to elicit certain responses that are relatively predictable for most drug recipients. However, some persons experience inadequate therapeutic effects, and others experience unusual or exaggerated effects, including increased toxicity. These interindividual variations in drug response are often attributed to genetic or ethnic differences in drug pharmacokinetics or pharmacodynamics. As a result, there is increased awareness that genetic and ethnic characteristics are important factors and that diverse groups must be included in clinical trials.

Pharmacogenetics

Pharmacogenetics is concerned with genetically related variability in responses to drugs. A person's genetic characteristics may influence drug action in several ways. For example, genes determine the types and amounts of proteins produced in the body. When most drugs enter the body, they interact with proteins (*e.g.,* in plasma, tissues, cell membranes, and drug-receptor sites) to reach their sites of action and with other proteins (*e.g.,* drug-metabolizing enzymes in the liver and other organs) to be biotransformed and eliminated from the body. Genetic characteristics that alter any of these proteins can alter drug pharmacokinetics or pharmacodynamics.

One of the earliest pharmacokinetic genetic variations to be identified was the observation that some people taking usual doses of isoniazid (an antitubercular drug), hydralazine (an antihypertensive agent), or procainamide (an antiarrhythmic) lacked therapeutic effects, while other people developed toxicity. Research established that these drugs are normally metabolized by acetylation, a chemical conjugation process in which the drug molecule combines with an acetyl group of acetyl coenzyme A. The reaction is catalyzed by a hepatic drug-metabolizing enzyme called acetyltransferase. It was further established that humans may acetylate the drug rapidly or slowly, depending largely on genetically controlled differences in acetyltransferase activity. Clinically, rapid acetylators may need larger-than-usual doses to achieve therapeutic effects, and slow acetylators may need smaller-than-usual doses to avoid toxic effects. In addition, several genetic variations of the cytochrome P-450 drug-metabolizing system have been identified. Specific variations may influence any of the chemical processes by which drugs are metabolized.

As another example of genetic variation in drug metabolism, some people lack the plasma pseudo-cholinesterase enzyme that normally inactivates succinylcholine, a potent muscle relaxant used in major surgical procedures. These people may experience prolonged paralysis and apnea if given succinylcholine.

Other people are deficient in glucose-6-phosphate dehydrogenase, an enzyme normally found in red blood cells and other body tissues. These people may develop hemolytic anemia when given antimalarial drugs, sulfonamides, analgesics, antipyretics, and other drugs.

Pharmacoanthropology

Pharmacoanthropology is concerned with racial and ethnic differences in responses to drugs. Most drug information has been derived from clinical drug trials using white men; few, if any, subjects of other ethnic groups are included. Interethnic variations became evident when drugs and dosages developed for white people produced unexpected responses, including toxicity, when given to other ethnic groups.

One common interethnic variation is that African-Americans are less responsive to some antihypertensive drugs than are white people. For example, angiotensin-converting enzyme (ACE) inhibitors and beta-adrenergic blocking drugs are less effective as single-drug therapy. Generally, African-American hypertensive patients respond better to diuretics or calcium channel blockers than to ACE inhibitors and beta-blockers. Another interethnic variation is that Asians generally require much smaller doses of some commonly used drugs, including beta-blockers and several psychotropic drugs (*e.g.*, alprazolam, an antianxiety agent, and haloperidol, an antipsychotic). Some documented interethnic variations are included in later chapters.

Gender

Except during pregnancy and lactation, gender has been considered a minor influence on drug action. Almost all research studies related to drugs have in-

volved men, and clinicians have extrapolated the findings to women. Several reasons have been advanced for excluding women from clinical drug trials, including the risks to a fetus if a woman becomes pregnant and the greater complexity in sample size and data analysis. However, because differences between males and females in responses to drug therapy are being identified, the need to include women in drug studies is evident.

Some gender-related differences in responses to drugs may stem from hormonal fluctuations in women during the menstrual cycle. Although this area has received little attention in research studies and clinical practice, altered responses have been demonstrated in some women taking clonidine, an antihypertensive; lithium, a mood-stabilizing agent; phenytoin, an anticonvulsant; propranolol, a beta-adrenergic blocking drug used in the management of hypertension, angina pectoris, and migraine; and antidepressants. For example, women with clinical depression may need higher doses of antidepressant medications premenstrually, when symptoms may exacerbate, and lower doses during the rest of the menstrual cycle.

Another example is that women with schizophrenia require lower dosages of antipsychotic medications than men. If given the higher doses required by men, women are likely to develop adverse drug reactions.

Pathologic Conditions

Pathologic conditions may alter pharmacokinetic processes. All pharmacokinetic processes are decreased in cardiovascular disorders characterized by decreased blood flow to tissues, such as hypotension, shock, low plasma volume, and congestive heart failure. In addition, the absorption of oral drugs is decreased with vomiting, diarrhea, intestinal malabsorption, and other gastrointestinal disorders. Distribution is altered in malnutrition, liver or kidney disease, and other conditions that decrease the number of plasma proteins providing drug-binding sites. Metabolism is decreased in malnutrition (*e.g.*, inadequate protein to synthesize drug-metabolizing enzymes) and severe liver disease; it may be increased in conditions that generally increase body metabolism, such as hyperthyroidism and fever. Excretion is decreased in kidney disease.

Psychological Considerations

Psychological considerations influence individual responses to drug administration, although specific mechanisms are unknown. An example is the "placebo response." A placebo is a pharmacologically inactive substance. Placebos are used in clinical drug trials to compare the medication being tested with a "dummy" medication. Interestingly, recipients often report both therapeutic and adverse effects from placebos.

Attitudes and expectations related to drugs in general, a particular drug, or a placebo influence client response. They also influence compliance or willingness to carry out the prescribed drug regimen, especially with long-term drug therapy.

Adverse Effects of Drugs

As used in this book, the term *adverse effects* refers to any undesired responses to drug administration, as opposed to *therapeutic effects*, which are desired responses. Most drugs produce a mixture of therapeutic and adverse effects; all drugs can produce adverse effects. Adverse effects may produce essentially any sign, symptom, or disease process and may involve any body system or tissue. They may be common or rare, mild or severe and life-threatening, localized or widespread, depending on the drug and the recipient.

Some adverse effects occur with usual therapeutic doses of drugs (often called side effects); others are more likely to occur and to be more severe with high doses. Common or serious adverse effects include the following:

1. *CNS effects* may result from CNS stimulation (*e.g.*, agitation, confusion, delirium, disorientation, hallucinations, psychosis, seizures) or CNS depression (dizziness, drowsiness, impaired level of consciousness, sedation, coma, impaired respiration and circulation). CNS effects may occur with many drugs, including most therapeutic groups, substances of abuse, and over-the-counter preparations.

2. *Gastrointestinal effects* (anorexia, nausea, vomiting, constipation, diarrhea) are among the most common adverse reactions to drugs. Nausea and vomiting occur with many drugs from local irritation of the gastrointestinal tract or stimulation of the vomiting center in the medulla oblongata. Diarrhea occurs with drugs that cause local irritation or increase peristalsis. More serious effects include bleeding or ulceration (most often with aspirin and nonsteroidal anti-inflammatory agents) and severe diarrhea/colitis (most often with antibiotics).

3. *Hematologic effects* (blood coagulation disorders, bleeding disorders, bone marrow depression, anemias, leukopenia, agranulocytosis, thrombocytopenia) are relatively common and potentially life-threatening. Excessive bleeding is most often associated with anticoagulants and thrombolytics; bone marrow depression is usually associated with antineoplastic drugs.

4. *Hepatotoxicity* (hepatitis, hepatic necrosis, biliary tract inflammation or obstruction) is relatively rare but potentially life-threatening. Because most drugs are metabolized by the liver, the liver is especially susceptible to drug-induced injury. Commonly used hepatotoxic drugs include acetaminophen (Tylenol), chlorpromazine (Thorazine), halothane (Fluothane), isoniazid (INH), methotrexate (Mexate), nitrofurantoin (Macrodantin), phenelzine (Nardil) and other MAO inhibitors, phenytoin (Dilantin), and aspirin and other salicylates. In the presence of drug- or disease-induced liver damage, the metabolism of many drugs is impaired. Consequently, drugs metabolized by the liver tend to accumulate in the body and cause adverse effects. Besides actual hepatotoxicity, many drugs produce abnormal values in liver function tests without producing clinical signs of liver dysfunction.

5. *Nephrotoxicity* (renal insufficiency or failure) occurs with several antimicrobial agents (*e.g.*, gentamicin and other aminoglycosides), nonsteroidal anti-inflammatory agents (*e.g.*, ibuprofen and related drugs), and others. It is potentially serious because it may interfere with drug excretion, thereby causing drug accumulation and increased adverse effects.

6. *Hypersensitivity* or *allergy* may occur with almost any drug in susceptible clients. It is largely unpredictable and unrelated to dose. It occurs in those who have previously been exposed to the drug or a similar substance (antigen) and who have developed antibodies. When readministered, the drug reacts with the antibodies to cause cell damage and the release of histamine and other intracellular substances. These substances produce reactions ranging from mild skin rashes to anaphylactic shock. Anaphylactic shock is a life-threatening hypersensitivity reaction characterized by respiratory distress and cardiovascular collapse. It occurs within a few minutes after drug administration and requires emergency treatment with epinephrine, antihistamines, and bronchodilator drugs. Some allergic reactions (*e.g.*, serum sickness) occur 1 to 2 weeks after the drug is given.

7. *Idiosyncrasy* refers to an unexpected reaction to a drug that occurs the first time it is given. These reactions are usually attributed to genetic characteristics that alter the person's drug-metabolizing enzymes.

8. *Drug dependence* may occur with mind-altering drugs, such as narcotic analgesics, sedative-hypnotic agents, antianxiety agents, and amphetamines. Dependence may be physiologic or psychological. Physiologic dependence produces unpleasant physical symptoms when the dose is reduced or the drug is withdrawn. Psychological dependence leads to excessive preoccupation with drugs and drug-seeking behavior. Drug dependence is discussed further in Chapter 15.

9. *Carcinogenicity* is the ability of a substance to cause cancer. Several drugs are carcinogens, including some hormones and anticancer drugs. Carcinogenicity apparently results from drug-induced alterations in cellular DNA.

10. *Teratogenicity* is the ability of a substance to cause abnormal fetal development when given to pregnant women. Drug groups considered teratogenic include analgesics, diuretics, antihistamines, antibiotics, antiemetics, and others.

Tolerance and Cross-Tolerance

Drug *tolerance* occurs when the body becomes accustomed to a particular drug over time so that larger doses must be given to produce the same effects. Tolerance may be acquired to the pharmacologic action of many drugs, especially narcotic analgesics, alcohol, and other CNS depressants. Tolerance to pharmacologically related drugs is called *cross-tolerance*. For example, a person who regularly drinks large amounts of alcohol becomes able to ingest even larger amounts before becoming intoxicated: this is tolerance to alcohol. If the person is then given sedative-type drugs or a general anesthetic, larger-than-usual doses are required to produce a pharmacologic effect: this is cross-tolerance.

Tolerance and cross-tolerance are usually attributed to activation of drug-metabolizing enzymes in the liver; these enzymes accelerate metabolism and excretion of the drug. They also are attributed to decreased sensitivity or numbers of receptor sites. Rapid development of tolerance after only a few doses of a drug is called *tachyphylaxis*.

REVIEW AND APPLICATION EXERCISES

1. What are some factors that decrease absorption of an oral drug?

2. Drug dosage is a major determinant of both therapeutic and adverse drug effects. How can you use this knowledge in monitoring a client's response to drug therapy?

3. Does protein binding speed or slow drug distribution to sites of action?

4. Are drugs equally distributed throughout the body? Why or why not?

5. What are the implications of hepatic enzyme induction and inhibition in terms of drug metabolism and elimination from the body?

6. For a drug in which biotransformation produces active metabolites, is drug action shortened or lengthened? What difference does this make in client care?

7. Which pharmacokinetic processes are likely to be impaired with severe cardiovascular disease and with severe renal disease?

8. What are the main elements of the receptor theory of drug action?

9. When drug–drug interactions occur, are drug actions increased or decreased?

10. Giving the same drug and dosage often results in differences in blood levels and other client responses. What are some reasons for individual differences in responses to drugs?

SELECTED REFERENCES

Benet, L.Z., Kroetz, D.L., & Sheiner, L.B. (1996). Pharmacokinetics: The dynamics of drug absorption, distribution, and elimination. In J.G. Hardman, L.E. Limbird, P.B. Molinoff, & R.W. Ruddon (Eds.), *Goodman & Gilman's The pharmacological basis of therapeutics*, 9th ed., pp. 3–27. New York: McGraw-Hill.

Haken, V. (1996). Interactions between drugs and nutrients. In L.K. Mahan & S. Escott-Stump, *Krause's Food, nutrition, and diet therapy*, 9th ed., pp. 387–402. Philadelphia: W.B. Saunders.

Nies, A.S., & Spielberg, S.P. (1996). Principles of therapeutics. In J.G. Hardman, L.E. Limbird, P.B. Molinoff, & R.W. Ruddon (Eds.), *Goodman & Gilman's The pharmacological basis of therapeutics*, 9th ed., pp. 43–62. New York: McGraw-Hill.

Ross, E.M. (1996). Pharmacodynamics: Mechanisms of drug action and the relationship between drug concentration and effect. In J.G. Hardman, L.E. Limbird, P.B. Molinoff, & R.W. Ruddon (Eds.), *Goodman & Gilman's The pharmacological basis of therapeutics*, 9th ed., pp. 29–41. New York: McGraw-Hill.

Williams, L., Davis, J.A., & Lowenthal, D.T. (1993). The influence of food on the absorption and metabolism of drugs. *Medical Clinics of North America*, 77(4), 815–829.

3 Administering Medications

Outline

Preventing Medication Errors

Medication Systems

Medication Orders

Drug Preparations and Dosage Forms

Calculating Drug Dosages
    commonly used systems of measurement
    mathematical calculations

Routes of Administration
    oral route
    parenteral routes
        drugs for injection
        equipment for injections
        subcutaneous route
        intramuscular route
        intravenous route
        other parenteral routes
    topical routes

Objectives

After studying this chapter, the student will be able to:

1 List the five rights of drug administration.

2 Discuss knowledge and skills needed to implement the five rights.

3 List requirements of a complete drug order or prescription.

4 Accurately interpret drug orders containing common abbreviations.

5 Discuss advantages and disadvantages of oral, parenteral, and topical routes of drug administration.

6 Identify supplies, techniques, and observations needed for safe and accurate administration by different routes.

Key Terms

Enteric-coated	**Topical**
Milliequivalents	**Transdermal**
Parenteral	

Drugs given for therapeutic purposes are usually called *medications*. Giving medications to clients is an important nursing responsibility in many health care settings, including ambulatory care, hospitals, long-term care facilities, and clients' homes. The basic requirements for accurate drug administration are often called the "five rights": giving the right *drug*, in the right *dose*, to the right *client*, by the right *route*, at the right *time*. Each "right" requires knowledge, skills, and specific nursing interventions:

1. Right drug
   a. Interpret the physician's order accurately (*i.e.*, name of drug).
   b. If the drug is unfamiliar, seek information from an authoritative source.
   c. Read labels of drug containers accurately.
   d. Question the prescribing physician about the order if the name of the drug is unclear or if the drug seems inappropriate for the client's condition.
2. Right dose
   a. Interpret abbreviations accurately.
   b. Interpret measurements accurately.
   c. Calculate doses accurately.
   d. Measure doses accurately.
3. Right client
   a. Check identification bands on institutionalized clients.
   b. Verify identity of ambulatory clients.
4. Right route
   a. Use correct techniques for all routes of administration.
   b. Always use appropriate anatomic landmarks to identify sites for intramuscular (IM) injections.
   c. For intravenous (IV) medications, follow manufacturers' instructions for preparation and administration.
5. Right time
   a. Schedule to maximize therapeutic effects and minimize adverse effects.
   b. Omit or delay doses as indicated by the client's condition.

Drug administration in children is potentially more problematic than in most other clients. One reason is that many drugs are prepared in dosage forms and concentrations suitable for adults. This often requires dilution (which may change the drug's stability and compatibility), calculation, preparation, and administration of minute doses (which are more likely to be inaccurate and possibly toxic than standard doses). In addition, children have limited sites for administration of IV drugs, and several may be given through the same site. In many cases, the need for small volumes of fluid precludes extensive flushing between drugs (which may produce undesirable interactions with other drugs and IV solutions).

Preventing Medication Errors

There are several steps and numerous people involved in getting each dose of a medication to the intended client. Each step or person has a potential for contributing to a medication error.

Physicians are usually very knowledgeable about disease processes. However, in relation to drug therapy, they may write orders illegibly; order a drug that is not indicated by the client's condition; fail to order a drug that is indicated; fail to consider the client's age, size, kidney function, liver function, and disease process when selecting a drug or dosage; fail to consider other medications the client is taking, including prescription and over-the-counter drugs; lack sufficient knowledge about the drug; fail to monitor for, or instruct others to monitor for, effects of administered drugs; and fail to discontinue drugs appropriately.

Pharmacists are usually very knowledgeable about drugs and their uses in various situations. However, in many instances, they do not have access to information about individual clients or they are not consulted and involved in patient care. As a result, they may not recognize an inappropriate or erroneous physician's order. They may dispense incorrect medications, mislabel containers, or fail to ask outpatients about other drugs being taken.

Nurses may have inadequate knowledge about a drug or about the client receiving the drug; not follow the "five rights;" not read drug labels sufficiently; give unfamiliar drugs; fail to question the physician's order when indicated; and assume that the physician has ordered and the pharmacist has dispensed the correct medication. In addition, nurses must be able to distinguish among drugs with similar names or similar packaging.

Clients/consumers may take drugs from several physicians; fail to inform one physician about drugs prescribed by another; get prescriptions filled at more than one pharmacy; fail to get prescriptions filled or refilled; underuse or overuse an appropriately prescribed drug; take drugs left over from a previous illness or prescribed for someone else; fail to follow instructions for drug administration or storage; fail to keep appointments for follow-up care; and fail to ask for information about prescribed and unprescribed drugs when needed.

All health care providers involved in drug therapy must be extremely vigilant in all phases of medication administration. The rest of this chapter emphasizes general information needed to fulfill nursing responsibilities related to drug administration.

Medication Systems

Each agency has a system for dispensing drugs. A widely used method is the unit-dose system, in which most drugs are dispensed in single-dose containers. Drug orders are checked by a pharmacist, who then places the indicated number of doses in the client's medication drawer at scheduled intervals. When a dose is due, the nurse removes the medication and takes it to the client. Unit-dose wrappings of oral drugs should be left in place until the medication is given at the client's bedside. Each dose of a drug must be recorded on a medication administration record (MAR), which becomes part of the client's permanent medical record.

Advantages of the unit-dose system include spending less time preparing drugs for administration, being able to identify most drugs until they are administered to the client, and having to calculate fewer doses. The major disadvantage is having to reorder or otherwise obtain a needed dose when it is not available in the client's medication drawer. This may lead to delayed or omitted doses.

Controlled drugs, such as narcotic analgesics, are usually kept as a stock supply in a locked drawer or cabinet and replaced as needed. Each dose is signed out on a special narcotic sheet and recorded on the client's MAR. Each nurse must comply with legal regulations and agency policies for dispensing and recording controlled drugs.

Medication Orders

Nurses administer medications from orders by licensed physicians and dentists. Drug orders should include the full name of the client; the generic or trade name of the drug; the dose, route, and frequency of administration; and the date, time, and signature of the prescribing physician.

For clients in a hospital or other health care agency, written orders are safer and much preferred, but occasionally verbal or telephone orders are acceptable. These are written on the client's order sheet, signed by the person taking the order, and later countersigned by the physician. Once the order is written, a copy is sent to the pharmacy, where the order is recorded and the drug is dispensed to the appropriate patient care unit. In many institutions, pharmacy staff prepare a computer-generated MAR for each 24-hour period.

For clients in ambulatory care settings, the procedure is essentially the same for drugs to be given immediately. For drugs to be taken at home, written prescriptions are given. In addition to the previous information, a prescription should include the client's address, instructions for taking the drug (*e.g.*, dose and frequency),

whether the prescription is to be labeled with the name of the drug, and whether the prescription can be refilled. Prescriptions for Schedule II controlled drugs cannot be refilled; a new prescription is required.

To interpret medication orders accurately, the nurse must know commonly used abbreviations for routes, dosages, and times of drug administration (Table 3-1). If the nurse cannot read the physician's order or if the order seems erroneous, he or she must question the order before giving the drug.

Drug Preparations and Dosage Forms

Drug preparations and dosage forms vary according to the drug's chemical characteristics, purpose, and route of administration. Some drugs are available in only one

TABLE 3-1   COMMON ABBREVIATIONS

Routes of Drug Administration

IM	intramuscular
IV	intravenous
OD	right eye
OS	left eye
OU	both eyes
PO	by mouth, oral
SC	subcutaneous
SL	sublingual

Drug Dosages

cc	cubic centimeter
g	gram
gr	grain
gt	drop*
mg	milligram
ml	milliliter
oz	ounce
tbsp	tablespoon
tsp	teaspoon

Times of Drug Administration

a.c.	before meals
ad lib	as desired
b.i.d.	twice daily
h.s.	bedtime
p.c.	after meals
PRN	when needed
q.d.	every day, daily
q4h	every four hours
q.i.d.	four times daily
q.o.d.	every other day
stat	immediately
t.i.d.	three times daily

*drops = gtt.

preparation or dosage form; others are available in several forms.

Dosage forms of systemic drugs include liquids, tablets, capsules, suppositories, and transdermal and pump delivery systems. Systemic liquids are given orally (PO) or parenterally. Those given by injection must be sterile.

Tablets and capsules are given PO. Tablets contain active drug plus binders, colorants, preservatives, and other substances. Capsules usually contain a powder or liquid form of active drug enclosed in a gelatin capsule. Most tablets and capsules dissolve in the acid fluids of the stomach and are absorbed in the alkaline fluids of the upper small intestine. Some (i.e., enteric-coated tablets and capsules) are coated with a substance that is insoluble in stomach acids. This delays dissolution until the medication reaches the intestine, usually to avoid gastric irritation or to keep the drug from being destroyed by gastric acid. Tablets for sublingual or buccal administration must be specifically formulated for such use.

Several controlled-release dosage forms or drug delivery systems have been developed to allow less frequent administration and more consistent serum drug levels. Newer formulations and mechanisms of release continue to be developed. Transdermal formulations include systemically absorbed clonidine, estrogen, fentanyl, nitroglycerin, and scopolamine. Pump delivery systems may be external or implanted under the skin and refillable or long-acting without refills. Pumps are used to administer insulin, narcotic analgesics, antineoplastics, and other drugs.

Ointments, creams, and suppositories are applied topically to skin or mucous membranes. They are usually specifically formulated for the intended route of administration.

Calculating Drug Dosages

Nurses in most practice settings are infrequently required to calculate drug doses because pharmacists usually perform the necessary calculations before dispensing drugs. Still, when calculations are needed, the importance of accuracy cannot be overemphasized. Accuracy requires basic skills in mathematics, knowledge of common units of measurement, and methods of using data in performing calculations.

COMMONLY USED SYSTEMS OF MEASUREMENT

The most commonly used system of measurement is the *metric system*, in which the meter is used for linear measure, the gram for weight, and the liter for volume. One milliliter (ml) equals one cubic centimeter (cc), and

both equal one gram (g) of water. The *apothecary system*, now obsolete and rarely used, has units called grains, minims, drams, ounces, pounds, pints, and quarts. The *household system*, with units of drops, teaspoons, tablespoons, and cups, is infrequently used in health care agencies but may be used at home. Table 3-2 lists equivalent measurements within and among these systems. Equivalents are approximate.

A few drugs are ordered and measured in terms of units or milliequivalents (mEq). Units express biologic activity in animal tests (i.e., the amount of drug required to produce a particular response). Units are unique for each drug. For example, concentrations of insulin and heparin are both expressed in units, but there is no relation between a unit of insulin and a unit of heparin. These drugs are usually ordered in the number of units per dose (e.g., NPH insulin 30 units subcutaneously [SC] every morning, or heparin 5000 units SC q12h) and labeled in number of units per milliliter (U 100 insulin contains 100 units/ml; heparin may have 1000, 5000, or 10,000 units/ml). Milliequivalents express the ionic activity of a drug. Drugs such as potassium chloride are ordered and labeled in the number of milliequivalents per dose, tablet, or milliliter.

MATHEMATICAL CALCULATIONS

Most physicians' drug orders and most drug labels are expressed in metric units of measurement. If the amount specified in the order is the same as that on the drug label, no calculations are required, and preparing the right dose is a simple matter. For example, if the order reads "acetaminophen 325 mg PO" and the drug label reads "acetaminophen 325-mg tablets," it is clear that one tablet is to be given.

TABLE 3-2	EQUIVALENTS	
Metric	**Apothecary**	**Household**
1 ml = 1 cc	= 15 or 16 minims	= 15 or 16 drops
4 or 5 ml	= 1 fluid dram	= 1 tsp
60 or 65 mg	= 1 gr	
30 or 32 mg	= ½ gr	
30 g = 30 ml	= 1 oz	= 2 tbsp
250 ml	= 8 oz	= 1 cup
454 g	= 1 lb	
500 ml = 500 cc	= 16 oz = 1 pint	= 1 pint
1 L = 1000 ml	= 32 oz = 1 quart	= 1 quart
1000 µg*	= 1 mg	
1000 mg	= 1 g	
1000 g = 1 kg	= 2.2 lb	= 2.2 lb
0.6 g = 600 mg or 650 mg	= 10 gr	

*µg = microgram

What happens if the order calls for a 650-mg dose and 325-mg tablets are available? The question is, "How many 325-mg tablets are needed to give a dose of 650 mg?" In this case, the answer can be readily calculated mentally to indicate two tablets. This is a simple example that also can be used to illustrate mathematical calculations. This problem can be solved by several acceptable methods; the following formula is presented because of its relative simplicity for students lacking a more familiar method.

$$\frac{D}{H} = \frac{X}{V}$$

D = desired dose (dose ordered by the physician, often in mg)
H = on-hand or available dose (dose on the drug label, often in mg/tablet, capsule, or milliliter)
X = unknown (number of tablets, in this example)
V = unit (one tablet, here)

$$\frac{650 \text{ mg}}{325 \text{ mg}} = \frac{X \text{ tablets}}{1 \text{ tablet}}$$

Cross multiply:

$$325X = 650$$

$$X = \frac{650}{325} = 2 \text{ tablets}$$

What happens if the order and the label are written in different units? For example, the order may read "amoxicillin 0.5 g" and the label may read "amoxicillin 500 mg/capsule." To calculate the number of capsules needed for the dose, the first step is to convert 0.5 g to the equivalent number of milligrams, or convert 500 mg to the equivalent number of grams. The desired or ordered dose and the available or label dose *must* be in the same units of measurement. Using the equivalents (*i.e.,* 1 g = 1000 mg) listed in Table 3-2, an equation can be set up as follows:

$$\frac{1 \text{ g}}{1000 \text{ mg}} = \frac{0.5 \text{ g}}{X \text{ mg}}$$

$$X = 0.5 \times 1000 = 500 \text{ mg}$$

The next step is to use the new information in the formula, which then becomes:

$$\frac{D}{H} = \frac{X}{V}$$

$$\frac{500 \text{ mg}}{500 \text{ mg}} = \frac{X \text{ capsules}}{1 \text{ capsule}}$$

$$500X = 500$$

$$X = \frac{500}{500} = 1 \text{ capsule}$$

The same procedure and formula can be used to calculate portions of tablets or dosages of liquids. These are illustrated in the following problems:

1. Order: 25 mg PO
   Label: 50-mg tablet

   $$\frac{25 \text{ mg}}{50 \text{ mg}} = \frac{X \text{ tablet}}{1 \text{ tablet}}$$

   $$50X = 25$$

   $$X = \frac{25}{50} = 0.5 \text{ tablet}$$

2. Order: 25 mg IM
   Label: 50 mg in 1 cc

   $$\frac{25 \text{ mg}}{50 \text{ mg}} = \frac{X \text{ cc}}{1 \text{ cc}}$$

   $$50X = 25$$

   $$X = \frac{25}{50} = 0.5 \text{ cc}$$

3. Order: 50 mg PO
   Label: 10 mg/cc

   $$\frac{50 \text{ mg}}{10 \text{ mg}} = \frac{X \text{ cc}}{1 \text{ cc}}$$

   $$10X = 50$$

   $$X = \frac{50}{10} = 5 \text{ cc}$$

4. Order: Heparin 5000 units
   Label: Heparin 10,000 units/ml

   $$\frac{5000 \text{ units}}{10,000 \text{ units}} = \frac{X \text{ ml}}{1 \text{ ml}}$$

   $$10,000X = 5000$$

   $$X = \frac{5000}{10,000} = 0.5 \text{ ml}$$

5. Order: KCl 20 mEq
   Label: KCl 10 mEq/5 ml

   $$\frac{20 \text{ mEq}}{10 \text{ mEq}} = \frac{X \text{ ml}}{5 \text{ ml}}$$

   $$10X = 100$$

   $$X = \frac{100}{10} = 10 \text{ ml}$$

Routes of Administration

Routes of administration depend largely on drug characteristics, client characteristics, and desired responses. The major routes are oral, parenteral, and topical. Each has advantages, disadvantages, indications for use, and specific techniques of administration.

ORAL ROUTE

The oral route of administration is most often used. It is simple, convenient, and relatively inexpensive, and it can be used by most people. The main disadvantages are relatively slower drug action and possible irritation of gastrointestinal mucosa, which may produce adverse effects such as anorexia, nausea, vomiting, diarrhea, and ulceration.

Drugs also may be given through tubes placed into the gastrointestinal tract, such as nasogastric or gastrostomy tubes. In people who cannot take drugs orally for prolonged periods, this route is preferable to injections.

PARENTERAL ROUTES

The term *parenteral* refers to any route other than gastrointestinal (enteral) but is commonly used to indicate SC, IM, and IV injections. Injections require special drug preparations, equipment, and techniques.

Drugs for Injection

Parenteral drugs must be prepared, packaged, and administered in ways to maintain sterility. Vials are closed glass or plastic containers with rubber stoppers through which a sterile needle can be inserted for withdrawing medication. Single-dose vials generally do not contain a preservative and must be discarded after a dose is withdrawn; multiple-dose vials contain a preservative and may be reused if aseptic technique is maintained.

Ampules are sealed glass containers, the tops of which must be broken off to allow insertion of a needle and withdrawal of the medication. Broken ampules and any remaining medication are discarded; they are no longer sterile and cannot be reused. When vials or ampules contain a powder form of the drug, a sterile solution of water or 0.9% sodium chloride must be added and the drug dissolved before withdrawal. Use a filter needle to withdraw the medication from an ampule because broken glass may need to be removed from the drug solution.

Many injectable drugs, including various concentrations of commonly used parenteral narcotic analgesics, are available in ready-to-use plastic or glass syringes with attached needles. These units are inserted into specially designed holders and used like other needle/syringe units.

Equipment for Injections

Sterile needles and syringes are used to contain, measure, and administer parenteral medications. They may be packaged together or separately. Needles are available in various gauges and lengths. The term *gauge* refers to lumen size, with larger numbers indicating smaller lumen sizes. For example, a 25-gauge needle is smaller than an 18-gauge needle. Choice of needle gauge and length depends on the route of administration, the viscosity of the solution to be given, and the size of the client. Usually, a 25-gauge, ⅝" needle is used for SC injections and a 22- or 20-gauge, 1.5" needle for IM injections. Other needle sizes are available for special uses, such as intradermal injections.

In many settings, needleless systems are being used. These involve a plastic cannula on the syringe instead of a needle and vials that can be entered with the cannula and then reseal themselves. They were developed because of the risk of injury and spread of blood-borne pathogens, such as the viruses that cause acquired immunodeficiency syndrome (AIDS) and hepatitis B. When needles are used, avoid recapping them, and dispose of them appropriately.

Syringes also are available in various sizes. The 3-ml size is probably used most often. It is usually plastic and is available with or without an attached needle. Syringes are calibrated so that drug doses can be measured accurately. However, the calibrations vary according to the size and type of syringe.

Insulin and tuberculin syringes are used for specific purposes. Insulin syringes are calibrated to measure up to 100 units of insulin. Safe practice requires that *only* insulin syringes be used to measure insulin and that they be used for no other drugs. Tuberculin syringes have a capacity of 1 ml. They should be used for small doses of any drug because measurements are more accurate than with larger syringes.

Subcutaneous Route

The SC route involves the injection of drugs under the skin. This route is used for a small volume (about 1 ml or less) of drug. Absorption is slower and drug action is generally longer with SC injections than with IV or IM injections. The SC route is commonly used for only a few drugs (*e.g.,* insulin). Many drugs cannot be given SC because they are irritating to tissues and may cause

Figure 3-1
Subcutaneous injection sites.

tissue necrosis and abscess formation. Common sites for SC injections are the upper arms, abdomen, back, and thighs (Fig. 3-1).

Intramuscular Route

The IM route involves the injection of drugs into certain muscles. This route is used for several drugs, usually in doses of 3 ml or less. Absorption is more rapid than from SC injections because muscle tissue has a greater blood supply. Site selection is especially important with IM injections because incorrect needle placement may damage blood vessels or nerves. Commonly used sites are the deltoid, dorsogluteal, ventrogluteal, and vastus lateralis. These sites must be selected by first identifying anatomic landmarks (Figs. 3-2 through 3-5).

Intravenous Route

The IV route involves the injection of a drug into the bloodstream. Drugs given IV act rapidly, and larger amounts can be given than by SC or IM injection. One way of giving drugs IV is to prepare the drug with a needle and syringe, insert the needle into a vein, and inject the drug. More often, however, drugs are given through an established IV line, intermittently or continuously. Direct injection is useful for emergency drugs, intermittent infusion is often used for antibiotics, and continuous infusion is used for potassium chloride and a few other drugs. The nurse should wear latex gloves to start IV infusions for protection against exposure to blood-borne pathogens.

Drug administration is usually more comfortable and convenient for the client through an IV line.

Disadvantages of this route include the time and skill required for venipuncture, the difficulty of maintaining an IV line, the greater potential for adverse reactions from rapid drug action, and possible complications of IV therapy (*i.e.*, bleeding, infection, fluid overload).

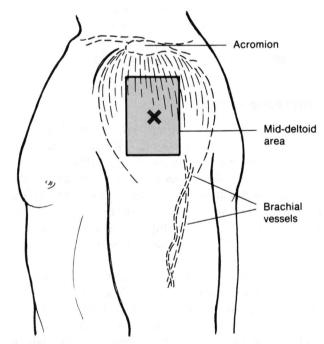

Figure 3-2
Placement of the needle for insertion into the deltoid muscle. The area of injection is bounded by the lower edge of the acromion on the top to a point on the side of the arm opposite the axilla on the bottom. The side boundaries of the rectangular site are parallel to the arm and one third and two thirds of the way around the side of the arm.

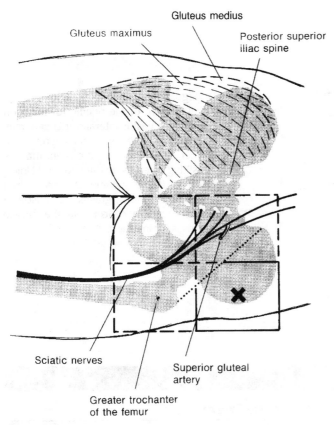

Figure 3-3
Proper placement of the needle for an IM injection into the dorsogluteal site. It is above and outside a diagonal line drawn from the greater trochanter of the femur to the posterior superior iliac spine. Notice how this site allows the nurse to avoid entering an area near the sciatic nerve and the superior gluteal artery.

Other Parenteral Routes

Other parenteral routes include injection into layers of the skin (intradermal), arteries (intra-arterial), joints (intra-articular), and cerebrospinal fluid (intrathecal). Nurses may administer drugs intradermally or intra-arterially (if an established arterial line is present); physicians administer intra-articular and intrathecal medications.

TOPICAL ROUTES

Topical administration involves the application of drugs to the skin or mucous membranes. Application to mucous membranes includes drugs given by inhalation or instillation into the lungs, eyes, nose, and ears, as well as those inserted under the tongue (sublingual), into the cheek (buccal), and into the vagina or rectum.

An advantage of topical administration is that many of the drugs act locally where applied; therefore, the likelihood of systemic adverse reactions is decreased. (However, several drugs are given topically for systemic effects.) A disadvantage is that specific drug preparations must be used for the various routes. Thus, only dermatologic preparations are safe to use on the skin, only ophthalmic drugs are used in the eyes, only a few drugs are given sublingually or buccally, and only vaginal or rectal preparations are given by those respective routes.

Figure 3-4
Placement of the needle for insertion into the ventrogluteal area. Notice how the nurse's palm is placed on the greater trochanter, and the index finger on the anterior superior iliac spine. The middle finger is spread posteriorly as far as possible along the iliac crest. The injection is made in the middle of the triangle formed by the nurse's fingers and the iliac crest.

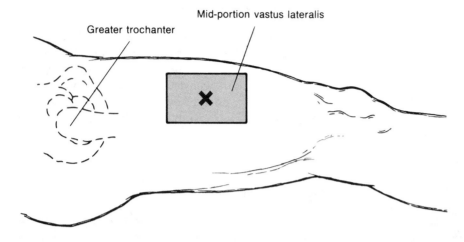

Greater trochanter

Mid-portion vastus lateralis

Figure 3-5
Placement of the needle for insertion into the vastus lateralis. It is generally easier to have the client lying on his or her back. However, the client may be sitting when using this site for IM injections. It is a suitable site for children when the nurse grasps the muscle in her hand to concentrate the muscle mass for injection.

NURSING ACTIONS

DRUG ADMINISTRATION

NURSING ACTIONS	*RATIONALE/EXPLANATION*
1. Follow general rules for administering medications safely and effectively.	
a. Prepare and give drugs in well-lighted areas, as free of interruptions and distractions as possible.	To prevent errors in selecting ordered drugs, calculating dosages, and identifying clients
b. Wash hands before preparing medications and, if needed, during administration.	To prevent infection and cross-contamination
c. Use sterile technique in preparing and administering injections.	To prevent infection. Sterile technique involves using sterile needles and syringes, using sterile drug solutions, not touching sterile objects to any unsterile objects, and cleansing injection sites with an antiseptic.
d. Read the medication administration record (MAR) carefully. Read the label on the drug container, and compare with the MAR in terms of drug, dosage or concentration, and route of administration.	For accurate drug administration. Most nursing texts instruct the nurse to read a drug label three times: when removing the container, while measuring the dose, and before returning the container.
e. Do not leave medications unattended.	To prevent accidental or deliberate ingestion by anyone other than the intended person. Also, to prevent contamination or spilling of medications.
f. Identify the client, preferably by comparing the identification wrist band to the medication sheet.	This is the best way to verify identity. Calling by name, relying on the name on a door or bed, and asking someone else are unreliable methods, although they must be used occasionally when the client lacks a name band.
g. Identify yourself, if indicated, and state your reason for approaching the client. For example, "I'm . . . I have your medication for you."	Explaining actions helps to decrease client anxiety and increase cooperation in taking prescribed medication.
h. Position the client appropriately for the intended route of administration.	To prevent complications, such as aspiration of oral drugs into the lungs

NURSING ACTIONS	RATIONALE/EXPLANATION
i. Provide water or other supplies as needed.	To promote comfort of the client and to ensure drug administration
j. Do not leave medications at the bedside as a general rule. Common exceptions are antacids, nitroglycerin, and eye medications.	To prevent omitting or losing the drug or hoarding of the drug by the client
k. Do not give a drug when signs and symptoms of toxicity are present. Notify the physician, and record that the drug was omitted and why.	Additional doses of a drug increase toxicity. However, drugs are not omitted without a careful assessment of the client's condition and a valid reason.
l. Record drug administration (or omission) as soon as possible and according to agency policies.	To maintain an accurate record of drugs received by the client
m. If it is necessary to omit a scheduled dose for some reason, the decision to give the dose later or omit it depends largely on the drug and frequency of administration. Generally, give drugs ordered once or twice daily at a later time. For others, omit the one dose, and give the drug at the next scheduled time.	Clients may be unable to take the drug at the scheduled time because of diagnostic tests or many other reasons. A temporary change in the time of administration—usually for one dose only—may be necessary to maintain therapeutic effects.
n. For medications ordered as needed (PRN), assess the client's condition; check the physician's orders or MAR for the name, dose, and frequency of administration; and determine the time of the most recently administered dose.	Administration of PRN medications is somewhat different from that of regularly scheduled drugs. Analgesics, antiemetics, and antipyretics are often ordered PRN.
o. For narcotics and other controlled substances, sign drugs out on separate narcotic records according to agency policies.	To meet legal requirements for dispensing controlled substances
p. If, at any time during drug preparation or administration, any question arises regarding the drug, the dose, or whether the client is supposed to receive it, check the original physician's order. If the order is not clear, call the physician for clarification before giving the drug.	To promote safety and prevent errors. The same procedure applies when the client questions drug orders at the bedside. For example, the client may state he has been receiving different drugs or different doses.
2. For oral medications: **a.** With adults	
(1) To give tablets or capsules, open the unit-dose wrapper, place medication in a medicine cup, and give the cup to the client. For solutions, hold the cup at eye level, and measure the dosage at the bottom of the meniscus. For suspensions, shake or invert containers to mix the medication before measuring the dose.	To maintain clean technique and measure doses accurately. Suspensions settle on standing, and if not mixed, diluent may be given rather than the active drug.
(2) Have the client in a sitting position when not contraindicated.	To decrease risks of aspirating medication into lungs. Aspiration may lead to difficulty in breathing and aspiration pneumonia.
(3) Give before, with, or after meals as indicated by the specific drug.	Food in the stomach usually delays drug absorption and action. It also decreases gastric irritation, a common side effect of oral drugs. Giving drugs at appropriate times in relation to food intake can increase therapeutic effects and decrease adverse effects.
(4) Give most oral drugs with a full glass (8 oz) of water or other fluid.	To promote dissolution and absorption of tablets and capsules. Also, to decrease gastric irritation by diluting drug concentration.

(continued)

NURSING ACTIONS	*RATIONALE/EXPLANATION*
b. With children, liquids or chewable tablets are usually given.	Children under 5 years of age are often unable to swallow tablets or capsules.
(1) Measure and give liquids to infants with a dropper or syringe, placing medication on the tongue or buccal mucosa and giving slowly.	For accurate measurement and administration. Giving slowly decreases risks of aspiration.
(2) Medications are often mixed with juice, applesauce, or other vehicle.	To increase the child's ability and willingness to take the medication. If this is done, use a small amount, and be sure the child takes all of it; otherwise, less than the ordered dose is given.
c. Do not give oral drugs if the client is:	
(1) NPO (receiving nothing by mouth)	Oral drugs and fluids may interfere with diagnostic tests or be otherwise contraindicated. Most drugs can be given after diagnostic tests are completed. If the client is having surgery, preoperative drug orders are cancelled. New orders are written postoperatively.
(2) Vomiting	Oral drugs and fluids increase vomiting. Thus, no benefit results from the drug. Also, fluid and electrolyte problems may result from loss of gastric acid.
(3) Excessively sedated or unconscious	To avoid aspiration of drugs into the lungs owing to impaired ability to swallow
3. For medications given by nasogastric tube: **a.** Use a liquid preparation when possible. If necessary, crush a tablet or empty a capsule into about 30 ml of water and mix well. **Do not crush enteric-coated or sustained-release products, and do not empty sustained-release capsules.**	Particles of tablets or powders from capsules may obstruct the tube lumen. Altering sustained-release products increases risks of overdosage and adverse effects.
b. Use a clean bulb syringe or other catheter-tipped syringe.	The syringe allows aspiration and serves as a funnel for instillation of medication and fluids into the stomach.
c. Before instilling medication, aspirate gastric fluid or instill 10 to 20 cc of air while listening with a stethoscope over the stomach.	To be sure the tube is in the stomach
d. Instill medication by gravity flow, and follow it with at least 50 ml of water. Do not allow the syringe to empty completely between additions.	Gravity flow is safer than applying pressure. Water "pushes" the drug into the stomach and rinses the tube, thereby maintaining tube patency. Additional water or other fluids may be given according to fluid needs of the client. Add fluids to avoid instilling air into the stomach unnecessarily, with possible client discomfort.
e. Clamp off the tube from suction or drainage for at least 30 minutes.	To avoid removing the medication from the stomach
4. For SC injections: **a.** Use only sterile drug preparations labeled or commonly used for SC injections.	Many parenteral drugs are too irritating to subcutaneous tissue for use by this route.
b. Use a 25-gauge, ⅝-inch needle for most SC injections.	This size needle is effective for most clients and drugs.
c. Select an appropriate injection site, based on client preferences, drug characteristics, and visual inspection of possible sites. In long-term therapy, such as with insulin, rotate injection sites. Avoid areas with lumps, bruises, or other lesions.	These techniques allow the client to participate in his or her care; avoid tissue damage and unpredictable absorption, which occur with repeated injections in the same location; and increase client comfort and cooperation.

NURSING ACTIONS	RATIONALE/EXPLANATION
d. Cleanse the site with an alcohol sponge.	To prevent infection
e. Tighten the skin or pinch a fold of skin and tissue between thumb and fingers.	Either is acceptable for most clients. If the client is obese, tightening the skin may be easier. If the client is very thin, the tissue fold may keep the needle from hitting bone.
f. Hold the syringe like a pencil, and insert the needle quickly at a 45-degree angle. Use enough force to penetrate the skin and subcutaneous tissue in one smooth movement.	To give the drug correctly with minimal client discomfort
g. Release the skin so that both hands are free to manipulate the syringe. Pull back gently on the plunger (aspirate). If no blood enters the syringe, inject the drug. If blood is aspirated into the syringe, remove the needle, and reprepare the medication.	To prevent accidental injection into the bloodstream. Blood return in the syringe is an uncommon occurrence.
h. Remove the needle quickly and apply gentle pressure for a few seconds.	To prevent bleeding
5. For IM injections:	
a. Use only drug preparations labeled or commonly used for IM injections. Check label instructions for mixing drugs in powder form.	Some parenteral drug preparations cannot be given safely by the IM route.
b. Use a 1½-inch needle for most adults and a ⅝- to 1½-inch needle for children, depending on the size of the client.	A long needle is necessary to reach muscle tissue, which underlies subcutaneous fat.
c. Use the smallest-gauge needle that will accommodate the medication. A 22-gauge is satisfactory for most drugs; a 20-gauge may be used for viscous medications.	To decrease tissue damage and client discomfort
d. Select an appropriate injection site, based on client preferences, drug characteristics, anatomic landmarks, and visual inspection of possible sites. Rotate sites if frequent injections are being given, and avoid areas with lumps, bruises, or other lesions.	To increase client comfort and participation and to avoid tissue damage. Identification of anatomic landmarks is mandatory for safe administration of IM drugs.
e. Cleanse the site with an alcohol sponge.	To prevent infection
f. Tighten the skin, hold the syringe like a pencil, and insert the needle quickly at a 90-degree angle. Use enough force to penetrate the skin and subcutaneous tissue into the muscle in one smooth motion.	To give the drug correctly with minimal client discomfort
g. Aspirate (see 4g, SC Injections).	
h. Remove the needle quickly and apply pressure for several seconds.	To prevent bleeding
6. For IV injections:	
a. Use only drug preparations that are labeled for IV use.	Others are not likely to be pure enough for safe injection into the bloodstream or are not compatible with the blood pH (7.35–7.45).
b. Check label instructions for the type and amount of fluid to use for dissolving or diluting the drug.	Some drugs require special preparation techniques to maintain solubility or pharmacologic activity. Most drugs in powder form can be dissolved in sterile water or sodium chloride for injection. Most drug solutions can be given with dextrose or dextrose and sodium chloride IV solutions.

(continued)

NURSING ACTIONS	RATIONALE/EXPLANATION
c. Prepare drugs just before use, as a general rule. Also, add drugs to IV fluids just before use.	Some drugs are unstable in solution. In some agencies, drugs are mixed and added to IV fluids in the pharmacy. This is the preferred method because sterility can be better maintained.
d. For venipuncture and direct injection into a vein, apply a tourniquet, select a site in the arm, cleanse the skin with an antiseptic (*e.g.*, povidone-iodine or alcohol), insert the needle, and aspirate a small amount of blood into the syringe to be sure that the needle is in the vein. Remove the tourniquet, and inject the drug slowly. Remove the needle and apply pressure until there is no evidence of bleeding.	For safe and accurate drug administration with minimal risk to the client. The length of time required to give the drug depends on the specific drug and the amount. Slow administration, over several minutes, allows immediate discontinuation if adverse effects occur.
e. For administration by an established IV line:	
(1) Check the infusion for patency and flow rate. Check the venipuncture site for signs of infiltration and phlebitis before each drug dose.	The solution must be flowing freely for accurate drug administration. If infiltration or phlebitis is present, do not give the drug until a new IV line is begun.
(2) For direct injection, cleanse an injection site on the IV tubing, insert the needle, and inject the drug slowly.	Most tubings have injection sites to facilitate drug administration.
(3) To use a volume-control set, fill it with 50 to 100 ml of IV fluid, and clamp it so that no further fluid enters the chamber and dilutes the drug. Inject the drug into an injection site after cleansing the site with an alcohol sponge and infuse, usually in 1 hour or less. Once the drug is infused, add solution to maintain the infusion.	This method is used for administration of antibiotics on an intermittent schedule. Dilution of the drug decreases adverse effects.
(4) To use a "piggyback" method, add the drug to 50 to 100 ml of IV solution in a separate container. Attach the IV tubing and a needle. Insert the needle in an injection site on the main IV tubing after cleansing the site. Infuse the drug over 15 to 60 minutes, depending on the drug.	This method is also used for intermittent administration of antibiotics and other drugs. Whether a volume-control or piggyback apparatus is used depends on agency policy and equipment available.
f. When more than one drug is to be given, flush the line between drugs. Do not mix drugs in syringes or in IV fluids unless the drug literature states that the drugs are compatible.	Physical and chemical interactions between the drugs may occur and cause precipitation, inactivation, or increased toxicity. Most nursing units have charts depicting drug compatibility, or information may be obtained from the pharmacy.
7. For application to skin: Use drug preparations labeled for dermatologic use. Cleanse the skin, remove any previously applied medication, and apply the drug in a thin layer. For broken skin or open lesions, use sterile gloves, tongue blade, or cotton-tipped applicator to apply the drug.	To promote therapeutic effects and minimize adverse effects
8. For instillation of eye drops: Use drug preparations labeled for ophthalmic use. Wash your hands, open the eye to expose the conjunctival sac, and drop the medication into the sac, not on the eyeball, without touching the dropper tip to anything. Provide a tissue for blotting any excess drug. If two or more eye drops are scheduled at the same time, wait 1 to 5 minutes between instillations.	Ophthalmic preparations must be sterile to avoid infection. Blot any excess drug from the inner canthus near the nose to decrease systemic absorption of the drug.
With children, prepare the medication, place the child in a head-lowered position, steady the hand holding the medication on the child's head, gently retract the lower lid, and instill the medication into the conjunctival sac.	Careful positioning and restraint to avoid sudden movements are necessary to decrease risks of injury to the eye.

NURSING ACTIONS	RATIONALE/EXPLANATION
9. For instillation of nose drops and nasal sprays: Have the client hold his or her head back, and drop the medication into the nostrils. Give only as ordered. With children, place in a supine position with the head lowered, instill the medication, and maintain the position for 2 to 3 minutes. Then, place the child in a prone position.	When nose drops are used for rhinitis and nasal congestion accompanying the common cold, overuse results in a rebound congestion that may be worse than the original symptom.
10. For instillation of ear medications: Open the ear canal by pulling the ear up and back for adults, down and back for children, and drop the medication on the side of the canal.	To straighten the canal and promote maximal contact between medication and tissue
11. For rectal suppositories: Lubricate the end with a water-soluble lubricant, wear a glove or finger cot, and insert into the rectum the length of the finger. Place the suppository next to the mucosal wall. If the client prefers and is able, provide supplies for self-administration.	To promote absorption. Allowing self-administration may prevent embarrassment to the client. Be sure the client knows the correct procedure.
12. For vaginal medications: Use gloves or an applicator for insertion. If an applicator is used, wash thoroughly with soap and water after each use. If the client prefers and is able, provide supplies for self-administration.	Some women may be embarrassed and prefer self-administration. Be sure the client knows the correct procedure.

REVIEW AND APPLICATION EXERCISES

1. When giving an oral medication, what are some interventions to aid absorption and hasten therapeutic effects?

2. What are the advantages and disadvantages of the oral route and the IV route of drug administration?

3. For a client who receives all medications through a nasogastric feeding tube, which dosage forms are acceptable? Which are unacceptable, and why?

4. Which dosage forms must be kept sterile during administration?

5. What are some legal factors that influence a nurse's administration of medications?

6. When administering medications, what safety precautions are needed with various routes?

7. What safety precautions must the nurse practice consistently to avoid self-injury and exposure to blood-borne pathogens?

8. With a client who refuses an important medication, what approaches or interventions might persuade the client to take the medication? Would the same approach be indicated if the medication were a vitamin supplement or a laxative?

SELECTED REFERENCES

Beyea, S.C., & Nicoll, L.H. (1996). Administering IM injections the right way. *American Journal of Nursing, 96*(1), 34–35.
Drug facts and comparisons. (1996). St. Louis: Facts and Comparisons.
Konick-McMahan, J. (1996). Full speed ahead—with caution: Pushing intravenous medications. *Nursing '96, 26*(6), 26–31.
Rosdahl, C.B. (1995). *Textbook of basic nursing,* 6th ed. Philadelphia: J.B. Lippincott.

4 Nursing Process in Drug Therapy

Objectives

After studying this chapter, the student will be able to:

1 Develop personal techniques for learning and using drug knowledge in client care.

2 Assess clients' conditions in relation to age, weight, health–illness status (especially renal and cardiovascular function), lifestyle habits likely to influence drug effects, and use of OTC and prescription drugs.

3 Obtain a medication history.

4 Identify nondrug interventions to prevent or decrease the need for drug therapy.

5 Discuss interventions to increase benefits and decrease hazards of drug therapy.

6 Discuss guidelines for rational choices of drugs, dosages, routes, and times of administration.

7 Observe clients for therapeutic and adverse responses to drug therapy.

8 Teach clients and family members safe and effective drug administration.

9 Discuss application of the nursing process in home care settings.

10 Discuss legal, ethical, and economic implications of drug therapy.

Key Terms

Drug classification	Maintenance doses
Chronologic age	Physiologic age
Clinical pathways	Quality of life
Loading doses	

Drug therapy involves the use of drugs to prevent or treat disease processes and manifestations. It may save lives, improve the quality of life, and otherwise benefit recipients. It also may cause adverse effects. Adverse effects and failure to achieve therapeutic effects may occur with correct use, but they are more likely to occur with incorrect use. Physicians, pharmacists, clients, and nurses all have important roles to play in the safe and effective use of drugs.

For the nurse, drug therapy is one of many responsibilities in client care. To fulfill this responsibility, the nurse must be knowledgeable about pharmacology (drugs and their effects on the body), physiology (normal body functions), and pathophysiology (alterations in mental and physical functions due to disease processes) and must be adept at using all steps of the nursing process.

Chapter 1 included general information about drugs and cellular physiology. Chapter 2 described concepts and processes essential to understanding drug effects in humans. Chapter 3 emphasized techniques of preparing and administering drugs safely and effectively. Although the importance of safe and accurate administration cannot be overemphasized, this is only one aspect of the nursing process in drug therapy. The nurse also must monitor responses to drug therapy, both therapeutic and adverse, and teach clients about drugs, both prescribed and over-the-counter. To help the nurse acquire knowledge and skills related to drug therapy, this chapter includes suggestions for studying pharmacology, legal responsibilities, nursing process guidelines, general principles of drug therapy, and general nursing actions.

Using the Prototype Approach to Study Pharmacology

The beginning student of pharmacology is faced with a bewildering number and variety of drugs. This number can be greatly reduced by concentrating initial study on therapeutic classifications or groups of drugs and prototypes of those groups. For example, narcotic analgesics is one classification or group, and morphine is the prototype of that group. Morphine and other narcotic analgesics have many common characteristics, including the following:

1. They are used primarily to relieve pain.
2. They produce central nervous system (CNS) depression ranging from slight drowsiness to unconsciousness, depending on dose.
3. A major adverse reaction is respiratory depression (depression of the respiratory center in the medulla oblongata as part of the CNS depression). Thus, the nurse must check rate and depth of respiration.

4. They have a high potential for abuse and dependence; therefore, their use is regulated by narcotic laws and requires special records and procedures.
5. They must be used with caution in people who already have respiratory depression or an impaired level of consciousness.

Understanding these characteristics makes studying all other narcotic analgesics easier because other drugs are compared to morphine, especially in their ability to relieve pain and their likelihood of causing respiratory depression.

Once you know the characteristics of the major drug groups, you must continue to study to add depth and scope to your drug knowledge. Most new or unfamiliar drugs fit into an established classification. For example, you may know that the unfamiliar drug is a thiazide diuretic. By recalling your knowledge of this drug classification, you have a base of information on which to build as you study the unfamiliar drug.

GUIDELINES FOR EFFECTIVE STUDY

When learning about an individual drug, you must assimilate a large amount of data. Although some people try to memorize drug information, this is not an effective way to learn, retain, and apply drug knowledge. Some guidelines for effective study include the following:

1. *Try to understand how the drug acts in the body.* This allows you to predict therapeutic effects and to predict, prevent, or minimize adverse effects by early detection and treatment.
2. *Concentrate your study efforts on major characteristics.* These include the main indications for use, common and potentially serious adverse effects, conditions in which the drug is contraindicated or must be used very cautiously, usual dosage ranges, and related nursing care needs.
3. *Compare the drug with a prototype when possible.* Relating the unknown to the known aids learning and retention of knowledge.
4. *Keep an authoritative, up-to-date drug reference readily available, preferably at work and home.* This is a much more reliable source of drug information than memory. Use the reference freely whenever you encounter an unfamiliar drug or when a question arises about a familiar one.
5. *Use your own words, when possible, when taking notes or writing drug information cards.* The mental processing required to put information in your own words aids learning and retention.
6. *Mentally practice applying drug knowledge in nursing care* by asking yourself, "What if I have a client who is receiving this drug? What must I do? For what must I observe? What if my client is an elderly person or a child?"

Legal Responsibilities of the Nurse

Registered and licensed practical nurses are legally empowered, under state nurse practice acts, to give medications ordered by licensed physicians and dentists. In some states, nurse practitioners may prescribe medications.

When giving medications, the nurse is legally responsible for safe and accurate administration (right drug, right dose, right client, right route, and right time). This means the nurse may be held liable for *not* giving a drug or for giving a wrong drug or a wrong dose. Also, *the nurse is expected to have sufficient drug knowledge to recognize and question erroneous orders*. If, after questioning the prescribing physician and seeking information from other authoritative sources, the nurse considers that giving the drug is unsafe, the nurse must refuse to give the drug. The fact that a physician wrote an erroneous order does not excuse the nurse from legal liability if he or she carries out that order. The nurse also is legally responsible for actions delegated to people who are inadequately prepared for or legally barred from administering medications (such as nursing assistants). However, certified medical assistants (CMAs) administer medications in physicians' offices and certified medication aides (nursing assistants with a short course of training, also called CMAs) often administer medications in long-term care facilities.

The nurse is responsible for storing narcotics and other controlled substances in locked containers, administering them only to people for whom they are prescribed, recording each dose given on appropriate narcotic sheets and on the client's medication administration record, counting the amount of each drug at the end of a work shift, and reporting any discrepancies to the proper authorities.

The nurse who follows safe practices in giving medications does not need to be concerned excessively about legal liability. The basic techniques and guidelines listed in Chapter 3 are aimed at safe and accurate preparation and administration; most errors result when these practices are not followed consistently.

Legal responsibilities in other aspects of drug therapy are less tangible and clear-cut. However, nurses are generally expected to observe clients for therapeutic and adverse effects and to teach clients safe and effective self-administration of drugs when indicated.

Applying the Nursing Process in Drug Therapy

The nursing process is a systematic way of gathering information and using that information to plan and provide client care and to evaluate the outcomes of care.

Knowledge and skill in the nursing process are required for drug therapy, as in other aspects of client care. Each of the five steps of the nursing process is described and illustrated below.

ASSESSMENT

The first step involves collecting data about client characteristics known to affect drug therapy. This can be done by observing and interviewing the client, interviewing family members or others involved in client care, completing a physical assessment, reviewing medical records for pertinent laboratory and diagnostic test reports, and other methods. Information is also sought about the ordered drugs, if needed. Data from all sources are then analyzed.

NURSING DIAGNOSES

These statements, as developed by the North American Nursing Diagnosis Association, describe client problems or needs and are based on assessment data. They should be individualized according to the client's condition and the drug or drugs prescribed. Thus, the nursing diagnoses chosen and the number needed to reflect adequately the client's condition vary considerably. Because almost any nursing diagnosis may apply in specific circumstances, this text emphasizes those diagnoses that generally apply to any course of drug therapy. These and others may be used to guide the nursing care of clients in relation to their drug therapy.

PLANNING/GOALS

This step involves stating the expected outcomes of the prescribed drug therapy. As a general rule, goals should be stated in terms of client behavior, not nurse behavior.

INTERVENTIONS

This step involves implementing the planned activities. General interventions include preventing the need for drug therapy and using nondrug measures to increase safety and effectiveness. Specific interventions include actions needed once a drug is ordered (*i.e.*, accurate administration, observing for therapeutic and adverse effects). In addition, teaching clients and family members is an important intervention in drug therapy.

EVALUATION

This step involves evaluating the client's status in relation to stated goals and expected outcomes. Some outcomes can be evaluated within a few minutes of drug administration (*e.g.*, relief of acute pain following administration of an analgesic). Most, however, require much longer periods of time, often extending from hospitalization and direct observation by the nurse to self-care at home and occasional contact with a health care provider.

With the current emphasis on outpatient treatment and short hospitalizations, the client is likely to experience brief contacts with many health care providers rather than more extensive contacts with a few health care providers. These factors, plus a client's usual reluctance to admit noncompliance, contribute to difficulties in evaluating outcomes of drug therapy. These difficulties can be managed by using appropriate techniques and criteria of evaluation.

Techniques include directly observing the client's status; interviewing the client, family members, or other health care providers; and checking medication records and laboratory and diagnostic test reports. With outpatients, "pill counts" may be done to compare doses remaining with the number prescribed during a designated time. These techniques may be used with every contact with a client, if appropriate.

General criteria include progress toward stated outcomes, such as relief of symptoms, accurate administration, avoidance of preventable adverse effects, compliance with instructions, and others. Specific criteria indicate the parameters that must be measured to evaluate responses to particular drugs (*e.g.*, blood sugar with antidiabetic drugs, blood pressure with antihypertensive drugs).

Each step of the nursing process is more specifically illustrated below.

Nursing Process

Assessment

Initially (before drug therapy is started or on first contact), assess the client regarding age, weight, health status (especially cardiovascular, renal, and hepatic function), acute or chronic disease processes, and ability to function in usual activities of daily living. The effects of these client-related factors on drug therapy are discussed in Chapter 2.

Assess for previous and current use of prescription, nonprescription, and nontherapeutic (*e.g.*, alcohol, caffeine, nicotine, cocaine, marijuana) drugs. A medication history (Box 4-1) is useful, or the information can be incorporated into any data collection tool. Some specific questions and areas of assessment include:

- What are current drug orders?
- What does the client know about current drugs? Is teaching needed?
- What drugs has the client taken before? Include any drugs taken regularly, such as those taken for chronic illnesses (*e.g.*, hypertension, diabetes mellitus, arthritis). It may be helpful to ask specifically about corticosteroids, oral contraceptives, and other hormonal drugs because they may have long-lasting effects. It also may be helpful to ask about nonprescription (over-the-counter, or OTC) drugs for headache, colds, indigestion, or constipation, because some people do not think of OTC preparations as drugs.

- Has the client ever had an allergic reaction to a drug? If so, what signs and symptoms occurred? This information is necessary because many people describe minor nausea and other symptoms as allergic reactions. Unless the reaction is further explored, the client may have therapy withheld inappropriately.
- What are the client's attitudes about drugs? Try to obtain information to help assess whether the client takes drugs freely or reluctantly, is likely to comply with a prescribed drug regimen, and is likely to abuse drugs.
- If long-term drug therapy is likely, can the client afford to buy medications?
- Can the client communicate his or her needs, such as requesting medication? Can he or she swallow oral medications? Are any other conditions present that influence drug therapy?

In addition to nursing assessment data, use progress notes, laboratory reports, and other sources as available and relevant. As part of the initial assessment, obtain baseline data on measurements to be used in monitoring therapeutic or adverse effects. Specific data to be acquired depend on the medication and the client's condition. Laboratory tests of liver, kidney, and bone marrow function are often helpful because some drugs may damage these organs. Also, if liver or kidney damage exists, drug metabolism or excretion may be altered. More specific laboratory tests include serum potassium levels before diuretic therapy, culture and susceptibility studies before antimicrobial therapy, and blood clotting tests before anticoagulant therapy. Other data that may be relevant include vital signs, weight, and urine output.

After drug therapy is begun, continue to assess the client's response in relation to therapeutic and adverse effects, ability and willingness to take the drugs as prescribed, and other aspects of safe and effective drug therapy.

Nursing Diagnoses

- Knowledge Deficit: Drug therapy regimen (*e.g.*, drug ordered, reason for use, expected effects, expected duration, and monitoring of response by health care providers, including diagnostic tests and office visits)
- Knowledge Deficit: Safe and effective self-administration (when appropriate)
- Risk for Injury: Adverse drug effects
- Noncompliance: Overuse
- Noncompliance: Underuse

Planning/Goals

The client will:
- Receive or take drugs as prescribed
- Experience relief of signs and symptoms
- Avoid preventable adverse drug effects
- Avoid unnecessary drug ingestion
- Self-administer drugs safely and accurately
- Verbalize essential drug information
- Keep appointments for monitoring and follow-up

Interventions

Use nondrug measures when appropriate to decrease the need for drugs, to enhance therapeutic effects, or to decrease adverse effects. General interventions include:
- Promoting healthful lifestyles in terms of nutrition, fluids, exercise, rest, and sleep

BOX 4-1. MEDICATION HISTORY

Name _____ Age _____

Health problems, acute and chronic

Are you allergic to any medications?

If yes, describe specific effects or symptoms.

Part 1: Prescription Medications

1. Do you take any prescription medications on a regular basis?

2. If yes, ask the following about each medication.

Name	Dose
Frequency	Specific times
How long taken	Reason for use

3. Are you able to take this medicine as prescribed?

4. Does anyone else help you take your medications?

5. What information or instructions were you given when the medications were first prescribed?

6. Do you think the medication is doing what it was prescribed to do?

7. Have you had any problems that you attribute to the medication?

8. Do you take any prescription medications on an irregular basis? If yes, ask the following about each medication.

Name	Reason
Dose	How long taken
Frequency	

Part 2: Nonprescription Medications

Do you take OTC medications?

		Medication		
Problem	*Yes/No*	*Name*	*Amount*	*Frequency*
Pain				
Headache				
Sleep				
Cold				
Indigestion				
Heartburn				
Diarrhea				
Constipation				
Other				

Part 3: Social Drugs

	Yes/No	*Amount*
Coffee		
Tea		
Cola drinks		
Alcohol		
Tobacco		

- Handwashing and other measures to prevent infection
- Positioning
- Assisting to cough and deep breathe
- Ambulating
- Applying heat or cold
- Increasing or decreasing sensory stimulation
- Scheduling activities to allow periods of rest or sleep
- Recording vital signs, fluid intake, urine output, and other assessment data
- Implementing specific interventions indicated by a particular drug or the client's condition

 Teach clients:

- Healthful lifestyle habits in relation to nutrition, exercise, rest, and sleep
- To avoid drug use when feasible and to use drugs cautiously when necessary
- Nondrug measures to prevent or relieve common health problems and prevent the need for drug therapy
- Nondrug measures to enhance beneficial effects and decrease adverse effects of drugs
- Not to take drugs prescribed for another person and not to share prescription drugs with anyone else. The likelihood of having the right drug in the right dose is extremely remote and the risk of adverse effects extremely high under such circumstances.
- To notify any physician or dentist of drugs being taken

Evaluation

Observe and interview clients and check appropriate medical records about drug usage, compliance with prescribed therapy, relief of symptoms, adverse effects, and drug knowledge.

Integrating Nursing Process, Drug Therapy, and Clinical Pathways

In an increasing number of circumstances, nursing responsibilities related to drug therapy are designated in clinical pathways (also called critical pathways or care maps). Clinical pathways are guidelines for patient care, developed primarily to control health care costs and shorten hospital lengths of stay. Additional characteristics include the following:

- Major components include a medical diagnosis, specific aspects of care related to the medical diagnosis, desired patient outcomes, and time frames (usually days) for achieving the desired outcomes during the expected length of stay.
- Medical diagnoses for which clinical pathways are usually developed are those often encountered in the agency, those that often result in complications or prolonged lengths of stay, and those for which the agency may lose money. In many agencies, clinical pathways have been developed for patients having coronary artery-

bypass grafts, myocardial infarction, or total hip replacement.

- Development and implementation of the clinical pathways should be an interdisciplinary, collaborative effort. Thus, all health care professionals usually involved in the care of a patient with a particular medical diagnosis should be represented.
- In hospital settings, case managers, who may be non-nurses, usually assess patients' conditions daily to evaluate progress toward the desired outcomes.
- Although clinical pathways are used mainly in hospitals, they are likely to be developed in ambulatory settings as well. Eventually, comprehensive patient pathways may be developed that extend from illness onset and initial contact with a health care provider through treatment and recovery. Such pathways could promote continuity of care among agencies, departments of agencies, and health care providers.

Depending on the medical diagnoses, many clinical pathways have very specific guidelines related to drug therapy. These guidelines may affect any step of the nursing process. With assessment, for example, the clinical pathway may state, "Assess for bleeding if on anticoagulant."

General Principles of Drug Therapy

GENERAL GUIDELINES

1. *The goal of drug therapy should be to maximize beneficial effects and minimize adverse effects.*
2. *Expected benefits should outweigh potential adverse effects.* Thus, drugs generally should not be prescribed for trivial problems or problems for which nondrug measures are effective. Nondrug measures are generally safer than drug therapy.
3. *Drug therapy should be individualized.* Many variables influence a drug's effects on the human body. Failure to consider these variables may decrease therapeutic effects or increase risks of adverse effects to an unacceptable level.
4. *Drug costs and effects on quality of life should be considered.* Pharmacoeconomic data that compare costs of pharmaceutical products are increasingly being considered a major factor in choosing medications. More specifically, for drugs of equal efficacy and toxicity, there is considerable pressure on prescribers to prescribe the less costly drug. There is also more emphasis on quality of life issues in current research, with greater expectations of measurable improvement as a result of drug therapy.

GENERAL DRUG SELECTION AND DOSAGE CONSIDERATIONS

Numerous factors must be considered when choosing a drug and dosage range for a particular client, including the following:

1. For the most part, use as few drugs in as few doses as possible. Minimizing the number of drugs and the frequency of administration increases client compliance with the prescribed drug regimen and decreases risks of serious adverse effects, including hazardous drug–drug interactions. There are notable exceptions to this basic rule. For example, multiple drugs are commonly used to treat severe hypertension or serious infections.
2. Individual drugs allow greater flexibility and individualization of dosage than fixed-dose combinations. However, fixed-dose combinations are commonly used because they are convenient and may promote compliance. Individualization may be accomplished by giving separate drugs initially. Then, if established dosages are similar to those in a combination product, the combination product may be given.
3. The least amount of the least potent drug that will yield therapeutic benefit should be given to decrease adverse reactions. For example, if a mild non-narcotic and a strong narcotic analgesic are both ordered, give the non-narcotic drug if it is effective in relieving pain.
4. Recommended dosages are listed in amounts likely to be effective for most people, but they are only guidelines to be interpreted according to the client characteristics discussed previously. For example, clients with serious illnesses may require larger doses of some drugs than clients with milder illnesses; clients with severe kidney disease often need much smaller doses of renally excreted drugs.
5. Treatment with a particular drug can be started rapidly or slowly. If a drug has a long half-life and maximal therapeutic effects do not usually occur for several days or weeks, the physician may give a limited number of relatively large (loading) doses followed by a regular schedule of smaller (maintenance) doses. When drug actions are not urgent, therapy may be initiated with a maintenance dose.
6. Different salts of the same drug rarely differ pharmacologically. Hydrochloride, sulfate, and sodium salts are often used. Pharmacists and chemists choose salts on the basis of cost, convenience, solubility, and stability. For example, solubility is especially important with parenteral drugs; taste is a factor with oral drugs.

DRUG THERAPY IN CHILDREN

Drug therapy during infancy (1 month to 1 year) and childhood (approximately 1–12 years) requires special consideration because of the child's changing size, developmental level, and organ function. Physiologic differences alter drug pharmacokinetics (Table 4-1), and drug therapy is less predictable than in adults. Most drug use in children is empirical in nature because few studies have been done in that population. For many drugs, manufacturers' literature states that "safety and effectiveness for use in children have not been established." Neonates (birth to 1 month) are especially vulnerable to adverse drug effects because of their immature liver and kidney function (see Table 4-1). Neonatal therapeutics are discussed further in Chapter 67.

Most drugs given to adults also are given to children, and general principles, techniques of drug administration, and nursing process guidelines apply. Additional principles and guidelines include the following:

1. All aspects of pediatric drug therapy must be guided by the child's age, weight, and level of growth and development.
2. Choice of drug is often restricted because many drugs commonly used in adult drug therapy have not been sufficiently investigated to ensure safety and effectiveness in children.
3. Safe therapeutic dosage ranges are less well defined for children than for adults. Some drugs are not recommended for use in children, and therefore dosages have not been established. For many drugs, doses for children are extrapolated from those established for adults. When pediatric dosage ranges are listed in drug literature, these should be used. Often, however, they are expressed in the amount of drug to be given per kilogram of body weight or square meter of body surface area, and the amount needed for a specific dose must be calculated as a fraction of the adult dose. The following methods are used for these calculations:
   A. Clark's rule is based on weight and is used for children at least 2 years old.

$$\frac{\text{Weight (in pounds)}}{150} \times \text{adult dose} = \text{child's dose}$$

   B. Calculating dosage based on body surface area is considered a more accurate method than those based on other characteristics. Body surface area, based on height and weight, is estimated using a nomogram (Fig. 4-1). Use the estimated body surface area in the following formula to calculate the child's dose:

$$\frac{\text{Body surface area (in square meters)}}{1.73 \text{ square meters (m}^2)}$$
$$\times \text{adult dose} = \text{child's dose}$$

   C. Dosages obtained from these calculations are approximate and must be individualized. These doses can be used initially and then increased or decreased according to the child's response.

| TABLE 4-1 | CHILDREN: PHYSIOLOGIC CHARACTERISTICS AND PHARMACOKINETIC CONSEQUENCES |

Physiologic Characteristics	Pharmacokinetic Consequences
Increased thinness and permeability of skin in neonates and infants	Increased absorption of topical drugs (*e.g.*, corticosteroids may be absorbed sufficiently to suppress adrenocortical function)
Immature blood-brain barrier in neonates and infants	Increased distribution of drugs into the central nervous system because myelinization (which creates the blood-brain barrier to the passage of drugs) is not mature until about 2 years of age
Increased percentage of body water (70% to 80% in neonates and infants, compared to 50% to 60% in children above 2 years of age and adults)	Usually increased volume of distribution in infants and young children, compared to adults. This would seem to indicate a need for larger doses. However, prolonged drug half-life and decreased rate of drug clearance may offset. The net effect is often a need for decreased dosage.
Altered protein binding until about 1 year of age, when it reaches adult levels	The amount and binding capacity of plasma proteins may be reduced. This may result in a greater proportion of unbound or pharmacologically active drug and greater risks of adverse drug effects. Dosage requirements may be decreased or modified by other factors. Drugs with decreased protein binding in neonates, compared with older children and adults, include ampicillin (Omnipen, others), diazepam (Valium), digoxin (Lanoxin), lidocaine (Xylocaine), nafcillin (Unipen), phenobarbital, phenytoin (Dilantin), salicylates (*e.g.*, aspirin), and theophylline (TheoDur).
Decreased glomerular filtration rate in neonates and infants, compared with older children and adults. Kidney function develops progressively during the first few months of life and is fairly mature by 1 year of age.	In neonates and infants, slowed excretion of drugs eliminated by the kidneys. Dosage of these drugs may need to be decreased, depending on the infant's age and level of growth and development.
Decreased activity of liver drug-metabolizing enzyme systems in neonates and infants	Decreased capacity for biotransformation of drugs. This results in slowed metabolism and elimination, with increased risks of drug accumulation and adverse effects.
Increased activity of liver drug-metabolizing enzyme systems in children	Increased capacity for biotransformation of some drugs. This results in a rapid rate of metabolism and elimination. For example, theophylline is cleared about 30% faster in a 7-year-old child than in an adult and about four times faster than in a neonate.

4. Use the oral route of drug administration when possible. Try to obtain the child's cooperation; never force oral medications, as forcing may lead to aspiration.

5. If intramuscular injections are required in infants, use the thigh muscles because the deltoid muscles are quite small and the gluteal muscles do not develop until the child is walking.

6. For safety, keep all medications in childproof containers, out of reach of children, and do not refer to medications as "candy."

DRUG THERAPY IN OLDER ADULTS

Aging is a continuum; precisely when a person becomes an "older adult" is not clearly established, but in this book people 65 years and older are so categorized. In this population, general nursing process guidelines

and principles of drug therapy apply. In addition, adverse effects are especially likely to occur due to physiologic changes associated with aging (Table 4-2), pathologic changes due to disease processes, multiple drug therapy for acute and chronic disorders, impaired memory and cognition, and difficulty in complying with drug orders. Overall, the goal of drug therapy may be "care" rather than "cure," with efforts to prevent or control symptoms and maintain the client's ability to function in usual activities of daily living. Additional principles are listed below.

1. Although age in years is an important factor, older adults are quite heterogeneous in their responses to drug therapy. Thus, responses differ widely within the same age group. Responses also differ in the same person over time. Physiologic age (*i.e.*, organ function) is more important than chronologic age.

Figure 4-1
Body-surface nomograms. To determine the surface area of the client, draw a straight line between the point representing his or her height on the left vertical scale to the point representing weight on the right vertical scale. The point at which this line intersects the middle vertical scale represents the client's surface area in square meters. (Courtesy of Abbott Laboratories)

2. It may be difficult to separate the effects of aging from the effects of disease processes or drug therapy, particularly long-term drug therapy. Symptoms attributed to aging or disease actually may be caused by medications. This occurs because older adults generally metabolize and excrete drugs less efficiently, and thus drugs are more likely to accumulate.

3. Medications—both prescription and nonprescription drugs—should be taken only when necessary.

4. Review current medications, including nonprescription drugs, before prescribing new drugs; discontinue unnecessary drugs.

5. When drug therapy is required, the choice of drug should be based on the available drug information regarding effects in older adults.

6. The basic principle of giving the smallest effective number of drugs applies especially to older adults.

A regimen of several drugs increases the incidence of adverse reactions and potentially hazardous drug interactions. In addition, many older adults are unable or unwilling to self-administer more than three or four drugs correctly.

7. All drugs should be given for the shortest effective time. This interval is not well established for most drugs, and many drugs are continued for years, whether they are needed or not. Health care providers must reassess drug regimens periodically to see whether drugs, dosages, or other aspects need to be revised. This is especially important when significant changes in health status have occurred.

8. The smallest number of effective doses should be prescribed. This allows less disruption of usual activities and promotes compliance with the prescribed regimen.

TABLE 4-2 OLDER ADULTS: PHYSIOLOGIC CHARACTERISTICS AND PHARMACOKINETIC CONSEQUENCES

Physiologic Characteristics	Pharmacokinetic Consequences
Decreased gastrointestinal secretions and motility	Slower absorption of oral drugs and delayed onset of action. However, total absorption may be increased because drug molecules have more contact with sites of absorption in the small intestine.
Decreased cardiac output	Slower absorption from sites of administration (*e.g.,* gastrointestinal tract, subcutaneous or muscle tissue). Decreased distribution to sites of action in tissues, with potential for delaying the onset and reducing the extent of therapeutic effects.
Decreased blood flow to the liver and kidneys	The resultant delays in metabolism and excretion may lead to drug accumulation and increased risks of adverse or toxic effects.
Decreased total body water and lean body mass per kg of weight; increased body fat	Water-soluble drugs (*e.g.,* ethanol, lithium) are distributed into a smaller area, with resultant higher plasma concentrations and higher risks of toxicity with a given dose. Fat-soluble drugs (*e.g.,* diazepam) are distributed to a larger area, accumulate in fat, and have a longer duration of action in the body.
Decreased serum albumin	Decreased availability of protein for binding and transporting drug molecules. This increases serum concentration of free, pharmacologically active drug, especially for those that are normally highly protein bound (*e.g.,* aspirin, warfarin). This may increase risks of adverse effects. However, the drug also may be metabolized and excreted more rapidly, thereby offsetting at least some of the risks.
Decreased blood flow to the liver; decreased number and activity of drug-metabolizing enzymes	Slowed metabolism and detoxification, with increased risks of drug accumulation and toxic effects
Decreased blood flow to the kidneys, decreased number of functioning nephrons, decreased glomerular filtration rate, and decreased tubular secretion	Impaired drug excretion, prolonged half-life, and increased risks of toxicity

9. When any drug is started, the dosage generally should be smaller than for younger adults. The dosage can then be increased or decreased according to response. If an increased dosage is indicated, increments should be smaller and made at longer intervals in older adults. This conservative, safe approach is sometimes called "start low, go slow."

10. Use nondrug measures to decrease the need for drugs and to increase their effectiveness or decrease their adverse effects. For example, insomnia is a common complaint among older adults. Preventing it (*e.g.,* by avoiding caffeine-containing beverages and excessive napping) is much safer than taking sedative-hypnotic drugs.

11. For people receiving long-term drug therapy at home, use measures to help them take drugs safely and effectively.

    A. If vision is impaired, label drug containers with large lettering for easier readability. A magnifying glass also may be useful.

    B. Be sure the client can open drug containers. For example, avoid childproof containers for an older adult with arthritic hands.

    C. Several devices may be used to schedule drug doses and decrease risks of omitting or repeating doses. These include written schedules, calendars, and charts. Also available are drug containers with doses prepared and clearly labeled as to the day and time each dose is to be taken. With the latter system, the client can tell at a glance whether a dose has been taken.

    D. Enlist family members or friends when necessary.

12. When a client develops new symptoms or becomes less able to function in usual activities of daily living, consider the possibility of adverse drug effects. Often, new signs and symptoms are attributed to aging or disease. They may then be ignored or treated by prescribing a new drug, when stopping or reducing the dose of an old drug is the indicated intervention.

HOME CARE

Home care is an expanding area of health care. This trend evolved from efforts to reduce health care costs, especially the costs of hospitalization. The consequences of this trend include increased outpatient care and brief hospitalizations for severe illness or major surgery. In both instances, clients of all age groups are often discharged to their homes for follow-up care and recovery. Skilled nursing care, such as managing medication regimens, is often required during follow-up. Most general principles and nursing responsibilities related to drug therapy apply in home care as in other health care settings. Some additional principles and factors include the following:

1. Clients may require short-term or long-term drug therapy. In most instances, the role of the nurse is to teach the client or caregiver to administer the medication and monitor its effects.

2. In a client's home, the nurse is a guest and must work within the environment to establish rapport, elicit cooperation, and provide nursing care. The initial contact is usually by telephone, and one purpose is to schedule a home visit. It is desirable to schedule the visit at a convenient time for the client and caregiver. In addition, state the main purpose of the visit and about how long the visit will be. Establish a method for contact in case the appointment must be canceled by either party.

3. Assess the client's attitude toward the prescribed medication regimen and his or her ability to provide self-care. If the client is unable, who will be the primary caregiver in terms of medication administration and observing for medication effects? What are the learning needs of the client or caregiver in relation to the medication regimen?

4. Ask to see all prescribed and OTC medications the client takes, and ask how and when the client takes each one. With this information, the nurse may be able to reinforce the client's compliance or identify potential problem areas (*e.g.*, differences between instructions and client usage of medications, drugs with opposing or duplicate effects, continued use of medications that were supposed to be discontinued, drugs discontinued because of adverse effects).

5. Assess the environment for potential safety hazards (*e.g.*, risk of infection with corticosteroids and other immunosuppressants, risk of falls and other injuries with narcotic analgesics and other drugs with sedating effects). In addition, assess the client's ability to obtain medications and keep appointments for follow-up visits to health care providers.

6. Areas of nursing intervention may include drug administration, teaching about medications, problem solving, promoting compliance, identifying barriers to compliance, identifying resources (*e.g.*, financial assistance for obtaining medications), and others.
   A. With administration of oral drugs, clients and caregivers may need information about timing in relation to food intake, whether a tablet can be crushed, when to omit the drug, and other aspects.
   B. With other routes, the nurse may initially need to demonstrate administration or coach the client or caregiver through each step. Demonstrating and having the client or caregiver practice and do a return demonstration is a good way to teach psychomotor skills such as giving a medication through a gastrointestinal tube, preparing and administering an injection, or manipulating an intravenous infusion pump.
   C. Clients and caregivers may feel anxious and overwhelmed, especially by complicated medication regimens. Try to decrease their anxiety and provide positive reinforcement for effort. Proceed slowly, in small steps, emphasize essential information, and provide ample opportunities to express concerns or ask questions.
   D. When teaching about medications, choose an appropriate time (*e.g.*, when the client is mentally alert and not in acute distress from pain, hypoxia, or other symptoms) and a place with minimal noise and distractions.
   E. In addition to safe and accurate administration, teach the client and caregiver to observe for beneficial and adverse effects. If side effects occur, teach them how to manage minor ones and which ones to report to a health care provider.
   F. Generally, a combination of verbal and written instructions is more effective than either alone. The nurse should minimize medical jargon and be aware that printed materials may be above the client's or caregiver's reading level. Even those with adequate education and reading skills may have difficulty understanding and retaining the material being taught because of the stress of the illness.

7. Assist in developing a medication schedule that minimally disrupts usual household activities. This promotes convenience and compliance. Also, help develop a plan for renewing or refilling prescriptions so that the medication supply does not run out when the prescribing physician is unavailable or the pharmacy is closed.

MONITORING DRUG THERAPY

Nursing Actions	*Rationale/Explanation*
1. **Prepare and administer drugs accurately** (see Chap. 3).	
a. Practice the five rights of drug administration (right *drug*, right *client*, right *dose*, right *route*, and right *time*).	These rights are ensured if the techniques described in Chapter 3 are consistently followed. The time may vary by about 30 minutes. For example, a drug ordered for 9 AM can be given between 8:30 AM and 9:30 AM. No variation is allowed in the other "rights."
b. Use correct techniques for different routes of administration.	For example, sterile equipment and techniques are required for injection of any drug.
c. Follow label instructions regarding mixing or other aspects of giving specific drugs.	Some drugs require specific techniques of preparation and administration.
2. **Observe for therapeutic effects**	Generally, the nurse should know the expected effects and when they are likely to occur. Specific observations depend on the specific drug or drugs being given.
3. **Observe for adverse effects**	All drugs are potentially harmful, although the incidence and severity of adverse reactions vary among drugs and clients. People most likely to suffer adverse reactions are those with severe liver or kidney disease, those who are very young or very old, those receiving several drugs, and those receiving large doses of any drug. Specific adverse effects for which to observe depend on the drugs being given.
4. **Observe for drug interactions**	The nurse must be knowledgeable about common and potentially significant drug interactions. Also, because interactions may occur whenever the client is receiving two or more drugs concurrently, they should be considered as a possible cause of unexpected responses to drug therapy.
5. **Teach clients about their drug therapy**	
a. General instructions	
(1) Take medications as directed.	Therapeutic effect greatly depends on taking medications correctly. Altering the dose or time may cause underdosage or overdosage.
(2) Do not start or stop drugs without consulting the physician.	Drug therapy is often a state of delicate balance. Altering this balance greatly increases risks of drug interactions, adverse effects, and loss of therapeutic effectiveness.
(3) Do not keep drugs for long periods.	The chemical composition of drugs tends to become altered over time. Manufacturers' drug labels often include a date after which the drug should be discarded. This information is not ordinarily included with prescription drugs dispensed to clients. Outdated drugs at best do no good and at worst may be harmful.
(4) Develop a routine for taking medications. For example, take them at the same time and place each day.	Having a routine helps clients remember to take medications as directed.
(5) Do not keep medications in the bathroom medicine cabinet.	Medications may deteriorate more rapidly owing to warmth and moisture.
(6) Never put several medications, such as different tablets, in one container	This is never a safe practice. The risk of taking the wrong medication or wrong dose is greatly increased if this is done. In addition, the drugs may interact chemically, altering drug composition.

(continued)

NURSING ACTIONS	*RATIONALE/EXPLANATION*
(7) Take medication in a well-lighted area.	To allow reading the label to ensure that the drug taken is the one intended
(8) Keep all medications out of reach of children, and never refer to medications as "candy."	To prevent accidental ingestion and poisoning
b. Instructions related to specific drugs	Many drugs are self-administered, and information is required to do this correctly, safely, and effectively.
(1) Name of the drug(s)	Knowledge of the drug name can be a safety measure, especially if the person has an allergic or other potentially serious adverse reaction or an overdose. It also may give the person a greater sense of control and responsibility regarding drug therapy.
(2) Purpose of the drug	People vary in the amount of drug information they want and need. For most, the purpose can be simply stated in terms of symptoms to be relieved or other expected benefits.
(3) Dosage schedule	This should be specific and as convenient as possible within the limitations imposed by the particular drugs. Working with the client to individualize drug therapy may help increase compliance with the prescribed regimen.
(4) Method of administration	Most people are accustomed to taking drugs orally, although they may need information about the amount or type of fluids to take with a particular drug or other instructions. For other routes of administration, instructions may need to be more specific and complete. Rectal suppositories and topical application of drugs to the eyes or skin are examples in which correct administration is essential to therapeutic effect.
(5) Adverse reactions or side effects to be reported	The goal is to provide needed information without causing unnecessary anxiety. Most drugs produce undesirable effects; some of these are minor, and others are potentially serious. Many people stop taking a drug rather than report adverse reactions. If reactions are reported, it may be possible to allow continued drug therapy by reducing dosage or by implementing other measures. The occurrence of severe reactions indicates that the drug should be stopped. In such cases the prescribing physician should be notified.
(6) Miscellaneous instructions, such as safety measures for taking certain drugs, storage, and others as indicated	

8. When the client visits a health care provider or experiences another illness that requires treatment, assess for changes in medication orders and teach as indicated. Clients are more likely to make medication errors with large numbers of medications or changes in the medication regimen.
9. Between home visits, the home care nurse can maintain telephone contact with clients and caregivers to monitor progress, answer questions, identify problems, and provide reassurance. Clients and caregivers should be given a telephone number to call with questions about medications, side effects, and so forth. The nurse may wish to schedule a daily time for receiving and making nonemergency calls.

 REVIEW AND APPLICATION EXERCISES

1. Why must nurses know the adverse effects of the drugs they give?

2. Given a newly assigned client, what information is needed about present and previous medications?

3. Anticipate the questions a client might ask about a drug and rehearse possible answers, including drugs that are well known to you and those that are not.

4. With children, what are some potential difficulties with drug administration, and how can they be prevented or minimized?

5. With older adults, what are some potential difficulties with drug administration, and how can they be prevented or minimized?

6. For older adults, explain what is meant by "start low, go slow" and why it is a good approach to drug therapy.

7. Why is client teaching about drug therapy needed, and what information should generally be included?

8. For the home care nurse assisting with a medication regimen, what are some likely differences between the nursing care needed by a child and an adult?

SELECTED REFERENCES

Bailey, A., Ferguson, E., & Voss, S. (1995). Factors affecting an individual's ability to administer medication. *Home Healthcare Nurse, 13*(5), 57–63.

Bressler, R. (1993). Adverse drug reactions. In R. Bressler & M.D. Katz (Eds.), *Geriatric pharmacology*, pp. 41–61. New York: McGraw-Hill.

Broussard, M.C., & Pitre, S. (1996). Medication problems in the elderly: A home healthcare nurse's perspective. *Home Healthcare Nurse, 14*(6), 441–443.

Lee, M. (1996). Drugs and the elderly: Do you know the risks? *American Journal of Nursing, 96*(7), 25–32.

Miller, C.A. (1995). *Nursing care of older adults: Theory and practice*, 2nd ed., pp. 427–459. Philadelphia: J.B. Lippincott.

Nies, A.S., & Spielberg, S.P. (1996). Principles of therapeutics. In J.G. Hardman, L.E. Limbird, P.B. Molinoff, & R.W. Ruddon (Eds.), *Goodman & Gilman's The pharmacological basis of therapeutics*, 9th ed., pp. 43–62. New York: McGraw-Hill.

Drugs Affecting the Central Nervous System

Physiology of the Central Nervous System

Objectives

After studying this chapter, the student will be able to:

1 Describe the process of neurotransmission.

2 Describe major neurotransmitters and their roles in nervous system functioning.

3 Discuss signs and symptoms of CNS depression.

4 Discuss general types and characteristics of CNS depressant drugs.

Terms and concepts

Acetylcholine	**Norepinephrine**
Dopamine	**Receptors**
Neuron	**Serotonin**
Neurotransmission systems	**Synapse**

The central nervous system (CNS), composed of the brain and spinal cord, acts as the control center for regulating physical and mental body processes. Afferent or sensory neurons carry messages to the CNS; efferent or motor neurons carry messages away from the CNS. More specifically, the CNS constantly receives information about blood levels of oxygen and carbon dioxide, body temperature, and sensory stimuli and sends messages to effector organs to adjust the environment toward homeostasis. It is also concerned with higher intellectual functions (*e.g.*, thought, learning, reasoning, problem solving, memory) and with muscle function, both skeletal and smooth.

The CNS has complex interactions with other parts of the body, and components of the CNS have complex interactions with each other. Although various components of brain function are often studied individually, it is the overall coordination of the "mind/body" connections that produces mental and physical health. A lack of coordination or imbalances among the components may lead to mental or physical disorders. Thus, emotions can strongly influence neural control of body function, and alterations in neural functions can strongly influence psychological behavior.

More specific characteristics are reviewed below to aid understanding of drugs that act by altering CNS functions.

Characteristics and Functions of the CNS

NEURONS

The CNS is composed mainly of two types of cells:. The *glia* protect, support, and nourish the neuron; the *neuron* is the basic functional unit. Most neurons are composed of a cell body, a dendrite, and an axon. Nerve cell bodies usually occur in groups or clusters, called ganglia or nuclei. A cluster of cell bodies or nuclei with the same function is called a center (*e.g.*, the vasomotor and respiratory centers in the medulla oblongata). A dendrite has a branching structure with many synapses or sites for receiving stimuli or messages, which are then conducted toward the cell body. An axon is a finger-like projection that carries impulses away from the cell body. The end of the axon branches into presynaptic fibers that end with small knob-like structures called vesicles. These structures project into the synapse and contain the granules where neurotransmitters are stored. Many axons are covered by a fatty substance called myelin. The myelin cover or sheath protects and insulates the axon. An axon together with its myelin sheath is called a nerve fiber. Nerve fibers involved in the transmission of the same type of impulses (*e.g.*, pain signals) are found together in a common pathway or tract.

Neurons must be able to communicate with other neurons and body tissues. This communication involves a complex network of electrical and chemical signals that receive, interpret or modify, and send messages. Characteristics that allow neurons to communicate with other cells include excitability (the ability to produce an action potential or be stimulated) and conductivity (the ability to convey electrical impulses). More specific components of the communication network include neurotransmitters, synapses, and receptors (described below).

NEUROTRANSMITTERS

Neurotransmitters are chemical substances that carry messages from one neuron to another, or from a neuron to other body tissues, such as cardiac or skeletal muscle. They are synthesized and stored in presynaptic nerve terminals and released in response to an electrical impulse (action potential) arriving at the end of the first neuron (presynaptic fiber). The basis for the action potential is the transient opening of ion channels. The entry of calcium ions is required for neurotransmitter release from storage sites in small sacs called synaptic vesicles. Storage of neurotransmitters allows them to be available quickly when needed and to avoid degradation by enzymes in the nerve terminal.

When released from the synaptic vesicles, molecules of neurotransmitter cross the synapse, bind to receptors in the cell membrane of the postsynaptic neuron (Fig. 5-1), and excite or inhibit postsynaptic neurons. Free neurotransmitter molecules (*i.e.*, those not bound to receptors) are rapidly removed from the synapse by three mechanisms: transportation back into the presynaptic nerve terminal (reuptake) for reuse, diffusion into surrounding body fluids, or destruction by enzymes (*e.g.*, acetylcholine is degraded by cholinesterase; norepinephrine is metabolized by monoamine oxidase and catecholo-methyl transferase).

The three types of neurotransmitters thus far identified are amines, amino acids, and peptides, all of which are derived from body proteins. Most acute CNS responses are caused by small-molecule, rapidly acting neurotransmitters, such as acetylcholine, the amines (dopamine, norepinephrine, serotonin), and amino acids (aspartate, gamma-aminobutyric acid [GABA], glutamate, and glycine). Most prolonged CNS responses are caused by large-molecule, slowly acting neurotransmitters, such as the neuropeptide hormones (*e.g.*, adrenocorticotropic hormone [ACTH or corticotropin] and antidiuretic hormone [ADH]). Prolonged effects are thought to involve closure of calcium channels, changes in cellular metabolism, changes in activation or deactivation of specific genes in the cell nucleus, and alterations in the numbers of excitatory or inhibitory postsynaptic membrane receptors. Some pep-

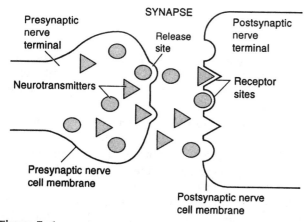

SYNAPSE

Presynaptic nerve terminal

Release site

Postsynaptic nerve terminal

Neurotransmitters

Receptor sites

Presynaptic nerve cell membrane

Postsynaptic nerve cell membrane

Figure 5–1

Neurotransmission in the central nervous system. Neurotransmitter molecules (*e.g.*, norepinephrine and acetylcholine), released by the presynaptic nerve, cross the synapse and bind with receptor proteins in the cell membrane of the postsynaptic nerve.

tides (*e.g.*, ADH) serve as chemical messengers in both the nervous system and the endocrine system.

Several factors affect the availability and function of neurotransmitters. One factor is the availability of precursor proteins and enzymes required to synthesize particular neurotransmitters. Another major factor is the number and binding capacity of *receptors* in the cell membranes of presynaptic and postsynaptic nerve endings. A particular neurotransmitter may interact with many different receptors. Other important factors include *acid–base imbalances* (acidosis decreases synaptic transmission; alkalosis increases synaptic transmission); *hypoxia*, which causes CNS depression (coma occurs within seconds without oxygen); and *drugs*, which may alter neurotransmitter synthesis, release, degradation, or binding to receptors to cause either CNS stimulation or depression.

SYNAPSES

Neurons in a chain are separated by a microscopic gap called a *synapse* or synaptic cleft. Synapses may be *electrical*, in which sodium and potassium ions can rapidly conduct an electrical impulse from one neuron to another, or *chemical*, in which a neurotransmitter conducts the message to the next neuron. The chemical synapse is more commonly used to communicate with other neurons or target cells. Neurotransmitter release and removal occur in the synapses.

RECEPTORS

Receptors are proteins embedded in the cell membranes of neurons. In the CNS, most receptors are on postsynaptic neurons, but some are on presynaptic

nerve terminals. For most receptors, several subtypes have been identified, for which specific characteristics and functions have not yet been delineated. A neurotransmitter must bind to receptors to exert an effect on the next neuron in the chain. Some receptors act rapidly to open ion channels; others interact with a variety of intracellular proteins to initiate a second messenger system. For example, when norepinephrine binds with alpha- or beta-adrenergic receptors, intracellular events include activation of the enzyme adenyl cyclase and the production of cyclic adenosine monophosphate (cAMP). In this case, the cAMP is a second messenger that activates cellular functions and the physiologic responses controlled by the alpha- and beta-adrenergic receptors. A neurotransmitter/receptor complex may have an excitatory or inhibitory effect on the postsynaptic neuron.

Receptors increase in number and activity (upregulation) when there is underactivity at the synapse. They decrease in number and activity (downregulation) when there is overactivity. Like other protein molecules in the body, receptors are constantly being synthesized and degraded. More specifically, it is believed that receptor proteins are constantly being formed by the endoplasmic reticulum–Golgi apparatus and inserted into presynaptic and postsynaptic membranes. If the synapses are overused and excessive amounts of neurotransmitter combine with receptor proteins, it is then postulated that many of the receptor proteins are inactivated and removed from the synaptic membrane. Thus, synaptic fatigue and downgrading or upgrading of receptors work with other control mechanisms of the nervous system to readjust abnormally stimulated or depressed nerve function toward normal.

NEUROTRANSMISSION SYSTEMS

Neurons function through communication networks that may be called neurotransmission systems, the major elements of which are neurotransmitters, synapses, and receptors. Although neurotransmitters, synapses, and receptors are discussed separately here, it is the interaction among these elements that promotes order or disorder in the body's physical and mental processes. Although many details of neuronal function remain elusive, a great deal of knowledge has been gained in recent years. For example, numerous neurotransmitters and subtypes of receptors have been identified and characterized. Major neurotransmission systems are the cholinergic, dopaminergic, GABA-ergic, noradrenergic, and serotonergic networks.

The **cholinergic system** uses acetylcholine as its neurotransmitter. *Acetylcholine*, the first substance to be designated as a neurotransmitter in the CNS, is located in many areas of the brain, with especially high concentrations in the motor cortex and basal ganglia. It is also a neurotransmitter in the autonomic nervous system and at peripheral neuromuscular junctions. Acetylcholine exerts excitatory effects at synapses and nerve–muscle junctions and inhibitory effects at some peripheral sites, such as organs supplied by the vagus nerves. In the CNS, acetylcholine is associated with level of arousal, memory, motor conditioning, and speech.

The **dopaminergic system** uses *dopamine* as its neurotransmitter. Dopamine is derived from tyrosine, an amino acid, and is a precursor substance in the synthesis of norepinephrine and epinephrine. Dopamine makes up more than half the catecholamine content in the brain and is found in the substantia nigra, the midbrain, and the hypothalamus, with high concentrations in the substantia nigra and basal ganglia. Much of the information about dopamine is derived from studies of antipsychotic drugs (see Chap. 9) and Parkinson's disease, a disorder caused by destruction of dopamine-producing neurons in the substantia nigra. Dopamine also occurs outside the brain, in renal and mesenteric blood vessels.

In the CNS, dopamine is thought to be inhibitory in the basal ganglia but may be excitatory in other areas. Repeated stimulation of dopamine receptors decreases their numbers (down-regulation) and their sensitivity to dopamine (desensitization). Prolonged blockade of dopamine receptors increases their numbers and sensitivity to dopamine. Some receptors (called autoreceptors) occur on the presynaptic nerve terminal. When released, dopamine stimulates these receptors and a negative feedback system is initiated that inhibits further dopamine synthesis and release.

Two groups of dopamine receptors have been identified. They are differentiated by the intracellular events that follow dopamine-receptor binding. One group includes D_1 and D_5 receptors, which activate adenyl cyclase to produce cAMP. The other group includes D_2, D_3, and D_4 receptors. D_2 receptors have been described most thoroughly; they are thought to inhibit activation of adenyl cyclase and subsequent production of cAMP, suppress calcium ion currents, and activate potassium ion currents. D_3 and D_4 receptor functions have not been delineated. Overall, dopamine actions at the cellular level depend on the subtype of receptor to which it binds and the simultaneous effects of other neurotransmitters at the same target neurons.

The **GABA-ergic system** uses *gamma-aminobutyric acid* (GABA) as its neurotransmitter. GABA is synthesized in the brain (cerebellum, basal ganglia, and cerebral cortex) and spinal cord in abundant amounts. It is the major inhibitory neurotransmitter in the CNS, with a role in many neuronal circuits (estimated at nearly one third of CNS synapses. GABA receptors have been divided into two main types, A and B.

$GABA_A$ receptor is a chloride ion channel that opens when GABA is released from presynaptic neurons. $GABA_B$ has not been delineated, but it is thought to function in regulation of ion channels and biochemical pathways. There is evidence of multiple subtypes of GABA receptors and important functional differences among them.

The **noradrenergic** (norepinephrine) **system** uses *norepinephrine* as its neurotransmitter and extends to virtually every area of the brain. Like dopamine, norepinephrine is a catecholamine synthesized from tyrosine. It is found in relatively large amounts in the hypothalamus and the limbic system and in smaller amounts in most areas of the brain, including the reticular formation. Norepinephrine is mainly an excitatory neurotransmitter that stimulates the brain to generalized increased activity. However, it is inhibitory in a few areas because of inhibitory receptors at some nerve synapses.

Norepinephrine receptors in the CNS, as in the sympathetic nervous system, are divided into alpha- and beta-adrenergic receptors and their subtypes. Activation of $alpha_1$ and $beta_1$ and $beta_2$ receptors is thought to stimulate activity of intracellular adenyl cyclase and the production of cAMP. Activation of $alpha_2$ receptors is associated with inhibition of adenyl cyclase activity and decreased production of cAMP. However, the effects of norepinephrine–$alpha_2$ receptor coupling are thought to stem mainly from activation of receptor-operated potassium ion channels and suppression of voltage-operated calcium ion channels. These effects on ion channels may increase membrane resistance to stimuli and inhibit the firing of CNS neurons. In addition, $alpha_2$ receptors on the presynaptic nerve ending are believed to regulate norepinephrine release. In other words, when high levels of extracellular norepinephrine act on presynaptic $alpha_2$ receptors, the effect is similar to a negative feedback system that inhibits the release of more norepinephrine. Overall, the noradrenergic system is associated with mood, motor activity, regulation of arousal, and reward. It is thought to play an important role in producing rapid-eye-movement (REM) sleep, during which dreaming occurs.

The **serotonergic system** uses *serotonin* (also called 5-hydroxytryptamine or 5-HT) as its neurotransmitter. Serotonin-synthesizing neurons are widely distributed in the CNS, beginning in the midbrain and projecting into the thalamus, hypothalamus, cerebral cortex, and spinal cord. Because serotonin is synthesized from the amino acid tryptophan, the amount of tryptophan intake in the diet controls the rate of serotonin production. CNS serotonin is usually an inhibitory neurotransmitter and is associated with mood, the sleep–wake cycle, habituation, and sensory perceptions, including inhibition of pain pathways in the spinal cord. Serotonin is thought to produce sleep by inhibiting CNS activity and arousal.

Serotonin receptors are found in regions of the CNS that are associated with mood and anxiety and are also thought to be involved in temperature regulation. Activation of some receptors leads to hyperpolarization and neuronal inhibition. Several subtypes of serotonin receptors have been identified, some of which are linked to inhibition of adenyl cyclase activity or to regulation of potassium or calcium ion channels.

Serotonin is also found outside the CNS, mainly in mast cells of the lungs and platelets. It plays a major role in the blood coagulation process, during which it is released from platelets and causes vasoconstriction. It may also be involved in the vascular spasm associated with some pulmonary allergic reactions (during which it is released from mast cells) and migraine headaches. However, peripheral serotonin cannot cross the blood-brain barrier.

Other systems of neurotransmission include several amino acids that may serve as both structural components for protein synthesis and neurotransmitters. Amino acids were recognized as neurotransmitters relatively recently, and their roles and functions in this regard have not been completely elucidated. A summary of their characteristics follows.

Aspartate is an excitatory neurotransmitter found in high concentrations in the brain. Aspartate and glutamate are considered the major fast-acting, excitatory neurotransmitters in the brain.

Glycine is an inhibitory neurotransmitter found in the brain stem and spinal cord. Glycine receptors have many of the features described for GABA$_A$ receptors; subtypes have been identified but their functions are unknown.

Glutamate is considered the most important excitatory neurotransmitter in the CNS. It occurs in high concentrations in virtually every area of the CNS, including the cerebral cortex, basal ganglia, limbic structures, and hippocampus. Several subtypes of glutamate receptors have been identified, each with a unique distribution in the CNS. The functions of these receptor subtypes have not been established, but research suggests that the N-methyl-D-aspartate (NMDA) glutamate-receptor subtype plays a role in memory.

Although some glutamate is apparently necessary for normal neurotransmission, brief exposure of neurons to high concentrations can lead to neuronal cell death. Events leading to neuronal death are triggered by excessive activation of NMDA receptors and movement of calcium ions into the neurons. This process may be similar to the neurotoxicity that occurs after ischemia or hypoglycemia in the brain, where increased release and impaired reuptake of glutamate lead to excessive stimulation of glutamate receptors and subsequent cell death.

NEUROTRANSMISSION SYSTEMS IN SELECTED CNS DISORDERS

Abnormalities in neurotransmission systems (*e.g.*, dysfunction or destruction of the neurons that normally produce neurotransmitters or altered receptor response to neurotransmitters) are implicated in many CNS disorders. For example, decreased acetylcholine is a characteristic of Alzheimer's disease; dopamine abnormalities occur in psychosis and Parkinson's disease; GABA abnormalities occur in anxiety, hyperarousal states, and seizure disorders; glutamate has been implicated in the pathogenesis of epilepsy, stroke, and Huntington's disease; and serotonin abnormalities are thought to be involved in mental depression and sleep disorders.

Although most research has focused on single neurotransmitters and their respective receptors, CNS function in both health and disease is probably determined by interactions among neurotransmission systems. In health, for example, complex mechanisms regulate the amounts and binding capacities of neurotransmitters and receptors, as well as the balance between excitatory and inhibitory forces. When abnormalities occur in any of these elements, the resulting dysregulation and imbalances lead to signs and symptoms of CNS disorders. Overall, then, neurotransmission systems function interdependently: One system may increase, decrease, or otherwise modify the effects of another system.

Except for mental depression, most psychiatric symptoms result from CNS stimulation and usually involve physical and mental hyperactivity. Such hyperactivity reflects a wide range of observable behaviors and nonobservable thoughts and feelings. In most people, manifestations may include pleasant feelings of mild euphoria and high levels of enthusiasm, energy, and productivity. In people with psychiatric illnesses, such as severe anxiety or psychosis, manifestations include unpleasant feelings of tension, psychomotor agitation, nervousness, and decreased ability to rest and sleep, even when very tired. Many psychiatric disorders, therapeutic drugs, and drugs of abuse may cause varying degrees of CNS stimulation. Generally, the pathogenesis of excessive CNS stimulation may involve one or more of the following mechanisms:

1. Excessive amounts of excitatory neurotransmitters (*e.g.*, norepinephrine)
2. Increased numbers or sensitivity of excitatory receptors
3. Insufficient amounts of inhibitory neurotransmitters (*e.g.*, GABA)
4. Decreased numbers or sensitivity of inhibitory receptors

CEREBRAL CORTEX

The cerebral cortex is involved in all conscious processes, such as learning, memory, reasoning, verbalization, and voluntary body movements. Some parts of the cortex receive incoming nerve impulses and are called *sensory areas*; other parts send impulses to peripheral structures and are called *motor areas*. Around the sensory and motor areas are the "association" areas, which occupy the greater portion of the cortex. These areas analyze the information received by the sensory areas and decide on the appropriate response. In some instances, the response may be to store the perception in memory; in others, it may involve stimulation of motor centers to produce movement or speech.

THALAMUS

The thalamus receives impulses carrying sensations such as heat, cold, pain, and muscle position sense. These sensations produce only a crude awareness at the thalamic level. They are relayed to the cerebral cortex, where they are interpreted regarding location, quality, intensity, and significance. The thalamus also relays motor impulses from the cortex to the spinal cord.

HYPOTHALAMUS

The hypothalamus has extensive neurologic and endocrine functions. In the CNS, it is connected with the thalamus, medulla oblongata, spinal cord, reticular activating system, and limbic system. In the autonomic nervous system, it is the center for motor control. In the endocrine system, the hypothalamus controls the secretion of all pituitary hormones. It is anatomically connected to the posterior pituitary gland, and it regulates the activity of the anterior pituitary. It constantly collects information about the internal environment of the body and helps maintain homeostasis by making continuous adjustments in water balance, body temperature, hormone levels, arterial blood pressure, heart rate, gastrointestinal motility, and other body functions. The hypothalamus is stimulated or inhibited by nerve impulses from different portions of the nervous system and by concentrations of nutrients, electrolytes, water, and hormones in the blood. Specific neuroendocrine functions include:

1. Producing oxytocin and ADH, which are stored in the posterior pituitary gland and released in response to nerve impulses from the hypothalamus. Oxytocin initiates uterine contractions to begin labor and delivery and helps to release milk from breast glands during breast-feeding. ADH helps maintain fluid balance by controlling water excretion. ADH secretion is controlled by the osmolarity of the extracellular fluid. When osmolarity is high, more ADH is secreted. This means that water is retained in the body to dilute the extracellular fluid and return it toward normal or homeostatic levels. When osmolarity is low, less ADH is secreted, and more water is excreted in the urine.
2. Regulating body temperature. When body temperature is elevated, sweating and dilation of blood vessels in the skin lower the temperature. When body temperature is low, sweating ceases and vasoconstriction occurs. When heat loss is decreased, the temperature is raised.
3. Assisting in regulation of arterial blood pressure by its effects on the vasomotor center. The vasomotor center in the medulla oblongata and pons maintains a state of partial contraction in blood vessels (vasomotor tone). The hypothalamus can exert excitatory or inhibitory effects on the vasomotor center, depending on which portions of the hypothalamus are stimulated. When nerve impulses from the hypothalamus excite the vasomotor center, vasomotor tone or vasoconstriction is increased, and blood pressure is raised. When the impulses from the hypothalamus inhibit the vasomotor center, vasomotor tone or vasoconstriction is decreased, with the overall effect of relative vasodilation and lowering of arterial blood pressure.
4. Regulating anterior pituitary hormones, including thyroid-stimulating hormone, ACTH, and growth hormone. The hypothalamus secretes "releasing factors," which cause the anterior pituitary to secrete these hormones. There is a hypothalamic releasing factor for each hormone. The hypothalamic factor called prolactin-inhibiting factor inhibits secretion of prolactin, another anterior pituitary hormone.
5. Regulating food and water intake by the hypothalamic thirst, appetite, hunger, and satiety centers
6. Regulating the physical changes associated with emotions (*e.g.,* increased blood pressure and heart rate). The hypothalamus, thalamus, and cerebral cortex interact to produce the feelings associated with emotions.

MEDULLA OBLONGATA

The medulla oblongata contains groups of neurons that form the vital cardiac, respiratory, and vasomotor centers. For example, if the respiratory center is stimulated, respiratory rate and depth are increased. If the respiratory center is depressed, respiratory rate and depth are decreased. The medulla also contains reflex centers for coughing, vomiting, sneezing, swallowing, and salivating.

The medulla and pons varolii also contain groups of neurons from which originate cranial nerves 5 through 12. Together with the midbrain, these structures form the brain stem.

RETICULAR ACTIVATING SYSTEM

The reticular activating system is a network of neurons that extends from the spinal cord through the medulla and pons to the thalamus and hypothalamus. It receives impulses from all parts of the body, evaluates the significance of the impulses, and decides which impulses to transmit to the cerebral cortex. It also excites or inhibits motor nerves that control both reflex and voluntary movement. Stimulation of these neurons produces wakefulness and mental alertness; depression causes sedation and loss of consciousness.

LIMBIC SYSTEM

The limbic system borders and interconnects with the thalamus, hypothalamus, basal ganglia, hippocampus, amygdala, and septum. It participates in regulation of feeding behavior, the sleep–wake cycle, emotions (*e.g.*, pleasure, fear, anger, sadness), and behavior (*e.g.*, aggression, laughing, crying). Many nerve impulses from the limbic system are transmitted through the hypothalamus; thus, physiologic changes in blood pressure, heart rate, respiration, and hormone secretion occur in response to the emotions.

CEREBELLUM

The cerebellum, which is connected with motor centers in the cerebral cortex and basal ganglia, coordinates muscular activity. When several skeletal muscles are involved, some are contracted and some are relaxed for smooth, purposeful movements. It also helps to maintain balance and posture by receiving nerve impulses from the inner ear that produce appropriate reflex responses.

BASAL GANGLIA

The basal ganglia are concerned with skeletal muscle tone and orderly activity. Normal function is influenced by dopamine, a neurotransmitter produced in several areas of the brain. Degenerative changes in one of these areas, the substantia nigra, cause dopamine to be released in decreased amounts. This process is a factor in the development of Parkinson's disease, which is characterized by rigidity and increased muscle tone.

PYRAMIDAL AND EXTRAPYRAMIDAL SYSTEMS

The pyramidal and extrapyramidal systems are pathways out of the cerebral cortex. In the pyramidal or corticospinal tract, nerve fibers originate in the cerebral cortex, go down the brain stem to the medulla, where the fibers cross, and continue down the spinal cord, where they end at various levels. Impulses are then carried from the spinal cord to skeletal muscle. Because the fibers cross in the medulla, impulses from the right side of the cerebral cortex control skeletal muscle movements of the left side of the body, and impulses from the left control muscle movements of the right side.

In the extrapyramidal system, fibers originate mainly in the premotor area of the cerebral cortex and travel to the basal ganglia and brain stem. The fibers are called extrapyramidal because they do not enter the medullary pyramids and cross over.

Pyramidal and extrapyramidal systems intermingle in the spinal cord; disease processes affecting higher levels of the CNS involve both tracts.

BRAIN METABOLISM

To function correctly, the brain must have an adequate and continuous supply of nutrients, especially oxygen, glucose, and thiamine.

Oxygen is carried to the brain by the carotid and vertebral arteries. The brain requires more oxygen than any other organ. Cerebral cortex cells are very sensitive to lack of oxygen (hypoxia), and interruption of blood supply causes immediate loss of consciousness. Brain stem cells are less sensitive to hypoxia. People in whom hypoxia is relatively prolonged may survive, although they may have irreversible brain damage.

Glucose is required as an energy source for brain cell metabolism. Hypoglycemia (low blood sugar) may cause mental confusion, dizziness, convulsions, loss of consciousness, and permanent damage to the cerebral cortex.

Thiamine is required for production and use of glucose. Thiamine deficiency can reduce glucose use by about half and can cause degeneration of the myelin sheaths of nerve cells. Such degeneration in central neurons leads to a form of encephalopathy known as Wernicke-Korsakoff syndrome. Degeneration in peripheral nerves leads to polyneuritis and muscle atrophy, weakness, and paralysis.

SPINAL CORD

The spinal cord is continuous with the medulla oblongata and extends down through the vertebral column to the sacral area. It consists of 31 segments, each of which is the point of origin for a pair of spinal nerves. The cord is a pathway between the brain and the peripheral nervous system. It carries impulses to and from the brain, along sensory and motor nerve fibers, and is a center for reflex actions. Reflexes are involuntary responses to certain nerve impulses received by the spinal cord (*e.g.*, the knee-jerk and pupillary reflexes).

Drugs Affecting the CNS

Drugs affecting the CNS, sometimes called centrally active drugs, are broadly classified as depressants or stimulants. CNS depressant drugs (*e.g.*, antipsychotics, narcotic analgesics, sedative-hypnotics) produce a general depression of the CNS when given in sufficient dosages. Mild CNS depression is characterized by lack of interest in surroundings and inability to focus on a topic (short attention span). As depression progresses, there is drowsiness or sleep, decreased muscle tone, decreased ability to move, and decreased perception of sensations such as pain, heat, and cold. Severe CNS depression produces unconsciousness or coma, loss of reflexes, respiratory failure, and death.

CNS stimulants produce a variety of effects. Mild stimulation is characterized by wakefulness, mental alertness, and decreased fatigue. Increasing stimulation produces hyperactivity, excessive talking, nervousness, and insomnia. Excessive stimulation can cause convulsive seizures, cardiac arrhythmias, and death. Because it is difficult to avoid excessive, harmful CNS stimulation by these drugs, CNS stimulants are less useful for therapeutic purposes than are CNS depressants.

REVIEW AND APPLICATION EXERCISES

1. Where are neurotransmitters synthesized and stored?

2. What events occur at the synapse between two neurons?

3. Once a neurotransmitter is released and acts on receptors, how are the remaining molecules inactivated?

4. What are the main functions of acetylcholine, dopamine, GABA, norepinephrine, and serotonin?

5. What part of the brain is concerned mainly with thoughts, reasoning, and learning?

6. What part of the brain contains vital respiratory and cardiovascular centers?

7. How would you expect a person with CNS depression to look and behave?

8. How would you expect a person with excessive CNS stimulation to look and behave?

SELECTED REFERENCES

Bloom, F.E. (1996) Neurotransmission and the central nervous system. In J.G. Hardman, L.E. Limbird, P.B. Molinoff, & R.W. Ruddon (Eds.), *Goodman and Gilman's The pharmacologic basic of therapeutics*, 9th ed., pp. 267–293. New York: McGraw-Hill.

Guyton, A.C. & Hall, J.E. (1996). *Textbook of medical physiology*, 9th ed. Philadelphia: W.B. Saunders.

Henn, F.A. (1994). The neurobiologic basis of psychiatric illnesses. In G. Winokur & P.J. Clayton (Eds.), *The medical basis of psychiatry*, 2nd ed., pp. 439–458. Philadelphia: W.B. Saunders.

McCrone, S.H. (1996). Physical dimensions of the journey: Neurobiological influences. In V.B. Carson & E.N. Arnold (Eds.), *Mental health nursing: The nurse-patient journey*, pp. 127–149. Philadelphia: W.B. Saunders.

Wilcox, R.E. & Gonzales, R.A. (1995). Introduction to neurotransmitters, receptors, signal transduction and second messengers. In A.F. Schatzberg & C.B. Nemeroff (Eds.), *The American Psychiatric Press Textbook of psychopharmacology*, pp. 3–29. Washington, D.C.: American Psychiatric Press.

Narcotic Analgesics and Narcotic Antagonists

Objectives

After studying this chapter, the student will be able to:

1 Discuss characteristics of pain.

2 Discuss the nurse's role in assessing and managing clients' pain.

3 List characteristics of narcotic analgesics in terms of mechanism of action, indications for use, and major adverse effects.

4 Describe morphine as the prototype of narcotic analgesics.

5 Discuss morphine dosage forms and dosage ranges for various clinical uses.

6 Explain why higher doses of narcotic analgesics are needed when the drugs are given orally.

7 Contrast the use of narcotic analgesics in "opiate-naive" and "opiate-tolerant" clients.

8 Assess level of consciousness and respiratory status before and after administering narcotics.

9 Discuss principles of therapy and nursing process for using narcotic analgesics in children and older adults.

10 Teach clients about safe, effective use of narcotic analgesics.

11 Discuss the clinical use of narcotic antagonists.

Key Terms

Analgesia	**Opiate**
Endogenous analgesia system	**Opioid receptors**
	Pain
Equianalgesia	**Patient-controlled analgesia**
Nociceptors	

Pain, the most common symptom prompting people to seek health care, is an unpleasant sensation that usually indicates tissue damage and impels the person to remove the cause of the damage. Narcotic analgesics are drugs that relieve moderate to severe pain. To aid understanding of drug actions, selected characteristics of pain and endogenous pain-relieving substances are described.

Pain

Pain occurs when tissue damage activates the free nerve endings (pain receptors or nociceptors) of peripheral nerves. Nociceptors are abundant in the skin and underlying soft tissue, joint surfaces, arterial walls, and periosteum; most internal organs, such as lung and uterine tissue, contain few nociceptors. Causes of tissue damage may be physical (e.g., heat, cold, pressure) or chemical (e.g., pain related to substances released from damaged cells and products of inflammation, including bradykinin, histamine, and prostaglandins). Bradykinin, one of the strongest pain-producing substances, is quickly metabolized and therefore may be involved mainly in acute pain. Prostaglandins increase bradykinin's pain-provoking effects by increasing the sensitivity of pain receptors. Several other substances are also thought to produce pain, including acetylcholine, adenosine triphosphate, histamine, leukotrienes, potassium, serotonin, and substance P. Overall, these chemical mediators produce pain by activating peripheral nociceptors, sensitizing peripheral endings of nociceptors, or stimulating the release of pain-producing substances.

When pain receptors are activated, the message of tissue damage is transmitted to the dorsal horn of the spinal cord by two groups of afferent nerve fibers. One group is the small, myelinated, A-delta fibers, which are activated by thermal and mechanical stimuli and transmit fast, sharp, well-localized pain signals. These fibers release glutamate and aspartate (neurotransmitter amino acids) at synapses in the spinal cord. The other group is unmyelinated C fibers that respond to thermal, mechanical, and chemical stimulation and mediate slow, burning, poorly localized pain signals. C fibers release somatostatin and substance P at synapses in the spinal cord. Substance P is a peptide neurotransmitter that is thought to play an important role in transmitting pain signals from peripheral tissues to the central nervous system (CNS).

The dorsal horn of the spinal cord is the control center or relay station for information from the A-delta and C nociceptive fibers, for local modulation of the pain impulse, and for descending influences from higher centers in the CNS (e.g., attention, emotion, memory). Here, nociceptive nerve fibers synapse with non-nociceptive

nerve fibers (neurons that carry information other than pain signals). The brain also contains powerful descending pathways that modify nociceptive input. Some brain nuclei are serotonergic and project to the dorsal horn of the spinal cord, where they suppress nociceptive transmission. Another major inhibitory pathway is noradrenergic and originates in the pons. Thus, increasing the concentration of norepinephrine and serotonin in the synapse interrupts or inhibits transmission of nerve impulses that carry pain signals to the brain and spinal cord. (This is thought to account for the pain-relieving effects of the tricyclic antidepressants, drugs that increase the amounts of serotonin and norepinephrine in the synapse by inhibiting their reuptake by presynaptic nerve endings.)

In the brain, the thalamus is a relay station for incoming sensory stimuli, including pain. Perception of pain is a primitive awareness in the thalamus, and sensation is not well localized or specific. From the thalamus, pain messages are relayed to the cerebral cortex, where they are perceived more specifically and analyzed to determine actions needed.

Pain is often described as acute or chronic and superficial or deep.

Acute pain is usually caused by tissue-damaging stimuli, and the duration is usually less than 6 months. It serves as a protective or warning system by demanding the sufferer's attention and compelling behavior to seek relief. It is often accompanied by anxiety and objective signs of discomfort, such as facial expressions of distress; moaning or crying; positioning to protect the affected part; tenderness, edema, and skin color or temperature changes in the affected part; and either restlessness and excessive movement or limited movement, if movement increases pain.

Chronic pain, usually defined as pain of 6 months or longer, demands attention less urgently, may not be characterized by visible signs, and is often accompanied by depression and changes in personality, lifestyle, and functional ability. It may occur with or without evidence of tissue damage and serves no useful purpose. It may include acute pain that persists beyond the normal healing time, pain related to a chronic disease, pain without an identifiable cause, and pain associated with cancer. It is important to differentiate between chronic pain and acute pain because they are managed quite differently.

Superficial pain originates in the skin or underlying structures and produces sharp pain with a burning quality that is readily localized by the sufferer. Superficial pain or pain of low to moderate intensity usually stimulates the sympathetic nervous system and produces increased blood pressure, pulse, and respiration; dilated pupils; and increased skeletal muscle tension, such as rigid posture or clenched fists.

Deep pain originates in bones and abdominal or thoracic organs and produces a dull, aching sensation that is hard to localize. Deep or severe pain stimulates the parasympathetic nervous system and produces decreased blood pressure and pulse, nausea and vomiting, weakness, syncope, and possibly loss of consciousness.

Endogenous Analgesia System

The CNS has its own system for suppressing the transmission of pain signals from peripheral nerves. The system can be activated by nervous signals entering the periaqueductal gray area of the brain or by morphine-like drugs. Important elements include opiate receptors and endogenous peptides with actions similar to those of morphine. Opiate receptors are highly concentrated in some regions of the CNS, including the ascending and descending pain pathways and portions of the brain essential to the endogenous analgesia system. The opioid peptides (*i.e.,* the enkephalins, dynorphins, and beta-endorphins) interact with opiate receptors to inhibit pain transmission. All are important in the endogenous opiate system, but the three types of peptides differ in precursors and anatomic locations. Enkephalins are believed to interrupt the transmission of pain signals at the spinal-cord level by inhibiting the release of substance P from C nerve fibers. The endogenous analgesia system probably can also inhibit pain signals at other points in the pain pathway.

Narcotic Analgesics

Narcotic analgesics are drugs that relieve moderate to severe pain by reducing the perception of pain sensation, producing sedation, and decreasing the emotional upsets often associated with pain. Most of these analgesics are Schedule II drugs under federal narcotic laws and may lead to drug abuse and dependence. *Morphine* is the prototype of these analgesics and the standard by which others are measured. These drugs are often called opioids (drugs that act like morphine in the body).

Morphine and other opioids exert widespread pharmacologic effects, especially in the CNS and the gastrointestinal (GI) system. These effects occur with usual doses and may be therapeutic or adverse, depending on the reason for use. CNS effects include analgesia, CNS depression ranging from drowsiness to sleep to unconsciousness, decreased mental and physical activity, respiratory depression, nausea and vomiting, and pupil constriction. Sedation and respiratory depression are major adverse effects and are potentially life-threatening. Most newer narcotic analgesics have been developed in an effort to find drugs as effective as morphine in relieving pain while causing less sedation, respiratory depression, and dependence. However, this effort has not been successful: *equianalgesic doses of these drugs produce sedative and respiratory depressant effects comparable to those of morphine.* In the GI system, narcotic analgesics slow motility and may cause smooth muscle spasms in the bowel and biliary tract.

MECHANISM OF ACTION

Opioids relieve pain by binding to opioid receptors in the brain and spinal cord and activating the endogenous analgesia system. Six major types of receptors have been identified (Table 6-1). Narcotic analgesics and narcotic antagonists bind to different receptors to varying degrees, and their pharmacologic actions can be differentiated and classified on this basis.

INDICATIONS FOR USE

The main indication for the use of opioids is to prevent or relieve acute or chronic pain. Specific conditions in which opioid drugs are used for analgesic effects include acute myocardial infarction, biliary colic, renal colic, burns and other traumatic injuries, postoperative states, and cancer. These drugs are usually given for chronic pain only when other measures and milder drugs are ineffective, as in terminal malignancy. Other clinical uses include:

1. Before and during surgery to promote sedation, decrease anxiety, facilitate induction of anesthesia, and decrease the amount of anesthesia required
2. Before and during invasive diagnostic procedures, such as angiograms and endoscopic examinations
3. During labor and delivery (obstetric analgesia)
4. Treating GI disorders, such as abdominal cramping and diarrhea
5. Treating acute pulmonary edema (morphine is used)
6. Treating severe, unproductive cough (codeine is generally used)

CONTRAINDICATIONS FOR USE

These drugs are contraindicated or must be used very cautiously in people with respiratory depression, chronic lung disease, liver or kidney disease, prostatic hypertrophy, increased intracranial pressure, or hypersensitivity reactions to opiates and related drugs.

Classifications and Individual Drugs

AGONISTS

Narcotic agonists include morphine and morphine-like drugs. These agents have activity at mu, kappa, and possibly delta opioid receptors and thus produce prototypical narcotic effects.

TABLE 6-1	OPIATE RECEPTORS AND THEIR EFFECTS

Drug Group	Receptor	Effects
Agonists (*e.g.*, morphine)	Mu-1	Analgesia
	Mu-2	Constipation
		Euphoria
		Physical dependence
		Respiratory depression
	Kappa	Analgesia
		Miosis
		Sedation
	Delta?	Analgesia
	Epsilon	Analgesia
Agonist/antagonists (*e.g.*, pentazocine)	Kappa	Analgesia
		Miosis
		Sedation
	Sigma	Dysphoria
		Hallucinations
		Respiratory stimulation
		Vasomotor stimulation

Morphine is a naturally occurring opium alkaloid used mainly to relieve acute or chronic severe pain. It is a Schedule II narcotic that is given orally and parenterally. Client response depends on route and dosage. After intravenous (IV) injection, maximal analgesia and respiratory depression usually occur within 10 to 20 minutes. After intramuscular (IM) injection, these effects occur in about 30 minutes. With subcutaneous (SC) injection, effects may be delayed up to 60 to 90 minutes.

Oral administration of morphine is common for chronic pain associated with cancer. When given orally, relatively high doses are required because part of each dose is metabolized in the liver and never reaches the systemic circulation. Concentrated solutions (*e.g.*, Roxanol, which contains 20 mg morphine/ml) and controlled-release tablets (*e.g.*, MS Contin, which contains 30 mg/tablet) have been developed for oral administration of these high doses. In some cases of severe pain that cannot be controlled by other methods, morphine is administered as a continuous IV infusion. Other routes of administration include epidural, in which the drug is instilled via a catheter placed in the epidural space and slowly diffuses into the spinal cord, and intrathecal, in which the drug is injected directly into the spinal cord. Epidural and intrathecal morphine provide pain relief with very small doses, once or twice daily. When clients cannot take oral medication and injections are undesirable, rectal suppositories are often given.

Morphine is primarily metabolized in the liver and excreted by the kidneys. Consequently, impaired liver and kidney function may cause prolonged drug action and accumulation, with a subsequent increase in the incidence and severity of adverse effects.

Routes and Dosage Ranges

Adults: PO 10–30 mg q4h PRN or as ordered by physician

PO controlled-release tablets, 30 mg q8–12h or as ordered by physician

IM, SC 5–20 mg/70 kg q4h PRN

IV injection, 2.5–15 mg/70 kg, diluted in 5 ml water for injection and injected slowly, for about 5 min, PRN

IV continuous infusion, 0.1–1 mg/ml in 5% dextrose in water, by controlled infusion pump

Epidural injection, 5 mg/24 h; continuous infusion, 2–4 mg/24 h

Intrathecal injection, 0.2–1 mg/24 h

Rectal, 10–20 mg q4h or as ordered by physician

Infants and children: IM, SC 0.1–0.2 mg/kg (up to 15 mg) q4h

Alfentanil (Alfenta), **fentanyl** (Sublimaze), and **sufentanil** (Sufenta) are potent drugs with a short duration of action. They are most often used in anesthesia (see Chap. 14) as analgesic adjuncts or primary anesthetic agents in open-heart surgery or complicated neurologic and orthopedic procedures. Fentanyl also is used for preanesthetic medication, postoperative analgesia, and chronic pain that requires an opioid analgesic. A transmucosal formulation (Fentanyl

Oralet, also called a lozenge or "lollipop") is available for conscious sedation or anesthesia premedication in children and adults. Because of a high risk of respiratory depression, recommended dosages must not be exceeded, and the drug should be given only in an area with staff and equipment for emergency care (*e.g.*, intensive care unit, operating room, emergency room). As with other routes of administration, dosage of the oral lozenge should be individualized according to age, weight, illness, other medications, type of procedure and anesthesia, and other factors. A transdermal formulation (Duragesic) is used in the treatment of chronic pain. The active drug is deposited in the skin and slowly absorbed systemically. Thus, the skin patches have a slow onset of action (about 12–24 hours), but they last about 3 days. When a patch is removed, the drug continues to be absorbed from the skin deposits for 24 hours or longer.

Alfentanil
Routes and Dosage Ranges

Adults: Analgesic adjunct in general anesthesia, IV initial dose 8–50 µg/kg; maintenance injection, 3–5 µg/kg; maintenance infusion, 0.5–1 µg/kg/min
Anesthesia induction, IV injection 130–245 µg/kg over 3 min or IV infusion 50–75 µg/kg
Anesthesia maintenance, IV infusion 0.5–3 µg/kg/min

Fentanyl
Routes and Dosage Ranges

Adults: Preanesthetic, IM 0.05–0.1 mg 30–60 min before surgery; oral lozenge, 200–400 µg, 20 to 40 min before a procedure, with instructions to suck, not chew, the medication. Maximum dose of oral lozenge, 400 µg.
Analgesic adjunct to general anesthesia, IV total dose of 0.002–0.05 mg/kg, depending on type and length of surgical procedure
Adjunct to regional anesthesia, IM or slow IV (over 1–2 min) 0.05–0.1 mg PRN
Postoperative analgesia, IM 0.05–0.1 mg, repeat in 1–2 h if needed
General anesthesia, IV 0.05–0.1 mg/kg with oxygen and a muscle relaxant (maximum dose 0.15 mg/kg with open-heart surgery, other major surgeries, and complicated neurologic or orthopedic procedures)
Chronic pain, transdermal system 2.5–10 mg every 72 h
Children <12 y: General anesthesia induction and maintenance, IV 1.7–3.3 mg/kg (20–30 µg/20–25 lb)
Children weighing at least 15 kg: Conscious sedation or preanesthetic sedation, 5–15 µg/kg of body weight (200–400 µg), depending on weight, type

of procedure, and other factors. Maximum dose, 400 µg, regardless of age and weight.

Sufentanil
Routes and Dosage Ranges

Adults: Analgesic adjunct to general anesthesia, IV initial dose 1–8 µg/kg; maintenance, 10–25 µg PRN
General anesthesia IV induction, 8–30 µg/kg; maintenance, 25–50 µg PRN
Children <12 y: General anesthesia, IV induction 10–25 µg with 100% oxygen; maintenance 25–50 µg PRN

Codeine is a naturally occurring opium alkaloid used for analgesic and antitussive effects. Codeine produces weaker analgesic and antitussive effects and milder adverse effects than morphine. Compared with other narcotic analgesics, codeine is more effective when given orally and is less likely to lead to abuse and dependence. Parenteral administration is more effective in relieving pain than oral administration, but onset (15–30 minutes) and duration of action (4–6 hours) are about the same. Larger doses are required for analgesic than for antitussive effects. Codeine is often given with aspirin or acetaminophen for additive analgesic effects.

Routes and Dosage Ranges

Adults: PO, SC, IM 15–60 mg q4–6h PRN
Cough, PO 10–20 mg q4h PRN
Children: PO, SC, IM 0.5 mg/kg q4–6h PRN
Cough, children 6–12 y, PO 5–10 mg q4–6h
Cough, children 2–6 y, PO 2.5–5 mg q4–6h

Hydrocodone, which is similar to codeine in its analgesic and antitussive effects, is a Schedule III drug. It is available only in combination products for cough (*e.g.*, Hycodan) and with acetaminophen for pain. Most products (*e.g.*, Hydrocet, Lortab, Vicodin) are analgesic combinations containing hydrocodone and acetaminophen.

Route and Dosage Ranges

Adults: PO 5–10 mg q6–8h
Children: PO 0.6 mg/kg/day in 3 or 4 divided doses

Hydromorphone (Dilaudid) is a semisynthetic derivative of morphine that has the same actions, uses, contraindications, and adverse effects as morphine. Hydromorphone is more potent on a milligram basis and is relatively more effective orally than morphine. Effects occur in 15 to 30 minutes, peak in 30 to 90 minutes, and last 4 to 5 hours.

Routes and Dosage Ranges

Adults: PO 2–4 mg q4–6h PRN
IM, SC, IV 1–1.5 mg q4–6h PRN (may be increased to 4 mg for severe pain)
Rectal suppository 3 mg q6–8h

Levorphanol (Levo-Dromoran) is a synthetic drug that is chemically and pharmacologically related to morphine. It has the same uses and produces the same adverse effects, although some reports indicate less nausea and vomiting. The average dose is probably equianalgesic with 10 mg of morphine. Maximal analgesia occurs 60 to 90 minutes after SC injection. Effects last 4 to 8 hours.

Routes and Dosage Range

Adults: PO, SC 2–3 mg q4–6h PRN

Meperidine (Demerol) is a frequently prescribed synthetic drug that is similar to morphine in pharmacologic actions. A parenteral dose of 80 to 100 mg is equivalent to 10 mg of morphine. Oral meperidine is only half as effective as a parenteral dose because about half is metabolized in the liver and never reaches the systemic circulation. Meperidine produces sedation and respiratory depression comparable to morphine. Meperidine differs from morphine as follows:

1. It has a shorter duration of action and requires more frequent administration. After parenteral administration, analgesia occurs in about 10 to 20 minutes, peaks in about 1 hour, and lasts about 2 to 4 hours.
2. It has little antitussive effect. However, excessive sedation with meperidine reduces the ability to cough effectively.
3. It causes less respiratory depression in the newborn when used for obstetric analgesia.
4. It causes less smooth muscle spasm and is preferred in renal and biliary colic.
5. With chronic use, toxic doses, or renal failure, meperidine may cause CNS stimulation characterized by tremors, hallucinations, and seizures. These effects are attributed to accumulation of a metabolite, normeperidine.

Routes and Dosage Ranges

Adults: IM, IV, SC, PO 50–100 mg q2–4h
Obstetric analgesia, IM, SC 50–100 mg q2–4h for three or four doses

Methadone (Dolophine) is a synthetic drug with the same pharmacologic actions as morphine. Compared with morphine, methadone has a longer duration of action and is relatively more effective when given orally. Analgesia occurs within 10 to 20 minutes after injection and 30 to 60 minutes after oral administration. Methadone is used for severe pain and in the detoxification and maintenance treatment of opiate addicts.

Routes and Dosage Ranges

Adults: IM, SC 2.5–10 mg q3–4h PRN
PO 5–20 mg q6–8h PRN

Oxycodone is a semisynthetic derivative of codeine used to relieve moderate pain. It is reportedly less potent and less likely to produce dependence than morphine but is more potent and more likely to produce dependence than codeine. It is a drug of abuse. Pharmacologic actions are similar to those of other narcotic analgesics. Oxycodone is available alone (Roxicodone) and in combination with aspirin (Percodan) or acetaminophen (Percocet, Tylox).

Route and Dosage Range

Adults: PO 5 mg q6h PRN
Children: Not recommended for children <12 y

Oxymorphone (Numorphan) is a semisynthetic derivative of morphine. Its actions, uses, and adverse effects are similar to those of morphine, except that it has little antitussive effect.

Routes and Dosage Ranges

Adults: IM, SC 1–1.5 mg q4–6h PRN
IV 0.5 mg q4–6h PRN
Rectal suppository, 5 mg q4–6h PRN
Obstetric analgesia, IM 0.5–1 mg

Propoxyphene (Darvon) is a synthetic drug chemically related to methadone. It is used for mild to moderate pain but is considered no more effective than 650 mg of aspirin or acetaminophen, with which it is usually given. It is not recommended for use in children or in patients at risk for suicide or addiction. Propoxyphene is abused (alone and with alcohol or other CNS depressant drugs), and deaths have occurred from overdoses. An overdose causes respiratory depression, excessive sedation, and circulatory failure. Despite these characteristics and dangers, the drug continues to be prescribed. Propoxyphene is a Schedule IV drug.

Propoxyphene Hydrochloride
Route and Dosage Range

Adults: PO 65 mg q4h PRN (maximal daily dose, 390 mg)
Children: Not recommended

Propoxyphene Napsylate
Route and Dosage Range

Adults: PO 100 mg q4h PRN (maximal daily dose, 600 mg)
Children: Not recommended

Tramadol (Ultram) is an oral, synthetic, centrally active analgesic for moderate to moderately severe pain. It is not chemically related to opioids. Its mechanism of action is unclear but includes binding to mu opioid receptors and inhibiting reuptake of norepinephrine and serotonin in the brain. Analgesia occurs within 1 hour after administration and peaks in about 2 to 3 hours. Tramadol causes significantly less respiratory depression than morphine but may cause other morphine-like adverse effects (*e.g.*, drowsiness, nausea, constipation, pruritus, orthostatic hypotension).

Tramadol is well absorbed after oral administration, even if taken with food. It is minimally bound (about 20%) to plasma proteins. It is extensively metabolized; about 30% of a dose is excreted unchanged in the urine and about 60% is excreted as metabolites. Dosage should be reduced in persons with severe renal impairment.

Route and Dosage Range

Adults: PO 50–100 mg q4–6h PRN (maximal daily dose, 400 mg)
  Adults with renal impairment (*i.e.*, creatinine clearance <30 ml/min): PO 50–100 mg q12h (maximal daily dose, 200 mg)
  Adults with hepatic impairment (cirrhosis): PO 50 mg q12h
  Elderly adults (65–75 y): Same as above, unless they also have renal or hepatic impairment
  Elderly adults (>75 y): <300 mg daily, in divided doses
Children: Dosage not established

Agonists/Antagonists

These agents have agonist activity at some receptors and antagonist activity at others. Because of their agonist activity, they are potent analgesics with a lower abuse potential than pure agonists; because of their antagonist activity, they may produce withdrawal symptoms in people with opiate dependence.

Buprenorphine (Buprenex) is a semisynthetic opioid with a long duration of action and a low incidence of causing physical dependence. These characteristics are attributed to its high affinity for and slow dissociation from mu receptors. With IM administration, analgesia onset occurs in 15 minutes, peaks in 60 minutes, and lasts about 6 hours. It is highly protein bound (about 96%) and has an elimination half-life of 2 to 3 hours. It is metabolized in the liver, and clearance is related to hepatic blood flow. It is excreted mainly in feces.

Routes and Dosage Range

Adults: IM or slow IV (over 2 min) 0.3 mg q6h PRN

Butorphanol (Stadol) is a synthetic agonist analgesic similar to morphine and meperidine in analgesic effects and ability to cause respiratory depression. It is used in moderate to severe pain and is given parenterally or topically to nasal mucosa by a metered spray (Stadol NS). After IM or IV administration, analgesia peaks in about 30 to 60 minutes. After nasal application, analgesia peaks within 1 to 2 hours. Butorphanol also has antagonist activity and therefore should not be given to people who have been receiving narcotic analgesics or who have narcotic dependence. Other adverse effects include drowsiness and nausea and vomiting. Butorphanol has not been established as a safe and effective drug for use in pregnancy, labor, delivery, or lactation or in children under age 18.

Routes and Dosage Ranges

Adults: IM, IV 1–4 mg q3–4h PRN
  Nasal spray 1 mg (one spray in one nostril) q3–4h PRN
Children: Not recommended

Dezocine (Dalgan) is a synthetic analgesic used for moderate to severe pain. It is given parenterally. It is similar to morphine in its effects. Onset of analgesia occurs within 15 minutes after IV administration and within 30 minutes after IM injection. Like other drugs in this group, dezocine may cause respiratory depression, sedation, nausea and vomiting, and other adverse effects. It also may cause allergic reactions, especially in people with asthma or allergy to sulfites because it contains metabisulfite.

Routes and Dosage Ranges

Adults: IM 5–20 mg q3–6h PRN
  IV 2.5–10 q2–4h PRN
Children: Not recommended

Nalbuphine (Nubain) is a synthetic analgesic used for moderate to severe pain. It is given parenterally. Onset, duration, and extent of analgesia and respiratory depression are comparable to those produced by morphine. Other adverse effects include sedation, sweating, headache, and psychotic symptoms, but these are reportedly minimal at doses of 10 mg or less.

Routes and Dosage Range

Adults: IM, IV, SC 10 mg/70 kg q3–6h PRN

Pentazocine (Talwin) is a synthetic analgesic drug of abuse and may produce physical and psychological dependence. It is a Schedule IV drug. Generally, pentazocine is used for the same clinical indications as other strong analgesics and causes similar adverse effects. Recommended doses for analgesia are less effective than usual doses of morphine or meperidine, but some people may tolerate pentazocine better than morphine or meperidine. Parenteral pentazocine usually produces analgesia within 10 to 30 minutes and lasts 2 to 3 hours. Adverse effects include hallucinations, bizarre dreams or nightmares, depression, nervousness, feelings of depersonalization, extreme euphoria, tissue damage with ulceration and necrosis or fibrosis at injection sites with long-term use, and respiratory depression.

Oral pentazocine tablets contain naloxone 0.5 mg, a narcotic antagonist that prevents the effects of pentazocine if the oral tablet is injected. It has no pharmacologic action if taken orally. Naloxone was added to prevent a method of abuse in which oral tablets of pentazocine and tripelennamine, an antihistamine, were dissolved and injected intravenously. The mixture caused such adverse effects as pulmonary emboli and stroke (from obstruction of blood vessels by talc and other insoluble ingredients in the tablets).

Routes and Dosage Ranges

Adults: PO 50–100 mg q3–4h (maximal daily dose, 600 mg)
  IM, SC, IV 30–60 mg q3–4h (maximal daily dose, 360 mg)
Children: Not recommended for children <12 years

Narcotic Antagonists

Narcotic antagonists reverse or block analgesia, CNS and respiratory depression, and other physiologic effects of narcotic agonists. They compete with narcotics for opioid receptor sites in the brain and thereby prevent narcotic binding with receptors or displace narcotics already occupying receptor sites. When an opioid cannot bind to receptor sites, it is "neutralized" and cannot exert its effects on body cells. Narcotic antagonists do not relieve the depressant effects of other drugs, such as sedative-hypnotic, antianxiety, and antipsychotic agents. The chief clinical use of these drugs is to relieve CNS and respiratory depression induced by therapeutic doses or overdoses of opioids. The drugs are also used to reverse postoperative opioid depression, and naltrexone is approved for the treatment of opioid and alcohol dependence. These drugs produce withdrawal symptoms when given to opiate-dependent people.

Naloxone (Narcan), **nalmefene** (Revex), and **naltrexone** (ReVia, formerly Trexan) are structurally and pharmacologically similar. Naloxone is the oldest of the three drugs and has long been the drug of choice in respiratory depression known or thought to be caused by a narcotic. Therapeutic effects occur within minutes after parenteral injection and last 1 to 2 hours. Naloxone has a shorter duration of action than narcotics, and repeated injections are usually needed. For a long-acting drug such as methadone, injections may be needed for 2 to 3 days. Naloxone produces few adverse effects, and repeated injections can be given safely. This drug should be readily available in all health care settings where narcotics are given. Nalmefene is a newer agent whose main difference from naloxone is a longer duration of action. It may be preferred when opioid depression results from long-acting drugs such as methadone, pentazocine, propoxyphene, or diphenoxylate. Nalmefene is available in two concentrations, one for use postoperatively and one for treatment of clients with opiate overdoses. Health care personnel must use the appropriate concentration for the intended purpose. Naltrexone is used in the maintenance of opiate-free states in opiate addicts. It is apparently effective in highly motivated, detoxified people. If given before the client is detoxified, acute withdrawal symptoms occur. Clients receiving naltrexone will not respond to analgesics if pain control is needed. The drug is recommended for use in conjunction with psychological and social counseling.

Naloxone
Routes and Dosage Ranges

Adults: IV, IM, SC 0.1–0.4 mg, repeated IV q2–3 min PRN
Children: IV, IM, SC 0.01 mg/kg initially, repeated IV q2–3 min PRN

Nalmefene
Route and Dosage Ranges

Adults, reversal of postoperative opioid depression: (Blue label, 1-ml ampules containing 100 μg), IV according to body weight (50 kg, 0.125 ml; 60 kg, 0.15 ml; 70 kg, 0.175 ml; 80 kg, 0.2 ml; 90 kg, 0.225 ml; 100 kg, 0.25 ml)
Adults, treatment of opioid overdose: (Green label, 2-ml ampules containing 1 mg), IV 0.5 mg/70 kg as initial dose for patients who are not opioid dependent, followed by 1 mg/70 kg in 2–5 min if necessary. For known or suspected opioid-dependent persons, give a test dose of 0.1 mg/70 kg. If no signs of opiate withdrawal occur within 2 min, proceed with the above dosage.

Naltrexone
Route and Dosage Range

Adults: PO 50 mg/day

Nursing Process

Assessment

Pain is a subjective experience (whatever the person says it is), and humans display a wide variety of responses. Although pain thresholds (the point at which a tissue-damaging stimulus produces a sensation of pain) are similar, people differ in their perceptions, behaviors, and tolerance of pain. Differences in pain perception may result from psychological components. Stressors such as anxiety, depression, fatigue, anger, and fear tend to increase pain; rest, mood elevation, and diversionary activities tend to decrease pain. Differences in behaviors may or may not indicate pain to observers, and overt signs and symptoms are not reliable indicators of the presence or extent of pain. Especially with chronic pain, overt signs and symptoms may be absent or minimal. Differences in tolerance of pain (the amount or duration of pain a person is willing to suffer before seeking relief) often reflect the person's concern about the meaning of the pain and the type or intensity of the painful stimulus. Thus, pain is a complex physiologic, psychological, and sociocultural phenomenon that must be thoroughly assessed if it is to be managed effectively.

The nurse must assess every client in relation to pain, initially to determine appropriate interventions and later to determine whether the interventions were effective in preventing or relieving pain. Although the client is usually the best source of data, other people may be questioned about the client's words and behaviors that indicate pain. This is especially important with young children. During assessment, keep in mind that acute pain may coexist with or be superimposed on chronic pain. Specific assessment data usually include:

- **Location.** Determining the location may assist in relieving the pain or identifying its underlying cause. Ask the client to show you where it hurts, if possible, and whether the pain stays in one place or radiates to other parts of the body. The term *referred pain* is used when pain arising from tissue damage in one area of the body is felt in another area. Patterns of referred pain may be helpful in diagnosis. For example, pain of cardiac origin may radiate to the neck, shoulders, chest muscles, and down the arms, often on the left side. This form of pain usually results from myocardial ischemia due to atherosclerosis of coronary arteries. Stomach pain is usually referred to the epigastrium and may indicate gastritis or peptic ulcer. Gallbladder and bile duct pain is usually localized in the midepigastrium or right upper quadrant of the abdomen. Uterine pain is usually felt as abdominal cramping or low back pain. Deep or chronic pain is usually more difficult to localize than superficial or acute pain.
- **Intensity or severity.** Because pain is a subjective experience and cannot be objectively measured, assessment of severity is based on the client's description and the nurse's observations. Various scales have been developed to measure and quantify pain. These include verbal descriptor scales in which the client is asked to rate pain as mild, moderate, or severe; numeric scales, with 0 representing no pain and 10 representing severe, intense pain; and visual analog scales, in which the client chooses the location indicating the level of pain on a continuum.
- **Relation to time, activities, and other signs and symptoms.** Specific questions include:
  - When did the pain start?
  - What activities were occurring when the pain started?
  - Does the pain occur with exercise or when at rest?
  - Do other signs and symptoms occur before, during, or after the pain?
  - Is this the first episode of this particular type of pain, or is this a repeated occurrence?
  - How long does the pain last?
  - What, if anything, decreases or relieves the pain?
  - What, if anything, aggravates the pain?
- **Other data.** For example, do not assume that postoperative pain is incisional and requires narcotic analgesics for relief. A person who has had abdominal surgery may have headache, musculoskeletal discomfort, or "gas pains." Also, restlessness may be caused by hypoxia or anxiety rather than pain.

Nursing Diagnoses

- Pain
- Impaired Gas Exchange related to sedation and decreased mobility
- Risk for Injury related to sedation and decreased mobility
- Constipation related to slowed peristalsis
- Altered Tissue Perfusion related to drug-induced decrease in cardiac output and blood pressure
- Urinary Retention related to decreased bladder contractility
- Knowledge Deficit: Effects and appropriate use of narcotic analgesics
- Noncompliance: Drug dependence related to overuse

Planning/Goals

The client will:
- Avoid or be relieved of pain
- Use narcotic analgesics appropriately
- Avoid preventable adverse effects
- Be closely monitored for excessive sedation and respiratory depression
- Be able to perform activities of daily living when feasible

Interventions

Use measures to prevent, relieve, or decrease pain when possible. General measures include those that promote optimal body functioning and those that prevent trauma, inflammation, infection, and other sources of painful stimuli. Specific measures include:

- Encourage pulmonary hygiene techniques (*e.g.,* coughing, deep breathing, ambulation) to promote respiration and prevent pulmonary complications, such as pneumonia and atelectasis.
- Use sterile technique when caring for wounds, urinary catheters, or IV lines.
- Use exercises, ambulation, and position changes to promote circulation and musculoskeletal function.
- Handle any injured tissue very gently to avoid further trauma.
- Prevent bowel or bladder distention.
- Apply heat or cold.
- Use relaxation or distraction techniques.
- If a client is in pain on initial contact, try to relieve the pain as soon as possible. Once pain is controlled, plan with the client to avoid or manage future episodes.
- If a client is not in pain initially but anticipates surgery or an uncomfortable diagnostic procedure, plan with the client ways to minimize and manage discomfort.

Teach clients:

- Personalized methods of pain prevention
- Personalized methods of pain management
- That use of a narcotic analgesic for acute pain is acceptable and unlikely to lead to addiction
- To use the least amount of the mildest drug that is likely to be effective in a particular situation
- **Preoperatively:**
  - How postoperative pain will be managed (*e.g.,* whether analgesics will be given orally or by injection; whether the medication will be nurse-administered or patient-controlled)
  - How to report pain or request pain medication
  - That it is better to take adequate medication to control pain and be able to cough, deep breathe, and ambulate than to avoid medication and be unable to perform activities that promote recovery and healing
- To avoid other CNS depressant drugs (*e.g.,* alcoholic beverages, antihistamines, sleeping pills) when taking narcotic analgesics as an outpatient and to report perceived adverse drug effects to a health care provider

Evaluation

- Ask clients about their levels of comfort or relief from pain.
- Observe behaviors that indicate the presence or absence of pain.
- Observe participation and ability to function in usual activities of daily living.
- Observe for presence or absence of sedation and respiratory depression.
- Observe for drug-seeking behavior (possibly indicating dependence).

Principles of Therapy

NEED FOR EFFECTIVE PAIN MANAGEMENT

Numerous studies have indicated ineffective management of patients' pain, especially moderate to severe pain associated with surgery or cancer. Much of the difficulty has been attributed to inadequate or improper use of narcotic analgesics, including administering the wrong drug, prescribing inadequate dosage, or leaving long intervals between doses. Even when ordered appropriately, nurses or patients and family members may not administer the drugs effectively. Traditionally, concerns about respiratory depression, excessive sedation, drug dependence, and other adverse effects have contributed to reluctance and delay in administering narcotic analgesics. Inadequate management of pain often leads to anxiety, depression, and other emotional upsets from anticipation of pain recurrence.

In recent years, a more humane approach to pain management has evolved. Basic assumptions of this approach are that no one should suffer pain needlessly; that pain occurs when the patient says it does and should be relieved by whatever means required, including pharmacologic and nonpharmacologic treatments; that doses of narcotics should be titrated to achieve maximal effectiveness and minimal toxicity; and that dependence rarely results from drugs taken for physical pain. Proponents of this view emphasize the need to assess and monitor all clients receiving narcotic analgesics.

DRUG SELECTION

1. Morphine is often the drug of first choice for severe pain. It is effective, is available in various dosage strengths and forms, and can be used on a short- or long-term basis, and its adverse effects are well known. In addition, it is a "non-ceiling" drug—there is no upper limit to the dosage that can be given to clients who have developed tolerance to previous dosages. This characteristic is especially valuable in cancer patients with severe pain, because drug dosage can be increased and titrated to relieve pain when pain increases or tolerance develops. Thus, some patients have safely received extremely large doses. Hydromorphone, levorphanol, and methadone are other non-ceiling drugs.

   In contrast, meperidine and pentazocine are "ceiling" drugs: Doses cannot be increased sufficiently or titrated to relieve increasing pain without greatly increasing the incidence and severity of adverse effects. These drugs are not recommended for the treatment of chronic cancer pain.

2. When more than one analgesic drug is ordered, use the least potent drug that is effective in relieving pain. For example, use a non-narcotic analgesic, such as acetaminophen, rather than a narcotic analgesic when feasible.

3. Non-narcotic analgesics may be alternated or given concurrently with narcotic analgesics, especially in chronic pain. This increases client comfort, reduces the likelihood of drug abuse and dependence, and decreases tolerance to the pain-relieving effects of the narcotic analgesics.

4. In many instances, the drug preparation of choice may be one that combines a narcotic and a non-narcotic. The drugs act by different mechanisms and therefore produce greater analgesic effects. Commonly used examples are Tylenol No. 3 (acetaminophen 325 mg and codeine 30 mg/tablet) and Percocet (acetaminophen 325 mg and oxycodone 5 mg/tablet).

ROUTE SELECTION

1. Oral drugs are preferred when feasible, especially for long-term use.

2. IV injection of a narcotic is usually preferred for rapid relief of acute pain. Small, frequent IV doses

are often effective in relieving pain with minimal risk of serious adverse effects. This is especially advantageous during a serious illness or after surgery.

A technique called patient-controlled analgesia allows self-administration. One device consists of a syringe of diluted drug connected to an IV line and infusion pump; another device uses a specially designed IV bag and special tubing. These devices deliver a dose when the patient pushes a button. The amount of drug delivered with each dose and the intervals between doses are preset and limited. Studies indicate that analgesia is more effective, patient satisfaction is high, and smaller amounts of drug are used than with conventional PRN administration.

3. Continuous IV infusion may be used to treat severe pain.
4. Two other routes of administration are used to manage acute pain. One route involves injection of narcotic analgesics directly into the CNS through a catheter placed into the epidural or intrathecal space by an anesthesiologist or other physician. This method provides effective analgesia while minimizing depressant effects. This type of pain control was developed after opioid receptors were found on neurons in the spinal cord. The other route involves the injection of local anesthetics to provide local or regional analgesia. Both of these methods interrupt the transmission of pain signals and are effective in relieving pain, but they also require special techniques and monitoring procedures for safe use.
5. For clients with chronic pain and contraindications for oral or injected medications, some narcotics are available in rectal suppositories or skin patches.

Dosage

Dosages of narcotic analgesics should be sufficient to relieve pain without causing unacceptable adverse effects. Thus, dosages should be individualized according to the type and severity of pain; the client's age, size, and health status; whether the client is "opiate-naive" (has not received narcotics enough to develop tolerance) or "opiate-tolerant" (has previously taken narcotics and developed drug tolerance, so that larger-than-usual doses are needed to relieve pain); whether the client has progressive or worsening disease; and other characteristics that influence responses to pain. Guidelines include:

1. Small to moderate doses relieve constant, dull pain; moderate to large doses relieve intermittent, sharp pain caused by trauma or conditions affecting the viscera.
2. When a narcotic analgesic is ordered in variable amounts (*e.g.*, 8–10 mg of morphine), give the smaller amount as long as it is effective in relieving pain.

3. Dosages of narcotic analgesics should be reduced for clients who also are receiving other CNS depressants, such as sedating antianxiety, antidepressant, antihistaminic, antipsychotic, or other sedative-type drugs.

Scheduling

Narcotic analgesics may be given as needed, within designated time limits, or on a regular schedule. Traditionally, the drugs have often been scheduled every 4 to 6 hours PRN. Numerous studies have indicated that such a schedule is often ineffective in managing patients' pain. Because narcotic analgesics are used for moderate to severe pain, they should generally be scheduled to provide effective and consistent pain relief. Some guidelines for scheduling drugs include:

1. When analgesics are ordered PRN, have a clear-cut system by which the client reports pain or requests medication. The client should know that analgesic drugs have been ordered and will be given promptly when needed. If a drug cannot be given or if administration must be delayed, explain this to the client. In addition, offer or give the drug when indicated by the client's condition rather than waiting for the client to request medication.
2. In acute pain, narcotic analgesics are most effective when given parenterally and at the onset of pain. In chronic, severe pain, narcotic analgesics are most effective when given on a regular schedule, around the clock.
3. When needed, analgesics should be given before coughing and deep-breathing exercises, dressing changes, and other therapeutic and diagnostic procedures.
4. Narcotics are not recommended for prolonged periods except for advanced malignant disease. Health care agencies usually have an automatic "stop order" for narcotics after 48 to 72 hours; this means that the drug is discontinued when the time limit expires if the physician does not reorder it.

Drug Use in Specific Situations
Cancer

When narcotic analgesics are required in chronic pain associated with malignancy, the main consideration is client comfort, not preventing drug addiction. Effective treatment requires that pain be relieved and prevented from recurring. With disease progression and the development of drug tolerance, extremely large doses and frequent administration may be required. Oral, rectal, and transdermal routes of administration are generally preferred over injections. When long-acting forms of narcotic analgesics are being given on a regular schedule, fast-acting forms also need to be ordered and available for "breakthrough" pain. If additional doses are needed frequently, the baseline dose of long-acting medication may need to be increased.

In addition to analgesics, other drugs may be used to increase client comfort. For example, tricyclic antidepressants have analgesic effects, antiemetics may be given for nausea and vomiting, and laxatives are usually needed to prevent or relieve constipation from the narcotics.

Biliary, Renal, or Ureteral Colic

When narcotic analgesics are used to relieve the acute, severe pain associated with various types of colic, an antispasmodic drug such as atropine may be needed as well. Narcotic analgesics may increase smooth muscle tone and cause spasm. Atropine does not have strong antispasmodic properties of its own in usual doses, but it reduces the spasm-producing effects of narcotic analgesics.

Postoperative Use

When analgesics are used postoperatively, the goal is to relieve pain without excessive sedation so that clients can do deep-breathing exercises, cough, ambulate, and implement other measures to promote recovery.

Burns

In severely burned clients, use narcotic analgesics cautiously. A common cause of respiratory arrest in burned clients is excessive administration of analgesics. Generally, agitation in a burned person should be interpreted as hypoxia or hypovolemia rather than pain, until proved otherwise. When narcotic analgesics are necessary, they are usually given IV in small doses. Drugs given by other routes are absorbed erratically in the presence of shock and hypovolemia and may not relieve pain. In addition, unabsorbed drugs may be rapidly absorbed when circulation is improved, with the potential for excessive dosage and toxic effects.

MANAGEMENT OF TOXICITY OR OVERDOSE

Acute toxicity or narcotic overdose can occur from therapeutic use or from abuse by drug-dependent people (see Chap. 15). The main goal of treatment is to restore and maintain adequate respiratory function. This can be accomplished by inserting an artificial airway, such as an endotracheal tube, and starting mechanical ventilation or by giving a narcotic antagonist, such as naloxone or nalmefene. Thus, emergency supplies should be readily available in any setting where narcotic analgesics are used, including ambulatory settings and clients' homes.

USE IN OPIATE-TOLERANT PERSONS

Whether opiate tolerance results from the use of prescribed, therapeutic drugs or the abuse of street drugs, there are two main considerations in using narcotic analgesics in this population. First, larger-than-usual doses are required to treat pain. Second, signs and symptoms of withdrawal (see Chap. 15) occur if adequate dosage is not maintained or if narcotic antagonists are given.

USE IN CHILDREN

There has generally been little understanding of the physiology, pathology, assessment, and management of pain in children. Many authorities indicate that children's pain is often ignored or undertreated, including children having surgical and other painful procedures for which adults routinely receive an anesthetic, an analgesic, or both. This is especially true in preterm and full-term neonates. One reason for inadequate prevention and management of pain in newborns has been a common belief that they did not experience pain because of immature nervous systems. However, research indicates that neonates have abundant C fibers and that A-delta fibers are developing during the first few months of life. These are the nerve fibers that carry pain signals from peripheral tissues to the spinal cord. In addition, brain pain centers and the endogenous analgesia system seem to be developed and functional. Endogenous opioids are released at birth and in response to fetal and neonatal distress such as asphyxia or other difficulty associated with the birth process.

Older infants and children may experience pain even when analgesics have been ordered and are readily available. For example, children may fear injections or may be unable to communicate their discomfort. Health care providers or parents may fear adverse effects of narcotic analgesics, including excessive sedation, respiratory depression, and addiction.

Generally, other than reduced dosage, there have been few guidelines about the use of narcotic analgesics in children. With increased knowledge about pain mechanisms and the recommendations prepared by the Acute Pain Management Guideline Panel in 1992, every nurse who works with children should be able to manage pain more effectively. Some specific considerations include the following:

1. Narcotic analgesics administered during labor and delivery may depress fetal and neonatal respiration.

The drugs cross the blood-brain barrier of the infant more readily than that of the mother. Therefore, doses that do not depress maternal respiration may profoundly depress the infant's respiration. Respiration should be monitored closely in neonates, and the narcotic antagonist naloxone should be readily available.

2. Expressions of pain may differ according to age and developmental level. Infants may cry and have muscular rigidity and thrashing behavior. Preschoolers may behave aggressively or complain verbally of discomfort. Young school-aged children may express pain verbally or behaviorally, often with regression to behaviors used at younger ages. Adolescents may be reluctant to admit they are uncomfortable or need help. With chronic pain, children of all ages tend to withdraw and regress to an earlier stage of development.

3. The Acute Pain Management Guideline Panel recommends that narcotic analgesics be given by routes (*e.g.*, PO, IV, epidurally) other than IM injections, because IM injections are painful and frightening for children. For any child receiving parenteral opioids, vital signs and level of consciousness must be assessed regularly.

4. Narcotic formulations specifically for children are not generally available. When children's doses are calculated from adult doses, the fractions and decimals that often result greatly increase the risk of a dosage error.

5. Narcotic rectal suppositories may be used more often in children than in adults. Although they may be useful when oral or parenteral routes are not indicated, there are disadvantages as well. Because drug absorption is erratic, the drug dose is unpredictable. Another disadvantage is that adult suppositories are sometimes cut in half or otherwise altered; this may lead to an unknown dose.

6. Narcotic effects in children may differ from those expected in adults because of physiologic and pharmacokinetic differences. Assess regularly and be alert for unusual signs and symptoms.

7. Hydromorphone, methadone, oxycodone, oxymorphone, and propoxyphene are not recommended for use in children, because safety, efficacy, or dosages have not been established.

8. Like adults, children seem more able to cope with pain when they are informed about what is happening to them and are assisted in developing coping strategies. Age-appropriate doll play, a favorite videotape, diversionary activities, and other techniques can be used effectively. However, such techniques should be used in conjunction with adequate analgesia, not as a substitute for pain medication.

USE IN OLDER ADULTS

Research studies and literature about the management of pain and the use of narcotic analgesics in older adults are limited. Generally, these drugs should be used cautiously in older adults, especially if they are debilitated, have respiratory disorders, or are receiving other drugs that depress the CNS. They also should be given in smaller doses and at longer intervals because the duration of action may be longer. Older adults are especially sensitive to respiratory depression, excessive sedation, confusion, and other adverse effects. However, they are entitled to and should receive adequate analgesia, along with vigilant monitoring. Older adults with short-term memory loss (common in this population) may be unable to self-administer narcotic analgesics safely.

HOME CARE

Narcotic analgesics are widely used in the home for both acute and chronic pain. With acute pain, such as postoperative recovery, the use of a narcotic analgesic is often limited to a short period and clients self-administer their medications. The need for strong pain medication recedes as healing occurs. The home care nurse may teach clients and caregivers safe usage of the drugs (*e.g.*, that the drugs decrease mental alertness and physical agility, so potentially hazardous activities should be avoided), nonpharmacologic methods of managing pain, and ways to prevent adverse effects of narcotics (*e.g.*, excessive sedation, constipation). Physical dependence is uncommon with short-term use of narcotic analgesics for acute pain.

With some types of chronic pain, such as that occurring with low back pain or osteoarthritis, narcotic analgesics are not indicated for long-term use. Treatment involves non-narcotic medications, physical therapy, and other measures. The home care nurse may need to explain the reasons for not using narcotics on a long-term basis and to help clients and caregivers learn alternative methods of relieving discomfort.

With cancer pain, as previously discussed, the goal of treatment is to prevent or relieve pain and keep clients comfortable, without concern about addiction. Consequently, the home care nurse must assist clients and caregivers in understanding the appropriate use of narcotic analgesics in cancer care, including administration on a regular schedule. The nurse also must be proficient in using and teaching various routes of drug administration and in arranging regimens with potentially very large doses and various combinations of drugs. In addition, an active effort is needed to prevent or manage adverse effects, such as a bowel program to prevent constipation.

NARCOTIC ANALGESICS

NURSING ACTIONS	RATIONALE/EXPLANATION
1. Administer accurately	
a. Check the rate, depth, and rhythm of respirations before each dose. If the rate is below 12 per minute, delay or omit the dose and report to the physician.	Respiratory depression is a major adverse reaction to strong analgesics. Assessing respirations before each dose can help prevent or minimize potentially life-threatening respiratory depression.
b. Have the client lie down to receive injections of narcotic analgesics and for at least a few minutes afterward.	To prevent or minimize hypotension, nausea, and vomiting. These side effects are more likely to occur in the ambulatory client. Also, the client may be sedated enough to make ambulation hazardous without help.
c. When injecting narcotic analgesics intravenously, give small doses; inject slowly over several minutes; and have narcotic antagonist drugs, artificial airways, and equipment for artificial ventilation readily available.	Large doses or rapid intravenous injection may cause severe respiratory depression and hypotension.
d. Give meperidine and pentazocine intramuscularly rather than subcutaneously.	Subcutaneous injections of these drugs may cause pain, tissue irritation, and possible abscess. This reaction is more likely with long-term use.
e. Put siderails up; instruct the client not to smoke or try to ambulate without help. Keep the call light within reach.	To prevent falls or other injuries.
f. When giving controlled-release tablets of morphine, do NOT crush them, and instruct the client not to chew them.	Crushing or chewing causes immediate release of drug, with a high risk of overdose and toxicity.
g. To apply transdermal fentanyl:	Correct preparation of the site and application of the medicated adhesive patch are necessary for drug absorption and effectiveness.
(1) Clip (do not shave) hair, if needed, on a flat surface of the upper trunk.	
(2) If necessary to cleanse the site, use plain water; do not use soaps, oils, lotions, alcohol, or other substances. Let the skin dry.	
(3) Apply the skin patch and press it in place for a few seconds.	
(4) Leave in place for 72 hours.	
(5) When a new patch is to be applied, remove the old one, fold it so that the medication is on the inside, and flush the patch down the toilet. Apply the new patch to a different skin site.	
2. Observe for therapeutic effects	Therapeutic effects depend on the reason for use, usually for analgesic effects, sometimes for antitussive or antidiarrheal effects.
a. A verbal statement of pain relief	
b. Decreased behavioral manifestations of pain or discomfort	
c. Sleeping	
d. Increased participation in usual activities of daily living, including interactions with other people in the environment	
e. Fewer and shorter episodes of nonproductive coughing when used for antitussive effects	Narcotic analgesics relieve cough by depressing the cough center in the medulla oblongata.
f. Lowered blood pressure, decreased pulse rate, slower and deeper respirations, and less dyspnea when morphine is given for pulmonary edema	Morphine may relieve pulmonary edema by causing vasodilation, which in turn decreases venous return to the heart and decreases cardiac work.

NURSING ACTIONS	RATIONALE/EXPLANATION
g. Decreased diarrhea when given for constipating effects	These drugs slow secretions and motility of the gastrointestinal tract. Constipation is usually an adverse effect. However, in severe diarrhea or with ileostomy, the drugs decrease the number of bowel movements and make the consistency more paste-like than liquid.

3. Observe for adverse effects

a. Respiratory depression—hypoxemia, restlessness, dyspnea, slow, shallow breathing, changes in blood pressure and pulse, decreased ability to cough	Respiratory depression is a major adverse effect of narcotic analgesics and results from depression of the respiratory center in the medulla oblongata. Respiratory depression occurs with usual therapeutic doses and increases in incidence and severity with large doses or frequent administration.
b. Hypotension	Hypotension stems from drug effects on the vasomotor center in the medulla oblongata that cause peripheral vasodilation and lowering of blood pressure. This is a therapeutic effect with pulmonary edema.
c. Excessive sedation—drowsiness, slurred speech, impaired mobility and coordination, stupor, coma	This is caused by depression of the CNS and is potentially life-threatening.
d. Nausea and vomiting	Narcotic analgesics stimulate the chemoreceptor trigger zone in the brain. Consequently, nausea and vomiting may occur with oral or parenteral routes of administration. They are more likely to occur with ambulation than with recumbency.
e. Constipation	This is caused by the drug's slowing effects on the gastrointestinal tract. Constipation may be alleviated by activity, adequate food and fluid intake, and regular administration of mild laxatives.

4. Observe for drug interactions
a. Drugs that *increase* effects of narcotic analgesics:

(1) CNS depressants—alcohol, general anesthetics, antianxiety agents, tricyclic antidepressants, antihistamines, antipsychotic agents, barbiturates, and other sedative-hypnotic drugs	All these drugs alone, as well as the narcotic analgesics, produce CNS depression. When combined, additive CNS depression results. If dosage of one or more interacting drugs is high, severe respiratory depression, coma, and death may ensue.
(2) Diuretics	Orthostatic hypotension, an adverse effect of strong analgesics and diuretics, may be increased if the two drug groups are given concurrently.
(3) Monoamine oxidase (MAO) inhibitors	These drugs interfere with detoxification of some narcotic analgesics, especially meperidine. They may cause additive CNS depression with hypotension and respiratory depression or CNS stimulation with hyperexcitability and convulsions. If an MAO inhibitor is necessary, dosage should be reduced because the combination is potentially life-threatening.

b. Drugs that *decrease* effects of narcotic analgesics:

(1) Narcotic antagonists	These drugs reverse respiratory depression produced by narcotic analgesics. This is their only clinical use, and they should not be given unless severe respiratory depresssion is present. They do not reverse respiratory depression caused by other CNS depressants.
(2) Butorphanol, nalbuphine, and pentazocine	These analgesics are weak antagonists of narcotic analgesics, and they may cause withdrawal symptoms in people who have been receiving opiates or who are physically dependent on narcotic analgesics.

(continued)

NURSING ACTIONS	RATIONALE/EXPLANATION
5. Teach clients	
a. Take only as prescribed. If desired effects are not achieved, report to the physician. Do not increase the dose, and do not take medication more often than prescribed.	Although these principles apply to all medications, they are especially important with analgesics because of potentially serious adverse reactions, including drug dependence, and because analgesics may mask or enable the client to tolerate pain for which medical attention is needed.
b. Correct techniques for using alternative dosage forms (*e.g.*, controlled-release tablets, concentrated liquids, rectal suppositories, skin patches) when indicated	Therapeutic effectiveness and avoiding or minimizing adverse effects depend largely on correct administration.
c. Do not drink alcohol or take other drugs without the physician's knowledge.	Alcohol and pain-relieving narcotics depress the nervous system; combining them can cause serious, even life-threatening problems. Numerous other drugs have depressant effects as well, and additive effects leading to excessive adverse reactions can result. For example, tranquilizers, sleeping pills, antihistamines, and cold remedies can all increase the risks of drug-induced problems that could be worse than the initial problem.
d. Do not drive a car or operate machinery when drowsy or dizzy or when vision is blurred from medication.	Automobiles and machinery should be operated only by fully alert people with good vision.
e. Do not smoke when drowsy from medication.	Smoking when less than alert is unsafe.
f. Stay in bed at least 30 to 60 minutes after receiving injection of an analgesic.	To prevent or minimize hypotension, nausea, and vomiting, which often occur with ambulation. Also, a sedated person is risking falls and traumatic injuries. An exception may be the person who has been receiving the drug for some time and who has developed tolerance to its sedative effects.
g. Do not object to having siderails up on the bed after an injection of analgesic.	Siderails promote safety by serving as a reminder to stay in bed or call for assistance.
h. If not contraindicated, eat high-fiber foods, such as whole-grain cereals, fruits, and vegetables, drink 2 to 3 quarts of fluid daily, and be as active as tolerated.	To prevent or minimize constipation.

REVIEW AND APPLICATION EXERCISES

1. When assessing a client for pain, what are the major guidelines?

2. What kinds of behaviors may indicate acute pain? Are similar behaviors associated with chronic pain?

3. What are some nonpharmacologic interventions for pain, and why should they be used instead of or along with analgesics?

4. What are the major adverse effects of narcotic analgesics? How do narcotic antagonists counteract adverse effects?

5. For a client who has had major surgery during the previous 24 to 72 hours, what type of analgesic is indicated? Why?

6. What are the potential differences in dosage between short-term (a few days) and long-term (weeks or months) administration of morphine?

7. Explain the rationale for using both narcotic analgesics and non-narcotic analgesics in the treatment of pain.

8. For a client with chronic cancer pain, what are the advantages and disadvantages of using narcotic analgesics?

9. Why is meperidine (Demerol) not recommended for the management of chronic cancer pain?

10. For a client with chronic cancer pain, should narcotic analgesics be given as needed or on a regular schedule? Why?

11. On a initial visit to a client with cancer who is receiving a narcotic analgesic, how would you assess the effectiveness of pain management?

SELECTED REFERENCES

Acute Pain Management Guideline Panel. (1992). *Acute pain management: Operative or medical procedures and trauma. Clinical practice guideline.* AHCPR Pub. No. 92-0032. Rockville, MD: Agency for Health Care Policy and Research, Public Health Service, U.S. Department of Health and Human Services for Health Care Policy and Research.

Baumann, T.J. (1993). Pain management. In J.T. DiPiro, R.L. Talbert, P.E. Hayes, G.C. Yee, G.R. Matzke, & L.M. Posey (Eds.), *Pharmacotherapy: A pathophysiologic approach*, 2d ed., pp. 924–941. Norwalk, CT: Appleton & Lange.

Cox, T.H. (1995). An evaluation of postoperative pain management in pediatric patients at a university teaching hospital. *Hospital Pharmacy, 30*(11):980–996.

Curtis, S.M. & Curtis, R.L. (1994). Somatosensory function and pain. In C.M. Porth (Ed.), *Pathophysiology: Concepts of altered health states*, 4th ed., pp. 973–1006. Philadelphia: J.B. Lippincott.

Drug facts and comparisons. (1996). St. Louis: Facts and Comparisons.

Guyton, A.C. & Hall, J.E. (1996). *Textbook of medical physiology*, 9th ed. Philadelphia: W.B. Saunders.

Holdsworth, M. & Forman, W.B. (1993). Pain control. In R. Bressler & M.D. Katz (Eds.), *Geriatric pharmacology*, pp. 207–229. New York: McGraw-Hill.

Hoyt, D.B., Winchell, R.J. & Ferris, N. (1996). Analgesia and sedation. In J.A. Weigelt & F.R. Lewis, Jr. (Eds.), *Surgical Critical Care.* Philadelphia: W.B. Saunders.

Levien, T.L. & Baker, D.E. (1996). Reviews of nalmefene and granisetron—oral. *Hospital Pharmacy, 31*(2):148–156.

Niles, R. (1995). Pharmacologic management of cancer pain. *Nursing Clinics of North America, 30*(4):745–763.

Reisine, T. & Pasternak, G. (1996). Opioid analgesics and antagonists. In J.G. Hardman, L.E. Limbird, P.B. Molinoff, & R.W. Ruddon (Eds.), *Goodman & Gilman's The pharmacological basis of therapeutics*, 9th ed., pp. 521–555. New York: McGraw-Hill.

7 Analgesic–Antipyretic–Anti-inflammatory and Related Drugs

Outline

Objectives

After studying this chapter, the student will be able to:

1 Discuss the role of prostaglandins in the etiology of pain, fever, and inflammation.

2 Discuss aspirin and other nonsteroidal anti-inflammatory drugs (NSAIDs) in terms of mechanism of action, indications for use, contraindications for use, nursing process, and principles of therapy.

3 Compare and contrast aspirin, other NSAIDs, and acetaminophen in terms of indications for use and adverse effects.

4 Differentiate among antiplatelet, analgesic, and anti-inflammatory doses of aspirin.

5 Teach clients interventions to prevent or decrease adverse effects of aspirin, other NSAIDs, and acetaminophen.

6 Identify factors influencing the use of aspirin, NSAIDs, and acetaminophen in children and older adults.

7 Discuss the use of acetylcysteine (Mucomyst) as an antidote for acetaminophen overdose.

8 Discuss nursing implications of drug therapy for gout and migraine.

Key Terms

Cyclooxygenase   Prostaglandins

Inflammation

Description

The analgesic–antipyretic–anti-inflammatory drugs relieve pain, fever, and inflammation. Acetylsalicylic acid (ASA, aspirin) is the prototype of the group. Except for acetaminophen, the drugs in this group also are called nonsteroidal anti-inflammatory drugs (NSAIDs). Several NSAIDs are used primarily for their analgesic and anti-inflammatory effects in various musculoskeletal disorders. Acetaminophen (Tylenol, others) is not an NSAID because it does not have anti-inflammatory effects. It is included in this chapter because of its extensive use as an analgesic and antipyretic.

With gout and migraine, an analgesic–antipyretic–anti-inflammatory drug is often used to treat pain associated with acute attacks. In addition, other drugs are used in the prevention and treatment of gout and migraine. (The adrenocorticosteroids, the most potent anti-inflammatory drugs, are discussed in Chap. 24.)

Aspirin and related drugs inhibit the synthesis of prostaglandins, and both therapeutic and adverse effects are attributed primarily to this action. To understand the effects of these drugs, an understanding of prostaglandins, pain, fever, inflammation, gout, and migraine is needed.

Prostaglandins

Prostaglandins are substances synthesized from arachidonic acid, a free fatty acid released from the phospholipids in cell membranes in response to various physical, chemical, hormonal, bacterial, and other stimuli. They are produced in specific body tissues, where they exert their effects and are then rapidly inactivated. The specific type of prostaglandin produced depends on the tissue involved, the stimulus, the hormonal environment, and other factors. Table 7-1 lists several physiologically important prostaglandins and their effects.

Prostaglandins are found in most body tissues and help regulate many cell functions, including:

1. In the inflammatory process, prostaglandins potentiate the pain and edema caused by bradykinin, histamine, and other substances released in areas of tissue damage.
2. They regulate smooth muscle in blood vessels, the gastrointestinal (GI) tract, respiratory system, and reproductive system.
3. They protect GI mucosa from the erosive effects of gastric acid.
4. They regulate renal blood flow and distribution.
5. They control platelet function.
6. They maintain a patent ductus arteriosus in the fetus.

TABLE 7-1 **PROSTAGLANDINS AND THEIR EFFECTS**

Prostaglandin	Effects
D_2	Bronchoconstriction
E_2	Vasodilation
	Bronchodilation
	Increased activity of gastrointestinal (GI) smooth muscle
	Increased sensitivity to pain
	Increased body temperature
F_2	Bronchoconstriction
	Increased uterine contraction
	Increased activity of GI smooth muscle
I_2 (Prostacyclin)	Vasodilation
	Decreased platelet aggregation
Thromboxane A_2	Vasoconstriction
	Increased platelet aggregation

PAIN, FEVER, INFLAMMATION, GOUT, AND MIGRAINE

Pain is the sensation of discomfort, hurt, or distress. It is a common human ailment and may be mild or severe, acute or chronic (see Chap. 6).

Fever is an elevation of body temperature above the normal range. Body temperature is controlled by a regulating center in the hypothalamus. Normally, there is a balance between heat production and heat loss so that a constant body temperature is maintained. When there is excessive heat production, mechanisms to increase heat loss are activated. As a result, blood vessels dilate, more blood flows through the skin, sweating occurs, and body temperature usually stays within normal range. When fever occurs, the heat-regulating center in the hypothalamus is reset so that it tolerates a higher body temperature. Fever may be produced by dehydration, inflammatory and infectious processes, some drugs, brain injury, or diseases involving the hypothalamus. Prostaglandin formation is stimulated by such circumstances and, along with bacterial toxins and other substances, prostaglandins act as pyrogens (fever-producing agents).

Inflammation is the normal body response to tissue damage from chemicals, microorganisms, trauma, foreign bodies, surgery, and ionizing radiation. It may occur in any tissue or organ. It is an attempt by the body to remove the damaging agent and repair the damaged tissue. The local manifestations of inflammation are redness, heat, edema, and pain. Redness and heat result from vasodilation and increased blood supply; edema results from leakage of blood plasma into the area; and pain is produced by the pressure of edema and secretions on nerve endings and by chemical irritation of bradykinin, histamine, and other substances released by the damaged cells. Prostaglandins also are released and increase the pain and edema caused by other substances. Systemic manifestations of inflammation include leukocytosis, increased erythrocyte sedimentation rate, fever, headache, loss of appetite, lethargy or malaise, and weakness. Both local and systemic manifestations vary according to the cause and extent of tissue damage. Like pain, inflammation may be acute or chronic.

Gout is a disorder characterized by an inability to metabolize uric acid, a waste product of protein metabolism. The resulting hyperuricemia may be asymptomatic or may lead to urate deposits in various tissues. In the musculoskeletal system, often in the feet, urate deposits produce periodic episodes of severe pain, edema, and inflammation (gouty arthritis). In the kidneys, urate deposits may form renal calculi or cause other damage.

Migraine is a type of vascular headache characterized by periodic attacks of severe pain, nausea and vomiting, and increased sensitivity to light and sound.

Mechanism of Action

Aspirin and NSAIDs inactivate cyclooxygenase (also called prostaglandin synthetase), the enzyme that initiates the formation of prostaglandins from arachidonic acid. This action prevents or inhibits prostaglandin formation and thereby prevents or inhibits its effects on body tissues. Although other factors may be involved, this antiprostaglandin effect is thought to be the primary mechanism of action for these drugs.

To relieve pain, aspirin acts both centrally and peripherally to block the transmission of pain impulses. Related analgesic–antipyretic–anti-inflammatory drugs act peripherally to prevent sensitization of pain receptors to various chemical substances released by damaged cells. To relieve fever, the drugs act on the hypothalamus to decrease its response to pyrogens and reset the "thermostat" at a lower level. For inflammation, they prevent prostaglandins from increasing the pain and edema produced by bradykinin and other substances released by damaged cells. Although these drugs relieve symptoms and contribute greatly to the client's comfort and quality of life, they do not cure the underlying disorders that cause the symptoms.

Antiplatelet effects of aspirin and other NSAIDs differ in mechanism and extent. When aspirin is absorbed into the bloodstream, the acetyl portion dissociates, then binds irreversibly to platelet cyclooxygenase. This action prevents synthesis of thromboxane A_2 and thereby inhibits platelet aggregation. A small single dose (325 mg or less) irreversibly acetylates circulating platelets within a few minutes, and effects last for the life span of the platelets (7–10 days). Other NSAIDs

bind reversibly with platelet cyclooxygenase so that antiplatelet effects occur only while the drug is present in the blood. Thus, aspirin has greater effects, but all the drugs inhibit platelet aggregation, cause hypoprothrombinemia, interfere with blood coagulation, and increase the risk of bleeding.

In addition to analgesic–antipyretic–anti-inflammatory and antiplatelet activity, aspirin and NSAIDs may cause gastric bleeding, irritation, and ulceration. Most of the newer drugs have been developed in an effort to retain the analgesic and anti-inflammatory properties of aspirin while decreasing the adverse effects. These efforts have been only partly successful.

Indications for Use

Despite many similarities, aspirin and other NSAIDs differ in their approved indications for use. Aspirin, a salicylate, has long been the drug of choice in many disorders characterized by pain, fever, or inflammation, and it may be used for one, two, or all three of these symptoms. It also is often prescribed for clients at high risk of myocardial infarction or stroke from thrombosis. This indication for use stems from its antiplatelet activity and resultant effects on blood coagulation (*i.e.*, decreased clot formation).

Acetaminophen, which differs chemically from aspirin, is commonly used as an aspirin substitute for pain and fever, but it lacks anti-inflammatory effects. It is increasingly used to relieve pain associated with osteoarthritis because the disease process is degenerative rather than inflammatory. Ibuprofen (Motrin, others) and other propionic acid derivatives are widely used as anti-inflammatory agents and analgesics. Ibuprofen, ketoprofen, and naproxen are available in prescription and over-the-counter (OTC) formulations. Ketorolac (Toradol), which can be given orally and parenterally, is used only as an analgesic. Most of the other NSAIDs are considered too toxic to use as analgesics and antipyretics. They are used primarily in rheumatoid arthritis and other musculoskeletal disorders that do not respond to safer drugs.

Some commonly used drugs and their indications for use are summarized in Table 7-2.

Contraindications for Use

Contraindications to clinical use of these drugs include peptic ulcer disease, GI or other bleeding disorders, history of hypersensitivity reactions, and impaired renal function. In people who are allergic to aspirin, nonaspirin NSAIDs also are contraindicated because hypersensitivity reactions may occur with any drugs that inhibit prostaglandin synthesis. In children and ado-

TABLE 7-2 CLINICAL INDICATIONS FOR COMMONLY USED ANALGESIC–ANTIPYRETIC–ANTI-INFLAMMATORY DRUGS

Generic/Trade Name	Pain	Fever	Osteoarthritis	Rheumatoid Arthritis	Juvenile Rheumatoid Arthritis	Dysmenorrhea	Acute Painful Shoulder	Ankylosing Spondylitis	Bursitis	Gout	Tendinitis
Acetaminophen (Tylenol, others)	✔	✔									
Acetylsalicylic Acid (Aspirin)	✔	✔	✔	✔	✔	✔	✔	✔	✔	✔	✔
Diclofenac (Voltaren)			✔	✔				✔			
Diflunisal (Dolobid)	✔		✔	✔							
Etodolac (Lodine)	✔		✔								
Fenoprofen (Nalfon)	✔		✔	✔							
Flurbiprofen (Ansaid)			✔	✔							
Ibuprofen (Motrin, others)	✔	✔	✔	✔		✔				✔	✔
Indomethacin (Indocin)			✔	✔			✔	✔	✔	✔	✔
Ketoprofen (Orudis)	✔		✔	✔		✔			✔	✔	✔
Ketorolac (Toradol)	✔										
Nabumetone (Relafen)			✔	✔							
Naproxen (Naprosyn)	✔		✔	✔	✔	✔		✔	✔	✔	✔
Oxaprozin (Daypro)			✔	✔							
Piroxicam (Feldene)			✔	✔							
Sulindac (Clinoril)			✔	✔			✔	✔	✔	✔	✔
Tolmetin (Tolectin)			✔	✔	✔						

lescents, aspirin is contraindicated in the presence of viral infections such as influenza or chickenpox because of its association with Reye's syndrome.

Individual Drugs

Aspirin is the prototype of the analgesic–antipyretic–anti-inflammatory drugs and is the most commonly used salicylate. Aspirin is effective in pain of low to moderate intensity, especially that involving the skin, muscles, joints, and other connective tissue. It is especially useful in disorders in which inflammation contributes to pain, such as rheumatoid arthritis.

Because aspirin is a nonprescription drug, it is a home remedy for headaches, colds, influenza and other respiratory infections, muscular aches, and fever. It also is prescribed by physicians for a variety of clinical conditions, including acute rheumatic fever, rheumatoid arthritis, and other musculoskeletal disorders.

Aspirin can be purchased in plain, chewable, enteric-coated, and effervescent tablets and rectal suppositories. It is not marketed in liquid form because it is unstable in solution. It also is available in combination with other analgesics, antacids, and antihistamines and is an ingredient in some nonprescription cold and allergy remedies.

Route and Dosage Ranges

Adults: Analgesia and antipyresis, PO 325–650 mg q4h PRN; usual single dose, 650 mg

   Arthritis and other rheumatic conditions, PO 3.2–6 g/d in divided doses

   Myocardial infarction prophylaxis, PO 325 mg/d

   Acute rheumatic fever, PO 5–8 g/d, initially, in divided doses

   Transient ischemic attacks in men, PO 1300 mg/d in divided doses (650 mg twice a day or 325 mg four times a day)

Children: Analgesia and antipyresis, PO 10–15 mg/kg q4h, up to 60–80 mg/kg/d. Recommended doses for specific weight ranges: 24–35 lb (10.6–15.9 kg), 162 mg; 36–47 lb (16–21.4 kg), 243 mg; 48–59 lb (21.5–26.8 kg), 324 mg; 60–71 lb (26.9–32.3 kg), 405 mg; 72–95 lb (32.4–43.2 kg) 486 mg; 96 lb or above (43.3 kg or above), 648 mg

   Juvenile rheumatoid arthritis, PO 60–110 mg/kg/d in divided doses q6–8h. Reduce amount for long-term use.

   Acute rheumatic fever, PO 100 mg/kg/d, in divided doses, for 2 wk, then 75 mg/kg/d for 4–6 wk

Diflunisal (Dolobid) is a salicylic acid derivative that differs chemically from aspirin. It is reportedly equal or superior to aspirin in mild to moderate pain, rheumatoid arthritis, and osteoarthritis. Compared to aspirin, it has less antipyretic effect and causes less gastric irritation; its longer duration of action allows for twice-daily administration.

Route and Dosage Ranges

Adults: Mild to moderate pain, PO 500–1000 mg initially, then 250–500 mg q8–12h
Rheumatoid arthritis, osteoarthritis PO 500–1000 mg/d, in two divided doses, increased to a maximum of 1500 mg/d if necessary

Acetaminophen USP (Tylenol, others) is a nonprescription drug commonly used as an aspirin substitute because it does not cause nausea, vomiting, or GI bleeding, and it does not interfere with blood clotting. It is equal to aspirin in analgesic and antipyretic effects, but it lacks anti-inflammatory activity.

Acetaminophen is well absorbed from oral administration and peak plasma concentrations are reached within 30 to 120 minutes. It is metabolized in the liver; about 94% is excreted in the urine as inactive glucuronate and sulfate conjugates. About 4% is metabolized to a toxic metabolite, which is normally inactivated by conjugation with glutathione and excreted in urine. Glutathione is important in liver detoxification of acetaminophen and an adequate supply is usually available in liver cells. In acute or chronic overdose situations, however, the supply of glutathione may become depleted. In the absence of glutathione, the toxic metabolite combines with liver cells and causes damage or fatal liver necrosis. In alcoholics, usual therapeutic doses may cause or increase liver damage. The probable mechanism for increased risk of hepatotoxicity in this population is that ethanol induces drug-metabolizing enzymes in the liver. The resulting rapid metabolism of acetaminophen produces enough toxic metabolite to exceed the available glutathione.

Acetaminophen is available in tablet, liquid, and rectal suppository forms and is in numerous combination products marketed as analgesics and cold remedies. It is often prescribed with codeine or oxycodone for added analgesic effects.

Routes and Dosage Ranges

Adults: PO 325–650 mg q4–6h, or 1000 mg three or four times per day; maximum 4 g/d
Rectal suppository 650 mg q4–6h, maximum of 6 in 24 h
Children: PO 10 mg/kg or according to age as follows: 0–3 mo, 40 mg; 4–11 mo, 80 mg; 1–2 y, 120 mg; 2–3 y, 160 mg; 4–5 y, 240 mg; 6–8 y, 320 mg; 9–10 y, 400 mg; 11 y, 480 mg. Doses may be given q4–6h to a maximum of 5 doses in 24 h.

Rectal suppository: age under 3 y, consult physician; age 3–6 y, 120 mg q4–6h, maximum 720 mg in 24 h; age 6–12 y, 325 mg q4–6h, maximum 2.6 g in 24 h

Fenoprofen (Nalfon), **flurbiprofen** (Ansaid), **ibuprofen** (Motrin, others), **ketoprofen** (Orudis), **naproxen** (Naprosyn, Anaprox), and **oxaprozin** (Daypro) are propionic acid derivatives that are chemically and pharmacologically similar. In addition to their use as anti-inflammatory agents in rheumatoid arthritis, gout, tendinitis, and bursitis, they are used as analgesics in conditions not necessarily related to inflammation (*e.g.,* dysmenorrhea, episiotomy, minor trauma) and as antipyretics. Ibuprofen, ketoprofen, and naproxen are available OTC, with recommended doses usually smaller than those for prescription formulations. Although these drugs are usually better tolerated than aspirin, they are much more expensive and may cause all the adverse effects associated with aspirin and other prostaglandin inhibitors.

Fenoprofen
Route and Dosage Ranges

Adults: Rheumatoid arthritis, osteoarthritis, PO 300–600 mg three or four times per day; maximum 3200 mg/d
Mild to moderate pain, PO 200 mg q4–6h PRN

Flurbiprofen
Route and Dosage Range

Adults: Rheumatoid arthritis, osteoarthritis, PO 200–300 mg/d in two, three, or four divided doses

Ibuprofen
Route and Dosage Ranges

Adults: Rheumatoid arthritis, osteoarthritis, PO 300–600 mg 3 or 4 times per day; maximum 2400 mg/d
Mild to moderate pain, PO 200–400 mg q4–6h PRN
Primary dysmenorrhea, PO 400 mg q4h PRN
Children: Fever, age 1–12 y, initial temperature 39.2°C (102.5° F) or less, PO 5 mg/kg q6–8 h; initial temperature above 39.2°C (102.5° F), PO 10 mg/kg q6–8h; maximum 40 mg/kg/d
Juvenile arthritis, PO 20–40 mg/kg/d, in three or four divided doses

Ketoprofen
Route and Dosage Ranges

Adults: Rheumatoid arthritis, osteoarthritis, PO 150–300 mg/d in three or four divided doses; maximum 300 mg/d. Sustained-release (Oruvail SR), 200 mg once daily

Mild to moderate pain, primary dysmenorrhea, PO 25–50 mg q6–8h PRN; maximum 300 mg/d

Naproxen
Route and Dosage Ranges

Adults: Rheumatoid arthritis, osteoarthritis, ankylosing spondylitis, PO 250–375 mg twice a day

Acute gout, PO 750 mg initially, then 250 mg q8h until the attack subsides

Mild to moderate pain, primary dysmenorrhea, acute tendinitis and bursitis, PO 500 mg initially, then 250 mg q6–8h

Children: Juvenile arthritis, PO 10 mg/kg/d in two divided doses; OTC preparation not recommended for children under 12 y

Naproxen Sodium
Route and Dosage Ranges

Adults: Rheumatoid arthritis, osteoarthritis, ankylosing spondylitis, PO 275 mg twice a day

Acute gout, PO 825 mg initially, then 275 mg q8h until the attack subsides

Mild to moderate pain, primary dysmenorrhea, acute tendinitis and bursitis, PO 550 mg initially, then 275 mg q6–8h

Oxaprozin
Route and Dosage Range

Adults: Rheumatoid arthritis, osteoarthritis, PO 600–1200 mg once daily; maximum, 1800 mg/d in divided doses

Indomethacin (Indocin), **sulindac** (Clinoril), and **tolmetin** (Tolectin) are acetic acid derivatives used for moderate to severe rheumatoid arthritis, osteoarthritis, ankylosing spondylitis, acute gouty arthritis, and acute painful shoulder (bursitis, tendinitis). These drugs have potent anti-inflammatory effects but are associated with a greater incidence and severity of adverse effects than aspirin and the propionic acid derivatives. Thus, they are not recommended for general use as analgesics or antipyretics. Uncommon but potentially serious adverse effects include GI ulceration, bone marrow depression, hemolytic anemia, mental confusion, depression, and psychosis. These adverse effects are especially associated with indomethacin; the other drugs were developed in an effort to find equally effective but less toxic derivatives of indomethacin. Although adverse reactions occur less often with sulindac and tolmetin, they are still common.

In addition to the uses listed above, tolmetin is approved for treatment of juvenile rheumatoid arthritis, and intravenous indomethacin is approved for treatment of patent ductus arteriosus in premature infants.

(The ductus arteriosus joins the pulmonary artery to the aorta in the fetal circulation. When it fails to close, blood is shunted from the aorta to the pulmonary artery, causing severe cardiopulmonary problems.)

Newer drugs related to this group are **etodolac** (Lodine), **ketorolac** (Toradol), and **nabumetone** (Relafen). Etodolac is used for pain and osteoarthritis and reportedly causes less gastric irritation, especially in older adults at high risk of GI bleeding. Ketorolac is used only for pain, and although it can be given orally, its unique characteristic is that it can be given by injection. Parenteral ketorolac is reportedly comparable to morphine and other opiates in analgesic effectiveness for moderate or severe pain. However, hematomas and wound bleeding have been reported with postoperative use, and its use is limited to 5 days. Nabumetone is approved for treatment of rheumatoid arthritis and osteoarthritis.

Etodolac
Route and Dosage Ranges

Adults: Osteoarthritis, PO 600–1200 mg/d in two to four divided doses; maximum dose, 1200 mg/d

Pain, PO 200–400 mg q6–8h PRN; maximum dose, 1200 mg/d

Indomethacin
Routes and Dosage Ranges

Adults: PO, rectal suppository 75 mg/d initially, increased by 25 mg/d at weekly intervals to a maximum of 150–200 mg/d if necessary

Acute gouty arthritis, acute painful shoulder, PO 75–150 mg/d in three or four divided doses until pain and inflammation are controlled (about 3–5 d for gout, 7–14 d for painful shoulder), then discontinued

Children: Premature infants with patent ductus arteriosus, IV 0.2–0.3 mg/kg q12h for a total of 3 doses

Ketorolac
Routes and Dosage Ranges

Adults: PO 10 mg q4–6h for limited duration; maximum dose, 40 mg/d

IM 30–60 mg initially, then 15–30 mg q6h on a regular schedule or as needed to control pain, up to 5 d

Nabumetone
Route and Dosage Range

Adults: Osteoarthritis, rheumatoid arthritis, PO 1000–2000 mg/d in one or two doses. For long-term treatment, use the lowest effective dose.

Sulindac
Route and Dosage Ranges

Adults: PO 150–200 mg twice a day; maximum 400 mg/d
  Acute gouty arthritis, acute painful shoulder, PO 200 mg twice a day until pain and inflammation are controlled (about 7–14 d), then discontinued

Tolmetin
Route and Dosage Ranges

Adults: PO 400 mg three times per day initially, increased to 1600 mg/d for osteoarthritis or 2000 mg/d for rheumatoid arthritis if necessary
Children: Rheumatoid arthritis, PO 20 mg/kg/d in three or four divided doses

Diclofenac sodium (Voltaren) is chemically different but pharmacologically similar to other NSAIDs. It is indicated for use in rheumatoid arthritis, osteoarthritis, and ankylosing spondylitis. **Diclofenac potassium** (Cataflam) may be given for pain and primary dysmenorrhea when rapid pain relief is desired.

Route and Dosage Ranges

Adults: Rheumatoid arthritis, PO 150–200 mg/d in three or four divided doses
  Osteoarthritis, PO 100–150 mg/d in three or four divided doses
  Ankylosing spondylitis, PO 100–125 mg/d in three or four divided doses
  Pain and primary dysmenorrhea (diclofenac potassium only), PO 150 mg/d, in three divided doses

Piroxicam (Feldene) is an oxicam NSAID that differs chemically from other agents but has similar pharmacologic properties. Approved for treatment of rheumatoid arthritis and osteoarthritis, it reportedly causes less GI irritation than aspirin. Its long half-life allows for once-daily dosing, but optimal efficacy may not occur for 1 to 2 weeks.

Route and Dosage Range

Adults: PO 20 mg/d

LESS COMMONLY USED NSAIDs

Meclofenamate (Meclomen) and **mefenamic acid** (Ponstel) are fenamate NSAIDs that are infrequently used because of a high incidence of GI and neurologic adverse effects.

Meclofenamate
Route and Dosage Range

Adults: Rheumatoid arthritis, osteoarthritis, PO 200–400 mg/d in three or four divided doses

Mefenamic Acid
Route and Dosage Ranges

Adults: Acute pain, PO 500 mg initially, then 250 mg q6h PRN for no longer than 1 wk
  Primary dysmenorrhea, PO 500 mg at start of menses, then 250 mg q6h PRN for 2 or 3 d
Children over 14 years: Acute pain, PO 500 mg initially, then 250 mg q6h PRN for no longer than 1 wk

DRUGS USED IN GOUT AND HYPERURICEMIA

Allopurinol (Zyloprim) is used to prevent or treat hyperuricemia, which occurs with gout and with antineoplastic drug therapy. Uric acid is formed by purine metabolism and an enzyme called xanthine oxidase. Allopurinol prevents formation of uric acid by inhibiting xanthine oxidase. It is especially useful in chronic gout characterized by tophi (deposits of uric acid crystals in the joints, kidneys, and soft tissues) and impaired renal function. The drug promotes resorption of urate deposits and prevents their further development. Acute attacks of gout may result when urate deposits are mobilized. These may be prevented by concomitant administration of colchicine until serum uric acid levels are lowered.

Route and Dosage Ranges

Adults: Mild gout, PO 200–400 mg/d
  Severe gout, PO 400–600 mg/d
  Hyperuricemia in clients with renal insufficiency, PO 100–200 mg/d
  Secondary hyperuricemia from anticancer drugs, PO 100–200 mg/d; maximum 800 mg/d
Children: Secondary hyperuricemia from anticancer drugs: <6 y, PO 150 mg/d; 6–10 y, PO 300 mg/d

Colchicine is an anti-inflammatory drug used to prevent or treat acute attacks of gout. In acute attacks, it is the drug of choice for relieving joint pain and edema. Colchicine decreases inflammation by decreasing the movement of leukocytes into body tissues containing urate crystals. It has no analgesic or antipyretic effects.

Routes and Dosage Ranges

Adults: Acute attacks, PO 0.5 mg q1h until pain is relieved or toxicity (nausea, vomiting, diarrhea) occurs; 3-d interval between courses of therapy

IV 1–2 mg initially, then 0.5 mg q3–6h until response is obtained; maximum total dose 4 mg
Prophylaxis, PO 0.5–1 mg/d

Probenecid (Benemid) increases the urinary excretion of uric acid. This uricosuric action is used therapeutically to treat hyperuricemia and gout. It is not effective in acute attacks of gouty arthritis but prevents hyperuricemia and tophi associated with chronic gout. Probenecid may precipitate acute gout until serum uric acid levels are within the normal range; concomitant administration of colchicine prevents this effect. (Probenecid also is used with penicillin, most often in treating sexually transmitted diseases. It increases blood levels and prolongs the action of penicillin by decreasing the rate of urinary excretion.)

Route and Dosage Ranges

Adults: PO 250 mg twice a day for 1 wk, then 500 mg twice a day
Children over 2 years: PO 40 mg/kg/d in divided doses

Sulfinpyrazone (Anturane) is a uricosuric agent similar to probenecid. It is not effective in acute gout but prevents or decreases tissue changes of chronic gout. Colchicine is usually given during initial sulfinpyrazone therapy to prevent acute gout.

Route and Dosage Range

Adults: PO 100–200 mg twice a day, gradually increased over 1 wk to a maximum of 400–800 mg/d

Drugs Used in Migraine

Ergotamine tartrate (Ergomar) is an ergot alkaloid used only in the treatment of migraine. Migraine is attributed to dilation of the extracerebral cranial arteries. Ergot preparations relieve migraine by constricting the vascular smooth muscle of blood vessels in the brain. Ergotamine is most effective when given sublingually or by inhalation at the onset of headache. When given orally, ergotamine is erratically absorbed, and therapeutic effects may be delayed for 20 to 30 minutes.

Ergotamine is contraindicated during pregnancy and in the presence of severe hypertension, peripheral vascular disease, coronary artery disease, renal or hepatic disease, and severe infections.

Routes and Dosage Ranges

Adults: PO, SL 1–2 mg at onset of acute migraine attack, then 2 mg q30 min, if necessary, to a maximum of 6 mg/24 h or 10 mg/wk

Inhalation, 0.36 mg (one inhalation) at onset of acute migraine, repeated in 5 min if necessary, to a maximum of 6 inhalations/24 h

Ergotamine tartrate and caffeine (Cafergot) is a commonly used antimigraine preparation. Caffeine reportedly increases the absorption and vasoconstrictive effects of ergotamine. The combination product is available in oral tablets containing ergotamine 1 mg and caffeine 100 mg and in rectal suppositories containing ergotamine 2 mg and caffeine 100 mg.

Routes and Dosage Ranges

Adults: PO 2 tablets at the onset of acute migraine, then 1 tablet every 30 min if necessary, up to 6 tablets per attack or 10 tablets/wk
Rectal suppository 0.5–1 suppository at the onset of acute migraine, repeated in 1 h if necessary, up to 2 suppositories per attack or 5 suppositories/wk
Children: PO 0.5–1 tablet initially, then 0.5 tablet every 30 min if necessary, to a maximum of 3 tablets

Dihydroergotamine mesylate (DHE 45) is a semisynthetic derivative of ergotamine that is less toxic and less effective than the parent drug.

Routes and Dosage Ranges

Adults: IM 1 mg at onset of acute migraine, repeated hourly if necessary to a total of 3 mg
IV 1 mg, repeated if necessary after 1 h; maximum dose 2 mg. Do not exceed 6 mg/wk.

Methysergide (Sansert) is an ergot derivative used only for prophylaxis of migraine; it is ineffective in acute migraine attacks. The drug is indicated only when migraine attacks are frequent or severe and for no longer than 4 consecutive months because of fibrosis in the aorta, heart, and lungs. Usage has declined because of adverse effects.

Route and Dosage Range

Adults: PO 4–8 mg/d in divided doses

Sumatriptan (Imitrex) increases serotonin in the brain and relieves acute migraine attacks by causing arterial vasoconstriction. Because of its vasoconstrictive properties, sumatriptan is contraindicated in patients with ischemic heart disease or uncontrolled hypertension. The drug produces fewer adverse effects than ergot alkaloids, and those that occur (discomfort at injection sites, anxiety, dizziness, and drowsiness) are usually mild and of short duration.

Routes and Dosage Ranges

Adults: PO 25–100 mg as a single dose; maximum dose, 300 mg/d

SC 6 mg as a single dose; maximum dose, 12 mg/d

Nursing Process

Assessment

- Assess for signs and symptoms of pain, such as location, severity, duration, and factors that cause or relieve the pain (see Chap. 6).
- Assess for fever (thermometer readings above 99.6°F [37.3°C] are usually considered fever). Hot, dry skin, flushed face, reduced urine output, and concentrated urine may accompany fever if the person also is dehydrated.
- Assess for inflammation. Local signs are redness, heat, edema, and pain or tenderness; systemic signs include fever, elevated white blood cell count (leukocytosis), and weakness.
- With arthritis or other musculoskeletal disorders, assess for limitations in activity and mobility.
- Ask about use of OTC analgesic, antipyretic, or anti-inflammatory drugs.
- Ask about allergic reactions to aspirin or NSAIDs.
- Assess for history of peptic ulcer disease, GI bleeding, or kidney disorders.

Nursing Diagnoses

- Pain
- Chronic Pain
- Activity Intolerance related to pain and impaired physical mobility
- Impaired Physical Mobility related to pain and inflammation
- Risk for Injury related to adverse drug effects (GI bleeding, renal insufficiency)
- Knowledge Deficit: Comparative characteristics of OTC and prescription drugs for pain, fever, and inflammation
- Knowledge Deficit: Therapeutic and adverse effects of commonly used drugs
- Knowledge Deficit: Correct use of OTC drugs for pain, fever, and inflammation

Planning/Goals

The client will:

- Experience relief of discomfort with minimal adverse drug effects
- Experience increased mobility and activity tolerance
- Inform health care providers if taking aspirin or an NSAID regularly
- Self-administer the drugs safely
- Verbalize signs and symptoms of adverse drug effects to be reported to health care providers
- Avoid overuse of the drugs
- Use measures to prevent accidental ingestion or overdose, especially in children

Interventions

Implement measures to prevent or minimize pain, fever, and inflammation:

- **Diagnosis and treatment of the underlying condition are very important.** Measures aimed at relief of the disorder, such as prevention or treatment of infections and improvement of the blood supply, may be helpful in alleviating symptoms.
- **Institute treatment measures as soon as they seem indicated.** Timing depends on thorough assessment and the ability to recognize early signs and symptoms. When drug therapy seems indicated, it generally should not be delayed any longer than necessary. With pain, for example, early treatment may prevent severe pain and allow the use of milder analgesic drugs. Other measures that may be used instead of or along with drug therapy include positioning, hygienic care, heat or cold applications, rest or exercise, and distraction or relaxation techniques. Assess response to various therapeutic approaches as carefully as initial signs and symptoms.

Teach clients:

- To inform any health care provider if they are taking aspirin, ibuprofen, or any other NSAID regularly
- That with inflammatory disorders, such as arthritis, improvement may take 1 to 2 weeks
- That if one drug is not effective, another one may work because people vary in responses to the drugs
- That because fever is one way the body fights infection, drug therapy may not be needed unless the fever is high or is accompanied by other uncomfortable signs and symptoms
- That aspirin is as effective as the more costly prescription NSAIDs
- That the main advantage of other NSAIDs over aspirin is decreased GI upset
- To avoid OTC aspirin or products containing aspirin (*e.g.,* Alka-Seltzer, Anacin, Arthritis Pain Formula, Ascriptin, Bufferin, Ecotrin, Excedrin, Midol, Vanquish) when taking aspirin or an NSAID regularly
- To avoid aspirin for about 2 weeks before and after major surgery or dental work to decrease the risk of excessive bleeding
- That acetaminophen is an effective aspirin substitute for pain or fever but not for inflammation or preventing heart attack or stroke
- That there are many trade names of OTC preparations of acetaminophen, and most contain 500 mg of drug per tablet or capsule. In addition, many OTC analgesics and cold remedies contain acetaminophen. Thus, all consumers should read product labels carefully to avoid duplicate sources and potential overdoses. Overuse may cause life-threatening liver damage.
- To avoid OTC products containing ibuprofen (*e.g.,* Advil, others), ketoprofen (Actron), or naproxen (Aleve) when taking any prescription NSAID.
- Correct scheduling and administration techniques to minimize the risk of adverse effects

Evaluation

- Interview and observe regarding relief of symptoms.
- Interview and observe regarding mobility and activity levels.

- Interview and observe regarding safe, effective use of the drugs.
- Select drugs appropriately.

Principles of Therapy

GUIDELINES FOR THERAPY WITH ASPIRIN

When pain, fever, or inflammation is present, aspirin is effective across a wide range of clinical conditions. Because it is a nonprescription drug and is widely available, people tend to underestimate its usefulness. Like any other drug, aspirin must be used appropriately to maximize therapeutic benefits and minimize adverse reactions. Some guidelines for correct usage include the following:

1. For *pain*, aspirin is useful alone when the discomfort is of low to moderate intensity. For more severe pain, aspirin may be combined with a narcotic or given between narcotic doses for better analgesia or to allow lower doses of the narcotic. Aspirin and narcotic analgesics act by different mechanisms, so such use is rational. Aspirin with codeine is especially effective. Aspirin may be used with other narcotics in clients who can take oral medications. For acute pain, aspirin is taken when the pain occurs and is often effective within a few minutes. For chronic pain, a regular schedule of administration, such as every 4 to 6 hours, is more effective.
2. For *fever*, aspirin is effective if drug therapy is indicated.
3. For *inflammation*, aspirin is useful in both short- and long-term therapy. It is especially useful in conditions characterized by pain and inflammation, such as rheumatoid arthritis.
4. Aspirin is usually the drug of choice when salicylate therapy is indicated. Sodium salicylate may be used for people who are hypersensitive to aspirin, but it is less effective, produces similar adverse reactions, and may be contraindicated because of its sodium content. Choline salicylate and a few other preparations are advertised as producing fewer GI adverse reactions but seem to offer little advantage over aspirin.
5. For most purposes, plain aspirin tablets are preferred. Enteric-coated tablets are more slowly absorbed and therefore take longer to exert their therapeutic effects. They may be better tolerated for long-term use of high doses in rheumatoid arthritis, however. Rectal suppositories are sometimes used when oral administration is contraindicated.
6. Aspirin dosage depends mainly on the condition being treated. Low doses are used for antiplatelet effects in preventing arterial thrombotic disorders such as myocardial infarction or stroke. Lower-than-

average doses are needed for clients with low serum albumin levels because a larger proportion of each dose is free to exert pharmacologic activity. Larger doses are needed for anti-inflammatory effects than for analgesic and antipyretic effects.
7. To decrease risks of toxicity, plasma salicylate levels should be measured periodically when large doses of aspirin are given for anti-inflammatory effects. Therapeutic levels are 150–300 µg/ml. Chronic administration of large doses saturates a major metabolic pathway, thereby slowing drug elimination, prolonging the serum half-life, and causing drug accumulation.
8. Salicylate intoxication may occur with an acute overdose or chronic use of therapeutic doses. Manifestations of salicylism include nausea, vomiting, fever, fluid and electrolyte deficiencies, tinnitus, decreased hearing, visual changes, drowsiness, confusion, hyperventilation, and others. Severe central nervous system dysfunction (*e.g.*, delirium, stupor, coma, seizures) indicates life-threatening toxicity. In children, metabolic acidosis develops rapidly and may be present on initial contact. In adults, metabolic acidosis develops more slowly and with severe overdosage.
9. In mild salicylism, stopping the drug or reducing the dose is usually sufficient. In severe salicylate overdose, treatment is symptomatic and aimed at preventing further absorption from the GI tract, increasing urinary excretion, and correcting fluid, electrolyte, and acid–base imbalances. When the drug may still be in the GI tract, emesis, gastric lavage, and activated charcoal, or a combination of these, help reduce absorption. IV sodium bicarbonate produces an alkaline urine in which salicylates are more rapidly excreted, and hemodialysis effectively removes salicylates from the blood. IV fluids are indicated when high fever or dehydration is present. The specific content of IV fluids depends on the serum electrolyte and acid–base status.

GUIDELINES FOR THERAPY WITH ACETAMINOPHEN

Acetaminophen is an effective aspirin substitute for the treatment of pain and fever when aspirin is contraindicated or not tolerated. It is the drug of choice for children with febrile illness (because of the association of aspirin with Reye's syndrome), elderly adults with impaired renal function (because aspirin and NSAIDs may cause further impairment), and pregnant women (because aspirin is associated with several maternal and fetal disorders, including bleeding).

The major drawback to acetaminophen is potential liver damage. Factors related to identification and treatment of hepatotoxicity include the following:

1. Acute hepatic failure may occur with a single large dose, usually about 10 to 15 g, but it has been reported with 6 g. Acute acetaminophen poisoning may be characterized by cyanosis, anemia, pancytopenia, jaundice, fever, vomiting, and central nervous system stimulation with excitement and delirium followed by vascular collapse, convulsions, coma, and death. Early symptoms (within 24 hours after ingestion) are nonspecific (*e.g.*, anorexia, nausea, vomiting). Peak hepatotoxicity occurs in 3 to 4 days, and recovery occurs in 7 to 8 days.

2. If overdose is detected soon after ingestion, activated charcoal can be given to inhibit absorption. However, the specific antidote is acetylcysteine (Mucomyst), a mucolytic agent given by inhalation in respiratory disorders (see Chap. 49). For acetaminophen poisoning, it is given orally. The drug provides cysteine, a precursor substance required for the synthesis of glutathione. Glutathione combines with a toxic metabolite and decreases hepatotoxicity if acetylcysteine is given within 24 hours of acetaminophen ingestion.

3. Hepatotoxicity also occurs with chronic ingestion of acetaminophen (5–8 g/d for several weeks or 3–4 g/d for 1 year) and short-term ingestion of usual therapeutic doses in alcoholics. Although no safe dosage range has been established for chronic alcohol abusers, it is recommended that they ingest no more than 2 g daily.

GUIDELINES FOR THERAPY WITH NSAIDs

Most NSAIDs are prescription drugs used primarily for analgesic and anti-inflammatory effects in arthritis and other musculoskeletal disorders. However, several are approved for more general use as an analgesic or antipyretic. Ibuprofen, ketoprofen, and naproxen are available by prescription and OTC. Clients must be instructed to avoid combined use of aspirin and an NSAID or prescription and nonprescription NSAIDs because of the high risk of adverse effects, especially GI ulceration and bleeding. Although NSAIDs may be no more effective than aspirin, they may cause fewer GI adverse effects than aspirin and thus may be better tolerated by some clients. These drugs are much more expensive than aspirin.

NSAIDs inhibit platelet activity only while drug molecules are in the bloodstream, not for the life of the platelet (about 1 week) as aspirin does. Thus, they are *not* prescribed therapeutically for antiplatelet effects.

GUIDELINES FOR TREATING RHEUMATOID ARTHRITIS AND RELATED DISORDERS

The primary goals of treatment are to control pain and inflammation and to minimize immobilization and disability. Rest, exercise, physical therapy, and drugs are used to attain these goals. None of these measures prevents joint destruction or related pathologic conditions.

Aspirin relieves pain and inflammation, and it is inexpensive, an important factor in the long-term treatment of chronic musculoskeletal disorders. Dosage should be individualized to relieve symptoms, maintain therapeutic salicylate blood levels, and minimize adverse effects. Regular administration of aspirin every 4 to 6 hours usually produces a therapeutic serum salicylate level of 150–300 µg/ml. For people who cannot take aspirin because of peptic ulcer disease, bleeding disorders, and other contraindications, another NSAID is usually ordered. The choice of a specific drug is largely empirical; one person may respond better to one NSAID than another. A drug may be given for 2 or 3 weeks on a trial basis. If therapeutic benefits occur, the drug may be continued; if no benefits seem evident or toxicity occurs, another drug may be tried.

Ibuprofen and other propionic acid derivatives are often used because they are associated with fewer GI adverse effects than most other NSAIDs. However, they cause significant toxicity in some cases and are quite expensive for long-term use.

Several other drugs also may be used to treat rheumatoid arthritis. These include adrenal corticosteroids and the disease-modifying antirheumatic drugs, such as gold, hydroxychloroquine (Plaquenil), penicillamine (Cuprimine, Depen), azathioprine (Imuran), cyclophosphamide (Cytoxan), and methotrexate. These drugs have anti-inflammatory and immunosuppressant effects and may cause significant toxicity. The disease-modifying drugs are used to slow tissue damage, which other drugs cannot do.

GUIDELINES FOR PERIOPERATIVE USE OF ASPIRIN AND OTHER NSAIDs

Aspirin should generally be avoided for 1 to 2 weeks before and after surgery. This precaution is indicated because aspirin increases the risk of bleeding. Most other NSAIDs should be discontinued about 3 days before surgery; nabumetone and piroxicam have long half-lives and must be discontinued about 1 week preoperatively. Postoperatively, especially after relatively minor procedures, such as dental extractions and episiotomies, several of the drugs are used to relieve pain. Caution is needed because of increased risks of bleeding, and the drugs should not be given if there are other risk factors for bleeding. In addition, ketorolac, the only injectable NSAID, has been used in more extensive surgeries. Although the drug has several advantages over narcotic analgesics, bleeding and hematomas may occur.

USE OF ASPIRIN, ACETAMINOPHEN, AND NSAIDS IN CHILDREN

Acetaminophen is usually the drug of choice for pain or fever in children, and children seem less susceptible to liver toxicity than adults. Ibuprofen also may be given for fever. Aspirin is not recommended because of its association with Reye's syndrome, a life-threatening illness characterized by encephalopathy, hepatic damage, and other serious problems. Reye's syndrome usually occurs after a viral infection, such as influenza B or chickenpox, during which aspirin was given for fever. For children with juvenile rheumatoid arthritis, aspirin, ibuprofen, naproxen, or tolmetin may be given. Pediatric indications for use and dosages have not been established for most of the other drugs. Ibuprofen (Children's Advil, Children's Motrin) is available in a liquid suspension containing 100 mg/5 ml.

USE OF ASPIRIN, ACETAMINOPHEN, AND NSAIDS IN OLDER ADULTS

Acetaminophen is generally safe in recommended doses unless liver damage is present or the person is a chronic alcohol abuser. Aspirin is generally safe in the small doses prescribed for prevention of myocardial infarction and stroke (antiplatelet effects). Aspirin and NSAIDs are probably safe in therapeutic doses for occasional use as an analgesic or antipyretic. However, older adults have a high incidence of musculoskeletal disorders (*e.g.*, rheumatoid arthritis, osteoarthritis), and an NSAID is often prescribed. Long-term use of the relatively high doses required for anti-inflammatory effects increases the risk of serious GI bleeding. Small doses, gradual increments, and

taking the drug with food or a full glass of water may decrease GI effects. In addition, misoprostol (Cytotec) may be given. Misoprostol can be used to prevent gastric ulcers in older adults, although its adverse effects of abdominal cramping and diarrhea may not be tolerated very well. Older adults also are more likely than younger adults to develop nephrotoxicity with NSAIDs.

GUIDELINES FOR TREATING HYPERURICEMIA AND GOUT

Opinions differ regarding treatment of asymptomatic hyperuricemia. Some authorities do not think drug therapy is indicated; others think that lowering serum uric acid levels may prevent joint inflammation and renal calculi. Allopurinol, probenecid, or sulfinpyrazone may be given for this purpose. Colchicine also should be given for several weeks to prevent acute attacks of gout while serum uric acid levels are being lowered. During initial administration of these drugs, a high fluid intake (to produce about 2000 ml of urine per day) and alkaline urine are recommended to prevent renal calculi. Urate crystals are more likely to precipitate in acid urine.

GUIDELINES FOR TREATING MIGRAINE

For treatment of migraine and similar disorders, ergot preparations should be given at the onset of headache, and the client should lie down in a quiet, darkened room. Help the client identify and avoid precipitating factors when possible. Sumatriptan may be preferred because it is effective and reportedly causes fewer adverse effects than ergot preparations.

NURSING ACTIONS

ANALGESIC–ANTIPYRETIC–ANTI-INFLAMMATORY AND RELATED DRUGS

NURSING ACTIONS	RATIONALE/EXPLANATION
1. Administer accurately **a.** Give aspirin and other nonsteroidal anti-inflammatory drugs (NSAIDs) with a full glass of water or other fluid and with or just after food.	To decrease gastric irritation. Even though food delays absorption and decreases peak plasma levels of some of the drugs, it is probably safer to give them with food.
b. Give antimigraine preparations at the onset of headache.	To prevent development of more severe symptoms
c. Give methysergide with meals.	To decrease nausea and vomiting

(continued)

NURSING ACTIONS	RATIONALE/EXPLANATION
2. Observe for therapeutic effects	
a. When drugs are given for pain, observe for decreased or absent manifestations of pain.	Pain relief is usually evident within 30 to 60 minutes.
b. When drugs are given for fever, record temperature every 2 to 4 hours, and observe for a decrease.	
c. When drugs are given for arthritis and other inflammatory disorders, observe for decreased pain, edema, redness, heat, and stiffness of joints. Also observe for increased joint mobility and exercise tolerance.	With aspirin, improvement is usually noted within 24 to 48 hours. With most of the NSAIDs, 1 to 2 weeks may be required before beneficial effects become evident.
d. When colchicine is given for acute gouty arthritis, observe for decreased pain and inflammation in involved joints.	Therapeutic effects occur within 4 to 12 hours after intravenous colchicine administration and 24 to 48 hours after oral administration. Edema may not decrease for several days.
e. When allopurinol, probenecid, or sulfinpyrazone is given for hyperuricemia, observe for normal serum uric acid level (about 2–8 mg/100 ml).	Serum uric acid levels usually decrease to normal range within 1 to 3 weeks.
f. When the above drugs are given for chronic gout, observe for decreased size of tophi, absence of new tophi, decreased joint pain and increased joint mobility, and normal serum uric acid levels.	
g. When ergot preparations are given in migraine headache, observe for relief of symptoms.	Therapeutic effects are usually evident within 15 to 30 minutes.
3. Observe for adverse effects	
a. With analgesic–antipyretic–anti-inflammatory and antigout agents, observe for:	
(1) *Gastrointestinal problems*—anorexia, nausea, vomiting, diarrhea, bleeding, ulceration	These are common reactions, more likely with aspirin, indomethacin, piroxicam, sulindac, tolmetin, colchicine, and sulfinpyrazone and less likely with acetaminophen, diflunisal, etodolac, fenoprofen, ibuprofen, and naproxen. A prostaglandin called misoprostol (Cytotec) may be given concurrently with aspirin and other NSAIDs to prevent gastric ulcers (see Chap. 60).
(2) *Hematologic problems*—petechiae, bruises, hematuria, melena, epistaxis, and bone marrow depression (leukopenia, thrombocytopenia, anemia)	Bone marrow depression is more likely to occur with colchicine.
(3) *Central nervous system effects*—headache, dizziness, fainting, ataxia, insomnia, confusion, drowsiness	These effects are relatively common with indomethacin and may occur with most of the other drugs, especially with high dosages.
(4) *Skin rashes, dermatitis*	
(5) *Hypersensitivity reactions* with dyspnea, bronchospasm, skin rashes	These effects may simulate asthma in people who are allergic to aspirin and aspirin-like drugs.
(6) *Tinnitus, blurred vision*	Tinnitus (ringing or roaring in the ears) is a classic sign of aspirin overdose (salicylate intoxication). It occurs with NSAIDs as well, especially with overdosage.
(7) *Nephrotoxicity*—decreased urine output, increased blood urea nitrogen (BUN), increased serum creatinine, hyperkalemia, retention of sodium and water with resultant edema	More likely to occur in people with pre-existing renal impairment, especially when fluid intake is decreased or fluid loss is increased. Elderly adults are at greater risk because of decreased renal blood flow and increased incidence of congestive heart failure and diuretic therapy. Renal damage is usually reversible when the drug is discontinued.

Nursing Actions	*Rationale/Explanation*
(8) *Cardiovascular and hepatic effects*	These are not common with usual therapeutic doses, but all vital organs may be adversely affected with overdoses.
b. With antimigraine preparations, observe for:	
(1) *Nausea, vomiting, diarrhea*	These drugs have a direct effect on the vomiting center of the brain and stimulate contraction of gastrointestinal smooth muscle.
(2) *Symptoms of ergot poisoning* (ergotism)—coolness, numbness, and tingling of the extremities, headache, vomiting, dizziness, thirst, convulsions, weak pulse, confusion, angina-like chest pain, transient tachycardia or bradycardia, muscle weakness and pain, cyanosis, gangrene of the extremities	The ergot alkaloids are highly toxic; poisoning may be acute or chronic. Acute poisoning is rare; chronic poisoning is usually a result of overdosage. Circulatory impairments may result from vasoconstriction and vascular insufficiency. Large doses also damage capillary endothelium and may cause thrombosis and occlusion. Gangrene of extremities rarely occurs with usual doses unless peripheral vascular disease or other contraindications are also present.
(3) *Hypertension*	Blood pressure may rise as a result of generalized vasoconstriction induced by the ergot preparation.
(4) *Hypersensitivity reactions*—local edema and pruritus, anaphylactic shock	Allergic reactions are relatively uncommon.
(5) With *methysergide*—inflammation followed by fibrosis in some body tissues. Retroperitoneal fibrosis can lead to urinary tract obstruction; fibrosis of lung tissue can lead to pulmonary complications. Cardiac valves and major arteries also may be affected by fibrotic thickening.	These growths usually regress if symptoms are detected and the drug is discontinued. The client is examined frequently during long-term therapy. A drug-free interval of several weeks is recommended between courses of therapy.
4. Observe for drug interactions	
a. Drugs that *increase* effects of aspirin and other NSAIDs:	
(1) Acidifying agents (*e.g.*, ascorbic acid)	Acidify urine and thereby decrease the urinary excretion rate of salicylates
(2) Alcohol	Increases gastric irritation and occult blood loss
(3) Anticoagulants, oral	Increase risk of bleeding substantially. People taking anticoagulants should not take aspirin or aspirin-containing products.
(4) Codeine, other narcotic analgesics, and some related analgesics such as methotrimeprazine (Levoprome) and pentazocine (Talwin)	Additive analgesic effects because of different mechanisms of action. Aspirin can be used with these drugs to provide adequate pain relief without excessive doses and sedation, in many cases.
(5) Corticosteroids (*e.g.*, prednisone)	Additive gastric irritation and ulcerogenic effects
b. Drugs that *decrease* effects of aspirin and other NSAIDs:	
(1) Alkalinizing agents (*e.g.*, sodium bicarbonate)	Increase rate of renal excretion
(2) Misoprostol (Cytotec)	This drug, a prostaglandin, was developed specifically to prevent aspirin and NSAID-induced gastric ulcers.
c. Drugs that *increase* effects of indomethacin:	
(1) Anticoagulants, oral	Increase risk of gastrointestinal bleeding. Indomethacin causes gastric irritation and is considered an ulcerogenic drug.
(2) Corticosteroids	Increase ulcerogenic effect
(3) Salicylates	Increase ulcerogenic effect

(continued)

NURSING ACTIONS	RATIONALE/EXPLANATION
(4) Heparin	Increases risk of bleeding. These drugs should not be used concurrently.
d. Drugs that *decrease* effects of indomethacin: Antacids	Delay absorption from the gastrointestinal tract
e. Drugs that *decrease* effects of allopurinol, probenecid, and sulfinpyrazone:	
(1) Alkalinizing agents (*e.g.*, sodium bicarbonate)	Decrease risks of renal calculi from precipitation of uric acid crystals. Alkalinizing agents are recommended until serum uric acid levels return to normal.
(2) Colchicine	Decreases attacks of acute gout. Recommended for concurrent use until serum uric acid levels return to normal.
(3) Diuretics	Decrease uricosuric effects
(4) Salicylates	Mainly at salicylate doses less than 2 g/d, decrease uricosuric effects of probenecid and sulfinpyrazone but do not interfere with the action of allopurinol. Salicylates are uricosuric at doses greater than 5 g/d.
f. Drugs that *increase* effects of ergot preparations: Vasoconstrictors (*e.g.*, ephedrine, epinephrine, phenylephrine)	Additive vasoconstriction with risks of severe, persistent hypertension and intracranial hemorrhage
5. Teach clients **a.** With analgesic–antipyretic–anti-inflammatory and antigout agents:	
(1) Take the drugs with a full glass of liquid and food.	To decrease stomach irritation and upset
(2) Drink 2½ to 3 quarts of fluid daily if not contraindicated.	To decrease gastric irritation. With long-term use of aspirin, adequate fluid intake is needed to prevent precipitation of salicylate crystals in the urinary tract. With allopurinol, probenecid, and sulfinpyrazone, fluids are needed to help prevent precipitation of urate crystals and formation of urate kidney stones. Fluid intake is especially important initially when serum uric acid levels are high and large amounts of uric acid are being excreted in the urine.
(3) Report signs of bleeding (nose bleed, vomiting blood, bruising, blood in urine or stools), difficulty breathing, skin rash or hives, ringing in ears, dizziness, or severe stomach upset.	
(4) Store aspirin in a closed childproof container and keep out of reach of children. *Never* call aspirin "candy."	A closed container reduces exposure of the drug to moisture and air, which cause chemical breakdown. Aspirin that is deteriorating smells like vinegar (acetic acid). Special precautions are needed with children because aspirin ingestion is a common cause of drug poisoning in children.
(5) With colchicine for chronic gout, carry the drug, and start taking it as directed (usually one pill every hour for several hours until relief is obtained or nausea, vomiting, and diarrhea occur) when joint pain starts.	To prevent or minimize an attack of gouty arthritis
b. With ergot preparations, report signs of vascular insufficiency, such as tingling sensation or coldness, numbness, or weakness of the extremities. Do not exceed recommended doses.	These are symptoms of ergot toxicity. To avoid potentially serious adverse reactions, do not exceed recommended doses.

HOME CARE

Home use of acetaminophen and NSAIDs is extremely widespread, and the drugs are usually self-administered. Many people are aware of the drugs' beneficial effects in relieving pain, but many do not seem adequately informed about potential problems associated with use of the drugs. Thus, the home care nurse may need to assist clients in perceiving a need for additional information and provide that information. Specific suggestions include reading and following instructions on labels of OTC analgesics, not exceeding recommended dosages without consulting a health care provider, and avoiding combinations of NSAIDs (*e.g.*, multiple OTC NSAIDs or an OTC and a prescription NSAID). In addition, adverse drug effects should be reviewed with clients, and clients should be assessed for characteristics (*e.g.*, older age group, renal impairment, overuse of the drugs) that increase the risks of adverse effects.

REVIEW AND APPLICATION EXERCISES

1. How do aspirin and other NSAIDs produce analgesic, antipyretic, anti-inflammatory, and antiplatelet effects?

2. What adverse effects occur with aspirin and other NSAIDs, especially with daily ingestion?

3. Compare and contrast the uses and effects of aspirin and acetaminophen.

4. For a 6-year-old child with fever, would aspirin or acetaminophen be preferred? Why?

5. For a 50-year-old adult with rheumatoid arthritis, would aspirin, another NSAID, or acetaminophen be preferred? Why?

6. For a 75-year-old adult with osteoarthritis and a long history of "stomach trouble," would aspirin, another NSAID, or acetaminophen be preferred? Why?

7. What are some nursing interventions to decrease the adverse effects of aspirin, other NSAIDs, and acetaminophen?

8. When teaching a client about home use of aspirin, other NSAIDs, and acetaminophen, what information must be included?

9. What is the rationale for using acetylcysteine in the treatment of acetaminophen toxicity?

10. What is the rationale for combining narcotic and non-narcotic analgesics in the treatment of moderate pain?

SELECTED REFERENCES

Aspirin for prevention of myocardial infarction. *The Medical Letter,* 37:14–16 (Feb. 17, 1995).

Boh, L.E. (1993). Osteoarthritis. In J.T. DiPiro, R.L. Talbert, P.E. Hayes, G.C. Yee, G.R. Matzke, & L.M. Posey (Eds.), *Pharmacotherapy: A pathophysiologic approach,* 2nd ed., pp. 1330–1342. Norwalk, CT: Appleton & Lange.

Courts, N.F. (1996). Salicylism in the elderly: "A little aspirin never hurt anybody." *Geriatric Nursing, 17*(2):55–59.

Drug facts and comparisons. (1996). St. Louis: Facts and Comparisons.

Gall, E.P. & Higbee, M. (1993). Pharmacologic therapy of rheumatic diseases. In R. Bressler & M.D. Katz (Eds.), *Geriatric pharmacology,* pp. 467–506. New York: McGraw-Hill.

Hawkins, D.W. (1993). Gout and hyperuricemia. In J.T. DiPiro, R.L. Talbert, P.E. Hayes, G.C. Yee, G.R. Matzke, & L.M. Posey (Eds.), *Pharmacotherapy: A pathophysiologic approach,* 2nd ed., pp. 1343–1348. Norwalk, CT: Appleton & Lange.

Insel, P.A. (1996). Analgesic-antipyretic and antiinflammatory agents and drugs employed in the treatment of gout. In J.G. Hardman, L.E. Limbird, P.B. Molinoff, & R.W. Ruddon (Eds.), *Goodman & Gilman's The pharmacological basis of therapeutics,* 9th ed., pp. 617–657. New York: McGraw-Hill.

Porth, C.M. (1994). *Pathophysiology: Concepts of altered health states,* 4th ed. Philadelphia: J.B. Lippincott.

Schuna, A.A., Coulter, L. & Lee, S.S. (1993). Rheumatoid arthritis and the seronegative spondyloarthropathies. In J.T. DiPiro, R.L. Talbert, P.E. Hayes, G.C. Yee, G.R. Matzke, & L.M. Posey (Eds.), *Pharmacotherapy: A pathophysiologic approach,* 2nd ed., pp. 1313–1329. Norwalk, CT: Appleton & Lange.

Antianxiety and Sedative-Hypnotic Drugs

Outline

Anxiety

Sleep and Insomnia

Drugs Used to Treat Anxiety and Insomnia
barbiturates
benzodiazepines
miscellaneous drugs

Mechanism of Action

Indications for Use

Contraindications for Use

Nursing Process
assessment
nursing diagnoses
planning/goals
interventions
evaluation

Principles of Therapy: Benzodiazepines
use in anxiety
use in insomnia
duration of therapy
dosage
scheduling
benzodiazepine withdrawal
benzodiazepine toxicity
use in liver disease
use in hypoalbuminemia
use in children
use in older adults
home care

Objectives

After studying this chapter, the student will be able to:

1 Discuss functions of sleep and consequences of sleep deprivation.

2 Discuss characteristics, sources, and signs and symptoms of anxiety.

3 Describe nondrug interventions to decrease anxiety and insomnia.

4 List characteristics of benzodiazepine antianxiety and hypnotic drugs in terms of mechanism of action, indications for use, nursing process implications, and potential for abuse and dependence.

5 Describe strategies for preventing, recognizing, or treating benzodiazepine withdrawal reactions.

6 Discuss characteristics of nonbenzodiazepine antianxiety and hypnotic agents.

7 Teach clients guidelines for rational, safe use of antianxiety and sedative/hypnotic drugs.

8 Discuss the use of flumazenil (Romazicon) and other treatment measures for overdose of benzodiazepines.

Key Terms

Anxiety

Benzodiazepine

GABA/benzodiazepine receptor complex

Insomnia

ntianxiety and sedative-hypnotic agents are central nervous system (CNS) depressants with similar effects. Antianxiety drugs and sedatives promote relaxation; hypnotics produce sleep. The difference between the effects depends largely on dosage: large doses of antianxiety and sedative agents produce sleep, and small doses of hypnotics produce antianxiety or sedative effects. In addition, therapeutic doses of hypnotics given at bedtime may have residual sedative effects ("morning hangover") the following day. Because these drugs produce varying degrees of CNS depression, some are also used as anticonvulsant and anesthetic agents.

To aid understanding of the uses and effects of these drugs, anxiety and insomnia are described below. The clinical manifestations of these disorders are similar and overlapping—that is, daytime anxiety may be manifested as nighttime difficulty in sleeping, as the person cannot "turn off" worries, and difficulty in sleeping may be manifested as anxiety, fatigue, and decreased ability to function during usual waking hours.

Anxiety

Anxiety may be called apprehension, fear, nervousness, tension, worry, or other terms that denote an unpleasant state of feeling. It occurs when a person perceives a situation as threatening to physical, emotional, social, or economic well-being. Causes of anxiety vary among people and in the same person at different times. Many occur with everyday events associated with home, work, school, social activities, and chronic illness. Others occur episodically, such as an acute illness, death, divorce, loss of a job, starting a new job, or taking a test. Thus, anxiety is a normal response to a stressful situation and may be beneficial when it motivates the person toward constructive, problem-solving, coping activities.

However, when anxiety is severe or prolonged, it impairs the ability to function in usual activities of daily living. The American Psychiatric Association delineates anxiety disorders as medical diagnoses in the *Diagnostic and Statistical Manual*, fourth edition, published in 1994. This classification includes phobias and panic, obsessive-compulsive, post-traumatic stress, and atypical anxiety disorders, as well as generalized anxiety disorder. *Generalized anxiety disorder* includes:

1. Excessive anxiety about two or more circumstances for 6 months or longer
2. Six of 18 symptoms related to motor tension (*e.g.*, muscle tension, restlessness, trembling, fatigue), overactivity of the autonomic nervous system (*e.g.*, dyspnea, palpitations, tachycardia, sweating, dry mouth, dizziness, nausea, diarrhea), and increased vigilance (feeling keyed up, startling easily, difficulty concentrating, irritability, insomnia)
3. Disease processes or other causative factors (*e.g.*, hyperthyroidism, excessive caffeine or other stimulants) ruled out

Sleep and Insomnia

Sleep is a recurrent period of decreased mental and physical activity during which the person is relatively unresponsive to sensory and environmental stimuli. Normal sleep allows rest, renewal of energy for performing activities of daily living, and alertness on awakening. When a person retires for sleep, there is an initial period of drowsiness or sleep latency, which lasts about 30 minutes. Once the person is asleep, cycles occur about every 90 minutes during the sleep period. During each cycle, the sleeper progresses from drowsiness (stage I) to deep sleep (stage IV). These stages are characterized by depressed body functions, nonrapid eye movements (non-REM), and nondreaming and are thought to be physically restorative. Stage IV is followed by a period of 5 to 20 minutes of rapid eye movements (REM), dreaming, and increased physiologic activity. REM sleep is thought to be mentally and emotionally restorative; REM deprivation can lead to serious psychological problems, including psychosis.

Insomnia, prolonged difficulty in going to sleep or staying asleep long enough to feel rested, is the most common sleep disorder. Insomnia has many causes, including such stressors as pain, anxiety, illness, changes in lifestyle or environment, and various drugs. Occasional sleeplessness is a normal response to many stimuli and is not usually harmful.

Drugs Used to Treat Anxiety and Insomnia

Drugs used to treat anxiety and insomnia include barbiturates, benzodiazepines, and others.

BARBITURATES

Barbiturates are the prototype sedative-hypnotic drugs, although they are rarely used (Table 8-1). They have similar pharmacologic actions but differ in onset and duration of action. They are usually described as ultrashort-, short-, intermediate-, and long-acting. The ultrashort-acting drugs are used mainly for anesthesia and are discussed in Chapter 14. Barbiturates are metabolized into water-soluble, inactive metabolites in the liver; the metabolites are excreted by the kidneys.

Before the introduction of the benzodiazepines about 1960, the barbiturates were widely used. Four major

| TABLE 8-1 | BARBITURATE SEDATIVE-HYPNOTICS |

Generic/Trade Name	Major Clinical Use	Routes and Dosage Ranges		Remarks
		Adults	*Children*	
Short-acting				
Pentobarbital sodium (Nembutal)	Hypnotic, preoperative sedation	*Sedative*: PO 30 mg 3–4 times daily; rectal 120–200 mg *Hypnotic*: PO 100 mg; rectal 120–200 mg; IM 150–200 mg; IV 100 mg	*Sedative*: PO rectal 2 mg/kg per day in 4 divided doses *Hypnotic*: IM 25–80 mg; rectal under 1 year, 30 mg; 1–4 years, 30 or 60 mg: 5-12 years, 60 mg; 12–14 years, 60 or 120 mg	Pentobarbital and secobarbital are Schedule II controlled substances. They lose effectiveness as hypnotics in about 2 weeks of continuous administration. Do not divide rectal suppositories.
Secobarbital sodium (Seconal)	Hypnotic, preoperative sedation	*Sedative*: PO rectal 120–200 mg *Hypnotic*: PO 100 mg; rectal 120–200 mg; IV 50–250 mg; IM 100–200 mg	*Sedative*: PO, rectal 6 mg/kg per day in 3 divided doses *Hypnotic*: IM 3–5 mg/kg; maximum dose, 100 mg	See pentobarbital
Intermediate-acting				
Amobarbital sodium (Amytal)	Hypnotic	*Sedative*: PO 50–300 mg daily in divided doses *Hypnotic*: PO 65-200 mg: IM, IV 65-500 mg	*Sedative*: over 12 years, same as adult dosage; under 12 years, PO 2 mg/kg per day in 4 divided doses *Hypnotic*: over 12 years, same as adult dosage	Schedule II drug
Aprobarbital (Alurate)	Sedative, hypnotic	*Sedative*: PO 40 mg 3 times daily *Hypnotic*: PO 40–160 mg		Schedule III drug
Butabarbital sodium (Butisol)	Sedative	*Sedative*: PO 50–120 mg/d in 3–4 divided doses *Hypnotic*: PO 50–100 mg	*Sedative*: PO 2 mg/kg per day in 3 divided doses	Schedule IV drug
Long-acting				
Mephobarbital (Mebaral)	Anticonvulsant	PO 200 mg at bedtime 600 mg daily in divided doses	*Over 5 years*: PO 32–64 mg 3–4 times daily *Under 5 years*: PO 16–32 mg 3–4 times daily	Serum levels of phenobarbital can be used as guidelines for adjusting dosage because mephobarbital is metabolized to phenobarbital
Phenobarbital (Luminal, others)	Sedative, anticonvulsant	*Sedative*: PO, IM, IV 30–120 mg daily in 2–3 divided doses *Hypnotic*: PO, IM, IV 100–300 mg *Anticonvulsant*: PO 100–300 mg daily in 2–3 divided doses	*Sedative*: PO rectal 1–2 mg/kg per day in 2–3 divided doses *Hypnotic*: PO 2–4 mg/kg *Anticonvulsant*: PO 5 mg/kg per day in 2–3 divided doses	Schedule IV drug. Not likely to produce abuse or dependence with chronic administration of anticonvulsant doses. Therapeutic plasma levels in seizure disorders are usually 10–25 μg/ml.

problems associated with their use were suppression of REM sleep, induction of drug-metabolizing enzymes in the liver, development of tolerance and cross-tolerance, and development of dependence and abuse.

Suppression of REM sleep occurs when barbiturates are given in hypnotic doses for insomnia. Decreased REM sleep is followed by a compensatory increase in REM sleep when the drug is discontinued, as though the mind must make up the lost dreaming time. This REM rebound effect can occur even when barbiturates are used for only 3 or 4 days. With longer drug use, REM rebound may be severe and accompanied by vivid dreams, nightmares, restlessness, and frequent awakening. This may promote dependence and abuse because people continue taking the drugs to avoid REM rebound. Normal sleep patterns may not return for several weeks after a barbiturate is discontinued, especially if it is stopped abruptly.

Enzyme induction means that barbiturates stimulate liver cells to produce larger amounts of drug-metabolizing enzymes. This allows larger amounts of a drug or other substance to be metabolized during a given period of time. Thus, barbiturates increase the liver's ability to metabolize themselves, several other drugs (*e.g.,* phenytoin, alcohol), and numerous substances that may be endogenous or administered as drugs (*e.g.,* adrenal corticosteroids, bile salts, sex hormones, vitamin K). Enzyme induction leads to tolerance, in which barbiturates lose their effectiveness as sedative-hypnotics in about 2 weeks of daily use, and cross-tolerance with other CNS depressants and other drugs metabolized by the same enzyme system in the liver. Barbiturate-induced enzyme induction disappears a few weeks after the drug is discontinued. Barbiturates have a high potential for dependence and abuse (see Chap. 15).

BENZODIAZEPINES

Benzodiazepines are the most widely used agents for anxiety and insomnia and are also used for several other indications (Table 8-2). They have several advan-

TABLE 8-2 BENZODIAZEPINES

Generic/Trade Name	Clinical Indications	Half-life (h)	Metabolite(s)	Routes and Dosage Ranges
Antianxiety Agents				
Alprazolam (Xanax)	Anxiety Panic attacks	Short (7–15)	Active	*Adults*: PO 0.25–0.5 mg 3 times daily; maximal dose, 4 mg daily in divided doses *Elderly or debilitated adults*: 0.25 mg 2–3 times daily, increased gradually if necessary
Chlordiazepoxide (Librium)	Anxiety Acute alcohol withdrawal	Long (5–30)	Active	*Adults*: PO 15–100 mg daily, once at bedtime or in 3–4 divided doses. IM, IV 50–100 mg, maximal daily dose 300 mg; for short-term use *Elderly or debilitated adults*: PO 5–10 mg 2–4 times daily *Children over 6 years*: PO, IM 0.5 mg/kg per day in 3–4 divided doses *Children under 6 years*: Not recommended
Clonazepam (Klonopin)	Seizure disorders	Long (20–40)	Inactive	*Adults*: PO 0.5 mg 3 times daily, increased by 0.5–1 mg every 3 days until seizures are controlled or adverse effects occur. Maximal daily dose, 20 mg
Clorazepate (Tranxene)	Anxiety Seizure disorders	Long (30–100)	Active	*Adults*: PO 7.5 mg 3 times daily, increased by no more than 7.5 mg/wk. Maximal daily dose, 90 mg *Children 9–12 years*: PO 7.5 mg 2 times daily, increased by no more than 7.5 mg/wk. Maximal daily dose, 60 mg *Children under 9 years*: Not recommended
Diazepam (Valium)	Anxiety Seizure disorders Acute alcohol withdrawals	Long (20–50)	Active	*Adults*: PO 2–10 mg 2–4 times daily; sustained release, PO 15–30 mg once daily; IM, IV 5–10 mg, repeated in 3–4 hours if necessary

TABLE 8-2	BENZODIAZEPINES (Continued)

Generic/Trade Name	Clinical Indications	Half-life (h)	Metabolite(s)	Routes and Dosage Ranges
	Muscle spasm Preoperative sedation Hypnotic			*Elderly or debilitated adults*: PO 2–5 mg once or twice daily, increased gradually if needed and tolerated. *Children*: PO 1–2.5 mg 3–4 times daily, increased gradually if needed and tolerated *Children over 30 days and under 5 years of age*: Seizures IM, IV 0.2–0.5 mg/2–5 min to a maximum of 5 mg *Children 5 years or older*: Seizures, IM, IV 1 mg/2–5 min to a maximum of 10 mg
Lorazepam (Ativan)	Anxiety Preoperative sedation	Short (8–15)	Inactive	*Adults*: PO 2–6 mg/d in 2–3 divided doses. IM 0.05 mg/kg to a maximum of 4 mg. IV 2 mg, diluted with 2 ml of sterile water, sodium chloride, or 5% dextrose injection, injected over 1 min or longer *Elderly or debilitated adults*: PO 1–2 mg/d in divided doses
Midazolam (Versed)	Preoperative sedation Sedation before short diagnostic tests and endoscopic examinations Induction of general anesthesia Supplementation of nitrous oxide/oxygen anesthesia for short surgical procedures	Short (1–12)	Active	*Adults*: Preoperative sedation, IM 0.05–0.08 mg/kg about 1 hour before surgery *Prediagnostic test sedation*. IV 0.1–0.15 mg/kg or up to 0.02 mg/kg initially; maintenance dose, about 25% of initial dose. Reduce dose by 25% to 30% if a narcotic is also given. *Induction of anesthesia*. IV 0.3–0.35 mg/kg initially, then reduce dose as above for maintenance. Reduce initial dose to 0.15–0.3 mg/kg if a narcotic is also given.
Oxazepam (Serax)	Anxiety Acute alcohol withdrawal	Short (5–15)	Inactive	*Adults*: PO 30–120 mg daily in 3–4 divided doses *Elderly or debilitated adults*: PO 30 mg daily in 3 divided doses, gradually increased to 45–60 mg daily if necessary
Prazepam (Centrax)	Anxiety	Long (30–100)	Active	*Adults*: PO 20–40 mg daily in divided doses *Elderly or debilitated adults*: PO 10–15 mg daily in divided doses
Estazolam (ProSom)	Hypnotic	Intermediate (10–24)	Inactive	*Adults*: PO 1–2 mg
Flurazepam (Dalmane)	Hypnotic	Long (47–100)	Active	*Adults*: PO 15–30 mg
Quazepam (Doral)	Hypnotic	Long (39)	Active	*Adults*: PO 7.5–15 mg
Temazepam (Restoril)	Hypnotic	Short (9–12)	Inactive	*Adults*: PO 15–30 mg
Triazolam (Halcion)	Hypnotic	Ultrashort (1.5–5.5)	Inactive	*Adults*: PO 0.125–0.25 mg

tages over the barbiturates. They have a wider margin of safety between therapeutic and toxic doses and are rarely fatal, even in overdose, unless combined with other CNS depressant drugs, such as alcohol. They do not induce drug-metabolizing enzymes or suppress REM sleep. When first marketed, benzodiazepines were considered nonaddictive. However, within a few years it became evident that the drugs were being abused and were causing physical and psychological dependence, although to a lesser extent than the barbiturates. Because of the physiologic dependence, withdrawal symptoms (see Chap. 15) occur if the drugs are stopped abruptly. To avoid withdrawal symptoms, the drugs should be gradually tapered and discontinued.

In addition to abuse and dependence, benzodiazepines may cause characteristic effects of CNS depression, including excessive sedation, impairment of physical and mental activities, and respiratory depression. Although the drugs are still widely used, they should be prescribed more selectively and for shorter periods. None of these drugs is recommended for long-term use.

These drugs are highly lipid-soluble, widely distributed in body tissues, and extensively bound to plasma proteins. Most are metabolized in the liver and excreted in the urine. They are Schedule IV drugs under the Controlled Substances Act. They are well absorbed with oral administration, and most are given orally; a few (*e.g.*, diazepam, lorazepam) are given both orally and parenterally.

Pharmacologically, all the benzodiazepines have similar characteristics and produce the same effects. However, they differ in clinical uses because the manufacturers developed and promoted them for particular purposes. The drugs also differ in serum half-lives, production of active metabolites, and duration of action. Several (*e.g.*, diazepam, flurazepam) have long half-lives and produce pharmacologically active metabolites that also have long half-lives. As a result, these drugs require about 5 to 7 days to reach steady-state serum levels. Therapeutic effects (*e.g.*, decreased anxiety or insomnia) and adverse effects (*e.g.*, sedation, ataxia) are more likely to occur after 2 or 3 days of therapy than initially. Such effects accumulate with chronic usage and persist for several days after the drugs are discontinued. Other drugs have short half-lives and produce inactive metabolites; thus, their durations of action are much shorter, and they do not accumulate.

MISCELLANEOUS DRUGS

Several nonbarbiturate, nonbenzodiazepine drugs of varied characteristics are also used as antianxiety and sedative-hypnotic agents. These include buspirone, clomipramine, and hydroxyzine as antianxiety agents and chloral hydrate and zolpidem as hypnotics. Selected characteristics of the drugs are described below; dosages are listed in Table 8-3.

Buspirone differs chemically and pharmacologically from other antianxiety drugs. Its mechanism of action is unclear, but it apparently interacts with serotonin and dopamine receptors in the brain. Compared to the benzodiazepines, buspirone lacks muscle relaxant and anticonvulsant effects, does not cause sedation or physical or psychological dependence, does not increase the CNS depression of alcohol and other drugs, and is not a controlled substance. Adverse effects include nervousness and excitement. Thus, clients wanting and accustomed to sedative effects may not like the drug or comply with instructions for its use. Its only clinical indication for use is the short-term treatment of anxiety. Because therapeutic effects may be delayed for a few weeks, it is not considered beneficial for immediate effects or occasional (PRN) use. Buspirone is rapidly absorbed following oral administration. Peak plasma levels occur within 45 to 90 minutes. It is metabolized by the liver to inactive metabolites, which are then excreted in the urine and feces. Its elimination half-life is 2 to 3 hours.

Clomipramine is a tricyclic antidepressant (see Chap. 10) used for the treatment of obsessive-compulsive disorder.

Hydroxyzine is an antihistamine with sedative and antiemetic properties. Clinical indications for use include anxiety, preoperative sedation, nausea and vomiting associated with surgery or motion sickness, and pruritus and urticaria associated with allergic dermatoses.

Chloral hydrate, the oldest sedative-hypnotic drug, is relatively safe, effective, and inexpensive in usual therapeutic doses. It reportedly does not suppress REM sleep. Tolerance develops after about 2 weeks of continual use. It is a drug of abuse and may cause physical dependence.

Zolpidem is a newer drug that is reportedly as effective as the benzodiazepines but is more likely to cause adverse effects (*e.g.*, excessive sedation, motor impairment). It is not recommended as a first-choice hypnotic.

In addition, several antihistamines cause drowsiness and are used as hypnotics, although they are not approved by the Food and Drug Administration for this purpose. **Diphenhydramine** (Benadryl) is used in hospitalized clients and is available over the counter. An antihistamine is the active ingredient in nonprescription sleep aids (*e.g.*, diphenhydramine in Compoz, Nytol, Sominex, Sleep-Eze; doxylamine in Unisom).

Mechanisms of Action

Barbiturates produce CNS depression by inhibiting functions of nerve cells, such as electrical stimulation, depolarization, impulse transmission, and neurotransmitter release. Neurons in the reticular formation,

TABLE 8-3 MISCELLANEOUS ANTIANXIETY AND SEDATIVE-HYPNOTIC AGENTS

Generic/Trade Name	Major Clinical Use	Routes and Dosage Ranges	
		Adults	*Children*
Antianxiety agents			
Buspirone (BuSpar)	Anxiety	PO 5 mg 3 times daily, increased by 5 mg/d at 2- to 3-day intervals if necessary. Usual maintenance dose 20–30 mg/d in divided doses; maximum dose 60 mg/d	Not recommended
Clomipramine (Anafranil)	Obsessive-compulsive disorder	PO 25 mg/d initially; increase to 100 mg/d during the first 2 weeks and to a maximum dose of 250 mg/d over several weeks if necessary	PO 25 mg/d initially; increase to 3 mg/kg or 100 mg, whichever is smaller, during the first 2 weeks and to 3 mg/kg or 200 mg, whichever is smaller, over several weeks if necessary
Hydroxyzine (Vistaril)	Anxiety, Sedative Pruritus	PO 75–400 mg/d in 3 or 4 divided doses. Pre- and postoperative and pre- and postpartum sedation, IM 25–100 mg in a single dose	PO 2 mg/kg per day in 4 divided doses. Pre- and postoperative sedation, IM 1 mg/kg in a single dose
Sedative-hypnotic agents			
Chloral hydrate	Sedative, Hypnotic	*Sedative*: PO, rectal suppository 250 mg 3 times per day, after meals *Hypnotic*: PO, rectal suppository 500–1000 mg at bedtime; maximum dose, 2 g/d	*Sedative*: PO, rectal suppository 25 mg/kg per day, in 3 or 4 divided doses. *Hypnotic*: PO, rectal suppository 50 mg/kg at bedtime; maximum single dose, 1 g
Zolpidem (Ambien)	Hypnotic	PO 10 mg	Not recommended

which control cerebral cortex activity and level of arousal or wakefulness, are especially sensitive to the depressant effects of barbiturates.

Benzodiazepines bind with a receptor complex in the nerve cells of the brain; this receptor complex also has binding sites for gamma-aminobutyric acid (GABA), an inhibitory neurotransmitter (see Chap. 5). This GABA/benzodiazepine receptor complex regulates the entry of chloride ions into the cell. When GABA binds to the receptor complex, chloride ions enter the cell and stabilize (hyperpolarize) the cell membrane so that it is less responsive to excitatory neurotransmitters, such as norepinephrine. Benzodiazepines bind at a different site on the receptor complex and enhance the inhibitory effect of GABA to relieve anxiety, tension, and nervousness and to produce sleep. Other antianxiety and sedative-hypnotic drugs have varied mechanisms of action.

Indications for Use

Major clinical uses of the benzodiazepines are as antianxiety, hypnotic, and anticonvulsant agents. They also are given for preoperative sedation, prevention of agitation and delirium tremens in acute alcohol withdrawal, and other uses. Not all benzodiazepines are approved for all uses; Table 8-2 lists indications for the use of individual benzodiazepines. Diazepam has been extensively studied and has more approved uses than others.

Clinical indications for the use of sedative-hypnotics include short-term treatment of insomnia and sedation before surgery or invasive diagnostic tests (*e.g.*, angiograms, endoscopies). Barbiturates also are used for their general anesthetic and anticonvulsant effects.

Contraindications for Use

Contraindications include severe respiratory disorders, severe liver or kidney disease, hypersensitivity reactions, and a history of alcohol or other drug abuse. The drugs must be used very cautiously when taken concurrently with any other CNS depressant drugs. In addition, barbiturates are contraindicated in acute intermittent porphyria (a rare hereditary metabolic disorder characterized by recurrent attacks of physical and mental disturbances).

Nursing Process

Assessment

Assess the client's need for antianxiety or sedative-hypnotic drugs, including intensity and duration of symptoms. Manifestations are more obvious with moderate to severe anxiety or insomnia. Some guidelines for assessment include the following:

- What is the client's statement of the problem? Does the problem interfere with usual activities of daily living? If so, how much and for how long?
- Try to identify factors that precipitate anxiety or insomnia in the client. Some common ones are physical symptoms; feeling worried, tense, or nervous; factors such as illness, death of a friend or family member, divorce, or job stress; and excessive CNS stimulation from caffeine-containing beverages or drugs such as bronchodilators and nasal decongestants. In addition, excessive daytime sleep and too little exercise and activity may cause insomnia, especially in older clients.
- Observe for behavioral manifestations of anxiety, such as psychomotor agitation, facial grimaces, tense posture, and others.
- Observe for physiologic manifestations of anxiety. These may include increased blood pressure and pulse rate, increased rate and depth of respiration, increased muscle tension, and pale, cool skin.
- If behavioral or physiologic manifestations seem to indicate anxiety, try to determine whether this is actually the case. Because similar manifestations may indicate pain or other problems rather than anxiety, the observer's perceptions must be validated by the client before appropriate action can be taken.
- If insomnia is reported, observe for signs of sleep deprivation such as drowsiness, slow movements or speech, and difficulty concentrating or focusing attention.
- Obtain a careful drug history, including the use of alcohol and sedative-hypnotic drugs, and assess the likelihood of drug abuse and dependence. People who abuse other drugs, including alcohol, are likely to abuse antianxiety and sedative-hypnotic drugs. Also assess for use of prescription and non-prescription CNS stimulants (*e.g.*, appetite suppressants, bronchodilators, nasal decongestants, excessive caffeine, cocaine).
- Identify coping mechanisms used in managing previous situations of stress, anxiety, and insomnia. These are very individualized. Reading, watching television, listening to music, or talking to a friend are examples. Some people are quiet and inactive; others participate in strenuous activity. Some prefer to be alone; others prefer being with a friend or family member or a group.
- Once drug therapy for anxiety or insomnia is begun, assess the client's level of consciousness and functional ability before each dose so that excessive sedation can be avoided.

Nursing Diagnoses

- Ineffective Individual Coping related to need for antianxiety or sedative-hypnotic drug
- Knowledge Deficit: Appropriate uses and effects of antianxiety or sedative-hypnotic drugs

- Knowledge Deficit: Nondrug measures for relieving anxiety and insomnia
- Noncompliance: Overuse
- Risk for Injury related to sedation, respiratory depression, impaired mobility, and other adverse effects
- Altered Thought Processes related to confusion (especially in older adults)
- Sleep Pattern Disturbance: Insomnia related to one or more causes (*e.g.*, anxiety, daytime sleep)

Planning/Goals

The client will:
- Feel more calm, relaxed, and comfortable with anxiety; experience improved quantity and quality of sleep with insomnia
- Be monitored for excessive sedation and impaired mobility to prevent falls or other injuries (in health care settings)
- Verbalize and demonstrate nondrug activities to reduce or manage anxiety or insomnia
- Demonstrate safe, accurate drug usage
- Notify a health care provider if he or she wants to stop taking a benzodiazepine; will not stop taking a benzodiazepine abruptly
- Avoid preventable adverse effects, including abuse and dependence

Interventions

Use nondrug measures to relieve anxiety or to enhance the effectiveness of antianxiety drugs.

- Support the client's usual coping mechanisms when feasible. Provide the opportunity for reading, exercising, listening to music, or watching television, promote contact with significant others, or simply allow the client to be alone and uninterrupted for a while.
- Use interpersonal and communication techniques to help the client manage anxiety. The degree of anxiety and the clinical situation largely determine which techniques are appropriate. For example, staying with the client, showing interest, listening, and allowing him or her to verbalize concerns may be beneficial.
- Providing information may be a therapeutic technique when anxiety is related to medical conditions. People vary in the amount and kind of information they want, but generally the following topics should be included:
  - The overall treatment plan, including medical or surgical treatment, choice of outpatient care or hospitalization, expected length of treatment, and expected outcomes in terms of health and ability to function in activities of daily living
  - Specific diagnostic tests, including preparation, after-effects if any, and how the client will be informed of results
  - Specific medication and treatment measures, including expected therapeutic results
  - What the client must do to carry out the plan of treatment
- When offering information and explanations, keep in mind that anxiety interferes with intellectual functioning. Thus, communication should be brief, clear, and repeated as necessary because clients may misunderstand or forget what is said.

- Modify the environment to decrease anxiety-provoking stimuli. Modifications may involve altering temperature, light, and noise levels.
- Use measures to increase physical comfort. These may include a wide variety of activities, such as positioning, helping the client bathe or ambulate, giving backrubs, or providing fluids of the client's choice.
- Consult with other services and departments on the client's behalf. For example, if financial problems were identified as a cause of anxiety, social services may be able to help.
- When a benzodiazepine is used with diagnostic tests or minor surgery, provide instructions for postprocedure care to the client or to family members, preferably in written form.

    Implement measures to decrease the need for or increase the effectiveness of sedative-hypnotic drugs, such as the following:
- Modify the environment to promote rest and sleep (*e.g.*, reduce noise and light).
- Plan care to allow uninterrupted periods of rest and sleep when possible.
- Relieve symptoms that interfere with rest and sleep. Drugs such as analgesics for pain or antitussives for cough are usually safer and more effective than sedative-hypnotic drugs. Nondrug measures, such as positioning, exercise, and backrubs, may be helpful in relieving muscle tension and other discomforts. Allowing the client to verbalize concerns, providing information so that he or she knows what to expect, or consulting other personnel (*e.g.*, social worker, chaplain) may be useful in decreasing anxiety.
- Help the client modify lifestyle habits to promote rest and sleep (*e.g.*, limiting intake of caffeine-containing beverages, limiting intake of fluids during evening hours if nocturia interferes with sleep, avoiding daytime naps, having a regular schedule of rest and sleep periods, increasing physical activity, and not trying to sleep unless tired or drowsy).

Teach clients:

- Nondrug measures to promote relaxation, rest, and sleep
- That antianxiety and sedative-hypnotic drugs help to relieve symptoms, but they do not relieve underlying psychological problems
- To consider psychotherapy or other counseling if symptoms are prolonged or impair the client's ability to function
- That all the benzodiazepines have similar characteristics and effects, including the potential to cause dependence
- That, in almost all cases, antianxiety and sedative-hypnotic drugs are recommended only for short-term use
- That drowsiness usually decreases within a few days after starting the drugs
- To avoid ingesting alcohol and other CNS depressants (*e.g.*, antihistamines, sleeping pills, narcotic analgesics)
- To avoid smoking, ambulating without help, driving a car, operating machinery, and other potentially hazardous tasks after taking a benzodiazepine or other drug that causes drowsiness. These activities may lead to falls or other injuries if undertaken while alertness is impaired.
- Not to take sedative-hypnotic drugs every night. These drugs lose their effectiveness in 2 to 4 weeks if taken nightly, and cause sleep disturbances when withdrawn.

Evaluation

- Decreased symptoms of anxiety or insomnia and increased rest and sleep are reported or observed.
- Excessive sedation and motor impairment are not observed.
- The client reports no serious adverse effects.
- Monitoring of prescriptions (*e.g.*, "pill counts") does not indicate excessive use.

Principles of Therapy: Benzodiazepines

USE IN ANXIETY

In general, antianxiety drugs should be used only if anxiety causes disability and interferes with job performance, interpersonal relationships, and other activities of daily living. The drugs are not recommended for treating everyday stress and anxiety. Some authorities believe such use promotes reliance on drugs and decreases development of healthier coping mechanisms. Chronic anxiety states are probably more effectively treated with psychotherapy. Because anxiety often accompanies pain, antianxiety agents are sometimes used to manage pain. In the management of chronic pain, antianxiety drugs have not demonstrated a definite benefit. Anxiety about recurrence of pain is probably better controlled by adequate analgesia than by antianxiety drugs.

USE IN INSOMNIA

In general, sedative-hypnotic drugs should be used only when insomnia causes significant distress and resists management by nonpharmacologic means; they should not be used for occasional sleeplessness. When drug therapy is required, the goal of treatment is to relieve anxiety or sleeplessness without permitting sensory perception, responsiveness to the environment, or alertness to drop below safe levels. Additional guidelines include the following:

1. Do not give sedative-hypnotic drugs every night unless necessary. Intermittent administration helps maintain drug effectiveness and decreases the risks of drug abuse and dependence. It also decreases disturbances of normal sleep patterns.
2. When sedative-hypnotic drugs are prescribed for outpatients, the prescription should limit the number of doses dispensed and the number of refills. This is one way of decreasing the risk of abuse and suicide.
3. In chronic insomnia, no hypnotic drug is recommended for long-term treatment. The benzodiazepine hypnotics lose their effectiveness in producing sleep after about 4 weeks of daily use. It is not

helpful to switch from one drug to another because cross-tolerance develops. To restore the sleep-producing effect, administration of the hypnotic drug must be interrupted for 1 to 2 weeks.

DURATION OF THERAPY

The drugs should be given for the shortest effective period to decrease the likelihood of drug abuse and physiologic and psychological dependence. Few problems develop with short-term use unless an overdose is taken or other CNS depressant drugs (*e.g.*, alcohol) are taken concurrently. Most problems occur with long-term use, especially of larger-than-usual doses.

DOSAGE

When benzodiazepines are used for anxiety or insomnia, the goal is to find the lowest effective dose that does not cause excessive daytime drowsiness or impaired mobility. Generally, start with the smallest dose likely to be effective, then evaluate the client's response and increase the dose only if necessary. Additional guidelines include the following:

1. Smaller-than-usual doses may be indicated in clients receiving cimetidine or several other drugs that decrease the hepatic metabolism of most benzodiazepines and in elderly or debilitated clients. In the elderly, most benzodiazepines are metabolized more slowly, and half-lives are longer than in younger adults. Exceptions are lorazepam and oxazepam, whose half-lives and dosages are the same for elderly adults as for younger ones.
2. Larger-than-usual doses may be needed for clients who are severely anxious or agitated. Also, large doses are usually required to relax skeletal muscle, control muscle spasm, control seizures, and provide sedation before surgery, cardioversion, endoscopy, and angiography.
3. When benzodiazepines are used with narcotic analgesics, the analgesic dose should be reduced initially and increased gradually to avoid excessive CNS depression.

SCHEDULING

The antianxiety benzodiazepines are often given in three or four daily doses. This is necessary for the short-acting agents, but there is no pharmacologic basis for multiple daily doses of the long-acting drugs. Because of their prolonged actions, all or most of the daily dose can be given at bedtime. This schedule promotes sleep, and there is usually enough residual sedation to maintain antianxiety effects throughout the next day. If necessary, one or two small supplemental doses may be given during the day.

BENZODIAZEPINE WITHDRAWAL

Physical dependence on benzodiazepines is indicated by withdrawal symptoms when the drugs are stopped. Mild symptoms occur in nearly half the clients taking therapeutic doses for 6 to 12 weeks; severe symptoms are most likely to occur when high doses of a short-acting drug are taken regularly for more than 4 months and then abruptly discontinued. Common manifestations include increased anxiety, psychomotor agitation, insomnia, irritability, headache, tremor, and palpitations. Less common but more serious manifestations include confusion, abnormal perception of movement, depersonalization, psychosis, and seizures. Symptoms may occur within 24 hours of stopping a short-acting drug such as alprazolam, but usually occur 4 to 5 days after stopping a long-acting drug such as diazepam. Symptoms can be relieved by administration of a benzodiazepine.

To prevent withdrawal symptoms, the drug should be tapered in dose and gradually discontinued. Generally, reducing the dose by 10% to 25% every 1 or 2 weeks over 4 to 16 weeks is effective. However, the rate may need to be slower with high doses or long-term use. Although the drugs have not been proven effective for more than 4 months of regular use, this period is probably exceeded quite often in clinical practice.

BENZODIAZEPINE TOXICITY

Flumazenil is a specific antidote that competes with benzodiazepines for benzodiazepine receptors and reverses sedation, coma, and respiratory depression. Clinical indications for use include benzodiazepine overdose and reversal of sedation after diagnostic or therapeutic procedures. The degree of sedation reversal depends on the plasma concentration of the ingested benzodiazepine and the flumazenil dose and frequency of administration. The drug acts rapidly, with onset within 2 minutes and peak effects within 6 to 10 minutes. However, the duration of action is short (serum half-life 60–90 minutes) compared to that of most benzodiazepines, so repeated doses are usually required. Adverse effects include precipitation of acute benzodiazepine withdrawal symptoms, agitation, confusion, and seizures. Resedation and hypoventilation may occur if flumazenil is not given long enough to coincide with the duration of action of the benzodiazepine.

The drug should be injected into a freely flowing intravenous line in a large vein. Dosage recommendations vary with use. For reversal of conscious sedation or general anesthesia, the initial dose is 0.2 mg over 15 seconds, then 0.2 mg every 60 seconds, if necessary, to a maximum of 1.0 mg (total of five doses). For overdose, the initial dose is 0.2 mg over 30 seconds, wait 30 seconds, then 0.3 mg over 30 seconds, then 0.5 mg every 60 seconds up to a total dose of 3 mg if necessary for the client to reach the desired level of consciousness. Slow administration and repeated doses are recommended to awaken the client gradually and decrease the risks of causing acute withdrawal symptoms. A client who does not respond within 5 minutes of administering the total recommended dose should be reassessed for other causes of sedation.

USE IN LIVER DISEASE

In the presence of liver disease (*e.g.*, cirrhosis, hepatitis), the metabolism of most benzodiazepines is slowed, with resultant accumulation and increased risk of adverse effects. If a benzodiazepine is deemed necessary, lorazepam or oxazepam is preferred because liver disease does not significantly affect drug elimination.

USE IN HYPOALBUMINEMIA

Benzodiazepines are highly bound to plasma proteins, especially those with long half-lives. If a benzodiazepine is given to clients with low serum albumin levels (*e.g.*, from malnutrition or liver disease), alprazolam or lorazepam is preferred because these drugs are less extensively bound to plasma proteins and less likely to cause adverse effects.

USE IN CHILDREN

Children may have unanticipated or variable responses to antianxiety and sedative-hypnotic drugs, including paradoxical CNS stimulation and excitement rather than CNS depression and calming. The drugs should be used only when clearly indicated and in the lowest effective dose. Of the benzodiazepines, only chlordiazepoxide and diazepam have been extensively used in children. Others do not have established dosages and are not recommended. Sedative-hypnotic drugs are rarely indicated in children.

USE IN OLDER ADULTS

Most antianxiety and sedative-hypnotic drugs are metabolized and excreted more slowly in older adults, so the effects of a given dose last longer. Also, several of the benzodiazepines produce pharmacologically active metabolites, prolonging drug actions. Thus, the drugs

may accumulate and increase adverse effects if dosages are not reduced. The initial dose of any antianxiety or sedative-hypnotic drug should be small and increments made gradually, according to response, to decrease the risks of adverse effects. Although hypotension is uncommon, the drugs should be used cautiously when a drop in blood pressure may cause cardiac complications. Other adverse effects include oversedation, dizziness, confusion, and impaired mobility, which may contribute to falls and other injuries unless clients are carefully monitored and safeguarded. Benzodiazepines should be tapered rather than discontinued abruptly in older adults, as in other populations. Withdrawal symptoms may occur within 24 hours after abruptly stopping a short-acting drug but may not occur for several days after stopping a long-acting agent.

For anxiety, short-acting benzodiazepines, such as alprazolam or lorazepam, are preferred over long-acting agents, such as diazepam. Buspirone may be preferred over a benzodiazepine because it does not cause sedation, psychomotor impairment, or increased risk of falls. However, it must be taken on a regular schedule and is not effective for PRN use.

For insomnia, sedative-hypnotic drugs should generally be avoided or their use minimized in older adults. Finding and treating the causes and using nondrug measures to aid sleep are much safer. If a sedative-hypnotic is used, shorter-acting benzodiazepines are preferred, because they are eliminated more rapidly and are therefore less likely to accumulate and cause adverse effects. In addition, dosages should be smaller than for younger adults, the drugs should not be used every night or for longer than a few days, and older adults should be monitored closely for adverse effects.

 HOME CARE

Although antianxiety and sedative-hypnotic drugs are not recommended for long-term use, they are often used at home. Previously described precautions and teaching needs related to safe use of the drugs apply in home care as in other settings. The home care nurse should encourage the client to use nondrug methods of reducing anxiety and insomnia and should review the risks of injuries if mental and physical responses are slowed by the drugs. In addition, assess the client for signs and symptoms of overuse, withdrawal, and use of other sedating drugs, including alcohol, sedating antihistamines, and other prescription drugs. Although the home care nurse is more likely to encounter these drugs as legal prescriptions, they are also commonly abused street drugs.

ANTIANXIETY AND SEDATIVE/HYPNOTIC DRUGS

NURSING ACTIONS	*RATIONALE/EXPLANATION*
1. Administer accurately	
a. If a client appears excessively sedated when a dose of an antianxiety or sedative-hypnotic drug is due, omit the dose and record the reason.	To avoid excessive sedation and other adverse effects
b. For oral sedative-hypnotics:	
(1) Prepare the client for sleep before giving hypnotic doses of any drug.	Most of the drugs cause drowsiness within 15 to 30 minutes. The client should be in bed when he or she becomes drowsy to increase the therapeutic effectiveness of the drug and to decrease the likelihood of falls or other injuries.
(2) Give with a glass of water or other fluid.	The fluid enhances dissolution and absorption of the drug for a quicker onset of action.
(3) Raise bedrails, and instruct the client to stay in bed or ask for help if necessary to get out of bed.	To avoid falls and other injuries related to sedation and impaired mobility.
c. For benzodiazepines:	
(1) Give orally, when feasible.	These drugs are well absorbed from the GI tract, and onset of action occurs within a few minutes. Diazepam is better absorbed orally than intramuscularly. When given IM, the drug crystallizes in tissue and is absorbed very slowly.
(2) Do not mix injectable diazepam with any other drug in a syringe or add to IV fluids.	Diazepam is physically incompatible with other drugs and solutions.
(3) Give IM benzodiazepines undiluted, deeply, into large muscle masses, such as the gluteus muscle of the hip.	These drugs are irritating to tissues and may cause pain at injection sites.
(4) With IV benzodiazepines, be very careful to avoid intra-arterial injection or extravasation into surrounding tissues. Have equipment available for respiratory assistance.	These drugs are very irritating to tissues and may cause venous thrombosis, phlebitis, local irritation, edema, and vascular impairment. They may also cause respiratory depression and apnea.
(5) Give IV **diazepam** slowly, over at least 1 minute for 5 mg (1 ml); into large veins (not hand or wrist veins); by direct injection into the vein or into IV infusion tubing as close as possible to the venipuncture site.	To avoid apnea and tissue irritation
(6) Give IV **lorazepam** slowly, over at least 1 minute for 2 mg, by direct injection into the vein or into IV infusion tubing. Immediately before injection, dilute with an equal volume of sterile water for injection, sodium chloride injection, or 5% dextrose injection.	To avoid apnea and tissue irritation
(7) Give IV **midazolam** slowly, over about 2 minutes, after diluting the dose with 0.9% sodium chloride injection or 5% dextrose in water.	Rapid IV injection may cause severe respiratory depression and apnea; dilution facilitates slow injection.
(8) Midazolam may be mixed in the same syringe with morphine sulfate, meperidine, and atropine sulfate.	No apparent chemical or physical incompatibilities occur with these substances.
d. When giving **barbiturates** parenterally, do not give solutions that are cloudy or contain a precipitate. Do not mix with any other drugs in the same syringe. Give IM injections deeply into a large muscle mass. Give IV injections slowly and have equipment available for	Parenteral barbiturate solutions are highly alkaline and irritating to tissues. These precautions are needed to ensure safe administration and minimize tissue irritation.

(continued)

NURSING ACTIONS	*RATIONALE/EXPLANATION*

artificial ventilation. Be very careful to avoid extravasation of the drug into surrounding tissues and accidental intra-arterial injection.

e. Give **hydroxyzine** orally or deep IM only. When given IM for preoperative sedation, it can be mixed in the same syringe with atropine, meperidine, and most other narcotic analgesics likely to be ordered at the same time.

IM hydroxyzine is very irritating to tissues.

f. Give **clomipramine** in divided doses, with meals, initially; after titration to a stable dose, give the total daily dose at bedtime.

Giving with meals decreases adverse effects on the GI tract; giving the total dose once daily at bedtime decreases daytime sedation.

2. Observe for therapeutic effects

a. When a drug is given for antianxiety effects, observe for:

Therapeutic effects depend largely on the reason for use. With benzodiazepines, decreased anxiety and drowsiness may appear within a few minutes.

(1) An appearance of being relaxed, perhaps drowsy, but easily aroused

With buspirone, antianxiety effects may occur within 7 to 10 days of regular use, with optimal effects in 3 to 4 weeks.

(2) Verbal statements, such as "less worried," "more relaxed," "resting better"

(3) Decrease or absence of manifestations of anxiety, such as rigid posture, facial grimaces, crying, elevated blood pressure and heart rate

b. When a drug is given for hypnotic effects, drowsiness should be evident within about 30 minutes, and the client usually sleeps for several hours.

c. When diazepam or lorazepam is given IV for control of acute convulsive disorders, seizure activity should decrease or stop almost immediately. When a drug is given for chronic anticonvulsant effects, lack of seizure activity is a therapeutic effect.

d. When hydroxyzine is given for nausea and vomiting, absence of vomiting and verbal statements of relief indicate therapeutic effects.

e. When hydroxyzine is given for antihistaminic effects in skin disorders, observe for decreased itching and fewer statements of discomfort.

3. Observe for adverse effects

a. Excessive sedation—drowsiness, stupor, difficult to arouse, impaired mental processes, impaired mobility, respiratory depression, confusion

Most adverse effects are caused by CNS depression.
These effects are more likely to occur with large doses or if the recipient is elderly, debilitated, or has liver disease that slows drug metabolism. Respiratory depression and apnea stem from depression of the respiratory center in the medulla oblongata; they are most likely to occur with large doses or rapid IV administration of diazepam, lorazepam, or midazolam. Excessive drowsiness is more likely to occur when drug therapy is begun, and it usually decreases within a week.

b. Hypotension

Hypotension probably results from depression of the vasomotor center in the brain and is more likely to occur with large doses or rapid IV administration of diazepam, lorazepam, or midazolam.

NURSING ACTIONS	RATIONALE/EXPLANATION
c. Pain and induration at injection sites	Parenteral solutions are irritating to tissues.
d. Paradoxical excitement, anger, aggression, and hallucinations	
e. Chronic intoxication—sedation, confusion, emotional lability, muscular incoordination, impaired mental processes, mental depression, GI problems, weight loss	These signs and symptoms may occur with benzodiazepines or barbiturates and are similar to those occurring with chronic alcohol abuse (see Chap. 15).
f. Withdrawal or abstinence syndrome—anxiety, insomnia, restlessness, irritability, tremors, postural hypotension, seizures	These signs and symptoms may occur when benzodiazepines or barbiturates are discontinued abruptly, especially after high doses or long-term use.
g. With buspirone, the most common adverse effects are headache, dizziness, nausea, nervousness, fatigue, and excitement. Less frequent effects include dry mouth, chest pain, tachycardia, palpitations, drowsiness, confusion, and depression.	
4. Observe for drug interactions	
a. Drugs that *increase* effects of antianxiety and sedative-hypnotic drugs:	
(1) CNS depressants—alcohol, narcotic analgesics, tricyclic antidepressants, antihistamines, phenothiazine and other antipsychotic agents	All these drugs produce CNS depression when given alone. Any combination increases CNS depression, sedation, and respiratory depression. Combinations of these drugs are hazardous and should be avoided. Ingesting alcohol with antianxiety or sedative-hypnotic drugs may cause respiratory depression, coma, and convulsions. Although buspirone does not appear to cause additive CNS depression, concurrent use with other CNS depressants is best avoided.
(2) Cimetidine, disulfiram, fluoxetine, isoniazid, ketoconazole, metoprolol, omeprazole, oral contraceptives, propranolol, valproic acid	These drugs interfere with the hepatic metabolism of diazepam and other benzodiazepines. They do not affect elimination of lorazepam or oxazepam.
b. Drugs that *decrease* effects of antianxiety and sedative-hypnotic agents:	
(1) CNS stimulants—appetite suppressants (*e.g.,* phenylpropanolamine), bronchodilators (*e.g.,* albuterol, theophylline), nasal decongestants (*e.g.,* phenylephrine, phenylpropanolamine, pseudoephedrine), and social drugs (*e.g.,* caffeine, nicotine)	Phenylpropanolamine is the active ingredient in OTC diet aids such as Dexatrim and a component of multisymptom cold remedies. Phenylephrine and pseudoephedrine are available alone or in multisymptom cold remedies. OTC asthma remedies are also CNS stimulants.
(2) Enzyme inducers (*e.g.,* barbiturates)	With chronic use, these drugs antagonize their own actions and the actions of other drugs metabolized in the liver. They increase the rate of drug metabolism and elimination from the body.
c. Drugs that *increase* effects of barbiturates (in addition to those that increase effects of antianxiety and sedative-hypnotic agents in general):	
(1) Acidifying agents (*e.g.,* ascorbic acid)	These agents increase absorption of barbiturates in the GI tract and increase drug reabsorption in renal tubules (except for phenobarbital).
(2) Benzodiazepines (*e.g.,* diazepam)	May potentiate sedative and respiratory effects of barbiturates

(continued)

NURSING ACTIONS	RATIONALE/EXPLANATION
d. Drugs that *decrease* effects of barbiturates: Alkalinizing agents (*e.g.*, sodium bicarbonate)	Increase renal excretion of phenobarbital; have been used in treating phenobarbital overdose
5. Teach clients	
a. Use nondrug measures to promote relaxation and sleep when possible.	Relaxation techniques are safer than any drug. Thus, it is a worthwhile endeavor to identify and use methods that promote rest and sleep (*e.g.*, physical exercise, reading).
b. Store drugs safely. Keep them out of reach of children and adults who are confused or less than alert. Do not keep at the bedside.	These mind-altering, brain depressant drugs should be taken only by those persons for whom they are prescribed. Accidental or intentional ingestion by others may lead to serious adverse effects. The drugs should not be left at the bedside because a person sedated by a previous dose may take addtional doses.
c. Do not drive a car or perform other tasks that require alertness if drowsy from medication.	The drugs often impair mental and physical functioning and thereby make routine activities potentially hazardous.
d. Avoid alcohol and other depressant drugs (*e.g.*, OTC antihistamines that cause drowsiness) while taking any antianxiety or sedative-hypnotic drugs (except buspirone).	To avoid excessive drowsiness, difficulty breathing, traumatic injuries, and other potentially serious adverse drug effects
e. Omit one or more doses if excessive drowsiness occurs.	To avoid difficulty breathing, falls, and other adverse drug effects
f. Use the drugs only when necessary. Do not increase dosage, do not increase frequency of administration, and do not take for prolonged periods.	Except for buspirone, these drugs are often misused and abused. They can produce psychological and physiologic dependence, which may eventually cause worse problems than the original anxiety or insomnia.
g. These drugs produce more beneficial effects and fewer adverse reactions when used in the smallest effective doses and for the shortest duration feasible in particular circumstances.	
h. Caffeine-containing beverages and stimulant drugs can cancel or decrease the antianxiety and sedative effects of these drugs	Caffeine is a stimulant. Other stimulant drugs include prescription and OTC asthma and cold remedies and appetite suppressants.
i. Buspirone causes little sedation, is not associated with abuse or physical dependence, and must be taken on a regular schedule for 3–4 weeks for optimal antianxiety effects.	This drug differs significantly from the Valium-related drugs and is not effective for occasional use.

REVIEW AND APPLICATION EXERCISES

1. What is anxiety, and how may it be manifested?

2. How do benzodiazepines act to relieve anxiety?

3. What are some nonpharmacologic interventions to decrease anxiety?

4. When assessing a client before giving an antianxiety benzodiazepine, what assessment data would cause you to omit the dose?

5. Why is sleep necessary? What functions does sleep fulfill?

6. Why are nonpharmacologic interventions to promote relaxation and sleep usually preferred over the use of sedative-hypnotic drugs?

7. What is the main difference between sedative drugs and hypnotic drugs?

8. What factors must be considered when planning care for an older adult who often takes a "sleeping pill"?

9. In terms of nursing care, what difference does it make whether a benzodiazepine is metabolized to active or inactive metabolites?

10. What are drug dependence, tolerance, and withdrawal symptoms in relation to the benzodiazepines?

11. For an ambulatory client beginning a prescription for a benzodiazepine antianxiety or hypnotic agent, what instructions must be emphasized for safe, effective, and rational drug use?

12. For a nurse assisting in home care of a client taking a benzodiazepine, what kinds of data would the nurse collect to evaluate whether the client is using the drug appropriately or abusing it?

SELECTED REFERENCES

Baldessarini, R.J. (1996). Drugs and the treatment of psychiatric disorders: Psychosis and anxiety. In J.G. Hardman, L.E. Limbird, P.B. Molinoff, & R.W. Ruddon (Eds.), *Goodman & Gilman's The pharmacological basis of therapeutics*, 9th ed., pp. 399–430. New York: McGraw-Hill.

Drug facts and comparisons. (1996). St. Louis: Facts and Comparisons.

Fankhauser, M.P. (1993). Anxiolytic drugs and sedative-hypnotics. In R. Bressler & M.D. Katz (Eds.), *Geriatric pharmacology*, pp. 165–205. New York: McGraw-Hill.

Hayes, P.E., & Kirkwood, C.K. (1993). Anxiety disorders. In J.T. DiPiro, R.L. Talbert, P.E. Hayes, G.C. Yee, G.R. Matzke, & L.M. Posey (Eds.), *Pharmacotherapy: A pathophysiologic approach*, 2nd ed., pp. 1092–1109. Norwalk, CT: Appleton & Lange.

Hobbs, W.R., Rall, T.W., & Verdoorn, T.A. (1996). Hypnotics and sedatives; ethanol. In J.G. Hardman, L.E. Limbird, P.B. Molinoff, & R.W. Ruddon (Eds.), *Goodman & Gilman's The pharmacological basis of therapeutics*, 9th ed., pp. 361–396. New York: McGraw-Hill.

Juergens, S.M. (1993). Problems with benzodiazepines in elderly patients. *Mayo Clinic Proceedings, 68,* 818–820.

Kirkwood, C.K. (1993). Sleep disorders. In J.T. DiPiro, R.L. Talbert, P.E. Hayes, G.C. Yee, G.R. Matzke, & L.M. Posey (Eds.), *Pharmacotherapy: A pathophysiologic approach*, 2nd ed., pp. 1110–1119. Norwalk, CT: Appleton & Lange.

Antipsychotic Drugs

Objectives

After studying this chapter, the student will be able to:

1 Discuss schizophrenia and common manifestations of psychotic disorders.

2 Discuss characteristics of phenothiazines and related antipsychotics in terms of mechanism of action, indications for use, adverse effects, nursing process implications, and principles of therapy.

3 Compare characteristics of clozapine, risperidone, and olanzapine with those of phenothiazines and related antipsychotic drugs.

4 List interventions to decrease adverse effects of antipsychotic drugs.

5 State interventions to promote compliance with outpatient use of antipsychotic drugs.

Key Terms

Akathisia	**Dystonia**
Chemoreceptor trigger zone (CTZ)	**Hallucinations**
	Parkinsonism
Delusions	**Tardive dyskinesia**
Dopamine	

Psychosis

Antipsychotic drugs are used mainly for the treatment of *psychosis*, a severe mental disorder characterized by disordered thought processes (disorganized and often bizarre thinking); blunted or inappropriate emotional responses; bizarre behavior ranging from hypoactivity to hyperactivity with agitation, aggressiveness, hostility, and combativeness; autism (self-absorption in which the person pays no attention to the environment or to other people); deterioration from previous levels of occupational and social functioning (poor self-care and interpersonal skills); hallucinations; and paranoid delusions. *Hallucinations* are sensory perceptions of people or objects that are not present in the external environment. More specifically, people see, hear, or feel (and occasionally taste or smell) stimuli that are not visible to external observers and cannot distinguish between these false perceptions and reality. Hallucinations occur with delirium, dementias, schizophrenia, and other psychotic states. Those occurring in schizophrenia or bipolar affective disorder are usually auditory, those in delirium are usually visual or tactile, and those in dementias are usually visual. *Delusions* are false beliefs that persist in the absence of reason or evidence. Deluded people often believe that other people control their thoughts, feelings, and behaviors or seek to harm them (paranoia). Delusions indicate severe mental illness. Although they are commonly associated with schizophrenia, delusions also occur with delirium, dementias, and other psychotic disorders.

Psychosis may be acute or chronic. Acute episodes, also called confusion or delirium, have a sudden onset over hours to days and may be precipitated by physical disorders (*e.g.,* brain damage related to cerebrovascular disease or head injury, metabolic disorders, infections), drug intoxication with adrenergics, antidepressants, some anticonvulsants, amphetamine, cocaine, and others, and drug withdrawal after chronic use (*e.g.,* alcohol, benzodiazepine antianxiety or sedative-hypnotic agents). In addition, acute psychotic episodes may be superimposed on chronic dementias and psychoses, such as schizophrenia. This chapter focuses primarily on schizophrenia as a chronic psychosis.

Schizophrenia

Although schizophrenia is often referred to as a single disease, it actually includes a variety of related disorders. Risk factors include a genetic predisposition and environmental stresses. Symptoms may begin gradually or suddenly, usually during adolescence or early adulthood. According to the American Psychiatric Association's *Diagnostic and Statistical Manual*, fourth edition, overt psychotic symptoms must be present for 6 months before schizophrenia can be diagnosed. Thus, schizophrenia is a chronic illness, and this characteristic helps distinguish schizophrenia from other psychotic states (*e.g.,* delirium, dementia).

In recent years, there has been an effort to categorize schizophrenia more specifically. One effort divides the behavioral manifestations into positive and negative symptoms. Positive symptoms are correlated with CNS stimulation and include agitation, delusions, hallucinations, insomnia, and paranoia. Negative symptoms are correlated with a lack of pleasure (anhedonia), a lack of motivation, a blunted affect, poor grooming and hygiene, poor social skills, and poverty of speech. However, all these symptoms may occur with other disorders.

ETIOLOGY

Although the etiology is unclear, there is evidence that schizophrenia results from dysfunction of the dopaminergic and other neurotransmission systems in the brain (see Chap. 5). The dopaminergic system has been more extensively studied than other systems because schizophrenia has long been attributed to increased dopamine activity in the brain. This etiology is supported by the findings that antipsychotic drugs exert their therapeutic effects by decreasing dopamine activity (*i.e.,* blocking dopamine receptors) and that drugs that increase dopamine levels in the brain (*e.g.,* bromocriptine, levodopa) can cause psychotic signs and symptoms. Another factor that increases the amount of dopamine available to bind with receptors is decreased activity of dopamine beta-hydroxylase. Because this enzyme normally converts dopamine to norepinephrine in adrenergic nerve endings, a decrease in its activity results in larger amounts of dopamine.

In addition to the increased amount of dopamine, dopamine receptors are also involved. Two groups of dopamine receptors have been differentiated, mainly by the effects of the dopamine/receptor complex on intracellular functions. One group consists of D_1 and D_5 receptors, which stimulate cellular functions. The other group consists of D_2, D_3, and D_4 receptors, which decrease cellular functions and alter the movement of calcium and potassium ions across neuronal cell membranes. The D_2 group of dopamine receptors is considered important in the pathophysiology of schizophrenia: Antipsychotic drugs bind to these receptors and block the action of dopamine.

Thus, at the cellular level, dopamine activity is determined by its interaction with various receptors and the simultaneous actions of other neurotransmitters at the same target neurons.

In addition to dopamine, other neurotransmitters and receptors may be involved in the production of psychosis. One indication of such involvement is the wide variety of drugs that may cause psychosis, including adrenergics (increase norepinephrine), antidepressants (affect norepinephrine, serotonin, or both), some anticonvulsants (increase the effects of gamma-aminobutyric acid), and others with unknown effects on neurotransmitters and receptors. Amino acid neurotransmitters, especially glutamate, are also receiving attention as possible etiologic factors.

Schizophrenia is a complex disorder and probably has multiple etiologies. Currently, emphasis is being placed on abnormalities in neurotransmission systems in the brain. In addition to the dopaminergic system, there is evidence of abnormalities in the glutamate and serotonin systems. There is also evidence of extensive interactions among neurotransmission systems whereby other systems can alter dopaminergic activity. The disease probably results from an upset in the balance and integration among neurotransmission systems.

Antipsychotic Drugs

Antipsychotic drugs are derived from several chemical groups and are broadly categorized as phenothiazines and nonphenothiazines. Despite chemical differences, their pharmacologic actions and antipsychotic effectiveness are similar.

The largest group of antipsychotic drugs is the phenothiazines, of which chlorpromazine (Thorazine) is the prototype. The phenothiazines are well absorbed after oral and parenteral administration. They are distributed to most body tissues and reach high concentrations in the brain. They are metabolized in the liver and excreted in urine. Some metabolites have pharmacologic activity similar to that of the parent compound. These drugs do not cause physical or psychological drug dependence.

Phenothiazines exert many pharmacologic effects in the body, including central nervous system (CNS) depression, autonomic nervous system depression (antiadrenergic and anticholinergic effects), antiemetic effects, lowering of body temperature, hypersensitivity reactions, and others. They differ mainly in potency and adverse effects. Differences in potency are demonstrated by the fact that some phenothiazines (piperazine subgroup) are as effective in doses of a few milligrams as others (aliphatic and piperadine subgroups) are in doses of several hundred milligrams. All phenothiazines produce the same kinds of adverse effects, but the subgroups differ in the incidence and severity of particular adverse effects.

Nonphenothiazine antipsychotic drugs represent several different chemical groups but are few in number. Their pharmacologic actions, clinical uses, and adverse effects are similar to those of the phenothiazines.

MECHANISM OF ACTION

Most antipsychotic drugs occupy or block dopamine receptors in brain tissue, thereby decreasing the effects of dopamine. However, drug binding to the receptors does not completely explain antipsychotic effects, as binding occurs within a few hours after a drug dose and antipsychotic effects may not occur until the drugs have been given for a few weeks. Manifestations of hyperarousal (*e.g.,* anxiety, agitation, hyperactivity, insomnia, aggressive or combative behavior) are relieved more quickly than hallucinations, delusions, and thought disorders. One view of the delayed effects is that the blockade of dopamine receptors leads to changes in the receptors and postreceptor effects on cell metabolism and function. With chronic drug administration (*i.e.,* chronic blockade of dopamine receptors in the synapse), there is an increased number of dopamine receptors on postsynaptic and possibly presynaptic nerve cell membranes (up-regulation). Clozapine and risperidone block both dopamine and serotonin receptors. Overall, the drugs apparently re-regulate the abnormal neurotransmission systems associated with psychosis.

INDICATIONS FOR USE

The major clinical indication for use of antipsychotic drugs is schizophrenia. The drugs also are used to treat psychotic symptoms associated with brain impairment induced by head injury, tumor, stroke, alcohol withdrawal, overdoses of CNS stimulant drugs, and other disorders. They may be useful in the manic phase of bipolar affective disorder to control manic behavior until lithium, the drug of choice, becomes effective.

Clinical indications not associated with psychiatric illness include prevention and treatment of nausea and vomiting and treatment of intractable hiccups. The drugs relieve nausea and vomiting by blocking dopamine receptors in the chemoreceptor trigger zone (CTZ). The CTZ is a group of neurons in the medulla oblongata that, when activated by physical or psychological stimuli, causes nausea and vomiting. The mechanism by which the drugs relieve hiccups is unclear.

CONTRAINDICATIONS FOR USE

Because of their wide-ranging adverse effects, antipsychotic drugs may cause or aggravate a number of conditions. Thus, they are contraindicated in clients with liver damage, coronary artery disease, cerebrovascular disease, parkinsonism, bone marrow depression, severe hypotension or hypertension, coma, or severely depressed states. They should be used cautiously in seizure disorders, diabetes mellitus, glaucoma, prostatic hypertrophy, peptic ulcer disease, and chronic respiratory disorders.

Individual Antipsychotic Drugs

PHENOTHIAZINES

Commonly used phenothiazine antipsychotic drugs are listed in Table 9-1. **Promethazine** (Phenergan) is a phenothiazine that is not used clinically for antipsychotic effects but is often used for sedative, antiemetic, and antihistaminic effects.

NONPHENOTHIAZINES

Chlorprothixene (Taractan) and **thiothixene** (Navane) are thioxanthenes chemically similar to phenothiazines. These potent and effective antipsychotic drugs are used clinically only for their antipsychotic effects, although they produce other effects similar to those of the phenothiazines. A 100-mg dose of chlorprothixene is therapeutically equivalent to 100 mg of chlorpromazine; a

| TABLE 9-1 | PHENOTHIAZINE ANTIPSYCHOTIC DRUGS |

Generic/ Trade Name	Routes of Administration and Dosage Ranges	Major Side Effects (Incidence)			Remarks
		Sedation	*Extrapyramidal Reactions*	*Hypotension*	
Acetophenazine (Tindal)	*Adults*: PO 60 mg daily in divided doses, may be gradually increased by 20 mg daily until therapeutic or adverse effects occur. Usual optimal dosage is 80–120 mg daily. *Elderly or debilitated adults*: one-third to one-half usual adult dose *Children*: 0.8–1.6 mg/kg per day in 3 divided doses (maximum, 80 mg daily)	Moderate	High	Low	20 mg is equivalent to 100 mg of chlorpromazine.
Chlorpromazine (Thorazine)	*Adults*: PO 200–600 mg daily in divided doses. Dose may be increased by 100 mg daily q2–3 days until symptoms are controlled, adverse effects occur, or a maximum daily dose of 2 g is reached. IM 25–100 mg initially for acute psychotic symptoms, repeated in 1–4 hours PRN until control is achieved. *Elderly or debilitated adults*: PO one-third to one-half usual adult dose, increased by 25 mg daily q2–3 days if necessary. IM 10 mg q6–8h until acute symptoms are controlled *Children*: PO, IM 0.5 mg/kg q4–8h. Maximum IM dose, 40 mg daily in children under 5 years of age and 75 mg for older children	High	Moderate	Moderate to high	Sustained-release capsules and liquid concentrates are available.
Fluphenazine decanoate and enanthate (Prolixin Decanoate; Prolixin Enanthate)	*Adults under 50 years*: IM, SC 12.5 mg initially followed by 25 mg every 2 weeks. Dosage requirements rarely exceed 100 mg q2–6 weeks.	Low to moderate	High	Low	

(continued)

| TABLE 9-1 | PHENOTHIAZINE ANTIPSYCHOTIC DRUGS (Continued) |

Generic/ Trade Name	Routes of Administration and Dosage Ranges	Major Side Effects (Incidence)			Remarks
		Sedation	Extrapyramidal Reactions	Hypotension	
Fluphenazine hydrochloride (Prolixin, Permitil)	*Adults over 50, debilitated clients, or clients with a history of extrapyramidal reactions*: 2.5 mg initially followed by 2.5–5 mg q10–14 days *Children*: No dosage established *Adults*: PO 2.5–10 mg initially, gradually reduced to maintenance dose of 1–5 mg (doses above 3 mg are rarely necessary). Acute psychosis: 1.25 mg initially, increased gradually to 2.5–10 mg daily in 3–4 divided doses *Elderly or debilitated adults*: PO 1–2.5 mg daily; IM one-third to one-half the usual adult dose *Children*: PO 0.75–10 mg daily in children 5 to 12 years. IM no dosage established	Low to moderate	High	Low	2 mg of the oral hydrochloride salt is equivalent to 100 mg of chlorpromazine.
Mesoridazine (Serentil)	*Adults and children over 12 years*: PO 150 mg daily in divided doses initially, increased gradually in 50-mg increments until symptoms are controlled. Usual dose range, 100–400 mg. IM 25–175 mg daily in divided doses *Elderly and debilitated adults*: one-third to one-half usual adult dose *Children under 12 years*: no dosage established	High	Low	Moderate	50 mg is equivalent to 100 mg of chlorpromazine.
Perphenazine (Trilafon)	*Adults*: PO 16–64 mg daily in divided doses. Acute psychoses: IM 5–10 mg initially, then 5 mg q6h if necessary. Maximum daily dose, 15 mg for ambulatory clients and 30 mg for hospitalized clients *Elderly or debilitated adults*: PO, IM one-third to one-half usual adult dose *Children*: PO dosages not established, but the following amounts have been given in divided doses: ages 1–6 years, 4–6 mg daily; 6–12 years, 6 mg daily; over 12 years, 6–12 mg daily	Low to moderate	High	Low	8 mg is equivalent to 100 mg of chlorpromazine.

TABLE 9-1 PHENOTHIAZINE ANTIPSYCHOTIC DRUGS (Continued)

Generic/ Trade Name	Routes of Administration and Dosage Ranges	Major Side Effects (Incidence)			Remarks
		Sedation	Extrapyramidal Reactions	Hypotension	
Prochlorperazine (Compazine)	*Adults*: PO 10 mg 3–4 times daily, increased gradually (usual daily dose, 100–150 mg). IM 10–20 mg; may be repeated in 2–4 hours. Switch to oral form as soon as possible. *Children over age 2 years*: PO, rectal 2.5 mg 2–3 times daily, IM 0.06 mg/lb	Moderate	High	Low	10 mg is equivalent to 100 mg of chlorpromazine.
Promazine (Sparine)	*Adults*: initially, 50–150 mg IM; maintenance, PO, IM 10–200 mg q4–6h *Children over 12 years*: 10–25 mg q4–6h	Moderate	Moderate	Moderate	200 mg is equivalent to 100 mg of chlorpromazine.
Thioridazine (Mellaril)	*Adults*: PO 150–300 mg daily in divided doses, gradually increased if necessary to a maximum daily dose of 800 mg *Elderly or debilitated adults*: PO one-third to one-half the usual adult dose *Children 2 years and over*: 1 mg/kg per day in divided doses. Maximum dose, 3 mg/kg per day *Children under 2 years*: no dosage established	High	Low	Moderate	Thioridazine is probably the most frequently used antipsychotic drug. It differs from other phenothiazines by lacking antiemetic effects. It also has little, if any, effect on seizure threshold; 100 mg is equivalent to 100 mg of chlorpromazine.
Trifluoperazine (Stelazine)	*Adults*: Outpatients PO 2–4 mg daily in divided doses. Hospitalized clients, PO 4–10 mg daily in divided doses. Acute psychoses: IM 1–2 mg q4–5h, maximum of 10 mg daily *Elderly or debilitated adults*: PO, IM one-third to one-half usual adult dose. If given IM, give at less frequent intervals than above. *Children 6 years and over*: PO, IM 1–2 mg daily, maximum daily dose 15 mg *Children under 6 years*: no dosage established	Moderate	High	Low	5 mg is equivalent to 100 mg of chlorpromazine.

4-mg dose of thiothixene is equivalent to 100 mg of chlorpromazine.

Chlorprothixene

Routes and Dosage Ranges

Adults: Acute psychosis, PO, IM 75–200 mg/d in divided doses, increased to a maximal oral dose of 600 mg/d if necessary

Elderly or debilitated adults: PO, IM 30–100 mg/d in divided doses, reduced when symptoms have been controlled

Children >12 y: IM, same as adults

Children 6–12 y: PO 30–100 mg/d in divided doses; IM dosage not established

Children <6 y: Dosage not established

Thiothixene

Routes and Dosage Ranges

Adults: PO 6–10 mg/d in divided doses; maximum 60 mg/d

Acute psychosis, IM 8–16 mg/d in divided doses; maximum 30 mg/d

Elderly or debilitated adults: PO, IM one-third to one-half the usual adult dosage

Children >12 y: Same as adults

Children <12 y: Dosage not established

Haloperidol (Haldol) is a butyrophenone compound and the only drug of this group available for use in psychiatric disorders; a related drug, droperidol (Inapsine), is used in anesthesia and as an antiemetic. Haloperidol is a frequently used antipsychotic agent that is chemically different but pharmacologically similar to the phenothiazines. A potent, long-acting drug, it is readily absorbed after oral or intramuscular administration, metabolized in the liver, and excreted in urine and bile. Haloperidol may cause adverse effects similar to those of other antipsychotic drugs. Usually, it produces a relatively low incidence of hypotension and sedation and a high incidence of extrapyramidal effects.

Haloperidol is used as the initial drug for treating psychotic disorders or as a substitute in clients who are hypersensitive or refractory to the phenothiazines. It also is used for some conditions in which other antipsychotic drugs are not used, including mental retardation with hyperkinesia (abnormally increased motor activity), Tourette syndrome (a rare disorder characterized by involuntary movements and vocalizations), and Huntington's disease (a rare genetic disorder that involves progressive psychiatric symptoms and involuntary movements). A 2-mg dose is therapeutically equivalent to 100 mg of chlorpromazine. For clients who are unable or unwilling to take the oral drug as prescribed, a slowly absorbed, long-acting formulation (haloperidol decanoate) may be given intramuscularly, once monthly.

Routes and Dosage Ranges

Adults: Acute psychosis, PO 1–15 mg/d initially in divided doses, gradually increased to 100 mg/d if necessary; usual maintenance dose, 2–8 mg daily; IM 2–10 mg q1–8h until symptoms are controlled (usually within 72 h)

Chronic schizophrenia, PO 6–15 mg/d; maximum 100 mg/d; dosage is reduced for maintenance, usually 15–20 mg/d. Haloperidol decanoate IM, initial dose up to 100 mg, depending on the previous dose of oral drug, then titrated according to response. Usually given every 4 weeks

Tourette syndrome, PO 6–15 mg/d; maximum 100 mg/d; usual maintenance dose, 9 mg/d

Mental retardation with hyperkinesia, PO 80–120 mg/d, gradually reduced to a maintenance dose of about 60 mg/d; IM 20 mg/d in divided doses, gradually increased to 60 mg/d if necessary. Oral administration should be substituted after symptoms are controlled.

Elderly or debilitated adults: Same as for children <12 years

Children >12 y: Acute psychosis, chronic refractory schizophrenia, Tourette syndrome, mental retardation with hyperkinesia: same as for adults

Children <12 y: Acute psychosis, PO 0.5–1.5 mg/d initially, gradually increased in increments of 0.5 mg; usual maintenance dose, 2–4 mg/d. IM dosage not established.

Chronic refractory schizophrenia, dosage not established

Tourette syndrome, PO 1.5–6 mg/d initially in divided doses; usual maintenance dose, about 1.5 mg/d

Mental retardation with hyperkinesia, PO 1.5 mg/d initially in divided doses, gradually increased to a maximum of 15 mg/d if necessary. When symptoms are controlled, dosage is gradually reduced to the minimum effective level. IM dosage not established.

Loxapine (Loxitane) and **clozapine** (Clozaril) are dibenzoxazepines pharmacologically similar to other antipsychotic drugs. They are recommended for use only in the treatment of schizophrenia, especially for clients who have not responded to other drugs. Clozapine may improve negative symptoms and does not cause the extrapyramidal effects (*e.g.*, acute dystonia, parkinsonism, akathisia, tardive dyskinesia) associated with most antipsychotic agents. However, there is a relatively high risk of agranulocytosis, a life-threatening decrease in white blood cells. Weekly white blood counts are recommended. Other adverse effects include sedation, orthostatic hypotension, and electrocardiographic (ECG) changes.

Loxapine
Route and Dosage Ranges

Adults and adolescents 16 years and older: PO 10 mg twice a day to a total of 50 mg/d in severe psychoses; usual maintenance dose 60–100 mg/d; maximum dose, 250 mg/d

Elderly or debilitated adults: One-third to one-half the usual adult dosage

Children <6 y: Dosage not established

Clozapine
Route and Dosage Range

Adults: PO 50–900 mg/d
Children: Dosage not established

Molindone (Moban) is an antipsychotic agent that differs chemically from other agents but has similar pharmacologic actions. A 20-mg dose is equivalent to 100 mg of chlorpromazine.

Route and Dosage Range

Adults: PO 50–75 mg/d, increased gradually if necessary up to 225 mg/d, then reduced for maintenance; usual maintenance dose, 15–40 mg/d

Elderly or debilitated adults: One-third to one-half the usual adult dosage

Children <12 y: Dosage not established

Olanzapine (Zyprexa) is a newer antipsychotic that blocks both dopamine and serotonin receptors. It is well absorbed after oral administration; its absorption is not affected by food. A steady-state concentration is reached in about 1 week of once daily administration. It is highly metabolized and excreted in urine and feces. Compared to clozapine, olanzapine may be more likely to cause extrapyramidal effects (*e.g.*, acute dystonia, parkinsonism, akathisia, tardive dyskinesia), but is less likely to cause agranulocytosis—a life-threatening decrease in white blood cells. Commonly reported adverse effects in clinical trials include agitation, dizziness, drowsiness, headache, and weight gain. Orthostatic hypotension may also occur.

Route and Dosage Range

Adults: PO 5–10 mg/d initially; given once daily at bedtime; increased over several weeks to 20 mg/d, if necessary
Children: Dosage not established

Pimozide (Orap) is an antipsychotic drug approved only for the treatment of Tourette syndrome in clients who fail to respond to haloperidol. Potentially serious adverse effects include tardive dyskinesia, major motor seizures, and sudden death.

Route and Dosage Range

Adults: PO 1–2 mg/d in divided doses initially, increased if necessary; usual maintenance dose, about 10 mg/d; maximum dose, 20 mg/d

Risperidone (Risperdal) is a newer drug that blocks both dopamine and serotonin receptors and relieves both positive and negative symptoms of psychosis. It is indicated for the treatment of schizophrenia in people who do not respond to other antipsychotic drugs. Risperidone is well absorbed with oral administration, is metabolized mainly in the liver by the cytochrome P450 enzyme system, and produces an active metabolite. Effects are attributed about equally to risperidone and the metabolite. Elimination half-life is 20 to 30 hours; 70% is excreted in urine and 14% in feces. Peak blood levels occur in 1 to 2 hours, but therapeutic effects are delayed for 1 to 2 weeks. Adverse effects include agitation, anxiety, headache, insomnia, dizziness, and hypotension. It may also cause parkinsonism and other movement disorders but is less likely to do so than other drugs.

Route and Dosage Range

Adults: PO, initially 1 mg twice daily (2 mg/d); increase to 2 mg twice daily on the second day (4 mg/d); increase to 3 mg twice daily on the third day (6 mg/d), if necessary. Usual maintenance dose, 4 to 8 mg/d. After initial titration, dosage increases or decreases should be made at a rate of 1 mg/wk.

Elderly or debilitated adults: PO, initially 0.5 mg twice daily (1 mg/d); increase in 0.5-mg increments to 1.5 mg twice daily (3 mg/d)

Renal impairment: PO, same as for elderly or debilitated adults

Children <12 y: Dosage not established

Nursing Process

Assessment

Assess the client's mental health status, need for antipsychotic drugs, and response to drug therapy. There is a wide variation in response to drug therapy. Close observation of physical and behavioral reactions is necessary to evaluate effectiveness and to individualize dosage schedules. Accurate assessment is especially important when starting drug therapy and when increasing or decreasing dosage. Some assessment factors include the following:

- Interview the client and family members. Attempts to interview an acutely psychotic person are likely to yield little useful information, due to the client's distorted perception of reality. The nurse may be able to assess the client's level of orientation and delusional and hallucinatory activity. If possible, try to determine from family members or others what the client was doing or experiencing when the acute episode began (*i.e.*, predisposing factors, such as increased environmental stress or a crisis situation); whether this is a first or a repeated episode of psychotic behavior; whether the person has physical illnesses, takes any drugs, or uses alcohol; whether the client seems to be a hazard to himself or herself or others; and some description of pre-illness personality traits, level of social interaction, and ability to function in usual activities of daily living.

- Observe the client for the presence or absence of psychotic symptoms such as agitation, hyperactivity, combativeness, and bizarre behavior.
- Obtain baseline data to help monitor the client's response to drug therapy. Some authorities advocate initial and periodic laboratory tests of liver, kidney, and blood functions, as well as ECGs. Although such tests do not help greatly in preventing adverse reactions, they may assist in earlier detection and treatment of adverse reactions. Baseline blood-pressure readings also may be helpful.
- Continue assessing the client's response to drug therapy and his or her ability to function in activities of daily living, whether the client is hospitalized or receiving outpatient treatment.

Nursing Diagnoses

- Altered Thought Processes related to the disease, especially during the first few weeks of antipsychotic drug therapy
- Self-Care Deficit related to the disease process or drug-induced sedation
- Impaired Physical Mobility related to sedation
- Decreased Cardiac Output related to cardiac arrhythmias and hypotension
- Altered Tissue Perfusion related to hypotension
- Risk for Injury related to excessive sedation and movement disorders (extrapyramidal effects)
- Risk for Violence: Self-Directed or Directed At Others
- Noncompliance related to underuse of prescribed drugs
- Knowledge Deficit: Expected recurrence of symptoms and hospitalization if drug therapy is not continued in chronic schizophrenia

Planning/Goals

The client will:

- Become less agitated within a few hours after drug therapy is started and less psychotic within a few days
- Be kept safe while sedated during early drug therapy
- Be cared for by staff in areas of nutrition, hygiene, exercise, and social interactions when unable to provide self-care
- Improve in ability to participate in self-care activities
- Avoid preventable adverse drug effects, especially those that impair safety
- Be helped to take medications as prescribed and return for follow-up appointments with health care providers

Interventions

Use nondrug measures when appropriate to increase the effectiveness of drug therapy and to decrease adverse reactions.

- Obviously, drug therapy will be ineffective if the client does not receive sufficient medication. For numerous reasons, many people are unable or unwilling to take medications as prescribed. Any nursing action aimed toward more accurate drug administration will increase the effectiveness of drug therapy.
  Specific nursing actions must be individualized to the client. Some general nursing actions that may be helpful

include emphasizing the therapeutic benefits expected from drug therapy, answering questions or providing information about drug therapy and other aspects of the treatment plan, devising a schedule of administration times that is as convenient as possible for the client, and giving the drug in the form (*e.g.*, syrup, capsule) most acceptable to the client.

- Supervise ambulation to prevent falls or other injuries if the client is drowsy or elderly or has postural hypotension.
- Several measures can help prevent or minimize hypotension, such as having the client lie down for about an hour after an injection of antipsychotic medication or a large oral dose, applying elastic stockings, and instructing the client to change positions gradually, elevate legs when sitting, avoid standing for prolonged periods, and avoid hot baths (hot baths cause vasodilation and increase the incidence of hypotension).
- Dry mouth and oral infections can be decreased by frequent brushing of the teeth, rinsing the mouth with water, or chewing sugarless gum or candy.
- The usual measures of increasing fluid intake, dietary fiber, and exercise can help prevent constipation.
- Support caregivers in efforts to maintain contact with inpatients and provide care for outpatients. One way is to provide caregivers with telephone numbers of health care providers and to make periodic telephone calls to caregivers.

Teach clients and caretakers:

- About the planned drug therapy regimen, including the desired therapeutic results and the length of time before therapeutic results can be expected. This is especially important to improve compliance in long-term drug therapy. Failure to take prescribed medications is a frequent reason for recurring episodes of acute illness and hospitalization.
- About the possible adverse effects of drug therapy. Emphasize those related to safety; for example, warn the client not to drive a car or operate machinery. Providing a detailed list of adverse effects is unnecessary and may confuse the client or increase anxiety. It may be helpful to note that drowsiness and impaired mental and motor activity are especially evident during the first 2 weeks of drug therapy but tend to decrease with time.
- To report unusual side effects and all physical illnesses, because changes in drug therapy may be indicated.
- To avoid using *any* nonprescribed drugs, such as those available without prescription or those prescribed for another person, to prevent undesirable drug interactions. Alcohol and sleeping pills should be avoided because they may cause excessive drowsiness and decreased awareness of safety hazards in the environment.
- To consult the physician who prescribed the medication before taking any drug prescribed by another physician. This also avoids undesirable drug interactions.

Evaluation

- Interview the client to determine the presence and extent of hallucinations and delusions.
- Observe the client for decreased signs and symptoms. Document abilities and limitations in self-care.

- Note whether any injuries have occurred during drug therapy.
- Interview the caregiver about the client's behavior and medication response (*i.e.*, during a home visit or telephone call).

Principles of Therapy

GOALS OF TREATMENT

Overall goals of treatment are to alleviate psychotic symptoms, increase the client's ability to cope with the environment, promote optimal functioning in self-care and activities of daily living, and prevent or shorten hospitalization. With drug therapy, clients often can participate in psychotherapy, group therapy, or other treatment modalities, return to community settings, and return to their pre-illness level of functioning.

DRUG SELECTION

The physician's choice of a particular antipsychotic drug is largely empirical because clear-cut guidelines have not been established. Some general factors to consider include the client's age and physical condition, the severity and duration of illness, the frequency and severity of adverse effects produced by each drug, the response to antipsychotic drugs in the past, the subjective response to the drugs (*e.g.*, the adverse reactions the client is willing to tolerate), the supervision available, and the physician's experience with a particular drug. Some specific factors include the following:

1. Antipsychotic drugs are apparently equally effective regardless of the client's symptoms. Drugs producing greater sedation are often prescribed for agitated, overactive clients, and drugs producing less sedation are prescribed for those who are apathetic and withdrawn.
2. Despite the similarities of antipsychotic drugs in therapeutic benefits and adverse effects, some clients who do not respond well to one type of antipsychotic drug may respond to another. Unfortunately, there is no way of predicting which drug is likely to be most effective for a particular client.
3. There is no logical basis for giving more than one antipsychotic agent at a time. There is no therapeutic advantage, and the risk of serious adverse reactions is increased.
4. If lack of therapeutic response requires that another antipsychotic drug be substituted for the one a client is currently receiving, this substitution must be done gradually; abrupt substitution may cause reappearance of symptoms. This can be avoided by gradually decreasing doses of the old drug while substituting equivalent doses of the new one.

5. Nonphenothiazine antipsychotic drugs are probably best used for clients with chronic schizophrenia whose symptoms have not been controlled by the phenothiazines and for clients with hypersensitivity reactions to the phenothiazines. Although adverse reactions to these agents are similar to those caused by phenothiazines, clients allergic to the phenothiazines can usually tolerate one of the other antipsychotic drugs.
6. Unless the choice of drug is dictated by the client's previous favorable response to a particular drug, the preferred drug should be available in both parenteral and oral forms for flexibility of administration.
7. Clients who are unable or unwilling to take daily doses of a maintenance antipsychotic drug may be given periodic injections of a long-acting form of fluphenazine or haloperidol.
8. Any person who has had an allergic or hypersensitivity reaction to an antipsychotic drug generally should not be given that drug again or any drug in the same chemical subgroup. Cross-sensitivity occurs, and the likelihood of another allergic reaction is high.

DOSAGE AND ADMINISTRATION

Dosage and route of administration must be individualized. Initial drug therapy for acute psychotic episodes usually requires high dosage, intramuscular administration, divided doses, and hospitalization. Symptoms are usually controlled within 48 to 72 hours, after which oral drugs can be given and dosage gradually reduced to the lowest effective amount. For maintenance therapy, drug dosages are usually much smaller, oral drugs are preferred, and a single bedtime dose is effective for most clients. This schedule increases compliance with prescribed drug therapy, allows better nighttime sleep, and decreases hypotension and daytime sedation. Effective maintenance therapy requires close supervision and contact with the client and family members.

DURATION OF THERAPY

In schizophrenia, antipsychotic drugs are usually given for years. There are no clear guidelines regarding the duration of drug therapy. There is a high rate of relapse (acute psychotic reactions) in schizophrenic clients when drug therapy is discontinued, most often by clients who become unwilling or unable to continue their medication regimen.

MANAGEMENT OF EXTRAPYRAMIDAL SYMPTOMS

For most clients receiving antipsychotic drugs, concurrent antiparkinsonism drug therapy should be given only after extrapyramidal symptoms (*e.g.*, abnormal rigidity and muscle movements) occur. Such neuro-muscular symptoms appear in fewer than half the clients taking antipsychotic drugs and are better handled by reducing dosage, if this does not cause recurrence of psychotic symptoms. If antiparkinsonism drugs are given, they should be gradually discontinued in about 3 months. Extrapyramidal symptoms do not usually recur despite continued administration of the same antipsychotic drug at the same dosage.

ETHNIC OR GENETIC CONSIDERATIONS

People of Asian heritage may have higher serum drug levels than white people given comparable doses, probably because of slower metabolism and elimination of the drugs. A cautious approach to antipsychotic drug therapy in this population would consist of lower initial doses (about half the usual dosage of white people) and titration of later doses according to clinical response and serum drug levels. Most studies have been done with haloperidol and with a limited number of Asian subgroups. Thus, it cannot be assumed that all antipsychotic drugs and all people of Asian heritage respond the same.

USE IN PERIOPERATIVE PERIODS

A major concern about giving antipsychotic drugs perioperatively is their potential for adverse interactions with other drugs. For example, the drugs potentiate the effects of general anesthetics and other CNS depressants that are often used before, during, and after surgery. As a result, risks of hypotension and excessive sedation are increased unless doses of other agents are reduced. If hypotension occurs and requires vasopressor drugs, phenylephrine (Neo-Synephrine) or norepinephrine (Levophed) should be used rather than epinephrine (Adrenalin) because antipsychotic drugs inhibit the vasoconstrictive (blood-pressure–raising) effects of epinephrine.

USE IN CHILDREN

Antipsychotic drugs are not generally recommended for children under 12 years of age. Thioridazine, prochlorperazine, trifluoperazine, and haloperidol may be used in children aged 2 to 12 years but are not recommended for children under 2 years. Extrapyramidal symptoms are more likely to occur in children than adults.

USE IN OLDER ADULTS

Antipsychotic drugs should be used cautiously in older adults. Before they are started, a thorough assessment is needed because psychiatric symptoms are often caused by organic disease or other drugs. If this is the case, treating the disease or stopping the offending drug may cancel the need for an antipsychotic drug. When the drugs are required, dosage should be reduced by 30% to 50% and increased gradually if necessary. Once symptoms are controlled, dosage should be reduced to the lowest effective level. Adverse effects are likely to occur because of slowed drug metabolism. These include cardiovascular (hypotension, arrhythmias), sedative, and anticholinergic effects that may be especially dangerous in older adults. Tardive dyskinesia may occur with long-term use of antipsychotic drugs.

In addition, older adults are more likely to have problems in which the drugs are contraindicated (*e.g.,* severe cardiovascular disease, liver damage, parkinsonism) or must be used very cautiously (diabetes mellitus, glaucoma, prostatic hypertrophy, peptic ulcer disease, chronic respiratory disorders).

For older adults in long-term care facilities, there is concern that antipsychotic drugs may be overused to control agitated or disruptive behavior that is caused by nonpsychotic disorders and for which other treatments are preferable. For example, clients with dementias may become agitated from environmental or medical problems. Alleviating such causes, when possible, is safer and more effective than administering antipsychotic drugs. Inappropriate use of the drugs exposes clients to adverse drug effects and does not resolve underlying problems. Because of the many implications for patient safety and welfare, federal regulations were established for the use of antipsychotics in facilities receiving Medicare and Medicaid funds. These regulations include appropriate (*e.g.,* psychotic disorders, delusions, schizophrenia, and dementia and delirium that meet certain criteria) and inappropriate (*e.g.,* agitation not thought to indicate potential harm to the resident or others, anxiety, depression, uncooperativeness, wandering) indications.

 ## HOME CARE

Chronically mentally ill clients, such as those with schizophrenia, are among the most challenging in a home care nurse's caseload. Major recurring problems include failure to take antipsychotic medications as prescribed and the concurrent use of alcohol and other drugs of abuse. Either problem is likely to lead to acute psychotic episodes and hospitalizations. The home care nurse must assist and support caregivers' efforts to maintain medications and manage adverse drug effects, other aspects of daily care, and follow-up psychiatric care. In addition, the home care nurse may need to coordinate the efforts of several health and social service agencies or providers.

NURSING ACTIONS

ANTIPSYCHOTIC DRUGS

NURSING ACTIONS	RATIONALE/EXPLANATION
1. Administer accurately **a.** When feasible, give oral antipsychotic drugs once daily, within 1 to 2 hours of bedtime.	Peak sedation occurs about 2 hours after administration and aids sleep. Hypotension, dry mouth, and other adverse reactions are less bothersome with this schedule. Although antipsychotic drugs are probably more often prescribed in two or three daily doses, their long duration of action usually allows once-daily dosage.
b. When preparing oral concentrated solutions or parenteral solutions, try to avoid contact with the solution. If contact is made, wash the area immediately.	These solutions are irritating to the skin and may cause contact dermatitis.
c. Mix liquid concentrates with at least 60 ml of fruit juice or water just before administration.	To mask the taste. If the client does not like juice or water, check the package insert for other diluents. Some of the drugs may be mixed with coffee, tea, milk, or carbonated beverages.
d. For intramuscular injections: (1) Give only those preparations labeled for intramuscular use.	
(2) Do not mix any other drugs in the same syringe with antipsychotic drugs.	These drugs are physically incompatible with many other drugs, and a precipitate may occur.
(3) Change the needle after filing the syringe for injection.	Parenteral solutions of these drugs are highly irritating to body tissues. Changing needles helps protect the tissues of the injection tract from unnecessary contact with the drug.
(4) Inject slowly and deeply into gluteal muscles.	Using a large muscle mass for the injection site decreases tissue irritation.
(5) Have the client lie down for 30 to 60 minutes after the injection.	To observe for adverse reactions. Orthostatic hypotension is likely if the client tries to ambulate.
e. Do not give antipsychotic drugs subcutaneously, except for fluphenazine decanoate and fluphenazine enanthate.	More tissue irritation occurs with subcutaneous administration than with intramuscular administration.
f. When parenteral fluphenazine is ordered, check the drug preparations very closely.	The hydrochloride solution of fluphenazine is given intramuscularly only. The decanoate and enanthate preparations (long-acting, sesame oil preparations) can be given intramuscularly or subcutaneously.
2. Observe for therapeutic effects **a.** When the drug is given for acute psychotic episodes, observe for decreased agitation, combativeness, and psychomotor activity.	The sedative effects of antipsychotic drugs are exerted within 48 to 72 hours. Sedation that occurs with treatment of acute psychotic episodes is a therapeutic effect. Sedation that occurs with treatment of nonacute psychotic disorders, or excessive sedation at any time, is an adverse reaction.
b. When the drug is given for acute or chronic psychosis, observe for decreased psychotic behavior, such as: (1) Decreased auditory and visual hallucinations (2) Decreased delusions	These therapeutic effects may not be evident for 3 to 6 weeks after drug therapy is begun.

(continued)

NURSING ACTIONS	RATIONALE/EXPLANATION

(3) Continued decrease in or absence of agitation, hostility, hyperactivity, and other behavior associated with acute psychosis

(4) Increased socialization

(5) Increased ability in self-care activities

(6) Increased ability to participate in other therapeutic modalities along with drug therapy.

c. When the drug is given for antiemetic effects, observe for decreased or absent nausea or vomiting.

3. Observe for adverse effects
  a. Excessive sedation—drowsiness, lethargy, fatigue, slurred speech, impaired mobility, and impaired mental processes

Excessive sedation is most likely to occur during the first few days of treatment of an acute psychotic episode, when large doses are usually given. Psychotic clients also seem sedated because the drug lets them catch up on psychosis-induced sleep deprivation. Sedation is more likely to occur in elderly or debilitated people. Tolerance to the drugs' sedative effects develops, and sedation tends to decrease with continued drug therapy.

  b. Extrapyramidal reactions:

  (1) *Akathisia*—compulsive, involuntary restlessness and body movements

Akathisia is the most common extrapyramidal reaction, and it may occur about 5 to 60 days after the start of antipsychotic drug therapy. The motor restlessness may be erroneously interpreted as psychotic agitation necessitating increased drug dosage. This condition can sometimes be controlled by substituting an antipsychotic drug that is less likely to cause extrapyramidal effects or by giving an anticholinergic antiparkinson drug.

  (2) *Parkinsonism*—loss of muscle movement (akinesia), muscular rigidity and tremors, shuffling gait, postural abnormalities, mask-like facial expression, hypersalivation, and drooling

These symptoms are the same as those occurring with idiopathic Parkinson's disease. They can be controlled with anticholinergic antiparkinson drugs, given along with the antipsychotic drug for about 3 months, then discontinued. This reaction may occur about 5 to 30 days after antipsychotic drug therapy is begun.

  (3) *Dyskinesias* (involuntary, rhythmic body movements) and *dystonias* (uncoordinated, bizarre movements of the neck, face, eyes, tongue, trunk, or extremities)

These are less common extrapyramidal reactions, but they may occur suddenly, about 1 to 5 days after drug therapy is started, and be very frightening to the client and healthcare personnel. The movements are caused by muscle spasms and result in exaggerated posture and facial distortions. These symptoms are sometimes misinterpreted as seizures, hysteria, or other disorders. Antiparkinson drugs are given parenterally during acute dystonic reactions, but continued administration is not usually required. These reactions occur most often in younger people.

  (4) *Tardive dyskinesia*—hyperkinetic movements of the face (sucking and smacking of lips, tongue protrusion, and facial grimaces) and choreiform movements of the trunk and limbs

This syndrome occurs after months or years of high-dose antipsychotic drug therapy. The drugs may mask the symptoms so that the syndrome is more likely to be diagnosed when dosage is decreased or the drug is discontinued for a few days. It occurs gradually and at any age but is more common in older people, women, and people with organic brain disorders. The condition is usually irreversible, and there is no effective treatment. Symptoms are not controlled and may be

NURSING ACTIONS	RATIONALE/EXPLANATION
	worsened by antiparkinson drugs. Low dosage and short-term use of antipsychotic drugs help prevent tardive dyskinesia; drug-free periods may aid early detection.
c. Antiadrenergic effects—hypotension, tachycardia, dizziness, faintness, and fatigue.	Hypotension is potentially one of the most serious adverse reactions to the antipsychotic drugs. It is most likely to occur when the client assumes an upright position after sitting or lying down (orthostatic or postural hypotension), but it does occur in the recumbent position. It is caused by peripheral vasodilation. Orthostatic hypotension can be assessed by comparing blood-pressure readings taken with the client in supine and standing positions.
	Tachycardia occurs as a compensatory mechanism in response to hypotension and as an anticholinergic effect in which the normal vagus nerve action of slowing the heart rate is blocked.
d. Anticholinergic effects—dry mouth, dental caries, blurred vision, constipation, paralytic ileus, urinary retention	These atropine-like effects are common with therapeutic doses and are increased with large doses of phenothiazines.
e. Respiratory depression—slow, shallow breathing and decreased ability to breathe deeply, cough, and remove secretions from the respiratory tract	This stems from general central nervous system (CNS) depression, which causes drowsiness and decreased movement. It may cause pneumonia or other respiratory problems, especially in people with hypercarbia and chronic lung disease.
f. Endocrine effects—menstrual irregularities, possibly impotence and decreased libido in the male, weight gain	These apparently result from drug-induced changes in pituitary and hypothalamic functions.
g. Hypothermia or hyperthermia	Antipsychotic drugs may impair the temperature-regulating center in the hypothalamus. Hypothermia is more likely to occur. Hyperthermia occurs with high doses and warm environmental temperatures.
h. Hypersensitivity reactions:	
(1) *Cholestatic hepatitis*—may begin with fever and influenza-like symptoms followed in about 1 week by jaundice	Cholestatic hepatitis results from drug-induced edema of the bile ducts and obstruction of the bile flow. It occurs most often in women and after 2 to 4 weeks of receiving the drug. It is usually reversible if the drug is discontinued.
(2) *Blood dyscrasias*—leukopenia, agranulocytosis (fever, sore throat, weakness)	Some degree of leukopenia occurs rather often and does not seem to be serious. Agranulocytosis, on the other hand, occurs rarely but is life-threatening. Agranulocytosis is most likely to occur during the first 4 to 10 weeks of drug therapy, in women, and in older people.
(3) *Skin reactions*—photosensitivity, dermatoses	Skin pigmentation and discoloration may occur with exposure to sunlight.
i. Electrocardiogram (ECG) changes	The mechanism and clinical significance of ECG changes are not completely clear. However, some antipsychotic drugs, especially thioridazine, alter normal impulse conduction through the ventricles. There is probably increased risk of cardiac arrhythmias, which may be serious in a person with cardiovascular disease.
j. Neuroleptic malignant syndrome—fever (may be confused with heatstroke), muscle rigidity, agitation, confusion, delirium, dyspnea, tachycardia, respiratory failure, acute renal failure	A rare but potentially fatal reaction that may occur hours to months after initial drug use. Symptoms usually develop rapidly over 24 to 72 hours. Treatment includes stopping the antipsychotic drug, giving supportive care related to fever

(continued)

NURSING ACTIONS	RATIONALE/EXPLANATION
	and other symptoms, and drug therapy (dantrolene, a skeletal muscle relaxant, and amantadine or bromocriptine, dopamine-stimulating drugs).
4. Observe for drug interactions	
a. Drugs that *increase* effects of antipsychotic drugs:	
(1) Anticholinergic drugs (*e.g.*, atropine)	Additive anticholinergic effects, especially with thioridazine
(2) Antidepressants, tricyclic	Potentiation of sedative and anticholinergic effects. Additive CNS depression, sedation, orthostatic hypotension, urinary retention, and glaucoma may occur unless dosages are decreased. Apparently these two drug groups inhibit the metabolism of each other, thus prolonging the actions of both groups if they are given concomitantly.
(3) Antihistamines	Additive CNS depression and sedation
(4) CNS depressants—alcohol, narcotic analgesics, antianxiety agents, barbiturates and other sedative-hypnotics	Additive CNS depression. Also, severe hypotension, urinary retention, seizures, severe atropine-like reactions, and others may occur, depending on which group of CNS depressant drugs is given.
(5) Propranolol (Inderal)	Additive hypotensive and ECG effects
(6) Thiazide diuretics, such as hydrochlorothiazide (HydroDIURIL)	Additive hypotension
(7) Lithium	Acute encephalopathy, including irreversible brain damage and dyskinesias, has been reported.
b. Drugs that *decrease* effects of antipsychotic drugs:	
(1) Antacids	Oral antacids, especially aluminum hydroxide and magnesium trisilicate, may inhibit gastrointestinal absorption of antipsychotic drugs.
(2) Barbiturates	By induction of drug-metabolizing enzymes in the liver
(3) Norepinephrine (Levophed), phenylephrine (Neo-Synephrine)	Antagonize the hypotensive effects of antipsychotic drugs
5. Teach clients	
a. Do not take antacids with these drugs. If an antacid is needed, take it 1 hour before or 2 hours after the antipsychotic drug.	Antacids may decrease absorption of these drugs from the intestine.
b. Lie down for about an hour after receiving medication when drug therapy is started or after any injection.	To avoid low blood pressure, dizziness, and faintness, which may occur with standing
c. If dizziness and faintness occur on standing, they can be minimized by changing positions slowly and sitting on the bedside a few minutes before standing. Do not try to stand or walk when feeling dizzy.	To avoid falls or other injuries
d. Practice good oral hygiene measures, including dental checkups, thorough and frequent toothbrushing, drinking fluids, and frequent mouth rinsing.	Mouth dryness is a common side effect of these drugs. Although more annoying than serious for the most part, it can predispose to mouth infections, dental cavities, and ill-fitting dentures.
e. If skin reactions occur, stay out of sunlight or wear protective clothing and use sunscreen lotions.	Sensitivity to sunlight is an adverse reaction of these drugs.
f. Avoid exposure to excessive heat.	Fever (hyperthermia) and heat prostration may occur with high environmental temperatures.

REVIEW AND APPLICATION EXERCISES

1. How do antipsychotic drugs act to relieve psychotic symptoms?

2. What are some uses of antipsychotic drugs other than the treatment of schizophrenia?

3. Do the phenothiazine, butyrophenone, and thioxanthene antipsychotic drugs differ significantly in therapeutic effects?

4. What are major adverse effects of antipsychotic drugs?

5. When instructing a client to lie down for a while or to rise slowly from a sitting or lying position, which adverse effect of an antipsychotic drug is the nurse trying to prevent?

6. In a client receiving an antipsychotic drug, what appearances or behaviors would lead you to suspect an extrapyramidal reaction?

7. Describe potential difficulties in getting psychotic clients to take their drugs as prescribed and interventions to overcome these difficulties.

8. Are antipsychotic drugs likely to be overused and abused? Why or why not?

9. In an older client taking an antipsychotic drug, what special safety measures are needed? Why?

10. How do clozapine and risperidone compare with older antipsychotic drugs in terms of therapeutic and adverse effects?

11. What can the home care nurse do to prevent acute psychotic episodes and hospitalization of chronically mentally ill clients?

SELECTED REFERENCES

American Psychiatric Association. (1994). *Diagnostic and statistical manual of mental disorders*, 4th ed. Washington, D.C.: American Psychiatric Association.

Avorn, J., Monane, M., Everitt, D.E., Beers, M.H., & Fields, D. (1994). Clinical assessment of extrapyramidal signs in nursing home patients given antipsychotic medication. *Archives of Internal Medicine*, 154:1113–1117.

Bendik, M.F. (1996). The schizophrenias. In K.M. Fortinash & P.A. Holoday-Worret (Eds.), *Psychiatric-mental health nursing*, pp. 284–316. St. Louis: Mosby.

Blair, D.T., & Dauner, A. (1993). Neuroleptic malignant syndrome: Liability in nursing practice. *Journal of Psychosocial Nursing*, 3(1): 5–12.

Coffey, C.E., & Cummings, J.L. (Eds.) (1994). *The American Psychiatric Press Textbook of geriatric neuropsychiatry*. Washington, D.C.: American Psychiatric Press.

Crismon, M.L., & Dorson, P.G. (1993). Schizophrenia. In J.T. DiPiro, R.L. Talbert, P.E. Hayes, G.C. Yee, G.R. Matzke, & L.M. Posey (Eds.), *Pharmacotherapy: A pathophysiologic approach*, 2nd ed., pp. 1020–1043. Norwalk, CT: Appleton & Lange.

Druckenbrod, R.W., Rosen, J., & Cluxton, R.J., Jr. (1993). As-needed dosing of antipsychotic drugs: Limitations and guidelines for use in the elderly agitated patient. *The Annals of Pharmacotherapy*, 27:645–648.

Drug facts and comparisons. (1996). St. Louis: Facts and Comparisons.

Dubovsky, S.L. (1994). Geriatric neuropsychopharmacology. In C.E. Coffey & J.L. Cummings (Eds.), *The American Psychiatric Press Textbook of geriatric neuropsychiatry*, pp. 596–631. Washington, D.C.: American Psychiatric Press.

Gelenberg, A.J., & Katz M.D. (1993). Antipsychotic agents. In R. Bressler & M.D. Katz (Eds.), *Geriatric pharmacology*, pp. 375–408. New York: McGraw-Hill.

Hirsch, S.R., & Weinverger, D.R. (1995). *Schizophrenia*. Cambridge, MA: Blackwell Science.

Lahti, A.C., & Tamminga, C.A. (1995). Recent developments in the neuropharmacology of schizophrenia. *American Journal of Health-System Pharmacy*, 52(Suppl 1):S5–S8.

Lehne, R.A., & Scott, D. (1996). Psychopharmacology. In V.B. Carson & E.L. Arnold (Eds.), *Mental health nursing: The nurse-patient journey*, pp. 523–569. Philadelphia: W.B. Saunders.

McBride, A.B., & Austin, J.K. (1996). *Psychiatric-mental health nursing*. Philadelphia: W.B. Saunders.

McCrone, S.H. (1996). Physical dimensions of the journey: Neurobiological influences. In V.B. Carson & E.L. Arnold (Eds.), *Mental health nursing: The nurse-patient journey*, pp. 127–149. Philadelphia: W.B. Saunders.

Perry, P.J. (1995). Clinical use of the newer antipsychotic drugs. *American Journal of Health-System Pharmacy*, 52(Suppl 1):S9–S14.

Tsuang, M.T., & Faraone, S.V. (1994). Schizophrenia. In G. Winokur & P.J. Clayton (Eds.), *The medical basis of psychiatry*, 2nd ed., pp. 87–114. Philadelphia: W.B. Saunders.

Ziring, B. (1993). Issues in the perioperative care of the patient with psychiatric illness. *Medical Clinics of North America*, 77(2) 443–452.

10 Antidepressants

Outline

Objectives

After studying this chapter, the student will be able to:

1 Define types and characteristics of depression.

2 Differentiate between mental depression and general central nervous system (CNS) depression.

3 Discuss characteristics of antidepressants in terms of mechanism of action, indications for use, adverse effects, principles of therapy, and nursing process implications.

4 Compare and contrast selective serotonin reuptake inhibitors (SSRIs) with tricyclic antidepressants (TCAs).

5 List limitations for use of monoamine oxidase (MAO) inhibitor antidepressants.

6 Describe the use of lithium in bipolar disorder.

7 Discuss interventions to increase safety of lithium therapy.

8 Describe the nursing role in preventing, recognizing, and treating overdoses of antidepressant drugs and lithium.

Key Terms

Bipolar disorder	**Serotonin**
Hypomania	**Tyramine**
Mania	**Unipolar disorder**
Monoamine oxidase	

Depression

Depression is an affective disorder often described as the most common mental illness. It is characterized by depressed mood, feelings of sadness, or emotional upset, and it occurs in all age groups. Numerous terms have been used to describe depression. Mild depression occurs in everyone as a normal response to life stresses and losses and usually does not require treatment; severe or major depression is a psychiatric illness and requires treatment. Depression also is categorized as unipolar, in which people of usually normal moods experience recurrent episodes of depression, and bipolar disorder, in which episodes of depression alternate with episodes of mania.

MAJOR DEPRESSION

The American Psychiatric Association's *Diagnostic and Statistical Manual*, fourth edition, lists two major categories of depression. One category is *major depression*, which consists of a depressed mood plus at least five of the following symptoms:

Loss of energy
Fatigue
Indecisiveness
Difficulty thinking and concentrating
Loss of interest in appearance, work, and leisure and sexual activities
Inappropriate feelings of guilt and worthlessness
Loss of appetite and weight loss, or excessive eating and weight gain
Sleep disorders (hypersomnia or insomnia)
Somatic symptoms (*e.g.,* constipation, headache, atypical pain)
Obsession with death, thoughts of suicide
Psychotic symptoms, such as hallucinations and delusions

DYSTHYMIA

The other category is *dysthymia*, a chronically depressed mood or loss of interest in usual activities that is not severe enough or does not last long enough to meet the criteria for major depression. Dysthymia is further described as primary or secondary. Primary depression cannot be related to an identifiable cause; secondary depression may be precipitated by the following:

Environmental stress (*e.g.,* job loss or dissatisfaction, financial worries)
Adverse life events (*e.g.,* divorce, death of a family member or friend)
Drugs (alcohol; antiarrhythmics, such as lidocaine, procainamide, and tocainide; antihypertensive drugs, such as clonidine, methyldopa, and prazosin; beta-blockers; corticosteroids; opiates; and oral contraceptives)
Concurrent disease states, including endocrine disorders (hypothyroidism and hyperthyroidism, diabetes mellitus, adrenal insufficiency or excess), central nervous system (CNS) disorders (stroke, tumors, or other brain lesions; Parkinson's disease), cardiovascular disorders (myocardial infarction, congestive heart failure, hypertension), and miscellaneous disorders (rheumatoid arthritis, infectious disease, malnutrition)

Differentiating between major depression and dysthymia is difficult because the symptoms are similar; the main differences are the severity and duration of symptoms.

Seasonal affective disorder, a type of depression that occurs during the winter, also has been described. Its classification and differentiation from major depression and dysthymia are unclear.

ETIOLOGY

Despite extensive study, the etiology of depression has not been clearly delineated. Generally, depression is attributed to neurotransmitter or receptor abnormalities in the brain, with much of the available information derived from studies about the actions of antidepressant drugs. Some possible etiologic factors are described below.

Neurotransmitters

One hypothesis was that depression results from a deficiency of norepinephrine, serotonin, or both. This theory was supported by studies demonstrating that antidepressant drugs increased the amounts of one or both of these neurotransmitters in the CNS synapse by inhibiting their reuptake into the presynaptic neuron. Since the advent of the selective serotonin reuptake inhibitor (SSRI) antidepressants, much research has been focused on the role of serotonin. Serotonin helps regulate several behaviors that are disturbed in depression and other psychiatric disorders, such as mood, sleep, appetite, energy level, and cognitive and psychomotor functions. Thus, a disturbance in the serotonin system may play a primary or secondary role in the etiology of depression. Other neurotransmitters, such as dopamine and acetylcholine, probably also play a role.

Receptors

Emphasis shifted toward receptors because the neurotransmitter hypothesis did not explain why the amounts of neurotransmitter were increased within minutes to hours after single doses of a drug, but relief of depression occurred only after several weeks of drug therapy. Researchers identified changes in norepinephrine and serotonin receptors with chronic antidepressant drug therapy. Studies demonstrated that chronic drug administration (*i.e.*, increased neurotransmitter in the synapse for several weeks) results in fewer receptors on the postsynaptic membrane. This down-regulation of receptors, first noted with beta-adrenergic receptors, corresponds with therapeutic drug effects. All known treatments for depression (including electroconvulsive shock) lead to the down-regulation of beta receptors and occur in the same time period as the behavioral changes associated with antidepressant drug therapy.

Alpha$_2$ adrenergic receptors, located on presynaptic nerve terminals, may also play a role in depression. When these receptors are stimulated, they inhibit the release of norepinephrine. There is evidence that alpha$_2$ receptors are also down-regulated by antidepressant drugs, thus allowing increased norepinephrine release. With serotonin receptors, available antidepressants may increase the sensitivity of postsynaptic receptors and decrease the sensitivity of presynaptic receptors.

Physiologically, presynaptic receptors regulate the release and reuptake of neurotransmitters; postsynaptic receptors participate in the transmission of nerve impulses. It seems apparent that long-term administration of antidepressant drugs produces complex changes in the sensitivities of both presynaptic and postsynaptic receptor sites.

Neurotransmission Systems

There is an increasing awareness that depression is a complex disorder and probably has multiple causes. Moreover, the balance, integration, and interactions among neurotransmission systems are probably more important etiologic factors than single neurotransmitter or receptor alterations. For example, disturbances in the norepinephrine or serotonin neurotransmission system (see Chap. 5) are often implicated in depression. One current view is that the serotonin and norepinephrine systems are related and in balance in the CNS and that depression may result from an imbalance or an alteration in their relationship

Genetic and Endocrine Factors

Genetic factors are considered important in depression, with close relatives of a depressed person more likely to experience depression. In addition, endocrine abnormalities are often present in people who are depressed. These include disturbances in the hypothalamic-pituitary-adrenal axis, excessive secretion of cortisol, and altered thyroid function.

In bipolar disorder, periods of depression alternate with periods of mania, an excited state characterized by

excessive CNS stimulation with physical and mental hyperactivity (*e.g.*, energetic and constant movement, decreased sleep, talkativeness, racing thoughts, short attention span, grandiose ideation). Hypomania is the term sometimes used to indicate a lesser state of CNS stimulation and hyperactivity than mania. Like depression, mania and hypomania may result from abnormal functioning of neurotransmitters or receptors, such as a relative excess of excitatory neurotransmitters (*e.g.*, norepinephrine) or a relative deficiency of inhibitory neurotransmitters (*e.g.*, serotonin and gamma-aminobutyric acid [GABA]). Drugs that stimulate the CNS can cause manic and hypomanic behaviors that are easily confused with schizophreniform psychoses.

Antidepressant Drugs

Antidepressant drugs are used in the pharmacologic management of depressive disorders (also called mood or affective disorders). They are derived from several chemical groups. Older or first-generation antidepressants include the tricyclic antidepressants (TCAs) and the monoamine oxidase inhibitors (MAOIs). Newer or second-generation drugs include serotonin enhancers and several other drugs, some of which differ chemically from the tricyclics but are similar in pharmacologic actions and antidepressant effectiveness. Characteristics of these drugs and lithium, an antimanic agent used for bipolar affective disorder, are described in the following section.

TRICYCLIC ANTIDEPRESSANTS

TCAs are chemically and pharmacologically similar drugs. They contain a triple-ring nucleus from which their name is derived. The drugs are structurally similar to phenothiazine antipsychotic agents (see Chap. 9) and have similar antiadrenergic and anticholinergic properties. They produce a relatively high incidence of sedation, orthostatic hypotension, cardiac arrhythmias, and other adverse effects, in addition to dry mouth and anticholinergic effects. TCAs are well absorbed after oral administration. However, first-pass metabolism by the liver results in blood-level variations of 10- to 30-fold among people given identical doses. Once absorbed, these drugs are widely distributed throughout body tissues and metabolized by the liver to active and inactive metabolites. Amitriptyline (Elavil) is a commonly used TCA.

SELECTIVE SEROTONIN REUPTAKE INHIBITORS

Selective serotonin reuptake inhibitors (SSRIs) are as effective as TCAs and have a similar onset of action. They are well absorbed with oral administration, undergo extensive first-pass metabolism in the liver, are highly protein bound (about 95%), and have a half-life of 24 to 72 hours, which may lead to accumulation with chronic administration. Fluoxetine also forms active metabolites with a half-life of 7 to 9 days. Thus, steady-state blood levels are achieved slowly, and drug effects decrease slowly when fluoxetine is discontinued. The drugs do not produce the sedation, anticholinergic effects, orthostatic hypotension, cardiac arrhythmias, and weight gain associated with TCAs. Their adverse effects include CNS stimulation (*e.g.*, anxiety, nervousness, insomnia), nausea, anorexia, weight loss, and a skin rash that sometimes requires stopping the drug. The currently available drugs in this group are given once daily.

MONOAMINE OXIDASE INHIBITORS

MAOIs are well absorbed after oral administration and produce maximal inhibition of MAO within 5 to 10 days. However, clinical improvement in depression may require 2 to 3 weeks.

MAOIs may interact with numerous foods and drugs to produce hypertensive crisis (*i.e.*, severe hypertension, severe headache, fever, possible myocardial infarction, or intracranial hemorrhage). Foods that interact with MAOIs are those containing tyramine, a monoamine precursor of norepinephrine. Normally, tyramine is deactivated in the gastrointestinal tract and liver so that large amounts do not reach the systemic circulation. However, when deactivation of tyramine is blocked by MAOIs, tyramine is absorbed systemically and transported to adrenergic nerve terminals, where it causes a sudden release of large amounts of norepinephrine. Hypertensive crisis may result. Several drugs also may interact with MAOIs to cause hypertensive crisis. Foods and drugs to be avoided during (and 2–3 weeks after) drug therapy with MAOIs are listed in Table 10-1.

MISCELLANEOUS ANTIDEPRESSANTS

Bupropion (Wellbutrin) inhibits the reuptake of dopamine, norepinephrine, and serotonin. It was marketed with warnings and precautions related to seizure activity. Seizures are most likely to occur with doses above 450 mg/d and in clients known to have a seizure disorder. Recommendations to prevent seizures are described below.

After an oral dose, peak plasma levels are reached in about 2 hours. The average drug half-life is about 14 hours. The drug is metabolized in the liver and excreted primarily in the urine. Several metabolites are pharmacologically active. Dosage should be reduced with impaired hepatic or renal function. Acute episodes

of depression usually require several months of drug therapy.

In addition to seizures, common adverse effects include agitation, dry mouth, insomnia, headache, nausea and vomiting, constipation, and tremor. The drug has CNS stimulant effects (excitement, increased motor activity, restlessness, agitation, insomnia, anxiety) that may require a sedative during the first few days of administration. These effects may increase the risk of abuse.

Maprotiline (Ludiomil) is a tetracyclic antidepressant that also has anxiolytic properties. It causes adverse effects similar to the TCAs and seems to have few, if any, advantages over the TCAs.

Mirtazapine (Remeron) is a newer antidepressant that blocks presynaptic alpha$_2$-adrenergic receptors, which increases the release of norepinephrine and serotonin. The drug is well absorbed after oral administration, and peak plasma levels occur in about 2 hours after an oral dose. It is metabolized in the liver, most often to inactive metabolites. Common adverse effects include drowsiness (with accompanying cognitive and motor impairment), increased appetite, weight gain, dizziness, dry mouth, and constipation. Agranulocytosis is a rare adverse effect. Mirtazapine should not be taken concurrently with other CNS depressants (*e.g.*, alcohol or benzodiazepine antianxiety or hypnotic agents) because of additive sedation. In addition, it should not be taken concurrently with an MAOI or for 14 days after

Foods to Avoid	**Drugs to Avoid**
Aged cheese (*e.g.*, cheddar, Camembert, Stilton, Gruyere)	Amphetamines
Alcoholic beverages (beer, Chianti and other red wines)	Antiallergy and antiasthmatic drugs (*e.g.*, ephedrine, epinephrine, phenylpropanolamine, pseudoephedrine)
Avocados and guacamole dip	
Bananas	
Caffeine-containing beverages (coffee, tea, cola drinks)	Antidepressants (tricyclic antidepressants, serotonin reuptake inhibitors)
Chicken livers	
Chocolate (in large amounts)	
Fava bean pods	Antihistamines (including over-the-counter cough and cold remedies)
Figs (canned)	
Meat tenderizers	
Pickled herring	Antihypertensive drugs (*i.e.*, methyldopa)
Raisins	
Sour cream	Levodopa
Soy sauce	Meperidine
Yogurt	

TABLE 10-1 **FOODS AND DRUGS TO BE AVOIDED DURING THERAPY WITH MAO INHIBITOR DRUGS**

stopping an MAOI. An MAOI should not be started until at least 14 days after stopping mirtazapine.

Nefazodone (Serzone) inhibits the neuronal reuptake of serotonin and norepinephrine. It is contraindicated in pregnancy and should be used with caution in persons with cardiovascular or cerebrovascular disorders, dehydration, hypovolemia, mania, hypomania, suicidal ideation, hepatic cirrhosis, electroconvulsive therapy, debilitation, and lactation. It has a long half-life (2–3 days) and crosses the placenta. It is metabolized in the liver and excreted in breast milk, urine, and feces.

Adverse effects include CNS (headache, nervousness, insomnia, drowsiness, anxiety, tremor, dizziness, agitation, sedation, abnormal gait, confusion), gastrointestinal (anorexia, nausea, vomiting, constipation, diarrhea, dysphagia, gastroenteritis, gingivitis), cardiovascular (postural hypotension), and dermatologic (sweating, rash, pruritus, acne, alopecia, contact dermatitis) manifestations. Potentially significant drug–drug interactions include the risk of severe toxic effects if taken with MAOIs or nonsedating antihistamines (*e.g.*, astemizole, terfenadine). These combinations should be avoided. If a client on nefazodone is to be transferred to an MAOI, the nefazodone should be discontinued at least 7 days before starting the MAOI; if a client on an MAOI is to be transferred to nefazodone, the MAOI should be discontinued at least 14 days before starting nefazodone. There is also a risk of increased CNS depression with general anesthetics.

Trazodone (Desyrel) represents a different chemical class of antidepressants. Oral trazodone is well absorbed, and peak plasma concentrations are obtained within 30 minutes to 2 hours. Trazodone is metabolized by the liver and excreted primarily by the kidneys. Although trazodone reportedly produces less anticholinergic activity than the TCAs, it causes a number of other adverse effects, including sedation, dizziness, edema, cardiac arrhythmias, and priapism (prolonged and painful penile erection).

Venlafaxine (Effexor), which is chemically related to bupropion, inhibits the reuptake of norepinephrine, serotonin, and dopamine, thereby increasing the activity of these neurotransmitters in the brain. The drug crosses the placenta and may enter breast milk. It is metabolized in the liver and excreted in urine. It is contraindicated during pregnancy, and women should use effective birth-control methods while taking this drug. Adverse effects include CNS (anxiety, dizziness, dreams, insomnia, nervousness, somnolence, tremors), gastrointestinal (anorexia, nausea, vomiting, constipation, diarrhea), cardiovascular (hypertension, tachycardia, vasodilation), genitourinary (abnormal ejaculation, impotence, urinary frequency), and dermatologic (sweating, rash, pruritus) symptoms. Venlafaxine should not be taken concurrently with MAOIs because of increased serum levels and risks of toxicity. If a client on venlafaxine is to be transferred to an MAOI, the venlafaxine should be discontinued at least 7 days before starting the MAOI; if a client on an MAOI is to be transferred to venlafaxine, the MAOI should be discontinued at least 14 days before starting venlafaxine.

MOOD-STABILIZING AGENT

Lithium carbonate (Eskalith) is a naturally occurring metallic salt used in the management of bipolar affective disorder. Lithium is more effective in the treatment and prevention of mania than in preventing depression. It is sometimes described as an "antimanic" drug.

Lithium is well absorbed after oral administration. Peak serum levels occur in 1 to 3 hours after a dose of lithium and steady-state concentrations are reached in 5 to 7 days. Because serum concentrations of lithium vary widely among clients taking comparable doses, frequent monitoring of the serum lithium concentration is required.

Lithium is not metabolized by the body; it is entirely excreted by the kidneys, so adequate renal function is a prerequisite for lithium therapy. About 80% of a lithium dose is reabsorbed in the proximal renal tubules. The amount of reabsorption depends on the concentration of sodium in the proximal renal tubules. A deficiency of sodium causes more lithium to be reabsorbed and increases the risk of lithium toxicity; excessive sodium intake causes more lithium to be excreted (*i.e.*, "lithium diuresis") and may lower serum lithium levels to nontherapeutic ranges.

Before lithium therapy is begun, baseline studies of renal, cardiac, and thyroid status should be obtained because adverse drug effects involve these organ systems. Baseline electrolyte studies are also necessary.

MECHANISMS OF ACTION

Antidepressant drugs probably exert their effects by re-regulating or normalizing abnormal neurotransmission systems in the brain. More specifically, the drugs increase the amount of norepinephrine or serotonin in the CNS synapse and alter the number or sensitivity of receptors. After neurotransmitters are released from presynaptic nerve endings, the molecules that are not bound to receptors are normally inactivated by reuptake into the presynaptic nerve fibers that released them or metabolized by the enzyme MAO. Most antidepressants prevent the reuptake of multiple neurotransmitters; SSRIs selectively inhibit the reuptake of serotonin. MAOIs prevent the metabolism of neurotransmitter molecules. These mechanisms thereby increase the amount of neurotransmitter available to bind to receptors.

With chronic drug administration, receptors apparently adapt to the presence of increased neurotransmitter by decreasing their number or sensitivity to the neurotransmitter. More specifically, norepinephrine receptors, especially postsynaptic beta receptors and presynaptic alpha$_2$ receptors, are down-regulated. The serotonin$_2$ receptor, a postsynaptic receptor, may also be down-regulated, whereas the serotonin$_1$ receptor is unaffected. Thus, antidepressant effects are attributed to changes in receptors rather than changes in neurotransmitters. Although some of the drugs act more selectively on one neurotransmission system than another initially, this selectivity seems to be lost with chronic administration.

With lithium, the exact mechanism of action is unknown. However, it is known to affect the synthesis, release, and reuptake of several neurotransmitters in the brain, including acetylcholine, dopamine, GABA, and norepinephrine. For example, the drug may increase the activity of GABA, an inhibitory neurotransmitter. It also stabilizes postsynaptic receptor sensitivity to neurotransmitters, probably by competing with calcium, magnesium, potassium, and sodium ions for binding sites.

INDICATIONS FOR USE

Antidepressant drug therapy may be indicated if depressive symptoms persist at least 2 weeks, impair social relationships or work performance, and occur independently of life events. In addition, some SSRIs are used for the treatment of obsessive-compulsive disorder and are being studied for possible use in numerous other disorders such as panic disorder, obesity, eating disorders, substance abuse, and chronic pain. TCAs may be used in children and adolescents in the management of enuresis (bed-wetting), involuntary urination resulting from a physical or psychological disorder. In this setting, a TCA may be given after physical causes (*e.g.*, urethral irritation, excessive intake of fluids) have been ruled out.

CONTRAINDICATIONS FOR USE

Antidepressant drugs are contraindicated or must be used with caution in clients with acute schizophrenia; mixed mania and depression; suicidal tendencies; severe renal, hepatic, or cardiovascular disease; narrow-angle glaucoma; and seizure disorders.

Individual Antidepressants

Table 10-2 lists the names, routes, and dosage ranges of individual antidepressants.

TABLE 10-2	ANTIDEPRESSANT AGENTS	
	Routes and Dosage Ranges	
Generic/Trade Name	*Adults*	*Children*
Tricyclic Antidepressants		
Amitriptyline (Elavil, Endep, others)	PO 75–100 mg daily in divided doses, gradually increased to 150–300 mg daily if necessary. Maintenance dose, 50–100 mg once daily at bedtime IM 80–120 mg daily in 4 divided doses *Older adults*: PO 10 mg 3 times daily and 20 mg at bedtime	Adolescents, PO 10 mg 3 times daily and 20 mg at bedtime Enuresis in children 5–14 years: PO 25 mg once daily at bedtime
Amoxapine (Asendin)	PO 50 mg 3 times daily, increased to 100 mg 3 times daily on the third day. Maintenance dose may be given in a single dose at bedtime.	Not recommended for children under age 16 years
Desipramine (Pertofrane, Norpramin)	PO 75 mg daily in divided doses, gradually increased to a maximum of 200–300 mg daily if necessary *Older adults*: PO 25–50 mg daily in divided doses, gradually increased to 100 mg daily if necessary	Not recommended
Doxepin (Sinequan, Adapin)	PO 75–150 mg daily, gradually increased to a maximum of 300 mg daily if necessary	Not recommended
Imipramine (Tofranil)	PO 75 mg daily in 3 divided doses, gradually increased to a maximum of 300 mg daily if necessary. Maintenance dose, 75–150 mg daily *Older adults*: PO 30–40 mg daily in divided doses, increased to 100 mg daily if necessary	Enuresis: PO 25–50 mg 1 hour before bedtime
Nortriptyline (Aventyl, Pamelor)	PO 40 mg daily in divided doses, gradually increased to 100–150 mg daily if necessary	Enuresis: PO 25 mg once daily at bedtime

(continued)

TABLE 10-2 **ANTIDEPRESSANT AGENTS** (Continued)

Generic/Trade Name	Routes and Dosage Ranges	
	Adults	*Children*
Protriptyline (Vivactil)	PO 15 mg daily in divided doses, increased to 60 mg daily if necessary	
Trimipramine maleate (Surmontil)	PO 75–100 mg daily, gradually increased to 300 mg daily if necessary	
Monoamine Oxidase Inhibitor Antidepressants		
Phenelzine (Nardil)	PO 60 mg daily in 3 divided doses, increased to 90 mg daily if necessary	Dosage not established
Tranylcypromine (Parnate)	PO 20 mg daily in 2 divided doses in the morning and afternoon for 2 weeks, then adjusted according to client's response. Maximal daily dose, 30 mg	Dosage not established
Selective Serotonin Reuptake Inhibitor Antidepressants		
Fluoxetine (Prozac)	PO 20 mg once daily in the morning, increased after several weeks if necessary. Divide doses larger than 20 mg, and give morning and noon; maximum daily dose. 80 mg.	Dosage not established
Fluvoxamine (Luvox)	PO 50 mg once daily at bedtime, increased in 50-mg increments every 4–7 days if necessary. For daily amounts above 100 mg, give in 2 divided doses. Maximum daily dose, 300 mg	Dosage not established
Paroxetine (Paxil)	PO 20 mg once daily in the morning, increased after 3–4 weeks if necessary; maximum dose, 50 mg daily (40 mg for older adults)	Dosage not established
Sertraline (Zoloft)	PO 50 mg once daily morning or evening, increased at 1-week or longer intervals to a maximum daily dose of 200 mg	Dosage not established
Miscellaneous Antidepressants		
Bupropion (Wellbutrin)	PO 100 mg twice daily, increased to 100 mg 3 times daily if necessary. Maximal single dose, 150 mg	Dosage not established
Maprotiline (Ludiomil)	PO 75 mg daily in single or divided doses, increased to a maximum of 300 mg daily if necessary	Not recommended for children under age 18 years
Mirtazapine (Remeron)	PO 15 mg/d, in a single dose, at bedtime	Dosage not established
Nefazodone (Serzone)	PO 200 mg daily in 2 divided doses; increase at 1-week intervals in increments of 100–200 mg/d; usual range, 300–600 mg/d. *Elderly or debilitated adults*: PO initially 100 mg/d in 2 divided doses	Not recommended in children under age 18 years
Trazodone (Desyrel)	PO 100–300 mg daily, increased to a maximum dose of 600 mg daily if necessary	
Venlafaxine (Effexor)	PO initially 75 mg/d in 2 or 3 divided doses, with food. May be increased slowly up to 225 mg/d if necessary. In hepatic or renal impairment, reduce dose by 50% and increase very slowly.	Not recommended in children under age 18 years
Mood-Stabilizing Agent		
Lithium carbonate (Eskalith)	Bipolar disorder (formerly called manic-depressive disorder), PO 900–1200 mg daily in divided doses, gradually increased in 300-mg increments if necessary, according to serum lithium levels and client's response	Not FDA-approved for use in children under 12 years but sometimes given PO 300–900 mg or 30 mg/kg per day, in divided doses

Nursing Process

Assessment

Assess the client's condition in relation to depressive disorders.

- Identify clients at risk for current or potential depression. Areas to assess include health status, family and social relationships, and work status. Severe or prolonged illness, impaired interpersonal relationships, inability to work, and job dissatisfaction may precipitate depression. Depression also occurs without a specific, discernible cause.
- Observe for the signs and symptoms of depression listed above. Manifestations may occur in any client, not just those who have or are suspected of having psychiatric illness. Clinical manifestations are nonspecific and vary in severity. For example, fatigue and insomnia may be caused by a variety of disorders and range from mild to severe. When symptoms are present, try to determine their frequency, duration, and severity.
- When a client appears depressed or has a history of depression, assess for suicidal thoughts and behaviors. Statements indicating a detailed plan, accompanied by the intent, ability, and method for carrying out the plan, place the client at high risk for suicide.
- Identify the client's usual coping mechanisms for stressful situations. Coping mechanisms vary widely, and behavior that may be helpful to one client may not be helpful to another. For example, one person may prefer being alone or having decreased contact with family and friends, whereas another may find increased contact desirable.

Nursing Diagnoses

- Dysfunctional Grieving related to loss (of health, ability to perform usual tasks, job, significant other, and so forth)
- Self-Care Deficit related to fatigue and self-esteem disturbance with depression or sedation with antidepressant drugs
- Sleep Pattern Disturbance related to depression or insomnia with SSRIs
- Impaired Physical Mobility related to sedation with TCAs and related antidepressants
- Altered Thought Processes related to confusion (especially in older adults)
- Knowledge Deficit: Effects and appropriate use of antidepressant drugs
- Decreased Cardiac Output related to cardiac arrhythmias and hypotension with TCAs and related antidepressants
- Altered Tissue Perfusion related to hypotension with TCAs and related antidepressants
- Risk for Injury related to sedation with TCAs and related antidepressants
- Risk for Violence: Self-Directed or Directed at Others

Planning/Goals

The client will:

- Experience improvement of mood and depressive state
- Receive or self-administer the drugs correctly
- Be kept safe while sedated during therapy with the TCAs and related drugs
- Be assessed regularly for suicidal tendencies. If present, caretakers will implement safety measures.
- Be cared for by staff in areas of nutrition, hygiene, exercise, and social interactions when unable to provide self-care

- Resume self-care and other usual activities
- Avoid preventable adverse drug effects

Interventions

Use measures to prevent or decrease the severity of depression. General measures include supportive psychotherapy and reduction of environmental stress. Specific measures include the following:

- Support the client's usual mechanisms for handling stressful situations, when feasible. Helpful actions may involve relieving pain or insomnia, scheduling rest periods, and increasing or decreasing socialization.
- Call the client by name, encourage self-care activities, allow him or her to participate in setting goals and making decisions, and praise efforts to accomplish tasks. These actions promote a positive self-image.
- When signs and symptoms of depression are observed, initiate treatment before depression becomes severe. Institute suicide precautions for clients at risk. These usually involve close observation, often on a one-to-one basis, and removal of potential weapons from the environment. For clients hospitalized on medical-surgical units, transfer to a psychiatric unit may be needed.

 Teach clients and caretakers:

- To take antidepressant drugs as directed to maximize therapeutic benefits and minimize adverse effects. Do not alter doses when symptoms subside. Antidepressants are usually given for several months; lithium therapy may be lifelong.
- That therapeutic effects (relief of symptoms) may not occur for 2 or 3 weeks after drug therapy is started. If clients do not know that therapeutic effects are delayed, they may think the drug is ineffective and stop taking it prematurely.
- Not to take any other drugs without the physician's knowledge, including over-the-counter cold remedies. Potentially serious drug interactions may occur with prescription or nonprescription drugs.
- To tell any other physician, surgeon, or dentist consulted about the antidepressant drugs being taken. Potentially serious adverse effects or drug interactions may occur if certain other drugs are prescribed.

Evaluation

- Observe for behaviors indicating lessened depression.
- Interview regarding feelings and mood.
- Observe and interview regarding adverse drug effects.
- Observe and interview regarding suicidal thoughts and behaviors.

Principles of Therapy

DRUG SELECTION

Because the available drugs seem similarly effective, the choice of an antidepressant depends on the patient's previous history of drug response, if any, and the specific drug's adverse effects, especially in relation to the client's medical conditions. Guidelines for choosing a drug include the following:

1. The SSRIs are the drugs of first choice. These drugs are effective and generally produce fewer and milder adverse effects than other drugs. Guidelines for choosing one SSRI over another have not been established.
2. With TCAs, initial selection may be based on the client's previous response or susceptibility to adverse effects. For example, if a client (or a close family member) responded well to a particular drug in the past, that is probably the drug of choice for repeated episodes of depression. The response of family members to individual drugs may be significant because there is a strong genetic component to depression and drug response. If therapeutic effects do not occur within 4 weeks, the TCA probably should be discontinued or changed, because some clients tolerate or respond better to one TCA than to another.
3. MAOIs are third-line drugs for the treatment of depression because of their potential interactions with other drugs and certain foods. An MAOI is most likely to be prescribed when the client does not respond to other antidepressant drugs or when electroconvulsive therapy is refused or contraindicated.
4. The benefits, risks, and roles of bupropion, mirtazapine, nefazodone, and venlafaxine are not yet clearly defined.
5. Lithium is the primary drug of choice for clients with bipolar disorder. When used therapeutically, lithium is effective in controlling mania in about 65% to 80% of clients. When used prophylactically, the drug decreases the frequency and intensity of manic cycles. Carbamazepine (Tegretol), an anticonvulsant, may be as effective as lithium as a mood-stabilizing agent. It is often used in clients who do not respond to lithium, although it is not approved by the Food and Drug Administration (FDA) for that purpose.

Dosage and Administration

Dosage of antidepressant drugs should be individualized according to clinical response. Antidepressant drug therapy is usually initiated with small, divided doses that are gradually increased until therapeutic or adverse effects occur. Specific guidelines for dosage include the following:

1. With SSRIs, nefazodone, and venlafaxine, therapy is begun with once-daily oral administration of the manufacturer's recommended dosage. Dosage may be increased after 3 or 4 weeks if depression is not relieved. As with most other drugs, smaller doses may be indicated in older adults and clients taking multiple medications.

2. With TCAs, therapy is begun with small doses, which are increased to the desired dose over 1 to 2 weeks. Minimal effective doses are about 150 mg/d of imipramine or its equivalent. TCAs can be administered once or twice daily because they have long elimination half-lives. Once dosage is established, TCAs are often given once daily at bedtime. This regimen is effective and well tolerated by most clients. Elderly clients may experience fewer adverse reactions if divided doses are continued.
3. With bupropion, seizures are more likely to occur with large single doses, large total doses, and large or abrupt increases in dosage. Recommendations to avoid these risk factors are:
   a. Give the drug in equally divided doses, preferably at least 6 hours apart.
   b. Single doses are usually 100 mg; the maximal single dose is 150 mg.
   c. The recommended initial dose is 200 mg, gradually increased to 300 mg. If no clinical improvement occurs after several weeks of 300 mg/d, dosage may be increased to 450 mg, the maximal daily dose.
   d. The recommended maintenance dose is the lowest amount that maintains remission.
4. With lithium therapy, dosage should be based on serum lithium levels, control of symptoms, and occurrence of adverse effects. Serum levels are required because therapeutic doses are only slightly lower than toxic doses and because clients vary widely in rates of lithium absorption and excretion. Thus, a dose that is therapeutic in one client may be toxic or lethal in another. Lower doses are indicated for older adults and for clients with conditions that impair lithium excretion (*e.g.*, diuretic drug therapy, dehydration, low-salt diet, renal impairment, decreased cardiac output).

   When lithium therapy is being initiated, the serum drug concentration should be measured two or three times weekly in the morning, 12 hours after the last dose of lithium. For most clients, the therapeutic range of serum levels is 0.5 to 1.2 mEq/L (SI units, 0.5–1.2 mmol/L). Serum lithium levels should not exceed 1.5 mEq/L because the risk of serious toxicity is increased at higher levels.

   Once symptoms of mania are controlled, lithium doses should be lowered. Serum lithium levels should be measured at least every 3 months during long-term maintenance therapy.

Duration of Drug Therapy

Guidelines for the duration of antidepressant drug therapy are not well established, and there are differences of opinion. However, evidence seems to be accumulating that about 6 months of treatment are needed for an acute episode of depression and that long-term maintenance therapy may be desirable. One argument for long-term maintenance therapy is that depression tends to relapse or recur, and successive episodes often are more severe and more difficult to treat.

Maintenance therapy for depression requires close supervision and periodic reassessment of the client's condition and response. With the use of TCAs for acute depression, maintenance therapy usually consists of low doses for about 3 to 6 months after recovery, followed by gradual tapering of the dose and drug discontinuation. However, recent studies indicate that full therapeutic doses (if clients can tolerate the adverse effects) for up to 5 years are effective in preventing recurrent episodes. The long-term effects (beyond 2–4 months) of SSRIs and newer agents have not been studied.

With lithium, long-term therapy is the usual practice because of a high recurrence rate if the drug is discontinued. When lithium is discontinued, most often because of adverse effects or the client's lack of adherence to the prescribed regimen, gradually tapering the dose over 2 to 4 weeks delays recurrence of symptoms.

ASSESSMENT AND MANAGEMENT OF TOXICITY

Some antidepressant drugs are highly toxic and potentially lethal when taken in large doses. Toxicity is most likely to occur in depressed clients who intentionally ingest large amounts of drug in suicide attempts and in young children who accidentally gain access to improperly stored medication containers. Measures to prevent acute poisoning from drug overdose include dispensing only a few days' supply (i.e., 5–7 days) to clients with suicidal tendencies and storing the drugs in places inaccessible to young children. General measures to treat acute poisoning include early detection of signs and symptoms, stopping the drug, and instituting treatment if indicated. Specific measures include the following:

1. **SSRI overdose:** Symptoms include nausea, vomiting, agitation, restlessness, hypomania, and other signs of CNS stimulation. Management includes symptomatic and supportive treatment, such as maintaining an adequate airway and ventilation and administering activated charcoal.
2. **TCA overdose:** Symptoms occur about 1 to 4 hours after drug ingestion and consist primarily of CNS depression and cardiovascular effects (e.g., nystagmus, tremor, restlessness, seizures, hypotension, arrhythmias, myocardial depression). Death usually results from cardiac, respiratory, and circulatory failure. Management of TCA toxicity consists of performing gastric lavage and giving activated charcoal to reduce drug absorption, giving cathartics to increase drug excretion, establishing and maintaining a patent airway, performing continuous electrocardiographic (ECG) monitoring of comatose clients or those with

respiratory insufficiency or wide QRS intervals, giving intravenous fluids and vasopressors for severe hypotension, and giving intravenous phenytoin or a parenteral benzodiazepine (e.g., diazepam, lorazepam) if seizures occur.
3. **MAOI overdose:** Symptoms occur 12 hours or more after drug ingestion and consist primarily of adrenergic effects (e.g., tachycardia, increased rate of respiration, agitation, tremors, convulsive seizures, sweating, heart block, hypotension, delirium, coma). Management consists of forced diuresis, acidification of urine, or hemodialysis to remove the drug from the body.
4. **Bupropion overdose:** Symptoms include agitation and other mental status changes, nausea and vomiting, and seizures. General treatment measures include hospitalization, decreasing absorption (e.g., inducing vomiting and giving activated charcoal to conscious clients), and supporting vital functions. If seizures occur, an intravenous benzodiazepine (e.g., lorazepam) is the drug of first choice.
5. **Nefazodone or venlafaxine overdose:** Symptoms include increased incidence or severity of adverse effects, with nausea, vomiting, and drowsiness most often reported. Hypotension and excessive sedation may occur with nefazodone, seizures and diastolic hypertension with venlafaxine. There are no specific antidotes; treatment is symptomatic and supportive.
6. **Lithium overdose:** Toxic manifestations occur with serum lithium levels above 2.5 mEq/L and include nystagmus, tremors, oliguria, confusion, impaired consciousness, visual or tactile hallucinations, choreiform movements, convulsions, coma, and death. Treatment involves supportive care to maintain vital functions, including correction of fluid and electrolyte imbalances. With severe overdoses, hemodialysis is preferred because it removes lithium from the body.

USE IN PERIOPERATIVE PERIODS

Antidepressants must be used very cautiously, if at all, perioperatively because of the risk of serious adverse effects and adverse interactions with anesthetics and other commonly used drugs. MAOIs are contraindicated and should be discontinued at least 10 days before elective surgery. TCAs should be discontinued several days before elective surgery and resumed several days postoperatively. SSRIs and miscellaneous antidepressants have not been studied in relation to perioperative use; however, it seems reasonable to discontinue the drugs when feasible because of potential adverse effects, especially on the cardiovascular system and CNS. It is generally recommended that antidepressants be tapered in dosage and gradually discontinued. Lithium should be stopped 1 to 2 days before surgery and resumed when full oral intake of food and fluids is allowed. Lithium may prolong the effects of anesthetics and neuromuscular blockers.

Use in Children

In children, antidepressant drugs should be used only when clearly indicated and then very cautiously. TCAs are not recommended for use in children under 12 years except for short-term treatment of enuresis in children over 6 years. With imipramine, the most commonly used drug, dosage should not exceed 2.5 mg/kg/d. ECG changes have occurred in children taking higher doses; the significance of the changes in terms of cardiac function is unknown. Effectiveness for enuresis may decrease with continued use, and no residual benefits continue once the drug is stopped. Common adverse effects include sedation, fatigue, nervousness, and sleep disorders.

Safety and effectiveness have not been established for amoxapine (Asendin) in children under 16 years, MAOIs in children under 16 years, and SSRIs, bupropion, maprotiline, nefazodone, or venlafaxine in children under 18 years. Lithium is not approved by the FDA for use in children under 12 years, but it has been used to treat bipolar disorder and aggressiveness. Children normally excrete lithium more rapidly than adults. As with adults, initial doses should be relatively low and gradually increased according to regular measurements of serum drug levels.

Use in Older Adults

SSRIs are probably the drugs of choice in older adults as in younger ones, because they cause fewer sedative, anticholinergic, cardiotoxic, and psychomotor adverse effects than the TCAs and related antidepressants. These drugs produce similar adverse effects in older adults as in younger adults. Although their effects in older adults are not well delineated, SSRIs may be eliminated more slowly, and smaller or less frequent doses may be prudent. If a TCA is chosen for an older adult, nortriptyline or desipramine is preferred. In addition, any TCA should be given in small doses initially and gradually increased over several weeks, if necessary, to achieve therapeutic effects. Initial and maintenance doses should be small because the drugs are metabolized and excreted more slowly than in younger adults. Dosage should be decreased by 30% to 50% to avoid serious adverse reactions. Impaired compensatory mechanisms make older adults more likely to experience anticholinergic effects, confusion, hypotension, and sedation. MAOIs may be more likely to cause hypertensive crises in older adults because cardiovascular, renal, and hepatic functions are often diminished. With nefazodone, smaller initial doses and increments are recommended. With venlafaxine, smaller doses are indicated in the presence of renal impairment, which commonly occurs in older adults. With lithium, initial doses should generally be low and increased gradually, according to regular measurements of serum drug levels.

Home Care

Whatever the primary problem for which a home care nurse is visiting a client, he or she must be vigilant for signs and symptoms of major depression. Depression often accompanies any serious physical illness and may occur in many other circumstances as well. The main role of the nurse may be in recognizing depressive states and referring clients for treatment. If antidepressant medications were recently started, the nurse may need to remind the client that it takes 2 or 3 weeks to feel better; the nurse should encourage the client to continue taking the medication. Also, observe the client's response and assess for suicidal thoughts or plans.

NURSING ACTIONS   ANTIDEPRESSANTS

NURSING ACTIONS	RATIONALE/EXPLANATION
1. Administer accurately a. Give fluoxetine and other SSRIs in the morning.	To prevent insomnia
b. Give venlafaxine and lithium with food.	To decrease gastrointestinal effects (*e.g.*, nausea and vomiting)
2. Observe for therapeutic effects a. With antidepressants, observe for statements of feeling better or being less depressed; increased appetite, physical activity, and interest in surroundings; improved sleep patterns; improved appearance; decreased anxiety; decreased somatic complaints.	Therapeutic effects usually do not occur for 2 to 3 weeks after drug therapy is started.

NURSING ACTIONS	*RATIONALE/EXPLANATION*

b. With lithium, observe for decreases in manic behavior and mood swings.

Therapeutic effects do not occur until about 7 to 10 days after therapeutic serum drug levels are attained. In severe mania, an antipsychotic drug is usually given to control behavior until the lithium takes effect.

3. Observe for adverse effects

a. With SSRIs, nefazodone, and venlafaxine, observe for headache, nervousness, insomnia, nausea, diarrhea, dry mouth, constipation, sedation, skin rash, palpitations, and dyspnea.

Although numerous adverse effects may occur, they are usually less serious than those occurring with most other antidepressants. Compared to the TCAs, SSRIs and other newer drugs are less likely to cause significant sedation, hypotension, and cardiac arrhythmias but are more likely to cause nausea, nervousness, and insomnia.

b. With TCAs, observe for:

(1) Dry mouth, constipation, blurred vision, tachycardia, orthostatic hypotension, drowsiness, dizziness, excessive sweating, weight gain

(2) Urinary retention, fainting, tremor, nausea, cardiac arrhythmias

(3) Confusion, delirium, seizures, skin rash, agranulocytosis, cholestatic jaundice, impotence, transition to mania in clients with bipolar disorder.

Most adverse effects result from anticholinergic or antiadrenergic activity. Symptoms listed in (1) commonly occur, especially when TCA therapy is initiated. Symptoms listed in (2) occur less frequently and those listed in (3) rarely occur.

c. With MAOIs, observe for hypotension, dizziness, increased incidence of angina, dry mouth, blurred vision, constipation, urinary retention, hypoglycemia.

Anticholinergic effects are common. Hypoglycemia results from a drug-induced reduction in blood sugar.

d. With bupropion, observe for seizure activity, central nervous system (CNS) stimulation (agitation, insomnia, hyperactivity, hallucinations, delusions), headache, nausea and vomiting, and weight loss.

Adverse effects are most likely to occur if recommended doses are exceeded.

e. With lithium observe for:

(1) Metallic taste, hand tremors, nausea, polyuria, polydipsia, diarrhea, muscular weakness, fatigue, edema, and weight gain

(2) More severe nausea and diarrhea, vomiting, ataxia, incoordination, dizziness, slurred speech, blurred vision, tinnitus, muscle twitching and tremors, increased muscle tone

Most clients who take lithium experience adverse effects. Symptoms listed in (1) are common, occur at therapeutic serum drug levels (0.8–1.2 mEq/L), and usually subside during the first few weeks of drug therapy. Symptoms listed in (2) occur at higher serum drug levels (1.5–2.5 mEq/L). Nausea may be decreased by giving lithium with meals. Propranolol (Inderal), 20–120 mg daily, may be given to control tremors. Severe or persistent adverse effects may be managed by decreasing lithium dosage, omitting a few doses, or discontinuing the drug temporarily. Toxic symptoms occur at serum drug levels above 2.5 mEq/L.

(3) Leukocytosis

Lithium mobilizes white blood cells (WBCs) from bone marrow to the bloodstream. Maximum increase in WBCs occurs in 7 to 10 days. The drug has been given therapeutically for this effect in cancer patients with neutropenia, but studies do not indicate decreased infections.

4. Observe for drug interactions

a. Drugs that *increase* effects of SSRIs:

(1) Cimetidine

(2) MAOIs

Drug interactions with the SSRIs vary with individual drugs.

May increase serum drug levels of SSRIs by slowing their metabolism

These two types of antidepressants should not be given concurrently or close together because serious and fatal reac-

(continued)

NURSING ACTIONS	*RATIONALE/EXPLANATION*
	tions have occurred. Signs and symptoms include hyperthermia, muscle rigidity or spasm, agitation, delirium, and coma. To avoid this reaction, an SSRI should not be started for at least 2 weeks after an MAOI is discontinued, and an MAOI should not be started for at least 5 weeks after an SSRI has been discontinued. The reaction is attributed to excessive serotonin and is sometimes called the "serotonin syndrome."
b. Drugs that *decrease* effects of SSRIs:	
Anticonvulsants (phenobarbital, phenytoin)	These drugs induce liver enzymes that accelerate the metabolism of the SSRIs.
c. Drugs that alter the effects of nefazodone and venlafaxine:	
MAOIs	See SSRIs, above. This combination should be avoided. Nefazodone or venlafaxine should be discontinued at least 7 days before starting an MAOI, and an MAOI should be stopped at least 14 days before starting nefazodone or venlafaxine.
d. Drugs that increase effects of TCAs:	
(1) Antiarrhythmics (*e.g.*, quinidine, disopyramide, procainamide)	Additive effects on cardiac conduction, increasing risk of heart block
(2) Antihistamines, atropine, and other drugs with anticholinergic effects	Additive anticholinergic effects (*e.g.*, dry mouth, blurred vision, urinary retention, constipation)
(3) Antihypertensives	Additive hypotension
(4) Cimetidine, fluoxetine	Increase risks of toxicity by decreasing hepatic metabolism and increasing blood levels of TCAs
(5) CNS depressants (*e.g.*, alcohol, benzodiazepine antianxiety and hypnotic agents, narcotic analgesics)	Additive sedation and CNS depression
(6) Urinary alkalizers (*e.g.*, sodium bicarbonate)	Decrease excretion of TCAs
e. Drugs that *decrease* effects of TCAs:	
(1) Barbiturates, chloral hydrate, nicotine (cigarette smoking)	These drugs decrease blood levels of TCAs by increasing the rate of hepatic metabolism of the antidepressant agent.
(2) Urinary acidifiers (*e.g.*, ascorbic acid)	Increase excretion of TCAs
f. Drugs that *increase* effects of MAOIs	
(1) Anticholinergic drugs (*e.g.*, atropine, antipsychotic agents, TCAs)	Additive anticholinergic effects
(2) Adrenergic agents (*e.g.*, epinephrine, isoproterenol, phenylephrine), alcohol (some beers and wines), levodopa, meperidine	Hypertensive crisis may occur.
g. Drugs that *increase* effects of lithium:	
(1) Angiotensin-converting enzyme inhibitors (*e.g.*, captopril)	These drugs decrease renal clearance of lithium and thus increase serum lithium levels.
(2) Diuretics (*e.g.*, ethacrynic acid, furosemide, hydrochlorothiazide)	Increase neurotoxicity and cardiotoxicity of lithium by increasing excretion of sodium and potassium and thereby decreasing excretion of lithium.
(3) Nonsteroidal anti-inflammatory drugs (NSAIDs)	These drugs decrease renal clearance of lithium and thus increase serum levels and risks of lithium toxicity.

NURSING ACTIONS	RATIONALE/EXPLANATION
(4) Phenothiazines	Increased risk of hyperglycemia
(5) Potassium iodide, TCAs	Increased risk of hypothyroidism
(6) TCAs	May increase antidepressant effects of lithium and are sometimes given in combination with lithium for this purpose. These drugs also may precipitate a manic episode.
h. Drugs that *decrease* effects of lithium.	
i. Acetazolamide (Diamox), sodium bicarbonate, sodium chloride (in excessive amounts), drugs with a high sodium content (*e.g.*, ticarcillin), theophylline compounds	Increase excretion of lithium

5. Teach clients
  a. With all antidepressants:

(1) Avoid activities that require high degrees of alertness and physical coordination (*e.g.*, operating a motor vehicle or other machinery) until reasonably sure the medication does not impair abilities.	For safety
(2) Avoid alcohol and other CNS depressants.	Additive CNS depression may occur.
(3) Do not take other prescription or over-the-counter drugs without consulting a health care provider	Potentially serious drug interactions may occur.
b. With SSRIs, nefazodone, and venlafaxine, notify a health care provider if a skin rash or other allergic reaction occurs.	An allergic reaction may require that the drug be discontinued.
c. With TCAs report urinary retention, fainting, irregular heartbeat, seizures, restlessness, and mental confusion.	These are potentially serious adverse drug effects. The physician may be able to alter drug therapy and decrease adverse effects.

  d. With MAOIs:

(1) Report severe headache to the physician.	Severe headache may be a symptom of a serious adverse effect.
(2) Avoid the foods and drugs listed in Table 10-1.	Severe hypertension and intracranial hemorrhage may occur.

  e. With lithium:

(1) Do not alter dietary salt intake.	Deceased salt intake (*e.g.*, low-salt diet) increases risk of adverse effects from lithium. Increased intake may decrease therapeutic effects.
(2) Drink 2 to 3 quarts of fluids daily; avoid excessive intake of caffeine-containing beverages.	Dehydration increases lithium toxicity; caffeine has a diuretic effect.
(3) Minimize activities that cause excessive perspiration.	Loss of salt in sweat increases risk of adverse effects from lithium.
(4) Report for measurements of lithium blood levels as instructed, and do not take the morning dose of lithium until the blood sample has been obtained.	Regular measurements of blood lithium levels are necessary for safe and effective lithium therapy. Accurate measurement of serum drug levels requires that blood be drawn 12 hours after the previous dose of lithium.

✔ REVIEW AND APPLICATION EXERCISES

1. During the initial assessment of any client, what kinds of appearances or behaviors may indicate depression?

2. Is antidepressant drug therapy indicated for most episodes of temporary sadness? Why or why not?

3. What are the major groups of antidepressant drugs?

4. How do the drugs act to relieve depression?

5. When a client begins antidepressant drug therapy, why is it important to explain that relief of depression may not occur for 2 to 3 weeks?

6. What are common adverse effects of TCAs, and how may they be minimized?

7. What is the advantage of giving a TCA at bedtime rather than in the early morning?

8. For a client taking an MAOI, what information would you provide for preventing a hypertensive crisis?

9. How do the SSRIs differ from TCAs?

10. How do the newer drugs, mirtazapine, nefazodone and venlafaxine, compare with the SSRIs in terms of adverse effects and adverse drug–drug interactions?

11. List the main elements of treatment for antidepressant overdoses.

12. What are common adverse effects of lithium, and how may they be minimized?

13. What is the nurse's role in assessing and managing depression in the home setting?

SELECTED REFERENCES

American Psychiatric Association. (1994). *Diagnostic and statistical manual of mental disorders,* 4th ed. Washington, D.C.: American Psychiatric Association.

Bressler, R. (1993). Depression. In R. Bressler & M.D. Katz (Eds.), *Geriatric pharmacology*, pp. 329–373. New York: McGraw-Hill.

Depression Guideline Panel. (1993). *Clinical practice guideline: Depression in primary care, 2: Treatment of major depression.* Rockville, MD: U.S. Department of Health and Human Services, Public Health Service, Agency for Health Care Policy and Research; AHCPR publication No. 93-0551.

Drug facts and comparisons. (1996). St. Louis: Facts and Comparisons.

Dubovsky, S.L. (1994). Geriatric neuropsychopharmacology. In C.E. Coffey & J.L. Cummings (Eds.), *The American Psychiatric Press Textbook of geriatric neuropsychiatry.* Washington, D.C.: American Psychiatric Press.

Faedda, G.L., Tondo, L., Baldessarini, R.J., Suppes, T., & Tohen, M. (1993). Outcome after rapid vs. gradual discontinuation of lithium treatment in bipolar disorders. *Archives of General Psychiatry, 50:*448–455.

Fankhauser, M.P. (1993). Bipolar disorder. In J.T. DiPiro, R.L. Talbert, P.E. Hayes, G.C. Yee, G.R. Matzke, & L.M. Posey (Eds.), *Pharmacotherapy: A pathophysiologic approach*, 2nd ed., pp. 1044–1064. Norwalk, CT: Appleton & Lange.

Perry, P.J. (1994). Clinical psychopharmacology and other somatic therapies. In G. Winokur & P.J. Clayton (Eds.), *The medical basis of psychiatry*, 2nd ed., pp. 545–588. Philadelphia: W.B. Saunders.

Schatzberg. A.F., & Nemeroff, C.B. (Eds.). (1995). *The American Psychiatric Press Textbook of psychopharmacology.* Washington, D.C.: American Psychiatric Press.

Shearer, S.L., & Adams, G.K. (1993). Nonpharmacologic aids in the treatment of depression. *American Family Physician, 47:*435–441.

Sherr, J. (1996). Psychopharmacology and other biologic therapies. In K.M. Fortinash & P.A. Holoday-Worret (Eds.), *Psychiatric-mental health nursing*, pp. 531–564. St. Louis: C.V. Mosby.

Stoudemire, A., Moran, M.G., & Fogel, B.S. (1995). Psychopharmacology in the medically ill patient. In A.F. Schatzberg & C.B. Nemeroff (Eds.), *The American Psychiatric Press Textbook of psychopharmacology*, pp. 783–801. Washington, D.C.: American Psychiatric Press.

Venlafaxine—A new antidepressant. *The Medical Letter, 36:*49–50 (June 10, 1994).

Wells, B.G., & Hayes, P.E. (1993). Depressive disorders. In J.T. DiPiro, R.L. Talbert, P.E. Hayes, G.C. Yee, G.R. Matzke, & L.M. Posey (Eds.), *Pharmacotherapy: A pathophysiologic approach*, 2nd ed., pp. 1065–1083. Norwalk, CT: Appleton & Lange.

Ziring, B. (1993). Issues in the perioperative care of the patient with psychiatric illness. *Medical Clinics of North America, 77*(2):443–452.

Anticonvulsants

Objectives

After studying this chapter, the student will be able to:

1 Define terms commonly used to describe seizure disorders.

2 Discuss major factors that influence choice of an anticonvulsant drug for a client with a seizure disorder.

3 Differentiate uses and effects of commonly used anticonvulsant drugs.

4 Apply the nursing process with clients experiencing selected seizure disorders.

Key Terms

Convulsion	**Seizure**
Epilepsy	**Status epilepticus**
Gingival hyperplasia	

Seizure Disorders

Anticonvulsant drugs (also called antiepileptic drugs or AEDs) are used to treat seizure disorders. The terms "seizure" and "convulsion" are often used interchangeably, although they are not the same. A *seizure* involves a brief episode of abnormal electrical activity in nerve cells of the brain that may or may not be accompanied by visible changes in appearance or behavior. A *convulsion* is a common, tonic-clonic type of seizure characterized by spasmodic contractions of involuntary muscles.

Seizures may occur as single events in response to hypoglycemia, fever, electrolyte imbalances, overdoses of numerous drugs (*e.g.*, cocaine, isoniazid, lidocaine, lithium, phenothiazine antipsychotic drugs, theophylline), and withdrawal of alcohol or sedative-hypnotic drugs. In these instances, treatment of the underlying problem or temporary use of an anticonvulsant drug may relieve the seizures.

EPILEPSY

When seizures occur in a chronic, recurrent pattern, the disorder is called *epilepsy*, and drug therapy is usually required. Epilepsy is characterized by abnormal and excessive electrical discharges of nerve cells. It is diagnosed by clinical signs and symptoms of seizure activity and by the presence of abnormal brain wave patterns on the electroencephalogram (EEG). The cause of most cases of epilepsy is unknown. When epilepsy begins in infancy, causes include developmental defects, metabolic disease, or birth injury. When it begins in adulthood, it is usually caused by an acquired brain disorder, such as head injury, disease or infection of the brain and spinal cord, cerebrovascular accident (stroke), metabolic disorder, primary or metastatic brain tumor, or other recognizable neurologic disease.

Epilepsy is classified as partial and generalized seizures. *Partial* or *focal seizures* begin in a specific area of the brain and produce symptoms ranging from simple motor and sensory manifestations to more complex abnormal movements and bizarre behavior. Movements are usually automatic, repetitive, and inappropriate to the situation, such as chewing, swallowing, or aversive movements. Behavior is sometimes so bizarre that the person is diagnosed as psychotic or schizophrenic.

Generalized seizures are bilateral and symmetric and have no discernible point of origin in the brain. The most common type is the tonic-clonic or major motor seizure, formerly called grand mal seizures. The tonic phase involves sustained contraction of skeletal muscles; abnormal postures, such as opisthotonos; and absence of respiration, during which the person becomes cyanotic. The clonic phase is characterized by rapid rhythmic and symmetric jerking movements of the body. Tonic-clonic seizures are sometimes preceded by an aura, a brief warning, such as a flash of light or a specific sound.

Another type of generalized seizure is the absence seizure, characterized by abrupt alterations in consciousness that last only a few seconds. The person may have a blank, staring expression with or without blinking of the eyelids, twitching of the head or arms, and other motor movements. Other types of generalized seizures include the myoclonic type (contraction of a muscle or group of muscles) and the akinetic type (absence of movement). Some people are subject to mixed seizures.

Status epilepticus is a life-threatening emergency characterized by generalized tonic-clonic convulsions occurring at close intervals. The client does not regain consciousness between seizures, and hypotension, hypoxia, and cardiac arrhythmias may occur. There is a high risk of permanent brain damage and death unless prompt, appropriate treatment is instituted. In a person taking medications for a diagnosed seizure disorder, the most common cause of status epilepticus is abruptly stopping anticonvulsant drugs. In other clients, whether they are known to have a seizure disorder or not, causes of status epilepticus include brain trauma or tumors, systemic or central nervous system (CNS) infections, alcohol withdrawal, and overdoses of drugs, such as cocaine, lidocaine, theophylline, and many others.

Anticonvulsant Drugs

Anticonvulsant drugs, which belong to several different chemical groups, can control seizure activity but do not cure the underlying disorder. Long-term administration is usually required. Most anticonvulsant drugs can be taken orally and are absorbed through the intestinal mucosa. The degree of absorption depends on drug solubility and other chemical or enzymatic conversions in the gastrointestinal tract. After absorption, the drugs pass through the liver and undergo transformation by liver enzymes, during which some of the drug is inactivated. Almost all anticonvulsant drugs are metabolized in the liver.

MECHANISM OF ACTION

Anticonvulsant drugs have similar antiseizure properties, but the precise mechanism and site of action are unclear. It is thought that the drugs act in two ways to control seizure activity. First, they may act directly on abnormal neurons to decrease neuronal excitability and responsiveness to stimuli. Consequently, the seizure threshold is raised, and seizure activity is decreased. Second, and more commonly, they prevent the spread of impulses to normal neurons surrounding the abnormal ones. This helps to prevent or minimize seizures by confining excessive electrical activity to a small portion of the brain.

The drugs' ability to reduce the responsiveness of neurons to stimuli may be related to alterations in the activity of sodium and other ions at the cell membrane. Such ionic activity is necessary for normal conduction of nerve impulses, and changes engendered by the anticonvulsant drugs result in stabilized, less responsive cell membranes. In addition, benzodiazepines and perhaps other AEDs may enhance the effects of gamma-aminobutyric acid (GABA), a major inhibitory neuro-transmitter in the brain.

INDICATIONS FOR USE

The major clinical indication for AEDs is the prevention or treatment of seizure activity, especially the chronic recurring seizures of epilepsy. Indications for particular drugs depend on the types of seizures involved. In addition to maintenance treatment of epilepsy, AEDs also are used to stop acute convulsions and status epilepticus. The drug of choice for this purpose is an intravenous (IV) benzodiazepine, such as diazepam (Valium) or lorazepam (Ativan). Once acute seizure activity is controlled, a longer-acting drug, such as phenytoin, is given to prevent recurrence. AEDs also are used prophylactically in clients with brain trauma from injury or surgery.

CONTRAINDICATIONS FOR USE

Anticonvulsants are contraindicated or must be used with caution in clients with CNS depression. Phenytoin, ethosuximide, and carbamazepine are contraindicated with hepatic or renal damage and bone marrow depression (*e.g.*, leukopenia, agranulocytosis). Valproic acid is contraindicated with liver disease.

Individual Anticonvulsant Drugs

Phenytoin (Dilantin) is one of the oldest and most widely used AEDs; it is generally considered the prototype drug. It is effective for generalized tonic-clonic and some partial seizures, such as psychomotor seizures. Phenytoin is often the initial drug of choice, especially in adults. It is also used to prevent seizures in people who have had brain surgery or brain injury. Phenytoin is ineffective in absence, myoclonic, or akinetic seizures. The drug also is used occasionally to treat cardiac arrhythmias.

The rate at which phenytoin is metabolized varies, but the average half-life is about 18 to 24 hours. The clinical significance of this relatively long half-life is that phenytoin can be given once or twice daily and that, when it is started at usual maintenance doses, a steady-state concentration in plasma is not reached for about 7 to 21 days. The therapeutic serum level is 5 to 20 µg/ml (SI units 40–80 µmol/L). Concentrations at or above the upper therapeutic level may be associated with clinical signs of toxicity.

Fosphenytoin (Cerebyx) is a prodrug formulation that is rapidly hydrolyzed to phenytoin after IV or IM injection. It is approved for treatment of status epilepticus and for short-term use in clients who cannot take oral phenytoin. In contrast to other preparations of injectable phenytoin, fosphenytoin causes minimal tissue irritation, can be diluted with 5% dextrose or 0.9% sodium chloride solution, and can be given IV more rapidly. The disadvantages of fosphenytoin include higher costs and potential confusion with dosage and administration. The manufacturer recommends that all dosages be expressed in phenytoin equivalents (PE). Fosphenytoin is available in 2-ml and 10-ml vials with 50 mg PE/ml (fosphenytoin 75 mg/ml). For IV administration, fosphenytoin can be diluted to a concentration of 1.5–25 mg PE/ml, and infused at a maximal rate of 150 mg PE/minute. The manufacturer of the Dilantin brand of parenteral phenytoin intended to stop production; it is unknown whether manufacturers of generic parenteral phenytoin will continue to market their products. Oral phenytoin preparations are not affected.

Phenytoin
Routes and Dosage Ranges

Adults: PO 100 mg three times daily initially; 300 mg (long-acting) once daily as maintenance
IV 100 mg q6–8h; maximum 50 mg/min
Children: PO 4–7 mg/kg/d in divided doses; maximum dose, 300 mg/d

Fosphenytoin
Routes and Dosage Ranges

Adults: Nonmergent seizures, IV, IM loading dose 1–20 mg PE/kg; maintenance dose 4–6 mg PE/kg/d; status epilepticus, IV 15–20 mg PE/kg, at a rate of 100–150 mg PE/min
Children: Dosage not established

Carbamazepine (Tegretol) is related chemically to the tricyclic antidepressants and pharmacologically to phenytoin. It is used mainly for psychomotor, generalized tonic-clonic, and mixed seizures. It is ineffective for absence, myoclonic, or akinetic seizures. The therapeutic range of serum drug levels is about 4 to 12 µg/ml (SI units, 17–51 µmol/L).

Carbamazepine is contraindicated in clients with previous bone marrow depression or hypersensitivity to carbamazepine or tricyclic antidepressants and in clients receiving monoamine oxidase inhibitors (MAOIs). MAOIs should be discontinued at least 14 days before carbamazepine is started. Carbamazepine also is used to treat facial pain associated with trigeminal neuralgia (tic douloureux).

Route and Dosage Ranges

Adults: Epilepsy, PO 200 mg twice a day initially, increased gradually to 600–1200 mg if needed, in three or four divided doses
Trigeminal neuralgia, PO 200 mg/d initially, increased gradually to 1200 mg if necessary
Children: PO 200 mg twice a day initially, gradually increased to 20–30 mg/kg/d if necessary to control seizures

Clonazepam (Klonopin), **diazepam** (Valium), and **lorazepam** (Ativan) are benzodiazepines (see Chap. 8) used in seizure disorders. Clonazepam may be used alone or with other anticonvulsant drugs in myoclonic or akinetic seizures. It is possibly effective in generalized tonic-clonic and psychomotor seizures. Its effectiveness in absence seizures is variable, but it may be helpful in some clients who do not respond to ethosuximide. Tolerance to anticonvulsant effects develops with long-term use. Clonazepam has a long half-life and may require weeks of continued administration to achieve therapeutic serum levels. As with other benzodiazepines, clonazepam produces physical dependence and withdrawal symptoms. Because of its long half-life, withdrawal symptoms may appear several days after administration is stopped. Abrupt withdrawal may precipitate seizure activity or status epilepticus.

Diazepam and lorazepam are used in seizure disorders to terminate acute convulsive seizures, especially the life-threatening seizures of status epilepticus. Diazepam has a short duration of action and must be given in repeated doses. In status epilepticus, it is followed with a long-acting anticonvulsant, such as phenytoin. Lorazepam has become the drug of choice for status epilepticus because its effects last longer than those of diazepam.

Clonazepam
Route and Dosage Ranges

Adults: PO 1.5 mg/d, increased by 0.5 mg/d every 3–7 d if necessary; maximum dose, 20 mg/d
Children: PO 0.01–0.03 mg/kg/d, increased by 0.25–0.5 mg/d every 3–7 d if necessary; maximum dose, 0.2 mg/kg/d

Diazepam
Route and Dosage Ranges

Adults: Acute convulsive seizures, status epilepticus, IV 5–10 mg at no more than 2 mg/min; repeat q5–10 min if needed; maximum dose, 30 mg. If necessary, repeat regimen in 2–4 h; maximum dose, 100 mg/24 h.
Children: Acute convulsive seizures, status epilepticus, IV (slowly as above), IM 2–5 mg in a single dose; repeat dose in 2–4 h if necessary

Lorazepam
Route and Dosage Ranges

Adults: Acute convulsive seizures, status epilepticus, IV 2–10 mg, diluted in an equal amount of sterile water for injection, 0.9% sodium chloride injection, or 5% dextrose in water and injected over 2 min

Ethosuximide (Zarontin) is the anticonvulsant of choice for absence seizures. It also may be effective in myoclonic and akinetic epilepsy. Ethosuximide may be used with other anticonvulsants for treatment of mixed types of seizures. The therapeutic range of serum drug levels is about 40 to 80 μg/ml, and about 5 days of drug administration are necessary to reach a steady-state serum concentration.

Route and Dosage Ranges

Adults: PO initially 500 mg/d, increased by 250 mg at weekly intervals until seizures are controlled or toxicity occurs; maximum dose, about 1500 mg/d
Children: PO initially 250 mg/d, increased as above; maximum dose, about 750–1000 mg/d

Gabapentin (Neurontin) is used with other AEDs for treatment of partial seizures that do not respond adequately to a single drug. Its mechanism of action is unknown. Gabapentin is about 60% absorbed from usual therapeutic doses, circulates largely in a free state because it does not bind significantly to plasma proteins, is not appreciably metabolized, and is eliminated by the kidneys as unchanged drug. The elimination half-life is about 5 to 7 hours with normal renal function and up to 50 hours with impaired renal function, depending on creatinine clearance.

Adverse effects include dizziness, drowsiness, fatigue, loss of muscle coordination, tremor, nausea, vomiting, constipation, abnormal vision, gingivitis, and pruritus. Most adverse effects subside spontaneously or with dosage reduction. As with all anticonvulsants, gabapentin should be discontinued gradually, over at least 1 week, to prevent seizure recurrence. Gabapentin reportedly does not cause significant drug–drug interactions. However, antacids taken within 2 hours of a gabapentin dose can decrease its absorption. Because gabapentin is eliminated only by the kidneys, dosage must be reduced in patients with renal impairment.

Route and Dosage Ranges

Adults: PO 300 mg first day, 300 mg twice on second day (600 mg), 300 mg three times on third day (900 mg), then increased by 250 mg at weekly intervals until seizures are controlled or toxicity occurs, up to 1800 mg/d if necessary. Usual maintenance dose, 900–1800 mg/d, in 3 doses.

Adults with renal impairment: Creatinine clearance >60 ml/min, 400 mg three times daily (1200 mg/d); creatinine clearance 30–60 ml/min, 300 mg twice daily (600 mg/d); creatinine clearance 15–30 ml/min, 300 mg once daily; creatinine clearance <15 ml/min, 300 mg every other day. For patients on hemodialysis, 200–300 mg after each 4 hours of hemodialysis.

Children >12 y: Same as adults

Children <12 y: Safety and dosage not established

Lamotrigine (Lamictal) is approved for combination with other anticonvulsants for treatment of adults with partial seizures. It is thought to act by stabilizing nerve cell membranes, thereby reducing the release of excitatory neurotransmitters (*e.g.*, glutamate) in the brain. It is well absorbed following oral administration, with peak plasma levels reached in about 1.5 to 4.5 hours. Lamotrigine is about 55% bound to plasma proteins. It is metabolized in the liver to an inactive metabolite and eliminated mainly in the urine.

Adverse effects include dizziness, drowsiness, headache, ataxia, blurred or double vision, nausea and vomiting, skin rash, and weakness. Lamotrigine apparently does not significantly affect the metabolism of other AEDs, but other AEDs affect lamotrigine's metabolism. Phenytoin, phenobarbital, and carbamazepine induce drug-metabolizing enzymes in the liver and accelerate lamotrigine's metabolism. Valproic acid inhibits those enzymes and thereby slows lamotrigine's metabolism by about 50%. If lamotrigine is combined with other AEDs plus valproic acid, dosage must be substantially reduced. To discontinue, taper dosage over at least 2 weeks.

Route and Dosage Ranges

Adults receiving AEDs other than valproic acid: PO 50 mg once daily for 2 wk, then 50 mg twice daily (100 mg/d) for 2 wk, then increase by 100 mg/d at weekly intervals to a maintenance dose. Usual maintenance dose, 300–500 mg/d in two divided doses.

Adults receiving AEDs plus valproic acid: PO 25 mg every other day for 2 wk, then 25 mg once daily for 2 wk, then increase by 25 to 50 mg/d every 1 to 2 wk to a maintenance dose. Usual maintenance dose, 100–150 mg/d in 2 divided doses.

Children <16 y: Safety and dosage not established

Phenobarbital is a long-acting barbiturate that has been widely used alone or with another anticonvulsant drug (most often phenytoin). It is most effective in generalized tonic-clonic epilepsy and temporal lobe and other partial seizures. It also may be used to treat status epilepticus. Use of phenobarbital has declined with the advent of other AEDs that cause less sedation and cognitive impairment. CNS depression and other adverse effects associated with barbiturates may occur, but drug dependence and barbiturate intoxication are unlikely with usual antiepileptic doses. Because phenobarbital has a long half-life, it takes about 2 to 3 weeks to reach therapeutic serum levels and about 3 to 4 weeks to reach a steady-state concentration. Serum drug levels of 15 to 40 µg/ml (SI units 65–172 µmol/L) are considered in the therapeutic range; higher concentrations are often accompanied by signs and symptoms of toxicity. For anticonvulsant doses of phenobarbital, see Table 8-1 in Chapter 8.

Primidone (Mysoline) is used for generalized tonic-clonic, psychomotor, or partial seizures, alone or with other anticonvulsants. Because it produces marked sedation, primidone is an alternative rather than a primary drug. Excessive sedation is minimized by increasing dosage gradually. Sedation decreases with continued administration of the drug. Primidone is converted to two metabolites, phenobarbital and phenylethylmalonamide (PEMA). The parent drug and both metabolites exert anticonvulsant effects. Therefore, measurements of plasma drug levels should include all three chemicals. The therapeutic ranges are phenobarbital, 10 to 20 µg/ml; primidone, 5 to 10 µg/ml; and PEMA, 7 to 15 µg/ml.

Route and Dosage Ranges

Adults: PO 500–1500 mg/d in divided doses

Children: PO 5–20 mg/kg/d

Valproic acid (Depakene) is used to treat absence and mixed seizures. It produces less sedation and cognitive impairment than phenytoin and phenobarbital. Although they are uncommon, potentially serious adverse effects include hepatotoxicity and pancreatitis. The drug's mechanism of action is unknown. Therapeutic plasma levels are about 50 to 100 µg/ml (SI units 350–700 µmol/L). Derivatives of valproic acid include sodium valproate and divalproex sodium (Depakote). Divalproex sodium contains equal parts of valproic acid and sodium valproate. Dosages of all formulations are expressed in valproic acid equivalents.

Route and Dosage Ranges

Adults: PO 1000–3000 mg/d in divided doses

Children: PO 15–30 mg/kg/d

Nursing Process

Assessment

Assess client status in relation to seizure activity and other factors:

- If the client has a known seizure disorder and is taking anti-convulsant drugs, helpful assessment data can be obtained by interviewing the client. Some questions and guidelines include the following:
  - How long has the client had the seizure disorder?
  - How long has it been since seizure activity occurred, or what is the frequency of seizures?
  - Does any particular situation or activity seem to cause a seizure?
  - How does the seizure affect the client? For example, what parts of the body are involved? Does he or she lose consciousness? Is he or she drowsy and tired afterward?
  - Which anticonvulsant drugs are taken? How do they affect the client? How long has the client taken the drugs? Is the currently ordered dosage the same as the client has been taking? Does the client usually take the drugs as prescribed, or does he or she find it difficult to do so?
  - What other drugs are taken? This includes both prescription and nonprescription drugs, as well as those taken regularly or periodically. This information is necessary because many drugs interact with anticonvulsant drugs to decrease seizure control or increase drug toxicity.
  - What is the client's attitude toward the seizure disorder? Clues to attitude may include terminology, willingness or reluctance to discuss the seizure disorder, compliance or rejection of drug therapy, and others.
- Check reports of serum drug levels for abnormal values.
- People without previous seizure activity may develop seizure disorders with brain surgery, head injury, hypoxia, hypoglycemia, drug overdosage (CNS stimulants, such as amphetamines, or local anesthetics, such as lidocaine), and withdrawal from CNS depressants, such as alcohol and barbiturates.
- To observe and record seizure activity accurately, note the location (localized or generalized); specific characteristics of abnormal movements or behavior; duration; concomitant events, such as loss of consciousness and loss of bowel or bladder control; and postseizure behavior.
- Assess for risk of status epilepticus. Risk factors include recent changes in anticonvulsant drug therapy, chronic alcohol ingestion, use of drugs known to cause seizures, and infection.

Nursing Diagnoses

- Ineffective Individual Coping related to anger or denial of the disease process and need for long-term drug therapy
- Self Esteem Disturbance related to having a seizure disorder
- Impaired Social Interaction related to perceived stigma of epilepsy
- Knowledge Deficit: Disease process
- Knowledge Deficit: Drug effects
- Risk for Injury: Trauma related to ataxia, drowsiness, confusion
- Risk for Injury: Seizure activity
- Noncompliance: Underuse of medications

Planning/Goals

The client will:

- Take medications as prescribed
- Experience control of seizures
- Avoid adverse drug effects
- Verbalize knowledge of the disease process and treatment regimen
- Avoid discontinuing anticonvulsant medications abruptly
- Keep follow-up appointments with health care providers

Interventions

Use measures to minimize seizure activity. Guidelines include the following:

- Help the client identify conditions under which seizures are likely to occur. These precipitating factors, to be avoided or decreased when possible, may include ingestion of alcoholic beverages or stimulant drugs, such as amphetamines; fever; severe physical or emotional stress; and sensory stimuli, such as flashing lights and loud noises.
- Teach the client such health-promotion measures as getting enough rest and exercise and eating a balanced diet.
- Help the client comply with prescribed drug therapy by:
  - Teaching the client and family members about the seizure disorder and the plan for treatment, including drugs
  - Involving the client in decision making when possible
  - Informing the client and family that seizure control is not gained immediately when drug therapy is started. The goal is to avoid unrealistic expectations and excessive frustration while drugs and dosages are being changed in an effort to determine the best combination for the client.
  - Discussing social and economic factors that promote or prevent compliance
- To protect a client experiencing a generalized tonic-clonic seizure:
  - Place a pillow or piece of clothing under the head if injury could be sustained from the ground or floor.
  - Do not restrain the client's movements; fractures may result.
  - Loosen tight clothing, especially around the neck and chest, to promote respiration.
  - When convulsive movements stop, turn the client to one side so that accumulated secretions can drain from the mouth and throat. The cyanosis, abnormal movements, and loss of consciousness that characterize a generalized tonic-clonic seizure can be quite alarming to witnesses. Most of these seizures, however, subside within 3 or 4 minutes, and the person starts responding and regaining normal skin color. If the person has one seizure after another (status epilepticus), has trouble breathing or continued cyanosis, or has sustained an injury, further care is needed, and a physician should be notified immediately.
- When risk factors for seizures, especially status epilepticus, are identified, try to prevent or minimize their occurrence.

Teach clients:

- To take drugs as prescribed. This is extremely important. These drugs must be taken regularly to maintain blood levels adequate to control seizure activity. At the same time, additional doses must not be taken because of increased risks of serious adverse reactions. Also, these drugs must not be stopped abruptly, or seizures are likely to result.

- To report any difficulties with drug therapy to the prescribing physician or other health care worker. These difficulties include seizure activity, excessive drowsiness, or other adverse effects. The physician may be able to adjust dosage or time of administration to relieve the problem.
- Not to drive a car, operate machinery, or perform other activities requiring physical and mental alertness when drowsy from anticonvulsant drugs. Drowsiness, sedation, decreased physical coordination, and decreased mental alertness increase the likelihood of injury.
- Not to take other drugs without the physician's knowledge, and to inform any other physician or dentist about taking anticonvulsant drugs. There are many potential drug interactions in which the effects of the anticonvulsant drug or other drugs may be altered when drugs are given concomitantly.
- To carry adequate identification, such as a card or a Medic-Alert device, that contains pertinent medical information. This is necessary for rapid and appropriate treatment in the event of a seizure, accidental injury, or other emergency situation.

Evaluation

- Interview and observe for decrease in or absence of seizure activity.
- Interview and observe for avoidance of adverse drug effects, especially those that impair safety.
- When available, check laboratory reports of serum drug levels for therapeutic ranges or evidence of under- or overdosing.

Principles of Therapy

DRUG SELECTION

With drug therapy for epilepsy, the goal is control of seizure activity without severe adverse drug effects. To meet this goal, therapy must be individualized.

1. The choice of drugs is determined largely by the type of seizure. Therefore, an accurate diagnosis is essential before drug therapy is started. For generalized convulsive and focal seizures, phenytoin, carbamazepine, phenobarbital, and valproic acid are effective. For absence seizures, ethosuximide is the drug of choice; clonazepam and valproic acid also are effective. For mixed seizures, a combination of drugs is usually necessary. Guidelines for optimal usage of the newer drugs, gabapentin and lamotrigine, have not been established.

   Because most types of seizures can be treated effectively by a variety of drugs, adverse effects of drugs are an important factor in drug selection. Numerous studies have documented cognitive and psychomotor impairment with the sedating anticonvulsants (*e.g.*, phenobarbital, phenytoin), so carba-

mazepine and valproic acid are increasingly used. However, carbamazepine and valproic acid may cause other potentially serious adverse effects. Other factors influencing drug choice include drug cost and client willingness to comply with the prescribed regimen.

2. A single drug (monotherapy) is recommended when possible. If effective in controlling seizures, monotherapy has the advantages of fewer adverse drug effects, fewer drug–drug interactions, lower costs, and usually greater client compliance. If adequate doses of a single drug do not control seizures, alternative interventions include reassessing the client for type of seizure or compliance with the prescribed drug therapy, adding a second drug, or substituting another anticonvulsant drug. When substituting, the second drug should be added and allowed to reach therapeutic blood levels before the first drug is gradually decreased in dosage and discontinued.

DRUG DOSAGE

1. Generally, larger doses are needed for a single drug than for multiple drugs, for people with a large body mass (assuming normal liver and kidney function), and in cases involving trauma, surgery, and emotional stress.
2. Smaller doses are usually required when liver disease is present and when multiple drugs are being given. Smaller doses of gabapentin must be given in the presence of renal impairment, and smaller doses of lamotrigine must be given when combined with valproic acid and another AED.
3. For most drugs, initial doses are relatively low; doses are gradually increased until seizures are controlled or adverse effects occur.
4. When fosphenytoin is substituted for oral phenytoin, the same total daily dosage (in PE) may be given IV or IM.

MONITORING DRUG THERAPY

1. The effectiveness of drug therapy is evaluated primarily by client response in terms of therapeutic or adverse effects. Measuring serum drug levels may be helpful in validating drug dosages, assessing client compliance with the prescribed drug regimen, and documenting toxicity or adverse drug effects. Serum drug levels must be interpreted in relation to clinical responses because there are wide variations among clients receiving similar doses, probably due to differences in hepatic metabolism. In other words, doses should not be increased or decreased solely to maintain a certain serum drug level.
2. Most anticonvulsant drugs have the potential for causing blood, liver, and kidney disorders. For this

reason, it is usually recommended that baseline blood studies (complete blood count, platelet count) and liver function tests (*e.g.*, bilirubin, serum protein, aspartate aminotransferase) be performed before drug therapy starts and periodically thereafter.

3. When drug therapy fails to control seizures, there are several possible reasons. Probably the most frequent one is the client's failure to take the anticonvulsant drug as prescribed. Other common causes include incorrect diagnosis of the type of seizure, use of the wrong drug for the type of seizure, inadequate drug dosage, and too-frequent changes or premature withdrawal of drugs (changing or withdrawing a drug before serum concentration has reached therapeutic levels and before the response can be evaluated properly). Additional causes may include drug overdoses (*e.g.*, theophylline) and severe electrolyte imbalances (*e.g.*, hyponatremia).

DURATION AND DISCONTINUATION OF THERAPY

Anticonvulsant drug therapy was formerly thought to be lifelong. Now, however, drugs may be discontinued for some clients, usually after a seizure-free period of at least 2 years. Although opinions differ about whether, when, and how the drugs should be discontinued, studies indicate that medications can be stopped in about two thirds of patients whose epilepsy is completely controlled with drug therapy. Advantages of discontinuation include avoiding adverse drug effects and decreasing costs; disadvantages include recurrence of seizures, with possible status epilepticus. Even if drugs cannot be stopped completely, periodic attempts to decrease the number or dosage of drugs are probably desirable to minimize adverse reactions. Discontinuing drugs, changing drugs, or changing dosage must be done gradually over 2 to 3 months for each drug and with close medical supervision because sudden withdrawal or dosage decreases may cause status epilepticus. Only one drug should be reduced in dosage or gradually discontinued at a time.

DRUG THERAPY FOR STATUS EPILEPTICUS

An IV benzodiazepine (*e.g.*, diazepam, lorazepam, midazolam) is the drug of choice for rapid control of tonic-clonic seizures. However, seizures often recur within 15 to 20 minutes unless the benzodiazepine is repeated or another, longer-acting drug is given (*e.g.*, IV phenytoin). Because there is a risk of significant respiratory depression with IV benzodiazepines, personnel and

supplies for emergency resuscitation must be readily available.

USE IN CHILDREN

Oral drugs are absorbed slowly and inefficiently in newborns. If an anticonvulsant drug is necessary during the first 7 to 10 days of life, IM phenobarbital is effective. Metabolism and excretion also are delayed during the first 2 weeks of life, but rates become more rapid than those of adults by 2 to 3 months of age. In infants and children, oral drugs are rapidly absorbed and have shorter half-lives. This produces therapeutic serum drug levels earlier in children than in adults. Rates of metabolism and excretion also are increased. Consequently, children require higher doses per kilogram of body weight than adults. The rapid rate of drug elimination persists until about 6 years of age, then decreases until it stabilizes around the adult rate by age 10 to 14. These drugs must be used cautiously to avoid excessive sedation and interference with learning and social development.

USE IN OLDER ADULTS

Anticonvulsants should be used cautiously in older adults because their liver and kidney functions may not be sufficient to metabolize and excrete the drugs. With impaired elimination, the drugs are more likely to accumulate and cause toxic effects unless dosage is reduced.

 ## HOME CARE

The home care nurse must work with clients and family members to implement and monitor AED therapy. When an AED is started, some time is usually required to titrate the dosage and determine whether the chosen drug is effective in controlling seizures. The nurse can play an important role by clinical assessment of the client, interviewing the family about the occurrence of seizures (a log of date, time, duration, and characteristics of seizures can be very helpful), ensuring that the client keeps appointments for serum drug levels and follow-up care, and encouraging compliance with the prescribed regimen. With long-term use of the drugs, the nurse must monitor the client for therapeutic and adverse drug effects, especially with changes in drugs or dosages. With any evidence that the client is not taking medication as directed, the nurse may need to review the potential loss of seizure control and status epilepticus.

ANTICONVULSANT DRUGS

NURSING ACTIONS	RATIONALE/EXPLANATION
1. Administer accurately	
a. Give on a regular schedule, about the same time each day.	To maintain therapeutic blood levels of drugs
b. Give oral anticonvulsant drugs after meals or with a full glass of water or other fluid.	Most anticonvulsant drugs cause some gastric irritation, nausea, or vomiting. Taking the drugs with food or fluid helps decrease gastrointestinal side effects.
c. To give phenytoin:	
(1) Shake oral suspensions of the drug vigorously before pouring, and always use the same measuring equipment.	When a drug preparation is called a *suspension*, it means that particles of drug are suspended or floating in water or other liquid. On standing, drug particles settle to the bottom of the container. Shaking the container is necessary to achieve a uniform distribution of drug particles in the liquid vehicle. If the contents are not mixed well every time a dose is given, the liquid vehicle will be given initially, and the concentrated drug will be given later. That is, underdosage will occur at first, and little if any therapeutic benefit will result. Overdosage will follow, and the risks of serious toxicity are greatly increased. Using the same measuring container ensures consistent dosage. Calibrated medication cups or measuring teaspoons or tablespoons are acceptable. Regular household teaspoons and tablespoons used for eating and serving are *not* acceptable because sizes vary widely.
(2) Do not mix parenteral phenytoin in the same syringe with any other drug.	Phenytoin solution is highly alkaline (pH approximately 12) and physically incompatible with other drugs. A precipitate occurs if mixing is attempted.
(3) Give phenytoin as an undiluted IV bolus injection at a rate not exceeding 50 mg/min, then flush the IV line with normal saline or dilute in 50 to 100 ml of normal saline (0.9% NaCl) and administer over approximately 30 to 60 minutes. If "piggybacked" into a primary IV line, the primary IV solution must be normal saline or the line must be flushed with normal saline before and after administration of phenytoin. An in-line filter is recommended.	Phenytoin cannot be diluted or given in IV fluids other than normal saline because it precipitates within minutes. Slow administration and dilution decrease local venous irritation from the highly alkaline drug solution. Rapid administration must be avoided because it may produce myocardial depression, hypotension, cardiac arrhythmias, and even cardiac arrest.
(4) Give IM phenytoin deeply into a large muscle mass, and rotate injection sites.	Phenytoin is absorbed slowly when given IM and causes local tissue irritation. Correct administration helps increase absorption and decrease pain.
d. To give IV fosphenytoin:	
(1) Check the physician's order and the drug concentration carefully.	Because the dose is expressed in phenytoin equivalents (75 mg of fosphenytoin is equivalent to 50 mg of phenytoin), there is a risk for error.
(2) Dilute the ordered dose in 5% dextrose or 0.9% sodium chloride solution to a concentration of 1.5 mg PE/ml to 25 mg PE/ml and infuse no faster than 150 mg PE/min.	The drug is preferably diluted in the pharmacy and labeled with the concentration and duration of the infusion. For a 100 mg PE dose, diluting with 4 ml yields the maximum concentration of 25 mg PE/ml; this amount could be infused in about 1 min at the maximal recommended rate. A 1 g load-

(continued)

NURSING ACTIONS	RATIONALE/EXPLANATION
	ing dose could be added to 50 ml of 0.9% sodium chloride and infused in about 10 min at the maximal recommended rate.
(3) Consult a pharmacist or the manufacturer's literature if any aspect of the dose or instructions for administration are unclear.	To avoid error until becoming accustomed to using this new parenteral dosage form of phenytoin
e. To give carbamazepine and phenytoin suspensions by nasogastric (NG) feeding tube, dilute with an equal amount of water, and rinse the NG tube before and after administration.	Absorption is slow and decreased, possibly because of drug adherence to the NG tube. Dilution and tube irrigation decrease such adherence.
2. Observe for therapeutic effects	
a. When the drug is given on a long-term basis to prevent seizures, observe for a decrease in or absence of seizure activity.	Therapeutic effects begin later with anticonvulsant drugs than with most other drug groups because the anticonvulsant drugs have relatively long half-lives. Optimum therapeutic benefits of phenytoin occur about 7 to 10 days after drug therapy is started. Those of phenobarbital occur in about 2 weeks; those of ethosuximide, in about 5 days.
b. When the drug is given to stop an acute convulsive seizure, seizure activity usually slows or stops within a few minutes.	Diazepam is the drug of choice for controlling an acute convulsion because it acts rapidly. Even when given IV, phenytoin and phenobarbital do not act for several minutes.
3. Observe for adverse effects	
a. CNS effects—drowsiness, sedation, ataxia, diplopia, nystagmus	These effects are common, especially during the first week or two of drug therapy.
b. Gastrointestinal effects—anorexia, nausea, vomiting	These common effects of oral drugs can be reduced by taking the drugs with food or a full glass of water.
c. Skin disorders—rash, urticaria, exfoliative dermatitis, Stevens-Johnson syndrome (a severe reaction accompanied by headache, arthralgia, and other symptoms in addition to skin lesions)	These may occur with almost all the anticonvulsant drugs. Some are mild; some are potentially serious but rare. Most skin reactions are apparently caused by hypersensitivity or idiosyncratic reactions and are usually sufficient reason to discontinue the drug.
d. Blood dyscrasias—anemia, leukopenia, thrombocytopenia, agranulocytosis	Most anticonvulsant drugs produce decreases in the levels of folic acid, which may progress to megaloblastic anemia. The other disorders indicate bone marrow depression and are potentially life-threatening. They do not usually occur with phenytoin, phenobarbital, or primidone but may infrequently occur with most other anticonvulsant drugs.
e. Respiratory depression	This is not likely to be a significant adverse reaction except when a depressant drug, such as diazepam or a barbiturate, is given IV to control acute seizures, such as status epilepticus. Even then, respiratory depression can be minimized by avoiding overdosage and rapid administration.
f. Liver damage—hepatitis symptoms, jaundice, abnormal liver function tests	Hepatic damage may occur with phenytoin, and fatal hepatotoxicity has been reported with valproic acid.
g. Gingival hyperplasia	Occurs often with phenytoin, especially in children. It may be prevented or delayed by vigorous oral hygiene or treated surgically by gingivectomy.
h. Hypocalcemia	May occur when anticonvulsant drugs are taken in high doses and over long periods
i. Lymphadenopathy resembling malignant lymphoma	This reaction has occurred with several anticonvulsant drugs, most often with phenytoin and other hydantoins.

NURSING ACTIONS	RATIONALE/EXPLANATION
4. Observe for drug interactions	
a. Drugs that *increase* effects of anticonvulsants:	
(1) CNS depressants	Additive CNS depression
(2) Other anticonvulsants	Additive or synergistic effects
b. Drugs that *decrease* effects of anticonvulsants:	
(1) Tricyclic antidepressants (TCAs), antipsychotic drugs	These drugs may lower the seizure threshold and precipitate seizures. Dosage of anticonvulsant drugs may need to be increased.
(2) Barbiturates and other enzyme inducers	These drugs inhibit themselves and other anticonvulsant drugs by activating liver enzymes and accelerating the rate of drug metabolism.
c. Additional drugs that alter effects of phenytoin and fosphenytoin:	
(1) Alcohol (acute ingestion), allopurinol, amiodarone, benzodiazepines, chloramphenicol, chlorpheniramine, cimetidine, disulfiram, fluconazole, ibuprofen, isoniazid, metronidazole, miconazole, omeprazole, phenothiazine antipsychotic drugs, salicylates, TCAs, and trimethoprim increase effects.	These drugs increase phenytoin toxicity by inhibiting hepatic metabolism of phenytoin or by displacing it from plasma protein-binding sites.
(2) Alcohol (chronic ingestion), antacids, antineoplastics, folic acid, loxapine, nitrofurantoin, pyridoxine, rifampin, sucralfate, and theophylline decrease effects.	These drugs decrease effects of phenytoin by decreasing absorption, accelerating metabolism, or by unknown mechanisms.
(3) Phenobarbital has variable interactions with phenytoin.	Phenytoin and phenobarbital have complex interactions with unpredictable effects. Interactions are considered separately because the two drugs are often used at the same time. Although phenobarbital induces drug metabolism in the liver and may increase the rate of metabolism of other anticonvulsant drugs, its interaction with phenytoin differs. Phenobarbital apparently decreases serum levels of phenytoin and perhaps its half-life. Still, the anticonvulsant effects of the two drugs together are greater than those of either drug given alone. The interaction apparently varies with dosage, route, time of administration, the degree of liver enzyme induction already present, and other factors. Thus, whether a significant interaction will occur in a client is unpredictable. Probably the most important clinical implication is that close observation of the client is necessary when either drug is being added or withdrawn.
d. Additional drugs that alter effects of carbamazepine:	
(1) Cimetidine, erythromycin, isoniazid, and valproic acid increase effects.	These drugs inhibit hepatic drug-metabolizing enzymes, thereby increasing blood levels of carbamazepine.
(2) Alcohol, phenytoin, phenobarbital, and primidone decrease effects.	These drugs increase activity of hepatic drug-metabolizing enzymes, thereby decreasing blood levels of carbamazepine.
e. Drugs that alter the effects of gabapentin:	
Antacids	Reduce absorption of gabapentin. Gabapentin should be given at least 2 hours after a dose of an antacid to decrease interference with absorption.

(continued)

NURSING ACTIONS	RATIONALE/EXPLANATION
f. Drugs that alter effects of lamotrigine:	
(1) Valproic acid increases effects.	Valproic acid inhibits the liver enzymes that metabolize lamotrigine, thereby increasing blood levels and slowing metabolism of lamotrigine. As a result, lamotrigine dosage must be substantially reduced when the drug is given in a multidrug regimen that includes valproic acid.
(2) Carbamazepine, phenytoin, phenobarbital decrease effects.	These drugs induce drug-metabolizing enzymes in the liver and thereby increase the rate of metabolism of themselves and of lamotrigine.
g. Additional drugs that alter effects of valproate:	
(1) Chlorpromazine, cimetidine, and salicylates increase effects.	These drugs decrease clearance and increase blood levels of valproic acid.
h. Interactions with phenobarbital:	
(1) Valproic acid	May increase plasma levels of phenobarbital as much as 40%, probably by inhibiting liver-metabolizing enzymes
(2) Other drugs	Many drugs interact with the barbiturates, the drug group of which phenobarbital is a member. These drug interactions are listed in Chapter 8.
i. Interactions with clonazepam, lorazepam, and diazepam	These drugs are benzodiazepines, discussed in Chapter 8.
5. Teach clients and parents of children **a.** Take anticonvulsant drugs with food or a full glass of fluid.	To avoid nausea, vomiting, and gastric distress, which are adverse reactions to most of these drugs
b. When taking phenytoin:	
(1) Ask for the same brand and form of the drug when renewing prescriptions.	There may be differences in drugs produced by different manufacturers. These differences, such as how fast and how completely the drug is absorbed into the bloodstream, influence seizure control and likelihood of adverse reactions.
(2) If taking or giving a liquid preparation of phenytoin, always mix thoroughly and use the same size medicine cup or measuring spoon. Do not use household teaspoons or tablespoons.	This is necessary to ensure accurate and consistent dosage. Household spoons vary widely in size, and using them leads to inaccurate dosages.

REVIEW AND APPLICATION EXERCISES

1. For a client with a newly developed seizure disorder, why is it important to verify the type of seizure by EEG before starting anticonvulsant drug therapy?

2. What are the indications for use of the major AEDs?

3. What are the major adverse effects of commonly used AEDs, and how can they be minimized?

4. What are the advantages and disadvantages of treatment with a single drug and of treatment with multiple drugs?

5. Which of the benzodiazepines (antianxiety agents and hypnotics) are used as anticonvulsants?

6. What are the advantages of carbamazepine and valproic acid in comparison with the benzodiazepines, phenytoin, and phenobarbital?

7. What is the treatment of choice for an acute convulsion or status epilepticus?

8. Why is it important when teaching clients to emphasize that none of the AEDs should be stopped abruptly?

9. How can a home care nurse monitor antiepileptic drug therapy during a home visit?

SELECTED REFERENCES

Armstrong, E.P. (1993). Epilepsy. In R. Bressler & M.D. Katz (Eds.), *Geriatric pharmacology*, pp. 289–308. New York: McGraw-Hill.

Asconape, J.J., Penry, J.K., Dreifuss, F.E., Riela, A., & Mirza, W. (1993). Valproate-associated pancreatitis. *Epilepsia, 34*(1):177–183.

Bader, M.K. (1993). A case study of two methods of administering phenytoin enterally and the subsequent serum phenytoin levels in head-injured patients. *Journal of Neuroscience Nursing, 25*(1):57–58.

Btaiche, I.F., & Woster, P.S. (1995). Gabapentin and lamotrigine: Novel antiepileptic drugs. *American Journal of Health-System Pharmacy, 52*:61–69.

Cascino, G.D. (1993). Antiepileptic drug management in patients with seizure disorders. *Hospital Formulary, 28*:154–172.

Chang, C.W.J., & Bleck, T.P. (1995). Status epilepticus. *Neurologic Clinics, 13*(3):529–548.

Dilorio, C., Faherty, B., & Manteuffel, B. (1993). Learning needs of persons with epilepsy: A comparison of perceptions of persons with epilepsy, nurses and physicians. *Journal of Neuroscience Nursing, 25*(1):22–29.

Drug facts and comparisons. (1996). St. Louis: Facts and Comparisons.

Garnett, W.R. (1993). Epilepsy. In J.T. DiPiro, R.L. Talbert, P.E. Hayes, G.C. Yee, G.R. Matzke, & L.M. Posey (Eds.), *Pharmacotherapy: A pathophysiologic approach*, 2d ed., pp. 879–903. Norwalk, CT: Appleton & Lange.

McNamara, J.O. (1996). Drugs effective in the therapy of the epilepsies. In J.G. Hardman, L.E. Limbird, P.B. Molinoff, & R.W. Ruddon (Eds.), *Goodman & Gilman's The pharmacological basis of therapeutics*, 9th ed., pp. 461–486. New York: McGraw-Hill.

Meador, K.J., Loring, D.W., Abney, O.L., et al. (1993). Effects of carbamazepine and phenytoin on EEG and memory in healthy adults. *Epilepsia, 34*(1):153–157.

Porth, C.M. (1994). *Pathophysiology: Concepts of altered health states*, 4th ed., pp. 1106–1110. Philadelphia: J.B. Lippincott.

Ramsay, R.E. (1993). Treatment of status epilepticus. *Epilepsia, 34*(Suppl. 1):S71–S81.

So, E.L. (1993). Update on epilepsy. *Medical Clinics of North America, 77*(1):203–214.

Antiparkinson Drugs

Objectives

After studying this chapter, the student will be able to:

1 Describe major characteristics of Parkinson's disease.

2 Differentiate the types of commonly used antiparkinson drugs.

3 Discuss therapeutic and adverse effects of dopaminergic and anticholinergic drugs.

4 Apply the nursing process with clients experiencing parkinsonism.

Key Terms

Anticholinergic	**Idiopathic**
Bradykinesia	**Spasticity**
Dopaminergic	**Tremors**

Parkinson's Disease

Parkinson's disease is a chronic, progressive, degenerative disorder of the central nervous system (CNS) characterized by abnormalities in movement and posture (tremor, bradykinesia, joint and muscular rigidity). It occurs equally in men and women, usually between 50 and 80 years of age. Classic parkinsonism probably results from destruction or degenerative changes in dopamine-producing nerve cells. Signs and symptoms of the disease also may occur with other CNS diseases or trauma and with the use of antipsychotic drugs.

The basal ganglia in the brain normally contain substantial amounts of the neurotransmitters dopamine and acetylcholine. The correct balance of dopamine and acetylcholine is important in regulating posture, muscle tone, and voluntary movement. People with Parkinson's disease suffer an imbalance in these neurotransmitters, resulting in a functional and absolute decrease in brain dopamine and a relative increase in acetylcholine. Other neurotransmitters (*e.g.*, norepinephrine, serotonin) may be involved as well, but their roles have not been elucidated.

Antiparkinson Drugs

Drugs used in Parkinson's disease act to increase levels of dopamine (dopaminergic agents) or inhibit the actions of acetylcholine (anticholinergic agents) in the brain. Thus, the drugs help adjust the balance of neurotransmitters.

DOPAMINERGIC DRUGS

Levodopa, carbidopa, amantadine, bromocriptine, pergolide, and selegiline increase dopamine concentrations in the brain and exert dopaminergic activity, directly or indirectly. Levodopa is the mainstay of drug therapy for classic or idiopathic parkinsonism. Carbidopa is used only in conjunction with levodopa. The other four drugs are used as adjunctive agents, usually with levodopa.

ANTICHOLINERGIC DRUGS

Anticholinergic drugs are discussed in Chapter 21 and listed in Table 12-1. They are described here only in relation to their use in the treatment of Parkinson's disease. Only anticholinergic drugs that are centrally active (*i.e.*, those that penetrate the blood-brain barrier) are useful in treating parkinsonism. Trihexyphenidyl (Artane) is often used. Atropine and scopolamine are centrally active but are not used because of a high incidence of adverse reactions. In addition to the primary anticholinergic drugs, a phenothiazine (ethopropazine) and an antihistamine (diphenhydramine) are used for parkinsonism because of their strong anticholinergic effects.

TABLE 12-1 ANTICHOLINERGIC ANTIPARKINSON DRUGS

Generic/Trade Name	Routes and Dosage Ranges (Adults)
Primary Agents	
Benztropine (Cogentin)	PO 0.5–1 mg at bedtime initially, gradually increased to 4–6 mg daily if necessary
Biperiden (Akineton)	Parkinsonism, PO 2 mg 3–4 times daily
	Drug-induced extrapyramidal reaction, PO 2 mg 1–3 times daily, IM 2 mg repeated q30 minutes if necessary to a maximum of 8 mg in 24 hours
Procyclidine (Kemadrin)	PO 5 mg twice daily initially, gradually increased to 5 mg 3–4 times daily if necessary
Trihexyphenidyl (Artane)	PO 1–2 mg daily initially, gradually increased to 12–15 mg daily, until therapeutic or adverse effects occur
	Drug-induced extrapyramidal reactions, PO 1 mg initially, gradually increased to 5–15 mg daily if necessary
Secondary Agents	
Diphenhydramine hydrochloride (Benadryl)	PO 25 mg 3 times daily, gradually increased to 50 mg 4 times daily if necessary
	Drug-induced extrapyramidal reactions, IM, IV 10–50 mg; maximal single dose, 100 mg; maximal daily dose, 400 mg
	Children: Drug-induced extrapyramidal reactions, IM 5 mg/kg per day; maximal daily dose, 300 mg
Ethopropazine hydrochloride (Parsidol)	PO 50 mg once or twice daily initially, gradually increased to a maximal daily dose of 600 mg if necessary

MECHANISMS OF ACTION

Dopaminergic drugs increase the amount of dopamine in the brain by different mechanisms. Amantadine increases dopamine release and decreases dopamine reuptake by presynaptic nerve fibers. Bromocriptine and pergolide are dopamine agonists that directly stimulate postsynaptic dopamine receptors. Levodopa is a precursor substance that enters the brain rapidly and is converted to dopamine. Selegiline blocks the enzyme (monoamine oxidase B, or MAO B) that normally inactivates dopamine. Anticholinergic drugs decrease the effects of acetylcholine. This decreases the apparent excess of acetylcholine in relation to the amount of dopamine.

INDICATIONS FOR USE

A common indication for use is idiopathic or acquired parkinsonism. Levodopa, pergolide, and selegiline are used only for parkinsonism; carbidopa is used only to decrease the peripheral biotransformation of levodopa. Most of the other drugs have additional uses. For example, amantadine is also used to prevent and treat influenza A viral infections. Bromocriptine is also used in the treatment of amenorrhea and galactorrhea associated with hyperprolactinemia.

Anticholinergic drugs are used in idiopathic parkinsonism to decrease salivation, spasticity, and tremors. They are used primarily for people who have minimal symptoms or who cannot tolerate levodopa, or in combination with other antiparkinson drugs. Anticholinergic agents also are used to relieve symptoms of parkinsonism that can occur with the use of antipsychotic drugs. If used for this purpose, a course of therapy of about 3 months is recommended, because symptoms usually subside by then even if the antipsychotic drug is continued.

CONTRAINDICATIONS FOR USE

Levodopa is contraindicated in clients with narrow-angle glaucoma, hemolytic anemia, severe angina pectoris, transient ischemic attacks, or a history of melanoma or undiagnosed skin disorders, and in clients taking MAO inhibitor drugs. In addition, levodopa must be used with caution in clients with severe cardiovascular, pulmonary, renal, hepatic, or endocrine disorders. Bromocriptine and pergolide are ergot derivatives and therefore are contraindicated in people hypersensitive to ergot alkaloids or those with uncontrolled hypertension. Selegiline is contraindicated in hypersensitive people.

Anticholinergic drugs are contraindicated in clients with glaucoma, gastrointestinal obstruction, prostatic hypertrophy, urinary bladder neck obstruction, and myasthenia gravis. The drugs must be used cautiously in clients with cardiovascular disorders (*e.g.,* tachycardia, arrhythmias, hypertension) and liver or kidney disease.

Individual Antiparkinson Drugs

DOPAMINERGIC AGENTS

Levodopa (Larodopa) is the most effective drug available for the treatment of Parkinson's disease. It relieves all major symptoms of parkinsonism, especially bradykinesia and rigidity. Although levodopa does not alter the underlying disease process, it may improve a client's quality of life.

Levodopa acts to replace dopamine in the basal ganglia of the brain. Dopamine cannot be used for replacement therapy because it does not enter the brain in sufficient amounts. Levodopa, in contrast, readily penetrates the CNS and is converted to dopamine by the enzyme L-aromatic amino acid decarboxylase. The concentration of decarboxylase is greater in peripheral tissues than in the brain. Consequently, most levodopa is biotransformed in peripheral tissues, and large amounts are required to obtain therapeutic levels of dopamine in the brain unless carbidopa also is given. Levodopa and carbidopa are often given together in a fixed-dose formulation called Sinemet, which is available in three dosages: 10 mg carbidopa/100 mg levodopa, 25 mg carbidopa/100 mg levodopa, and 25 mg carbidopa/250 mg levodopa.

Levodopa is well absorbed from the small intestine after oral administration and has a short serum half-life (1–3 hours). Absorption is decreased by delayed gastric emptying, hyperacidity of gastric juice, and competition with amino acids (from digestion of protein foods) for sites of absorption in the small intestine. Levodopa is metabolized to 30 or more metabolites, some of which are pharmacologically active and probably contribute to drug toxicity; the metabolites are excreted primarily in the urine, usually within 24 hours.

Because of side effects and recurrence of parkinsonian symptoms after a few years of levodopa therapy, levodopa is often reserved for clients with significant symptoms and functional disabilities. In addition to treating Parkinson's disease, levodopa also may be useful in other CNS disorders in which symptoms of parkinsonism occur (*e.g.,* juvenile Huntington's chorea, chronic manganese poisoning). Levodopa relieves only parkinsonian symptoms in these conditions.

Route and Dosage Range

Adults: PO 0.5–1 g/d initially in three or four divided doses, increased gradually by increments of 100–500 mg/d, every 3–7 d. The rate of dosage increase depends primarily on the client's tolerance of adverse effects, especially nausea and vomiting. Average daily maintenance dose is 3–6 g/d; maximum dose is 8 g/d. Dosage must be reduced when carbidopa is also given (see carbidopa, below). Therapeutic effects may be increased and adverse effects decreased by frequent administration of small doses.

Carbidopa (Lodosyn) inhibits the enzyme L-aromatic amino acid decarboxylase. As a result, less levodopa is decarboxylated in peripheral tissues, more levodopa reaches the brain, where it is decarboxylated to dopamine, and much smaller doses of levodopa can be given. Carbidopa does not penetrate the blood-brain barrier. A levodopa/carbidopa fixed-dose combination product (Sinemet) is available (see levodopa, above).

Route and Dosage Range

Adults: PO initially levodopa 400 mg and carbidopa 40 mg/d in divided doses. This dosage can be gradually increased if necessary to a daily maximum of 2000 mg levodopa and 200 mg carbidopa. When carbidopa is added to a regimen of levodopa, the levodopa should be withheld at least 8 h before Sinemet therapy is begun, and dosage should be about 25% of the previous levodopa dosage.

Amantadine (Symmetrel) is a synthetic antiviral agent initially used to prevent infection from influenza A virus. Amantadine increases the release and inhibits the reuptake of dopamine in the brain, thereby increasing dopamine levels. The drug relieves symptoms rapidly, within 1 to 5 days, but it loses efficacy with about 6 to 8 weeks of continuous administration. Consequently, it is usually given for 2- to 3-week periods during initiation of drug therapy with longer-acting agents (*e.g.*, levodopa), or when symptoms worsen. Amantadine is often given in conjunction with levodopa. Compared with other antiparkinson drugs, amantadine is considered less effective than levodopa but more effective than anticholinergic agents.

Amantadine is well absorbed from the gastrointestinal tract and has a relatively long duration of action. It is excreted unchanged in the urine. Dosage must be reduced with impaired renal function to avoid drug accumulation.

Route and Dosage Range

Adults: PO 100 mg twice a day

Bromocriptine (Parlodel) and **pergolide** (Permax) are ergot derivatives that directly stimulate dopamine receptors in the brain. They are used in the treatment of idiopathic Parkinson's disease, with levodopa/carbidopa, to prolong effectiveness and allow reduced dosage of levodopa. Pergolide has a longer duration of action than bromocriptine and may be effective in some patients unresponsive to bromocriptine. Adverse effects are similar for the two drugs.

Bromocriptine
Route and Dosage Range

Adults: PO 1.25 mg twice a day with meals, increased by 2.5 mg/d every 2–4 wk if necessary for therapeutic benefit. Reduce dose gradually if severe adverse effects occur.

Pergolide
Route and Dosage Range

Adults: PO 0.05–0.1 mg/d at bedtime, increased by 0.05–0.15 mg every 3 d to a maximum dose of 6 mg/d if necessary

Selegiline (Eldepryl) increases dopamine in the brain by inhibiting its metabolism by MAO B. MAO has long been known as an important enzyme. In recent years, two types have been differentiated. MAO A metabolizes catecholamines, such as norepinephrine, serotonin, and tyramine; MAO B metabolizes dopamine. Within the brain, most MAO activity is due to type B. The drug's ability to inhibit MAO B selectively may not be evident at higher doses. Selegiline is added when clients experience decreased responsiveness with levodopa/carbidopa. Its addition aids symptom control and allows the dosage of levodopa/carbidopa to be reduced. Overall, therapeutic effects are limited in extent and duration.

Route and Dosage Range

Adults: PO 5 mg twice daily, morning and noon

Nursing Process

Assessment

Assess for signs and symptoms of Parkinson's disease and drug-induced extrapyramidal reactions. These may include the following, depending on the severity and stage of progression:
- Slow movements (bradykinesia) and difficulty in changing positions, assuming an upright position, eating, dressing, and other self-care activities
- Stooped posture
- Accelerating gait with short steps
- Tremor at rest (*e.g.*, "pill rolling" movements of fingers)
- Rigidity of arms, legs, and neck
- Mask-like, immobile facial expression
- Speech problems (*e.g.*, low volume, monotonous tone, rapid, difficult to understand)
- Excessive salivation and drooling

- Dysphagia
- Excessive sweating
- Constipation from decreased intestinal motility
- Mental depression from self-consciousness and embarrassment over physical appearance and activity limitations. The intellect is usually intact until the late stages of the disease process.

Nursing Diagnoses

- Self Care Deficit: Total, related to tremors and impaired motor function
- Impaired Physical Mobility related to alterations in balance and coordination
- Body Image Disturbance related to disease and disability
- Knowledge Deficit: Safe usage and effects of antiparkinson drugs
- Altered Thought Processes related to impaired mentation
- Altered Nutrition: Less Than Body Requirements related to difficulty in chewing and swallowing food
- Risk for Injury: Dizziness, hypotension related to adverse drug effects

Planning/Goals

The client will:
- Experience relief of excessive salivation, muscle rigidity, spasticity, and tremors
- Experience improved motor function, mobility, and self-care abilities
- Experience improvement of self-concept and body image
- Increase knowledge of the disease process and drug therapy
- Take medications as instructed
- Avoid falls and other injuries from the disease process or drug therapy

Interventions

Use measures to assist the client and family in coping with symptoms and maintaining function. These include the following:
- Provide physical therapy for heel-to-toe gait training, widening stance to increase balance and base of support, other exercises.
- Encourage ambulation and frequent changes of position, assisted if necessary.
- Help with active and passive range-of-motion exercises.
- Encourage self-care as much as possible. Cutting meat, opening cartons, giving frequent small meals, and allowing privacy during mealtime may be helpful. If the client has difficulty chewing or swallowing, chopped or soft foods may be necessary. Velcro-type fasteners or zippers are easier to handle than buttons. Slip-on shoes are easier to manage than laced ones.
- Spend time with the client and encourage socialization with other people. Victims of Parkinson's disease tend to become withdrawn, isolated, and depressed.
- Schedule rest periods. Tremor and rigidity are aggravated by fatigue and emotional stress.
- Provide facial tissues if drooling is a problem.

 Teach clients:
- Not to take other drugs without the physician's knowledge and consent. This is necessary to avoid adverse drug interactions. Prescription and nonprescription drugs may interact with antiparkinson drugs to increase or decrease effects.
- To avoid driving an automobile or operating other potentially hazardous machinery if vision is blurred or drowsiness occurs with levodopa
- To change positions slowly, especially when assuming an upright position, and to wear elastic stockings if needed

Evaluation

- Interview and observe for relief of symptoms.
- Interview and observe for increased mobility and participation in activities of daily living.
- Interview and observe regarding correct usage of medications.

Principles of Therapy

GOAL OF TREATMENT

The goal of antiparkinson drug therapy is to control symptoms and improve the client's ability to perform activities of daily living.

DRUG SELECTION

The choice of antiparkinson drug depends on the type of parkinsonism (idiopathic or drug-induced) and the severity of symptoms.

1. Anticholinergic agents may be the drugs of choice for early idiopathic parkinsonism, when symptoms are relatively mild, and for drug-induced symptoms. These agents are most effective in decreasing salivation and tremor.
2. Levodopa and carbidopa are the drugs of choice in idiopathic parkinsonism when bradykinesia and rigidity are prominent symptoms.
3. Combination drug therapy may be preferred for many clients. Two advantages of combination therapy are better control of symptoms and reduced dosage of individual drugs. Anticholinergic drugs may be given with levodopa alone or with a levodopa/carbidopa combination. Amantadine, bromocriptine, pergolide, and selegiline are usually used as adjuncts to levodopa/carbidopa.

DRUG DOSAGE

The dosage of antiparkinson drugs is highly individualized. The general rule is to start with a low initial dose and gradually increase the dosage until therapeutic effects, adverse effects, or the maximum drug dosage is achieved. Optimal dosage may not be established for 6 to 8 weeks with levodopa. When combinations of drugs are used, dosage adjustments of individual components are sometimes necessary. When levodopa is added to a regimen of anticholinergic drug therapy, for example, the anticholinergic drug need not be discontinued or reduced in dosage. However, when carbidopa is given with levodopa, the dosage of levodopa must be reduced by about 75%. Dosage of levodopa/carbidopa is also reduced when adjunctive dopaminergic drugs are added.

USE IN CHILDREN

Safety and effectiveness for use in children have not been established for most antiparkinson drugs, including the centrally acting anticholinergics (all ages), levodopa (under 12 years), and bromocriptine (under 15 years).

Because parkinsonism is a degenerative disorder of adults, antiparkinson drugs are most likely to be used for other purposes in children. Amantadine, for influenza A prevention or treatment, is not recommended for neonates or infants under 1 year old but may be given to children 9 to 12 years old.

USE IN OLDER ADULTS

When amantadine is given to older adults, the dosage may need to be reduced. Because about 90% of a dose is excreted unchanged in the urine and renal function is usually decreased in older adults, there is a risk of accumulation and toxicity. Dosage reduction is recommended for people with creatinine clearance under 80 ml/min.

Anticholinergic drugs may cause dry mouth, tachycardia, urinary retention, blurred vision, mental confusion, and delirium. They also decrease sweating and the ability to adapt to high environmental temperatures; consequences may be fever or heatstroke. Fever may occur in any age group, but heatstroke is more likely to occur in older adults, especially with cardiovascular disease, strenuous activity, and high environmental temperatures.

When centrally active anticholinergics, such as trihexyphenidyl and benztropine (Cogentin), are given for Parkinson's disease, mental confusion, agitation, hallucinations, and psychotic-like symptoms may occur. The dosage should be carefully regulated and supervised.

In addition to the primary anticholinergic agents, many other drugs have significant anticholinergic activity. These include many antihistamines (histamine-1 receptor antagonists), tricyclic antidepressants, and phenothiazine antipsychotic drugs.

HOME CARE

The home care nurse must help clients and caregivers understand that the purpose of drug therapy is to control symptoms and that noticeable improvement may not occur for several weeks. In addition, teaching may be needed about preventing or managing adverse drug effects.

NURSING ACTIONS

ANTIPARKINSON DRUGS

NURSING ACTIONS	RATIONALE/EXPLANATION
1. Administer accurately **a.** Give levodopa and bromocriptine with or just after food intake.	To prevent or reduce anorexia, nausea, and vomiting
b. Give selegiline in the morning and at noon.	To decrease central nervous system (CNS) stimulating effects that may interfere with sleep if the drug is taken in the evening
2. Observe for therapeutic effects **a.** With anticholinergic agents, observe for decreased tremor, salivation, drooling, and sweating.	Decreased salivation and sweating are therapeutic effects when these drugs are used in Parkinson's disease, but they are adverse effects when the drugs are used in other disorders.
b. With levodopa, observe for improvement in mobility, balance, posture, gait, speech, handwriting, and self-care ability. Drooling and seborrhea may be abolished, and mood may be elevated.	Therapeutic effects are usually evident within 2 to 3 weeks, as dosage approaches 2 to 3 g/d, but may not reach optimum levels for 6 months.

(continued)

Nursing Actions   *Rationale/Explanation*

3. Observe for adverse effects

a. With anticholinergic drugs, observe for atropine-like effects, such as:

(1) Tachycardia and palpitations

These effects may occur with usual therapeutic doses but are not likely to be serious except in people with underlying heart disease.

(2) Excessive CNS stimulation (tremor, restlessness, confusion, hallucinations, delirium)

This effect is most likely to occur with large doses of trihexyphenidyl (Artane) or benztropine (Cogentin). It may occur with levodopa.

(3) Sedation and drowsiness

These are most likely to occur with benztropine. The drug has antihistaminic and anticholinergic properties, and sedation is attributed to the antihistamine effect.

(4) Constipation, impaction, paralytic ileus

These effects result from decreased gastrointestinal motility and muscle tone. They may be severe because decreased intestinal motility and constipation also are characteristics of Parkinson's disease; thus, additive effects may occur.

(5) Urinary retention

This reaction is caused by loss of muscle tone in the bladder and is most likely to occur in elderly men who have enlarged prostate glands.

(6) Dilated pupils (mydriasis), blurred vision, photophobia

Ocular effects are due to paralysis of accommodation and relaxation of the ciliary muscle and the sphincter muscle of the iris.

b. With levodopa, observe for:

(1) Anorexia, nausea, and vomiting

These symptoms usually disappear after a few months of drug therapy. They may be minimized by giving levodopa with food, gradually increasing dosage, administering smaller doses more frequently, or adding carbidopa so that dosage of levodopa can be reduced.

(2) Orthostatic hypotension—check blood pressure in both sitting and standing positions q4h while the client is awake.

This effect is common during the first few weeks but usually subsides eventually. It can be minimized by arising slowly from supine or sitting positions and by wearing elastic stockings.

(3) Cardiac arrhythmias (tachycardia, premature ventricular contractions) and increased myocardial contractility

Levodopa and its metabolites stimulate beta-adrenergic receptors in the heart. People with pre-existing coronary artery disease may need a beta-adrenergic blocking agent (*e.g.*, propranolol) to counteract these effects.

(4) Dyskinesia—involuntary movements that may involve only the tongue, mouth, and face or the whole body

Dyskinesia eventually develops in most people who take levodopa. It is related to duration of levodopa therapy rather than dosage. Carbidopa may heighten this adverse effect, and there is no way to prevent it except by decreasing levodopa dosage. Many people prefer dyskinesia to lowering drug dosage and subsequent return of the parkinsonism symptoms.

(5) CNS stimulation—restlessness, agitation, confusion, delirium

This is more likely to occur with levodopa/carbidopa combination drug therapy.

(6) Abrupt swings in motor function (on–off phenomenon)

This fluctuation may indicate progression of the disease process. It often occurs after long-term levodopa use.

c. With amantadine, observe for:

(1) CNS stimulation—insomnia, hyperexcitability, ataxia, dizziness, slurred speech, mental confusion, hallucinations

Compared with other antiparkinson drugs, amantadine produces few adverse effects. The ones that occur are mild, transient, and reversible. However, adverse effects increase if daily dosage exceeds 200 mg.

NURSING ACTIONS	RATIONALE/EXPLANATION
(2) Livedo reticularis—patchy, bluish discoloration of skin on the legs	This is a benign but cosmetically unappealing condition. It usually occurs with long-term use of amantadine and disappears when the drug is discontinued.
d. With bromocriptine and pergolide, observe for: (1) Nauseà (2) Confusion and hallucinations (3) Hypotension	These symptoms are usually mild and can be minimized by starting with low doses and increasing the dose gradually until the desired effect is achieved. If adverse effects do occur, they usually disappear with a decrease in dosage.
e. With selegiline, observe for: (1) CNS effects—agitation, ataxia, bradykinesia, confusion, dizziness, dyskinesias, hallucinations, insomnia (2) Nausea, abdominal pain	
4. Observe for drug interactions **a.** Drugs that *increase* effects of anticholinergic drugs: Antihistamines, disopyramide (Norpace, an antiarrhythmic agent), phenothiazines, thioxanthene agents, and tricyclic antidepressants	These drugs have anticholinergic properties and produce additive anticholinergic effects.
b. Drugs that *decrease* effects of anticholinergic drugs: Cholinergic agents	These drugs counteract the inhibition of gastrointestinal motility and tone, which is a side effect of anticholinergic drug therapy.
c. Drugs that *increase* effects of levodopa: (1) Amantadine, anticholinergic agents, bromocriptine, carbidopa, pergolide, selegiline	These drugs are often used in combination for treatment of Parkinson's disease.
(2) Tricyclic antidepressants	These drugs potentiate levodopa effects and increase the risk of cardiac arrhythmias in people with heart disease.
(3) MAO-A inhibitors, including isocarboxazid (Marplan), phenelzine (Nardil), and tranylcypromine (Parnate)	The combination of a catecholamine precursor (levodopa) and MAO-A inhibitors that decrease metabolism of catecholamines can result in excessive amounts of dopamine, epinephrine, and norepinephrine. Heart palpitations, headache, hypertensive crisis, and stroke may occur. Levodopa and MAO-A inhibitors should not be given concurrently. Also, levodopa should not be started within 3 weeks after an MAO-A inhibitor is discontinued. Effects of MAO-A inhibitors persist for 1 to 3 weeks after their discontinuation. These effects are unlikely to occur with selegiline, an MAO-B inhibitor, which more selectively inhibits the metabolism of dopamine. However, selectivity may be lost at doses higher than the recommended 10 mg/d. Selegiline is used with levodopa.
d. Drugs that *decrease* effects of levodopa: (1) Anticholinergics	Although anticholinergics are often given with levodopa for increased antiparkinson effects, they also may decrease effects of levodopa by delaying gastric emptying. This causes more levodopa to be metabolized in the stomach and decreases the amount available for absorption from the intestine.

(continued)

NURSING ACTIONS	RATIONALE/EXPLANATION
(2) Alcohol, antianxiety agents (*e.g.*, diazepam [Valium] and probably other benzodiazepines), antiemetics, antipsychotic agents (phenothiazines, butyrophenones, thioxanthenes)	The mechanisms by which most of these drugs decrease effects of levodopa are not clear. Phenothiazines block dopamine receptors in the basal ganglia.
(3) Oral iron preparations	Iron binds with levodopa and reduces levodopa absorption, possibly as much as 50%.
(4) Pyridoxine (vitamin B_6)	Pyridoxine stimulates decarboxylase, the enzyme that converts levodopa to dopamine. As a result, more levodopa is metabolized in peripheral tissues, and less reaches the CNS, where antiparkinson effects occur. This interaction does not occur when carbidopa is given with levodopa.
e. Drugs that *decrease* effects of dopaminergic antiparkinson drugs:	
(1) Antipsychotic drugs	These drugs are dopamine antagonists and therefore inhibit the effects of dopamine agonists.
(2) Metoclopramide	
5. Teach clients	
a. Excessive mouth dryness can be minimized by maintaining an adequate fluid intake (2000–3000 ml daily if not contraindicated) and using sugarless chewing gum and hard candies.	Both anticholinergics and levodopa may cause mouth dryness. This is usually a therapeutic effect in Parkinson's disease. However, excessive mouth dryness (xerostomia) causes discomfort and dental caries.
b. Limit intake of alcohol and high-protein foods (*e.g.*, meat, poultry, fish, milk, eggs, cheese, nuts). Do not take multivitamin preparations that contain vitamin B_6.	Alcohol, protein, and vitamin B_6 decrease the therapeutic effects of levodopa alone but not the effects of levodopa/carbidopa in combination. Larobec is a multivitamin preparation available without vitamin B_6.
c. Report adverse effects.	Adverse effects can often be reduced by changing drugs or dosages. However, some adverse effects usually must be tolerated for control of disease symptoms.

REVIEW AND APPLICATION EXERCISES

1. Which neurotransmitter is deficient in idiopathic and drug-induced parkinsonism?

2. How do the antiparkinson drugs act to alter the level of the deficient neurotransmitter?

3. What are the advantages and disadvantages of the various drugs used to treat parkinsonism?

4. What are the major adverse effects of antiparkinson drugs, and how can they be minimized?

5. What is the rationale for combining carbidopa with levodopa?

SELECTED REFERENCES

Drug facts and comparisons. (1996). St. Louis: Facts and Comparisons.

Erwin, W.G. (1993). Parkinson's disease. In J.T. DiPiro, R.L. Talbert, P.E. Hayes, G.C. Yee, G.R. Matzke, & L.M. Posey (Eds.), *Pharmacotherapy: A pathophysiologic approach*, 2d ed., pp. 913–923. Norwalk, CT: Appleton & Lange.

Montgomery, E.B. & Lipsy, R.J. (1993). Treatment of Parkinson's disease. In R. Bressler & M.D. Katz (Eds.), *Geriatric pharmacology.* New York: McGraw-Hill.

Porth, C.M. (1994). *Pathophysiology: Concepts of altered health states*, 4th ed., pp. 1182–1185. Philadelphia: J.B. Lippincott.

13

Skeletal Muscle Relaxants

Outline

Skeletal Muscle Relaxants
mechanism of action
indications for use
contraindications for use

Nursing Process
assessment
nursing diagnoses
planning/goals
interventions
evaluation

Principles of Therapy
goal of treatment
drug selection
use in children
use in older adults

Objectives

After studying this chapter, the student will be able to:

1 Discuss common symptoms/disorders for which skeletal muscle relaxants are used.

2 Differentiate uses and effects of selected drugs.

3 Describe nonpharmacologic interventions to relieve muscle spasm and spasticity.

4 Apply the nursing process with clients experiencing muscle spasm or spasticity.

Key Terms

Clonic

Malignant hyperthermia

Muscle spasm

Spasticity

Tonic

Skeletal Muscle Relaxants

Skeletal muscle relaxants are used to decrease muscle spasm or spasticity that occurs in certain neurologic and musculoskeletal disorders. (Neuromuscular blocking agents used as adjuncts to general anesthesia for surgery are discussed in Chap. 14.)

Muscle spasm is sudden movement that may involve alternating contraction and relaxation (clonic) or sustained contraction (tonic). Muscle spasm may occur with musculoskeletal trauma or inflammation (*e.g.,* sprains, strains, bursitis, arthritis). It is also encountered with acute or chronic low back pain, a common condition that is primarily a disorder of posture.

Spasticity involves increased muscle tone or contraction, which produces stiff, awkward movements. Spasticity results from neurologic disorders such as cerebral palsy, stroke, paraplegia, spinal cord injury, and multiple sclerosis.

MECHANISM OF ACTION

Almost all skeletal muscle relaxants are centrally active agents. Pharmacologic action is probably caused by general depression of the central nervous system (CNS) but may result from blockage of nerve impulses that cause increased muscle tone and contraction. It is unclear whether relief of pain results from sedative effects, muscular relaxation, or a placebo effect. In addition, although parenteral administration of some drugs (*e.g.,* diazepam [Valium], methocarbamol [Robaxin]) relieves pain associated with acute musculoskeletal trauma or inflammation, it is uncertain whether oral administration of usual doses exerts a beneficial effect in acute or chronic disorders. Dantrolene (Dantrium) is the only skeletal muscle relaxant that acts peripherally on the muscle itself.

INDICATIONS FOR USE

Skeletal muscle relaxants are recommended for use primarily as adjuncts to other treatment measures. Occasionally, parenteral agents are given to facilitate various orthopedic procedures and examinations. In spastic disorders, skeletal muscle relaxants are not generally indicated for use only to relieve spasticity. However, they may be indicated when spasticity causes severe pain or inability to tolerate physical therapy, sit in a wheelchair, or participate in self-care activities of daily living (*e.g.,* eating, dressing). Drugs should not be given if they cause excessive muscle weakness and impair rather than facilitate mobility and function.

Dantrolene also is indicated for prevention and treatment of malignant hyperthermia, a rare but life-threatening complication of anesthesia characterized by hypercarbia, metabolic acidosis, skeletal muscle rigidity, fever, and cyanosis. For preoperative prophylaxis in people with previous episodes of malignant hyperthermia, the drug is given orally for 1 to 2 days before surgery. For intraoperative malignant hyperthermia, the drug is given intravenously. Postoperatively, after occurrences, the drug is given orally for 1 to 3 days to prevent recurrence of symptoms.

CONTRAINDICATIONS FOR USE

Most skeletal muscle relaxants cause CNS depression and have the same contraindications as other CNS depressants. They should be used cautiously in clients with impaired renal or hepatic function or respiratory depression, and in clients who must be alert for activities of daily living (*e.g.,* driving a car, operating potentially hazardous machinery). Orphenadrine and cyclobenzaprine have high levels of anticholinergic activity and therefore should be used cautiously with glaucoma, urinary retention, cardiac arrhythmias, or tachycardia.

Individual skeletal muscle relaxants are listed in Table 13-1.

Nursing Process

Assessment

Assess for muscle spasm and spasticity.
- With muscle spasm, assess for:
  - **Pain.** This is a prominent symptom of muscle spasm and is usually aggravated by movement. Try to determine the location as specifically as possible, as well as the intensity, duration, and precipitating factors (*e.g.,* traumatic injury, strenuous exercise).
  - **Accompanying signs and symptoms,** such as bruises (ecchymoses), edema, or signs of inflammation (redness, heat, edema, tenderness to touch)
- With spasticity, assess for pain and impaired functional ability in self-care (*e.g.,* eating, dressing). In addition, severe spasticity interferes with physical therapy exercises to maintain joint and muscle mobility.

Nursing Diagnoses

- Pain related to muscle spasm
- Impaired Physical Mobility related to spasm and pain
- Self Care Deficit related to spasm and pain
- Knowledge Deficit: Nondrug measures to relieve muscle spasm, pain, and spasticity
- Knowledge Deficit: Safe usage and effects of skeletal muscle relaxants
- Risk for Injury: Dizziness, sedation related to CNS depression

Planning/Goals

The client will:
- Experience relief of pain and spasm
- Experience improved motor function
- Increase self-care abilities in activities of daily living
- Take medications as instructed
- Use nondrug measures appropriately
- Be safeguarded when sedated from drug therapy

TABLE 13-1 SKELETAL MUSCLE RELAXANTS

| Generic/Trade Name | Routes and Dosages Ranges | |
	Adults	*Children*
Baclofen (Lioresal)	PO 5 mg 3 times daily initially, increased to 10 mg 3 times daily after 3 days, then gradually increased further if necessary; maximal dose, 20 mg 4 times daily Dosage must be reduced in the presence of impaired renal function.	Under age 12 years, not recommended)
Carisoprodol (Rela, Soma)	PO 350 mg 4 times daily	Age 5 years and over, PO 25 mg/kg per day in 4 divided doses
Chlorphenesin (Maolate)	PO 800 mg 3 times daily until desired effect attained, then 400 mg 4 times daily or less for maintenance as needed	Dosage not established
Cyclobenzaprine (Flexeril)	PO 10 mg 3 times daily. Maximal recommended duration, 3 weeks; maximal recommended dose, 60 mg daily	
Dantrolene (Dantrium)	PO 25 mg daily initially, gradually increased weekly (by increments of 50–100 mg/d) to a maximal dose of 400 mg daily in 4 divided doses Preoperative prophylaxis of malignant hyperthermia: PO 4–8 mg/kg per day in 3–4 divided doses for 1 or 2 days before surgery Intraoperative malignant hyperthermia: IV push 1 mg/kg initially, continued until symptoms are relieved or a maximum total dose of 10 mg/kg has been given Postcrisis follow-up treatment: PO 4–8 mg/kg per day in 4 divided doses for 1–3 days	PO 1 mg/kg per day initially, gradually increased to a maximal dose of 3 mg/kg 4 times daily, not to exceed 400 mg daily Same as adult
Diazepam (Valium)	PO 2–10 mg 3 or 4 times daily IM, IV 5–10 mg repeated in 3–4 hours if necessary	PO 0.12–0.8 mg/kg per day in 3 or 4 divided doses IM, IV 0.04–0.2 mg/kg in a single dose, not to exceed 0.6 mg/kg within an 8-hour period
Metaxalone (Skelaxin)	PO 800 mg 3 or 4 times daily for not more than 10 consecutive days	
Methocarbamol (Robaxin)	PO 1.5–2 g 4 times daily for 48–72 hours, reduced to 1.0 g 4 times daily for maintenance IM 500 mg q8h IV 1–3 g daily at a rate not to exceed 300 mg/minute (3 ml of 10% injection). Do not give IV more than 3 days.	PO, IM, IV 60–75 mg/kg per day in 4 divided doses
Orphenadrine citrate (Norflex)	PO 100 mg twice daily IM, IV 60 mg twice daily	

Interventions

Use adjunctive measures for muscle spasm and spasticity:
- Physical therapy (massage, moist heat, exercises)
- Bed rest for acute muscle spasm
- Relaxation techniques

- Correct posture and lifting techniques (*e.g.*, stooping rather than bending to lift objects, holding heavy objects close to the body, *not* lifting excessive amounts of weight)
- Regular exercise and use of warm-up exercises. Strenuous exercise performed on an occasional basis (*e.g.*, weekly or monthly) is more likely to cause acute muscle spasm.

Teach clients:
- How to use nondrug measures, such as exercises and applications of heat and cold, to decrease muscle spasm and spasticity
- To avoid activities that require mental alertness or physical coordination (*e.g.*, driving an automobile, operating potentially dangerous machinery) if drowsy from medication
- Not to take other drugs without the physician's knowledge, including nonprescription drugs. The major risk occurs with concurrent use of alcohol, antihistamines, sleeping aids, or other drugs that cause drowsiness.

Evaluation
- Interview and observe for relief of symptoms.
- Interview and observe regarding correct usage of medications and nondrug therapeutic measures.

Principles of Therapy

GOAL OF TREATMENT

The goal of treatment is to relieve pain, muscle spasm, and muscle spasticity without impairing the ability to perform self-care activities of daily living.

DRUG SELECTION

Choice of a skeletal muscle relaxant depends primarily on the disorder being treated:

1. For acute muscle spasm and pain, a drug that can be given parenterally (*e.g.*, diazepam, methocarbamol) is usually the drug of choice.

2. Parenteral agents are preferred for orthopedic procedures because they have greater sedative and pain-relieving effects.
3. Baclofen (Lioresal) is approved for treatment of spasticity in people with multiple sclerosis. It is variably effective, and its clinical usefulness may be limited by adverse reactions. Baclofen is not recommended for pregnant women or children under 12 years of age.
4. None of the skeletal muscle relaxants has been established as safe for use during pregnancy and lactation.
5. Many of the skeletal muscle relaxants have not been established as safe for use in children. Choice of drug should be limited to those with established pediatric dosages.

USE IN CHILDREN

For most of the drugs, safety and effectiveness for use in children 12 years and younger have not been established. The drugs should be used only when clearly indicated, for short periods of time, when close supervision is available for monitoring drug effects (especially sedation), and when mobility and alertness are not required.

USE IN OLDER ADULTS

Any CNS depressant or sedating drugs should be used cautiously in older adults. Risks of falls, mental confusion, and other adverse effects are generally higher in older adults because of impaired drug metabolism and excretion.

NURSING ACTIONS

SKELETAL MUSCLE RELAXANTS

NURSING ACTIONS	*RATIONALE/EXPLANATION*
1. Administer accurately **a.** Give baclofen, chlorphenesin, metaxalone with milk or food.	To decrease gastrointestinal distress
b. Do not mix parenteral diazepam in a syringe with any other drugs.	Diazepam is physically incompatible with other drugs.
c. Inject IV diazepam directly into a vein or the injection site nearest the vein (during continuous IV infusions) at a rate of about 2 mg/min.	Diazepam may cause a precipitate if diluted. Avoid contact with IV solutions as much as possible. A slow rate of injection minimizes the risks of respiratory depression and apnea.
d. Avoid extravasation with IV diazepam, and inject IM diazepam deeply into a gluteal muscle.	To prevent or reduce tissue irritation
e. With IV methocarbamol, inject or infuse slowly.	Rapid administration may cause bradycardia, hypotension, and dizziness.

NURSING ACTIONS	RATIONALE/EXPLANATION
f. With IV methocarbamol, have the client lie down during and at least 15 minutes after administration.	To minimize orthostatic hypotension and other adverse drug effects
g. Avoid extravasation with IV methocarbamol, and give IM methocarbamol deeply into a gluteal muscle. (Dividing the dose and giving two injections is preferred.)	Parenteral methocarbamol is a hypertonic solution that is very irritating to tissues. Thrombophlebitis may occur at IV injection sites, and sloughing of tissue may occur at sites of extravasation or IM injections.
2. Observe for therapeutic effects **a.** When the drug is given for acute muscle spasm, observe for: (1) Decreased pain and tenderness (2) Increased mobility (3) Increased ability to participate in activities of daily living **b.** When the drug is given for spasticity in chronic neurologic disorders, observe for: (1) Increased ability to maintain posture and balance (2) Increased ability for self-care (*e.g.*, eating and dressing) (3) Increased tolerance for physical therapy and exercises	Therapeutic effects usually occur within 30 minutes after IV injection of diazepam or methocarbamol.
3. Observe for adverse effects **a.** With centrally active agents, observe for: (1) Drowsiness and dizziness	These are the most common adverse effects.
(2) Blurred vision, lethargy, flushing	These effects occur more often with IV administration of drugs. They are usually transient.
(3) Nausea, vomiting, abdominal distress, constipation or diarrhea, ataxia, areflexia, flaccid paralysis, respiratory depression, tachycardia, hypotension	These effects are most likely to occur with large oral doses.
(4) Hypersensitivity—skin rash, pruritus	The drug should be discontinued if hypersensitivity reactions occur. Serious allergic reactions (*e.g.*, anaphylaxis) are rare.
(5) Psychological or physical dependence with diazepam and other antianxiety agents	Most likely to occur with long-term use of large doses
b. With a peripherally active agent (dantrolene), observe for:	Adverse effects are usually transient.
(1) Drowsiness, fatigue, lethargy, weakness, nausea, vomiting	These effects are the most common.
(2) Headache, anorexia, nervousness	Less common effects
(3) Hepatotoxicity	This potentially serious adverse effect is most likely to occur in people more than 35 years of age who have taken the drug 60 days or longer. Women over age 35 who take estrogens have the highest risk. Hepatotoxicity can be prevented or minimized by administering the lowest effective dose, monitoring liver enzymes (aspartate aminotransferase [AST], alanine aminotransferase [ALT] during therapy, and discontinuing the drug if no beneficial effects occur within 45 days.

(continued)

NURSING ACTIONS   *RATIONALE/EXPLANATION*

4. Observe for drug interactions

    a. Drugs that *increase* effects of skeletal muscle relaxants:

        (1) CNS depressants (alcohol, antianxiety agents, antidepressants, antihistamines, antipsychotic drugs, sedative-hypnotics) | Additive CNS depression with increased risks of excessive sedation and respiratory depression or apnea

        (2) MAO inhibitors | May potentiate effects by inhibiting metabolism of muscle relaxants

5. Teach clients

    a. Take the drugs with milk or food. | To avoid nausea and gastric irritation

    b. Do not stop drugs abruptly. Dosage should be decreased gradually, especially with baclofen, carisoprodol, and cyclobenzaprine | Abrupt withdrawal of baclofen may cause hallucinations; abrupt withdrawal of the other drugs may cause headache, nausea, and malaise.

REVIEW AND APPLICATION EXERCISES

1. How do skeletal muscle relaxants act to relieve spasm and pain?

2. What are the indications for the use of skeletal muscle relaxants?

3. What are the contraindications for the use of these drugs?

4. What are the major adverse effects of these drugs, and how can they be minimized?

5. What are some nonpharmacologic interventions to use instead of or along with the drugs?

SELECTED REFERENCES

Drug facts and comparisons. (1996). St. Louis: Facts and Comparisons.

Guyton, A.C., & Hall, J.E. (1996). *Textbook of medical physiology*, 9th ed. Philadelphia: W.B. Saunders.

Anesthetics

Outline

Objectives

After studying this chapter, the student will be able to:

1 Discuss factors considered when choosing an anesthetic agent.

2 Describe characteristics of general and regional anesthetic agents.

3 Compare general and local anesthetics in terms of administration, client safety, and nursing care.

4 Discuss the rationale for using adjunctive drugs before and during surgical procedures.

5 Describe the nurse's role in relation to anesthetics and adjunctive drugs.

Key Terms

Adjunctive drugs	**Perioperative**
Epidural anesthesia	**Regional anesthesia**
General anesthesia	

Anesthesia means loss of sensation with or without loss of consciousness. Anesthetic drugs are given to prevent pain and promote relaxation during surgery, childbirth, some diagnostic tests, and some treatments. They interrupt the conduction of painful nerve impulses from a site of injury to the brain. The two basic types of anesthesia are general and regional.

General Anesthesia

General anesthesia is a state of profound central nervous system (CNS) depression, during which there is complete loss of sensation, consciousness, pain perception, and memory. It has three components: hypnosis, analgesia, and muscle relaxation. Several different drugs are usually combined to produce desired levels of these components without excessive CNS depression. This so-called balanced anesthesia also allows lower dosages of potent general anesthetics.

The four stages of general anesthesia are analgesia (I), excitement and hyperactivity (II), surgical anesthesia (III), and medullary paralysis (IV). General anesthesia is administered so that stage III anesthesia is maintained as long as necessary and stage IV is avoided. Spontaneous breathing stops with stage IV; death follows unless the anesthetic is discontinued and resuscitative measures are undertaken. These stages were described in relation to ether, an obsolete anesthetic, and may not be discernible with newer agents. Knowing the stages is important for the nurse because clients recovering from anesthesia progress through the same stages in reverse. Thus, analgesia or hyperactivity may extend into the postanesthesia recovery period.

General anesthesia is usually induced with an ultra-short-acting barbiturate given intravenously (IV) and is maintained with a gas mixture of an anesthetic agent and oxygen given by inhalation. The IV agent produces rapid loss of consciousness, is not explosive, and provides a pleasant induction and recovery. Its rapid onset of action is attributed to rapid circulation to the brain and accumulation in the neuronal tissue of the cerebral cortex. Duration of action is also very short with a single dose but can be prolonged with continuous IV infusion. These drugs also may be used alone for anesthesia during brief diagnostic tests or surgical procedures.

Inhalation anesthetics vary in the degree of CNS depression produced and thereby vary in the rate of induction, anesthetic potency, degree of muscle relaxation, and analgesic potency. CNS depression is determined by the concentration of the drug in the CNS. Drug concentration, in turn, depends on the rate at which the drug is transported from the alveoli to the blood, transported past the blood-brain barrier to reach the CNS, redistributed by the blood to other body tissues, and eliminated by the lungs. Depth of anesthesia can be regulated readily by varying the concentration of the inhaled anesthetic gas. General inhalation anesthetics should be given only by specially trained people, such as anesthesiologists and nurse anesthetists, and only with appropriate equipment.

Regional Anesthesia

Regional anesthesia involves loss of sensation and motor activity in localized areas of the body. It is induced by application or injection of local anesthetic drugs. The drugs act to decrease the permeability of nerve cell membranes to ions. This action stabilizes the cell membrane, prevents initiation and transmission of nerve impulses, and therefore prevents the cells from responding to pain impulses and other sensory stimuli.

Regional anesthesia is usually categorized according to the site of application. The area anesthetized may be the site of application, or it may be distal to the point of injection. Specific types of anesthesia attained with local anesthetic drugs include the following:

1. Topical or surface anesthesia involves applying local anesthetic agents to skin or mucous membrane. Such application makes sensory receptors unresponsive to pain, itching, and other stimuli. Local anesthetics for topical use are usually ingredients of various ointments, solutions, or lotions designed for use at particular sites. For example, preparations are available for use on eyes, ears, nose, oral mucosa, perineum, hemorrhoids, and skin.
2. Infiltration involves injecting the local anesthetic solution directly into or very close to the area to be anesthetized.
3. Peripheral nerve block involves injecting the anesthetic solution into the area of a larger nerve trunk or a nerve plexus at some access point along the course of a nerve distant from the area to be anesthetized.
4. Field block anesthesia involves injecting the anesthetic solution around the area to be anesthetized.
5. Spinal anesthesia involves injecting the anesthetic agent into the cerebrospinal fluid, usually in the lumbar spine. The anesthetic blocks sensory impulses at the root of peripheral nerves as they enter the spinal cord. Spinal anesthesia is especially useful for surgery involving the lower abdomen and legs.

The body area anesthetized is determined by the level to which the drug solution rises in the spinal canal. This, in turn, is determined by the site of injection, the position of the client, and the specific gravity, amount, and concentration of the injected solution.

Solutions of local anesthetic drugs used for spinal anesthesia are either hyperbaric or hypobaric. *Hyperbaric* or heavy solutions are diluted with dextrose, have a higher specific gravity than cerebrospinal fluid, and gravitate toward the head when the client is tilted in a head-down position. *Hypobaric* or light solutions are diluted with distilled water, have a lower specific gravity than cerebrospinal fluid, and gravitate toward the lower (caudal) end of the spinal canal when the client is tilted in a head-down position.

6. Epidural or caudal anesthesia involves injecting the anesthetic into the epidural space. In lumbar epidural anesthesia, the injection is usually made between the second lumbar and the first sacral vertebrae to avoid injuring the spinal cord, which ends at the first lumbar vertebra in 95% of people. In caudal anesthesia, the drug solution is injected into the caudal canal through the sacral area. Epidural or caudal anesthesia is used most often in obstetrics during labor and delivery and occasionally is used in surgery of the perineal or rectal areas.

Generally, the area anesthetized is determined by the site of injection (lumbar or caudal), the position of the client, the volume and concentration of the anesthetic solution, the age of the client, whether the client is pregnant, and the extent of arteriosclerosis. A smaller area is anesthetized if the recipient is in a sitting position. A larger area is anesthetized if high volumes and high concentrations of drug solutions are used, if the client is a child or is elderly, if the client is pregnant and at full term, and if occlusive arterial disease is present.

The extent and duration of anesthesia produced by injection of local anesthetics depend on several factors. Generally, large amounts, high concentrations, or injections into highly vascular areas (*e.g.,* head and neck, intercostal and paracervical sites) produce rapid peak plasma levels. Duration depends on the chemical characteristics of the drug used and the rate at which it leaves nerve tissue. When a vasoconstrictor drug, such as epinephrine, has been added, onset and duration of anesthesia are prolonged due to slowed absorption of the anesthetic agent.

Adjuncts to Anesthesia

Several nonanesthetic drugs are used as adjuncts or supplements to anesthetic drugs. Most are discussed elsewhere and are described here only in relation to anesthesia. Drug groups include antianxiety agents and sedative-hypnotics (see Chap. 8), anticholinergics (see Chap. 21), and narcotic analgesics (see Chap. 6). The neuromuscular blocking agents are described in this chapter.

ANTIANXIETY AGENTS AND SEDATIVE-HYPNOTICS

Antianxiety agents and *sedative-hypnotics* are given to decrease anxiety, promote rest, and increase client safety by allowing easier induction of anesthesia and smaller doses of anesthetic agents. These drugs may be given the night before to aid sleep and 1 or 2 hours before the scheduled procedure. Hypnotic doses are usually given for greater sedative effects. Some commonly used drugs are diazepam (Valium) and hydroxyzine (Vistaril).

ANTICHOLINERGICS

Anticholinergic drugs are given to prevent excessive activity of the parasympathetic nervous system (vagal stimulation). Vagal stimulation occurs with some inhalation anesthetics, such as halothane; with succinylcholine, a commonly used muscle relaxant; and with surgical procedures in which there is manipulation of the pharynx, trachea, peritoneum, stomach, intestine, or other viscera and procedures in which pressure is exerted on the eyeball. If not blocked by anticholinergic drugs, vagal stimulation may cause excessive bradycardia, hypotension, and cardiac arrest. Useful drugs are atropine and glycopyrrolate (Robinul).

Anticholinergic drugs also have been widely used to decrease secretions in the respiratory tract. Because newer inhalation anesthetics produce less respiratory tract irritation and fewer secretions, anticholinergic drugs are not routinely indicated. However, the drugs may be useful with bronchoscopy or head and neck surgery.

NARCOTIC ANALGESICS

Narcotic analgesics, such as morphine and meperidine, induce relaxation and pain relief in the preanesthetic period. These drugs potentiate the CNS depression produced by other drugs, and less anesthetic agent is required. Morphine and fentanyl may be given in anesthetic doses in certain circumstances.

NEUROMUSCULAR BLOCKING AGENTS

Neuromuscular blocking agents cause muscle relaxation, the third component of general anesthesia, and allow the use of smaller amounts of anesthetic agent. Artificial ventilation is necessary because these drugs paralyze muscles of respiration as well as other skeletal muscles. The drugs do not cause sedation; therefore, unless the recipients are unconscious, they can see and hear environmental activities and conversations.

There are two types of neuromuscular blocking agents: depolarizing and nondepolarizing. Succinylcholine is the only commonly used depolarizing drug. Like acetylcholine, the drug combines with cholinergic receptors at the motor endplate to produce depolarization and muscle contraction initially. Repolarization and further muscle contraction are then inhibited as long as an adequate concentration of drug remains at the receptor site.

Muscle paralysis is preceded by muscle spasms, which may damage muscles. Injury to muscle cells may cause postoperative muscle pain and release potassium into the circulation. If hyperkalemia develops, it is usually mild and insignificant but may cause cardiac arrhythmias or even cardiac arrest in some situations. Succinylcholine is normally deactivated by plasma pseudocholinesterase. There is no antidote except reconstituted fresh-frozen plasma that contains pseudocholinesterase.

Nondepolarizing neuromuscular blocking agents prevent acetylcholine from acting at neuromuscular junctions. Consequently, the nerve cell membrane is not depolarized, the muscle fibers are not stimulated, and skeletal muscle contraction does not occur. The prototype drug is tubocurarine, the active ingredient of curare, a naturally occurring plant alkaloid that causes skeletal muscle relaxation or paralysis. Most of the newer drugs are synthetic preparations. Anticholinesterase drugs, such as neostigmine (Prostigmin; see Chap. 20), are antidotes and are used to reverse muscle paralysis.

Individual Anesthetic Agents

General anesthetics are listed in Table 14-1, neuromuscular blocking agents in Table 14-2, and local anesthetics in Table 14-3.

TABLE 14-1 GENERAL ANESTHETICS

Generic/Trade Name	Characteristics	Remarks
General Inhalation Anesthetics		
Desflurane (Suprane)	Similar to isoflurane	Used for induction and maintenance of general anesthesia
Enflurane (Ethrane)	Nonexplosive, nonflammable volatile liquid; similar to halothane but may produce better analgesia and muscle relaxation; sensitizes heart to catecholamines—increases risks of cardiac arrhythmias; renal or hepatic toxicity not reported	A frequently used agent
Halothane (Fluothane)	Nonexplosive, nonflammable volatile liquid. Advantages: 1. Produces rapid induction with little or no excitement; rapid recovery with little excitement or nausea and vomiting 2. Does not irritate respiratory tract mucosa; therefore does not increase saliva and tracheobronchial secretions 3. Depresses pharyngeal and laryngeal reflexes, which decreases risk of laryngospasm and bronchospasm. Disadvantages: 1. Depresses contractility of the heart and vascular smooth muscle, which causes decreased cardiac output, hypotension, and bradycardia 2. Circulatory failure may occur with high doses. 3. Causes cardiac arrhythmias. Bradycardia is common; ventricular arrhythmias are uncommon unless ventilation is inadequate. 4. Sensitizes heart to catecholamines; increases risk of cardiac arrhythmias 5. Depresses respiration and may produce hypoxemia and respiratory acidosis (hypercarbia) 6. Depresses functions of the kidneys, liver, and immune system	Halothane has largely been replaced by newer agents with increased efficacy, decreased adverse effects, or both. It may be used in balanced anesthesia with other agents. Although quite potent, it may not produce adequate analgesia and muscle relaxation at a dosage that is not likely to produce significant adverse effects. Therefore, nitrous oxide is given to increase analgesic effects; a neuromuscular blocking agent is given to increase muscle relaxation; and an IV barbiturate is used to produce rapid, smooth induction, after which halothane is given to maintain anesthesia.

TABLE 14-1   GENERAL ANESTHETICS (Continued)

Generic/Trade Name	Characteristics	Remarks
	7. May cause jaundice and hepatitis 8. May cause malignant hyperthermia	
Isoflurane (Forane)	Similar to halothane in action; less likely to cause cardiovascular depression and ventricular arrhythmias than halothane. Isoflurane may cause malignant hyperthermia but apparently does not cause hepatotoxicity.	Used for induction and maintenance of general anesthesia
Methoxyflurane (Penthrane)	Nonexplosive, nonflammable volatile liquid; similar to halothane in most respects but is more analgesic when inhaled at low concentrations, has slower induction and recovery, does not sensitize the heart to catecholamines, and causes renal damage and failure. Renal failure is dose-related and increases with drug concentration and length of time administered. It is attributed to metabolites of methoxyflurane.	Use as a general anesthetic is limited because of renal toxicity. It is used in dentistry, childbirth, or other procedures in which small amounts can be given for brief periods. This does not allow enough accumulation of the drug or its metabolites to cause renal damage.
Nitrous oxide	Nonexplosive gas; good analgesic, weak anesthetic; one of oldest and safest anesthetics; causes no appreciable damage to vital organs unless hypoxia is allowed to develop and persist; administered with oxygen to prevent hypoxia; rapid induction and recovery. *Note*: Nitrous oxide is an incomplete anesthetic; that is, by itself, it cannot produce stage III anesthesia.	Often used in balanced anesthesia with IV barbiturates, neuromuscular blocking agents, narcotic analgesics, and more potent inhalation anesthetics, such as halothane. It is safer for prolonged surgical procedures (see "Characteristics"). It is used alone for analgesia in dentistry, obstetrics, and brief surgical procedures.
Sevoflurane (Ultane)	Similar to isoflurane	Used for induction and maintenance of general anesthesia
General Intravenous Anesthetics		
Alfentanil (Alfenta)	Opioid analgesic-anesthetic related to fentanyl and sufentanil. Rapid-acting.	May be used as a primary anesthetic or an analgesic adjunct in balanced anesthesia
Etomidate (Amidate)	A nonanalgesic hypnotic used for induction and maintenance of general anesthesia	May be used with nitrous oxide and oxygen in maintenance of general anesthesia for short operative procedures such as uterine dilation and curettage
Fentanyl and droperidol combination (Innovar)	Droperidol (Inapsine) is related to the antipsychotic agent haloperidol. It produces sedative and antiemetic effects. Fentanyl citrate (Sublimaze) is a very potent narcotic analgesic whose actions are similar to those of morphine but of shorter duration. Innovar is a fixed-dose combination of the two drugs. Additional doses of fentanyl are often needed because its analgesic effect lasts about 30 minutes, while droperidol's effects last 3–6 hours.	Either drug may be used alone, but they are most often used together for neuroleptanalgesia and combined with nitrous oxide for neuroleptanesthesia. Neuroleptanalgesia is a state of reduced awareness and reduced sensory perception during which a variety of diagnostic tests or minor surgical procedures can be done, such as bronchoscopy and burn dressings. Neuroleptanesthesia can be used for major surgical procedures. Consciousness returns rapidly, but respiratory depression may last 3–4 hours into the postoperative recovery period.
Ketamine (Ketalar)	Rapid-acting, nonbarbiturate anesthetic; produces marked analgesia, sedation, immobility, amnesia, and a lack of awareness of surroundings	Used most often for brief surgical, diagnostic, or therapeutic procedures. It also may be used to induce anesthesia.

(continued)

TABLE 14-1   GENERAL ANESTHETICS (Continued)

Generic/Trade Name	Characteristics	Remarks
	(called dissociative anesthesia); may be given IV or IM; awakening may require several hours; during recovery, unpleasant psychic symptoms may occur, including dreams and hallucinations; vomiting, hypersalivation, and transient skin rashes also may occur during recovery.	If used for major surgery, it must be supplemented by other general anesthetics. It is generally contraindicated in individuals with increased intracranial pressure, severe coronary artery disease, hypertension, or psychiatric disorders. Hyperactivity and unpleasant dreams occur less often with children than adults. See thiamylal, thiopental, below.
Methohexital sodium (Brevital)	An ultrashort-acting barbiturate similar to thiamylal and thiopental	
Midazolam (Versed)	Short-acting benzodiazepine. May cause respiratory depression, apnea, death with IV administration. Smaller doses are needed if other CNS depressants (e.g., narcotic analgesics, general anesthetics) are given concurrently.	Given IM for preoperative sedation. Given IV for conscious sedation during short endoscopic or other diagnostic procedures; induction of general anesthesia; and maintenance of general anesthesia with nitrous oxide and oxygen for short surgical procedures
Propofol (Diprivan)	A rapid-acting hypnotic used with other agents in balanced anesthesia. May cause hypotension, apnea, and other signs of CNS depression. Recovery is rapid, occurring within minutes after the drug is stopped.	Given by IV bolus or infusion for induction or maintenance of general anesthesia
Sufentanil (Sufenta)	A synthetic opioid analgesic-anesthetic related to fentanyl. Compared to fentanyl, it is more potent and faster-acting and may allow a more rapid recovery.	May be used as a primary anesthetic or an analgesic adjunct in balanced anesthesia
Thiamylal sodium Thiopental sodium (Surital, Pentothal)	Ultrashort-acting barbiturates, used almost exclusively in general anesthesia; excellent hypnotics but do not produce significant analgesia or muscle relaxation; given IV by intermittent injection or by continuous infusion of a dilute solution.	Thiopental is commonly used. A single dose produces unconsciousness in less than 30 seconds and lasts 20–30 minutes. Usually given to induce anesthesia. It is used alone only for brief procedures. For major surgery, it is usually supplemented by inhalation anesthetics and muscle relaxants.

Nursing Process

Preoperative Assessment

- Assess nutritional status.
- Assess use of prescription and nonprescription drugs, especially those taken within the past 3 days. Ask if corticosteroids have been taken within the past 3 months.
- Ask about drug allergies. If use of local or regional anesthesia is anticipated, ask if the client has ever had an allergic reaction to a local anesthetic.
- Assess for risk factors for complications of anesthesia and surgery (cigarette smoking, obesity, limited exercise or activity, chronic cardiovascular, respiratory, renal, or other disease processes).
- Assess the client's understanding of the intended procedure, attitude toward anesthesia and surgery, and degree of anxiety and fear.
- Assess ability and willingness to participate in postoperative activities to promote recovery.

- Assess vital signs, laboratory data, and other data as indicated to establish baseline measurements for monitoring changes.

Postoperative Assessment

- During the immediate postoperative period, assess vital signs and respiratory and cardiovascular function every 5 to 15 minutes until reactive and stabilizing.
- Continue to assess vital signs, fluid balance, and laboratory and other data.
- Assess for signs of complications (e.g., fluid and electrolyte imbalance, respiratory problems, thrombophlebitis, wound infection).

Nursing Diagnoses

- Risk for Injury: Trauma related to impaired sensory perception and impaired physical mobility from anesthetic
- Risk for Injury: CNS depression with premedications and general anesthetics

TABLE 14-2 NEUROMUSCULAR BLOCKING AGENTS (SKELETAL MUSCLE RELAXANTS)

Generic/Trade Name	Characteristics	Uses
Depolarizing Type		
Succinylcholine (Anectine)	Short-acting after single dose; action can be prolonged by repeated injections or continuous IV infusion. Malignant hyperthermia may occur.	All types of surgery and brief procedures, such as endoscopy and endotracheal intubation
Nondepolarizing Type		
Atracurlum (Tracrium)	Intermediate-acting*	Adjunct to general anesthesia
Cisatracurium (Nimbex)	Intermediate-acting*	Same as rocuronium, below
Doxacurium (Nuromax)	Long-acting*	Adjunct to general anesthesia
Gallamine (Flaxedil)	Long-acting*	Adjunct to general anesthesia
Metocurine (Metubine)	Long-acting; more potent than tubocurarine*	Same as vecuronium, below
Mivacurium (Mivacron)	Short-acting*	Adjunct to general anesthesia
Pancuronium (Pavulon)	Long-acting*	Mainly during surgery after general anesthesia has been induced; occasionally to aid endotracheal intubation or mechanical ventilation
Pipecuronium (Arduan)	Long-acting*	Adjunct to general anesthesia; recommended only for procedures expected to last 90 minutes or longer
Rocuronium (Zemuron)	Intermediate-acting*	Adjunct to general anesthesia to aid endotracheal intubation and provide muscle relaxation during surgery or mechanical ventilation
Tubocurarine	Long-acting; the prototype of nondepolarizing drugs*	Adjunct to general anesthesia; occasionally to facilitate mechanical ventilation
Vecuronium (Norcuron)	Intermediate-acting*	Adjunct to general anesthesia; to facilitate endotracheal intubation and mechanical ventilation

*All the nondepolarizing agents may cause hypotension; effects of the drugs can be reversed by neostigmine (Prostigmin).

- Pain related to operative procedure
- Decreased Cardiac Output related to effects of anesthetics, other medications, and surgery
- Impaired Gas Exchange related to effects of anesthetics, other medications, and surgery
- Anxiety or Fear related to anticipated surgery and possible outcomes

Planning/Goals

The client will:

- Receive sufficient emotional support and instruction to facilitate a smooth preoperative and postoperative course
- Be protected from injury and complications while self-care ability is impaired
- Have emergency supplies and personnel available if needed
- Have postoperative discomfort managed appropriately

Interventions

Preoperatively, assist the client to achieve optimal conditions for surgery. Some guidelines include the following:

- Provide foods and fluids to improve or maintain nutritional status (e.g., those high in protein, vitamin C and other vitamins, and electrolytes to promote healing).

- Help the client maintain exercise and activity, when feasible. This helps promote respiratory and cardiovascular function and decreases anxiety.
- Explain the expected course of events of the perioperative period (e.g., specific preparations for surgery, close observation and monitoring during postanesthesia recovery, approximate length of stay).
- Teach clients measures to facilitate recovery postoperatively (e.g., coughing and deep-breathing exercises, leg exercises and early ambulation, maintaining fluid balance and urine output). Some of these will initially be performed or assisted by staff; others are best performed by the client when able.
- Explain how pain will be managed postoperatively. This is often a major source of anxiety.

Postoperatively, the major focus is to maintain a safe environment and vital functions. Specific interventions include:

- Observe and record vital signs, level of consciousness, respiratory and cardiovascular status, wound status, and elimination frequently until sensory and motor functions return, then periodically until discharge.

TABLE 14-3	LOCAL ANESTHETICS	

Generic/Trade Name	Characteristics	Clinical Uses
Benzocaine (Americaine)	Poorly water soluble and poorly absorbed; thus, anesthetic effects are relatively prolonged, and systemic absorption is minimal; available in many prescription and nonprescription preparations, including aerosol sprays, throat lozenges, rectal suppositories, lotions, and ointments	Topical anesthesia of skin and mucous membrane to relieve pain and itching of sunburn, other minor burns and wounds, skin abrasions, earache, hemorrhoids, sore throat, and other conditions. Caution: may cause hypersensitivity reactions.
Bupivacaine (Marcaine)	Given by injection; has a relatively long duration of action; may produce systemic toxicity	Regional anesthesia by infiltration, nerve block, and epidural anesthesia during childbirth. It is not used for spinal anesthesia.
Butamben (Butesin)	Applied topically to skin only	Used mainly in minor burns and skin irritations
Chloroprocaine (Nesacaine)	Chemically and pharmacologically related to procaine, but its potency is greater and duration of action is shorter; rapidly metabolized and less likely to cause systemic toxicity than other local anesthetics; given by injection	Regional anesthesia by infiltration, nerve block, and epidural anesthesia
Cocaine	One of the oldest local anesthetics; a naturally occurring plant alkaloid; readily absorbed through mucous membranes; a Schedule II controlled substance with high potential for abuse, largely because of euphoria and other CNS stimulatory effects; produces psychic dependence and tolerance with prolonged use; too toxic for systemic use	Topical anesthesia of ear, nose, and throat
Dibucaine (Nupercaine, Nupercainal)	Potent agent; onset of action slow but duration relatively long; rather high incidence of toxicity	Topical or spinal anesthesia
Dyclonine (Dyclone)	Rapid onset of action and duration comparable to procaine; absorbed through skin and mucous membrane	Topical anesthesia in otolaryngology
Etidocaine (Duranest)	A derivative of lidocaine that is more potent and more toxic than lidocaine; long duration of action	Regional nerve blocks and epidural anesthesia
Lidocaine (Xylocaine)	Given topically and by injection; more rapid in onset, intensity, and duration of action than procaine, also more toxic; acts as an antiarrhythmic drug by decreasing myocardial irritability. One of the most widely used local anesthetic drugs.	Topical anesthesia and regional anesthesia by local infiltration, nerve block, spinal, and epidural anesthesia. It also is used intravenously to prevent or treat cardiac arrhythmias (see Chap. 52). (Caution: do not use preparations containing epinephrine for arrhythmias.)
Mepivacaine (Carbocaine)	Chemically and pharmacologically related to lidocaine; action slower in onset and longer in duration than lidocaine; effective only in large doses; not used topically	Infiltration, nerve block, and epidural anesthesia
Pramoxine (Tronothane)	Not injected or applied to nasal mucosa because it irritates tissues	Topical anesthesia for skin wounds, dermatoses, hemorrhoids, endotracheal intubation, sigmoidoscopy
Prilocaine (Citanest)	Pharmacologically similar to lidocaine with about the same effectiveness but slower onset, longer duration, and less toxicity because it is more rapidly metabolized and excreted	Regional anesthesia by infiltration, nerve block, and epidural anesthesia
Procaine (Novocain)	Most widely used local anesthetic for many years, but it has largely been replaced by lidocaine and other newer drugs. It is rapidly metabolized, which increases safety but shortens duration of action.	Regional anesthesia by infiltration, nerve block, and spinal anesthesia. Not used topically.

TABLE 14-3	LOCAL ANESTHETICS (Continued)	
Generic/Trade Name	**Characteristics**	**Clinical Uses**
Proparacaine (Alcaine)	Causes minimal irritation of the eye but may cause allergic contact dermatitis of the fingers	Topical anesthesia of the eye for tonometry and for removal of sutures, foreign bodies, and cataracts
Tetracaine (Pontocaine)	Applied topically or given by injection	Topical and spinal anesthesia mainly; can be used for local infiltration or nerve block

- Maintain IV infusions. Monitor the site and amount and type of fluids. If potential problems are identified (*e.g.,* hypovolemia or hypervolemia), intervene to prevent them from becoming actual problems.
- Give pain medication appropriately as indicated by the client's condition.
- Help the client to turn, cough, deep breathe, exercise legs, ambulate, and perform other self-care activities until he or she can perform them independently.
- Use sterile technique in wound care.
- Teach clients about the effects of narcotic analgesics on gastrointestinal and urinary functions.
- Teach clients ways to prevent postoperative complications, including respiratory and wound infections.
- Initiate discharge planning for a smooth transition to home care.

Evaluation

- Observe for absence of injury and complications (*e.g.,* no fever or other signs of infection).
- Observe for improved ability in self-care activities.
- The client states that pain has been managed satisfactorily.

Principles of Therapy

1. Principles for using adjunctive drugs (antianxiety agents, anticholinergics, narcotic analgesics) are the same when these drugs are given preoperatively as at other times. They are usually ordered by an anesthesiologist and sometimes by the surgeon. Many drugs are available for use as anesthetics and adjunctive agents. The anesthesiologist is usually responsible for choosing particular drugs, and the choice depends on several factors. Some client-related factors include age; the specific procedure to be performed and its anticipated duration; the client's physical condition, including severity of illness, presence of chronic diseases, and any other drugs being given; and the client's mental status. Severe anxiety, for example, may be a contraindication for regional anesthesia, and the client may require larger doses of preanesthetic sedative-type medication.
   a. General anesthesia can be used for almost any surgical, diagnostic, or therapeutic procedure. If a medical disorder of a vital organ system (cardiovascular, respiratory, renal) is present, it should be corrected before anesthesia is induced when possible. General anesthesia and major surgical procedures have profound effects on normal body functioning. When alterations due to other disorders are also involved, the risks of anesthesia and surgery are greatly increased.
   b. Regional or local anesthesia is usually safer than general anesthesia because it produces fewer systemic effects. For example, spinal anesthesia is often the anesthesia of choice for surgery involving the lower abdomen and lower extremities, especially in people who are elderly or have chronic lung disease. A major advantage of spinal anesthesia is that it causes less CNS and respiratory depression.
2. Anesthetics should be given *only* by people with special training in correct usage. This applies especially to general anesthetics and neuromuscular blocking agents, but it is also important with local anesthetics when they are injected. In addition, general and local anesthetics should be given only in locations where personnel, equipment, and drugs are available for emergency use or cardiopulmonary resuscitation.
3. Choice of a local anesthetic drug depends mainly on the reason for use or the type of regional anesthesia desired. Lidocaine, one of the most widely used, is available in topical and injectable forms.

GUIDELINES FOR ADMINISTRATION OF A LOCAL ANESTHETIC

When local anesthetic solutions are injected, some guidelines for safe use include the following:

1. Local anesthetic solutions must not be injected into blood vessels because of the high risk of serious adverse reactions involving the cardiovascular system and CNS. To prevent accidental injection into a blood vessel, needle placement must be verified by

aspirating before injecting the local anesthetic solution. If blood is aspirated into the syringe, another injection site must be selected.

2. Local anesthetics given during labor cross the placenta and may depress muscle strength, muscle tone, and rooting behavior in the newborn. Apgar scores are usually normal. If excessive amounts are used (*e.g.,* in paracervical block), local anesthetics may cause fetal bradycardia, increased movement, and expulsion of meconium before birth and marked depression after birth. Dosage used for spinal anesthesia during labor is too small to depress the fetus or the newborn.

3. For spinal or epidural anesthesia, use only local anesthetic solutions that have been specifically prepared for spinal anesthesia and are in single-dose containers. Multiple-dose containers are not used because of the risk of injecting contaminated solutions.

4. Use of local anesthetic solutions containing epinephrine requires some special considerations, such as the following:

   a. This combination of drugs should not be used for nerve blocks in areas supplied by end arteries (fingers, ears, nose, toes, penis) because it may produce ischemia and gangrene.

   b. This combination should not be given IV or in excessive dosage because the local anesthetic and epinephrine can cause serious systemic toxicity, including cardiac arrhythmias.

   c. This combination should not be used with inhalation anesthetic agents that increase myocardial sensitivity to catecholamines. Severe ventricular arrhythmias may result.

   d. These drugs should probably not be used in clients with severe cardiovascular disease or hyperthyroidism.

   e. If used in obstetrics, the concentration of epinephrine should be no greater than 1:200,000 because of the danger of producing vasoconstriction in uterine blood vessels. Such vasoconstriction may cause decreased placental circulation, decreased intensity of uterine contractions, and prolonged labor.

For topical anesthesia of mucous membranes of the nose, mouth, pharynx, larynx, trachea, bronchi, and urethra, local anesthetics are effective but should be given in reduced dosage. Because drug absorption from these areas is rapid, no more than one fourth to one third of the dose used for infiltration should be given to minimize systemic adverse reactions.

NURSING ACTIONS
ANESTHETIC DRUGS

NURSING ACTIONS	RATIONALE/EXPLANATION
1. Administer accurately	Drug administration in relation to anesthesia refers primarily to preanesthetic or postanesthetic drugs because physicians, dentists, and nurse anesthetists administer anesthetic drugs.
a. Schedule the administration of preanesthetic medications so that their peak effects are reached at the optimal time, if possible.	Timing is important. It is probably better if these medications are administered so that peak sedative effects occur before administration of anesthetics to avoid excessive central nervous system (CNS) depression. If they are given too early, the client may be sedated longer than necessary, and the risk of postanesthetic respiratory and circulatory complications is increased. Also, the medication effects may wear off before induction of anesthesia. If they are given too late, the client may suffer needless anxiety and not be relaxed and drowsy when anesthesia is being initiated. Preanesthetic medications are often ordered "on call" rather than for a specific time, and the client may or may not become sedated before being transported to the surgery suite.
b. When a combination of two or three preanesthetic medications is ordered, do *not* mix in the same syringe and give as one injection unless the drugs are known to be compatible and the total volume is about 2 ml.	A precipitate may develop, or one of the drugs may be inactivated or altered when combined. Although larger amounts are sometimes given, probably no more than 2 to 3 ml should be given intramuscularly (IM) for both drug absorption and client comfort. About 1¼ ml (20 minims) is the upper limit for subcutaneous injections.

Nursing Actions	*Rationale/Explanation*
(1) Morphine and meperidine (Demerol) mix with promethazine (Phenergan) and hydroxyzine (Vistaril) and may be combined in the same syringe.	These are commonly used drugs.
(2) Atropine and scopolamine mix with all the above drugs.	
(3) Glycopyrrolate (Robinul) is often ordered instead of atropine or scopolamine. It is compatible with morphine, meperidine, Innovar, and hydroxyzine.	
(4) Do *not* mix injectable pentobarbital (Nembutal) or other barbiturates with any other drug.	Parenteral barbiturates are physically incompatible with other parenteral drugs.
(5) If there is any doubt about the compatibility of a drug combination, *do not mix.* Instead, give two or more injections if necessary.	
c. If assisting a physician in injecting a local anesthetic solution, show the drug container to the physician and verbally verify the name of the drug, the percentage concentration, and whether the solution is plain or contains epinephrine.	Although the physician is responsible for drugs he or she administers, the nurse often assists by obtaining and perhaps holding the drug vial while the physician aspirates drug solution into a syringe.
	Accuracy of administration is essential so that adverse reactions can be avoided or treated appropriately if they do occur. The incidence of adverse reactions increases with the amount and concentration of local anesthetic solution injected. Also, adverse reactions to epinephrine may occur.
d. Have drugs and equipment for resuscitation readily available in any location where local anesthetics are given.	
e. When applying local anesthetics for topical or surface anesthesia, be certain to use the appropriate preparation of the prescribed drug.	Most preparations are used in particular conditions or bodily locations. For example, lidocaine viscous is used only as an oral preparation for anesthesia of the mouth and throat. Other preparations are used only on the skin.
2. Observe for therapeutic effects	Therapeutic effects depend on the type of drug and the reason for use.
a. When adjunctive drugs are given for preanesthetic medication, observe for relaxation, drowsiness, and relief of pain.	Depending on dose and client condition, these effects are usually evident within 20 to 30 minutes after the drugs are given.
b. When local anesthetic drugs are applied for surface anesthesia, observe for relief of the symptom for which the drug was ordered, such as sore mouth or throat, pain in skin or mucous membrane, and itching of hemorrhoids.	Relief is usually obtained within a few minutes. Ask the client if the symptom has been relieved, and if not, assess the situation to determine whether further action is needed.
3. Observe for adverse effects	Serious adverse effects are most likely to occur during and within a few hours after general anesthesia and major surgery. During general anesthesia, the anesthesiologist monitors the client's condition constantly to prevent, detect, or treat hypoxia, hypotension, cardiac arrhythmias, and other problems. The nurse observes for adverse effects in the preanesthetic and postanesthetic periods.
a. With preanesthetic drugs, observe for excessive sedation.	The often-used combination of a narcotic analgesic and a sedative-type drug produces additive CNS depression.

(continued)

NURSING ACTIONS	*RATIONALE/EXPLANATION*
b. After general anesthesia, observe for:	
(1) Excessive sedation—delayed awakening, failure to respond to verbal or tactile stimuli	The early recovery period is normally marked by a progressive increase in alertness, responsiveness, and movement.
(2) Respiratory problems—laryngospasm, hypoxia, hypercarbia	Laryngospasm may occur after removal of the endotracheal tube used to administer general anesthesia. Hypoxia and hypercarbia indicate inadequate ventilation and may result from depression of the respiratory center in the medulla oblongata, prolonged paralysis of respiratory muscles with muscle relaxant drugs, or retention of respiratory tract secretions due to a depressed cough reflex.
(3) Cardiovascular problems—hypotension, tachycardia and other cardiac arrhythmias, fluid and electrolyte imbalances	Vital signs are often unstable during the early recovery period and therefore need to be checked frequently. Extreme changes must be reported to the surgeon or the anesthesiologist. These problems are most likely to occur while general anesthesia is being administered and progressively less likely as the patient recovers or awakens.
(4) Other problems—restlessness, nausea, and vomiting. With ketamine, unpleasant dreams or hallucinations also may occur.	Restlessness may be caused by the anesthetic, pain, or hypoxia and should be assessed carefully before action is taken. For example, if caused by hypoxia but interpreted as being caused by pain, administration of analgesics would aggravate hypoxia.
c. After regional anesthesia, observe for:	
(1) CNS stimulation at first (hyperactivity, excitement, seizure activity) followed by CNS depression	These symptoms are more likely to occur with large doses, high concentrations, injections into highly vascular areas, or accidental injection into a blood vessel.
(2) Cardiovascular depression—hypotension, arrhythmias	Local anesthetics depress myocardial contractility and the cardiac conduction system. These effects are most likely to occur with high doses. Doses used for spinal or epidural anesthesia usually have little effect on cardiovascular function.
(3) Headache and urinary retention with spinal anesthesia	Headache is more likely to occur if the person does not lie flat for 8 to 12 hours after spinal anesthesia is given. Urinary retention may occur in anyone but is more likely in older men with enlarged prostate glands.
4. Observe for drug interactions	For interactions involving preanesthetic medications, see Sedative-Hypnotics and Antianxiety Drugs (Chap. 8), Anticholinergic Drugs (Chap. 21), and Narcotic Analgesics (Chap. 6).
a. Drugs that *increase* effects of general anesthetic agents:	
(1) Antibiotics—bacitracin, aminoglycosides (gentamicin and related drugs), polymyxin B	These antibiotics inhibit neuromuscular transmission. When they are combined with general anesthetics, additive muscle relaxation occurs with increased likelihood of respiratory paralysis and apnea.
(2) Antihypertensives	Additive hypotension, shock, and circulatory failure may occur.
(3) Catecholamines—dopamine, epinephrine, isoproterenol, levarterenol	Increased likelihood of cardiac arrhythmias. Halothane, cyclopropane, and a few rarely used general anesthetics sensitize the myocardium to the effects of catecholamines. If they are combined, ventricular tachycardia or ventricular fibrillation may occur. Such a combination is contraindicated.

NURSING ACTIONS	RATIONALE/EXPLANATION
(4) CNS depressants—alcohol, antianxiety agents, anticonvulsants, antidepressants, antihistamines, antipsychotics, barbiturates, narcotic analgesics, sedative-hypnotics	CNS depressants include many different drug groups and hundreds of individual drugs. Some are used therapeutically for their CNS depressant effects; others are used mainly for other purposes, and CNS depression is a side effect. Any combination of these drugs with each other or with general anesthetic agents produces additive CNS depression. Extreme caution must be used to prevent excessive CNS depression.
(5) Corticosteroids	Additive hypotension may occur during and after surgery due to adrenocortical atrophy and reduced ability to respond to stress. For clients who have been receiving corticosteroids, most physicians recommend administration of hydrocortisone before, during, and, in decreasing doses, after surgery.
(6) Monoamine oxidase (MAO) inhibitors—isocarboxazid, isoniazid, procarbazine, tranylcypromine, others	Additive CNS depression. These drugs should be discontinued at least 10 days to 3 weeks before elective surgery. If emergency surgery is required, clients taking MAO inhibitors should not be given general anesthesia. Although they may be given spinal anesthesia, there is increased risk of hypotension. They should not be given local anesthetic solutions to which epinephrine has been added.
(7) Muscle relaxants—succinylcholine, tubocurarine, others	Additive relaxation of skeletal muscles. These drugs are given for this therapeutic effect so that smaller amounts of general anesthetics may be given.
b. Drugs that *decrease* effects of general anesthetics:	Few drugs actually decrease effects of general anesthetics. When clients are excessively depressed and develop hypotension, cardiac arrhythmias, respiratory depression, and other problems, the main treatment is stopping the anesthetic and supporting vital functions rather than giving additional drugs. Effects of general inhalation anesthetics decrease rapidly once administration is discontinued. Effects of IV anesthetics decrease more slowly.
(1) Alcohol	Alcohol is a CNS depressant, and acute ingestion has an additive CNS depressant effect with general anesthetic agents. With chronic ingestion, however, tolerance to the effects of alcohol and general anesthetics develops; that is, larger amounts of general anesthetic agents are required in clients who have developed tolerance to alcohol.
(2) Atropine	Atropine is often given as preanesthetic medication to prevent reflex bradycardia, which may occur with halothane, and other general anesthetics.
c. Drugs that *increase* effects of local anesthetics:	
(1) Cardiovascular depressants—general anesthetics, propranolol (Inderal)	Additive depression and increased risk of hypotension and arrhythmias
(2) CNS depressants	Additive CNS depression with high doses
(3) Epinephrine	Epinephrine is often used in dental anesthesia to prolong anesthetic effects by delaying systemic absorption of the local anesthetic drug. It is contraindicated for this use, however, in clients with hyperthyroidism or severe heart disease or those receiving adrenergic blocking agents such as guanethidine (Ismelin) for hypertension.
(4) Succinylcholine (Anectine)	Apnea may be prolonged by the combination of a local anesthetic agent and succinylcholine.

(continued)

NURSING ACTIONS	*RATIONALE/EXPLANATION*
d. Drugs that *decrease* effects of local anesthetics:	These are seldom necessary or desirable. If overdosage of local anesthetics occurs, treatment is mainly symptomatic and supportive.
Succinylcholine (Anectine)	This drug may be given to treat acute convulsions resulting from toxicity of local anesthetic drugs.
e. Drugs that *increase* effects of neuromuscular blocking agents (muscle relaxants):	
(1) Aminoglycoside antibiotics (*e.g.,* gentamicin), colistin (Coly-Mycin) and related antibiotics	Additive neuromuscular blockade, apnea, and respiratory depression
(2) Diuretics, potassium-losing (*e.g.,* furosemide, hydrochlorothiazide)	Diuretics that produce hypokalemia potentiate skeletal muscle relaxants.
(3) General anesthetics	Additive muscle relaxation
(4) Local anesthetics	Prolong apnea from succinylcholine
(5) MAO inhibitors	Additive respiratory depression
(6) Narcotic analgesics	Additive respiratory depression
(7) Procainamide (Pronestyl) and quinidine	Additive neuromuscular blockade
f. Drugs that *decrease* effects of neuromuscular blocking agents:	
Anticholinesterase drugs (*e.g.,* neostigmine)	These drugs often are used to reverse the effects of the nondepolarizing agents. They do not reverse the effects of succinylcholine and may potentiate them instead.
5. Teach clients	
a. With preanesthetic, sedative-type medications:	The medications cause drowsiness and relaxation.
(1) Stay in bed with siderails up.	Lying quietly helps the drugs to act. Activities are generally unsafe unless another person is available to provide assistance.
(2) Use call light if help is needed.	
(3) Do not smoke.	
b. With local anesthetics applied topically:	
(1) Use the drug preparation only on the part of the body for which it was prescribed.	Most preparations are specifically made to apply on certain areas, and they cannot be used effectively and safely on other body parts.
(2) Use the drug only for the condition for which it was prescribed.	For example, a local anesthetic prescribed to relieve itching may aggravate an open wound.
(3) Apply local anesthetics to clean areas. If needed, wash skin areas or take a sitz bath to cleanse the perineal area.	To enhance drug effectiveness. The drug must have direct contact with the affected area.
(4) Do *not* apply more often than directed.	Local irritation, skin rash, and hives can develop.
(5) With spray preparations, do not inhale vapors, spray near food, or store near any heat source.	
(6) Use local anesthetic preparations for only a short period. If the condition for which it is being used persists, report the condition to the physician.	
(7) Inform dentists or other physicians if allergic to any local anesthetic drug.	To prevent further reactions. Allergic reactions are rare, but if they have occurred, another type of local anesthetic can usually be substituted safely.

REVIEW AND APPLICATION EXERCISES

1. When assessing a client before, during, or after general anesthesia, what are important factors to consider?

2. What are major adverse effects of general anesthetics and neuromuscular blocking agents?

3. What interventions are needed to ensure client safety during recovery from general anesthesia?

4. When assessing a client before, during, or after local or regional anesthesia, what are important factors to consider?

5. What are major adverse effects of local anesthetic agents?

6. What interventions are needed to ensure client safety during recovery from local or regional anesthesia?

SELECTED REFERENCES

Catterall, W.A., & Mackie, K. (1996). Local anesthetics. In J.G. Hardman, L.E. Limbird, P.B. Molinoff, & R.W. Ruddon (Eds.), *Goodman & Gilman's The pharmacological basis of therapeutics*, 9th ed., pp. 331–347. New York: McGraw-Hill.

Drug facts and comparisons. (1996). St. Louis: Facts and Comparisons.

Marshall, B.E., & Longnecker, D.E. (1996). General anesthetics. In J.G. Hardman, L.E. Limbird, P.B. Molinoff, & R.W. Ruddon (Eds.), *Goodman & Gilman's The pharmacological basis of therapeutics*, 9th ed., pp. 307–330. New York: McGraw-Hill.

15 Alcohol and Other Drug Abuse

Outline

Objectives

After studying this chapter, the student will be able to:

1 Identify risk factors for developing drug dependence.

2 Describe the effects of alcohol, cocaine, and marijuana on selected body organs.

3 Compare and contrast characteristics of dependence associated with alcohol, benzodiazepines, cocaine, and opiates.

4 Describe specific antidotes for overdoses of central nervous system (CNS) depressant drugs and the circumstances indicating their use.

5 Outline major elements of treatment for overdoses of commonly abused drugs that do not have antidotes.

6 Describe interventions to prevent or manage withdrawal reactions associated with benzodiazepines, cocaine and other CNS stimulants, ethanol, and opiates.

Key Terms

Alcohol abuse	**Hallucinogen**
Drug abuse	**Physical dependence**
Drug withdrawal reactions	**Psychological dependence**

Abuse and Dependence

Abuse of alcohol and other drugs is a significant health, social, economic, and legal problem. Substance abuse is often associated with substantial damage to the individual abuser and with numerous social ills (*e.g.*, crime, child and spouse abuse, traumatic injury, death). As used in this chapter, *drug abuse* is defined as self-administration of a drug for prolonged periods or in excessive amounts to the point of producing physical or psychological dependence and reduced ability to function as a productive member of society. Thus, alcohol and drug abuse denote excessive or inappropriate use of alcohol and other drugs. Most drugs of abuse are those that affect the central nervous system (CNS) and alter the state of consciousness. These include prescription and nonprescription and legal and illegal drugs. Commonly abused drugs include CNS depressants (*e.g.*, alcohol, antianxiety/sedative-hypnotic agents, narcotic analgesics), CNS stimulants (*e.g.*, amphetamines, cocaine, nicotine), and other mind-altering drugs (*e.g.*, marijuana).

Drug dependence involves compulsive drug-seeking behavior. *Psychological dependence* involves feelings of satisfaction and pleasure from taking the drug. These feelings, perceived as extremely desirable by the drug-dependent person, contribute to acute intoxication, development and maintenance of drug abuse patterns, and return to drug-taking behavior after periods of abstinence.

Physical dependence involves physiologic adaptation to chronic use of a drug so that unpleasant signs and symptoms occur when the drug is stopped or its action is antagonized by another drug. The withdrawal or abstinence syndrome produces specific manifestations according to the type of drug and does not occur as long as adequate dosage is maintained. Attempts to avoid withdrawal symptoms reinforce psychological dependence and promote continuing drug use and relapses to drug-taking behavior. Tolerance is often an element of drug dependence, and increasing doses are therefore required to obtain psychological effects or avoid physical withdrawal symptoms. A person may be dependent on more than one drug.

Drug dependence is a complex phenomenon. The cause is unknown, although various reasons and influencing factors have been postulated. One view is that drugs stimulate or inhibit neurotransmitters in the brain to produce pleasure and euphoria or to decrease unpleasant feelings such as anxiety. The specific drug and the amount, frequency, and route of administration are also important. In addition to drug effects, other influencing factors include a person's psychological and physiologic characteristics, and environmental or circumstantial characteristics. Peer pressure seems to be an important factor in initial and continuing drug ingestion. A genetic factor seems evident in alcohol abuse: Studies indicate that children of abusers are at risk of becoming abusers themselves, even if reared away from the abusing parent. Additional general characteristics of substance abuse and dependence are listed below.

- Substance abuse involves all socioeconomic levels and almost all age groups, from school-age children to elderly adults. Patterns of abuse may vary in age groups. For example, adolescents and young adults may be more likely to use illicit drugs and elderly adults are more likely to abuse alcohol and prescription drugs. Health care professionals (*e.g.*, physicians, pharmacists, nurses) are also considered at high risk of developing substance abuse disorders, at least partly because of easy access.
- A person who abuses one drug is at risk of abusing others.
- Multiple drugs are often abused concomitantly. Alcohol, for example, is often used with other drugs of abuse, probably because it is legal and readily available. In addition, alcohol, marijuana, opioids, and sedatives are often used to combat the anxiety and nervousness induced by cocaine and other CNS stimulants.
- Drug effects vary according to the type of substance being abused, the amount, route of administration, duration of use, and phase of substance abuse (*e.g.*, acute intoxication, withdrawal syndromes, organ damage and medical illness). Thus, acute intoxication often produces profound behavioral changes and chronic abuse often leads to serious organ damage and impaired ability to function in work, family or social settings. Withdrawal symptoms are characteristic for particular types of drugs and are usually opposite the effects originally produced. For example, withdrawal symptoms of alcohol and sedative-type drugs are mainly agitation, nervousness, and hyperactivity.
- Alcohol and other drug abusers are not reliable sources of information about the types or amounts of drugs used. Most abusers understate the amount and frequency of using abused substances; heroin addicts may overstate the amount used in attempts to obtain higher doses of methadone. In addition, those who use illegal street drugs may not know what they have taken because of varying purity, potency, additives, and names.
- Substance abusers rarely seek health care unless circumstances force the issue. Thus, most substance abuse comes to the attention of health care professionals when the abuser experiences a complication such as acute intoxication, with-

drawal, or serious medical problems resulting from chronic drug overuse, misuse, or abuse.

- Smoking or inhaling drug vapors is a preferred route of administration for cocaine, marijuana, and nicotine because the drugs are rapidly absorbed from the large surface area of the lungs. Then, they rapidly circulate to the heart and brain without dilution by the systemic circulation or metabolism by enzymes. With crack cocaine, inhaling vapors from the heated drug produces blood levels comparable to those obtained with IV administration.
- Substance abusers who inject their drugs intravenously are prey to serious problems because they use impure drugs of unknown potency, contaminated needles, poor hygiene, and other dangerous practices. Specific problems include overdoses, death, and numerous infections (*e.g.,* hepatitis, human immunodeficiency virus [HIV] infection, endocarditis, phlebitis, and cellulitis at injection sites).

Many drugs are abused for their mind-altering properties. Most of these have clinical usefulness and are discussed elsewhere in this text: Antianxiety Drugs and Sedative-Hypnotics (see Chap. 8), Narcotic Analgesics and Narcotic Antagonists (see Chap. 6), and Central Nervous System Stimulants (see Chap. 16). This chapter describes commonly abused substances, characteristics of substance-related disorders, and drugs used to treat substance-related disorders (Table 15-1).

CNS Depressants

CNS depressant drugs include alcohol, antianxiety and sedative-hypnotic agents, and opiates.

ALCOHOL (ETHANOL)

Alcohol is the most abused drug in the world. It is legal and readily available, and its use is accepted in most societies. There is no clear-cut dividing line between use and abuse, but rather a continuum of progression over several years. Alcohol exerts profound metabolic and physiologic effects on all organ systems (Box 15-1). Some of these effects are evident with acute alcohol intake, whereas others become evident with chronic intake of substantial amounts. Alcohol is thought to exert its effects on the CNS by enhancing the activity of gamma aminobutyric acid (GABA), an inhibitory neu-

TABLE 15-1	DRUGS USED TO TREAT SUBSTANCE ABUSE DISORDERS		
Generic/Trade Name	**Indications for Use**	**Routes and Dosage Ranges**	**Comments**
Chlordiazepoxide (Librium)	Alcohol detoxification; benzodiazepine withdrawal	PO 50 mg q6–8h initially, then tapered over 1–2 wk	
Clonidine (Catapres)	Alcohol withdrawal; opiate withdrawal	Alcohol withdrawal PO 0.3–0.6 mg q6h Opiate withdrawal PO 2 µg/kg 3 times daily for 7–10 days	Unlabeled uses May cause hypotension
Disulfiram (Antabuse)	Chronic alcohol abuse, to prevent continued alcohol ingestion	PO 125–500 mg daily	Limited effectiveness because many alcoholics will not take the drug; should not be given until at least 12 h after alcohol ingestion
Flumazenil (Romazicon)	Acute intoxication or overdose of benzodiazepine antianxiety or sedative-hypnotic drugs	IV 0.1–0.2 mg/min up to 1 mg	May precipitate acute withdrawal symptoms
Haloperidol (Haldol)	Psychotic symptoms associated with acute intoxication with cocaine and other CNS stimulants	IM 2–5 mg every 30 min to 6 h PRN for psychotic behavior	Other antipsychotic agents may also be used
Levo-alpha-acetylmethadol (LAAM) (Orlaam)	Maintenance therapy of heroin addiction	PO 60–100 mg 3 times weekly	Reportedly as effective and well accepted by heroin addicts as methadone

TABLE 15-1	DRUGS USED TO TREAT SUBSTANCE ABUSE DISORDERS (Continued)		
Generic/Trade Name	**Indications for Use**	**Routes and Dosage Ranges**	**Comments**
Lorazepam (Ativan)	Excessive CNS stimulation associated with acute intoxication with cocaine and other CNS stimulants, hallucinogens, marijuana, inhalants, and phencyclidine; alcohol withdrawal	*Agitation,* IM q30 min–6 h PRN; *alcohol withdrawal* hallucinations or seizures, IM 2 mg, repeated if necessary; *benzodiazepine withdrawal,* PO 2 mg q6–8h initially, then tapered over 1–2 wk	1 wk of tapering usually adequate for withdrawal from short-acting benzodiazepines; 2 wk needed for long-acting benzodiazepines
Methadone	Opiate withdrawal; maintenance therapy of heroin addiction	*Withdrawal,* PO 20–80 mg daily initially, reduced by 5–10 mg daily over 7–10 days; *maintenance* PO 20–80 mg daily	Maintenance doses of 60–80 mg daily more effective than 20–30 mg daily in decreasing heroin use
Naloxone (Narcan)	Acute intoxication or overdose of opiates (heroin, morphine, others)	IV 0.4–2 mg q3min	May precipitate acute withdrawal symptoms
Naltrexone (ReVia, Trexan)	Opiate dependence; alcohol dependence	PO 50 mg daily	With opiate dependence, should not be started until patient opioid-free for at least 7 d
Nicotine (Habitrol, Nicotrol, Nicoderm, ProStep, Nicorette)	Aid smoking cessation by relieving nicotine withdrawal symptoms	*Transdermal patches, Habitrol, Nicotrol,* 21 mg/d for 6 wk; 14 mg/d for 2 wk; 7 mg/d for 2 wk *Nicotrol,* 15 mg/d for 12 wk; 10 mg/d for 2 wk; 5 mg/d for 2 wk *ProStep,* 22 mg/d for 4–8 wk; 11 mg/d for 2–4 wk *Chewing gum,* 4 mg 9–12 pieces daily (maximum of 20 pieces); 2 mg 9–12 pieces daily (maximum of 30 pieces)	Should not be used while continuing to smoke because of high risk of serious adverse effects; used patches contain enough nicotine to be toxic to children and pets; they should be discarded in a safe manner.

rotransmitter, or by inhibiting the activity of glutamate, an excitatory neurotransmitter.

When alcohol is ingested orally, a portion is inactivated in the stomach (by the enzyme alcohol dehydrogenase) and not absorbed systemically. Women have less enzyme activity than men and therefore absorb about 30% more alcohol than men when comparable amounts are ingested according to weight and size. As a result, women are especially vulnerable to adverse effects of alcohol, including more rapid intoxication from smaller amounts of alcohol and earlier development of hepatic cirrhosis and other complications of alcohol abuse.

In men and women, alcohol is absorbed partly from the stomach but mostly from the upper small intestine. It is rapidly absorbed when the stomach and small intestine are empty. Food delays absorption by diluting the alcohol and delaying gastric emptying. Once absorbed, alcohol is quickly distributed to all body tissues, partly because it is lipid soluble and crosses cell membranes easily. The alcohol concentration in the brain rapidly approaches that in the blood, and CNS effects usually occur within a few minutes. These effects depend on the amount ingested, how rapidly it was ingested, whether the stomach was empty, and other factors. Generally, effects with acute intoxication progress from a feeling of relaxation to impaired mental and motor functions to stupor and sleep. Excited behavior may occur, due to depression of the cerebral cortex, which normally controls behavior. The person may seem more relaxed, talkative, and outgoing or more impulsive and aggressive because inhibitions have been lessened.

The rate of alcohol metabolism largely determines the duration of CNS effects. Most alcohol is oxidized in the liver to acetaldehyde, a substance that can be used for energy or converted to fat and stored. When metabolized to acetaldehyde, alcohol no longer exerts

---

BOX 15-1. EFFECTS OF ALCOHOL ABUSE

Central and Peripheral Nervous System Effects

Sedation ranging from drowsiness to coma; impaired memory, learning, and thinking processes; impaired motor coordination, with ataxia or staggering gait, altered speech patterns, poor task performance, and hypoactivity or hyperactivity; mental depression, anxiety, insomnia; impaired interpersonal relationships; brain damage; polyneuritis and Wernicke-Korsakoff syndrome.

Hepatic Effects

Induces drug-metabolizing enzymes that accelerate metabolism of alcohol and many other drugs and produces tolerance and cross-tolerance; eventually damages the liver enough to slow drug metabolism, leading to accumulation and toxic effects; decreases use and increases production of lactate, leading to lactic acidosis, decreased renal excretion of uric acid, and secondary hyperuricemia; decreases use and increases production of lipids, leading to hyperlipidemia and fatty liver. Fatty liver may be a precursor to hepatic cirrhosis and hepatitis; causes accumulation of fat and protein, leading to hepatomegaly; eventually produces severe liver injury characterized by necrosis and inflammation (alcoholic hepatitis) or by fibrous bands of scar tissue that irreversibly alter structure and function (cirrhosis).

The incidence of liver disease correlates with the amount of alcohol consumed, and the progression of liver damage, from early and mild to late and severe, is attributed directly to ethanol or indirectly to the metabolic changes produced by ethanol.

Gastrointestinal Effects

Slowed gastric emptying time; increased intestinal motility, which probably contributes to the diarrhea that often occurs with alcoholism; damage to the epithelial cells of the intestinal mucosa; multiple nutritional deficiencies, including protein and water-soluble vitamins, such as thiamine, folic acid, and vitamin B_{12}; pancreatic disease, which contributes to malabsorption of fat, nitrogen, and vitamin B_{12}.

Cardiovascular Effects

Damage to myocardial cells; cardiomyopathy manifested by cardiomegaly, edema, dyspnea, abnormal heart sounds, and ECG changes indicating left ventricular hypertrophy, abnormal T waves, and conduction disturbances; possible impairment of coronary blood flow and myocardial contractility.

Hematologic Effects

Bone marrow depression due to alcohol or associated conditions, such as malnutrition, infection, and liver disease; several types of anemia including *megaloblastic anemia* from folic acid deficiency, *sideroblastic anemia* (sideroblasts are precursors of red blood cells) probably from nutritional deficiency, *hemolytic anemia* from abnormalities in the structure of red blood cells, *iron deficiency anemia* usually from gastrointestinal bleeding, and anemias from hemodilution, chronic infection, and fatty liver and bone marrow failure associated with cirrhosis; thrombocytopenia and decreased platelet aggregation from folic acid deficiency, hypersplenism, and other factors; decreased numbers and impaired function of white blood cells, which lead to decreased resistance to infection.

Endocrine Effects

Increased release of cortisol and catecholamines and decreased release of aldosterone from the adrenal glands; hypogonadism, gynecomastia, and feminization in men with cirrhosis due to decreased secretion of male sex hormones; degenerative changes in the anterior pituitary gland; decreased secretion of antidiuretic hormone from the posterior pituitary; hypoglycemia due to impaired glucose synthesis or hyperglycemia due to glycogenolysis.

Skeletal Effects

Impaired growth and development, which is most apparent in children born to alcoholic mothers. Fetal alcohol syndrome is characterized by low birth weight and length and by birth defects, such as cleft palate and cardiac septal defects. Impairment of growth and motor development persists in the postnatal period, and mental retardation becomes apparent. Other effects include decreased bone density, osteoporosis, and increased susceptibility to fractures; osteonecrosis due to obstructed blood supply; hypocalcemia, which leads to bone resorption and decreased skeletal mass; hypomagnesemia, which may further stimulate bone resorption; hypophosphatemia, probably from inadequate dietary intake of phosphorus.

Muscular Effects

Acute myopathy, which may be manifested by acute pain, tenderness, edema, and hyperkalemia; chronic myopathy, which may involve muscle weakness, atrophy, episodes of acute myopathy associated with a drinking spree, and elevated creatine phosphokinase (CPK).

---

depressant effects on the CNS. Although the rate of metabolism differs with acute ingestion or chronic intake and some other factors, it is generally about 120 mg/kg of body weight or about 10 ml/h. This is the amount of alcohol contained in about ⅔ oz of whiskey,

3 to 4 oz of wine, or 8 to 12 oz of beer. *Alcohol is metabolized at the same rate regardless of the amount present in body tissues.*

Alcohol may cause several potentially significant interactions when used with other drugs. These interactions often differ between acute and chronic ingestion. *Acute ingestion* inhibits drug-metabolizing enzymes. This slows the metabolism of some drugs, thereby increasing their effects and the likelihood of toxicity. *Chronic ingestion* induces metabolizing enzymes. This increases the rate of metabolism and decreases drug effects. Note, however, that long-term ingestion of large amounts of alcohol causes liver damage and impaired ability to metabolize drugs.

Because so many variables influence alcohol's interactions with other drugs, it is difficult to predict effects of interactions in particular people. However, some important interactions include those with other CNS depressants, antihypertensive agents, antidiabetic agents, oral anticoagulants, and disulfiram. With other CNS depressants (*e.g.*, sedative-hypnotics, narcotic analgesics, antianxiety agents, antipsychotic agents, general anesthetics, and tricyclic antidepressants), alcohol potentiates CNS depression and increases risks of excessive sedation, respiratory depression, impaired mental and physical functioning, and other effects. Combining alcohol with these drugs may be lethal and should be avoided. With antihypertensive agents, alcohol potentiates vasodilation and hypotensive effects. With oral antidiabetic drugs, alcohol potentiates hypoglycemic effects. With oral anticoagulants (*e.g.*, warfarin), alcohol interactions vary. Acute ingestion increases anticoagulant effects and the risk of bleeding. Chronic ingestion decreases anticoagulant effects by inducing drug-metabolizing enzymes in the liver and increasing the rate of warfarin metabolism. However, if chronic ingestion has caused liver damage, metabolism of warfarin may be slowed. This increases the risk of excessive anticoagulant effect and bleeding. With disulfiram (Antabuse), alcohol produces significant distress. This reaction may be used to treat alcohol dependence. A disulfiram-like reaction also may occur with other drugs, such as chlorpropamide (Diabinese), tolbutamide (Orinase), and metronidazole (Flagyl).

Alcohol Dependence

Alcohol dependence involves acute or chronic consumption of alcohol in excess of the limits accepted by the person's culture, at times considered inappropriate by that culture, and to the extent that physical health and social relationships are impaired. Psychological dependence, physical dependence, tolerance, and cross-tolerance (with other CNS depressants) are prominent characteristics.

Acute intoxication impairs thinking, judgment, and psychomotor coordination. These impairments lead to poor work performance, accidents, and disturbed relationships with other people. Conscious control of behavior is lost, and exhibitionism, aggressiveness, and assaultiveness often result. Chronic ingestion affects essentially all body systems and may cause severe organ damage and mental problems. Effects are summarized in Box 15-1.

Signs and symptoms of alcohol withdrawal include agitation, anxiety, tremors, sweating, nausea, tachycardia, fever, hyperreflexia, postural hypotension, and, if severe, convulsions and delirium. Delirium tremens (DTs), the most serious form of alcohol withdrawal, is characterized by confusion, disorientation, delusions, visual hallucinations, and other signs of acute psychosis. The intensity of the alcohol withdrawal syndrome varies with the duration and amount of alcohol ingestion. Withdrawal symptoms start within a few hours after a person's last drink and last for several days.

Treatment of Alcohol Dependence

Alcohol dependence is a progressive illness and early recognition and treatment are desirable. The alcohol-dependent person is unlikely to seek treatment for alcohol abuse unless an acute situation forces the issue. He or she is likely, however, to seek treatment for other disorders, such as nervousness, anxiety, depression, insomnia, and gastroenteritis. Thus, health professionals may recognize alcohol abuse in its early stages if they are aware of indicative assessment data.

If the first step of treatment is recognition of alcohol abuse, the second step is probably confronting the client with evidence of alcohol abuse and trying to elicit cooperation. Unless the client admits that alcohol abuse is a problem and agrees to participate in a treatment program, success is unlikely. The client may fail to make return visits or may seek treatment elsewhere. If the client agrees to treatment, the three primary approaches are psychological counseling, referral to a self-help group such as Alcoholics Anonymous, and drug therapy.

Acute intoxication with alcohol does not usually require treatment. If the client is hyperactive and combative, a sedative-type drug may be given. The client must be closely observed because sedatives potentiate alcohol, and excessive CNS depression may occur. If the client is already sedated and stuporous, he or she can be allowed to sleep off the alcohol effects. If the client is comatose, supportive measures are indicated. For example, respiratory depression may require insertion of an artificial airway and mechanical ventilation.

Benzodiazepine antianxiety agents are usually the drugs of choice for treating alcohol withdrawal syndromes. They can help the client participate in rehabilitation programs and can be gradually reduced in dosage and discontinued. They provide adequate sedation and have a significant anticonvulsant effect.

Seizures require treatment if they are repeated or continuous. Anticonvulsant drugs need not be given for more than a few days unless the person has a pre-existing seizure disorder. Clonidine may be given to reduce symptoms (*e.g.,* hyperactivity, tremors) associated with excessive stimulation of the sympathetic nervous system.

Drug therapy for maintenance of sobriety is limited, mainly because of poor compliance. The two drugs approved for this purpose are *disulfiram* (Antabuse) and *naltrexone* (ReVia). Disulfiram interferes with hepatic metabolism of alcohol and allows accumulation of acetaldehyde. If alcohol is ingested during disulfiram therapy, acetaldehyde causes nausea and vomiting, dyspnea, hypotension, tachycardia, syncope, blurred vision, headache, and confusion. Severe reactions include respiratory depression, cardiovascular collapse, cardiac arrhythmias, myocardial infarction, congestive heart failure, unconsciousness, convulsions, and death. The severity of reactions varies but is usually proportional to the amounts of alcohol and disulfiram taken. The duration of the reaction varies from a few minutes to several hours, as long as alcohol is present in the blood. Ingestion of prescription and over-the-counter medications that contain alcohol may cause a reaction in the disulfiram-treated alcoholic. Disulfiram alone may produce adverse reactions of drowsiness, fatigue, impotence, headache, and dermatitis. These are more likely to occur during the first 2 weeks of treatment, after which they usually subside. Disulfiram also interferes with the metabolism of phenytoin and warfarin, which may increase blood levels of the drugs and increase their toxicity. Because of these reactions, disulfiram must be given only with the client's full consent, cooperation, and knowledge. Naltrexone is an opiate antagonist that reduces alcohol consumption and supports abstinence by an unknown mechanism. A possible mechanism is blockade of the endogenous opioid system, which is thought to reinforce alcohol craving and consumption.

BARBITURATES AND BENZODIAZEPINES

Barbiturates are old drugs that are rarely used therapeutically but remain drugs of abuse; benzodiazepines are widely used for antianxiety and sedative-hypnotic effects (see Chap. 8) and are also widely abused.

Barbiturate and Benzodiazepine Dependence

This type of dependence resembles alcohol dependence in symptoms of intoxication and withdrawal. Other characteristics include physical dependence, psychological dependence, tolerance, and cross-tolerance. Signs and symptoms of withdrawal include anxiety, tremors and muscle twitching, weakness, dizziness, distorted visual perceptions, nausea and vomiting, insomnia, weight loss, postural hypotension, generalized tonic-clonic (grand mal) seizures, and delirium that resembles the delirium tremens of alcoholism or a major psychotic episode. Convulsions are more likely to occur during the first 48 hours of withdrawal and delirium after 48 to 72 hours. Signs and symptoms of withdrawal are less severe with the benzodiazepines than with the barbiturates.

Treatment of Barbiturate or Benzodiazepine Abuse

Treatment may involve overdose and withdrawal syndromes. Overdose produces intoxication similar to that produced by alcohol. There may be a period of excitement and emotional lability followed by progressively increasing signs of CNS depression (*e.g.,* impaired mental function, muscular incoordination, and sedation). Treatment is unnecessary for mild overdose if vital functions are adequate. The client usually sleeps off the effects of the drug. The rate of recovery depends primarily on the amount of drug ingested and its rate of metabolism. More severe overdoses cause respiratory depression and coma. There is no antidote for barbiturate overdose; treatment is symptomatic and supportive. The goals of treatment are to maintain vital functions until the drug is metabolized and eliminated from the body. Insertion of an artificial airway and mechanical ventilation often are necessary. Gastric lavage may help if started within about 3 hours of drug ingestion. If the person is comatose, a cuffed endotracheal tube should be inserted and the cuff inflated before lavage to prevent aspiration. Diuresis helps to eliminate the drugs and can be induced by intravenous (IV) fluids or diuretic drugs. Hemodialysis also removes most of these drugs and may be used with high serum drug levels or failure to respond to other treatment measures. Hypotension and shock are usually treated with IV fluids.

Until recently, these treatments also were used for benzodiazepine overdoses and may still be needed in some cases (*e.g.,* overdoses involving multiple drugs). However, a specific antidote is now available to reverse sedation, coma, and respiratory depression. Flumazenil (Romazicon) competes with benzodiazepines for benzodiazepine receptors. The drug has a short duration of action, and repeated IV injections are usually needed. Recipients must be closely observed because symptoms of overdose may recur when the effects of a dose of flumazenil subside and because the drug may precipitate acute withdrawal symptoms (*e.g.,* agitation, confusion, seizures) in benzodiazepine abusers.

Treatment of withdrawal may involve administration of a benzodiazepine or phenobarbital to relieve acute signs and symptoms, then tapering the dose until the drug can be discontinued. Barbiturate and benzodiazepine withdrawal syndromes can be life-threatening. The person may experience cardiovascular collapse, generalized tonic-clonic (grand mal) seizures, and acute psychotic episodes. These can be prevented by gradually withdrawing the offending drug. If they do occur, each situation requires specific drug therapy and supportive measures. Withdrawal reactions should be supervised and managed by experienced people, such as health care professionals or staff at detoxification centers.

OPIATES

Opiates are potent analgesics and extensively used in pain management (see Chap. 6). They are also commonly abused. Because therapeutic opiates are discussed elsewhere, the focus here is heroin. Heroin, a semisynthetic derivative of morphine, is a common drug of abuse. It is a Schedule I drug in the United States and is not used therapeutically.

Heroin may be taken by IV injection, smoking, or nasal application (snorting). IV injection produces intense euphoria, which occurs within seconds, lasts a few minutes, and is followed by a period of sedation. Effects diminish over about 4 hours, depending on the dose. Addicts may inject several times daily, cycling between desired effects and symptoms of withdrawal. Tolerance to euphoric effects develops rapidly, leading to dosage escalation and continued use to avoid withdrawal. Like other opiates, heroin causes severe respiratory depression with overdose and produces a characteristic abstinence syndrome.

Opiate Dependence

Opiates produce tolerance and high degrees of psychological and physical dependence. Most other drugs that produce dependence do so with prolonged usage of large doses, but morphine-like drugs produce dependence with repeated administration of small doses. Medical usage of these drugs produces physical dependence and tolerance but rarely leads to use or abuse for mind-altering effects. Thus, "addiction" should not be an issue when the drugs are needed for pain management in patients with cancer or other severe illnesses.

Acute effects of opiate administration vary according to dosage, route of administration, and physical and mental characteristics of the user. They may produce euphoria, sedation, analgesia, respiratory depression, postural hypotension, vasodilation, pupil constriction, and constipation.

Abstinence from opiates following chronic use produces a withdrawal syndrome characterized by anxiety; aggressiveness; restlessness; generalized body aches; insomnia; lacrimation; rhinorrhea; perspiration; pupil dilation; piloerection (goose flesh); anorexia, nausea, and vomiting; diarrhea; elevation of body temperature, respiratory rate, and systolic blood pressure; abdominal and other muscle cramps; dehydration; and weight loss. Withdrawal symptoms vary in time of onset, peak intensity, and duration, depending on the specific drug involved. With morphine, symptoms begin within a few hours of the last dose, reach peak intensity in 24 to 48 hours, and subside spontaneously. The more severe symptoms usually disappear within 10 days, but some residual symptoms may persist much longer. If a narcotic antagonist, such as naloxone (Narcan), is given, withdrawal symptoms occur rapidly and are more intense but of shorter duration.

Treatment of Opiate Dependence

Treatment may be needed for overdose or withdrawal syndromes. Overdose may produce severe respiratory depression and coma. Insertion of an endotracheal tube and mechanical ventilation may be required. Drug therapy consists of a narcotic antagonist to reverse opioid effects. Giving a narcotic antagonist can precipitate withdrawal symptoms. If there is no response to the narcotic antagonist, the symptoms may be caused by depressant drugs other than opiates. In addition to profound respiratory depression, pulmonary edema, hypoglycemia, pneumonia, cellulitis, and other infections often accompany narcotic overdose and require specific treatment measures. Signs and symptoms of withdrawal from opiates and related drugs can be reversed immediately by giving the drug producing the dependence. Therapeutic withdrawal, which is more comfortable and safer, can be managed by gradually reducing dosage over several days. Clonidine, an antihypertensive drug, is sometimes used to relieve withdrawal symptoms associated with sympathetic nervous system overactivity.

Ideally, the goal of treatment for opiate abuse is abstinence from further opiate usage. Because this goal is rarely met, long-term drug therapy may be used to treat heroin dependence. One method uses opioid substitutes to prevent withdrawal symptoms and improve a lifestyle that revolves around obtaining, using, and recovering from a drug. Methadone has long been used for this purpose, usually a single, daily, oral dose given in a methadone clinic. Proponents say that methadone blocks euphoria produced by heroin, acts longer, and reduces preoccupation with drug use. This allows a more normal lifestyle for the client and reduces morbidity and mortality associated with the use of illegal and injected drugs. Also, because methadone is free, the heroin addict does not commit crimes to obtain drugs. Opponents say that methadone maintenance only substitutes one type of drug dependence for another. In addition, a substantial percentage of those receiving methadone maintenance therapy abuse other drugs, including cocaine. Another drug approved for maintenance therapy is levo-alpha-acetylmethadol, also called LAAM. LAAM (Orlamm) is a synthetic opioid analgesic that is metabolized to long-acting, potent metabolites. After oral administration, effects occur within 90 minutes, peak in about 4 hours, and last about 72 hours. Its main advantage over methadone is that it can be given three times weekly rather than daily. However, if given on a Monday, Wednesday, Friday schedule, the Friday dose may need to be larger to prevent withdrawal symptoms until the Monday dose can be given. Also, initial dosage needs careful titration to prevent withdrawal symptoms but avoid overdosage when peak effects occur. Patients must be informed about the delayed effects of the drug and the risks of overdosage if they take other opiates. Another treatment modality is naltrexone (Trexan, ReVia), a narcotic antagonist that prevents opiates from occupying receptor sites and thereby prevents their physiologic effects. Used to maintain opiate-free states in the opiate addict, it is recommended for use in conjunction with psychological counseling to promote client motivation and compliance.

CNS Stimulants

AMPHETAMINES AND RELATED DRUGS

Amphetamines and related drugs (see Chap. 16) are used for appetite suppression and other effects. However, the drugs are probably more important as drugs of abuse than therapeutic agents.

Amphetamine-Type Dependence

Amphetamines and related drugs (*e.g.,* methylphenidate, phenmetrazine) produce stimulation and euphoria, effects often sought by drug users. The user may increase the amount and frequency of administration to reach or continue the state of stimulation. One of the drugs, methamphetamine, may be chemically treated to produce potent crystals (called "ice"), which are then heated and the vapors smoked or inhaled. Psychological effects of amphetamines are similar to those produced by cocaine and are largely dose-related. Small amounts produce mental alertness, wakefulness, and increased energy. Large amounts may produce psychotic behavior (*e.g.,* hallucinations and paranoid delusions). Tolerance develops to amphetamines.

Acute ingestion of these drugs masks underlying fatigue or depression; withdrawal allows these conditions to emerge in an exaggerated form. The resulting exhaustion and depression reinforce the compulsion to continue using the drugs. Users may take them alone or

to counteract the effects of other drugs. In the latter case, these drugs may be part of a pattern of polydrug use in which CNS depressants, such as alcohol or sedative-type drugs ("downers"), are alternated with CNS stimulants, such as amphetamines ("uppers").

Treatment of Amphetamine-Type Abuse

Treatment of amphetamine-type abuse is mainly concerned with overdosage because these drugs supposedly do not produce physical dependence and withdrawal, at least in the sense that alcohol, opiates, and sedative-hypnotic drugs do. Because amphetamines delay gastric emptying, gastric lavage may be helpful even if several hours have passed since drug ingestion. The client is likely to be hyperactive, agitated, and hallucinating (toxic psychosis) and may have tachycardia, fever, and other symptoms. Symptomatic treatment includes sedation, lowering of body temperature, and administration of an antipsychotic drug. Sedative-type drugs must be used with great caution, however, because depression and sleep usually follow amphetamine use, and these after-effects can be aggravated by sedative administration.

COCAINE

Cocaine is a popular drug of abuse. It produces powerful CNS stimulation by preventing reuptake of neurotransmitters (*e.g.,* dopamine, norepinephrine), which increases and prolongs neurotransmitter effects. Cocaine is commonly inhaled (snorted) through the nose; "crack" is heated and the vapors inhaled. Acute use of cocaine or "crack" produces euphoria, tachycardia, increased blood pressure, and restlessness followed by depression, fatigue, and drowsiness as drug effects wear off. Overdosage can cause cardiac arrhythmias, convulsions, myocardial infarction, respiratory failure, stroke, and death, even in young, healthy adults and even with initial exposure. Both acute and chronic use produce numerous physiologic effects (Box 15-2).

Cocaine Dependence

Cocaine-induced euphoria is intense but brief and often leads to drug ingestion every few minutes as long as the drug is available. Cocaine is not thought to produce physical dependence, although fatigue, depression, and drowsiness occur as drug effects dissipate. "Crack" is a a strong, inexpensive, extremely addicting, and widely used form of cocaine. It is prepared by altering cocaine hydrochloride with chemicals and heat to form rock-like formations of cocaine base. The process removes impurities and results in a very potent drug. When the drug is heated and the vapors inhaled, crack acts within a few seconds. It re-

---

BOX 15-2. PHYSIOLOGIC AND BEHAVIORAL EFFECTS OF COCAINE ABUSE

Central Nervous System Effects

Cerebral infarct; subarachnoid and other hemorrhages; excessive CNS stimulation, manifested by anxiety, agitation, delirium, hyperactivity, irritability, insomnia; anorexia and weight loss; psychosis with paranoid delusions and hallucinations that may be indistinguishable from schizophrenia; seizures.

Cardiovascular Effects

Arrhythmias, including tachycardia, premature ventricular contractions, ventricular tachycardia and fibrillation, and asystole; cardiopathy; myocardial ischemia and acute myocardial infarction; hypertension; stroke; rupture of the aorta; constriction of coronary and peripheral arteries.

Respiratory Effects

Ulceration and perforation of the nasal septum; rhinitis, rhinorrhea; pneumonitis, pulmonary edema.

Gastrointestinal Effects

Nausea; weight loss; intestinal ischemia, possible necrosis.

Genitourinary Effects

Delayed orgasm for men and women; difficulty in maintaining erection.

Effects of IV Use

Hepatitis; human immunodeficiency virus (HIV) infection; endocarditis; cellulitis; abscesses.

---

portedly can cause psychological dependence with one use.

Treatment of Cocaine Abuse

Treatment is largely symptomatic. Thus, agitation and hyperactivity may be treated with a benzodiazepine antianxiety agent; psychosis may be treated with haloperidol or other antipsychotic agent; cardiac arrhythmias may be treated with usual antiarrhythmic drugs; myocardial infarction may be treated by standard methods; and so forth. Initial detoxification and long-term treatment are best accomplished in centers or units that specialize in substance abuse disorders.

NICOTINE

Nicotine, one of many active ingredients in tobacco products, is the ingredient that promotes compulsive use, abuse, and dependence. Inhaling smoke from a cigarette produces CNS stimulation in a few seconds. The average cigarette contains about 8 to 9 mg of nicotine and delivers about 1 mg of nicotine systemically to the smoker (most is burned or dissipated as "sidestream" smoke). Nicotine obtained from chewing tobacco produces longer-lasting effects because it is more slowly absorbed than inhaled nicotine. Nicotine produces its effects by increasing levels of dopamine and other substances in the brain.

Nicotine is readily absorbed through the lungs, skin, and mucous membranes. It is extensively metabolized, mainly in the liver, and its metabolites are eliminated by the kidneys. It is also excreted in breast milk of nursing mothers. Adverse effects include nausea in new smokers at low blood levels and in experienced smokers at blood levels higher than their accustomed levels. Nicotine poisoning can occur in infants and children from ingestion of tobacco products, skin contact with used nicotine transdermal patches, or chewing nicotine gum. Poisoning may also occur with accidental ingestion of insecticide sprays containing nicotine. Oral ingestion usually causes vomiting, which limits the amount of nicotine absorbed. Toxic effects of a large dose may include hypertension, cardiac arrhythmias, convulsions, coma, respiratory arrest, and paralysis of skeletal muscle. With chronic tobacco use, nicotine is implicated in the vascular disease and sudden cardiac death associated with smoking. However, the role of nicotine in the etiology of other disorders (*e.g.,* cancer and pulmonary disease) associated with chronic use of tobacco is unknown. Effects are summarized in Box 15-3.

Nicotine Dependence

Like alcohol and opiate dependence, nicotine dependence is characterized by compulsive use and the development of tolerance and physical dependence. Mental depression is also associated with nicotine dependence. It is unknown whether depression leads to smoking or develops concomitantly with nicotine dependence. Cigarette smokers may smoke to obtain the perceived pleasure of nicotine's effects, avoid the discomfort of nicotine withdrawal, or both. Evidence indicates a compulsion to smoke when blood levels of nicotine become low. Abstinence from smoking leads to signs and symptoms of withdrawal (*e.g.,* anxiety, irritability, difficulty concentrating, restlessness, headache, increased appetite, weight gain, sleep disturbances), which usually begin within 24 hours of the last exposure to nicotine.

BOX 15-3. EFFECTS OF NICOTINE

Central Nervous System Effects
CNS stimulation with increased alertness, possibly feelings of enjoyment, decreased appetite, tremors, convulsions at high doses.

Cardiovascular Effects
Cardiac stimulation with tachycardia, vasoconstriction, increased blood pressure, increased force of myocardial contraction, and increased cardiac workload.

Gastrointestinal Effects
Increases secretion of gastric acid; increases muscle tone and motility; nausea and vomiting; aggravates gastroesophageal and peptic ulcer disease.

Treatment of Nicotine Dependence

Most tobacco users who quit do so on their own. For those who are strongly dependent and unable or unwilling to quit on their own, drug formulations of nicotine may be used to initiate smoking cessation. These products prevent or reduce withdrawal symptoms, but they do not produce the subjective effects or peak blood levels seen with cigarettes.

Nicotine is available in transdermal patches and chewing gum. Pieces of the gum may be chewed several times daily; the transdermal patch is applied once daily. Transdermal patches produce a steady blood level of nicotine and patients seem to use them more consistently than they use the chewing gum. These products formerly required prescriptions but are now available over the counter. They are contraindicated in people with significant cardiovascular disease (angina pectoris, arrhythmias, or recent myocardial infarction). Adverse effects include soreness of mouth and throat (with gum), nausea, vomiting, dizziness, hypertension, arrhythmias, confusion, and skin irritation at sites of transdermal patch application.

Although nicotine products are effective in helping smokers achieve abstinence, about three fourths resume smoking within a year. Treatment regimens that combine counseling and behavioral therapy with drug therapy are more successful than those using nicotine replacement therapy alone.

Marijuana

Marijuana and other cannabis preparations are obtained from *Cannabis sativa*, the hemp plant, which grows in most parts of the world, including the entire United States. Marijuana and hashish are the two cannabis preparations used in the United States. Marijuana is obtained from leaves and stems; hashish, prepared from plant resin, is five to ten times as potent as commonly available marijuana. These cannabis preparations contain several related compounds called *cannabinoids*. Delta-9-tetrahydrocannabinol (Δ-9-THC) is the main psychoactive ingredient, but metabolites and other constituents also may exert pharmacologic activity. The mechanism of action is unknown, although specific cannibinoid receptors have been identified in several regions of the brain. The endogenous substances that react with these receptors have not yet been determined.

Cannabis preparations are difficult to classify. Some people call them depressants, some call them stimulants, and others label them as mind-altering, hallucinogenic, psychotomimetic, or unique in terms of fitting into drug categories. It is also difficult to predict the effects of these drugs. Many factors apparently influence a person's response. One factor is the amount of active ingredients, which varies with the climate and soil where the plants are grown and with the method of preparation. Other factors include dose, route of administration, personality variables, and the environment in which the drug is taken.

Marijuana can be taken orally but is more often smoked and inhaled through the lungs. It is more potent and more rapid in its actions when inhaled. After smoking, subjective effects begin in minutes, peak in about 30 minutes, and last 2 to 3 hours. Low doses are mildly intoxicating and similar to small amounts of alcohol. Large doses can produce panic reactions and hallucinations similar to acute psychosis. Effects wear off as THC is metabolized to inactive products. Many physiologic effects (Box 15-4) and adverse reactions have been reported with marijuana use, including impaired ability to drive an automobile and perform other common tasks of everyday life.

Except for dronabinol (Marinol), marijuana and other cannabis preparations are illegal and not used

BOX 15-4. EFFECTS OF MARIJUANA

Central Nervous System Effects
Impaired memory; perceptual and sensory distortions; disturbances in time perception; mood alteration; restlessness; depersonalization; panic reactions; paranoid ideation; impaired performance on cognitive, perceptual, and psychomotor tasks; drowsiness with high doses.

Cardiovascular Effects
Hypertension; bradycardia; peripheral vasoconstriction; orthostatic hypotension and tachycardia at high doses.

Respiratory Effects
Irritation of bronchial mucosa; mild bronchoconstriction followed by bronchodilation.

Musculoskeletal Effects
Ataxia, impaired coordination, increased reaction time.

Miscellaneous Effects
Constipation, decreased libido, thirst, decreased intraocular pressure.

---

therapeutically in the United States. Dronabinol, a formulation of Δ-9-THC, is used to treat nausea and vomiting associated with anticancer drugs and to stimulate appetite in patients with acquired immunodeficiency syndrome (AIDS). The risks of abuse are high, and the drug may cause physical and psychological dependence. It is a Schedule II controlled drug. Cannabinoids can also decrease intraocular pressure and may be useful in treating glaucoma. Some people promote legalization of marijuana for medical uses. However, clinicians state that such usage is no more effective than available legal treatments with less abuse potential.

MARIJUANA DEPENDENCE

Tolerance and psychic dependence do not usually develop with occasional use but may occur with chronic use; physical dependence rarely occurs. There is no specific treatment other than abstinence.

Hallucinogens

Hallucinogenic drugs include a variety of substances that cause mood changes, anxiety, distorted sensory perceptions, hallucinations, delusions, depersonalization, pupil dilation, elevated body temperature, and elevated blood pressure.

LSD is a synthetic derivative of lysergic acid, a compound in ergot and some varieties of morning glory seeds. It is very potent, and small doses can alter normal brain functioning. LSD is usually distributed as a soluble powder and ingested in capsule, tablet, or liquid form. The exact mechanism of action is unknown, and effects cannot be predicted accurately. Generally, LSD alters sensory perceptions and thought processes; impairs most intellectual functions, such as memory and problem-solving ability; distorts perception of time and space; and produces sympathomimetic reactions, including increased blood pressure, heart rate, body temperature, and pupil dilation. Adverse reactions include self-injury and possibly suicide, violent behavior, psychotic episodes, "flashbacks" (a phenomenon characterized by psychological effects and hallucinations that may recur days, weeks, or months after the drug is taken), and possible chromosomal damage resulting in birth defects.

Mescaline is an alkaloid of the peyote cactus. It is the least active of the commonly used psychotomimetic agents but produces effects similar to those of LSD. It is usually ingested in the form of a soluble powder or capsule.

Phencyclidine (PCP) produces excitement, delirium, hallucinations and other profound psychological and physiologic effects, including a state of intoxication similar to that produced by alcohol; altered sensory perceptions; impaired thought processes; impaired motor skills; psychotic reactions; sedation and analgesia; nystagmus and diplopia; and pressor effects that can cause hypertensive crisis, cerebral hemorrhage, convulsions, coma, and death. Death from overdose also has occurred as a result of respiratory depression. Bizarre murders, suicides, and self-mutilations have been attributed to the schizophrenic reaction induced by PCP, especially in high doses. The drug also produces flashbacks.

PCP is usually distributed in liquid or crystal form and can be ingested, inhaled, or injected. It is usually sprayed or sprinkled on marijuana or herbs and smoked. Probably because it is cheap, easily synthesized, and readily available, PCP is often sold as LSD, mescaline, cocaine, or THC (the active ingredient in marijuana). It is also added to low-potency marijuana without the user's knowledge. Consequently, the drug user may experience severe and unexpected reactions, including death.

HALLUCINOGEN DEPENDENCE

Tolerance develops, but there is no apparent physical dependence or abstinence syndrome. Psychological dependence probably occurs but is usually not intense. Users may prefer one of these drugs, but they apparently do without or substitute another drug if the one they favor is unavailable. A major danger with these drugs is their ability to impair judgment and insight, which can lead to panic reactions in which users may try to injure themselves (*e.g.*, by running into traffic).

TREATMENT OF HALLUCINOGEN ABUSE

There is no specific treatment for hallucinogen dependence. Those who experience severe panic reactions may be kept in a safe, supportive environment until drug effects wear off or may be given a sedative-type drug.

Volatile Solvents (Inhalants)

These drugs include acetone, toluene, and gasoline. These solvents may be constituents of some types of glue, plastic cements, aerosol sprays, and other products. Some general inhalation anesthetics, such as nitrous oxide, have also been abused to the point of dependence. Volatile solvents are most often abused by preadolescents and adolescents who squeeze glue into a plastic bag, for example, and sniff the fumes. Suffocation sometimes occurs when the sniffer loses consciousness while the bag covers the face.

These substances produce symptoms somewhat comparable to acute intoxication with alcohol, including initial mild euphoria followed by ataxia, confusion, and disorientation. Some substances in gasoline and toluene also may produce symptoms similar to those produced by the hallucinogens, including euphoria, hallucinations, recklessness, and loss of self-control. Large doses may cause convulsions, coma, and death. Substances containing gasoline, benzene, or carbon tetrachloride are especially likely to cause serious damage to the liver, kidneys, and bone marrow.

These substances produce psychological dependence, and some produce tolerance. There is some question about whether physical dependence occurs. If it does occur, it is considered less intense than the physical dependence associated with alcohol, barbiturates, and opiates.

Nursing Process

Assessment

Assess clients for signs of alcohol and other drug abuse, including abuse of prescription drugs, such as antianxiety agents, narcotics, and sedative-hypnotics. Some general screening-type questions are appropriate for any initial nursing assessment. The overall purpose of these questions is to determine whether a current or potential problem exists and whether additional information is needed. Some clients may refuse to answer or will give answers that contradict other assessment data. Denial of excessive drinking and of problems resulting from alcohol use is a prominent characteristic of alcoholism; underreporting the extent of drug use is common in other types of drug abuse as well. Useful information includes each specific drug, the amount, the frequency of administration, and the duration of administration. If answers to general questions reveal problem areas, such as long-term use of alcohol or psychotropic drugs, more specific questions can be formulated to assess the scope and depth of the problem. It may be especially difficult to obtain needed information about illegal "street drugs," most of which have numerous, frequently changed names. For nurses who often encounter substance abusers, efforts to keep up with drug names and terminology may be helpful.

- Interview the client regarding alcohol and other drug use to help determine immediate and long-term nursing needs. For example, information may be obtained that would indicate the likelihood of a withdrawal reaction, the risk of increased or decreased effects of a variety of drugs, and the client's susceptibility to drug abuse. People who abuse one drug are likely to abuse others, and abuse of multiple drugs is a more common pattern than abuse of a single drug. These and other factors aid effective planning of nursing care.
- Assess behavior that may indicate drug abuse, such as alcohol on the breath, altered speech patterns, staggering gait, hyperactivity or hypoactivity, and other signs of excessive CNS depression or stimulation. Impairments in work performance and in interpersonal relationships also may be behavioral clues.
- Assess for disorders that may be caused by alcohol or drug abuse. These disorders may include infections, liver disease, accidental injuries, and psychiatric problems of anxiety or depression. These disorders may be caused by other factors, of course, and are nonspecific.
- Check laboratory reports, when available, for abnormal liver function tests, indications of anemia, abnormal white blood cell counts, abnormal electrolytes (hypocalcemia, hypomagnesemia, and acidosis are common in alcoholics), and alcohol and drug levels in the blood.

Nursing Diagnoses

- Ineffective Individual Coping related to reliance on alcohol or other drugs
- Risk for Injury: Adverse drug effects
- Risk for Violence related to altered thought processes, impaired judgment, and impulsive behavior
- Altered Nutrition: Less Than Body Requirements related to drug effects and drug-seeking behavior
- Altered Thought Processes related to use of psychoactive drugs
- Risk for Injury: Infection, hepatitis, acquired immunodeficiency syndrome related to use of contaminated needles and syringes for IV drugs

Planning/Goals

- Safety will be maintained for clients impaired by alcohol and drug abuse.

- Information will be provided regarding drug effects and treatment resources.
- The client's efforts toward stopping drug usage will be recognized and reinforced.

Interventions

- Administer prescribed drugs correctly during acute intoxication or withdrawal.
- Decrease environmental stimuli for the person undergoing drug withdrawal.
- Record vital signs; cardiovascular, respiratory, and neurologic functions; mental status; and behavior at regular intervals.
- Support use of resources for stopping drug abuse (psychotherapy, treatment programs).
- Request patient referrals to psychiatric/mental health physicians, nurse clinical specialists, or self-help programs when indicated.
- Use therapeutic communication skills to discuss alcohol or other drug-related health problems, health-related benefits of stopping substance use or abuse, and available services or treatment options.
- Teach nondrug techniques for coping with stress and anxiety.
- Provide positive reinforcement for efforts toward quitting substance abuse.
- Inform smokers with young children in the home that cigarette smoke can precipitate or aggravate asthma and upper respiratory disorders in children.
- Inform smokers with nonsmoking spouses or other members of the household that "second-hand" smoke can increase the risks of cancer and lung disease in the nonsmokers as well as the smoker.
- For smokers who are concerned about weight gain if they quit smoking, emphasize that the health benefits of quitting far outweigh the disadvantages of gaining a few pounds, and discuss ways to control weight without smoking.

Evaluation

- Observe for improved behavior (*e.g.*, less impulsiveness, improved judgment and thought processes, commits no injury to self or others).
- Observe for use or avoidance of nonprescribed drugs while hospitalized.
- Interview to determine the client's insight into personal problems stemming from drug abuse.
- Verify enrollment in a treatment program.
- Observe for appropriate use of drugs to decrease abuse of other drugs.

Principles of Therapy

PREVENTION OF ALCOHOL AND OTHER DRUG ABUSE

Use measures to prevent development of alcohol and drug abuse. Although there are difficulties in trying to prevent conditions for which causes are not known, some of the following community-wide and individual measures may be helpful:

1. Decrease the supply or availability of commonly abused drugs. Most efforts at prevention have tried to reduce the supply of drugs. For example, laws designate certain drugs as illegal and provide penalties for possession or use of these drugs. Other laws regulate circumstances in which legal drugs, such as narcotic analgesics and barbiturates, may be used. Also, laws regulate the sale of alcoholic beverages.

2. Decrease the demand for drugs. Because this involves changing attitudes, it is likely to be very difficult but more effective in the long run. Many current attitudes seem to promote drug use, misuse, and abuse, including:

   a. The belief that a drug is available for every mental and physical discomfort and should be taken in preference to tolerating even minor discomfort. Consequently, society has a permissive attitude toward taking drugs, and this attitude is probably perpetuated by physicians who are quick to prescribe drugs and nurses who are quick to administer them. Of course, there are many appropriate uses of drugs, and clients certainly should not be denied their benefits. The difficulties emerge when there is excessive reliance on drugs as chemical solutions to problems that are not amenable to chemical solutions.

   b. The widespread acceptance and use of alcohol. In some groups, every social occasion is accompanied by alcoholic beverages of some kind.

   c. The apparently prevalent view that drug abuse refers only to the use of illegal drugs and that using alcohol or prescription drugs, however inappropriately, does not constitute drug abuse.

   d. The acceptance and use of illegal drugs in certain subgroups of the population. This is especially prevalent in high school and college students.

   Efforts to change attitudes and decrease demand for drugs can be made through education and counseling about such topics as drug effects and nondrug ways to handle the stresses and problems of daily life.

3. Each person must take personal responsibility for drinking alcoholic beverages and taking mind-altering drugs. Initially, conscious, voluntary choices are made to drink or not to drink, to take a drug or not to take it. This period varies somewhat, but drug dependence develops in most instances only after prolonged use. When mind-altering drugs are prescribed for a legitimate reason, the client must use them in prescribed doses and preferably for a short time.

4. Physicians can help prevent drug abuse by prescribing drugs appropriately, prescribing mind-altering drugs in limited amounts and for limited periods, using nondrug measures when they are likely to be effective, educating clients about the drugs prescribed for them, participating in drug education

programs, and recognizing, as early as possible, clients who are abusing or are likely to abuse drugs.

5. Nurses can help prevent drug abuse by administering drugs appropriately, using nondrug measures when possible, teaching clients about drugs prescribed for them, and participating in drug education programs.

6. Parents can help prevent drug abuse in their children by minimizing their own use of drugs and by avoiding heavy cigarette smoking. Children are more likely to use illegal drugs if their parents have a generally permissive attitude about drug taking, if either parent takes mind-altering drugs regularly, and if either parent is a heavy cigarette smoker.

7. Pregnant women should avoid alcohol, nicotine, and other drugs of abuse because of potentially harmful effects on the fetus.

TREATMENT MEASURES FOR ALCOHOL AND OTHER DRUG ABUSE

Treatment measures for alcohol and other drug abuse have not been especially successful. Even people who have been institutionalized and achieved a drug-free state for prolonged periods are apt to resume their drug-taking behavior when released from the institution. So far, voluntary, self-help groups, such as Alcoholics Anonymous and Narcotics Anonymous, have been more successful than health professionals in dealing with drug abuse. Health professionals are more likely to be involved in acute situations, such as intoxication or overdose, withdrawal syndromes, or various medical-surgical conditions. As a general rule, treatment depends on the type, extent, and duration of drug-taking behavior and the particular situation for which treatment is needed. Some general management principles include the following:

1. Psychological rehabilitation efforts should be part of any treatment program for a drug-dependent person. Several approaches may be useful, including psychotherapy, voluntary groups, and other types of emotional support and counseling.

2. Drug therapy is relatively limited in treating drug dependence for several reasons. First, specific antidotes are available only for benzodiazepines (flumazenil) and opioid narcotics (naloxone). Second, there is a high risk of substituting one abused drug for another. Third, there are significant drawbacks to giving CNS stimulants to reverse effects of CNS depressants, and vice versa. Fourth, there is often inadequate information about the types and amounts of drugs taken.

   Despite these drawbacks, however, there are some clinical indications for drug therapy, including treatment of overdose or withdrawal syndromes.

Even when drug therapy is indicated, there are few guidelines for optimal use. Doses, for example, must often be estimated initially and then titrated according to response.

3. General care of clients with drug overdose is primarily symptomatic and supportive. The aim of treatment is usually to support vital functions, such as respiration and circulation, until the drug is metabolized and eliminated from the body. For example, respiratory depression from an overdose of a CNS depressant drug may be treated by inserting an artificial airway and mechanical ventilation. Removal of some drugs can be hastened by hemodialysis or hemoperfusion.

4. Treatment of substance abuse may be complicated by the presence of other disorders. For example, depression is common and may require antidepressant drug therapy.

REVIEW AND APPLICATION EXERCISES

1. Why is it important to assess each client in relation to alcohol or other substance abuse?

2. What are signs and symptoms of overdose with alcohol, benzodiazepine antianxiety or hypnotic agents, cocaine, and opiates?

3. What are general interventions for treatment of drug overdoses?

4. What are specific antidotes for opiate and benzodiazepine overdoses, and how are they administered?

5. Which commonly abused drugs may produce life-threatening withdrawal reactions if stopped abruptly?

6. How can severe withdrawal syndromes be prevented, minimized, or safely managed?

7. What are the advantages of treating substance abuse disorders in centers established for that purpose?

SELECTED REFERENCES

Acute reactions to drugs of abuse (1996). *The Medical Letter, 38* (Issue 974), May 10, pp. 43–46.

Adams, I.B. & Martin, B.R. (1996). Cannabis: Pharmacology and toxicology in animals and humans. *Addiction, 91*(11), 1585–1614.

Antai-Otong, D. (1995). Helping the alcoholic patient recover. *American Journal of Nursing, 95*(8), 22–29.

Cornish, J.W., McNicholas, L.F., & O'Brien, C.P. (1995). Treatment of substance-related disorders. In A.F. Schatzberg & C.B. Nemeroff

(Eds.), *The American Psychiatric Press textbook of psychopharmacology*, pp. 707–724. Washington, DC: American Psychiatric Press, Inc.

Crabtree, B.L. & Polles, A. (1997). Substance-related disorders. In J.T. DiPiro, R.L. Talbert, G.C. Yee, G.R. Matzke, B.G. Wells, & L.M. Posey (Eds.), *Pharmacotherapy: A pathophysiologic approach*, 3rd ed., pp. 1345–1365. Stamford, CT: Appleton & Lange.

Kosten, T.R. (1997). Generic substance and polydrug use disorders. In A. Tasman, J. Kay, & J.A. Lieberman (Eds.), *Psychiatry*, pp. 743–754. Philadelphia: W.B. Saunders.

Ling, W., Rawson, R.A., & Compton, M.A. (1994). Substitution pharmacotherapies for opioid addiction: From methadone to LAAM and buprenorphine. *Journal of Psychoactive Drugs, 17*(3), 119–128.

Munzer, A. (1996). Smoking and smoking cessation. In W.N. Kelley (Ed.), *Textbook of internal medicine*, 3rd ed., pp. 163–167. Philadelphia: Lippincott-Raven.

O'Brien, C.P. (1996). Drug addiction and drug abuse. In J.G. Hardman, L.E. Limbird, P.B. Molinoff, & R.W. Ruddon (Eds.), *Goodman & Gilman's The pharmacological basis of therapeutics*, 9th ed., pp. 557–577. New York: McGraw-Hill.

Rawson, R.A., McCann, M.J., Hasson, A.J., & Ling, W. (1994). Cocaine abuse among methadone maintenance patients: Are there effective treatment strategies? *Journal of Psychoactive Drugs, 26*(2), 129–136.

Sullivan, E.J. (1995). *Nursing care of clients with substance abuse.* St. Louis: Mosby-Year Book.

Central Nervous System Stimulants

Objectives

After studying this chapter, the student should be able to:

1 Describe general characteristics of central nervous system (CNS) stimulant drugs.

2 Discuss reasons for decreased use of amphetamines for therapeutic purposes.

3 Discuss the rationale for treating attention deficit-hyperactivity disorder (ADHD) with CNS stimulant drugs.

4 Describe characteristics and effects of xanthine drugs.

Key Terms

Attention deficit-hyperactivity disorder (ADHD)

Narcolepsy

Uses

Many drugs stimulate the central nervous system (CNS), but only a few are used therapeutically, and their indications for use are limited. Two disorders treated with CNS stimulants are narcolepsy and attention deficit-hyperactivity disorder (ADHD; formerly called attention deficit disorder and hyperkinetic syndrome).

Narcolepsy is a rare disorder characterized by periodic "sleep attacks" in which the victim has an uncontrollable feeling of drowsiness and goes to sleep at any place or any time. In addition to excessive daytime drowsiness and fatigue, nighttime sleep patterns are disturbed. The hazards of suddenly going to sleep in unsafe environments restrict activities of daily living.

ADHD occurs in children and is characterized by hyperactivity, a short attention span, difficulty completing assigned tasks or schoolwork, restlessness, and impulsive behavior. Drug therapy may be indicated if the symptoms are severe and present for several months.

Types of Stimulants

Most CNS stimulants act by facilitating initiation and transmission of nerve impulses that excite other cells. The drugs are somewhat selective in their actions at lower doses but tend to involve the entire CNS at higher doses. The major groups of CNS stimulants are amphetamines and related drugs, analeptics, and xanthines.

Amphetamines increase the amounts of norepinephrine, dopamine, and possibly serotonin in the brain, thereby producing mood elevation or euphoria, increasing mental alertness and capacity for work, decreasing fatigue and drowsiness, and prolonging wakefulness. Larger doses, however, produce signs of excessive CNS stimulation, such as restlessness, hyperactivity, agitation, nervousness, difficulty concentrating on a task, and confusion. Overdoses can produce convulsions and psychotic behavior. Amphetamines also stimulate the sympathetic nervous system, resulting in increases in heart rate and blood pressure, mydriasis, slowed gastrointestinal motility, and other symptoms. In ADHD, the drugs reduce behavioral symptoms and may improve cognitive performance.

These drugs produce tolerance and psychological dependence. They are Schedule II drugs under the Controlled Substances Act, and prescriptions for them are nonrefillable. These drugs are widely sold on the street and commonly abused (see Chap. 15).

Analeptics stimulate respiration but do not reverse the effects of CNS depressant drugs. A major drawback to their clinical use is that doses sufficient to stimulate

respiration often cause convulsive seizures. Respiratory depression can be more safely and effectively treated with endotracheal intubation and mechanical ventilation than with analeptic drugs.

Xanthines stimulate the cerebral cortex, increasing mental alertness and decreasing drowsiness and fatigue. Other effects include myocardial stimulation with increased cardiac output and heart rate, diuresis, and increased secretion of pepsin and hydrochloric acid. Large doses can impair mental and physical functions by producing restlessness, nervousness, anxiety, agitation, insomnia, and cardiac arrhythmias.

Indications for Use

Amphetamines are used in the treatment of narcolepsy, ADHD, and obesity. Methylphenidate is indicated only for ADHD and narcolepsy. Analeptics are used occasionally to treat respiratory depression. Caffeine (a xanthine) is often an ingredient in nonprescription analgesics and stimulants (*e.g.*, No-Doz). A combination of caffeine and sodium benzoate is occasionally used as a respiratory stimulant in neonates.

Contraindications for Use

CNS stimulants cause cardiac stimulation and thus are contraindicated in clients with cardiovascular disease (*e.g.*, angina, arrhythmias, hypertension) that is likely to be aggravated by the drugs. They also are contraindicated in clients with anxiety or agitated states, glaucoma, or hyperthyroidism. They are generally contraindicated in clients with a history of drug abuse.

Individual CNS Stimulants

AMPHETAMINES AND RELATED DRUGS

Amphetamine, **dextroamphetamine** (Dexedrine), and **methamphetamine** (Desoxyn) are closely related drugs that share characteristics of the amphetamines as a group. They are more important as drugs of abuse than as therapeutic agents.

Amphetamine and dextroamphetamine
Route and Dosage Ranges

Adults: Narcolepsy, PO 5–60 mg/d in divided doses
Children >6 y: Narcolepsy, PO 5 mg/d to start therapy; raise by 5 mg/wk to effective dose
ADHD, PO 5 mg once or twice daily initially, increased by 5 mg/d at weekly intervals until optimal response is obtained (usually no greater

than 40 mg/d). Do not initiate dosage with a long-acting preparation.

Children 3–5 y: ADHD, PO 2.5 mg/d initially, increased by 2.5 mg/d at weekly intervals until optimal response is obtained. Do not initiate dosage with a long-acting preparation.

Methamphetamine
Route and Dosage Ranges

Adults: Narcolepsy, same as amphetamine

Children >6 y: Narcolepsy, no dosage established
ADHD, same as amphetamine

Children <6 y: No dosage established

Methylphenidate (Ritalin) is chemically related to amphetamines and is used to treat ADHD in children and narcolepsy in adults. The drug has actions and adverse effects similar to those produced by amphetamines. As a CNS stimulant, methylphenidate is considered less potent than amphetamines and more potent than caffeine. Methylphenidate is a Schedule II drug because it produces psychic dependence and is a drug of abuse.

Route and Dosage Ranges

Adults: Narcolepsy, PO 10–60 mg/d in two or three divided doses (average dose 20–30 mg/d)

Children 6 years or older: ADHD, PO 5 mg twice a day initially, increased by 5–10 mg at weekly intervals to a maximum of 60 mg/d

Pemoline (Cylert) differs chemically from amphetamines and methylphenidate but exerts similar pharmacologic actions. A Schedule IV controlled drug, it is used only in treating ADHD in children.

Route and Dosage Range

Children >6 y: PO 37.5 mg/d initially in the morning; increase by 18.75 mg at weekly intervals until desired response is obtained; maximum dose 112.5 mg/d

ANALEPTIC AGENT

Doxapram (Dopram) has limited clinical usefulness as a respiratory stimulant. Although it does increase tidal volume and respiratory rate, it also increases oxygen consumption and carbon dioxide production. Limitations include a short duration of action (5–10 minutes after a single intravenous [IV] dose) and therapeutic dosages near or overlapping those that produce convulsions. Mechanical ventilation is safer and more effective in relieving respiratory depression from depressant drugs or other causes. Doxapram is occasionally used by anesthesiologists and pulmonary specialists.

Route and Dosage Range

Adults: IV 0.5–1.5 mg/kg in single or divided doses; IV continuous infusion 5 mg/min initially, decreased to 2.5 mg/min or more. Dose by infusion should not exceed 3 g.

XANTHINES

Caffeine is commercially prepared from tea leaves. Pharmaceutical preparations include an oral preparation and a solution for injection. Caffeine is usually prescribed as caffeine citrate for oral use and caffeine and sodium benzoate for parenteral use because these forms are more soluble than caffeine itself. Caffeine has limited therapeutic usefulness. It is an ingredient in some nonprescription analgesic preparations (Anacin, A.P.C., Excedrin, Vanquish) and may increase analgesia. It is also an ingredient in nonprescription stimulant (antisleep) preparations (*e.g.*, No-Doz). It is sometimes combined with an ergot alkaloid to treat migraine headaches (*e.g.*, Cafergot). A combination of caffeine and sodium benzoate is used as a respiratory stimulant in neonatal apnea unresponsive to other therapies.

Most caffeine is consumed in beverages, such as coffee, tea, cocoa, and cola drinks. One cup of coffee contains about 100 to 150 mg of caffeine, analgesic preparations contain 30 to 60 mg, and antisleep preparations contain 100 to 200 mg. Thus, the stimulating effects of caffeine can be obtained as readily with coffee as with a drug preparation. Caffeine produces tolerance to its stimulating effects, and psychological dependence or habituation occurs.

Theophylline and theophylline salts are xanthine derivatives used therapeutically in the treatment of respiratory disorders, such as asthma and bronchitis. In these conditions, the desired effect is bronchodilation and improvement of breathing; CNS stimulation is then an adverse reaction. For additional information, see Chapter 47.

Nursing Process

Assessment

- Assess use of stimulant and depressant drugs (prescribed, over-the-counter, or street drugs).
- Assess for conditions that would be aggravated by CNS stimulants.
- For a child with possible ADHD, assess behavior as specifically and thoroughly as possible. Interview the child, parents or caretakers, and teachers to document baseline symptoms before drug therapy is started. Some authorities believe that this condition is overdiagnosed and that stimulant drugs are prescribed unnecessarily.
- For any client receiving amphetamines or methylphenidate, assess behavior for signs of tolerance and abuse.

Nursing Diagnoses

- Sleep Pattern Disturbance related to hyperactivity, nervousness, insomnia
- Risk for Injury: Adverse drug effects (excessive cardiac and CNS stimulation, drug dependence)
- Knowledge Deficit: Drug effects on children and adults
- Noncompliance: Overuse of drug

Planning/Goals

The client will:
- Take drugs safely and accurately
- Improve attention span and task performance and decrease hyperactivity (for children with ADHD)
- Have fewer sleep episodes during normal waking hours (for clients with narcolepsy)

Interventions

- For a child receiving CNS stimulants, assist parents in scheduling drug holidays (*e.g.*, weekends, summers) to help prevent drug dependence and stunted growth.
- Teach parents to give drugs on school days or when high levels of attention and task performance are required.
- Teach clients to avoid other CNS stimulants, including caffeine.
- Teach clients to avoid doses within 6 to 8 hours of bedtime to avoid interference with sleep.
- Record weight at least weekly.
- Teach clients about their nutritional needs while receiving these drugs.
- Teach clients about their drug therapy.

Evaluation

- Reports of improved behavior and academic performance from parents and teachers of children with ADHD
- Reports of decreased inappropriate sleep episodes with narcolepsy

Principles of Therapy

1. Counseling and psychotherapy are recommended along with drug therapy for clients with narcolepsy and ADHD. With narcolepsy, for example, clients must be informed about the risks of driving an automobile and other activities. With ADHD, parental counseling or family therapy is indicated for effective treatment and realistic expectations of outcomes.

2. Stimulant drugs are often misused and abused by people who want to combat fatigue and delay sleep, such as long-distance drivers, students, and athletes. Use of amphetamines or other stimulants for this purpose is not justified. These drugs are dangerous for drivers and those involved in similar activities, and they have no legitimate use in athletics.

3. When an amphetamine or methylphenidate is prescribed, giving the smallest effective dose and limiting the number of doses obtained with one prescription decrease the likelihood of drug dependence.

4. Analeptics are not indicated for most clients with depression of the CNS or the respiratory system. Anesthesiologists, if they use analeptic drugs at all, use them only in carefully selected circumstances and with great caution. Doxapram generally should not be used to stimulate ventilation in clients with drug-induced coma or exacerbations of chronic lung disease. Respiration can be more effectively and safely controlled with mechanical ventilation than with drugs.

USE IN CHILDREN

CNS stimulants are not recommended for ADHD in children under 6 years of age or as anorexiants in children under 12 years. When used, dosage should be carefully monitored to avoid excessive CNS stimulation, anorexia, and insomnia. Suppression of weight and height have been reported and growth should be monitored at regular intervals during drug therapy. When possible, children with ADHD should have reduced dosage or no drug when they are not in school. In children with psychosis or Tourette syndrome, CNS stimulants may exacerbate symptoms.

USE IN OLDER ADULTS

CNS stimulants should be used cautiously in older adults. As with most other drugs, slowed metabolism and excretion increase the risks of accumulation and toxicity. Older adults are likely to experience anxiety, nervousness, insomnia, and mental confusion from excessive CNS stimulation. In addition, older adults often have cardiovascular disorders (*e.g.*, angina, arrhythmias, hypertension) that may be aggravated by the cardiac-stimulating effects of the drugs.

NURSING ACTIONS

CENTRAL NERVOUS SYSTEM STIMULANTS

NURSING ACTIONS	*RATIONALE/EXPLANATION*
1. Administer accurately	
a. Give amphetamines and methylphenidate early in the day, at least 6 hours before bedtime.	To avoid interference with sleep. If insomnia occurs, give the last dose of the day at an earlier time or decrease the dose.
b. For children with ADHD, give amphetamines and methylphenidate after meals.	To minimize the drugs' appetite-suppressing effects and risks of interference with nutrition and growth.
2. Observe for therapeutic effects	Therapeutic effects depend on the reason for use.
a. Fewer "sleep attacks" with narcolepsy	
b. Improved behavior and performance of cognitive and psychomotor tasks with ADHD	
c. Increased mental alertness and decreased fatigue	
3. Observe for adverse effects	Adverse effects may occur with acute or chronic ingestion of excessive amounts of coffee and with other forms of central nervous system (CNS) stimulant drugs.
a. Excessive CNS stimulation—hyperactivity, nervousness, insomnia, anxiety, tremors, convulsions, psychotic behavior	These reactions are more likely to occur with large doses.
b. Cardiovascular effects—tachycardia, other arrhythmias, hypertension	These reactions are caused by the sympathomimetic effects of the drugs.
c. Gastrointestinal effects—anorexia, weight loss, nausea, diarrhea, constipation	
d. Increased liver enzymes and potential hepatic failure with pemoline	Hepatic effects are associated with long-term use.
4. Observe for drug interactions	
a. Drugs that *increase* effects of amphetamines:	
(1) Alkalinizing agents (sodium bicarbonate, antacids, some diuretics)	Drugs that increase the alkalinity of the gastrointestinal tract increase intestinal absorption of amphetamines, and urinary alkalinizers decrease urinary excretion. Increased absorption and decreased excretion serve to potentiate drug effects.
(2) Monoamine oxidase (MAO) inhibitors	Potentiate amphetamines by slowing drug metabolism. These drugs thereby increase the risks of headache, subarachnoid hemorrhage, and other signs of a hypertensive crisis. A variety of neurologic toxic effects and malignant hyperpyrexia may occur. The combination may cause death.
b. Drugs that *decrease* effects of amphetamines:	
(1) Acidifying agents	Urinary acidifying agents (*e.g.*, ammonium chloride) increase urinary excretion and lower blood levels of amphetamines. Decreased absorption and increased excretion serve to decrease drug effects.
(2) Antipsychotic agents	Decrease or antagonize the excessive CNS stimulation produced by amphetamines. Chlorpromazine (Thorazine) or haloperidol (Haldol) is sometimes used in treating amphetamine overdose.

NURSING ACTIONS	*RATIONALE/EXPLANATION*
c. Drugs that *increase* effects of doxapram:	
MAO inhibitors; sympathomimetic or adrenergic drugs (*e.g.*, epinephrine, norepinephrine)	Synergistic vasopressor effects may occur.
d. Drugs that *decrease* effects of doxapram:	
Barbiturates	These CNS depressant drugs (sedative-hypnotics) may be used to manage excessive CNS stimulation caused by doxapram overdosage.
5. Teach clients	
a. Take amphetamines and methylphenidate only as prescribed by a physician.	These drugs have a high potential for abuse. The risks of drug dependence are lessened if the drugs are taken correctly.
b. Do not take stimulant drugs to delay fatigue and sleep.	Fatigue and sleep are normal resting mechanisms for the body.
c. Get adequate rest and sleep.	This is a much safer and more effective way to function than preventing rest and sleep by taking drugs or drinking large amounts of coffee or other caffeine-containing beverages.
d. Prevent nervousness, anxiety, tremors, and insomnia from excessive caffeine intake by decreasing consumption of coffee and other caffeine-containing beverages or by drinking decaffeinated coffee, tea, and cola.	Brewed coffee generally has more caffeine than instant coffee, tea, and other beverages.

REVIEW AND APPLICATION EXERCISES

1. What kinds of behaviors may indicate narcolepsy?

2. What kinds of behaviors may indicate ADHD?

3. What is the rationale for treating narcolepsy and ADHD with CNS stimulants?

4. What are the major adverse effects of CNS stimulants, and how may they be minimized?

5. Why is it important that children taking CNS stimulants for ADHD have drug-free periods when feasible?

SELECTED REFERENCES

Drug facts and comparisons. (1996). St. Louis: Facts and Comparisons.

Hoffman, B.B., & Lefkowitz, R.J. (1996). Catecholamines, sympathomimetic drugs, and adrenergic receptor antagonists. In J.G. Hardman, L.E. Limbird, P.B. Molinoff, & R.W. Ruddon (Eds.), *Goodman & Gilman's The pharmacological basis of therapeutics*, 9th ed., pp. 199–248. New York: McGraw-Hill.

Theesen, K.A., & Stimmel, G.L. (1993). Disorders of infancy and childhood. In J.T. DiPiro, R.L. Talbert, P.E. Hayes, G.C. Yee, G.R. Matzke, & L.M. Posey (Eds.), *Pharmacotherapy: A pathophysiologic approach*, 2nd ed., pp. 953–961. Norwalk, CT: Appleton & Lange.

Drugs Affecting the Autonomic Nervous System

Physiology of the Autonomic Nervous System

Outline

The Autonomic Nervous System
the sympathetic nervous system
adrenergic receptors
the parasympathetic nervous system
cholinergic receptors

Characteristics of Autonomic Drugs

Objectives

After studying this chapter, the student will be able to:

1 Identify physiologic effects of the sympathetic nervous system.

2 Differentiate subtypes and functions of sympathetic nervous system (SNS) receptors.

3 Identify physiologic effects of the parasympathetic nervous system.

4 Differentiate subtypes and functions of parasympathetic nervous system (PNS) receptors.

5 State names and general characteristics of drugs affecting the autonomic nervous system.

Key Terms

Acetylcholine	**Cholinergic**
Adrenergic	**Norepinephrine**
Alpha adrenergic receptors	**Parasympatholytic**
Anticholinergic	**Parasympatho-mimetic**
Beta adrenergic receptors	**Sympatholytic**
	Sympathomimetic
Catecholamines	

The Autonomic Nervous System

The autonomic nervous system (ANS) is a branch of the central nervous system (CNS) regulated mainly by centers in the hypothalamus, brain stem, and spinal cord. These centers serve to alter and integrate activities of the ANS, which has both central and peripheral components. The ANS automatically, without conscious thought or effort, regulates many body functions. These functions can be described broadly as mechanisms designed to maintain a constant internal environment (homeostasis), to respond to stress or emergencies, and to repair body tissues.

Nerve impulses are generated and transmitted in the ANS as they are in the CNS (see Chap. 5). Autonomic nerve impulses are transmitted to body tissues through two major subdivisions of the ANS: the *sympathetic nervous system* (SNS) and the *parasympathetic nervous system* (PNS). More specifically, nerve impulses are carried through preganglionic fibers, ganglia, and postganglionic fibers. Preganglionic impulses travel from the CNS to ganglia (clusters of cell bodies of postganglionic fibers located outside the brain and spinal cord); postganglionic impulses travel from ganglia to effector tissues of the heart, blood vessels, glands, other visceral organs, and smooth muscle.

The main neurotransmitters of the ANS are acetylcholine and norepinephrine (see Chap. 5). Acetylcholine is synthesized from acetylcoenzyme A and choline and released at preganglionic fibers of both the SNS and PNS and at postganglionic fibers of the PNS. The nerve fibers that secrete acetylcholine are called cholinergic fibers. Norepinephrine is synthesized from the amino acid tyrosine by a series of enzymatic conversions that also produce dopamine and epinephrine (*i.e.*, tyrosine → dopamine → norepinephrine → epinephrine). Norepinephrine is the end product, except in the adrenal medulla, where most of the norepinephrine is converted to epinephrine. Norepinephrine is released at postganglionic fibers of the SNS. Nerve fibers secreting norepinephrine are called adrenergic fibers.

Acetylcholine and norepinephrine act on body organs and tissues to cause parasympathetic or sympathetic effects, respectively. Stimulation of both systems causes excitatory effects in some organs but inhibitory effects in others. However, most organs are predominantly controlled by one system. Also, when the sympathetic system excites a particular organ, the parasympathetic system often inhibits it. For example, sympathetic stimulation of the heart causes an increased rate and force of myocardial contraction. Parasympathetic stimulation decreases rate and force of contraction, thereby resting the heart.

THE SYMPATHETIC NERVOUS SYSTEM

The SNS is stimulated by physical or emotional stress, such as strenuous exercise or work, pain, hemorrhage, intense emotions, and temperature extremes. Increased capacity for vigorous muscle activity in response to a perceived threat, whether real or imaginary, is often called the "fight or flight" reaction. Specific body responses include:

1. Increased arterial blood pressure and cardiac output
2. Increased blood flow to the brain, heart, and skeletal muscles; decreased blood flow to viscera, skin, and other organs not needed for "fight or flight"
3. Increased rate of cellular metabolism—increased oxygen consumption and carbon dioxide production
4. Increased breakdown of muscle glycogen for energy
5. Increased blood sugar
6. Increased mental activity and ability to think clearly
7. Increased muscle strength
8. Increased rate of blood coagulation
9. Increased rate and depth of respiration
10. Pupil dilation to aid vision

These responses are protective mechanisms designed to help the person cope with the stress or get away from it. The intensity and duration of responses depend on the amounts of norepinephrine and epinephrine present. Norepinephrine is synthesized in adrenergic nerve endings and released into the synapse (the gap between nerve cells in a chain) when adrenergic nerve endings are stimulated. It exerts intense but brief effects on pre- and postsynaptic adrenergic receptors. Then, most of the norepinephrine is taken up again by the nerve endings and reused as a neurotransmitter; the remainder diffuses into surrounding tissue fluids and blood, or it is metabolized by monoamine oxidase (MAO) or catechol-O-methyl transferase (COMT).

Norepinephrine also functions as a hormone, along with epinephrine. In response to adrenergic nerve stimulation, norepinephrine and epinephrine are secreted into the bloodstream by the adrenal medullae and transported to all body tissues. They are continually present in arterial blood in amounts that vary according to the degree of stress present and the ability of the adrenal medullae to respond to stimuli. The larger proportion of the circulating hormones (about 80%) is epinephrine. These catecholamines exert the same effects as those caused by direct stimulation of the SNS. However, the effects last longer because the hormones are removed from the blood more slowly. These hormones are metabolized mainly in the liver by the enzymes MAO and COMT.

Dopamine is also an adrenergic neurotransmitter and catecholamine. In the brain, dopamine is essential for normal function (see Chap. 5); in peripheral tissues, its main effects are on the heart and blood vessels.

Adrenergic Receptors

When norepinephrine and epinephrine act on body cells that respond to sympathetic nerve or catecholamine stimulation, they interact with two distinct adrenergic receptors, alpha and beta. Norepinephrine acts mainly on alpha receptors; epinephrine acts on both alpha and beta receptors. These receptors have been further subdivided into alpha$_1$, alpha$_2$, beta$_1$, and beta$_2$ receptors. A beta$_3$ receptor has recently been cloned, but its functions are unclear.

When dopamine acts on body cells that respond to adrenergic stimulation, it can activate alpha$_1$ and beta$_1$ receptors as well as dopaminergic receptors. Only dopamine can activate dopaminergic receptors. Dopamine receptors are located in the brain, in blood vessels of the kidneys and other viscera, and probably in presynaptic sympathetic nerve terminals. Activation (agonism) of these receptors may result in stimulation or inhibition of cellular function. Like alpha and beta receptors, dopamine receptors are divided into several subtypes (D$_1$–D$_5$), and specific effects depend on which subtype of receptor is activated.

Intracellular events following stimulation of adrenergic receptors are thought to include the following mechanisms:

Alpha$_1$ receptors: The binding of adrenergic substances to receptor proteins in the cell membrane of smooth muscle cells is thought to open ion channels, allow calcium ions to move into the cell, and produce muscle contraction (*e.g.*, vasoconstriction, gastrointestinal and bladder sphincter contraction).

Alpha$_2$ receptors: In the brain, some of the norepinephrine released into the synaptic cleft between neurons returns to the nerve endings from which it was released and stimulates presynaptic alpha$_2$ receptors. This negative feedback causes less norepinephrine to be released by subsequent nerve impulses. The result is decreased sympathetic outflow and an antiadrenergic effect. The probable mechanism is that the calcium required for neurotransmitter release from storage vesicles is prevented from entering the presynaptic nerve cell. In peripheral tissues, alpha$_2$ receptors are probably postsynaptic and have a variety of functions when

stimulated by norepinephrine, epinephrine, or dopamine. However, their specific effects on the intracellular mechanisms of body cells have not been clearly elucidated.

Beta$_1$ and beta$_2$ receptors: Activation of these receptors stimulates activity of adenyl cyclase, an enzyme in cell membranes. Adenyl cyclase, in turn, stimulates formation of cyclic adenosine monophosphate (cAMP). The cAMP can initiate any of several different intracellular actions, with specific actions depending on the type of cell.

Dopaminergic receptors D$_1$ and D$_5$: Activation of these receptors is thought to stimulate the production of cAMP, as does activation of beta$_1$ and beta$_2$ receptors.

Dopaminergic receptor D$_2$: Activation of this receptor is thought to inhibit formation of cAMP and to alter calcium and potassium ion currents. D$_3$ and D$_4$ receptors are subgrouped with D$_2$ receptors, but the effects of their activation have not been clearly delineated.

The number and the binding activity of receptors may be altered. These phenomena are most clearly understood with beta receptors. For example, when chronically exposed to high concentrations of substances that stimulate their function, the receptors decrease in number and become less efficient in stimulating adenyl cyclase. The resulting decrease in beta-adrenergic responsiveness is called desensitization or down-regulation of receptors.

Conversely, when chronically exposed to substances that block their function, the receptors may increase in number and become more efficient in stimulating adenyl cyclase. The resulting increase in beta-adrenergic responsiveness (called hypersensitization or up-regulation) may lead to an exaggerated response when the blocking substance is withdrawn.

The types of adrenergic receptors, their locations, and their effects on body tissues are summarized in Table 17-1.

THE PARASYMPATHETIC NERVOUS SYSTEM

Functions stimulated by the PNS are often described as resting, reparative, or vegetative functions. They include digestion, excretion, cardiac deceleration, anabolism, and near vision.

About 75% of all parasympathetic nerve fibers are in the vagus nerves. These nerves supply the thoracic and abdominal organs; their branches go to the heart, lungs, esophagus, stomach, small intestine, the proximal half of the colon, the liver, gallbladder, pancreas, and the upper portions of the ureters. Other parasympathetic fibers supply pupillary sphincters and ciliary muscles;

TABLE 17-1	ADRENERGIC RECEPTORS	
Type	**Location**	**Effects of Stimulation**
Alpha$_1$	Blood vessels	Vasoconstriction
	Heart	Increased force of contraction; arrhythmias
	Intestinal smooth muscle	Relaxation
	Liver	Glycogenolysis, gluconeogenesis
	Genitourinary smooth muscle	Contraction
	Eye	Blinking, mydriasis
Alpha$_2$	Nerve endings	Inhibit release of norepinephrine
	Vascular smooth muscle	Vasoconstriction
	Pancreatic beta cells	Inhibit insulin secretion
	Platelets	Aggregation
Beta$_1$	Heart	Increased heart rate, force of contraction, automaticity, and rate of AV conduction
	Kidney	Increased renin release
Beta$_2$	Bronchioles	Bronchodilation
	Blood vessels	Vasodilation
	Gastrointestinal tract	Decreased motility and tone
	Liver	Glycogenolysis, gluconeogenesis
	Urinary bladder	Relaxed detrusor muscle
	Pregnant uterus	Relaxation
Dopamine	Blood vessels of heart, kidney, other viscera	Vasodilation

lacrimal, nasal, submaxillary, and parotid glands; descending colon and rectum; lower portions of the ureters and bladder; and genitalia.

Specific body responses to parasympathetic stimulation include:

1. Dilation of blood vessels in the skin; no particular effect on systemic blood vessels
2. Decreased heart rate, possibly bradycardia
3. Increased secretion of digestive enzymes and motility of the gastrointestinal tract
4. Constriction of smooth muscle of bronchi
5. Increased secretions from glands in the lungs, stomach, intestines, and skin (sweat glands)
6. Constricted pupils (from contraction of the sphincter muscle of the iris) and accommodation to near vision (from contraction of the ciliary muscle of the eye)
7. Contraction of smooth muscle in the urinary bladder
8. Contraction of skeletal muscle
9. No apparent effects on blood coagulation, blood sugar, mental activity, or muscle strength

These responses are regulated by acetylcholine, a neurotransmitter in the brain, ANS, and neuromuscular junctions. Acetylcholine is formed in cholinergic nerve endings from choline and acetylcoenzyme A; the reaction is catalyzed by choline acetyltransferase. After its release from the nerve ending, acetylcholine acts briefly (milliseconds), then is rapidly metabolized by acetylcholinesterase (an enzyme present in the nerve ending and on the surface of the receptor organ). Acetylcholinesterase splits the active acetylcholine into inactive acetate and choline; the choline is taken up again by the presynaptic nerve terminal and reused. Acetylcholine exerts excitatory effects at nerve synapses and nerve/muscle junctions and inhibitory effects at some peripheral sites such as the heart.

Cholinergic Receptors

When acetylcholine acts on body cells that respond to parasympathetic nerve stimulation, it interacts with two types of cholinergic receptors, *nicotinic* and *muscarinic*. Nicotinic receptors are located in motor nerves and skeletal muscle. When they are activated by acetylcholine, the cell membrane depolarizes and produces muscle contraction. Muscarinic receptors are located in most internal organs, including the cardiovascular, respiratory, gastrointestinal, and genitourinary systems. When muscarinic receptors are activated by acetylcholine, the affected cells may be excited or inhibited in their functions. These receptors have been further subdivided, with two types of nicotinic and five types of muscarinic receptors identified.

Although the subtypes of cholinergic receptors have not been as well characterized as those of the adrenergic receptors, intracellular events following stimulation are thought to include the following mechanisms:

Muscarinic₁ receptors: Activation of these receptors results in a series of processes during which phospholipids in the cell membrane and inside the cell are broken down. One of the products of phospholipid metabolism is inositol phosphate. The inositol phosphate acts as a "second messenger" to increase the intracellular concentration of calcium. Calcium also acts as a second messenger and functions to activate several intracellular enzymes, initiate contraction of smooth muscle cells, and increase secretions of exocrine glands.

Muscarinic₂ receptors: Activation of these receptors results in inhibition of adenyl cyclase in the heart, smooth muscle, and brain. As a result, less cAMP is formed to act as a second messenger and stimulate intracellular activity. The overall consequence is inhibition of affected cells.

Muscarinic₃ receptors: Activation apparently causes the same cascade of intracellular processes as the muscarinic₁ receptors.

Muscarinic₄ and muscarinic₅ receptors: These two subtypes have been identified, but their locations and functions have not been delineated.

Nicotinic₁ receptors: These receptors are located on presynaptic nerve fibers. Their activation promotes the release of acetylcholine in the cerebral cortex and enhances the transmission of nerve impulses at all parasympathetic and sympathetic ganglia (clusters of nerve cell bodies outside the brain and spinal cord). They also promote the release of epinephrine from the adrenal medullae.

Nicotinic₂ receptors: These are located at neuromuscular junctions in skeletal muscle. Their activation causes muscle contraction.

Characteristics of Autonomic Drugs

Many drugs are used clinically because of their ability to stimulate or block activity of the SNS or PNS. Drugs that stimulate activity act like endogenous neurotransmitter substances; drugs that block activity prevent the action of both endogenous substances and stimulating drugs.

Drugs that act on the ANS generally affect the entire body rather than certain organs and tissues. Drug effects depend on which branch of the ANS is involved and whether it is stimulated or inhibited by drug therapy. Thus, knowledge of the physiology of the ANS is required if drug effects are to be understood and predicted. In addition, it is becoming increasingly important to understand receptor activity and the consequences of stimulation or inhibition. More drugs are being developed to stimulate or inhibit particular subtypes of receptors. This is part of the continuing effort to design drugs that act more selectively on particular body tissues and decrease adverse effects on other body tissues. For example, drugs such as terbutaline have been developed to stimulate beta₂ receptors in the respiratory tract and produce bronchodilation (a desired effect) with decreased stimulation of beta₁ receptors in the heart (an adverse effect).

The terminology used to describe autonomic drugs is often confusing because different terms are used to refer to the same phenomenon. Thus, *sympathomimetic, adrenergic,* and *alpha-* and *beta-adrenergic agonists* are used to describe a drug that has the same effects on the human body as stimulation of the SNS. *Parasympathomimetic, cholinomimetic,* and *cholinergic* are used to describe a drug that has the same effects on the body as stimulation of the PNS. There are also drugs that oppose or block stimulation of these systems. *Sympatholytic, antiadrenergic,* and *alpha-* and *beta-adrenergic blocking drugs* inhibit sympathetic stimulation. *Parasympatholytic, anticholinergic,* and *cholinergic blocking drugs* inhibit parasympathetic stimulation. This book uses the terms *adrenergic, antiadrenergic, cholinergic,* and *anticholinergic.*

REVIEW AND APPLICATION EXERCISES

1. What are the major differences between the sympathetic and parasympathetic branches of the ANS?

2. What are the major SNS and PNS neurotransmitters?

3. What are the locations and functions of SNS receptors?

4. What is meant when drugs are described as adrenergic, sympathomimetic, antiadrenergic, sympatholytic, cholinergic, or anticholinergic?

SELECTED REFERENCES

Guyton, A.C., & Hall, J.E. (1996). *Textbook of medical physiology,* 9th ed. Philadelphia: W.B. Saunders.

Lefkowitz, R.J., Hoffman, B.R., & Taylor, P. (1996). Neurotransmission: The autonomic and somatic motor nervous systems. In J.G. Hardman, L.E. Limbird, P.B. Molinoff, & R.W. Ruddon (Eds.), *Goodman & Gilman's The pharmacological basis of therapeutics,* 9th ed., pp. 105–139. New York: McGraw-Hill.

Porth, C.M., & Curtis, R.L. (1994). Normal and altered autonomic nervous system function. In C.M. Porth (Ed.), *Pathophysiology: Concepts of altered health states,* 4th ed., pp. 1007–1026. Philadelphia: J.B. Lippincott.

Adrenergic Drugs

Outline

Description
mechanisms of action and effects
indications for use
contraindications for use

Individual Adrenergic Drugs
epinephrine
ephedrine
pseudoephedrine
isoproterenol
phenylephrine
phenylpropanolamine

Nursing Process
assessment
nursing diagnoses
planning/goals
interventions
evaluation

Principles of Therapy
drug selection and administration
use in specific situations
anaphylaxis
cardiopulmonary resuscitation
hypotension and shock
nasal congestion
use in children
use in older adults
home care

Objectives

After studying this chapter, the student will be able to:

1 Differentiate effects of stimulation of alpha- and beta-adrenergic receptors.

2 List characteristics of adrenergic drugs in terms of effects on body tissues, indications for use, adverse effects, nursing process implications, principles of therapy, and observation of client responses.

3 Discuss use of epinephrine to treat anaphylactic shock, acute bronchospasm, and cardiac arrest.

4 Identify clients at risk of experiencing adverse effects with adrenergic drugs.

5 List commonly used over-the-counter (OTC) preparations that contain adrenergic drugs.

Key Terms

Alpha-adrenergic receptors

Beta-adrenergic receptors

Bronchoconstriction

Bronchospasm

Dopamine

Norepinephrine

Vasoconstriction

Vasodilation

Description

Adrenergic (sympathomimetic) drugs produce effects similar to those produced by stimulation of the sympathetic nervous system (see Chap. 17) and therefore have widespread effects on body tissues. Some of the drugs are exogenous formulations of the naturally occurring neurotransmitters and hormones (*e.g.*, norepinephrine, epinephrine, dopamine); others are chemical relatives.

Specific effects depend mainly on the client's health status when a drug is given and the drug's activation of particular adrenergic receptors. Major therapeutic uses and adverse effects stem from drug effects on the heart, blood vessels, and lungs. The drugs discussed in this chapter are those with multiple effects and clinical uses (epinephrine, ephedrine and pseudoephedrine, isoproterenol, phenylephrine, and phenylpropanolamine). Because epinephrine, ephedrine, and phenylpropanolamine stimulate both alpha- and beta-adrenergic receptors, these drugs have widespread effects on body tissues and multiple clinical uses. Isoproterenol stimulates beta-adrenergic receptors (both $beta_1$ and $beta_2$) and may be used in the treatment of several clinical conditions. Phenylephrine stimulates alpha-adrenergic receptors and is used to induce vasoconstriction in several conditions.

Other adrenergic drugs act mainly on specific adrenergic receptors or are given topically to produce more selective therapeutic effects and fewer adverse effects. These drugs have relatively restricted clinical indications and are discussed more extensively elsewhere (Drugs Used in Hypotension and Shock, Chap. 54; Bronchodilating and Antiasthmatic Drugs, Chap. 47; Nasal Decongestants, Antitussives, Mucolytics, and Cold Remedies, Chap. 49; and Drugs Used in Ophthalmic Conditions, Chap. 65). Table 18-1 lists commonly used adrenergic drugs in relation to adrenergic receptor activity and clinical use.

MECHANISMS OF ACTION AND EFFECTS

For the most part, adrenergic drugs combine with postsynaptic alpha- or beta-adrenergic receptors on the surface membrane of body cells. The drug/receptor complex then alters the cell membrane's permeability to ions or intracellular enzymes to stimulate intracellular metabolism and production of other enzymes, structural proteins, energy, and other products required for cell function and reproduction. An exception is that activation of $alpha_2$ receptors on presynaptic nerve fibers inhibits the release of additional norepinephrine.

Because most body tissues have both alpha and beta receptors, the effects of adrenergic drugs depend

TABLE 18-1	ADRENERGIC DRUGS
Generic/Trade Name	**Major Clinical Uses**
Alpha and Beta Activity	
Dopamine (Intropin)	Hypotension and shock
Epinephrine (Adrenalin)	Allergic reactions, cardiac arrest, hypotension and shock, local vasoconstriction, bronchodilation, cardiac stimulation, ophthalmic conditions
Ephedrine	Bronchodilation, cardiac stimulation, nasal decongestion
Alpha Activity	
Levarterenol (Levophed)	Hypotension and shock
Metaraminol (Aramine)	Hypotension and shock
Methoxamine (Vasoxyl)	Hypotension and shock
Naphazoline hydrochloride (Privine)	Nasal decongestion
Oxymetazoline hydrochloride (Afrin)	Nasal decongestion
Phenylephrine (Neo-Synephrine)	Hypotension and shock, nasal decongestion, ophthalmic conditions
Phenylpropanolamine hydrochloride (Propagest, Dexatrim)	Nasal decongestion, appetite suppression
Propylhexedrine (Benzedrex)	Nasal decongestion
Tetrahydrozoline hydrochloride (Tyzine, Visine)	Nasal decongestion, local vasoconstriction in the eye
Tuaminoheptane (Tuamine)	Nasal decongestion
Xylometazoline hydrochloride (Otrivin)	Nasal decongestion
Beta Activity	
Albuterol (Proventil)	Bronchodilation
Bitolterol (Tornalate)	Bronchodilation
Dobutamine (Dobutrex)	Cardiac stimulation
Isoproterenol (Isuprel)	Brochodilation, cardiac stimulation
Isoetharine (Bronkosol)	Bronchodilation
Metaproterenol (Alupent)	Bronchodilation
Pirbuterol (Maxair)	Bronchodilation
Salmeterol (Serevent)	Bronchodilation
Terbutaline (Brethine)	Bronchodilation

largely on each drug's activation of particular receptors and the number of affected receptors in a particular body tissue. Some drugs act on both types of receptors; some act more selectively on certain subtypes of receptors. Activation of $alpha_1$ receptors in blood vessels results in vasoconstriction, which then raises blood pressure and decreases nasal congestion. Activation of beta$_1$ receptors in the heart results in cardiac stimulation (increased force of myocardial contraction and increased heart rate). Activation of beta$_2$ receptors in the lungs results in bronchodilation, and activation of beta$_2$ receptors in blood vessels results in vasodilation (increased blood flow to the heart, brain, and skeletal muscles, the tissues needed to aid the "fight or flight" response). Many newer adrenergic drugs (*e.g.,* beta$_2$-receptor agonists used as bronchodilators in asthma and other bronchoconstrictive disorders) were developed specifically to be more selective.

In addition to the cardiac, vascular, and pulmonary effects, other effects of adrenergic drugs include contraction of gastrointestinal (GI) and urinary sphincters, lipolysis, decrease in GI tone, changes in renin secretion, uterine relaxation, hepatic glycogenolysis and gluconeogenesis, and decreased secretion of insulin.

INDICATIONS FOR USE

Clinical indications for the use of adrenergic drugs stem mainly from their effects on the heart, blood vessels, and bronchi. They are often used as emergency drugs in the treatment of acute cardiovascular, respiratory, and allergic disorders.

In cardiac arrest and Stokes-Adams syndrome (heart block), they may be given as cardiac stimulants. In hypotension and shock, they may be given to increase blood pressure. In hemorrhagic or hypovolemic shock, the drugs are second-line agents that may be used if adequate fluid volume replacement does not restore sufficient blood pressure and circulation to maintain organ perfusion.

In bronchial asthma and other obstructive pulmonary diseases, the drugs are given as bronchodilators to relieve bronchoconstriction and bronchospasm. In upper respiratory infections, including the common cold and sinusitis, they may be given orally or topically (nasal mucosa) for decongestant effects.

In allergic disorders, the drugs are given for vasoconstricting or decongestant effects to relieve edema in the respiratory tract, skin, and other tissues. Thus, they may be used to treat allergic rhinitis, acute hypersensitivity (anaphylactoid reactions to drugs, animal serums, insect stings, and other allergens), serum sickness, urticaria, and angioneurotic edema.

Other clinical uses include relaxation of uterine musculature and inhibition of uterine contractions in preterm labor. They may be added to intraspinal and local anesthetics to prolong anesthesia. Topical uses include application to skin and mucous membranes for vasoconstriction and hemostatic effects, and to the eyes for vasoconstriction and mydriasis.

CONTRAINDICATIONS FOR USE

Contraindications for using adrenergic drugs include cardiac arrhythmias, angina pectoris, hypertension, hyperthyroidism, cerebrovascular disease, narrow-angle glaucoma, and hypersensitivity to the drug or any component (some preparations contain sulfites, to which some persons are allergic). They are also contraindicated with local anesthesia of distal areas (*e.g.,* fingers, toes, nose, ears) because of potential tissue damage and sloughing from vasoconstriction. They should not be given during the second stage of labor because they may delay progression. The drugs should be used with caution in clients with anxiety, insomnia, and psychiatric disorders because of their stimulant effects on the central nervous system (CNS) and in older adults because of their cardiac and CNS stimulating effects.

Individual Adrenergic Drugs

Epinephrine (Adrenalin) is the prototype of adrenergic drugs. When given systemically, the effects may be therapeutic or adverse, depending on the reason for use and route of administration. Specific effects include:

1. Increased systolic blood pressure, due primarily to increased force of myocardial contraction and vasoconstriction in skin, mucous membranes, and kidneys
2. Vasodilation and increased blood flow to skeletal muscles, heart, and brain
3. Vasoconstriction in peripheral blood vessels. This allows shunting of blood to the heart and brain, with increased perfusion pressure in the coronary and cerebral circulations. This action is thought to be the main beneficial effect in cardiac arrest and cardiopulmonary resuscitation.
4. Increased heart rate and possibly arrhythmias due to stimulation of conducting tissues in the heart. Reflex bradycardia may occur when blood pressure is raised.
5. Relaxation of GI smooth muscle
6. Relaxation or dilation of bronchial smooth muscle
7. Increased glucose, lactate, and fatty acids in the blood due to metabolic effects
8. Inhibition of insulin secretion
9. Miscellaneous effects, including increased total leukocyte count, increased rate of blood coagulation, and decreased intraocular pressure in wide-angle glaucoma. When given locally, the main effect is vasoconstriction.

Epinephrine stimulates both alpha and beta receptors. At usual doses, beta-adrenergic effects on the heart and vascular and other smooth muscles predominate. However, at high doses, alpha-adrenergic effects (*e.g.*, vasoconstriction) predominate. As the prototype of adrenergic drugs, effects and clinical indications for epinephrine are the same as for adrenergic drugs. In addition, epinephrine is the adrenergic drug of choice for relieving the acute bronchospasm and laryngeal edema of anaphylactic shock, the most serious allergic reaction. Epinephrine is used in cardiac arrest for its cardiac stimulant and peripheral vasoconstrictive effects. It also is added to local anesthetics for vasoconstrictive effects, which prolong the action of the local anesthetic drug and minimize bleeding.

Epinephrine should be used with caution in infants and children; syncope has occurred with use in asthmatic children. Epinephrine is the active ingredient in over-the-counter (OTC) inhalation products for asthma (AsthmaNefrin, Asthma-Meter Mist, microNefrin, Primatene Mist, Bronkaid Mist, others). These products should not be used on a regular basis, especially by people who have heart disease or are elderly. These preparations have a short duration of action, which promotes frequent and excessive use. They also lose their effectiveness with prolonged use and may cause adverse effects.

Epinephrine is not given orally because it is destroyed by enzymes in the GI tract and liver. It may be given by inhalation, injection, or topical application. Numerous epinephrine solutions are available for various uses and routes of administration. Solutions vary widely in the amount of drug they contain. They must be used correctly to avoid potentially serious hazards. When given by intravenous (IV) injection, epinephrine raises blood pressure, stimulates the heart to increase the force and rate of ventricular contraction, relaxes smooth muscle of the bronchi, and constricts arterioles in skin, mucosa, and most viscera. It also increases blood sugar and liver glycogenolysis.

Epinephrine crosses the placenta but not the blood-brain barrier. When given by injection, it acts rapidly but has a short duration of action. For acute asthma attacks, subcutaneous (SC) administration usually produces bronchodilation within 5 to 10 minutes; maximal effects may occur within 20 minutes. Most epinephrine is rapidly metabolized in the liver to inactive metabolites, which are then excreted in the urine. The small amount that is not metabolized is deactivated by reuptake at synaptic receptor sites. Epinephrine is excreted in breast milk.

Sus-Phrine is an aqueous suspension of epinephrine that is given SC only. Some of the epinephrine is in solution and acts rapidly; some is suspended in crystalline form for slower absorption and relatively prolonged activity.

Epinephrine Injection, 1:1000 (1 mg/ml) Aqueous Solution
Routes and Dosage Ranges

Adults: IM, SC 0.3–0.5 mg q2h if necessary; IV 1 mg diluted to 10 ml with sodium chloride injection; final concentration 1:10,000 (0.1 mg/ml)
Children: SC 0.01 mg/kg q4h if necessary

Epinephrine Inhalation, 1:100 (1%) Aqueous Solution
Route and Dosage Ranges

Adults: Oral inhalation by aerosol, nebulizer, or intermittent positive-pressure breathing machine (not a preferred route of administration for epinephrine)

Epinephrine Nasal Solution, 1:1000 Solution
Routes and Dosage Ranges

Adults: Topical application to nasal mucosa, 1 or 2 drops per nostril q4–6h
  Topical application to skin and mucous membranes for hemostasis, nasal solution diluted to 1:50,000–1:2000

Sus-Phrine Injection, 1:200 Suspension
Route and Dosage Ranges

Adults: SC only, 0.1 ml initially, maximum dose 0.3 ml; do not repeat for at least 6 h
Children: SC 0.005 ml/kg, maximum dose 0.15 ml

Ephedrine is an adrenergic drug that acts by stimulating alpha and beta receptors and causing release of norepinephrine. Its actions are less potent but longer-lasting than those of epinephrine. Ephedrine produces more CNS stimulation than other adrenergic drugs. It may be used in the treatment of bronchial asthma to prevent bronchospasm, but it is less effective than epinephrine for acute bronchospasm and respiratory distress.

Ephedrine can be given orally or parenterally. When given orally, therapeutic effects occur within 1 hour and last 3 to 5 hours. When given SC, it acts in about 20 minutes and effects last about 60 minutes; with intramuscular administration, it acts in about 10 to 20 minutes and effects last less than 60 minutes.

Ephedrine is a common ingredient in OTC anti-asthma tablets (Bronkaid, Primatene, others). The tablets contain 12.5 to 25 mg of ephedrine and 100 to 130 mg of theophylline, a xanthine bronchodilator. Other clinical uses include shock associated with spinal or epidural anesthesia, Stokes-Adams syndrome (sudden attacks of unconsciousness caused by heart block), allergic disorders, nasal congestion, and eye disorders.

Pseudoephedrine (Sudafed) is a related drug with similar actions. It is used for bronchodilating and nasal decongestant effects. Pseudoephedrine is available OTC alone and as an ingredient in several multi-ingredient sinus, allergy, and cold remedies.

Ephedrine
Route and Dosage Ranges

Adults: Asthma, PO 25–50 mg q4h

    Hypotension, SC, IM 25–50 mg; IV 20 mg; do not exceed 150 mg/24 h

    Mydriasis, eye drops of 0.1% solution

    Nasal congestion, nose drops of 0.5%, 1%, or 3% solutions; PO 25–50 mg q4h

Children 6–12 y: PO 6.25–12.5 mg q4–6h

Children 2–6 y: PO 0.3–0.5 mg/kg q4–6h

Pseudoephedrine
Route and Dosage Ranges

Adults: PO 60 mg three or four times a day

Children 6–12 y: PO 30 mg q6h

Children 2–6 y: PO 15 mg q6h

Isoproterenol (Isuprel) is a synthetic catecholamine that acts on beta$_1$- and beta$_2$-adrenergic receptors. Its main actions are to stimulate the heart, dilate blood vessels in skeletal muscle, and relax bronchial smooth muscle. Compared to epinephrine, its cardiac stimulant effects are similar, but it does not affect alpha receptors and therefore does not cause vasoconstriction. It is well absorbed when given by injection or as an aerosol. However, absorption is unreliable with sublingual and oral preparations, so their use is not recommended. Isoproterenol may be used as a cardiac stimulant in heart block and cardiogenic shock and as a bronchodilator in respiratory conditions characterized by bronchospasm. However, beta$_2$-selective agonists (*e.g.*, albuterol, others) are preferred for bronchodilating effects because they cause less cardiac stimulation. Too-frequent use may lead to tolerance and decreased bronchodilating effects.

Routes and Dosage Ranges

Adults: Bradycardia and heart block, IV 1–2 mg (5–10 ml of 1:5000 solution), diluted in 5% dextrose injection, infused at 0.5–5 µg/min initially, then changed according to heart rate as indicated by continuous electrocardiogram monitoring

    Hypotension and shock, IV 1–2 mg (5–10 ml of 1:5000 solution) diluted in 5% dextrose injection, infused at 1–10 µg/min

    Bronchospasm during anesthesia, IV 0.01–0.02 mg or 0.5–1 ml of diluted solution initially (1 ml of 1:5000 solution, diluted to 10 ml with sodium chloride or 5% dextrose injection for a final concentration of 1:50,000), repeated PRN

    Bronchodilation, inhalation by nebulizer, 5–15 deep inhalations of a mist of 1:200 solution,

repeated in 10–30 min if necessary; by oxygen aerosol, up to 0.5 ml of 1:200 solution or 0.3 ml of 1:100 solution with oxygen flow at 4 L/min for 15–20 min; by measured-dose inhalers (Mistometer, Medihaler), 1 or 2 inhalations (second inhalation is given 2–5 min after first). These treatments should generally be given no more often than q4h.

    Sublingual tablets, 10–15 mg 3 or 4 times a day, maximum 60 mg/d; not a recommended route because absorption is unpredictable

Children: Bronchodilation, inhalation, generally the same as above, with adult supervision; sublingual, 5–10 mg 3 or 4 times a day, maximum 30 mg/d; not a preferred route because of erratic absorption

Phenylephrine (Neo-Synephrine, others) is a synthetic drug that acts on alpha-adrenergic receptors to produce vasoconstriction. Vasoconstriction decreases cardiac output and renal perfusion and increases peripheral vascular resistance and blood pressure. There is little cardiac stimulation because phenylephrine does not activate beta$_1$ receptors in the heart or beta$_2$ receptors in blood vessels. Phenylephrine may be given to raise blood pressure in hypotension and shock. Compared with epinephrine, phenylephrine produces longer-lasting elevation of blood pressure (20–50 minutes with injection). When given systemically, phenylephrine produces a reflex bradycardia; this effect may be used therapeutically to relieve paroxysmal atrial tachycardia. Other uses include local application for nasal decongestant and mydriatic effects. Various preparations are available for different uses. Phenylephrine is often an ingredient in prescription and nonprescription cold and allergy remedies.

Routes and Dosage Ranges

Adults: Hypotension and shock, IM, SC 5–10 mg; IV 0.25–0.5 mg diluted in sodium chloride injection and given slowly, or 10 mg diluted in 500 ml 5% dextrose injection and infused slowly, according to blood-pressure readings

    Orthostatic hypotension, PO 20 mg 3 times per day

    Nasal congestion, nasal solutions of 0.125%, 0.25%, 0.5%, or 1.0%

    Mydriasis, ophthalmic solutions of 2.5% or 10%

Phenylpropanolamine (Propagest, Dexatrim) stimulates both alpha and beta receptors, causing vasoconstriction, increased blood pressure, and cardiac stimulation. Its clinical uses stem mainly from its nasal decongestant and appetite-suppressing actions. It is a common ingredient in OTC cold and allergy remedies and is the active ingredient in most OTC appetite suppressants. For obesity, phenylpropanolamine should be used no longer than 8 to 12 weeks, and calorie restriction and safety precautions should be strictly followed. Severe hypertension and stroke may occur with overuse.

Phenylpropanolamine is readily absorbed from the GI tract; peak plasma levels and half-life depend on the drug formulation (immediate- versus sustained-release). Most is excreted unchanged in urine. Most OTC preparations are long-acting.

Route and Dosage Ranges

Adults: PO immediate-release formulations, 25 mg 3 times daily 30 min before meals
PO timed-release, 75 mg once daily in morning
PO precision-release (16-h duration), 75 mg after breakfast

Nursing Process

Assessment

Assess the client's status in relation to the following conditions:

- **Allergic disorders.** It is standard procedure to question a client about allergies on initial contact or admission to a health care agency. If the client reports a previous allergic reaction, try to determine what caused it and what specific symptoms occurred. It may be helpful to ask if swelling, breathing difficulty, or hives (urticaria) occurred. With anaphylactic reactions, severe respiratory distress (from bronchospasm and laryngeal edema) and profound hypotension (from vasodilation) may occur.
- **Asthma.** If the client is known to have asthma, assess the frequency of attacks, the specific signs and symptoms experienced, the precipitating factors, the actions taken to obtain relief, and the use of bronchodilators or other medications on a long-term basis. With acute bronchospasm, respiratory distress is clearly evidenced by loud, rapid, gasping, wheezing respirations. Acute asthma attacks may be precipitated by exposure to allergens or respiratory infections. When available, check arterial blood gas reports for the adequacy of oxygen–carbon dioxide gas exchange. Hypoxemia ($\downarrow$po$_2$), hypercarbia ($\uparrow$pco$_2$), and acidosis ($\downarrow$pH) may occur with acute bronchospasm.
- **Chronic obstructive pulmonary disorders.** Emphysema and chronic bronchitis are characterized by bronchoconstriction and dyspnea with exercise or at rest. Check arterial blood gas reports when available. Hypoxemia, hypercarbia, and acidosis are likely with chronic bronchoconstriction. Acute bronchospasm may be superimposed on the chronic bronchoconstrictive disorder, especially with a respiratory infection.
- **Cardiovascular status.** Assess for conditions that are caused or aggravated by adrenergic drugs (*e.g.,* angina, hypertension, tachyarrhythmias).

Nursing Diagnoses

- Impaired Gas Exchange related to bronchoconstriction
- Altered Tissue Perfusion related to hypotension and shock or vasoconstriction with drug therapy
- Altered Nutrition: Less than Body Requirements related to anorexia
- Sleep Pattern Disturbance: Insomnia, nervousness
- Noncompliance: Overuse
- Risk for Injury related to cardiac stimulation (arrhythmias, hypertension)
- Knowledge Deficit: Drug effects and safe usage

Planning/Goals

The client will:
- Receive or self-administer drugs accurately
- Experience relief of symptoms for which adrenergic drugs are given
- Comply with instructions for safe drug use
- Demonstrate knowledge of adverse drug effects to be reported
- Avoid preventable adverse drug effects
- Avoid combinations of adrenergic drugs

Interventions

Use measures to prevent or minimize conditions for which adrenergic drugs are required:
- Decrease exposure to allergens. Allergens include cigarette smoke, foods, drugs, air pollutants, plant pollens, insect venoms, and animal dander. Specific allergens must be determined for each person.
- For clients with chronic lung disease, use measures to prevent respiratory infections. These include interventions to aid removal of respiratory secretions, such as adequate hydration, ambulation, deep-breathing and coughing exercises, and chest physiotherapy. Immunizations with pneumococcal pneumonia vaccine (a single dose) and influenza vaccine (annually) are also strongly recommended.
- When administering substances known to produce hypersensitivity reactions (penicillin and other antibiotics, allergy extracts, vaccines, local anesthetics), observe the recipient carefully for at least 30 minutes after administration. Have adrenergic and other emergency drugs and equipment readily available in case a reaction occurs.

 Teach clients:

- To use these drugs only as directed. The potential for abuse is high, especially for the client with asthma or other chronic lung disease who is seeking relief from labored breathing. Some of these drugs are prescribed for long-term use, but excessive use does not increase therapeutic effects. Instead, it causes tolerance and decreased benefit from usual doses and increases the incidence and severity of adverse reactions.
- To take no other medications without the physician's knowledge and approval. Many OTC cold remedies and appetite suppressants contain adrenergic drugs. Use of these along with prescribed adrenergic drugs can result in overdose and serious cardiovascular or CNS problems. In addition, adrenergic drugs interact with numerous other drugs to increase or decrease effects; some of these interactions may be life-threatening.

Evaluation

- Observe for increased blood pressure and improved tissue perfusion when a drug is given for hypotension and shock or anaphylaxis.

- Interview and observe for improved breathing and arterial blood gas reports when a drug is given for bronchoconstriction or anaphylaxis.
- Interview and observe for decreased nasal congestion.

Principles of Therapy

DRUG SELECTION AND ADMINISTRATION

The choice of drug, dosage, and route of administration depends largely on the reason for use. IV or SC epinephrine is the drug of choice in anaphylactic shock. Isoproterenol by oral inhalation may be used for producing bronchodilation. However, a selective beta$_2$ agonist is preferred because it causes less cardiac stimulation. Adrenergic drugs are given IV only for emergencies, such as cardiac arrest, severe arterial hypotension, circulatory shock, and anaphylactic shock. No standard doses of individual adrenergic drugs are always effective; the dosage must be individualized according to the client's response. This is especially true in emergencies, but it also applies to long-term use.

USE IN SPECIFIC SITUATIONS

Because adrenergic drugs are often used in crises, they must be readily available in all health care settings (e.g., hospitals, long-term care facilities, physicians' offices). All health care personnel should know where emergency drugs are stored.

Anaphylaxis

Epinephrine is the drug of choice for the treatment of anaphylaxis. It relieves bronchospasm, laryngeal edema, and hypotension. In conjunction with its alpha (vasoconstriction) and beta (cardiac stimulation, bronchodilation) effects, epinephrine acts as a physiologic antagonist of histamine and other bronchoconstricting and vasodilating substances released during anaphylactic reactions. Persons susceptible to severe allergic responses should carry a syringe of epinephrine at all times. Antihistamines are not very useful because histamine plays a minor role in causing anaphylaxis, compared to leukotrienes and other inflammatory mediators.

Victims of anaphylaxis who have been taking beta-adrenergic blocking drugs (e.g., propranolol [Inderal]) do not respond as readily to epinephrine as those not taking a beta-blocker. Larger doses of epinephrine and large amounts of IV fluids may be required.

Cardiopulmonary Resuscitation

Epinephrine is one of the first drugs administered during CPR and is the adrenergic drug of choice. Its most important action is constriction of peripheral blood vessels. This shunts blood to the central circulation and increases blood flow to the heart and brain. It is also given for asystole to stimulate electrical and mechanical activity to produce myocardial contraction. This effect is also thought to result from its vasoconstrictive action. The specific effects of epinephrine depend largely on the dose and route of administration. The optimal dose in CPR has not been established. Traditional doses are relatively conservative (e.g., 0.5–1 mg q3–5 min). In recent years, some studies and some authorities indicate that higher doses (e.g., 2–5 mg or up to 0.1 mg/kg q3–5 min) may be more effective, possibly because of a more intense vasopressor response.

Hypotension and Shock

In hypotension and shock, initial efforts involve identifying and treating the cause when possible. Such treatments include blood transfusions, fluid and electrolyte replacement, and treatment of infection. If these measures are ineffective in raising blood pressure enough to maintain tissue perfusion, vasopressor drugs may be used. The usual goal of vasopressor drug therapy is to maintain tissue perfusion and a systolic blood pressure of at least 80 to 100 mm Hg.

Nasal Congestion

Adrenergic drugs are given topically and systemically to constrict blood vessels in nasal mucosa and decrease the nasal congestion associated with the common cold, allergic rhinitis, and sinusitis. Topical agents are effective, undergo little systemic absorption, are available OTC, and are widely used. However, overuse leads to decreased effectiveness, irritation of nasal mucosa, and rebound congestion. These effects can be minimized by using small doses only when necessary and for no longer than 3 to 5 days.

Oral agents have a slower onset of action than topical ones but may last longer. They also may cause more adverse effects. Adverse effects may occur with usual therapeutic doses and are especially likely with high doses. Most worrisome are cardiac and CNS stimulation. Commonly used oral agents are pseudoephedrine, phenylpropanolamine, and ephedrine. Pseudoephedrine seems to be the safest of the three in relation to risks of hypertension and cerebral hemorrhage (stroke). Phenylpropanolamine and ephedrine may cause hypertension even in normotensive persons, with higher risks in hypertensive persons. Hypertensive patients should avoid these drugs if possible.

USE IN CHILDREN

Guidelines for safe and effective use of adrenergic drugs in children are not well established. Children are very sensitive to drug effects, including cardiac and CNS stimulation, and recommended doses generally should not be exceeded.

The main use of epinephrine in children is for treatment of bronchospasm due to asthma or allergic reactions. Parenteral epinephrine may cause syncope when given to asthmatic children. Isoproterenol is rarely given parenterally, but if given, the first dose should be about half that of an adult, and later doses should be based on the response to the first dose. There is little reason to use the inhalation route because in children, as in adults, selective beta₂ agonists such as albuterol are preferred for bronchodilation in asthma.

Phenylephrine is most often used to relieve congestion of the upper respiratory tract and may be given topically, as nose drops. Doses must be carefully measured. Rebound nasal congestion occurs with overuse. Phenylpropanolamine is a common ingredient in OTC cold remedies. Dosage guidelines should be followed carefully, and the drugs should be inaccessible to young children. Phenylpropanolamine also is the active ingredient in OTC appetite suppressants. These should not be used for weight reduction in children.

Use in Older Adults

Adrenergic drugs stimulate the heart to increase rate and force of contraction and blood pressure. Older adults often have chronic cardiovascular conditions (*e.g.*, angina, arrhythmias, congestive heart failure, coronary artery disease, hypertension, peripheral vascular disease) that are aggravated by the drugs. Adrenergics are often prescribed as bronchodilators and decongestants in older adults. Therapeutic doses increase the workload of the heart and may cause symptoms of impaired cardiovascular function; overdoses may cause severe cardiovascular dysfunction, including life-threatening arrhythmias.

The drugs also cause CNS stimulation. With therapeutic doses, anxiety, restlessness, nervousness, and insomnia often occur in older adults. Overdoses may cause hallucinations, convulsions, CNS depression, and death.

Adrenergics are ingredients in OTC asthma remedies, cold remedies, nasal decongestants, and appetite suppressants. Cautious use of these preparations is required for older adults. They should not be taken concurrently with prescription adrenergic drugs because of the high risk of overdose and toxicity.

Ophthalmic preparations of adrenergic drugs also should be used cautiously. For example, phenylephrine is used as a vasoconstrictor and mydriatic. Applying larger-than-recommended doses to the normal eye or usual doses to the traumatized, inflamed, or diseased eye may result in enough systemic absorption of the drug to cause increased blood pressure and other adverse effects.

Home Care

Adrenergic drugs are often used in the home setting. Frequently prescribed drugs include bronchodilators and nasal decongestants. OTC drugs with the same effects are also commonly used for asthma, allergic rhinitis, cold symptoms, and appetite suppression for weight control. A major function of the home care nurse is to teach clients to use the drugs correctly (especially metered-dose inhalers), to report excessive CNS or cardiac stimulation to a health care provider, and not to take OTC drugs with the same or similar ingredients as prescription drugs.

Excessive adverse effects are probably most likely to occur in children and older adults. Older adults often have other illnesses that may be aggravated by adrenergic drugs or take other drugs, the effects of which may be altered by concomitant use of adrenergics.

NURSING ACTIONS

ADRENERGIC DRUGS

NURSING ACTIONS	RATIONALE/EXPLANATION
1. Administer accurately **a.** Check package inserts or other references if not absolutely sure about the preparation or concentration and method of administration for an adrenergic drug.	The many different preparations and concentrations available for various routes of administration increase the risk of medication error unless extreme caution is used. Preparations for intravenous, subcutaneous, inhalation, ophthalmic, or nasal routes must be used by the designated route only.
b. To give epinephrine subcutaneously, use a tuberculin syringe, aspirate, and massage the injection site.	The tuberculin syringe is necessary for accurate measurement of the small doses usually given (often less than 0.5 ml).

(continued)

NURSING ACTIONS	RATIONALE/EXPLANATION
	Aspiration is necessary to avoid inadvertent IV administration of the larger, undiluted amount of drug intended for subcutaneous use. Massaging the injection site accelerates drug absorption and thus relief of symptoms.
c. Give Sus-Phrine subcutaneously only, and shake well before using (both vial and syringe).	Sus-Phrine is a suspension preparation of epinephrine, and suspensions must not be given IV. Rotating or shaking the container ensures that the medication is evenly distributed throughout the suspension.
d. For inhalation, be sure to use the correct drug concentration, and use the nebulizing device properly.	Inhalation medications are often administered by clients themselves or by respiratory therapists if intermittent positive-pressure breathing is used. The nurse may need to demonstrate and supervise self-administration initially.
e. Do *not* give epinephrine and isoproterenol at the same time or within 4 hours of each other.	Both of these drugs are potent cardiac stimulants, and the combination could cause serious cardiac arrhythmias. However, they have synergistic bronchodilating effects, and doses can be alternated and given safely if the drugs are given no more closely together than 4 hours.
f. For IV injection of epinephrine, dilute 1 ml of 1:1000 solution to a total volume of 10 ml with sodium chloride injection, or use a commercial preparation of 1:10,000 concentration. Use parenteral solutions of epinephrine only if clear.	Dilution increases safety of administration. A solution that is brown or contains a precipitate should not be used. Discoloration indicates chemical deterioration of epinephrine.
g. For IV infusion of isoproterenol and phenylephrine:	
(1) Administer in an intensive care unit when possible.	These drugs are given IV in emergencies, during which the client's condition must be carefully monitored. Frequent recording of blood pressure and pulse and continuous electrocardiographic monitoring are needed.
(2) Use only clear drug solutions	A brownish color or precipitate indicates deterioration, and such solutions should not be used.
(3) Dilute the drugs in 500 ml of 5% dextrose injection. Do not add the drug until ready to use.	A 5% dextrose solution is compatible with the drugs. Mixing solutions when ready for use helps to ensure drug stability. Note that drug concentration varies with the amount of drug and the amount of dextrose solution to which it is added.
(4) Use an infusion device to regulate flow rate accurately.	Flow rate usually requires frequent adjustment according to blood pressure measurements. An infusion device helps to regulate drug administration, so wide fluctuations in blood pressure are avoided.
(5) Use a "piggyback" IV apparatus.	Only one bottle contains an adrenergic drug, and it can be regulated or discontinued without disruption of the primary IV line.
(6) Start the adrenergic drug solution slowly and increase flow rate according to the client's response (*e.g.*, blood pressure, color, mental status). Slow or discontinue gradually as well.	To avoid abrupt changes in circulation and blood pressure
h. When giving adrenergic drugs as eye drops or nose drops, do not touch the dropper to the eye or nose.	Contaminated droppers can be a source of bacterial infection.
2. Observe for therapeutic effects	These depend on the reason for use.
a. When the drug is used as a bronchodilator, observe for absence or reduction of wheezing, less labored breathing, and decreased rate of respirations.	Indicates prevention or relief of bronchospasm. Acute bronchospasm is usually relieved within 5 minutes by injected or inhaled epinephrine or inhaled isoproterenol.

NURSING ACTIONS	RATIONALE/EXPLANATION
b. When epinephrine is given in anaphylactic shock, observe for decreased tissue edema and improved breathing and circulation.	Epinephrine injection usually relieves laryngeal edema and bronchospasm within 5 minutes and lasts for about 20 minutes.
c. When isoproterenol or phenylephrine is given in hypotension and shock, observe for increased blood pressure, stronger pulse, and improved urine output, level of consciousness, and color.	These are indicators of improved circulation.
d. When a drug is given nasally for decongestant effects, observe for decreased nasal congestion and ability to breathe through the nose.	The drugs act as vasoconstrictors to reduce engorgement of nasal mucosa.
e. When given as eye drops for vasoconstrictor effects, observe for decreased redness. When giving for mydriatic effects, observe for pupil dilation.	
3. Observe for adverse effects	Adverse effects depend to some extent on the reason for use. For example, cardiovascular effects are considered adverse reactions when the drugs are given for bronchodilation. Adverse effects occur with usual therapeutic doses and are more likely to occur with higher doses.
a. Cardiovascular effects—cardiac arrhythmias, hypertension	Tachycardia and hypertension are common; if severe or prolonged, myocardial ischemia or heart failure may occur. Premature ventricular contractions and other serious arrhythmias may occur. Propranolol (Inderal) or another beta-blocker may be given to decrease heart rate and hypertension resulting from overdosage of adrenergic drugs. Phentolamine (Regitine) may be used to decrease severe hypertension.
b. Excessive CNS stimulation—nervousness, anxiety, tremor, insomnia	These effects are more likely to occur with ephedrine or high doses of other adrenergic drugs. Sometimes, a sedative-type drug is given concomitantly to offset these effects.
c. Rebound nasal congestion, rhinitis, possible ulceration of nasal mucosa	These effects occur with excessive use of nasal decongestant drugs.
4. Observe for drug interactions **a.** Drugs that *increase* effects of adrenergic drugs:	Most of these drugs increase incidence or severity of adverse reactions.
(1) Anesthetics, general (*e.g.,* halothane)	Increased risk of cardiac arrhythmias. Potentially hazardous.
(2) Anticholinergics (*e.g.,* atropine)	Increased bronchial relaxation. Also increased mydriasis and therefore contraindicated with narrow-angle glaucoma.
(3) Antidepressants, tricyclic (*e.g.,* amitriptyline [Elavil])	Increased pressor response with intravenous epinephrine
(4) Antihistamines	May increase pressor effects
(5) Cocaine	Increases pressor and mydriatic effects by inhibiting uptake of norepinephrine by nerve endings. Cardiac arrhythmias, convulsions, and acute glaucoma may occur.
(6) Digitalis	Sympathomimetics, especially beta-adrenergics like epinephrine and isoproterenol, increase the likelihood of cardiac arrhythmias due to ectopic pacemaker activity.
(7) Doxapram (Dopram)	Increased pressor effect
(8) Ergot alkaloids (*e.g.,* Gynergen)	Increased vasoconstriction. Extremely high blood pressure may occur. There also may be decreased perfusion of fingers and toes.

(continued)

NURSING ACTIONS	RATIONALE/EXPLANATION
(9) Monoamine oxidase (MAO) inhibitors (*e.g.*, isocarboxazid [Marplan])	Contraindicated. The combination may cause death. When these drugs are given concurrently with adrenergic drugs, there is danger of cardiac arrhythmias, respiratory depression, and acute hypertensive crisis with possible intracranial hemorrhage, convulsions, coma, and death. Effects of MAO inhibitors may not occur for several weeks after treatment is started and may last up to 3 weeks after the drug is stopped. Every client taking MAO inhibitors should be warned against taking any other medication without the advice of a physician or pharmacist.
(10) Methylphenidate (Ritalin)	Increased pressor and mydriatic effects. The combination may be hazardous in glaucoma.
(11) Thyroid preparations (*e.g.*, Synthroid)	Increased adrenergic effects, resulting in increased likelihood of arrhythmias
(12) Xanthines (in caffeine-containing substances, such as coffee, tea, cola drinks; theophylline)	Synergistic bronchodilating effect. Sympathomimetics with CNS-stimulating properties (*e.g.*, ephedrine, isoproterenol) may produce excessive CNS stimulation with cardiac arrhythmias, emotional disturbances, and insomnia.
(13) Beta-adrenergic blocking agents (*e.g.*, propranolol [Inderal])	May augment hypertensive response to epinephrine (see also b[4] below)
b. Drugs that *decrease* effects of adrenergics:	
(1) Anticholinesterases (*e.g.*, neostigmine [Prostigmin], pyridostigmine [Mestinon]) and other cholinergic drugs	Decrease mydriatic effects of adrenergics; thus, the two groups should not be given concurrently in ophthalmic conditions
(2) Antihypertensives (*e.g.*, methyldopa [Aldomet])	Generally antagonize pressor effects of adrenergics, which act to increase blood pressure while antihypertensives act to lower it
(3) Antipsychotic drugs (*e.g.*, haloperidol [Haldol], chlorpromazine [Thorazine])	Block the vasopressor action of epinephrine. Therefore, epinephrine should not be used to treat hypotension induced by these drugs.
(4) Beta-adrenergic blocking agents (*e.g.*, propranolol [Inderal])	Decrease bronchodilating effects of adrenergics and may exacerbate asthma. Contraindicated with asthma.
(5) Phentolamine (Regitine)	Antagonizes vasopressor effects of adrenergics
5. Teach clients **a.** Inhaled solutions of isoproterenol may turn saliva and sputum pink.	This harmless discoloration is caused by the medication, not by bleeding.
b. Report adverse reactions, such as fast pulse, palpitations, chest pain.	So that drug dosage can be reevaluated and therapy changed if needed
c. Report if previously effective dose becomes ineffective.	This may indicate that drug tolerance has developed. This is more likely to occur with long-term use of ephedrine and isoproterenol for bronchodilation. Tolerance can be prevented or treated by discontinuing the individual drug for a few days or by substituting another adrenergic drug.
d. For clients receiving intravenous adrenergic drugs for cardiac stimulation or vasopressor effects, explain the necessity for cardiac monitoring, frequent checks of flow rate, blood pressure, urine output, and so on.	An explanation may help decrease anxiety in a seriously ill patient. He or she should know that these measures increase the safety and benefits of drug therapy rather than indicate the presence of a critical condition.

REVIEW AND APPLICATION EXERCISES

1. How do adrenergic drugs act to relieve symptoms of acute bronchospasm, anaphylaxis, cardiac arrest, hypotension and shock, and nasal congestion?

2. Which adrenergic receptors are stimulated by administration of epinephrine?

3. Why is it important to have epinephrine and other adrenergic drugs readily available in all health care settings?

4. Which adrenergic drug is the drug of choice to treat acute anaphylactic reactions?

5. Why is inhaled epinephrine not a drug of choice for long-term treatment of asthma and other bronchoconstrictive disorders?

6. What are the major adverse effects of adrenergic drugs?

7. Why are clients with cardiac arrhythmias, angina pectoris, hypertension, or diabetes mellitus especially likely to experience adverse reactions to adrenergic drugs?

8. For a client who reports frequent use of OTC asthma remedies and cold remedies, what teaching is needed to increase client safety?

9. Mentally rehearse nursing interventions for various emergency situations (anaphylaxis, acute respiratory distress, cardiac arrest) in terms of medications and equipment needed and how to obtain them promptly.

SELECTED REFERENCES

Drug facts and comparisons. (1996). St. Louis: Facts and Comparisons.

Gonzalez, E.R., Jones, L.A., & Durso, M.H. (1993). Pharmacotherapy of cardiopulmonary resuscitation. In J.T. DiPiro, R.L. Talbert, P.E. Hayes, Yee, G.C., G.R. Matzke, & L.M. Posey (Eds.), *Pharmacotherapy: A pathophysiologic approach*, 2nd ed., pp. 128–138. Norwalk, CT: Appleton & Lange.

Guyton, A.C., & Hall, J.E. (1996). *Textbook of medical physiology*, 9th ed. Philadelphia: W.B. Saunders.

Hoffman, B.B., & Lefkowitz, R.J. (1996). Catecholamines, sympathomimetic drugs, and adrenergic receptor antagonists. In J.G. Hardman, L.E. Limbird, P.B. Molinoff, & R.W. Ruddon (Eds.), *Goodman and Gilman's The pharmacological basis of therapeutics*, 9th ed., pp. 199–248. New York: McGraw-Hill.

Kelly, H.W., & Hill, M.R. (1993). Asthma. In J.T. DiPiro, R.L. Talbert, P.E. Hayes, Yee, G.C., G.R. Matzke, & L.M. Posey (Eds.), *Pharmacotherapy: A pathophysiologic approach*, 2nd ed., pp. 408–449. Norwalk, CT: Appleton & Lange.

Lefkowitz, R.J., Hoffman, B.B., & Taylor, P. (1996). Neurotransmission: The autonomic and somatic motor nervous systems. In J.G. Hardman, L.E. Limbird, P.B. Molinoff, & R.W. Ruddon (Eds.), *Goodman and Gilman's The pharmacological basis of therapeutics*, 9th ed., pp. 105–139. New York: McGraw-Hill.

19 Antiadrenergic Drugs

Objectives

After studying this chapter, the student will be able to:

1 List characteristics of antiadrenergic drugs in terms of effects on body tissues, indications for use, nursing process implications, principles of therapy, and observation of client response.

2 Discuss alpha$_1$-adrenergic blocking agents and alpha$_2$-adrenergic agonists in terms of indications for use, adverse effects, and selected other characteristics.

3 Compare and contrast beta-adrenergic blocking agents in terms of cardioselectivity, indications for use, adverse effects, and selected other characteristics.

4 Discuss teaching needs of clients taking antiadrenergic drugs.

Key Terms

Alpha-adrenergic blocking agents

Beta-adrenergic blocking agents

Cardioselective

Description

Antiadrenergic or sympatholytic drugs decrease or block the effects of sympathetic nerve stimulation, endogenous catecholamines (*e.g.*, epinephrine), and adrenergic drugs. The drugs are chemically diverse and have a wide spectrum of pharmacologic activity, with specific effects depending mainly on the client's health status when a drug is given and the drug's binding with particular adrenergic receptors. Included here are clonidine and related centrally active antiadrenergic drugs, which are used primarily in the treatment of hypertension, and peripherally active agents (alpha- and beta-adrenergic blocking agents), which are used to treat various cardiovascular and other disorders. A few uncommonly used antiadrenergic drugs are included in Chapter 55.

A basal level of sympathetic tone is necessary to maintain normal body functioning, including regulation of blood pressure, blood glucose, and stress response. Therefore, the goal of antiadrenergic drug therapy is to suppress pathologic stimulation, not the normal, physiologic response to activity, stress, and other stimuli.

MECHANISMS OF ACTION AND EFFECTS

Most antiadrenergic drugs have antagonist (blocking) effects in which they combine with $alpha_1$, $beta_1$, $beta_2$, or a combination of receptors in peripheral tissues and prevent adrenergic (sympathomimetic) effects. Clonidine and related drugs have agonist effects at presynaptic $alpha_2$ receptors in the brain. This means that some of the norepinephrine released by the presynaptic nerve cell into the synapse returns to the presynaptic site and activates $alpha_2$ receptors. This results in a negative feedback type of mechanism that decreases the release of additional norepinephrine. Thus, the overall effect is decreased sympathetic outflow from the brain and antiadrenergic effects on peripheral tissues (*i.e.*, decreased activation of alpha and beta receptors by norepinephrine throughout the body).

Alpha-Adrenergic Agonists and Blocking Agents

Alpha$_2$-adrenergic agonists inhibit the release of norepinephrine in the brain, thereby decreasing the effects of sympathetic nervous system stimulation throughout the body. A major clinical effect is decreased blood pressure. Although clinical effects are attributed mainly to drug action at presynaptic $alpha_2$ receptors in the brain, postsynaptic $alpha_2$ receptors in the brain and peripheral tissues (*e.g.*, vascular smooth muscle) may also be involved. Activation of $alpha_2$ receptors in the pancreatic islets suppresses insulin secretion.

Alpha$_1$-adrenergic blocking agents occupy $alpha_1$-adrenergic receptor sites in smooth muscles and glands innervated by sympathetic nerve fibers. These drugs act primarily in the skin, mucosa, intestines, and kidneys to prevent alpha-mediated vasoconstriction. Specific effects include dilation of arterioles and veins, increased local blood flow, decreased blood pressure, constriction of pupils, and increased motility of the gastrointestinal tract. Alpha-adrenergic antagonists may activate reflexes that oppose the fall in blood pressure by increasing heart rate and cardiac output and causing fluid retention.

The drugs also can prevent alpha-mediated contraction of smooth muscle in nonvascular tissues. For example, benign prostatic hyperplasia (BPH) is characterized by obstructed urine flow because the enlarged prostate gland presses on the urethra. The drugs can decrease urinary retention and improve urine flow by inhibiting contraction of muscles in the prostate and urinary bladder.

Nonselective alpha-adrenergic blocking agents occupy peripheral $alpha_1$ receptors to cause vasodilation and $alpha_2$ receptors to cause cardiac stimulation. Consequently, decreased blood pressure is accompanied by tachycardia and perhaps other arrhythmias.

Beta-Adrenergic Blocking Drugs

Beta-adrenergic blocking agents occupy beta-adrenergic receptor sites and prevent the receptors from responding to sympathetic nerve impulses, circulating catecholamines, and beta-adrenergic drugs (Fig. 19-1). Specific effects include:

1. Decreased heart rate (negative chronotropy)
2. Decreased force of myocardial contraction (negative inotropy)
3. Decreased cardiac output at rest and with exercise
4. Slowed conduction through the atrioventricular (AV) node
5. Decreased automaticity of ectopic pacemakers
6. Decreased blood pressure in supine and standing positions
7. Bronchoconstriction from blockade of $beta_2$ receptors in bronchial smooth muscle. This effect occurs primarily in people with asthma or other chronic lung diseases.
8. Less effective metabolism of glucose (decreased glycogenolysis) when needed by the body, especially in persons taking beta-blocking agents along with antidiabetic drugs. These clients may experience more severe and prolonged hypoglycemia. In addition, early symptoms of hypoglycemia (*e.g.*, tachycardia) may be blocked, delaying recognition of the hypoglycemia.

Figure 19-1
Beta-adrenergic blocking agents prevent epinephrine and norepinephrine from occupying receptor sites on cell membranes. This action alters cell functions normally stimulated by epinephrine and norepinephrine, according to the number of receptor sites occupied by the beta-blocking drugs. (Adapted by J. Harley from Encyclopedia Britannica Medical and Health Annual. Chicago, Encyclopedia Britannica, 1983)

INDICATIONS FOR USE

Alpha-Adrenergic Agonists and Blocking Agents

Alpha$_2$ agonists are used in the treatment of hypertension. Clonidine has been tested for numerous other indications, including treatment of alcohol withdrawal and opioid dependence, but is not approved by the Food and Drug Administration for these purposes. Alpha$_1$-blocking agents are used in the treatment of hypertension and BPH. Nonselective alpha-blocking agents are not used as antihypertensive drugs except in hypertension caused by excessive catecholamines. Excessive catecholamines may result from overdosage of adrenergic drugs or from pheochromocytoma, a rare tumor of the adrenal medulla that secretes epinephrine and norepinephrine and causes hypertension, tachycardia, and cardiac arrhythmias. Although the treatment of choice for pheochromocytoma is surgical excision, alpha-adrenergic blocking drugs are useful adjuncts. They are given before and during surgery, usually in conjunction with beta-blockers. Alpha-blockers also are used in vascular diseases characterized by vasospasm,

such as Raynaud's disease and frostbite, in which they improve blood flow. Phentolamine also can be used to prevent tissue necrosis from extravasation of potent vasoconstrictors (*e.g.*, norepinephrine, dopamine) into subcutaneous tissues.

Beta-Adrenergic Blocking Drugs

Clinical indications for use of beta-blocking agents are mainly cardiovascular disorders (*i.e.*, angina pectoris, cardiac tachyarrhythmias, hypertension, and myocardial infarction) and glaucoma. In angina, beta-blockers decrease myocardial contractility, cardiac output, heart rate, and blood pressure. These effects decrease myocardial oxygen demand (cardiac workload), especially in response to activity, exercise, and stress. In arrhythmias, drug effects depend on the sympathetic tone of the heart (that is, the degree of adrenergic stimulation of the heart that the drug must block or overcome). The drugs slow the sinus rate and prolong conduction through the AV node, thereby slowing the ventricular response rate to supraventricular tachyarrhythmias.

In hypertension, the actions by which the drugs lower blood pressure are unclear. Possible mechanisms include reduced cardiac output, inhibition of renin, and inhibition of sympathetic nervous system stimulation in the brain. However, the drugs effective in hypertension do not consistently demonstrate these effects—in other words, a drug may lower blood pressure without reducing cardiac output or inhibiting renin, for example. After myocardial infarction, the drugs help protect the heart from reinfarction and decrease mortality rates over several years. A possible mechanism is preventing or decreasing the incidence of catecholamine-induced arrhythmias.

In glaucoma, the drugs reduce intraocular pressure by binding to beta-adrenergic receptors in the ciliary body of the eye and decreasing formation of aqueous humor.

Propranolol (Inderal) is the prototype of beta-adrenergic blocking agents. It is also the oldest, most widely used, and most extensively studied beta-blocker. In addition to its use in the treatment of hypertension, arrhythmias, angina pectoris, and myocardial infarction, propranolol is used in hypertrophic obstructive cardiomyopathies, in which it improves exercise tolerance; pheochromocytoma, in which it decreases tachycardia and arrhythmias but must be used along with an alpha-adrenergic blocking agent; hyperthyroidism, in which it decreases heart rate, cardiac output, and tremor; and prevention of migraine headaches by an unknown mechanism (it is not helpful in acute attacks of migraine). The drug also relieves palpitation and tremor associated with anxiety, but it is not approved for clinical use as an antianxiety drug.

CONTRAINDICATIONS FOR USE

Alpha$_2$ agonists are contraindicated in clients with hypersensitivity to the drugs, and methyldopa is also contraindicated in clients with active liver disease. Alpha-adrenergic blocking agents are contraindicated in angina pectoris, myocardial infarction, and stroke. Beta-adrenergic blocking agents are contraindicated in bradycardia, heart block, congestive heart failure, and asthma and other allergic or pulmonary conditions characterized by bronchoconstriction.

Individual Antiadrenergic Drugs

These drugs are described below; trade names, clinical indications, and dosage ranges are listed in Tables 19-1 and 19-2.

ALPHA-ADRENERGIC AGONISTS AND BLOCKING AGENTS

Alpha$_2$-adrenergic agonists include clonidine, guanabenz, guanfacine, and methyldopa. These drugs produce similar therapeutic and adverse effects but differ in their pharmacokinetics and frequency of administration. Oral **clonidine** reduces blood pressure within 1 hour, reaches peak plasma levels in 3 to 5 hours, and has a plasma half-life of about 12 to 16 hours (longer with renal impairment). About half the oral dose is metabolized in the liver; the remainder is excreted unchanged in urine. With transdermal clonidine, therapeutic plasma levels are reached in 2 to 3 days and last 1 week. **Guanabenz** action occurs within 1 hour, peaks within 2 to 4 hours, and lasts 6 to 8 hours. It is metabolized extensively; very little unchanged drug is excreted in urine. **Guanfacine** is well absorbed and widely distributed, with about 70% bound to plasma proteins. Peak plasma levels occur in 1 to 4 hours and the half life is 10 to 30 hours. About half is metabolized and the metabolites and unchanged drug are excreted in urine. Because of its longer half-life, guanfacine can be given once daily. **Methyldopa** is an older drug with low to moderate absorption, peak plasma levels in 2 to 4 hours, and peak antihypertensive effects in about 2 days. When discontinued, blood pressure rises in about 2 days. Intravenous administration reduces blood pressure in 4 to 6 hours and lasts 10 to 16 hours. Methyldopa is metabolized to some extent in the liver but is largely excreted in urine. In clients with renal impairment, blood-pressure–lowering effects may be pronounced and prolonged because of slower excretion. In addition to the adverse effects that occur with all these drugs, methyldopa also may cause hemolytic anemia and hepatotoxicity (*e.g.,* jaundice, hepatitis).

Alpha$_1$-adrenergic antagonists include doxazosin, prazosin, and terazosin. **Prazosin**, the prototype, is well absorbed after oral administration and reaches peak plasma concentrations in 1 to 3 hours; action lasts about 4 to 6 hours. The drug is highly bound to plasma proteins and the plasma half-life is about 2 to 3 hours. It is extensively metabolized in the liver and its metabolites are excreted by the kidneys. **Doxazosin** and **terazosin** are similar to prazosin but have longer half-lives (doxazosin, 10–20 hours; terazosin, about 12 hours) and durations of action (doxazosin, up to 36 hours; terazosin, 18 hours or longer). Prazosin must be taken in multiple doses; doxazosin and terazosin may usually be taken once daily to control hypertension.

Nonselective alpha-adrenergic blocking agents include phenoxybenzamine and phentolamine. **Phenoxybenzamine** is long-acting; effects of a single dose persist for 3 to 4 days. **Phentolamine** is similar to phenoxybenzamine but more useful clinically. Phentolamine is short-acting; effects last only a few hours and can be reversed by an alpha-adrenergic stimulant drug, such as norepinephrine (Levophed).

BETA-ADRENERGIC BLOCKING DRUGS

Numerous beta-blocking agents are marketed in the United States. Although they produce similar effects, they differ in several characteristics, including clinical indications for use, receptor selectivity, intrinsic sympathomimetic activity, membrane-stabilizing ability, lipid solubility, routes of excretion, routes of administration, and duration of action.

Clinical Indications

Most beta-blockers are approved for the treatment of hypertension. A beta-blocker may be used alone or with another antihypertensive drug, such as a diuretic. Labetalol is also approved for treatment of hypertensive emergencies. Atenolol, metoprolol, nadolol, and propranolol are approved as antianginal agents; acebutolol, esmolol, propranolol, and sotalol are approved as antiarrhythmic agents. Atenolol, metoprolol, propranolol, and timolol are used to prevent myocardial infarction or reinfarction. Betaxolol, carteolol, and timolol (Timoptic) are used for hypertension and glaucoma; levobunolol and metipranolol are used only for glaucoma.

Receptor Selectivity

Carteolol, levobunolol, metipranolol, penbutolol, nadolol, pindolol, propranolol, sotalol, and timolol are nonselective beta-blockers. The term *nonselective* indicates that the drugs block both beta$_1$ (cardiac) and beta$_2$ (mainly smooth muscle in the bronchi and blood vessels) receptors. Blockade of beta$_2$ receptors is asso-

TABLE 19-1	ALPHA-ADRENERGIC AGONISTS AND BLOCKING AGENTS

Generic / Trade Name	Clinical Indications	Routes and Dosage Ranges
Alpha₂ agonists		
Clonidine (Catapres)	Hypertension	PO 0.1 mg 2 times daily initially, gradually increased if necessary. Average maintenance dose, 0.2–0.8 mg/d. Transdermal 0.1-mg patch every 7 d initially; increase every 7–14 d to 0.2 mg or 0.3 mg if necessary. Maximum dose, two 0.3-mg patches every 7 d.
Guanabenz (Wytensin)	Hypertension	PO 4 mg twice daily, increased by 4–8 mg/d every 1–2 wk if necessary to a maximal dose of 32 mg twice daily.
Guanfacine (Tenex)	Hypertension	PO 1 mg daily at bedtime, increased to 2 mg after 3–4 wk, then to 3 mg if necessary.
Methyldopa (Aldomet)	Hypertension	*Adults:* PO 250 mg 2 or 3 times daily initially, increased gradually at intervals of not less than 2 d until blood pressure is controlled or a daily dose of 3 g is reached. *Children:* PO 10 mg/kg/d in 2 to 4 divided doses initially, increased or decreased according to response. Maximal dose, 65 mg/kg/d or 3 g daily, whichever is less.
Alpha₁-blocking agents		
Doxazosin (Cardura)	Hypertension Benign prostatic hyperplasia (BPH)	PO 1 mg once daily initially, increased to 2 mg, then to 4, 8, and 16 mg if necessary.
Prazosin (Minipress)	Hypertension BPH	PO 1 mg 2 to 3 times daily initially, increased if necessary to a total daily dose of 20 mg in divided doses. Average maintenance dose, 6–15 mg/d.
Terazosin (Hytrin)	Hypertension BPH	PO 1 mg at bedtime initially, increased gradually to maintenance dose, usually 1–5 mg once daily
Nonselective alpha-blocking agents		
Phenoxybenzamine (Dibenzyline)	Hypertension caused by pheochromocytoma Raynaud's disorder Frostbite	PO 10 mg daily initially, gradually increased by 10 mg every 4 d until therapeutic effects are obtained or adverse effects become intolerable; optimum dosage level usually reached in 2 wk; usual maintenance dose 20–60 mg/d
Phentolamine (Regitine)	Hypertension caused by pheochromocytoma Prevention of tissue necrosis from extravasation of vasoconstrictive drugs	*Before and during surgery for pheochromocytoma:* IV, IM 5–20 mg as needed to control blood pressure *Prevention of tissue necrosis:* IV 10 mg in each liter of IV solution containing a potent vasoconstrictor *Treatment of extravasation:* SC 5–10 mg in 10 ml saline, infiltrated into the area within 12 h

ciated with adverse effects, such as bronchoconstriction, peripheral vasoconstriction, and interference with glycogenolysis.

Acebutolol, atenolol, betaxolol, bisoprolol, esmolol, and metoprolol are cardioselective agents, which means they have more effect on beta₁ receptors than on beta₂ receptors. As a result, they may cause less bronchospasm, less impairment of glucose metabolism, and less peripheral vascular insufficiency. These drugs are preferred when beta-blockers are needed by

TABLE 19-2	BETA-ADRENERGIC BLOCKING AGENTS

Generic / Trade Name	Clinical Indications	Routes and Dosage Ranges
Nonselective blocking agents		
Carteolol (Cartrol, Ocupress)	Hypertension Glaucoma	PO: Initially, 2.5 mg once daily, gradually increased to a maximum daily dose of 10 mg if necessary. Usual maintenance dose, 2.5–5 mg once daily. Extend dosage interval to 48 h for a creatinine clearance of 20–60 ml/min and to 72 h for a creatinine clearance below 20 ml/min.
Levobunolol (Betagan)	Glaucoma	Topically to affected eye, 1 drop twice daily
Metipranolol (OptiPranolol)	Glaucoma	Topically to each eye, 1 drop once or twice daily
Penbutolol (Levatol)	Hypertension	Topically to affected eye(s), 1 drop twice daily
Propranolol (Inderal)	Hypertension Angina pectoris Cardiac arrhythmias Myocardial infarction Hypertrophic obstructive cardiomyopathy Migraine prophylaxis Thyrotoxicosis Pheochromocytoma	PO 20 mg, once daily Hypertension, PO 40 mg twice daily, gradually increased to 160–480 mg daily in divided doses; maximal daily dose, 960 mg Angina pectoris, dysrhythmias, PO 10–30 mg in divided doses, q4–6h Migraine prophylaxis, PO 40 mg daily in divided doses Life-threatening arrhythmias, IV 1–3 mg at a rate not to exceed 1 mg/min with electrocardiographic and blood-pressure monitoring
Nadolol (Corgard)	Hypertension Angina pectoris	Hypertension, PO 40 mg once daily initially, gradually increased. Usual daily maintenance dose, 80–320 mg Angina, PO 40 mg once daily initially, increased by 40–80 mg at 3- to 7-d intervals. Usual daily maintenance dose, 80–240 mg
Pindolol (Visken)	Hypertension	PO 5 mg twice daily initially, increased by 10 mg every 3–4 wk, to a maximal daily dose of 60 mg
Sotalol (Betapace)	Cardiac arrhythmias	PO 80–160 mg twice daily
Timolol (Blocadren, Timoptic)	Hypertension Myocardial infarction Glaucoma	Hypertension, PO 10 mg twice daily initially, increased at 7-d intervals to a maximum of 60 mg/d in 2 divided doses; usual maintenance dose, 20–40 mg daily Myocardial infarction, PO 10 mg twice daily Glaucoma, topically to eye, 1 drop of 0.25% or 0.5% solution (Timoptic) in each eye twice daily
Cardioselective blocking agents		
Acebutolol (Sectral)	Hypertension Ventricular arrhythmias	Hypertension, PO 400 mg daily in 1 or 2 doses; usual maintenance dose, 400–800 mg daily Arrhythmias, PO 400 mg daily in 2 divided doses; usual maintenance dose, 600–1200 mg daily
Atenolol (Tenormin)	Hypertension Angina pectoris Myocardial infarction	Hypertension, PO 50–100 mg daily Angina, PO 50–100 mg daily, increased to 200 mg daily if necessary Myocardial infarction, IV 5 mg over 5 min, then 5 mg 10 min later, then 50 mg PO 10 min later, then 50 mg 12 h later. Thereafter, PO 100 mg daily, in 1 or 2 doses, for 6–9 d or until discharge from hospital
Betaxolol (Betoptic, Kerlone)	Glaucoma Hypertension	Topically to each eye, 1 drop twice daily Hypertension, PO 10–20 mg daily
Bisoprolol (Zebeta)	Hypertension	PO 5–20 mg once daily
Esmolol (Brevibloc)	Supraventricular tachyarrhythmias	IV 50–200 µg/kg per minute; average dose, 100 µg/kg per minute, titrated to effect with close monitoring of client's condition

(continued)

TABLE 19-2	BETA-ADRENERGIC BLOCKING AGENTS (Continued)	
Generic / Trade Name	**Clinical Indications**	**Routes and Dosage Ranges**
Metoprolol (Lopressor)	Hypertension Myocardial infarction	Hypertension, PO 100 mg daily in single or divided doses, increased at 7-d or longer intervals; usual maintenance dose, 100–450 mg/d Myocardial infarction, early treatment, IV 5 mg every 2 min for total of 3 doses (15 mg), then 50 mg PO q6h for 48 h, then 100 mg PO twice daily. MI, late treatment, PO 100 mg twice daily, at least 3 months, up to 1–3 y
Alpha–beta blocking agents **Carvedilol** (Coreg)	Hypertension	PO 6.25 mg twice daily for 7–14 d, then increase to 12.5 mg twice daily if necessary for 7–14 d, then increase to 25 mg twice daily if necessary (maximum dose).
Labetalol (Trandate, Normodyne)	Hypertension, including hypertensive emergencies	PO 100 mg twice daily IV 20 mg over 2 min then 40–80 mg every 10 min until desired blood pressure achieved or 300 mg given IV infusion 2 mg/min (*e.g.*, add 200 mg of drug to 250 ml 5% dextrose solution for a 2 mg/3 ml concentration)

clients with asthma or other bronchospastic pulmonary disorders, with diabetes mellitus, and with peripheral vascular disorders. However, cardioselectivity is lost at higher doses, because most organs have both beta$_1$ and beta$_2$ receptors rather than one or the other exclusively.

Labetalol and carvedilol block alpha$_1$ receptors to cause vasodilation and beta$_1$ and beta$_2$ receptors to cause all the effects of the nonselective agents. Both alpha- and beta-adrenergic blocking actions contribute to antihypertensive effects, but it is unclear whether these drugs have any definite advantage over other beta-blockers. They may cause less bradycardia but more postural hypotension than other beta-blocking agents, and they may cause less reflex tachycardia than other vasodilators.

Intrinsic Sympathomimetic Activity

Drugs with this characteristic (*i.e.*, acebutolol, carteolol, penbutolol, and pindolol) have a chemical structure similar to catecholamines. As a result, they can block some beta receptors and stimulate others. Consequently, these drugs are less likely to cause bradycardia and may be useful for clients experiencing bradycardia with other beta-blockers.

Membrane-Stabilizing Activity

Several beta-blockers have a membrane-stabilizing effect sometimes described as quinidine-like (*i.e.*, producing myocardial depression). Because the doses re-

quired to produce this effect are much higher than those used for therapeutic effects, this characteristic is considered clinically insignificant.

Lipid Solubility

The more lipid-soluble beta-blockers were thought to penetrate the central nervous system (CNS) more extensively and cause adverse effects, such as confusion, depression, hallucinations, and insomnia. Some clinicians state that this characteristic is important only in terms of drug usage and excretion in certain disease states. Thus, a water-soluble, renally excreted beta-blocker may be preferred in clients with liver disease, and a lipid-soluble, hepatically metabolized drug may be preferred in clients with renal disease.

Routes of Elimination

Most beta-blocking agents are metabolized in the liver. Atenolol, carteolol, nadolol, and an active metabolite of acebutolol are excreted by the kidneys, and dosage must be reduced in the presence of renal failure.

Routes of Administration

Most beta-blockers can be given orally. Atenolol, esmolol, labetalol, metoprolol, and propranolol also can be given intravenously, and ophthalmic solutions are applied topically to the eye. Betaxolol, carteolol, and timolol are available in oral and ophthalmic forms.

Duration of Action

Acebutolol, atenolol, bisoprolol, carteolol, penbutolol, and nadolol have long serum half-lives and can usually be given once daily. Carvedilol, labetalol, metoprolol, pindolol, sotalol, and timolol are usually given twice daily. Propranolol required administration several times daily until development of a sustained-release capsule allowed once-daily dosing.

Nursing Process

Assessment

- Assess the client's condition in relation to disorders in which antiadrenergic drugs are used. Because most of the drugs are used to treat hypertension, assess blood-pressure patterns over time, when possible, including antihypertensive drugs used and the response obtained. With other cardiovascular disorders, check blood pressure for elevation and pulse for tachycardia or arrhythmia, and determine the presence or absence of chest pain, migraine headache, or hyperthyroidism. If the client reports or medical records indicate one or more of these disorders, assess for specific signs and symptoms. With BPH, assess for signs and symptoms of urinary retention and difficulty voiding.
- Assess for conditions that contraindicate the use of antiadrenergic drugs.
- Assess vital signs to establish a baseline for later comparisons.
- Assess for use of prescription and nonprescription drugs that are likely to increase or decrease effects of antiadrenergic drugs.
- Assess for lifestyle habits that are likely to increase or decrease effects of antiadrenergic drugs (*e.g.*, ingestion of caffeine or nicotine).

Nursing Diagnoses

- Decreased Cardiac Output related to drug-induced postural hypotension (alpha₂ agonists, alpha₁ and nonselective alpha-blocking agents, and beta-blockers) and congestive heart failure (beta-blockers)
- Impaired Gas Exchange related to drug-induced bronchoconstriction with beta-blockers
- Sexual Dysfunction in males related to impotence and decreased libido
- Fatigue related to decreased cardiac output
- Noncompliance related to adverse drug effects or inadequate understanding of drug regimen
- Risk for Injury related to hypotension, dizziness, sedation
- Knowledge Deficit: Drug effects and safe usage

Planning/Goals

The client will:
- Receive or self-administer drugs accurately
- Experience relief of symptoms for which antiadrenergic drugs are given
- Comply with instructions for safe drug usage
- Avoid stopping antiadrenergic drugs abruptly
- Demonstrate knowledge of adverse drug effects to be reported
- Avoid preventable adverse drug effects
- Keep appointments for blood-pressure monitoring and other follow-up activities

Interventions

Use measures to prevent or decrease the need for antiadrenergic drugs. Because the sympathetic nervous system is stimulated by physical and emotional stress, efforts to decrease stress may indirectly decrease the need for drugs to antagonize sympathetic effects. Such efforts may include the following:
- Helping the client stop or decrease cigarette smoking. Nicotine stimulates the CNS and the sympathetic nervous system to cause tremors, tachycardia, and elevated blood pressure.
- Teaching measures to relieve pain, anxiety, and other stresses
- Counseling regarding relaxation techniques
- Helping the client avoid temperature extremes
- Helping the client avoid excessive caffeine in coffee or other beverages
- Helping the client develop a reasonable balance among rest, exercise, work, and recreation
- Recording vital signs at regular intervals in hospitalized clients to monitor for adverse effects
- Helping with activity or ambulation as needed to prevent injury from dizziness

Teach clients:
- Stress management techniques (*e.g.*, relaxation, imagery)
- Not to take other drugs without the physician's knowledge and consent. Many drugs may interact to increase or decrease effects of the antiadrenergic drug.
- To inform any health care provider from whom treatment is sought when taking these drugs
- Not to stop antiadrenergic drugs abruptly. Suddenly stopping an alpha₂ agonist may lead to rebound hypertension; suddenly stopping a beta-blocker may cause or aggravate angina. To avoid serious problems, these drugs must be tapered and discontinued gradually, with supervision.
- How to count pulse rate (to monitor for tachycardia with alpha agonists and antagonists and bradycardia with beta-blockers)
- To record pulse rate daily and take the record to appointments with health care providers

Evaluation

- Observe for decreased blood pressure when antiadrenergic drugs are given for hypertension.
- Interview regarding decreased chest pain when beta-blockers are given for angina.
- Interview and observe for signs and symptoms of adverse drug effects (*e.g.*, edema, tachycardia with alpha agonists and blocking agents; bradycardia, congestive heart failure, bronchoconstriction with beta-blockers).
- Interview regarding knowledge and use of drugs.

Principles of Therapy

ALPHA-ADRENERGIC AGONISTS AND BLOCKING AGENTS

1. When an alpha₁-blocking agent (doxazosin, prazosin, or terazosin) is given for hypertension, "first-dose syncope" may occur from hypotension. This reaction

can be prevented or minimized by starting with a low dose, increasing the dose gradually, and giving the first dose at bedtime. In addition, the decreased blood pressure stimulates reflex mechanisms to raise blood pressure (increase heart rate and cardiac output, fluid retention) so that a diuretic may be needed.

2. A client diagnosed with BPH should be evaluated for prostatic cancer before starting drug therapy, because the signs and symptoms of the two conditions are similar. The two conditions may also co-exist.

3. When an alpha$_2$ agonist is given for hypertension, it is very important not to stop the drug abruptly because of the risk of rebound hypertension. To discontinue clonidine, for example, the dose should be gradually reduced over 2 to 4 days.

4. When phenoxybenzamine is given on a long-term basis, dosage must be carefully individualized. Because the drug is long-acting and accumulates in the body, dosage is small initially and gradually increased at intervals of about 4 days. Several weeks may be required for full therapeutic benefit, and drug effects persist for several days after the drug is discontinued. If circulatory shock develops from overdosage or hypersensitivity, norepinephrine (Levophed) can be given to overcome the blockade of alpha-adrenergic receptors in arterioles and to raise blood pressure. Epinephrine is contraindicated because it stimulates both alpha- and beta-adrenergic receptors, with a result of increased vasodilation and hypotension.

BETA-ADRENERGIC BLOCKING DRUGS

1. For most people, a nonselective beta-blocker that can be taken once or twice daily is acceptable. For others, the choice of a beta-blocking agent depends largely on the client's condition and response to the drugs. For example, cardioselective drugs are preferred for clients with pulmonary disorders and diabetes mellitus; a drug with intrinsic sympathomimetic activity may be preferred for those who experience significant bradycardia with beta-blockers lacking this property.

2. Dosage of beta-blocking agents must be individualized because of wide variations in plasma levels from comparable doses. Variations are attributed to initial metabolism in the liver, the extent of binding to plasma proteins, and the degree of beta-adrenergic stimulation that the drugs must overcome. Generally, low doses should be used initially and increased gradually until therapeutic or adverse effects occur. Adequacy of dosage or extent of beta blockade can be assessed by determining whether the heart rate increases in response to exercise.

3. When a beta-blocker is used to prevent myocardial infarction, it should be started as soon as the client is hemodynamically stable after a definite or suspected acute myocardial infarction. The drug should be continued at least 3 months and possibly 1 to 3 years.

4. Beta-blocking drugs should not be discontinued abruptly. Long-term blockade of beta-adrenergic receptors increases the receptors' sensitivity to epinephrine and norepinephrine when the drugs are discontinued. There is a risk of severe hypertension, angina, arrhythmias, and myocardial infarction from the increased or excessive sympathetic nervous system stimulation. Thus, dosage should be tapered and gradually discontinued to allow beta-adrenergic receptors to return to predrug density and sensitivity. An optimal tapering period has not been defined. Some authorities recommend 1 to 2 weeks; others recommend reducing dosage over about 10 days to 30 mg/d of propranolol (or an equivalent amount of other drugs) and continuing this amount at least 2 weeks before the drug is stopped completely.

5. Opinions differ regarding use of beta-blockers before anesthesia and major surgery. On one hand, the drugs block arrhythmogenic properties of some general inhalation anesthetics; on the other hand, there is a risk of excessive myocardial depression. If feasible, the drug may be tapered gradually and discontinued (at least 48 hours) before surgery. If the drug is continued, the lowest effective dosage should be given. If emergency surgery is necessary, the effects of beta-blockers can be reversed by administration of beta-receptor stimulants, such as dobutamine or isoproterenol.

6. Various drugs may be used to treat adverse effects of beta-blockers. Atropine can be given for bradycardia, digoxin and diuretics for congestive heart failure, vasopressors for hypotension, and bronchodilator drugs for bronchoconstriction.

7. In the presence of hepatic disease (*e.g.*, cirrhosis) or impaired blood flow to the liver (*e.g.*, reduced cardiac output from any cause), dosage of propranolol, metoprolol, and timolol should be substantially reduced because these drugs are extensively metabolized in the liver. The use of atenolol or nadolol is preferred in liver disease because both are eliminated primarily by the kidneys.

8. In renal failure, dosage of acebutolol, atenolol, carteolol, and nadolol must be reduced because they are eliminated mainly through the kidneys. Dosage of acebutolol and nadolol should be reduced if creatinine clearance is under 50 ml/min; dosage of atenolol should be decreased if creatinine clearance is under 35 ml/min.

   With carteolol, the same amount is given per dose, but the interval between doses is extended to 48 hours for a creatinine clearance of 20 to 60 ml/min and to 72 hours for a creatinine clearance below 20 ml/min.

GENETIC OR ETHNIC CONSIDERATIONS

Most studies involve adults with hypertension and compare drug therapy responses between African-American and white people. Findings indicate that monotherapy with alpha$_1$-blockers and combined alpha- and beta-blockers is equally effective in the two groups. However, monotherapy with beta-blockers is less effective in African-Americans than in whites. When beta-blockers are used in African-Americans, they should generally be part of a multidrug treatment regimen, and higher doses may be required.

Several studies indicate that Asians achieve higher blood levels of beta-blockers with given doses and generally need much smaller doses than white people. This increased sensitivity to the drugs may result from slower metabolism and excretion.

USE IN CHILDREN

Alpha-adrenergic agonists and blocking agents have not been established as safe and effective in children.

Beta-adrenergic blocking agents are used in children for disorders similar to those occurring in adults. However, safety and effectiveness have not been established, and manufacturers of most of the drugs do not recommend pediatric use or doses. The drugs are probably contraindicated in young children with resting heart rates below 60 beats per minute.

When a beta-blocker is given, general guidelines include the following:

1. Dosage should be adjusted for body weight.
2. Monitor responses closely. Children are more sensitive to adverse drug effects than adults.
3. If given to infants (up to 1 year old) with immature liver function, blood levels may be higher and accumulation is more likely even when doses are based on weight.
4. When monitoring responses, remember that heart rate and blood pressure vary among children according to age and level of growth and development. They also differ from those of adults.
5. Children are more likely to have asthma than adults. Thus, they may be at greater risk of drug-induced bronchoconstriction.

Propranolol is probably the most frequently used beta-blocker in children. Intravenous administration is not recommended. The drug is given orally for hypertension, and dosage should be individualized. The usual dosage range is 2 to 4 mg/kg/d in two equal doses. Dosage calculated from body surface area is not recommended because of excessive blood levels of drug and greater risk of toxicity. As with adults, dosage should be tapered gradually over 1 to 3 weeks. The drug should not be stopped abruptly.

USE IN OLDER ADULTS

Alpha$_2$-adrenergic agonists (clonidine and related drugs) may be used to treat hypertension in older adults; alpha$_1$-adrenergic antagonists (prazosin and related drugs) may be used to treat hypertension and BPH. Dosage of these drugs should be reduced because older adults are more likely to experience adverse drug effects, especially with impaired renal or hepatic function. As with other populations, these drugs should not be stopped suddenly. Instead, they should be tapered in dosage and discontinued gradually, over 1 to 2 weeks.

Beta-adrenergic blocking agents are commonly used in older adults for angina, arrhythmias, hypertension, and glaucoma. With hypertension, beta-blockers are not recommended for monotherapy because older adults may be less responsive than younger adults. Thus, the drugs are probably most useful as second drugs (with diuretics) in clients who require multidrug therapy and clients who also have angina pectoris or another disorder for which a beta-blocker is indicated.

Whatever the circumstances for using beta-blockers in older adults, use them cautiously and monitor responses closely. Older adults are likely to have disorders that place them at high risk of adverse drug effects, such as congestive heart failure and other cardiovascular conditions, renal or hepatic impairment, and chronic pulmonary disease. Thus, they may experience bradycardia, bronchoconstriction, and hypotension to a greater degree than younger adults. Dosage generally should be reduced because of decreased hepatic blood flow and subsequent slowing of drug metabolism. As with other populations, beta-blockers should be tapered in dosage and discontinued over 1 to 3 weeks to avoid myocardial ischemia and other potentially serious adverse cardiovascular effects.

 ## HOME CARE

Antiadrenergic drugs are commonly used in the home setting, mainly to treat chronic disorders in adults. With alpha$_1$-adrenergic blocking agents, the home care nurse may need to teach clients ways to avoid orthostatic hypotension. Most clients probably take these medications for hypertension. However, some older men with BPH take one of these drugs to aid urinary elimination. For an older man taking one of these drugs, the home care nurse must assess the reason for use to teach the client and monitor for drug effects.

With beta-adrenergic blocking agents, the home care nurse may need to assist clients and caregivers in assessing for therapeutic and adverse drug effects. It is helpful to have the client or someone else in the household count and record the radial pulse daily, preferably about the same time interval before or after taking a beta-blocker. Several days of a slow pulse should probably be reported to the health care provider who prescribed the beta-blocker, especially if the client also has excessive fatigue or signs of congestive heart failure.

If a client taking a nonselective beta-blocker develops wheezing respirations (indicating bronchoconstriction), the client or the home care nurse must consult the prescribing physician about changing to a cardioselective beta-blocker. If a client has diabetes mellitus, the home care nurse must interview and observe the client for alterations in blood-sugar control, especially increased episodes of hypoglycemia. If a client has hypertension, the home care nurse must teach the client to avoid over-the-counter (OTC) asthma and cold remedies, decongestants, and appetite suppressants because these drugs act to increase blood pressure and may reduce the benefits of antiadrenergic medications. In addition, OTC analgesics such as ibuprofen, ketoprofen, and naproxen may raise blood pressure by causing retention of sodium and water.

NURSING ACTIONS   ANTIADRENERGIC DRUGS

NURSING ACTIONS	RATIONALE/EXPLANATION
1. Administer accurately	
a. With alpha$_2$ agonists:	
(1) Give all or most of a dose at bedtime, when possible.	To minimize daytime drowsiness and sedation
(2) Apply the clonidine skin patch to a hairless, intact area on the upper arm or torso; then apply adhesive overlay securely. Do not cut or alter the patch. Remove a used patch and fold its adhesive edges together before discarding. Apply a new patch in a new site.	To promote effectiveness and safe usage
b. With alpha$_1$-blocking agents:	
(1) Give the first dose of doxazosin, prazosin, or terazosin at bedtime.	To prevent fainting from severe orthostatic hypotension
c. With beta-adrenergic blocking agents:	
(1) Check blood pressure and pulse frequently, especially when dosage is being increased.	To monitor therapeutic effects and the occurrence of adverse reactions. Some clients with heart rates between 50 and 60 beats per minute may be continued on a beta-blocker if they do not develop hypotension or escape arrhythmias.
(2) See Table 19-2 and manufacturers' literature regarding IV administration.	Specific instructions vary with individual drugs.
2. Observe for therapeutic effects	
a. With alpha$_2$ agonists and alpha-blocking agents:	
(1) With hypertension, observe for decreased blood pressure.	With most of the drugs, blood pressure decreases within a few hours. However, antihypertensive effects with clonidine skin patches occur 2–3 days after initial application (overlap with oral clonidine or other antihypertensive drugs may be needed) and persist 2–3 days when discontinued.
(2) With benign prostatic hyperplasia, observe for improved urination.	The client may report a larger stream, less nocturnal voiding, and more complete emptying of the bladder.
(3) In pheochromocytoma, observe for decreased pulse rate, blood pressure, sweating, palpitations, and blood sugar.	Because symptoms of pheochromocytoma are caused by excessive sympathetic nervous system stimulation, blocking stimulation with these drugs produces a decrease or absence of symptoms.
(4) In Raynaud's disease or frostbite, observe affected areas for improvement in skin color and temperature and in the quality of peripheral pulses.	These conditions are characterized by vasospasm, which diminishes blood flow to the affected part. The drugs improve blood flow by vasodilation.

NURSING ACTIONS	RATIONALE/EXPLANATION
3. Observe for adverse effects a. With alpha₂ agonists and alpha-blocking agents:	Adverse effects are usually extensions of therapeutic effects.
(1) Hypotension	Hypotension may range from transient postural hypotension to a more severe hypotensive state resembling shock. "First-dose syncope" may occur with prazosin and related drugs.
(2) Sedation, drowsiness	Sedation can be minimized by increasing dosage slowly and giving all or most of the daily dose at bedtime.
(3) Tachycardia	Tachycardia occurs as a reflex mechanism to increase blood supply to body tissues in hypotensive states.
(4) Edema	These drugs promote retention of sodium and water. Concomitant diuretic therapy may be needed to maintain antihypertensive effects with long-term use.
b. With beta-blocking agents:	
(1) Bradycardia and heart block	These are extensions of the therapeutic effects, which slow conduction of electrical impulses through the AV node, particularly in clients with compromised cardiac function.
(2) Congestive heart failure—edema, dyspnea, fatigue	Caused by reduced force of myocardial contraction
(3) Bronchospasm—dyspnea, wheezing	Caused by drug-induced constriction of bronchi and bronchioles. It is more likely to occur in people with bronchial asthma or other obstructive lung disease.
(4) Fatigue and dizziness, especially with activity or exercise	These symptoms occur because the usual sympathetic nervous system stimulation in response to activity or stress is blocked by drug action.
(5) CNS effects—depression, insomnia, vivid dreams, and hallucinations	The mechanism by which these effects are produced is unknown.
4. Observe for drug interactions a. Drugs that *increase* effects of alpha antiadrenergic agents:	
(1) Other antihypertensive drugs	Additive antihypertensive effects
(2) CNS depressants	Additive sedation and drowsiness
(3) Nonsteroidal antiinflammatory drugs	Additive sodium and water retention, possible edema.
(4) Epinephrine	Epinephrine increases the hypotensive effects of phenoxybenzamine and phentolamine and should not be given to treat shock caused by these drugs. Because epinephrine stimulates both alpha- and beta-adrenergic receptors, the net effect is vasodilation and a further drop in blood pressure.
b. Drugs that *decrease* effects of alpha antiadrenergic agents	
(1) Alpha adrenergics (*e.g.*, norepinephrine [Levophed]).	Norepinephrine is a strong vasoconstricting agent and is the drug of choice for treating shock caused by overdosage of, or hypersensitivity to, phenoxybenzamine or phentolamine.
(2) Estrogens, oral contraceptives, nonsteroidal antiinflammatory drugs	These drugs may cause sodium and fluid retention and thereby decrease antihypertensive effects of alpha antiadrenergic drugs.

(continued)

NURSING ACTIONS	RATIONALE/EXPLANATION
c. Drugs that *increase* effects of beta-adrenergic blocking agents (*e.g.*, propranolol):	
(1) Other antihypertensives	Synergistic antihypertensive effects. Clients who do not respond to beta-blockers or vasodilators alone may respond well to the combination. Also, beta-blockers prevent reflex tachycardia, which usually occurs with vasodilator antihypertensive drugs.
(2) Phenoxybenzamine or phentolamine	Synergistic effects to prevent excessive hypertension before and during surgical excision of pheochromocytoma
(3) Chlorpromazine, cimetidine, furosemide	Increase plasma levels by slowing hepatic metabolism
(4) Digoxin	Additive bradycardia, heart block
(5) Phenytoin	Potentiates cardiac depressant effects of propranolol
(6) Quinidine	The combination may be synergistic in treating cardiac arrhythmias. However, additive cardiac depressant effects also may occur (bradycardia, decreased force of myocardial contraction (negative inotropy), decreased cardiac output.
(7) Verapamil, IV	IV verapamil and IV propranolol should never be used in combination because of additive bradycardia and hypotension.
d. Drugs that *decrease* effects of beta-adrenergic blocking agents:	
(1) Antacids	Decrease absorption of several oral beta blockers from the GI tract
(2) Atropine	Increases heart rate and may be used to counteract excessive bradycardia caused by beta blockers
(3) Isoproterenol	Stimulates beta-adrenergic receptors and therefore antagonizes effects of beta-blocking agents. Isoproterenol also can be used to counteract excessive bradycardia.
5. Teach clients **a.** With alpha$_2$ agonists and alpha-blocking agents:	
(1) The adverse reactions of palpitations, weakness, and dizziness usually disappear with continued use. However, they may recur with conditions promoting vasodilation (dosage increase, exercise, high environmental temperatures, ingesting alcohol or a large meal).	These are symptoms of orthostatic hypotension and reflex tachycardia.
(2) If the above reactions occur, sit down or lie down immediately and flex arms and legs. Change positions slowly, especially from supine to standing.	To prevent falls and injuries from hypotension and syncope
(3) Do not drive a car or operate machinery if drowsy or dizzy from medication.	For safety. Sedation may be minimized by taking all or most of the prescribed dose at bedtime.
(4) Do *not* stop the drugs abruptly.	Hypertension, possibly severe, may develop.
b. With beta-adrenergic blocking agents:	
(1) Take the drug at the same time each day.	To maintain therapeutic blood levels and adequate blockade of beta-adrenergic receptors
(2) Count pulse daily: report to a healthcare provider if under 50 for several days in succession.	To determine if the drug therapy regimen needs to be altered to avoid more serious adverse effects

NURSING ACTIONS	RATIONALE/EXPLANATION
(3) Report weight gain (more than 2 lb within a week), ankle edema, shortness of breath, or excessive fatigue.	These are signs of congestive heart failure. If they occur, the drug will be stopped.
(4) Report fainting spells, excessive weakness, or difficulty in breathing.	Beta-blocking drugs decrease the usual adaptive responses to exercise or stress. Syncope may result from hypotension or bradycardia and heart block. Occurrence will probably indicate stopping or decreasing the dose of the drug.
(5) Do *not* stop the drugs abruptly.	Stopping the drugs suddenly may cause or aggravate chest pain (angina).

REVIEW AND APPLICATION EXERCISES

1. How do alpha$_2$ agonists and alpha$_1$-blocking agents decrease blood pressure?

2. What are safety factors in administering and monitoring the effects of alpha$_2$ agonists and alpha$_1$-blocking agents?

3. Why should a client be cautioned against stopping alpha$_2$ agonists and alpha$_1$-blocking agents abruptly?

4. What are the main mechanisms by which beta-blockers relieve angina pectoris?

5. How are beta-blockers thought to be "cardioprotective" in preventing repeat myocardial infarctions?

6. What are some noncardiovascular indications for the use of propranolol?

7. What are the main differences between cardioselective and nonselective beta-blockers?

8. Why are cardioselective beta-blockers preferred for clients with asthma or diabetes mellitus?

9. List at least five adverse effects of beta-blockers.

10. Explain the drug effects that contribute to each adverse reaction.

11. What signs, symptoms, or behaviors would lead you to suspect adverse drug effects?

12. Do the same adverse effects occur with beta-blocker eye drops that occur with systemic drugs? If so, how may they be prevented or minimized?

13. What information needs to be included in teaching clients about beta-blocker therapy?

14. What is the risk of abruptly stopping a beta-blocker drug rather than tapering the dose and gradually discontinuing, as recommended?

SELECTED REFERENCES

Drug facts and comparisons. (1996). St. Louis: Facts and Comparisons.

Hawkins, D.W., Bussey, H.I., & Prisant, L.M. (1993). Hypertension. In J.T. DiPiro, R.L. Talbert, P.E. Hayes, G.C. Yee, G.R. Matzke, & L.M. Posey (Eds.), *Pharmacotherapy: A pathophysiologic approach*, 2d ed., pp. 139–159. Norwalk, CT: Appleton & Lange.

Hoffman, B.B., & Lefkowitz, R.J. (1996). Catecholamines, sympathomimetic drugs, and adrenergic receptor antagonists. In J.G. Hardman, L.E. Limbird, R.B. Molinoff, & R.W. Ruddon (Eds.), *Goodman and Gilman's The pharmacological basis of therapeutics*, 9th ed., pp. 199–248. New York: McGraw-Hill.

Joint National Committee on Detection, Evaluation, and Treatment of High Blood Pressure. (1993). The Fifth Report. *Archives of Internal Medicine, 153*:154–183.

Porth, C.M., & Curtis, R.L. (1994). Normal and altered autonomic nervous system function. In C.M. Porth (Ed.), *Pathophysiology: Concepts of altered health states*, 4th ed., pp. 1007–1026. Philadelphia: J.B. Lippincott.

Sorenson, S.J., & Abel, S.R. (1996). Comparison of the ocular beta-blockers. *Annals of Pharmacotherapy, 30*:43–54.

Stewart, S.M. (1994). Alterations in structure and function of the male genitourinary system. In C.M. Porth (Ed.), *Pathophysiology: Concepts of altered health states*, 4th ed., pp. 727–743. Philadelphia: J.B. Lippincott.

20 Cholinergic Drugs

Outline

Objectives

After studying this chapter, the student will be able to:

1 Describe effects and indications for use of selected cholinergic drugs.

2 Discuss drug therapy of myasthenia gravis.

3 Discuss atropine as an antidote for cholinergic drugs.

4 Describe major nursing care needs of clients receiving cholinergic drugs.

Key Terms

Acetylcholine

Acetylcholinesterase

Cholinergic

Myasthenia gravis

Urinary retention

Description

Cholinergic drugs, also called parasympathomimetics and cholinomimetics, stimulate the parasympathetic nervous system in the same manner as acetylcholine (see Chap. 17). Some drugs act directly to stimulate cholinergic receptors; others act indirectly by slowing acetylcholine metabolism at autonomic nerve synapses and terminals. Selected drugs are discussed here in relation to their use in urinary retention, myasthenia gravis, and primary degenerative dementia, Alzheimer's type.

In normal neuromuscular function, acetylcholine is released from nerve endings and binds to receptors on cell membranes of muscle cells to cause muscle contraction. Myasthenia gravis is an autoimmune disorder in which autoantibodies are thought to destroy receptors for acetylcholine. As a result, acetylcholine is less able to stimulate muscle contraction, and muscle weakness occurs.

In normal brain function, acetylcholine is an essential neurotransmitter and plays an important role in cognitive functions, including memory storage and retrieval. Alzheimer's disease, the most common type of dementia in adults, is characterized by abnormalities in the cholinergic, serotonergic, noradrenergic, and glutamatergic neurotransmission systems (see Chap. 5). In the cholinergic system, there is a substantial loss of neurons that secrete acetylcholine in the brain and decreased activity of choline acetyltransferase, the enzyme required for synthesis of acetylcholine.

MECHANISMS OF ACTION AND EFFECTS

Direct-acting cholinergic drugs are synthetic derivatives of choline. These drugs can exert their therapeutic effects because they are highly resistant to metabolism by acetylcholinesterase, the enzyme that normally metabolizes acetylcholine. Their action is longer than the action of acetylcholine. They have widespread systemic effects when they combine with receptors in cardiac muscle, smooth muscle, and glands. Specific effects include:

1. Decreased heart rate, vasodilation, and unpredictable changes in blood pressure
2. Increased tone and contractility in gastrointestinal (GI) smooth muscle, relaxation of sphincters, increased salivary gland and GI secretions
3. Increased tone and contractility of smooth muscle (detrusor) in the urinary bladder and relaxation of the sphincter
4. Increased tone and contractility of bronchial smooth muscle
5. Increased respiratory secretions
6. Constriction of pupils and contraction of ciliary muscle

Indirect-acting cholinergic or *anticholinesterase drugs* decrease the inactivation of acetylcholine in the synapse by the enzyme acetylcholinesterase. Acetylcholine can then accumulate in the synapse and enhance the activation of postsynaptic receptors. This improves cholinergic neurotransmission in the brain and improves the force of muscle contraction in peripheral tissues.

INDICATIONS FOR USE

Cholinergic drugs have limited but varied uses. A direct-acting drug, bethanechol, is used to treat urinary retention. The anticholinesterase agents are used in the diagnosis and treatment of myasthenia gravis and to reverse the action of nondepolarizing neuromuscular blocking agents (*e.g.*, tubocurarine and related drugs) used in surgery. The drugs do not reverse the neuromuscular blockade produced by depolarizing agents, such as succinylcholine (Anectine). In addition, tacrine is an anticholinesterase agent approved for treatment of Alzheimer's disease. Cholinergic drugs may also be used to treat glaucoma (see Chap. 65).

CONTRAINDICATIONS FOR USE

These drugs are contraindicated in urinary or GI tract obstruction, asthma, peptic ulcer disease, coronary artery disease, hyperthyroidism, pregnancy, and inflammatory abdominal conditions. Tacrine is also contraindicated in previous users who developed jaundice or a serum bilirubin level above 3 mg/dl.

Individual Cholinergic Drugs

DIRECT-ACTING CHOLINERGICS

Bethanechol (Urecholine) is a synthetic derivative of choline used to relieve urinary retention. Because the drug produces smooth muscle contractions, it should not be used in obstructive conditions. Because oral bethanechol is not well absorbed from the GI tract, oral doses are much larger than subcutaneous doses. Because severe adverse effects may occur with IM or IV administration, the drug is not given by these routes.

Routes and Dosage Ranges

Adults: PO 10–30 mg two to four times per day; maximum dose 120 mg/d, SC 2.5–5 mg three or four times per day

Children: PO 0.2 mg/kg three times per day, SC 0.05 mg/kg three times per day

INDIRECT-ACTING CHOLINERGICS (ANTICHOLINESTERASES)

Neostigmine (Prostigmin) is the prototype anticholinesterase agent. It is used for long-term treatment of myasthenia gravis and as an antidote for tubocurarine and other nondepolarizing skeletal muscle relaxants used in surgery. Neostigmine is poorly absorbed from the GI tract; consequently, oral doses are much larger than parenteral doses. When it is used for long-term treatment of myasthenia gravis, resistance to its action may occur, and larger doses may be required.

Routes and Dosage Ranges

Adults: Myasthenia gravis, PO 15–30 mg q4h while awake

Exacerbation of myasthenia gravis, IM, SC 0.25–2 mg q2–3h

Prevention and treatment of urinary retention, IM, SC 0.25–0.5 mg q4–6h (up to 2 or 3 d)

Children: Myasthenia gravis, PO 0.3–0.6 mg/kg q3–4h while awake

Exacerbation of myasthenia gravis, IM, SC 0.01–0.04 mg/kg q2–3h

Donepezil (Aricept) is a newer drug for the treatment of mild to moderate Alzheimer's disease. Like tacrine (see below), donepezil increases acetylcholine in the brain by inhibiting its metabolism. The drug is well absorbed after oral administration and absorption is unaffected by food. It is highly bound (96%) to plasma proteins. It is metabolized in the liver to several metabolites, some of which are pharmacologically active; metabolites and some unchanged drugs are excreted mainly in urine. Adverse effects include nausea, vomiting, diarrhea, bradycardia, and possible aggravation of asthma and chronic obstructive pulmonary disease.

Route and Dosage Ranges

Adults: PO 5 mg daily at bedtime for 4–6 wk, then increase to 10 mg once daily if necessary

Edrophonium (Tensilon) is a short-acting cholinergic drug used to diagnose myasthenia gravis, to differentiate between myasthenic crisis and cholinergic crisis, and to reverse the neuromuscular blockade produced by nondepolarizing skeletal muscle relaxants. It is given IM or IV by a physician who remains in attendance. Atropine, an antidote, and life-support equipment, such as ventilators and endotracheal tubes, must be available when the drug is given.

Routes and Dosage Ranges

Adults: Diagnosis of myasthenia gravis, IV 2–4 mg initially; may be repeated and increased up to a total dose of 10 mg if no response is elicited by smaller amounts after 45 sec; or IM 10 mg as a single dose

Differential diagnosis of myasthenic crisis or cholinergic crisis, IV 1–2 mg

Children: Diagnosis of myasthenia gravis, IV 0.2 mg/kg

Diagnosis in infants, IM 0.1 mg/kg

Ambenonium (Mytelase) is a long-acting drug used for the treatment of myasthenia gravis. It is used less often than neostigmine and pyridostigmine. It may be useful in clients who are allergic to bromides, however, because the other drugs are both bromide salts. Ambenonium may be useful for myasthenic clients on ventilators because it is less likely to increase respiratory secretions than other anticholinesterase drugs.

Route and Dosage Range

Adults: PO 5 mg initially, increased to 10–30 mg q3–4h while awake. Dosage varies considerably, depending on client; dosage range, 5–75 mg/d

Children: PO 0.1 mg/kg initially, increased if necessary to 0.4 mg/kg q4h while awake

Physostigmine salicylate (Antilirium) is sometimes used as an antidote for overdosage of anticholinergic drugs ("atropine poisoning"), including tricyclic antidepressants. However, its potential for causing serious adverse effects limits its usefulness. Some preparations of physostigmine are used in the treatment of glaucoma.

Routes and Dosage Range

Adults: IV, IM 0.5–2 mg; give slowly IV, no faster than 1 mg/min

Pyridostigmine (Mestinon) is similar to neostigmine in actions, uses, and adverse effects. It may have a longer duration of action than neostigmine and is the maintenance drug of choice for clients with myasthenia gravis. An added advantage is the availability of a slow-release form, which is effective for 8 to 12 hours. When this form is taken at bedtime, the client does not have to take other medication during the night and does not awaken too weak to swallow.

Routes and Dosage Ranges

Adults: PO 60–120 mg q3–4h when awake; maximal single dose, 180 mg; or one Timespan tablet (180 mg) at bedtime. Up to 1500 mg daily may be necessary.

IM (exacerbations of myasthenia gravis or when oral administration is contraindicated) 2 mg

Children: PO 1–2 mg/kg q3–4h when awake

Newborns whose mothers have myasthenia gravis, IM 0.05–0.15 mg/kg

Tacrine (Cognex) is a centrally acting anticholinesterase agent approved for treatment of clients with mild to moderate Alzheimer's disease. The drug does not cure the disease, but it may delay progression in some clients. Tacrine is well absorbed following oral administration and reaches peak plasma levels in 1 to 2 hours. It is about 50% protein bound, is extensively metabolized in the liver, is excreted in the urine, and has an elimination half-life of 2 to 4 hours. The initial enthusiasm for tacrine has declined because of inconsistent clinical trial results and the occurrence of hepatotoxicity.

Route and Dosage Ranges

Adults: PO 40 mg/d (10 mg qid) for 6 wk, during which transaminase levels are monitored weekly; after 6 wk, increase dose to 80 mg/d (20 mg qid). If the client tolerates the drug and transaminase levels are within normal limits, increase the daily dose by 10 mg every 6 wk to a total of 120–160 mg/d.

Nursing Process

Assessment

Assess the client's condition in relation to disorders for which cholinergic drugs are used:

- In clients known to have myasthenia gravis, assess for muscle weakness. This may be manifested by ptosis (drooping) of the upper eyelid and diplopia (double vision) caused by weakness of the eye muscles. More severe disease may be indicated by difficulty in chewing, swallowing, and speaking; accumulation of oral secretions, which the client may be unable to expectorate or swallow; decreased skeletal muscle activity, including impaired chest expansion; and eventual respiratory failure.
- In clients with possible urinary retention, check for bladder distention and time and amount of previous urination, and assess fluid intake.
- In clients with Alzheimer's disease, assess for abilities and limitations in relation to memory, cognitive functioning, self-care activities, and pre-existing conditions that may be aggravated by a cholinergic drug.

Nursing Diagnoses

- Altered Urinary Elimination: Incontinence
- Ineffective Breathing Pattern related to bronchoconstriction
- Ineffective Airway Clearance related to increased respiratory secretions
- Self-Care Deficit related to muscle weakness or cognitive impairment
- Knowledge Deficit: Drug administration and effects
- Risk for Injury related to adverse drug effects

Planning/Goals

The client will:

- Verbalize or demonstrate correct drug administration
- Improve in self-care abilities
- Regain usual patterns of urinary elimination
- Maintain effective oxygenation of tissues

- Report adverse drug effects
- For clients with myasthenia gravis, at least one family member will verbalize or demonstrate correct drug administration, symptoms of too much or too little drug, and emergency care procedures.
- For clients with dementia, a caregiver will verbalize or demonstrate correct drug administration and knowledge of adverse effects to be reported to a health care provider.

Interventions

- Use measures to prevent or decrease the need for cholinergic drugs. Ambulation, adequate fluid intake, and judicious use of narcotic analgesics or other sedative-type drugs help prevent postoperative urinary retention. In myasthenia gravis, muscle weakness is aggravated by exercise and improved by rest. Therefore, scheduling activities to avoid excessive fatigue and to allow adequate rest periods may be beneficial.
- With tacrine, assist and teach caregivers to:
  - Maintain a quiet, stable environment and daily routines to decrease confusion (*e.g.*, verbal or written reminders and simple directions, adequate lighting, calendars, personal objects within view and reach).
  - Avoid altering dosage or stopping the drug without consulting the prescribing physician.
  - Be sure that clients keep appointments for supervision and blood tests.
  - Report signs and symptoms (*i.e.*, skin rash, jaundice, light-colored stools) that may indicate hepatotoxicity.
  - Notify surgeons about tacrine therapy. Exaggerated muscle relaxation may occur if succinylcholine-type drugs are given.
- Before giving cholinergic drugs for bladder atony and urinary retention, be sure there is no obstruction in the urinary tract.
- For long-term use, assist clients and families to establish a schedule of drug administration that best meets the client's needs.
- With myasthenia gravis, recommend that one or more family members be trained in cardiopulmonary resuscitation.

 Teach clients and family:

- That when the drugs are taken for urinary retention, they usually act within about 60 minutes. Therefore, bathroom facilities need to be nearby.
- That with long-term use (*e.g.*, hypotonic bladder or myasthenia gravis), the client should wear a Medic-Alert identification device with the name of the drug
- Signs and symptoms of underdosage and overdosage
- How to inject atropine intramuscularly

Evaluation

- Observe and interview about the adequacy of urinary elimination.
- Observe abilities and limitations in self-care.
- Question the client and at least one family member of clients with myasthenia gravis about correct drug usage, symptoms of underdosage and overdosage, and emergency care procedures.
- Question caregivers of clients with dementia about the client's level of functioning and response to medication.

Principles of Therapy

USE IN MYASTHENIA GRAVIS

Guidelines for the use of anticholinesterase drugs in myasthenia gravis include the following:

1. Drug dosage should be increased gradually until maximal benefit is obtained. Larger doses are often required with increased physical activity, with emotional stress, with infections, and sometimes premenstrually.
2. Some clients with myasthenia gravis cannot tolerate optimal doses of anticholinesterase drugs unless atropine is given to decrease the severity of adverse reactions. However, atropine should be given only if necessary because it may mask the sudden increase of side effects. This increase is the first sign of overdose.
3. Drug dosage in excess of the amount needed to maintain muscle strength and function can produce a cholinergic crisis. A cholinergic crisis is characterized by excessive stimulation of the parasympathetic nervous system. If early symptoms are not treated, hypotension and respiratory failure may occur. At high doses, anticholinesterase drugs weaken rather than strengthen skeletal muscle contraction because excessive amounts of acetylcholine accumulate at motor endplates and reduce nerve impulse transmission to muscle tissue.
   a. *Treatment for cholinergic crisis* includes withdrawal of anticholinesterase drugs, administration of atropine, and measures to maintain respiration. Endotracheal intubation and mechanical ventilation may be necessary due to profound skeletal muscle weakness (including muscles of respiration), which is not counteracted by atropine.
   b. *Differentiating myasthenic crisis from cholinergic crisis* may be difficult because both are characterized by respiratory difficulty or failure. It is necessary to differentiate between them, however, because they require *opposite* treatment measures. Myasthenic crisis requires more anticholinesterase drug, whereas cholinergic crisis requires discontinuing any anticholinesterase drug the client has been receiving. The physician may be able to make an accurate diagnosis from signs and symptoms and their timing in relation to medication; that is, signs and symptoms having their onset within about 1 hour after a dose of anticholinesterase drug are more likely to be caused by cholinergic crisis (too much drug). Signs and symptoms beginning 3 hours or more after a drug dose are more likely to be caused by myasthenic crisis (too little drug).
   c. If the differential diagnosis cannot be made on the basis of signs and symptoms, the client can be intubated, mechanically ventilated, and observed closely until a diagnosis is possible. Still another way to differentiate between the two conditions is for the physician to inject a small dose of edrophonium intravenously. If the edrophonium causes a dramatic improvement in breathing, the diagnosis is myasthenic crisis; if it makes the patient even weaker, the diagnosis is cholinergic crisis. Note, however, that edrophonium or any other pharmacologic agent should be administered only after endotracheal intubation and controlled ventilation have been instituted.
4. Some people develop partial or total resistance to anticholinesterase drugs after taking them for months or years. Therefore, do not assume that drug therapy that is effective initially will continue to be effective over the long-term course of the disease.

USE IN ALZHEIMER'S DISEASE

When tacrine is started, serum alanine aminotransferase (ALT) should be monitored weekly for 18 weeks. Then, if values are within normal limits and signs of liver damage do not occur, the test can be done every 3 months.

ANTIDOTE TO CHOLINERGIC AGENTS

Atropine, an anticholinergic drug, is a specific antidote to cholinergic agents. The drug and equipment for injection should be readily available whenever cholinergic drugs are given.

USE IN CHILDREN

Bethanechol is occasionally used, but safety and effectiveness for children under 8 years old have not been established. Neostigmine is used to treat myasthenia gravis and to reverse neuromuscular blockade after general anesthesia but is not recommended for urinary retention. Other indirect-acting cholinergic drugs are used only in the treatment of myasthenia gravis. Precautions and adverse effects are the same for children as for adults.

USE IN OLDER ADULTS

Indirect-acting cholinergic drugs may be used in myasthenia gravis, Alzheimer's disease, or overdoses of atropine and other centrally acting anticholinergic drugs (*e.g.,* those used for parkinsonism). Older adults are more likely to experience adverse drug effects because of age-related physiologic changes and superimposed pathologic conditions.

CHOLINERGIC DRUGS

NURSING ACTIONS	RATIONALE/EXPLANATION
1. Administer accurately	
a. Give oral bethanechol before meals.	If given after meals, nausea and vomiting may occur because the drug stimulates contraction of muscles in the gastrointestinal (GI) tract.
b. Give parenteral bethanechol by the subcutaneous route *only*.	Intramuscular and intravenous injections may cause acute, severe hypotension and circulatory failure. Cardiac arrest may occur.
c. With pyridostigmine and other drugs for myasthenia gravis, give at regularly scheduled intervals.	For consistent blood levels and control of symptoms
d. Give tacrine on an empty stomach, 1 hour before or 2 hours after a meal, if possible, at regular intervals around the clock (*e.g.,* q6h). Give with meals if GI upset occurs.	Food decreases absorption and decreases serum drug levels by 30% or more. Regular intervals increase therapeutic effects and decrease adverse effects.
2. Observe for therapeutic effects	
a. When the drug is given for postoperative hypoperistalsis, observe for bowel sounds, passage of flatus through the rectum, or a bowel movement.	These are indicators of increased GI muscle tone and motility.
b. When bethanechol or neostigmine is given for urinary retention, micturition usually occurs within about 60 minutes. If it does not, urinary catheterization may be necessary.	
c. When the drug is given in myasthenia gravis, observe for increased muscle strength as shown by:	With neostigmine, onset of action is 2–4 hours after oral administration and 10–30 minutes after injection. Duration is about 3–4 hours. With pyridostigmine, onset of action is about 30–45 minutes after oral use, 15 minutes after intramuscular (IM) injection, and 2–5 minutes after intravenous (IV) injection. Duration is about 4–6 hours. The long-acting form of pyridostigmine lasts 8–12 hours.
(1) Decreased or absent ptosis of eyelids	
(2) Decreased difficulty with chewing, swallowing, and speech	
(3) Increased skeletal muscle strength, increased tolerance of activity, less fatigue	
d. With tacrine and donepezil, observe for improvement in memory and cognitive functioning in activities of daily living.	Improved functioning is most likely to occur in patients with mild to moderate dementia.
3. Observe for adverse effects	Adverse effects occur with usual therapeutic doses but are more likely with large doses. They are caused by stimulation of the parasympathetic nervous system.
a. CNS effects—convulsions, dizziness, drowsiness, headache, loss of consciousness	
b. Respiratory effects—increased secretions, bronchospasm, laryngospasm, respiratory failure	
c. Cardiovascular effects—arrhythmias (bradycardia, tachycardia, AV block), cardiac arrest, hypotension, syncope	These may be detected early by regular assessment of blood pressure and heart rate. Bradycardia is probably the most likely arrhythmia to occur.
d. GI effects—nausea and vomiting, diarrhea, increased peristalsis, abdominal cramping, increased secretions (*i.e.,* saliva, gastric and intestinal secretions)	GI effects commonly occur.

(continued)

NURSING ACTIONS	RATIONALE/EXPLANATION
e. Other effects—increased frequency and urgency of urination, increased sweating, miosis, skin rash	Skin rashes are most likely to occur from formulations of neostigmine or pyridostigmine that contain bromide.
4. Observe for drug interactions **a.** Drug that *increases* effects of tacrine:	
(1) Cimetidine	Slows metabolism of tacrine in the liver, thereby increasing risks of accumulation and adverse effects
b. Drugs that *decrease* effects of cholinergic agents:	
(1) Anticholinergic drugs (*e.g.,* atropine)	Antagonize effects of cholinergic drugs (miosis, increased tone and motility in smooth muscle of the GI tract, bronchi, and urinary bladder, bradycardia). Atropine is the specific antidote for overdosage with cholinergic drugs.
(2) Antihistamines	Most antihistamines have anticholinergic properties that antagonize effects of cholinergic drugs.
5. Teach clients with myasthenia gravis and at least one responsible family member to:	Cholinergic drugs are not prescribed for long-term therapeutic use except for clients with myasthenia gravis, certain types of hypotonic bladder disorders, and glaucoma.
a. Take drugs as directed on a regular schedule.	To maintain consistent blood levels and control of symptoms. Underdosage will not relieve muscle weakness enough for adequate function; overdosage can cause severe, even life-threatening reactions.
b. Record symptoms of myasthenia and effects of drug therapy, especially when drug therapy is initiated and medication doses are being titrated.	Clients vary widely in the amounts of medication required. The physician usually aims for the lowest effective dose to minimize adverse drug reactions. Information provided by the client can allow the physician to prescribe more effectively.
c. Rest between activities; do not carry on activities to the point of extreme fatigue or exhaustion.	Although the dose of medication may be increased during periods of increased activity, spacing activities is probably more desirable to obtain optimal benefit from the drug while avoiding adverse reactions.
d. Have atropine readily available.	Atropine (0.6 mg IM or IV) is a specific antidote for overdosage with cholinergic drugs.
e. Report increased muscle weakness or recurrence of myasthenic symptoms to the physician.	Drug dosage may need to be increased or other alterations made in treatment.
f. Report adverse reactions, including abdominal cramps, diarrhea, excessive oropharyngeal secretions, difficulty in breathing, and muscle weakness.	These are signs of drug overdosage (cholinergic crisis) and require immediate discontinuation of drugs and treatment by the physician. Respiratory failure can result if this condition is not recognized and treated appropriately.

REVIEW AND APPLICATION EXERCISES

1. What are the actions of cholinergic drugs?

2. Which neurotransmitter is involved in cholinergic (parasympathetic) stimulation?

3. When a cholinergic drug is given to treat myasthenia gravis, what is the expected effect?

4. When tacrine is given to treat Alzheimer's disease, what is the desired effect?

5. Is a cholinergic drug the usual treatment of choice for urinary bladder atony or hypotonicity? Why or why not?

6. What are the adverse effects of cholinergic drugs?

7. What drug is an antidote for an overdose of a cholinergic drug?

SELECTED REFERENCES

Drug facts and comparisons. (1996). St. Louis: Facts and Comparisons.

Ereshefsky, L., & Anderson, C.B. (1993). Organic brain syndromes. In J.T. DiPiro, R.L. Talbert, P.E. Hayes, G.C. Yee, G.R. Matzke, & L.M. Posey (Eds.), *Pharmacotherapy: A pathophysiologic approach*, 2nd ed., pp. 973–1000. Norwalk, CT: Appleton & Lange.

Malseed, R.T., Goldstein, F.J., & Balkon N. (1995). *Pharmacology: Drug therapy and nursing considerations*, 4th ed., pp. 70–84. Philadelphia: J.B. Lippincott.

Porth, C.M., & Curtis, R.L. (1994). Normal and altered autonomic nervous system function. In C.M. Porth (Ed.), *Pathophysiology: Concepts of altered health states*, 4th ed., pp. 1007–1026. Philadelphia: J.B. Lippincott.

21 Anticholinergic Drugs

Outline

Objectives

After studying this chapter, the student will be able to:

1 List characteristics of anticholinergic drugs in terms of effects on body tissues, indications for use, nursing process implications, observation of client response, and teaching clients.

2 Discuss atropine as the prototype of anticholinergic drugs.

3 Discuss clinical disorders/symptoms for which anticholinergic drugs are used.

4 Describe the mechanism by which atropine relieves bradycardia.

5 Review anticholinergic effects of antipsychotics, tricyclic antidepressants, and antihistamines.

Key Terms

Acetylcholine	**Mydriasis**
Antispasmodic	**Parasympatholytic**
Cycloplegia	**Vagal stimulation**
Heat stroke	

Description

Anticholinergic drugs, also called cholinergic blocking and parasympatholytic agents, block the action of acetylcholine on the parasympathetic nervous system (PNS). Usual doses block muscarinic cholinergic receptors in the brain, secretory glands, and smooth muscle; large doses may block nicotinic receptors in skeletal muscle (see Chap. 17). The prototype drug is *atropine*, and this drug class includes belladonna alkaloids, their derivatives, and many synthetic substitutes.

MECHANISM OF ACTION AND EFFECTS

These drugs act by occupying receptor sites at parasympathetic nerve endings, thereby leaving fewer receptor sites free to respond to acetylcholine. Parasympathetic response is absent or decreased, depending on the number of receptors blocked by anticholinergic drugs, and the underlying degree of parasympathetic activity. Overall, anticholinergic drugs have widespread effects on the body, including smooth muscle relaxation, decreased glandular secretions, and mydriasis. Specific effects on body tissues and organs include:

1. **Central nervous system (CNS) stimulation followed by depression,** which may result in coma and death. This is most likely to occur with large doses of anticholinergic drugs that cross the blood-brain barrier (atropine, scopolamine, and antiparkinson agents).
2. **Decreased cardiovascular response to parasympathetic (vagal) stimulation that slows heart rate.** Atropine is the anticholinergic drug most used for its cardiovascular effects. Usual clinical doses may produce a slight and temporary decrease in heart rate; moderate to large doses (0.5–1 mg) increase heart rate. This effect may be therapeutic in bradycardia or an adverse effect in other types of heart disease. Atropine usually has little or no effect on blood pressure. Large doses cause facial flushing due to dilation of blood vessels in the neck.
3. **Bronchodilation and decreased respiratory tract secretions.** Bronchodilating effects result from blocking the bronchoconstrictive effects of acetylcholine.
4. **Antispasmodic effects in the gastrointestinal (GI) tract due to decreased muscle tone and motility.** The drugs have little inhibitory effect on gastric acid secretion with usual doses, and insignificant effects on pancreatic and intestinal secretions.
5. **Mydriasis and cycloplegia in the eye.** Normally, anticholinergics do not change intraocular pressure, but with glaucoma, they may increase intraocular pressure. When the pupil is fully dilated, photophobia may be bothersome, and reflexes to light and accommodation may disappear.
6. **Miscellaneous effects** include decreased secretions from salivary and sweat glands; relaxation of ureters, urinary bladder, and the detrusor muscle; and relaxation of smooth muscle in the gallbladder and bile ducts.

The clinical usefulness of anticholinergic drugs is limited by their widespread effects. Consequently, numerous synthetic drugs have been developed in an effort to increase selectivity of action on particular body tissues, especially to retain the antispasmodic and antisecretory effects of atropine while eliminating its adverse effects. This effort has been less than successful: All the synthetic drugs produce atropine-like adverse effects when given in sufficient dosage.

One group of synthetic drugs is used for antispasmodic effects in GI disorders (Table 21-1). They are quaternary ammonium compounds, which do not readily cross the blood-brain barrier. Therefore, they are less likely to cause CNS effects than the natural alkaloids, which readily enter the CNS.

Another group of synthetic drugs includes centrally active anticholinergics used in the treatment of Parkinson's disease (see Chap. 12). They balance the relative cholinergic dominance that causes the movement disorders associated with parkinsonism.

INDICATIONS FOR USE

Clinical indications for use of anticholinergic drugs include GI, genitourinary, ophthalmic and respiratory disorders, bradycardia, and Parkinson's disease. They also are used preoperatively and before bronchoscopy.

GI disorders in which anticholinergics have been used include peptic ulcer disease, gastritis, pylorospasm, diverticulitis, ileitis, and ulcerative colitis. These conditions are often characterized by excessive gastric acid and abdominal pain due to increased motility and spasm of GI smooth muscle. In peptic ulcer disease, more effective drugs have been developed, and anticholinergics are rarely used. The drugs are weak inhibitors of gastric acid secretion even in maximal doses (which usually produce intolerable adverse effects). Although they do not heal peptic ulcers, they may relieve abdominal pain by relaxing GI smooth muscle.

Anticholinergics may be helpful in treating irritable colon or colitis, but they may be contraindicated in chronic inflammatory disorders (*e.g.,* diverticulitis, ulcerative colitis) or acute intestinal infections (*e.g.,* bacterial, viral, amebic). Other drugs are used to decrease diarrhea and intestinal motility in these conditions.

In genitourinary disorders, anticholinergic drugs may be given for their antispasmodic effects on smooth muscle. In infections such as cystitis, urethritis, and prostatitis, the drugs decrease the frequency and pain

TABLE 21-1 SYNTHETIC ANTICHOLINERGIC-ANTISPASMODICS USED IN GASTROINTESTINAL DISORDERS

	Routes and Dosage Ranges	
Generic/Trade Name	*Adults*	*Children*
Anisotropine methylbromide (Valpin)	PO 50 mg 3 times daily	Dosage not established
Clidinium bromide (Quarzan)	PO 2.5–5 mg 3–4 times daily Geriatric: PO 2.5 mg TID before meals	Dosage not established
Dicyclomine hydrochloride (Bentyl)	PO, IM 10–20 mg 3–4 times daily	PO, IM 10 mg 3–4 times daily Infants: 5 mg 3–4 times daily
Glycopyrrolate (Robinul)	PO 1–2 mg 3 times daily initially, 1 mg 2 times daily for maintenance IM, IV, SC 0.1–0.2 mg 3–4 times daily at 4-h intervals	Dosage not established
Isopropamide chloride (Darbid)	PO 5–10 mg q12h	Not recommended for children under 12 y
Mepenzolate bromide (Cantil)	PO 25 mg 4 times daily with meals and at bedtime, increased gradually to 50 mg if necessary	Dosage not established
Methantheline bromide (Banthine)	PO 50–100 mg q6h initially, reduced to 25–50 mg q6h for maintenance IM 50 mg q6h	PO, IM 6 mg/kg per day in 4 divided doses
Oxyphencyclimine bromide (Daricon)	PO 10 mg 2 times daily (morning and at bedtime), gradually increased to 50 mg if no adverse effects	Dosage not established
Propantheline bromide (Pro-Banthine)	PO 15 mg 3 times daily before meals and 30 mg at bedtime IM, IV 30 mg q6h	PO 1.5 mg/kg per day in 4 divided doses
Tridihexethyl (Pathilon)	PO 25–50 mg 3 or 4 times daily, before meals and at bedtime	Dosage not established

of urination. The drugs are also given to increase bladder capacity in enuresis, paraplegia, or neurogenic bladder.

In ophthalmology, anticholinergic drugs are applied topically for mydriatic and cycloplegic effects to aid examination or surgery. They are also used to treat some inflammatory disorders. Anticholinergic preparations used in ophthalmology are discussed further in Chapter 65.

In respiratory disorders characterized by broncho-constriction (*i.e.,* asthma, chronic bronchitis), ipratropium (Atrovent) may be given by inhalation for bronchodilating effects (see Chap. 47).

In cardiology, atropine may be given to increase heart rate in bradycardia and heart block characterized by hypotension and shock.

In Parkinson's disease, anticholinergic drugs are given for their central effects in decreasing salivation, spasticity, and tremors. They are used mainly in clients who have minimal symptoms, who do not respond to levodopa, or who cannot tolerate levodopa because of

adverse reactions or contraindications. An additional use of anticholinergic drugs is to relieve Parkinson-like symptoms that occur with older antipsychotic drugs.

Preoperatively, anticholinergics are given to prevent vagal stimulation and potential bradycardia, hypotension, and cardiac arrest. They are also given to reduce respiratory tract secretions, especially in head and neck surgery and bronchoscopy.

CONTRAINDICATIONS FOR USE

Contraindications to the use of anticholinergic drugs include any condition characterized by symptoms that would be aggravated by the drugs. Some of these are prostatic hypertrophy, glaucoma, tachyarrhythmias, myocardial infarction, and congestive heart failure unless bradycardia is present. They should not be given in hiatal hernia or other conditions contributing to reflux esophagitis because the drugs delay gastric emptying, relax the cardioesophageal sphincter, and increase esophageal reflux.

Individual Anticholinergic Drugs

BELLADONNA ALKALOIDS AND DERIVATIVES

Atropine, the prototype of anticholinergic drugs, produces the same effects and has the same clinical indications for use and the same contraindications as those described earlier. In addition, it is used as an antidote for an overdose of cholinergic drugs and exposure to insecticides that have cholinergic effects.

Atropine is a naturally occurring belladonna alkaloid that can be extracted from the belladonna plant or prepared synthetically. It is usually prepared as atropine sulfate, a salt that is very soluble in water. It is well absorbed from the GI tract and distributed throughout the body. It crosses the blood-brain barrier to enter the CNS, where large doses produce stimulant effects, and toxic doses produce depressant effects. Atropine is also absorbed systemically when applied locally to mucous membranes. The drug is rapidly excreted in the urine. Pharmacologic effects are of short duration except for ocular effects, which may last for several days.

Routes and Dosage Ranges

Adults: GI disorders, PO, SC 0.3–1.2 mg q4–6h
  Preoperatively, IM 0.4–0.6 mg in a single dose 45–60 min before anesthesia
  Bradyarrhythmias, IV 0.4–1 mg q1–2h PRN
  Bronchoconstriction, 0.025 mg/kg diluted with 3–5 ml saline and given by nebulizer three or four times per day
  Topically to eye, one drop of 1% or 2% ophthalmic solution
Children: GI disorders, SC 0.01 mg/kg of body weight q4–6h
  Preoperatively, IM 0.4 mg for children 3–14 y, less for younger children and infants
  Bradyarrhythmias, IV 0.01–0.03 mg/kg of body weight
  Bronchoconstriction, 0.05 mg/kg diluted with 3–5 ml saline and given by nebulizer three or four times per day
  Topically to eye, one drop of 0.5% or 1% ophthalmic solution

Belladonna tincture is a mixture of alkaloids in an aqueous-alcohol solution. It is most often used in GI disorders for antispasmodic effect. It is an ingredient in several drug mixtures.

Route and Dosage Range

Adults: PO 0.6–1 ml three or four times per day
Children: PO 0.03 ml/kg per day in three or four divided doses

Homatropine hydrobromide (Homapin) is a semisynthetic derivative of atropine used as eye drops to produce mydriasis and cycloplegia. Homatropine may be preferable to atropine because ocular effects do not last as long.

Route and Dosage Ranges

Adults: Topically to eye, 1 drop of 5% ophthalmic solution every 5 min for two or three doses for refraction; 1 drop of 2% to 5% solution two or three times per day for uveitis

Hyoscyamine (Anaspaz) is a belladonna alkaloid used in GI and genitourinary disorders characterized by spasm, increased secretion, and increased motility. It has the same effects as other atropine-like drugs.

Routes and Dosage Ranges

Adults: PO 0.125–0.25 mg q64–8h until symptoms are controlled; IM, SC, IV 0.25–0.5 mg q6–12h until symptoms are controlled
Children: PO 0.062–0.125 mg q6–8h for children 2–10 y; half this dosage for children under <2 y

Methscopolamine (Pamine) is a belladonna derivative used occasionally to treat peptic ulcer disease. It lacks the central action of scopolamine and is less potent and longer-acting than atropine.

Route and Dosage Ranges

Adults: PO 2.5–5 mg four times per day
Children: PO 0.2 mg/kg/d in four divided doses

Scopolamine is similar to atropine in uses, adverse effects, and peripheral effects but different in central effects. When given parenterally, scopolamine depresses the CNS and causes amnesia, drowsiness, euphoria, relaxation, and sleep. Effects of scopolamine appear more quickly and disappear more readily than those of atropine. Scopolamine also is used in motion sickness. It is available as oral tablets and as a transdermal adhesive disc that is placed behind the ear. The disc (Transderm-V) protects against motion sickness for 72 hours.

Routes and Dosage Ranges

Adults: Preoperatively, IM 0.4 mg
  Motion sickness, PO 0.25–0.8 mg 1 h before travel; transdermally 1 disc q72h
  Mydriasis, topically to the eye, 1 drop of 0.2% to 0.25% ophthalmic solution, repeated PRN
Children: Preoperatively, 6 months–3 y, IM 0.1–0.15 mg; 3–6 y, IM 0.15–0.2 mg; 6–12 y, 0.2–0.3 mg
  Mydriasis, same as for adults

SYNTHETIC ANTICHOLINERGICS USED IN PARKINSON'S DISEASE

Trihexyphenidyl (Artane) is used in the treatment of parkinsonism and extrapyramidal reactions caused by some antipsychotic drugs. Trihexyphenidyl relieves smooth muscle spasm by a direct action on the muscle and by inhibiting the PNS. The drug supposedly has fewer side effects than atropine, but about half the recipients report mouth dryness, blurring of vision, and other side effects common to anticholinergic drugs. Trihexyphenidyl requires the same precautions as other anticholinergic drugs and is contraindicated in glaucoma. **Biperiden** (Akineton) and **procyclidine** (Kemadrin) are chemical derivatives of trihexyphenidyl and have similar actions, uses, and adverse effects.

Trihexyphenidyl
Route and Dosage Ranges

Adults: Parkinsonism, PO 2 mg two or three times per day initially, gradually increased until therapeutic effects or severe adverse effects occur
Drug-induced extrapyramidal reactions, PO 1 mg initially, gradually increased to 5–15 mg/d in divided doses

Biperiden
Routes and Dosage Ranges

Adults: Parkinsonism, PO 2 mg three or four times per day
Drug-induced extrapyramidal reactions, IM 2 mg, repeated q30 min if necessary; maximum of four consecutive doses in 24 h
Children: Drug-induced extrapyramidal reactions, IM 0.04 mg/kg, repeated as above if necessary

Procyclidine
Route and Dosage Ranges

Adults: Parkinsonism, PO 5 mg twice daily initially, gradually increased to 5 mg three or four times per day if necessary
Drug-induced extrapyramidal reactions, PO 2–2.5 mg three times per day, gradually increased to 10–20 mg/d if necessary

Benztropine (Cogentin) is a synthetic drug with both anticholinergic and antihistaminic effects. Its anticholinergic activity approximates that of atropine. A major clinical use is to treat acute dystonic reactions caused by antipsychotic drugs and to prevent their recurrence in clients receiving long-term antipsychotic drug therapy. It also may be given in small doses to supplement other antiparkinson drugs. In full dosage, adverse reactions are common.

Routes and Dosage Ranges

Adults: PO 0.5–1 mg at bedtime, initially, gradually increased to 4–6 mg/d if required and tolerated
Drug-induced extrapyramidal reactions PO, IM, IV 1–4 mg once or twice per day

URINARY ANTISPASMODICS

Flavoxate (Urispas) was developed specifically to counteract spasm in smooth muscle tissue of the urinary tract. It has anticholinergic, local anesthetic, and analgesic effects. Thus, the drug relieves dysuria, urgency, frequency, and pain with genitourinary infections, such as cystitis and prostatitis.

Route and Dosage Range

Adults and children >12 y: PO 100–200 mg three or four times per day. Reduce dose when symptoms improve.
Children <12 y: Dosage not established

Oxybutynin (Ditropan) has direct antispasmodic effects on smooth muscle and anticholinergic effects. It increases bladder capacity and decreases frequency of voiding in clients with neurogenic bladder.

Route and Dosage Range

Adults: PO 5 mg two or three times per day; maximum dose 5 mg 4 times per day
Children >5 y: PO 5 mg twice a day; maximum dose 5 mg three times per day

Nursing Process

Assessment

- Assess the client's condition in relation to disorders for which anticholinergic drugs are used (*i.e.,* check for bradycardia or heart block, diarrhea, dysuria, abdominal pain, and other disorders). If the client reports or medical records indicate a specific disorder, assess for signs and symptoms of that disorder (*e.g.,* Parkinson's disease).
- Assess for disorders in which anticholinergic drugs are contraindicated (*e.g.,* glaucoma, prostatic hypertrophy, reflux esophagitis).
- Assess use of other drugs with anticholinergic effects, such as antihistamines (histamine-1 receptor antagonists [see Chap. 48], antipsychotic agents, and tricyclic antidepressants).

Nursing Diagnoses

- Altered Urinary Elimination: Decreased bladder tone and urine retention

- Constipation related to slowed GI function
- Altered Thought Processes: Confusion, disorientation, especially in older adults
- Knowledge Deficit: Drug effects and accurate usage
- Risk for Injury related to drug-induced blurred vision and photophobia
- Risk for Noncompliance related to adverse drug effects

Planning/Goals

The client will:
- Receive or self-administer the drugs correctly
- Experience relief of symptoms for which anticholinergic drugs are given
- Be assisted to avoid or cope with adverse drug effects on vision, thought processes, and bowel and bladder elimination

Interventions

Use measures to decrease the need for anticholinergic drugs. For example, with peptic ulcer disease, teach the client to avoid factors known to increase gastric secretion and GI motility (alcohol; cigarette smoking; caffeine-containing beverages, such as coffee, tea, and cola drinks; ulcerogenic drugs, such as aspirin). Late evening snacks also should be avoided because increased gastric acid secretion occurs about 90 minutes after eating and may cause pain and awakening from sleep. Although milk was once considered an "ulcer food," it contains protein and calcium, which promote acid secretion, and is a poor buffer of gastric acid. Thus, drinking large amounts of milk should be avoided.

Teach clients:
- Not to take other drugs without the physician's knowledge. In addition to prescribed antidepressants, antihistamines and antipsychotic drugs with anticholinergic properties, over-the-counter sleeping pills and antihistamines have anticholinergic effects. Taking any of these concurrently could cause overdosage or excessive anticholinergic effects.
- Measures to minimize risks of heat exhaustion and heat stroke:
  - Wear light, cool clothing in warm climates or environments.
  - Maintain fluid and salt intake if not contraindicated.
  - Limit exposure to direct sunlight.
  - Limit physical activity.
  - Take frequent cool baths.
  - Ensure adequate ventilation, with fans or air conditioners if necessary.
  - Avoid alcoholic beverages.

Evaluation

- Interview and observe in relation to safe, accurate drug administration.
- Interview and observe for relief of symptoms for which the drugs are given.
- Interview and observe for adverse drug effects.

Principles of Therapy

USE IN SPECIFIC CONDITIONS

Renal or Biliary Colic

Atropine is sometimes given with morphine or meperidine to relieve the severe pain of renal or biliary colic. It acts mainly to decrease the spasm-producing effects of the narcotic analgesics. It has little antispasmodic effect on the involved muscles and is not used alone for this purpose.

Preoperative Use in Clients With Glaucoma

Glaucoma is usually listed as a contraindication for anticholinergic drugs because the drugs impair outflow of aqueous humor and may cause an acute attack of glaucoma (increased intraocular pressure). However, anticholinergic drugs can be given safely preoperatively to clients with open-angle glaucoma (80% of clients with primary glaucoma) if they are receiving miotic drugs, such as pilocarpine. If anticholinergic preoperative medication is needed in clients predisposed to angle closure, the hazard of causing acute glaucoma can be minimized by also giving pilocarpine eye drops and acetazolamide (Diamox).

Gastrointestinal Disorders

When anticholinergic drugs are given for GI disorders, larger doses may be given at bedtime to prevent pain and awakening during sleep.

Parkinsonism

When these drugs are used in parkinsonism, small doses are given initially and gradually increased. This regimen decreases adverse reactions.

Extrapyramidal Reactions

When used in drug-induced extrapyramidal reactions (parkinson-like symptoms), these drugs should be prescribed only if symptoms occur. They should not be used routinely to prevent extrapyramidal reactions because fewer than half the clients taking antipsychotic drugs experience such reactions. Most drug-induced reactions last about 3 months and do not recur if anticholinergic drugs are discontinued at that time. (An exception is tardive dyskinesia, which does not respond to anticholinergic drugs and may be aggravated by them.)

Treatment of Atropine or Anticholinergic Overdosage

Overdosage of atropine or other anticholinergic drugs produces the usual pharmacologic effects in a severe and exaggerated form. Physostigmine salicylate (Antilirium) is a specific antidote. It is usually given intravenously at a slow rate of injection. Adult dosage is 2 mg (no more than 1 mg/min); child dosage is 0.5 to 1 mg (no more than 0.5 mg/min). Rapid administration may cause bradycardia, hypersalivation (with subsequent respiratory distress), and seizures. Repeated doses may be given if life-threatening arrhythmias, convulsions, or coma occur. Diazepam (Valium) or a similar drug may be given for excessive CNS stimulation (delirium, excitement). Cardiopulmonary resuscitative measures are used if excessive depression of the CNS causes coma and respiratory failure.

USE IN CHILDREN

Systemic anticholinergics, including atropine, glycopyrrolate (Robinul), and scopolamine are given to children of all ages for essentially the same effects as for adults. The antispasmodic agents are also used. Flavoxate is not recommended for children under 12 years, and oxybutynin is not recommended for children under 5 years.

The drugs cause the same adverse effects in children as in adults. However, they may be more severe because children are especially sensitive to the drugs. Facial flushing is common in children, and a skin rash may occur.

Ophthalmic anticholinergic drugs are used for cycloplegia and mydriasis before eye examinations and surgical procedures. They should be used only with close medical supervision. Cyclopentolate (Cyclogyl) and tropicamide (Mydriacyl) have been associated with behavioral disturbances and psychotic reactions in children. Tropicamide also has been associated with cardiopulmonary collapse.

USE IN OLDER ADULTS

Anticholinergic drugs are given for the same purposes as in younger adults. In addition to the primary anticholinergic drugs, many others that are commonly prescribed for older adults have high anticholinergic activity. These include many antihistamines (histamine-1 receptor antagonists), tricyclic antidepressants, and antipsychotic drugs.

Older adults are especially likely to have significant adverse reactions because of slowed drug metabolism and the frequent presence of several disease processes. Some common adverse effects and suggestions for reducing their impact are:

1. **Blurred vision.** The client may need help with ambulation, especially with stairs or other potentially hazardous environments. Remove obstacles and hazards when possible.
2. **Confusion.** Provide whatever assistance is needed to prevent falls and other injuries.
3. **Heat stroke.** Help to avoid precipitating factors, such as strenuous activity and high environmental temperatures.
4. **Constipation.** Encourage or assist with an adequate intake of high-fiber foods and fluids and adequate exercise when feasible.
5. **Urinary retention.** Encourage adequate fluid intake and avoid high doses of the drugs. Men should be examined for prostatic hypertrophy.
6. **Hallucinations and other psychotic symptoms.** These are most likely to occur with the centrally active anticholinergics given for Parkinson's disease or drug-induced extrapyramidal effects, such as trihexyphenidyl or benztropine. Dosage of these drugs should be carefully regulated and supervised.

 HOME CARE

Anticholinergic medications are commonly used in home care with children and adults. Children and elderly adults are probably most likely to experience adverse effects of these drugs and should be monitored carefully. With elderly clients, the home care nurse needs to assess medication regimens for combinations of drugs with anticholinergic effects, especially if mental confusion develops or worsens. The home care nurse may also need to teach elderly clients or caregivers that the drugs prevent sweating and heat loss and increase risks of heat stroke if precautions to avoid overheating are not taken.

ANTICHOLINERGIC DRUGS

NURSING ACTIONS	*RATIONALE/EXPLANATION*
1. Administer accurately	
a. For gastrointestinal disorders, give most oral anticholinergic drugs about 30 min before meals and at bedtime.	To allow the drugs to reach peak antisecretory effects by the time ingested food is stimulating gastric acid secretion. Bedtime administration helps prevent awakening with abdominal pain.
b. When given preoperatively, parenteral preparations of atropine can be mixed in the same syringe with several other common preoperative medications, such as meperidine (Demerol), morphine, oxymorphone (Numorphan), and promethazine (Phenergan).	The primary reason for mixing medications in the same syringe is to decrease the number of injections and thus decrease client discomfort. Note, however, that extra caution is required when mixing drugs to be sure that the dosage of each drug is accurate. Also, if any question exists regarding compatibility with another drug, it is safer not to mix the drugs, even if two or three injections are required.
c. When applying topical atropine solutions or ointment to the eye, be sure to use the correct concentration and blot any excess from the inner canthus.	Atropine ophthalmic preparations are available in several concentrations (usually 1%, 2%, and 3%). Excess medication should be removed so the drug will not enter the nasolacrimal (tear) ducts and be absorbed systemically through the mucous membrane of the nasopharynx or be carried to the throat and swallowed.
d. If propantheline is to be given intravenously, dissolve the 30-mg dose of powder in no less than 10 ml of sterile water for injection.	Parenteral administration is reserved for clients who cannot take the drug orally.
e. Instruct clients to swallow oral propantheline tablets, not to chew them.	The tablets have a hard sugar coating to mask the bitter taste of the drug.
f. Parenteral glycopyrrolate can be given through the tubing of a running IV infusion of physiologic saline or lactated Ringer's solution.	
2. Observe for therapeutic effects	Therapeutic effects depend primarily on the reason for use. Thus, a therapeutic effect in one condition may be a side effect or an adverse reaction in another condition.
a. When a drug is given for *peptic ulcer disease* or other gastrointestinal disorders, observe for decreased abdominal pain.	Relief of abdominal pain is due to the smooth muscle relaxant or antispasmodic effect of the drug.
b. When the drug is given for *diagnosing or treating eye disorders*, observe for pupil dilation (mydriasis) and blurring of vision (cycloplegia).	Note that these ocular effects are side effects when the drugs are given for problems not related to the eyes.
c. When the drug is given for *symptomatic bradycardia*, observe for increased pulse rate.	These drugs increase heart rate by blocking action of the vagus nerve.
d. When the drug is given for *urinary tract disorders*, such as cystitis or enuresis, observe for decreased frequency of urination. When the drug is given for *renal colic due to stones*, observe for decreased pain.	Anticholinergic drugs decrease muscle tone and spasm in the smooth muscle of the ureters and urinary bladder.
e. When the centrally acting anticholinergics are given for *Parkinson's disease*, observe for decrease in tremor, salivation, and drooling.	Decreased salivation is a therapeutic effect with parkinsonism but an adverse reaction in most other conditions.

(continued)

NURSING ACTIONS	*RATIONALE/EXPLANATION*
3. Observe for adverse effects **a**. Tachycardia	These depend on reasons for use and are dose related. Tachycardia may occur with usual therapeutic doses because anticholinergic drugs block vagal action, which normally slows heart rate. Tachycardia is not likely to be serious except in clients with underlying heart disease. For example, in clients with angina pectoris, prolonged or severe tachycardia may increase myocardial ischemia to the point of causing an acute attack of angina (chest pain) or even myocardial infarction. In clients with congestive heart failure, severe or prolonged tachycardia can increase the workload of the heart to the point of causing acute heart failure or pulmonary edema.
b. Excessive central nervous system (CNS) stimulation, (tremor, restlessness, confusion, hallucinations, delirium) followed by excessive CNS depression (coma, respiratory depression)	These effects are more likely to occur with large doses of atropine because atropine crosses the blood-brain barrier. Large doses of trihexyphenidyl (Artane) also may cause CNS stimulation.
c. Sedation and amnesia with scopolamine or benztropine (Cogentin)	This may be a therapeutic effect but becomes an adverse reaction if severe or if the drug is given for another purpose. Benztropine has anticholinergic and antihistaminic properties. Apparently, drowsiness and sedation are caused by the antihistaminic component.
d. Constipation or paralytic ileus	These effects are the result of decreased gastrointestinal motility and muscle tone. Constipation is more likely with large doses or parenteral administration. Paralytic ileus is not likely unless the drugs are given to clients who already have decreased gastrointestinal motility.
e. Decreased oral and respiratory tract secretions, which cause mouth dryness and thick respiratory secretions	Mouth dryness is more annoying than serious in most cases and is caused by decreased salivation. However, clients with chronic lung disease, who usually have excessive secretions, tend to retain them with the consequence of frequent respiratory tract infections.
f. Urinary retention	This reaction is caused by loss of bladder tone and is most likely to occur in elderly men with enlarged prostate glands. Thus, the drugs are generally contraindicated with prostatic hypertrophy.
g. Hot, dry skin; fever; heat stroke	These effects are due to decreased sweating and impairment of the normal heat loss mechanism. Fever may occur with any age group. Heat stroke is more likely to occur with cardiovascular disease, strenuous physical activity, and high environmental temperatures, especially in elderly people.
h. Ocular effects—mydriasis, blurred vision, photophobia	These are adverse effects when anticholinergic drugs are given for conditions not related to the eyes.
4. Observe for drug interactions **a.** Drugs that *increase* effects of anticholinergic drugs: Antihistamines, disopyramide, phenothiazines, thioxanthene agents, and tricyclic antidepressants	These drugs have anticholinergic properties and produce additive anticholinergic effects.
b. Drugs that *decrease* effects of anticholinergic drugs: Cholinergic drugs	These drugs counteract the inhibition of gastrointestinal motility and tone induced by atropine. They are sometimes used in atropine overdose.
5. Teach clients **a.** Mouth dryness commonly occurs. Use sugarless chewing gum and hard candy if not contraindicated.	To relieve mouth dryness

NURSING ACTIONS	RATIONALE/EXPLANATION
b. The importance of dental hygiene (*e.g.*, regular brushing of teeth)	Dental caries and loss of teeth may result from drug-induced xerostomia (dry mouth from decreased saliva production). This is more likely to occur with long-term use of these drugs.
c. Blurring of vision is also common. Avoid potentially hazardous activities (*e.g.*, driving a car or operating machinery) when this occurs.	To prevent injury
d. Dark glasses can be worn outdoors in strong light.	To reduce sensitivity to light (photophobia)

REVIEW AND APPLICATION EXERCISES

1. How do anticholinergic drugs exert their therapeutic effects?

2. What are indications for use and contraindications for anticholinergic drugs?

3. What is the effect of anticholinergic drugs on heart rate, and what is the mechanism for this effect?

4. Under what circumstances is it desirable to administer atropine preoperatively and why?

5. What are adverse effects of anticholinergic drugs?

6. What treatment measures are indicated for a client with an overdose of a drug with anticholinergic effects?

7. Name two other commonly used drug groups that have anticholinergic effects.

8. What nursing observations and interventions are needed to increase client safety and comfort during anticholinergic drug therapy?

SELECTED REFERENCES

Brown, J.H. & Taylor, P. (1996). Muscarinic receptor agonists and antagonists. In J.G. Hardman, L.E. Limbird, P.B. Molinoff, & R.W. Ruddon (Eds.), *Goodman & Gilman's The pharmacological basis of therapeutics*, 9th ed., pp. 141-160. New York: McGraw-Hill.

Drug facts and comparisons. (1996). St. Louis: Facts and Comparisons.

Guyton, A.C. & Hall, J.E. (1996). *Textbook of medical physiology*, 9th ed. Philadelphia: W.B. Saunders.

Porth, C.M. & Curtis, R.L. (1994). Normal and altered autonomic nervous system function. In C.M. Porth (Ed.), *Pathophysiology: Concepts of altered health states*, 4th ed., pp. 1007–1026. Philadelphia: J.B. Lippincott.

Drugs Affecting the Endocrine System

Physiology of the Endocrine System

Outline

Objectives

After studying this chapter, the student will be able to:

1 Discuss the relationship between the endocrine system and the central nervous system (CNS).

2 Describe general characteristics and functions of hormones.

3 Differentiate steroid and protein hormones in relation to site of action and pharmacokinetics.

4 Discuss hormonal action at the cellular level.

5 Describe the second messenger roles of cyclic adenosine monophosphate (cAMP) and calcium within body cells.

6 Differentiate between physiologic and pharmacologic doses of hormonal drugs.

Key Terms

Hormone

Hypothalamic-
Pituitary-
Adrenocortical
(HPA) axis

Negative feedback
system

Second
messenger

The Endocrine System

The endocrine system participates in the regulation of essentially all body activities, including metabolism of nutrients and water, reproduction, growth and development, and adapting to changes in internal and external environments. The major organs of the endocrine system are the hypothalamus, pituitary, thyroid, parathyroids, pancreas, adrenals, ovaries, and testes. These tissues function through *hormones*, substances that are synthesized and secreted into body fluids by one group of cells and have physiologic effects on other body cells. Hormones act as chemical messengers to transmit information between body cells. Most hormones from the traditional endocrine glands are secreted into the bloodstream and act on distant organs.

In addition to the major endocrine organs, other tissues also produce hormones. These endocrine-like cells intermingle with nonendocrine cells in various organs. Their hormones are secreted into tissue fluids and act locally on nearby cells, as in the following examples:

Gastrointestinal mucosa produces hormones that are important in the digestive process (*e.g.,* gastrin, enterogastrone, secretin, and cholecystokinin).

The kidneys produce erythropoietin, a hormone that stimulates the bone marrow to produce red blood cells.

White blood cells produce cytokines that function as messengers among leukocytes in inflammatory and immune processes.

Most body tissues produce prostaglandins, which have a variety of physiologic effects.

Neoplasms also may produce hormones. In endocrine tissues, neoplasms may be an added source of the hormone normally produced by the organ. In nonendocrine tissues, various hormones may be produced. For example, lung tumors may produce corticotropin, antidiuretic hormone, or parathyroid hormone; kidney tumors may produce parathyroid hormone. The usual effects are those of excess hormone secretion.

This chapter focuses on the traditional endocrine organs and their hormones. Specific organs are discussed in the following chapters; some general characteristics of the endocrine system and hormones are described below.

Endocrine System–Nervous System Interactions

The endocrine and nervous systems are closely connected, anatomically and physiologically, and work in harmony to integrate and regulate body functions.

Generally, the nervous system regulates rapid muscular and sensory activities by secreting substances that act as neurotransmitters, circulating hormones, and local hormones (*e.g.,* norepinephrine, epinephrine). The endocrine system regulates slow metabolic activities by secreting hormones that control cellular metabolism, transport of substances across cell membranes, and other functions (*e.g.,* reproduction, growth and development, secretion).

The main connecting link between the nervous system and the endocrine system is the hypothalamus, which responds to nervous system stimulation by producing hormones. Thus, secretion of almost all hormones from the pituitary gland is controlled by the hypothalamus. Special nerve fibers originating in the hypothalamus and ending in the posterior pituitary gland control secretions of the posterior pituitary. The hypothalamus secretes hormones called *releasing* and *inhibitory factors,* which regulate functions of the anterior pituitary. The anterior pituitary, in turn, secretes hormones that act on target tissues, usually to stimulate production of other hormones. One example is that hypothalamic corticotropin-releasing factor (CRH) stimulates the anterior pituitary to produce corticotropin (ACTH), and the corticotropin, in turn, stimulates the adrenal cortex to produce cortisol. This complex interrelationship is often referred to as the *hypothalamic-pituitary-adrenocortical (HPA) axis.* It functions by a *negative feedback* system, in which hormone secretion is stimulated when hormones are needed and inhibited when they are not needed. The hypothalamic-pituitary-thyroid axis also functions by a negative feedback mechanism.

General Characteristics of Hormones

Hormones are extremely important in regulating body activities. Their normal secretion and function help to maintain the internal environment and determine response and adaptation to the external environment. Hormones participate in complex interactions with other hormones and nonhormone chemical substances in the body to influence every aspect of life. Although hormones are usually studied individually, virtually all endocrine functions are complex processes that are influenced by more than one hormone.

Although hormones circulating in the bloodstream reach essentially all body cells, some (*e.g.,* growth hormone, thyroid hormone) affect almost all cells, whereas others affect specific "target" tissues (*e.g.,* corticotropin stimulates the adrenal cortex). In addition, *one hormone can affect different tissues* (*e.g.,* ovarian estrogen can act on ovarian follicles to promote their maturation, on the endometrial lining of the uterus to stimulate its growth and cyclic changes, on breast tissue to stimulate growth of milk ducts, and on the hypothalamic-pituitary system to regulate its own secretion), or *several hormones can affect a single tissue or function* (*e.g.*, catecholamines, glucagon, secretin, and prolactin regulate lipolysis [release of fatty acids from adipose tissue]).

Several hormones are secreted in cyclic patterns. For example, ACTH, cortisol and growth hormone are secreted in 24-hour (circadian) cycles, whereas estrogen and progestin secretion is related to the 28-day menstrual cycle.

HORMONE PHARMACOKINETICS

Protein-derived hormones (amines, amino acids, peptides and polypeptides) are synthesized, stored and released into the bloodstream in response to a stimulus. The steroid hormones, which are synthesized in the adrenal cortex and gonads from cholesterol, are released as they are synthesized. Most hormones are constantly present in the blood; plasma concentrations vary according to body needs, the rate of synthesis and release, and the rate of metabolism and excretion.

Protein-derived hormones generally circulate in an unbound, active form. Steroid and thyroid hormones are transported by specific carrier proteins synthesized in the liver. (Some drugs may compete with a hormone for binding sites on the carrier protein. If this occurs, hormone effects are enhanced because more unbound, active molecules are available to act on body cells.)

Hormones must be continuously inactivated to prevent their accumulation and excessive effects. Several mechanisms operate to eliminate hormones from the body. The water-soluble, protein-derived hormones have a short duration of action and are inactivated by enzymes mainly in the liver and kidneys. The lipid-soluble steroid and thyroid hormones have a longer duration of action because they are bound to plasma proteins. Once released by the plasma proteins, these hormones are conjugated in the liver to inactive forms, and then excreted in bile or urine. A third, less common mechanism is inactivation by enzymes at receptor sites on target cells.

HORMONE ACTION AT THE CELLULAR LEVEL

Hormones modify rather than initiate cellular reactions and functions. Once hormone molecules reach a responsive cell, they bind with receptors in the cell membrane (*e.g.*, catecholamines and protein hormones) or inside the cell (*e.g.*, steroid and thyroid hormones). The number of hormone receptors and the affinity of the receptors for the hormone are the major determinants of target cell response to hormone action. The main target organs for a given hormone contain large numbers of receptors. However, the number of receptors may be altered by various conditions. For example, receptors may be increased (called up regulation) when there are low levels of hormone. This allows the cell to obtain more of the needed hormone than it can obtain with fewer receptors. Receptors may be decreased (called down regulation) when there are excessive amounts of hormone. This mechanism protects the cell by making it less responsive to excessive hormone levels. Receptor up regulation and down regulation occur with chronic exposure to abnormal levels of hormones. In addition, receptor proteins may be decreased by inadequate formation or antibodies that destroy them. It seems clear that receptors are constantly being synthesized and degraded so the number of receptors may change within hours. Receptor affinity for binding with hormone molecules probably changes as well.

After binding occurs, the resulting hormone-receptor complex initiates intracellular biochemical reactions, depending on the particular hormone and the type of cell. Many hormones act as a "first messenger" to the cell, and the hormone-receptor complex activates a "second messenger." The second messenger then activates intracellular structures to produce characteristic cellular functions and products. Steroid hormones from the adrenal cortex, ovaries, and testes stimulate target cells to synthesize various proteins (*e.g.*, enzymes, transport and structural proteins) needed for normal cellular function.

Second Messenger Systems

Second messengers for several hormones are unknown; however, three major systems are fairly well understood. These are cyclic adenosine monophosphate (cAMP), calcium-calmodulin, and phospholipid products, which are described below.

Cyclic AMP is the second messenger for many hormones, including adrenocorticotropin, catecholamines, glucagon, thyroid-stimulating hormone, follicle-stimulating hormone, luteinizing hormone, parathyroid hormone, secretin, and vasopressin. It is formed by the action of the enzyme adenyl cyclase on adenosine triphosphate, a component of all cells and the main source of energy for cellular metabolism. Once formed, cAMP activates a series of enzyme reactions that alter cell function. The amount of intracellular cAMP is increased by hormones that activate adenyl cyclase (*e.g.*, the pituitary hormones, calcitonin, glucagon, parathyroid hormone) and decreased by hormones that inactivate adenyl cyclase (*e.g.*, angiotensin, somatostatin). Cyclic AMP is inactivated by phosphodiesterase enzymes.

Calcium is the second messenger for angiotensin II, a strong vasoconstrictor that participates in control of arterial blood pressure, and for gonadotropin-releasing hormone. The postulated sequence of events is that hormone binding to receptors increases intracellular calcium. The calcium binds with an intracellular regulatory protein called calmodulin. The calcium-calmodulin complex activates protein kinases, which then regulate contractile structures of the cell, cell membrane permeability, and intracellular enzyme activity. Specific effects include contraction of smooth muscle, changes in the secretions produced by secreting cells, changes in ciliary action in the lungs, and others.

Phospholipid products are mainly involved with local hormones. Phospholipids are major components of the cell membrane portion of all body cells. Some local hormones activate cell membrane receptors and transform them into phospholipase C, an enzyme that causes some of the phospholipids in cell membranes to split into smaller molecules (*e.g.,* inositol triphosphate and diacylglycerol). These products then act as second messengers to intracellular structures. The inositol triphosphate mobilizes intracellular calcium ions and the calcium ions then fulfill their functions as second messengers as described above. The diacylglycerol activates an enzyme, protein kinase C, which is important in cell reproduction. Also, the lipid component of diacylglycerol is arachidonic acid, the precursor for prostaglandins, leukotrienes, and other local hormones with extensive effects.

Steroid Stimulation of Protein Synthesis

Steroid hormones are lipid soluble and therefore cross cell membranes easily. Once inside the cell cytoplasm, the hormone molecules bind with specific receptor proteins. The hormone-receptor complex then enters the nucleus of the cell where it activates nucleic acids (DNA and RNA) and the genetic code to synthesize new proteins.

MAJOR HORMONES AND THEIR GENERAL FUNCTIONS

1. Anterior pituitary hormones are growth hormone (also called somatotropin), corticotropin, thyroid-stimulating hormone, follicle-stimulating hormone, luteinizing hormone, and prolactin. Most of these hormones function by stimulating secretion of other hormones.
2. Posterior pituitary hormones are antidiuretic hormone (ADH or vasopressin) and oxytocin. ADH helps maintain fluid balance; oxytocin stimulates uterine contractions during childbirth.
3. Adrenal cortex hormones, commonly called corticosteroids, include the glucocorticoids, such as cortisol, and the mineralocorticoids, such as aldosterone. Glucocorticoids influence carbohydrate storage, exert anti-inflammatory effects, suppress

corticotropin secretion, and increase protein catabolism. Mineralocorticoids help regulate electrolyte balance, mainly by promoting sodium retention and potassium loss. The adrenal cortex also produces sex hormones. Adrenal medulla hormones are epinephrine and norepinephrine (see Chap. 17).
4. Thyroid hormones include triiodothyronine (T_3 or liothyronine) and tetraiodothyronine (T_4 or thyroxine). These hormones regulate the metabolic rate of the body and greatly influence growth and development.
5. Parathyroid hormone, also called parathormone or PTH, regulates calcium and phosphate metabolism.
6. Pancreatic hormones are insulin and glucagon, which regulate the metabolism of glucose, lipids, and proteins.
7. Ovarian hormones (female sex hormones) are estrogens and progesterone. Estrogens promote growth of specific body cells and development of most secondary sexual characteristics in females. Progesterone helps prepare the uterus for pregnancy and the mammary glands for lactation.
8. Testicular hormone (male sex hormone) is testosterone, which regulates development of masculine characteristics.
9. Placental hormones are chorionic gonadotropin, estrogen, progesterone, and human placental lactogen, all of which are concerned with reproductive functions.

HORMONAL DISORDERS

Abnormal secretion and function of hormones, even minor alterations, can impair physical and mental health. Malfunction of an endocrine organ is usually associated with hyposecretion, hypersecretion, or inappropriate secretion of its hormones. Any malfunction can produce serious disease or death.

Hypofunction

Hypofunction may be associated with a variety of circumstances, including the following:

1. A congenital defect may result in the absence of an endocrine gland, the presence of an abnormally developed gland, or the absence of an enzyme required for glandular synthesis of its specific hormone.
2. The endocrine gland may be damaged or destroyed by impaired blood flow, infection or inflammation, autoimmune disorders, or neoplasms.
3. The endocrine gland may atrophy and become less able to produce its hormone because of aging, drug therapy, disease, or unknown reasons.
4. The endocrine gland may produce adequate hormone, but the hormone may not be able to function

normally because of receptor defects (not enough receptors or the receptors present are unable to bind with the hormone).

5. Even if there is adequate hormone and adequate binding to receptors, intracellular metabolic processes (*e.g.*, enzyme function, protein synthesis, energy production) may not respond appropriately.

Hyperfunction

Hyperfunction is usually characterized by excessive hormone production. Excessive amounts of hormone may occur from excessive stimulation and enlargement of the endocrine gland, from a hormone-producing tumor of the gland, or from a hormone-producing tumor of nonendocrine tissues (*e.g.*, some primary lung tumors produce antidiuretic hormone and adrenocorticotropic hormone).

General Characteristics of Hormonal Drugs

1. Hormone preparations given for therapeutic purposes include natural hormones from human or animal sources and synthetic hormones. Many of the most important hormones have been synthesized, and these preparations may have more potent and prolonged effects than the naturally occurring hormones.

2. Hormones are given for physiologic or pharmacologic effects. Physiologic use involves giving small doses as a replacement or substitute for the amount ordinarily secreted by a normally functioning endocrine gland. Such usage is indicated only when a gland cannot secrete an adequate amount of hormone. Examples of physiologic use include insulin administration in diabetes mellitus and adrenal corticosteroid administration in Addison's disease. Pharmacologic use involves relatively large doses for effects greater than physiologic effects. For example, adrenal corticosteroids are widely used for anti-inflammatory effects in endocrine and nonendocrine disorders.

3. Hormones are powerful drugs that produce widespread therapeutic and adverse effects.

4. Administration of one hormone may alter effects of other hormones. These alterations result from the complex interactions among hormones.

5. Hormonal drugs are more often given for disorders resulting from endocrine gland hypofunction than for those related to hyperfunction.

 REVIEW AND APPLICATION EXERCISES

1. How do hormones function in maintaining homeostasis?

2. What is the connection between the nervous system and the endocrine system?

3. What is meant by a negative feedback system?

4. Because classic hormones are secreted into blood and circulated to essentially all body cells, why do they not affect all body cells?

5. What are the functions and characteristics of the pituitary gland?

SELECTED REFERENCES

Guyton, A.C. & Hall, J.E. (1996). *Textbook of medical physiology,* 9th ed. Philadelphia: W.B. Saunders.

Malseed, R.T., Goldstein, F.J. & Balkon, N. (1995). *Pharmacology: Drug therapy and nursing considerations,* 4th ed., pp. 423–435. Philadelphia: J.B. Lippincott.

Porth, C.M. (1994). *Pathophysiology: Concepts of altered health states,* 4th ed., pp. 897–905. Philadelphia: J.B. Lippincott.

23 Hypothalamic and Pituitary Hormones

Objectives

After studying this chapter, the student will be able to:

1 Describe clinical uses of major pituitary hormones.

2 Differentiate characteristics and functions of anterior and posterior pituitary hormones.

3 Discuss limitations of hypothalamic and pituitary hormones as therapeutic agents.

4 State major nursing considerations in the care of clients receiving specific hypothalamic and pituitary hormones.

Key Terms

Adrenocorticotropic hormone (ACTH)

Antidiuretic hormone (ADH)

Corticotropin

Gonadotropin

Growth hormone

Oxytocin

Releasing hormone

Somatotropin

Thyroid-stimulating hormone (TSH)

Thyrotropin

Description

The hypothalamus and pituitary gland (hypophysis) interact to control most metabolic functions of the body and to maintain homeostasis. They are anatomically connected by the hypophyseal stalk. The hypothalamus controls secretions of the pituitary gland. The pituitary gland, in turn, regulates secretions or functions of other body tissues, called "target" tissues. The pituitary gland is actually two glands, each with different structures and functions. The anterior pituitary (adenohypophysis) is composed of different types of glandular cells that synthesize and secrete different hormones. The posterior pituitary (neurohypophysis) is anatomically an extension of the hypothalamus and is composed largely of nerve fibers. It does not manufacture any hormones itself but stores and releases hormones synthesized in the hypothalamus.

HYPOTHALAMIC HORMONES

The hypothalamus produces a releasing hormone (also called factor) or an inhibiting hormone that corresponds to each of the major hormones of the anterior pituitary gland. Specifically, they are:

1. **Corticotropin-releasing hormone,** which causes release of corticotropin in response to stress and threatening stimuli.
2. **Growth hormone-releasing factor,** which causes release of growth hormone in response to low blood levels of the hormone.
3. **Growth hormone release-inhibiting hormone** (somatostatin), which inhibits release of growth hormone.
4. **Thyrotropin-releasing hormone** (TRH), which causes release of thyroid-stimulating hormone (TSH or thyrotropin) in response to stress, such as exposure to cold.
5. **Gonadotropin-releasing hormone** (GnRH), which causes release of follicle-stimulating hormone (FSH) and luteinizing hormone (LH).
6. **Prolactin-releasing factor,** which is active during lactation after childbirth.
7. **Prolactin-inhibitory factor** (PIF), which is active at times other than during lactation.
8. **Melanocyte-stimulating hormone releasing factor,** which stimulates release of melanocyte stimulating hormone.
9. **Melanocyte-stimulating hormone inhibiting factor,** which inhibits release of melanocyte-stimulating hormone.

PITUITARY HORMONES

The anterior pituitary gland produces seven hormones. Two of these, growth hormone and prolactin, act directly on their target tissues; the other five act indirectly by stimulating target tissues to produce other hormones.

1. **Corticotropin,** also called adrenocorticotropic hormone (ACTH), stimulates the adrenal cortex to produce adrenocorticosteroids. Secretion is controlled by the hypothalamus and by plasma levels of cortisol, the major adrenocorticosteroid. When plasma levels are adequate for body needs, the anterior pituitary does not release corticotropin (negative feedback mechanism).
2. **Growth hormone,** also called somatotropin, stimulates growth of all body tissues that are capable of responding. It promotes an increase in cell size and number, largely by affecting metabolism of carbohydrate, protein, fat, and bone tissue. Deficient growth hormone in children produces dwarfism, a condition marked by severely decreased linear growth and frequently, severely delayed mental, emotional, dental, and sexual growth as well. Excessive growth hormone in preadolescent children produces gigantism, marked by heights of 8 or 9 ft if untreated. Excessive growth hormone in adults produces acromegaly.
3. **Thyrotropin,** also called TSH, regulates secretion of thyroid hormones. Thyrotropin secretion is controlled by a negative feedback mechanism in proportion to metabolic needs. Thus, increased thyroid hormones in body fluids inhibit secretion of thyrotropin by the anterior pituitary and of TRH by the hypothalamus.
4. **FSH,** one of the gonadotropins, stimulates functions of sex glands. It is produced by the anterior pituitary gland of males and females beginning at puberty. FSH acts on the ovaries in a cyclical fashion during the reproductive years, stimulating growth of ovarian follicles. These follicles then produce estrogen, which prepares the endometrium for implantation of a fertilized ovum. FSH acts on the testes to stimulate the production and growth of sperm (spermatogenesis), but it does not stimulate secretion of male sex hormones.
5. **LH** (also called *interstitial cell-stimulating hormone*), is another gonadotropin that stimulates hormone production by the gonads of both sexes. LH is important in the maturation and rupture of the ovarian follicle (ovulation). After ovulation, LH acts on the cells of the collapsed sac to produce the corpus luteum, which then produces progesterone during the last half of the menstrual cycle. When blood progesterone levels rise, a negative feedback effect is exerted on hypothalamic and anterior pituitary secretion of gonadotropins. Decreased pituitary secretion of LH causes the corpus luteum to die and stop producing progesterone. Lack of progesterone causes slough and discharge of the endometrial lining as

menstrual flow. (Of course, if the ovum has been fertilized and attached to the endometrium, menstruation does not occur.)

In males, LH stimulates the Leydig's cells in the spaces between the seminiferous tubules. These cells then secrete androgens, mainly testosterone.

6. **Prolactin** plays a part in milk production by nursing mothers. It is not usually secreted in nonpregnant women because of the hypothalamic hormone PIF. During late pregnancy and lactation, various stimuli, including suckling, inhibit the production of PIF, and thus prolactin is synthesized and released.

7. **Melanocyte-stimulating hormone** plays a role in skin pigmentation, but its function in humans is not clearly delineated.

The posterior pituitary gland stores and releases two hormones that are synthesized by nerve cells in the hypothalamus:

1. **Antidiuretic hormone** (ADH), also called vasopressin. It functions to regulate water balance. When ADH is secreted, it makes renal tubules more permeable to water. This allows water in renal tubules to be reabsorbed into the plasma and so conserves body water. In the absence of ADH, little water is reabsorbed, and large amounts are lost in the urine.

ADH is secreted when body fluids become concentrated (high amounts of electrolytes in proportion to the amount of water) and when blood volume is low. In the first instance, ADH causes reabsorption of water, dilution of extracellular fluids, and restoration of normal osmotic pressure. In the second instance, ADH raises blood volume and arterial blood pressure toward homeostatic levels.

2. **Oxytocin,** which functions in childbirth and lactation. It initiates uterine contractions at the end of gestation to induce childbirth, and it causes milk to move from breast glands to nipples so the infant can obtain the milk by suckling.

Therapeutic Limitations

There are few approved clinical uses for hypothalamic hormones and pituitary hormones. Drug formulations of some hypothalamic hormones are relatively new and clinical experience with their use is limited and there are several reasons why pituitary hormones are not used extensively. First, other effective agents are available for some potential uses. When there is a deficiency of target gland hormones (*e.g.,* adrenocorticosteroids, thyroid hormones, male or female sex hormones), it is usually more convenient and effective to administer those hormones than the anterior pituitary hormones that stimulate their secretion. Second, some pituitary

hormones must be obtained from natural sources, which tends to be inconvenient and expensive. For example, corticotropin, thyrotropin, and ADH are obtained from the pituitary glands of domestic animals slaughtered for food; gonadotropins are obtained from the urine of pregnant or menopausal women. A third reason for the infrequent use of pituitary hormones is that most conditions in which pituitary hormones are indicated are uncommon.

Despite their limitations, hypothalamic and pituitary hormones perform important functions when indicated for clinical use.

Individual Hormonal Agents

HYPOTHALAMIC HORMONES

Gonadorelin acetate (Lutrepulse), gonadorelin hydrochloride (Factrel), and nafarelin (Synarel) are synthetic equivalents of GnRH. The acetate salt is used to induce ovulation in women with hypothalamic amenorrhea. The hydrochloride salt is used in diagnostic tests of gonadotropic functions of the anterior pituitary. Nafarelin is used in the treatment of endometriosis. For specific instructions regarding administration, consult current literature from the drug manufacturer.

Gonadorelin Acetate
Route and Dosage Range

Adults: IV using special pump 5 µg every 90 min for about 21 d

Gonadorelin Hydrochloride
Route and Dosage Range

Adults: SC, IV 100 µg

Nafarelin
Route and Dosage Range

Adults: One spray (200 µg) in one nostril in the morning and one spray in the other nostril in the evening (total daily dose, 400 µg), starting between the second and fourth days of the menstrual cycle

Protirelin (Thypinone) is a synthetic equivalent of natural TRH. It is used for diagnostic tests of thyroid, pituitary, and hypothalamic function. For specific test methodology and interpretation, consult the drug manufacturers' instructions.

Routes and Dosage Ranges

Adults: IV 200–500 µg, injected over 15–30 sec, with patient supine and remaining supine for at least 15 min

Children, 6–16 y of age: 7 µg/kg, up to a maximum dose of 500 µg

Infants and children up to 6 y of age: Dosage not established

ANTERIOR PITUITARY HORMONES

Corticotropin (ACTH, Acthar) is obtained from pituitary glands of cattle and hogs, then purified and standardized. Corticotropin is composed of 39 amino acids, 24 of which exert the characteristic physiologic effects. Because it is a protein substance, corticotropin is destroyed by proteolytic enzymes in the digestive tract and must therefore be given parenterally. Corticotropin has a short duration of action and must be administered frequently. There are, however, repository preparations (Cortrophin-Gel, Cortrophin-Zinc) that are slowly absorbed, have a longer duration of action, and can be given once daily.

Corticotropin is given to stimulate synthesis of hormones by the adrenal cortex (glucocorticoids, mineralocorticoids, sex hormones). It is not effective unless the adrenal cortex can respond. Adrenocortical response is variable, and dosage of corticotropin must be individualized. When corticotropin therapy is being discontinued, dosage is gradually reduced to avoid the steroid withdrawal syndrome characterized by muscle weakness, fatigue, and hypotension. Corticotropin is also used in laboratory tests of adrenal function.

Cosyntropin (Cortrosyn) is a synthetic drug with biologic activity similar to that of corticotropin. It is used as a diagnostic test in suspected adrenal insufficiency.

Corticotropin
Routes and Dosage Ranges

Adults: Therapeutic use, IM, SC 20 units four times per day
Diagnostic use, IM 40–80 units daily for 1–3 d; IV 10–25 units in 500 ml of 5% dextrose or 0.9% sodium chloride solution, infused over 8 h once a day. A continuous infusion with 40 units q12h for 48 h may also be used.

Cortrophin-Gel
Route and Dosage Range

Adults: Therapeutic use, IM 40–80 units q24–72h
Diagnostic use, IM 40–80 units/d for 1–3 d

Cosyntropin
Routes and Dosage Ranges

Adults: Diagnostic use, IM, IV 0.25 mg (equivalent to 25 units ACTH)

Growth hormone is synthesized from bacteria by recombinant DNA technology. Two forms are available.

Somatropin (Humatrope) contains the same number and sequence of amino acids as pituitary-derived human growth hormone. Somatrem (Protropin) is the same except it contains one additional amino acid, methionine. The drugs are therapeutically equivalent to endogenous growth hormone produced by the pituitary gland. The only clinical use of the drugs is for children whose growth is impaired by a deficiency of endogenous growth hormone. The drugs are ineffective when impaired growth results from other causes or after puberty, when epiphyses of the long bones have closed. Dosage should be individualized according to response. Excessive administration can cause excessive growth (gigantism).

Somatrem
Route and Dosage Range

Children: IM, up to 0.1 mg/kg three times per week

Somatropin
Route and Dosage Range

Children: IM, up to 0.06 mg/kg three times per week

Human chorionic gonadotropin (HCG [Follutein]) is a placental hormone obtained from the urine of pregnant women. In men, HCG produces physiologic effects similar to those of the naturally occurring LH. HCG is used clinically to evaluate the ability of the Leydig's cells to produce testosterone and to treat cryptorchidism (undescended testicle) in preadolescent boys. Excessive doses or prolonged administration can lead to sexual precocity, edema, and breast enlargement caused by oversecretion of testosterone and possibly estrogen. In women, HCG is used in combination with menotropins to induce ovulation in the treatment of infertility.

Route and Dosage Ranges

Adults and preadolescent boys: Cryptorchidism and hypogonadism in males, IM 500–4000 units two or three times per week for several weeks
To induce ovulation, IM 5000–10,000 units in one dose, 1 d after treatment with menotropins

Menotropins (Pergonal), a gonadotropin preparation obtained from the urine of postmenopausal women, contains both FSH and LH. It is usually combined with HCG to induce ovulation in the treatment of infertility caused by lack of pituitary gonadotropins.

Route and Dosage Range

Adults: IM 1 ampule (75 units FSH and 75 units LH) daily for 9–12 d, followed by HCG to induce ovulation

Thyrotropin (Thytropar) is obtained from the anterior pituitary glands of cattle. It is used as a diagnostic agent to distinguish between primary hypothyroidism (caused by a thyroid disorder) and secondary hypothyroidism (caused by pituitary malfunction). If thyroid hormones in serum are elevated after the administration of thyrotropin, then the hypothyroidism is secondary to inadequate pituitary function. Thyrotropin must be used cautiously in clients with coronary artery disease, congestive heart failure, or adrenocortical insufficiency.

Routes and Dosage Ranges

Adults: IM, SC 10 units daily for 1–3 d, followed by ^{131}I in 18–24 h. Thyroid uptake of iodine is measured 24 h after iodine administration. Accumulation is greater in hypopituitarism than in primary hypothyroidism.

POSTERIOR PITUITARY HORMONES

Desmopressin acetate (DDAVP, Stimate) is a synthetic analogue of ADH. A major clinical use is the treatment of neurogenic diabetes insipidus, a disorder characterized by a deficiency of ADH and the excretion of large amounts of dilute urine. Diabetes insipidus may be idiopathic, hereditary, or acquired as a result of trauma, surgery, tumor, infection, or other conditions that impair the function of the hypothalamus or posterior pituitary. Parenteral desmopressin is also used as a hemostatic in clients with hemophilia A or mild-to-moderate von Willebrand's disease (type 1). The drug is effective in controlling spontaneous or trauma-induced bleeding and intraoperative and postoperative bleeding when given 30 minutes before the procedure.

Routes and Dosage Ranges

Adults: Diabetes insipidus, intranasally 0.1–0.4 ml/d, usually in two divided doses
Hemophilia A, von Willebrand's disease, IV 0.3 µg/kg in 50 ml sterile saline, infused over 15–30 min
Children 3 months–2 y: Diabetes insipidus, intranasally 0.05–0.3 ml/d in one or two doses
Children weighing over 10 kg: Hemophilia A, von Willebrand's disease, same as adult dosage
Children weighing 10 kg or less: Hemophilia A, von Willebrand's disease, IV 0.3 µg/kg in 10 ml of sterile saline

Lypressin is a synthetic vasopressin that has several advantages over the natural product. Because it is free of oxytocin impurity and foreign proteins, it is less likely to produce allergic reactions and other side effects than vasopressin, which is derived from animal sources. Lypressin is also advantageous in that it is given intranasally rather than by injection. It is used only for controlling the excessive water loss of diabetes insipidus caused by inadequate function of the posterior pituitary gland.

Route and Dosage Range

Adults: Intranasal spray, one or two sprays to one or both nostrils, three or four times per day

Vasopressin (Pitressin) is available as an extract derived from animal pituitary glands and as a synthetic preparation. The synthetic preparation is preferred because it contains no oxytocin. Until lypressin was developed, vasopressin was the most widely used drug for diabetes insipidus caused by hypofunction of the posterior pituitary gland. Vasopressin has a short duration of action (a few hours). This short action is sometimes an advantage (*e.g.,* when acutely ill patients require precise control of fluid balance after brain surgery or trauma), but it is a disadvantage when long-term treatment of diabetes insipidus is necessary. Vasopressin tannate is a long-acting oil suspension that also must be injected; its effects last 1 to 3 days. Vasopressin has a vasoconstrictor effect and is used in the treatment of bleeding esophageal varices.

Vasopressin
Routes and Dosage Ranges

Adults: IM, SC, intranasally on cotton pledgets, 0.25–0.5 ml (5–10 units) two or three times per day
Children: IM, SC, intranasally on cotton pledgets, 0.125–0.5 ml (2.5–10 units) three or four times per day

Oxytocin (Pitocin) is a synthetic drug that exerts the same physiologic effects as the posterior pituitary hormone. Thus, it promotes uterine contractility and is used clinically to induce labor and in the postpartum period to control bleeding. Oxytocin must be used only when clearly indicated and when the recipient can be supervised by well-trained personnel. It is usually given in a hospital.

Routes and Dosage Ranges

Adults: Induction of labor, IV 1-ml ampule (10 units) in 1000 ml of 5% dextrose injection (10 units/1000 ml = 10 milliunits/ml), infused at 0.2–2 milliunits/min initially, then regulated according to frequency and strength of uterine contractions
Prevention or treatment of postpartum bleeding, IV 10–40 units in 1000 ml of 5% dextrose injection, infused at 125 ml/h (40 milliunits/min) or 0.6–1.8 units (0.06–0.18 ml) diluted in 3–5 ml sodium chloride injection and injected slowly IM 0.3–1 ml (3–10 units)

Nursing Process

Assessment

Assess for disorders for which hypothalamic and pituitary hormones are given:

- For children with impaired growth, assess height and weight (actual and in comparison with growth charts) and diagnostic x-ray reports of bone age.
- For clients with diabetes insipidus, assess baseline blood pressure, weight, fluid intake to urine output ratio, urine specific gravity, and laboratory reports of serum electrolytes.

Nursing Diagnoses

- Knowledge Deficit: Drug administration and effects
- Altered Growth and Development
- Anxiety related to multiple injections
- Risk for Injury: Adverse drug effects

Planning/Goals

The client will:

- Experience relief of symptoms without serious adverse effects
- Take or receive the drug accurately
- Comply with procedures for monitoring and follow-up

Interventions

- For children receiving growth hormone, assist the family to set reasonable goals for increased height and weight and to comply with accurate drug administration and follow-up procedures (periodic x-rays to determine bone growth and progress toward epiphyseal closure, recording height and weight at least weekly).
- For clients with diabetes insipidus, teach them to weigh themselves daily, monitor their fluid intake and urine output for approximately equal amounts, or to check urine specific gravity daily (should be at least 1.015) and replace fluids accordingly.

Evaluation

- Interview and observe for compliance with instructions for taking the drug(s).
- Observe for relief of symptoms for which pituitary hormones were prescribed.

Principles of Therapy

1. Hypothalamic hormones are rarely used in most clinical practice settings. Generally, the drugs should be prescribed by physicians who are knowledgeable about endocrinology and administered according to current manufacturers' literature.
2. Most drug therapy with pituitary hormones is given to replace or supplement naturally occurring hormones in situations involving inadequate function of the pituitary gland (hypopituitarism). Conditions resulting from excessive amounts of pituitary hormones (hyperpituitarism) are more often treated with surgery or irradiation.
3. Diagnosis of suspected pituitary disorders should be as complete and as specific as possible. This promotes more specific and more effective treatment measures, including drug therapy.
4. Even though manufacturers recommend corticotropin for treatment of diseases that respond to glucocorticoids, corticotropin is less predictable and less convenient than glucocorticoids and has no apparent advantages over them.
5. Dosage of any pituitary hormone must be individualized because responsiveness of affected tissues varies.

 HYPOTHALAMIC AND PITUITARY HORMONES

NURSING ACTIONS	*RATIONALE/EXPLANATION*
1. Administer accurately Read the manufacturer's instructions and drug labels carefully before drug preparation and administration.	These hormone preparations are given infrequently and often require special techniques of administration.
2. Observe for therapeutic effects	Therapeutic effects vary widely, depending on the particular pituitary hormone given and the reason for use.
a. With gonadorelin, observe for ovulation or decreased symptoms of endometriosis and absence of menstruation.	Therapeutic effects depend on the reason for use. Note that different formulations are used to stimulate ovulation and treat endometriosis.
b. With corticotropin, therapeutic effects stem largely from increased secretion of adrenal cortex hormones, especially the glucocorticoids, and include anti-inflammatory effects (see Chap. 24).	Corticotropin is usually not recommended for the numerous nonendocrine inflammatory disorders that respond to glucocorticoids. Administration of glucocorticoids is more convenient and effective than administration of corticotropin.

(continued)

NURSING ACTIONS	RATIONALE/EXPLANATION
c. With chorionic gonadotropin and menotropins given in cases of female infertility, ovulation and conception are therapeutic effects.	
d. With chorionic gonadotropin given in cryptorchidism, the therapeutic effect is descent of the testicles from the abdomen to the scrotum.	
e. With growth hormone, observe for increased skeletal growth and development.	Indicated by appropriate increases in height and weight
f. With antidiuretics (desmopressin, lypressin, and vaso-pressin), observe for decreased urine output, increased urine-specific gravity, decreased signs of dehydration, decreased thirst.	These effects indicate control of diabetes insipidus.
g. With oxytocin given to induce labor, observe for the beginning or the intensifying of uterine contractions.	
h. With oxytocin given to control postpartum bleeding, observe for a firm uterine fundus and decreased vaginal bleeding.	
3. Observe for adverse effects	
a. With gonadorelin, observe for headache, nausea, lightheadedness, and local edema, pain and pruritus after subcutaneous injections.	Systemic reactions occur infrequently.
b. With protirelin, observe for hypotension, nausea, headache, lightheadedness, anxiety, drowsiness.	Although adverse effects occur in about 50% of patients, they are usually minor and of short duration.
c. With corticotropin, observe for sodium and fluid retention, edema, hypokalemia, hyperglycemia, osteoporosis, increased susceptibility to infection, myopathy, behavioral changes.	These adverse reactions are generally the same as those produced by adrenal cortex hormones. Severity of adverse reactions tends to increase with dosage and duration of corticotropin administration.
d. With human chorionic gonadotropin given to preadolescent boys, observe for sexual precocity, breast enlargement, and edema.	Sexual precocity results from stimulation of excessive testosterone secretion at an early age.
e. With growth hormone, observe for mild edema, headache, localized muscle pain, weakness, hyperglycemia.	Adverse effects are not common. Another adverse effect may be development of antibodies to the drug, but this does not prevent its growth-stimulating effects.
f. With menotropins, observe for symptoms of ovarian hyperstimulation, such as abdominal discomfort, weight gain, ascites, pleural effusion, oliguria, and hypotension.	Adverse effects can be minimized by frequent pelvic examinations to check for ovarian enlargement and by laboratory measurement of estrogen levels. Multiple gestation (mostly twins) is a possibility and is related to ovarian overstimulation.
g. With desmopressin, observe for headache, nasal congestion, nausea, and occasionally a slight increase in blood pressure. A more serious adverse reaction is water retention and hyponatremia.	Adverse reactions usually occur only with high dosages and tend to be relatively mild. Water intoxication (headache, nausea, vomiting, confusion, lethargy, coma, convulsions) may occur with any antidiuretic therapy if excessive fluids are ingested.
h. With lypressin, observe for headache and congestion of nasal passages, dyspnea and coughing (if the drug is inhaled), and water intoxication if excessive amounts of lypressin or fluid are taken.	Adverse effects are usually mild and occur infrequently with usual doses.
i. With vasopressin, observe for water intoxication; allergic reactions; chest pain, myocardial infarction, increased blood pressure; abdominal cramps, nausea, and diarrhea.	Adverse reactions to vasopressin are likely to be more widespread and to occur more often than reactions to the synthetic agents, desmopressin and lypressin. With high doses,

Nursing Actions	*Rationale/Explanation*
	vasopressin constricts blood vessels, especially coronary arteries, and stimulates smooth muscle of the gastrointestinal tract. Special caution is necessary in clients with heart disease, asthma, or epilepsy.
j. With oxytocin, observe for excessive stimulation or contractility of the uterus, uterine rupture, and cervical and perineal lacerations.	Severe adverse reactions are most likely to occur when oxytocin is given to induce labor and delivery.
4. Observe for drug interactions **a.** Drugs that *decrease* effects of protirelin (*i.e.,* TSH response): Aspirin (2 g or more per day), glucocorticoids (pharmacologic doses), levodopa, thyroid hormones	
b. Drugs that *increase* effects of vasopressin:	
(1) General anesthetics, chlorpropamide (Diabinese)	Potentiate vasopressin
(2) Ganglionic blocking agents (*e.g.,* trimethaphan [Arfonad])	Markedly increase the pressor effects of vasopressin
c. Drugs that *decrease* effects of vasopressin:	
Lithium	Inhibits the renal tubular reabsorption of water normally stimulated by vasopressin
d. Drugs that *increase* effects of oxytocin:	
(1) Estrogens	With adequate estrogen levels, oxytocin increases uterine contractility. When estrogen levels are low, the effect of oxytocin is reduced.
(2) Vasoconstrictors or vasopressors (*e.g.,* ephedrine, epinephrine, norepinephrine)	Severe, persistent hypertension with rupture of cerebral blood vessels may occur because of additive vasoconstrictor effects. This is a potentially lethal interaction and should be avoided.
5. Teach clients **a.** Take the drug as directed.	To increase therapeutic effects and decrease potentially serious adverse reactions
b. Report adverse effects.	The drug may need to be discontinued or reduced in dosage.
c. With corticotropin:	
(1) Follow a low-sodium, high-potassium diet.	To decrease sodium retention and potassium loss
(2) Weigh regularly.	Weight gain may indicate fluid retention. Edema may occur.
(3) Avoid exposure to infections, when possible.	Corticotropin increases susceptibility to infections.
(4) Follow instructions when the drug is being discontinued.	Corticotropin is gradually reduced in dosage to avoid symptoms such as fatigue, muscle weakness, and hypotension, which may occur with abrupt withdrawal.
(5) Test urine for glycosuria.	This is probably not indicated for all clients but may be helpful in those who have family histories of diabetes mellitus or who are obese. Corticotropin may cause hyperglycemia, activate latent diabetes mellitus, or aggravate existing diabetes mellitus.
d. With antidiuretics:	
(1) Reduce fluid intake when starting an antidiuretic drug.	To avoid water intoxication
(2) Regulate dosage in accordance with physician's instructions and with occurrence of excessive urination and thirst.	The purpose of the drugs is to control symptoms of diabetes insipidus. The amount of drug necessary to achieve this purpose varies among clients.

REVIEW AND APPLICATION EXERCISES

1. What hormones are secreted by the hypothalamus and pituitary, and what are their functions?

2. What are the functions and clinical uses of ADH, growth hormone, and oxytocin?

3. What are adverse effects of the hypothalamic and pituitary hormones used in clinical practice?

SELECTED REFERENCES

Ascoli, M. & Segaloff, D.L. (1996). Adenohypophyseal hormones and their hypothalamic releasing factors. In J.G. Hardman, L.E. Limbird, P.B. Molinoff, & R.W. Ruddon (Eds.), *Goodman & Gilman's The pharmacological basis of therapeutics*, 9th ed., pp. 1363–1382. New York: McGraw-Hill.

Drug facts and comparisons. (1996). St. Louis: Facts and Comparisons.

Guyton, A.C. & Hall. J.E. (1996). *Textbook of medical physiology*, 9th ed. Philadelphia: W.B. Saunders.

Porth, C.M. (1994). *Pathophysiology: Concepts of altered health states*, 4th ed. Philadelphia: J.B. Lippincott.

24

Corticosteroids

Objectives

After studying this chapter, the student will be able to:

1 Review physiologic effects of endogenous corticosteroids.

2 List at least five clinical indications for use of exogenous corticosteroids.

3 Differentiate between physiologic and pharmacologic doses of corticosteroids.

4 Differentiate between short-term and long-term corticosteroid therapy.

5 List at least ten adverse effects of long-term corticosteroid therapy.

6 Explain the pathophysiologic basis of adverse effects.

7 State the rationale for giving corticosteroids topically when possible rather than systemically.

8 Use other drugs and interventions to decrease the need for corticosteroids.

9 Apply the nursing process with a client receiving long-term systemic corticosteroid therapy, including teaching needs.

Key Terms

Addison's disease

Adrenocortical insufficiency

Cushing's disease

Glucocorticoid

Hyperglycemia

Immunosuppressive

Mineralocorticoid

Osteoporosis

Corticosteroids, also called glucocorticoids or steroids, are hormones produced by the adrenal cortex. These hormones are extremely important in maintaining homeostasis when secreted in normal amounts. Disease results from inadequate or excessive secretion. Exogenous corticosteroids are used as drugs in a variety of endocrine and nonendocrine disorders. Few drug groups produce such profound therapeutic or adverse effects as the corticosteroids. Consequently, their use must be carefully regulated and their effects closely monitored. To understand the effects of corticosteroids used as drugs, one needs to understand physiologic effects and other characteristics of the endogenous hormones.

Endogenous Corticosteroids

The adrenal cortex produces about 30 steroid hormones, which are divided into glucocorticoids, mineralocorticoids, and adrenal sex hormones. Glucocorticoids have important roles in inflammatory and immune responses and in the metabolism of carbohydrates, proteins, and fats. Mineralocorticoids are important in maintaining fluid and electrolyte balance. The adrenal sex hormones are secreted in small amounts and are considered relatively unimportant in normal body function.

Chemically, all corticosteroids are derived from cholesterol and have similar chemical formulas. Despite their similarities, however, very slight differences in structure cause them to have different functions.

SECRETION OF CORTICOSTEROIDS

Corticosteroid secretion is controlled by the hypothalamus, anterior pituitary, and adrenal cortex (the hypothalamic-pituitary-adrenal, or HPA, axis). Various stimuli (*e.g.,* low plasma levels of corticosteroids, pain, anxiety, trauma, illness, anesthesia) activate the system. These stimuli cause the hypothalamus to secrete corticotropin-releasing hormone (CRH). CRH stimulates the anterior pituitary to secrete corticotropin, and corticotropin stimulates the adrenal cortex to secrete corticosteroids.

The rate of corticosteroid secretion is usually maintained within relatively narrow limits but changes according to need. When plasma corticosteroid levels rise to an adequate level, secretion of corticosteroids slows or stops. The mechanism by which the hypothalamus and anterior pituitary are informed that no more corticosteroids are currently needed is called a *negative feedback mechanism.*

This negative feedback mechanism is normally very important, but it does not work during stress responses. The stress response activates the sympathetic nervous system (SNS) to produce more epinephrine and norepinephrine and the adrenal cortex to produce as much as ten times the normal amount of cortisol. The synergistic interaction of these hormones increases the person's ability to respond to stress. However, the increased SNS activity continues to stimulate cortisol production and overrules or inhibits the negative feedback mechanism. Excessive and prolonged corticosteroid secretion damages body tissues.

Corticosteroids are secreted directly into the bloodstream and have a plasma half-life of about 1½ h. They are metabolized in the liver. Most metabolites (about 75%) are excreted in the urine, the remainder in bile and feces. Major secretory products can be measured in the urine.

Metabolism is slowed by severe hepatic disease, and excretion is slowed by renal disease. In these conditions, corticosteroids may accumulate and cause signs and symptoms of hypercorticism.

GLUCOCORTICOIDS

The term *corticosteroids* actually means all secretions of the adrenal cortex, but it is most often used to designate the glucocorticoids. Glucocorticoids include cortisol, corticosterone, and cortisone. *Cortisol* accounts for at least 95% of glucocorticoid activity, and about 15 to 25 mg are secreted daily. Corticosterone has a small amount of activity, and about 1.5 to 4 mg are secreted daily. *Cortisone* has little activity and is secreted in minute quantities. *Glucocorticoids* are secreted cyclically, with the largest amount being produced in the early morning and the smallest amount during the evening hours (in people with a normal day–night schedule). At the cellular level, glucocorticoids account for most of the effects ascribed to the corticosteroids as a group, including the following:

1. Effects on carbohydrate metabolism
   a. **Stimulated formation of glucose (gluconeogenesis) by causing the breakdown of protein into amino acids.** The amino acids are then transported to the liver, where they are acted on by enzymes that convert them to glucose. The glucose is then returned to the circulation for use by body tissues or storage in the liver as glycogen.
   b. **Moderate decrease in cell use of glucose,** especially in muscle cells. This is attributed to a decreased effect of insulin on the proteins that normally transport glucose into cells and by decreased numbers and functional capacity of insulin receptors.
   c. Both the increased production and decreased use of glucose promote higher levels of glucose in the blood (hyperglycemia) and may lead to diabetes mellitus. These actions also increase the amount

of glucose stored as glycogen in the liver, skeletal muscles, and other tissues.

2. Effects on protein metabolism
   a. **Increased breakdown of protein into amino acids** (catabolic effect). They further increase the rate at which amino acids are transported to the liver and converted into glucose.
   b. **Decreased rate at which new proteins are formed** from dietary and other amino acids (antianabolic effect).
   c. Both the increased breakdown of cell protein and decreased protein synthesis produce protein depletion in virtually all body cells except those of the liver. Thus, glycogen stores in the body are increased, whereas protein stores are decreased.

3. Effects on lipid metabolism
   a. **Increased breakdown of adipose tissue into fatty acids** in much the same way as they increase catabolism of protein into amino acids. These fatty acids are transported in the plasma and used as a source of energy by body cells.
   b. **Stimulated oxidation of fatty acids within body cells.**

4. Effects on inflammatory and immune responses
   a. **Suppressed inflammatory response.** Inflammation is the normal bodily response to tissue damage and involves three stages. First, a large amount of plasma-like fluid leaks out of capillaries into the damaged area and becomes clotted. Second, leukocytes migrate into the area. Third, tissue healing occurs, largely by growth of fibrous scar tissue. Normal or physiologic amounts of glucocorticoids probably do not significantly affect inflammation and healing, but large amounts of glucocorticoids inhibit all three stages of the inflammatory process.

      More specifically, corticosteroids stabilize lysosomal membranes (and thereby prevent the release of inflammatory proteolytic enzymes), decrease capillary permeability (and thereby decrease leakage of fluid and proteins into the damaged tissue), inhibit the accumulation of neutrophils and macrophages at sites of inflammation (and thereby impair phagocytosis of pathogenic microorganisms and waste products of cellular metabolism), and inhibit production of inflammatory chemicals, such as interleukin-1, prostaglandins, and leukotrienes, by injured cells.
   b. **Suppressed immune response.** The immune system normally protects the body from foreign invaders, and several immune responses overlap inflammatory responses, including phagocytosis. In addition, the immune response stimulates the production of antibodies and activated lymphocytes to destroy the foreign substance. Glucocorticoids impair protein synthesis, including the production of antibodies; decrease the numbers of circulating lymphocytes, eosinophils, and macrophages; and decrease amounts of lymphoid tissue. These effects influence immune and allergic responses and help to account for the immunosuppressive and antiallergic actions of the glucocorticoids.

5. Effects on the nervous system
   a. Physiologic levels help to *maintain normal nerve excitability*; increased or pharmacologic amounts decrease nerve excitability, slow activity in the cerebral cortex, and alter brain wave patterns.
   b. **Suppressed secretion of CRH by the hypothalamus and of corticotropin by the anterior pituitary gland.** This results in suppression of further glucocorticoid secretion by the adrenal cortex.

6. Effects on the musculoskeletal system
   a. **Maintenance of muscle strength** when present in physiologic amounts but muscle atrophy (from protein breakdown) when present in excessive amounts.
   b. **Inhibition of bone formation and growth and increased bone breakdown.** Glucocorticoids also decrease intestinal absorption and increase renal excretion of calcium. These effects contribute to bone demineralization (osteoporosis) in adults and to decreased linear growth in children.

7. Effects on the respiratory system
   a. **Maintenance of open airways.** Glucocorticoids do not have direct bronchodilating effects, but they probably help to maintain responsiveness to the bronchodilating effects of endogenous catecholamines, such as epinephrine.
   b. **Stabilize mast cells** and other cells to inhibit the release of bronchoconstrictive and inflammatory substances, such as histamine.

8. Effects on the gastrointestinal system
   a. **Decreased viscosity of gastric mucus.** This effect may decrease protective properties of the mucus and contribute to the development of peptic ulcer disease.

9. Effects on fluid and electrolyte balance
   a. **Retention of sodium and water.**
   b. **Excretion of potassium and calcium.**

MINERALOCORTICOIDS

Mineralocorticoids play a vital role in maintaining fluid and electrolyte balance. *Aldosterone* is the main mineralocorticoid and is responsible for about 90% of mineralocorticoid activity. Characteristics and physiologic effects of aldosterone include the following:

1. The overall physiologic effects are to conserve sodium and water and eliminate potassium. Aldosterone increases sodium reabsorption from kidney

tubules, and water is reabsorbed along with the sodium. When sodium is conserved, another cation must be excreted to maintain electrical neutrality of body fluids; thus, potassium is excreted. This is the only potent mechanism for controlling the concentration of potassium ions in extracellular fluids.

2. Secretion of aldosterone is controlled by several factors, most of which are related to kidney function. Generally, secretion is increased when the potassium level of extracellular fluid is high, the sodium level of extracellular fluid is low, the renin-angiotensin system of the kidneys is activated, or the anterior pituitary gland secretes corticotropin.

3. Inadequate secretion of aldosterone causes hyperkalemia, hyponatremia, and extracellular fluid volume deficit (dehydration). Hypotension and shock may result from decreased cardiac output. Absence of mineralocorticoids causes death.

4. Excessive secretion of aldosterone produces hypokalemia, hypernatremia, and extracellular fluid volume excess (water intoxication). Edema and hypertension may result.

ADRENAL SEX HORMONES

The adrenal cortex secretes male (androgens) and female (estrogens and progesterone) sex hormones. The adrenal sex hormones are insignificant compared with those produced by the testes and ovaries. Adrenal androgens, secreted continuously in small quantities by both men and women, are responsible for most of the physiologic effects exerted by the adrenal sex hormones. They increase protein synthesis (anabolism), which increases the mass and strength of muscle and bone tissue; they affect development of male secondary sex characteristics; and they increase hair growth and libido in women. Excessive secretion of adrenal androgens in women causes masculinizing effects (*e.g.,* hirsutism, acne, breast atrophy, deepening of the voice, and amenorrhea). Female sex hormones are secreted in small amounts and normally exert few physiologic effects. Excessive secretion may produce feminizing effects in men (*e.g.,* breast enlargement, decreased hair growth, voice changes).

Disorders of the Adrenal Cortex

Disorders of the adrenal cortex involve increased or decreased production of corticosteroids, especially cortisol as the primary glucocorticoid and aldosterone as the primary mineralocorticoid. These disorders include:

1. **Primary adrenocortical insufficiency (Addison's disease)** is associated with destruction of the adrenal cortex by disorders such as tuberculosis, cancer, or hemorrhage; with atrophy of the adrenal cortex caused by autoimmune disease or excessive and prolonged administration of exogenous corticosteroids; and with surgical excision of the adrenal glands. In this condition, there is inadequate production of both cortisol and aldosterone.

2. **Secondary adrenocortical insufficiency,** produced by inadequate secretion of corticotropin, is most often caused by prolonged administration of corticosteroids. This condition is largely a glucocorticoid deficiency. Mineralocorticoid secretion is not significantly impaired.

3. **Congenital adrenogenital syndromes and adrenal hyperplasia** result from deficiencies in one or more enzymes required for cortisol production. Low plasma levels of cortisol lead to excessive corticotropin secretion, which then leads to excessive adrenal secretion of androgens and hyperplasia.

4. **Androgen-producing tumors** of the adrenal cortex, which are usually benign, produce masculinizing effects.

5. **Adrenocortical hyperfunction** (Cushing's disease) may result from excessive corticotropin or a primary adrenal tumor. Adrenal tumors may be benign or malignant. Benign tumors often produce one corticosteroid normally secreted by the adrenal cortex, but malignant tumors often secrete several corticosteroids.

6. **Hyperaldosteronism** is a rare disorder caused by adenoma or hyperplasia of the adrenal cortex cells that produce aldosterone. It is characterized by hypokalemia, hypernatremia, hypertension, thirst, and polyuria.

Exogenous Corticosteroids (Glucocorticoids)

When corticosteroids are administered from sources outside the body, they are given for replacement, therapeutic, or diagnostic purposes. When given to replace or substitute for the endogenous hormones, they are given in relatively small doses to correct a deficiency state, and their purpose is to restore normal function. When given for therapeutic purposes, they are given in relatively large doses to exert pharmacologic effects. Drug effects involve extension of the physiologic effects of endogenous corticosteroids and new effects that do not occur with small, physiologic doses. The most frequently desired effects are antiinflammatory, immunosuppressive, antiallergic, and antistress. These are glucocorticoid effects. Mineralocorticoid and androgenic effects are usually considered adverse reactions.

All adrenal corticosteroids are commercially available for use as drugs, as are many synthetic derivatives.

The newer corticosteroids have been developed by chemically altering the basic steroid molecule in efforts to increase therapeutic effects while minimizing adverse effects. These efforts have been most successful in decreasing mineralocorticoid activity. Despite considerable progress, however, synthetic corticosteroids can produce all the adverse reactions associated with the natural corticosteroids.

Exogenous corticosteroids are palliative. They control many symptoms but do not cure the underlying disease process. In chronic disorders, for example, they may enable a client to continue the usual activities of daily living and delay disability. However, the disease may continue to progress. Long-term use of corticosteroids inevitably produces adverse effects.

Exogenous corticosteroids have widely different actions on body tissues and fluids, so a specific effect may be considered therapeutic in one client but adverse in another. For example, an increased blood sugar level is therapeutic for the client with adrenocortical insufficiency or an islet cell adenoma of the pancreas, but this is an adverse reaction for most clients, especially for those with diabetes mellitus. In addition, some clients respond more favorably or develop adverse reactions more readily than others taking equivalent doses. This is partially caused by individual differences in the rate at which corticosteroids are metabolized.

Administration of exogenous corticosteroids suppresses the HPA axis. This decreases secretion of corticotropin, which, in turn, causes atrophy of the adrenal cortex and decreased production of endogenous adrenal corticosteroids. Daily administration of physiologic doses (about 20 mg of hydrocortisone or its equivalent) or administration of pharmacologic doses (more than 20 mg of hydrocortisone or its equivalent) for about 2 weeks suppresses the HPA axis. Recovery may take 6 months or longer after corticosteroids are discontinued. During that time, supplemental corticosteroids are usually needed during stressful situations (*e.g.*, fever, illness, surgical procedures) to improve the client's ability to respond to stress and prevent acute adrenocortical insufficiency.

Hydrocortisone, the exogenous equivalent of endogenous cortisol, is the prototype of corticosteroid drugs. When a new corticosteroid is developed, it is compared with hydrocortisone to determine its potency in producing anti-inflammatory and antiallergic responses, increasing deposition of liver glycogen, and suppressing secretion of corticotropin.

Exogenous mineralocorticoid drugs are infrequently used for therapeutic purposes. Even with adrenocortical insufficiency in Addison's disease or adrenalectomy, many physicians prefer to use a glucocorticoid with high mineralocorticoid activity rather than separate drugs.

MECHANISMS OF ACTION AND OTHER CHARACTERISTICS OF GLUCOCORTICOID DRUGS

Glucocorticoids are the largest subgroup of corticosteroids and they account for almost all clinical usage of corticosteroid drugs. Specific characteristics of the glucocorticoids include the following:

1. Like endogenous glucocorticoids, exogenous drug molecules act at the cellular level by binding to glucocorticoid receptors in target tissues. The receptors are small proteins located in intracellular cytoplasm. The drug-receptor complex then moves to the cell nucleus where it influences genetically controlled aspects of cellular synthesis. Because the genes vary in different types of body cells, glucocorticoid effects also vary, depending on the specific cells being targeted.
2. Pharmacologic effects sought from glucocorticoid drugs are largely antiallergic, anti-inflammatory, antistress, and immunosuppressive. The mechanisms by which glucocorticoids produce these effects are not clearly understood but may include:
   a. Strengthening or stabilizing biologic membranes. This inhibits capillary permeability and thus prevents leakage of fluid into the injured area and development of edema. It further inhibits release of bradykinin, histamine, lysosomal enzymes, and perhaps other substances that normally cause vasodilation and tissue irritation.
   b. Impaired ability of phagocytic cells to migrate into the injured area from the blood
   c. Interference with lymphocyte function and antibody production
   d. Shrinkage of lymphoid tissues
   e. Decreased growth of new capillaries, fibroblasts, and collagen
3. Important differences among glucocorticoid drugs are duration of action, relative glucocorticoid potency, and relative mineralocorticoid potency. Anti-inflammatory potency of the various glucocorticoids is approximately equal when the drugs are given in equivalent doses. Mineralocorticoid activity is intermediate to high in the older drugs, cortisone and hydrocortisone, and low in newer agents.
4. Many glucocorticoid preparations are available for use in different clinical problems, and routes of administration vary. Several of these drugs can be given by more than one route; others can be given only orally or topically. For intramuscular (IM) or intravenous (IV) injections, sodium phosphate or sodium succinate salts are used because they are most soluble in water. For intra-articular or intralesional injections, acetate salts are used because they have low solubility in water and provide prolonged local action.

INDICATIONS FOR USE

Corticosteroids are used to treat many different disorders that have few characteristics in common and produce a vast array of clinical signs and symptoms. Corticosteroid preparations applied topically in ophthalmic and dermatologic disorders are discussed in Chapters 65 and 66, respectively. The corticosteroids discussed in this chapter (Table 24-1) are primarily those given systemically, topically to nasal and oral mucosa, or by local injection in potentially serious or disabling disorders. These disorders are as follows:

1. **Allergic** disorders, such as allergic reactions to drugs, serum and blood transfusions, and dermatoses with an allergic component
2. **Collagen** disorders, such as systemic lupus erythematosus, scleroderma, and periarteritis nodosa. Collagen is the basic structural protein of connective tissue, tendons, cartilage, and bone, and it is therefore present in almost all body tissues and organ systems. The collagen disorders are characterized by inflammation of various body tissues. Signs and symptoms depend on which body tissues or organs are affected and the severity of the inflammatory process.
3. **Dermatologic** disorders, such as pemphigus, exfoliative dermatitis, and severe psoriasis
4. **Endocrine** disorders, such as adrenocortical insufficiency and congenital adrenal hyperplasia. Corticosteroids are given to replace or substitute for the natural hormones (both glucocorticoids and mineralocorticoids) in cases of insufficiency and to suppress corticotropin when excess secretion causes adrenal hyperplasia. These conditions are rare and account for only a small percentage of corticosteroid usage.

(text continues on page 283)

TABLE 24-1 **CORTICOSTEROIDS***

Generic/Trade Name	Routes and Dosage Ranges	Anti-inflammatory Dose Equivalent to 20 mg of Hydrocortisone (mg)	Mineralocorticoid Activity	Duration of Action (h)
Glucocorticoids				
Beclomethasone Oral inhalation (Beclovent, Vanceril)	*Adults:* 2 oral inhalations (84 μg) 3–4 times daily (maximal daily dose is 20 inhalations or 840 μg) *Children 6–12 y:* 1–3 oral inhalations (42–84 μg) 3–4 times daily (maximal daily dose is 10 inhalations or 420 μg)			
Nasal inhalation (Beconase, Vancenase)	*Adults and children 12 y or older:* 1 nasal inhalation (42 μg) in each nostril 2–4 times daily (total dose 168–336 μg/d) *Children 6–12 y:* 1 nasal inhalation in each nostril 3 times daily (252 μg/d) *Children <6 y:* Not recommended			
Betamethasone (Celestone)	*Adults:* PO 6–7.2 mg daily initially, depending on the disease being treated, gradually reduced to lowest effective maintenance dose	0.6	Low	48
Betamethasone acetate and sodium phosphate (Celestone Soluspan)	*Adults:* IM 1–2 ml (3–6 mg each of betamethasone acetate and betamethasone phosphate) Intra-articular injection 0.25–2 ml Soft-tissue injection 0.25–1.0 ml			
Budesonide (Rhinocort) Nasal inhalation	*Adults and children 6 y and older:* Initially 256 μg daily (2 sprays each nostril morning and evening or 4 sprays each nostril every morning). When symptoms are controlled, reduce dosage to lowest effective maintenance dose.			

TABLE 24-1   **CORTICOSTEROIDS*** (Continued)

Generic/Trade Name	Routes and Dosage Ranges	Anti-inflammatory Dose Equivalent to 20 mg of Hydrocortisone (mg)	Mineralocorticoid Activity	Duration of Action (h)
Cortisone (Cortone)	Chronic adrenocortical insufficiency, PO 15–30 mg daily Congenital adrenal hyperplasia, PO 15–50 mg daily Anti-inflammatory effects, PO 25–50 mg daily for mild, chronic disorders; 125–300 mg daily in 4 or more doses for acute, life-threatening disease Anti-inflammatory effects, IM 75–300 mg daily for serious disease	25	High	12
Dexamethasone (Decadron)	PO 0.75–9 mg daily in 2–4 doses. Dosages in higher ranges are used for serious disease (leukemia, pemphigus)	0.75	Low	48
Dexamethasone acetate	IM 8–16 mg (1–2 ml) in single dose, repeated every 1–3 wk if necessary Intralesional 0.8–1.6 mg (0.1–0.2 ml) Intra-articular or soft-tissue injection, 4–16 mg (0.5–2 ml), repeated every 1–3 wk if necessary			
Dexamethasone sodium phosphate	IM, IV 0.5–9 mg, depending on severity of the disease Intra-articular, soft-tissue injection 0.2–6 mg, depending on size of affected area or joint			
(Decadron Turbinaire)	Intranasal, 2 sprays in each nostril 2–3 times daily			
(Decadron Respihaler)	2–3 inhalations 3–4 times daily			
Dexamethasone/ lidocaine (Decadron with Xylocaine)	Soft-tissue injection, 0.5–0.75 ml			
Flunisolide Oral inhalation (Aerobid) Nasal inhalation (Nasalide)	*Adults:* 2 oral inhalations (500 µg) twice daily *Children 6–15 y:* Same as adults *Adults:* 2 sprays (50 µg) in each nostril 2 times daily (total dose 200 µg/d); maximal daily dose is 8 sprays in each nostril (400 µg/d) *Children 6–14 y:* 1 spray (25 µg) in each nostril 3 times daily or 2 sprays (50 µg) in each nostril 2 times daily (total dose 150–200 µg/d); maximal daily dose 4 sprays in each nostril (200 µg/d)			
Fluticasone (Flonase) Nasal inhalation	*Adults:* Initially 200 µg daily (2 sprays each nostril once daily or 1 spray each nostril twice daily). After a few days, reduce dosage to 100 µg daily (1 spray each nostril once daily) for maintenance therapy. *Adolescents 12 y and older:* 100 µg daily (1 spray per nostril once daily)			

(continued)

TABLE 24-1 CORTICOSTEROIDS* (Continued)

Generic/Trade Name	Routes and Dosage Ranges	Anti-inflammatory Dose Equivalent to 20 mg of Hydrocortisone (mg)	Mineralocorticoid Activity	Duration of Action (h)
Hydrocortisone (Hydrocortone, Cortef)	Chronic adrenocortical insufficiency, PO 10–20 mg daily in 3–4 doses Chronic nonfatal diseases, PO 20–40 mg daily in 3–4 doses Congenital adrenal hyperplasia, PO 10–30 mg daily in 3–4 doses Chronic, potentially fatal diseases, PO 60–120 mg daily in 3–4 doses Acute, nonfatal diseases, PO 60–120 mg daily in 3–4 doses Acute life-threatening diseases, PO 100–240 mg daily in at least 4 divided doses Disorders other than shock, IV 100–500 mg initially, repeated if necessary Intra-articular injections, 5–50 mg depending on size of joint Soft-tissue injection, 25–75 mg Rectally, one enema (100 mg) nightly for 21 d or until optimal response is obtained	20	Intermediate	18
Methylprednisolone (Medrol) **Methylprednisolone sodium succinate** (Solu-Medrol)	PO 4–48 mg daily initially, gradually reduced to lowest effective level IM 40–120 mg as needed IV 100–250 mg q4–6h for shock; 10–40 mg as needed for other conditions Intra-articular and soft-tissue injection, 4–80 mg as needed, depending on size of the affected area Intralesional injection, 20–60 mg Rectally, 40 mg as retention enema 3–7 times weekly for 2 or more wk	4	Low	18–36
Prednisolone (Sterane, Delta-Cortef) **Prednisolone acetate** (Fernisolone, others) **Prednisolone sodium phosphate** (Hydeltrasol) **Prednisolone sodium succinate** (Meticortelone soluble)	PO 5–60 mg daily initially, adjusted for maintenance IM 4–60 mg daily initially, adjusted for maintenance Intra-articular or soft-tissue injection, 4–60 mg daily, depending on the disease IM 4–60 mg daily initially, adjusted for maintenance Emergencies, IV 20–100 mg, repeated if necessary, to a maximal daily dose of 400 mg. When the client's condition improves, 10–20 mg in single doses may be given. Intra-articular or soft-tissue injection, 2–30 mg from once every 3–5 d to once every 2–3 wk IM 4–60 mg daily initially, adjusted for maintenance Emergencies, IV 20–100 mg, repeated if necessary to a maximal daily dose of 480 mg. When the client's condition	5	Intermediate	18–36

TABLE 24-1   CORTICOSTEROIDS* (Continued)

Generic/Trade Name	Routes and Dosage Ranges	Anti-inflammatory Dose Equivalent to 20 mg of Hydrocortisone (mg)	Mineralocorticoid Activity	Duration of Action (h)
	improves, 10–20 mg in single doses may be given.			
Prednisolone tebutate (Hydeltra-TBA)	Intra-articular or soft-tissue injection, 4–60 mg daily, depending on the disease			
Prednisone (Deltasone)	PO 5–60 mg daily initially, reduced for maintenance	5	Intermediate	18–30
Triamcinolone (Aristocort, Kenacort)	PO 4–48 mg daily initially; dosage reduced for maintenance	4	Low	18–36
Triamcinolone acetonide (Kenalog-40)	IM (deep) 2.5–60 mg daily, depending on the disease. When the client's condition improves, dosage should be reduced and oral therapy instituted when feasible			
	Intra-articular or intrabursal injection, 2.5–15 mg every 1–8 wk depending on the size of the joint and the disease being treated			
	Soft-tissue injection, 5–48 mg			
Oral inhalation (Azmacort)	*Adults:* 2 oral inhalations (200 µg) 3 times daily *Children:* 1–2 oral inhalations (100–200 µg) 3 times daily			
Nasal inhalation (Nasacort)	*Adults and children >12 y:* 2 sprays (110 µg) in each nostril once daily (total dose 220 µg/d). May increase to maximal daily dose of 440 µg.			
Triamcinolone diacetate (Aristocort diacetate, Kenacort diacetate)	PO 4–48 mg daily initially; dosage reduced for maintenance IM (deep) 20–80 mg initially Intra-articular injection, 2.5–80 mg every 1–8 wk, depending on size of joint or affected area Soft-tissue injection, 5–48 mg			
Triamcinolone hexacetonide (Aristospan)	Intra-articular injection, 2.5–80 mg every 1–8 wk, depending on size of joint or affected area			
Mineralocorticoid				
Fludrocortisone (Florinef)	Chronic adrenocortical insufficiency, PO 0.05–0.1 mg daily Salt-losing adrenogenital syndromes, PO 0.1–0.2 mg daily			

*Ophthalmic and dermatologic preparations are discussed in Chapters 65 and 66, respectively

5. **Gastrointestinal** disorders, such as ulcerative colitis and regional enteritis (Crohn's disease)
6. **Hematologic** disorders, such as idiopathic thrombocytopenic purpura or acquired hemolytic anemia
7. **Liver** disorders characterized by edema, such as cirrhosis and ascites

8. **Neoplastic** disease, such as acute and chronic leukemias, Hodgkin's disease, other lymphomas, and multiple myeloma. The effectiveness of corticosteroids in these conditions probably stems from their ability to suppress lymphocytes and other lymphoid tissue.

9. **Neurologic** conditions, such as cerebral edema, brain tumor, and myasthenia gravis

10. **Ophthalmic** disorders, such as optic neuritis, sympathetic ophthalmia, and chorioretinitis

11. **Organ or tissue transplants and grafts** (*e.g.,* kidney, heart, bone marrow). Corticosteroids suppress cellular and humoral immune responses (see Chap. 42) and help prevent rejection of transplanted tissue. Drug therapy is continued as long as the transplanted tissue is in place (usually lifelong).

12. **Renal** disorders characterized by edema, such as the nephrotic syndrome

13. **Respiratory** disorders, such as asthma, status asthmaticus, chronic obstructive pulmonary disease (COPD), and inflammatory disorders of nasal mucosa (rhinitis). In asthma, corticosteroids increase the number of beta-adrenergic receptors and increase or restore responsiveness of beta receptors to beta-adrenergic bronchodilating drugs. In asthma, COPD, and rhinitis, the drugs decrease mucus secretion and inflammation.

14. **Rheumatic** disorders, such as ankylosing spondylitis, acute and chronic bursitis, acute gouty arthritis, rheumatoid arthritis, and some types of osteoarthritis.

15. **Shock.** Corticosteroids are clearly indicated only for shock resulting from adrenocortical insufficiency (addisonian crisis); their use in other types of shock is controversial. Maximal levels of corticosteroids are already being produced in hemorrhagic or cardiogenic shock and in other forms of severe stress, and giving exogenous corticosteroids probably has little therapeutic effect. On the other hand, in anaphylactic shock resulting from an allergic reaction, corticosteroids may increase or restore cardiovascular responsiveness to adrenergic drugs.

CONTRAINDICATIONS FOR USE

Corticosteroids are contraindicated in systemic fungal infections and in people who are hypersensitive to drug formulations. They should be used with caution in clients at risk of infections (they may decrease resistance), clients with infections (they may mask signs and symptoms so that infections become more severe before they are recognized and treated), diabetes mellitus (they cause or increase hyperglycemia), peptic ulcer disease, inflammatory bowel disorders, hypertension, congestive heart failure, and renal insufficiency.

Nursing Process

Assessment Related to Initiation of Corticosteroid Therapy

- Each client should be thoroughly assessed before long-term, systemic corticosteroid therapy is initiated. Assessment may include diagnostic tests for diabetes mellitus, tuberculosis,

and peptic ulcer disease because these conditions may develop from or be exacerbated by administration of corticosteroid drugs. If one of these conditions is present, corticosteroid therapy must be altered and other drugs given concomitantly.

- If acute infection is found on initial assessment, it should be treated with appropriate antibiotics either before corticosteroid drugs are started or concomitantly with corticosteroid therapy. This is necessary because corticosteroids may mask symptoms of infection and impair healing. Thus, even minor infections can become serious if left untreated during corticosteroid therapy. If infection occurs during long-term corticosteroid therapy, appropriate antibiotic therapy (as determined by culture of the causative microorganism and antibiotic sensitivity studies) is again indicated. Also, increased doses of corticosteroids are usually indicated to cope with the added stress of the infection.

Assessment Related to Previous or Current Corticosteroid Therapy

Initial assessment of every client should include information about previous or current treatment with systemic corticosteroids. This can usually be determined by questioning the client or reviewing medical records.

- If the nurse determines that the client has taken corticosteroids in the past, additional information is needed about the specific drug and dosage taken, the purpose and length of therapy, and when therapy was stopped. Such information is necessary for planning nursing care. If the client had an acute illness and received an oral or injected corticosteroid for 1 to 2 weeks or received corticosteroids by local injection or application to skin lesions, no special nursing care is likely to be required. If, however, the client took systemic corticosteroids for more than 1 to 2 weeks during the past year (approximately), nursing observations must be especially vigilant. Such a client may be at higher risk for developing acute adrenocortical insufficiency during stressful situations. If the client is having surgery, corticosteroid therapy is restarted either before or on the day of surgery and continued, in decreasing dosage, for a few days after surgery. In addition to anesthesia and surgery, potentially significant sources of stress include hospitalization, various diagnostic tests, concurrent infection or other illnesses, and family problems.

- If the client is currently taking a systemic corticosteroid drug, again the nurse must identify the drug, the dosage and schedule of administration, the purpose for which the drug is being taken, and the length of time involved. Once this basic information is obtained, the nurse can further assess client status and plan nursing care. Some specific factors include the following:
  - If the client will undergo anesthesia and surgery, expect that higher doses of corticosteroids will be given for several days. This may be done by changing the drug, the route of administration, and the dosage. Specific regimens vary according to type of anesthesia, surgical procedure, client condition, physician preference, and other variables. A client having major abdominal surgery may be given 300 to 400 mg of hydrocortisone (or the equivalent dosage of other agents) on the day of surgery and then be tapered back to maintenance dosage within a few days.

- Note that additional corticosteroids may be given in other situations as well. One extra dose may be adequate for a short-term stress situation, such as an angiogram or other invasive diagnostic test.
- Using all available data, assess the likelihood of the client's having acute adrenal insufficiency (sometimes called adrenal crisis).
- Assess for signs and symptoms of adrenocortical excess (hypercorticism, Cushing's disease).
- Assess for signs and symptoms of the disease for which long-term corticosteroid therapy is being given.

Nursing Diagnoses

- Body Image Disturbance related to cushingoid changes in appearance
- Altered Nutrition: Less Than Body Requirements related to protein and potassium losses
- Altered Nutrition: More Than Body Requirements related to sodium and water retention and hyperglycemia
- Altered Tissue Perfusion related to atherosclerosis and hypertension
- Fluid Volume Excess related to sodium and water retention
- Risk for Injury related to adverse drug effects of impaired wound healing; increased susceptibility to infection; weakening of skin and muscles; osteoporosis, gastrointestinal ulceration, diabetes mellitus, hypertension, and acute adrenocortical insufficiency
- Ineffective Individual Coping related to chronic illness and long-term drug therapy
- Ineffective Individual Coping related to drug-induced mood changes, irritability, insomnia
- Knowledge Deficit related to disease process and corticosteroid drug therapy

Planning/Goals

The client will:

- Receive or take the drug correctly
- Receive and practice measures to decrease the need for corticosteroids and minimize adverse effects
- Be monitored regularly for adverse drug effects
- Keep appointments for follow-up care
- Be assisted to cope with body image changes
- Verbalize or demonstrate essential drug information

Interventions

Use supplementary drugs as ordered and nondrug measures to decrease dosage and side effects of corticosteroid drugs. Some specific measures include the following:

- Help clients to set reasonable goals of drug therapy. For example, partial relief of symptoms may be better than complete relief if the latter requires larger doses or longer periods of treatment with systemic drugs.
- In clients with bronchial asthma and COPD, bronchodilating drugs and other treatment measures should be continued during corticosteroid therapy.
- In clients with rheumatoid arthritis, rest, physical therapy, salicylates or other nonsteroid anti-inflammatory drugs, and local injections of corticosteroid drugs into joints when only one or two are involved are continued during systemic corticosteroid therapy.
- Help clients to identify stressors and to find ways to modify or avoid stressful situations when possible. For example,

most clients probably do not think of extreme heat or cold or minor infections as significant stressors. They can be, however, for people taking corticosteroid drugs. This assessment of potential stressors must be individualized because a situation viewed as stressful by one client may not be stressful to another.

- Encourage activity, if not contraindicated, to slow demineralization of bone (osteoporosis). This is especially important in postmenopausal women who are not taking replacement estrogens, because they are very susceptible to osteoporosis. Walking is preferred if the client is able. Range-of-motion exercises are indicated in immobilized or bedfast people. Also, bedfast clients taking corticosteroid drugs should have their positions changed frequently because these drugs thin the skin and increase the risk of pressure ulcers. This risk is further increased if edema also is present.
- Dietary changes may be beneficial in some clients. Salt restriction may help prevent hypernatremia, fluid retention, and edema. Foods high in potassium may help prevent hypokalemia. A diet high in protein, calcium, and vitamin D may help to prevent osteoporosis. Increased intake of vitamin C may help to decrease bleeding in the skin and soft tissues.
- Avoid exposing the client to potential sources of infection by washing hands frequently, using aseptic technique when changing dressings, keeping health care personnel and visitors with colds or other infections away from the client, and following other appropriate measures. Reverse or protective isolation of the client is sometimes indicated, commonly for those who have had organ transplants and are receiving corticosteroids to help prevent rejection of the transplanted organ.

 Teach clients on long-term systemic corticosteroid therapy to:

- Wear a special alert bracelet or tag or carry an identification card stating the drug being taken; the dosage; the physician's name, address, and telephone number; and instructions for emergency treatment. If an accident or emergency situation occurs, health care providers must know about corticosteroid drug therapy to give additional amounts during the stress of the emergency.
- Report to all health care providers consulted that corticosteroid drugs are being taken or have been taken within the past year. Current or previous corticosteroid therapy can influence treatment measures. Such knowledge increases the ability to provide appropriate treatment.
- Maintain regular medical supervision. This is extremely important so that the physician can detect adverse reactions, evaluate disease status, and evaluate drug response and indications for dosage change, as well as other responsibilities that can be carried out only with personal contact between the physician and the client. Periodic blood tests, x-ray studies, and other tests may be performed during long-term corticosteroid therapy.
- Take no other drugs, prescription or nonprescription, without notifying the physician who is supervising corticosteroid therapy. Corticosteroid drugs influence reactions to many other drugs, and many other drugs interact with corticosteroids to either increase or decrease their effects. Thus, taking other

drugs can decrease the expected therapeutic benefits or increase the incidence or severity of adverse reactions.

- Ask the physician about the amount and kind of activity or exercise needed. As a general rule, being as active as possible helps to prevent or delay osteoporosis, a common adverse reaction. However, increased activity may not be desirable for everyone. A client with rheumatoid arthritis, for example, may become too active when drug therapy relieves joint pain and increases mobility.
- Follow instructions for other measures used in treatment of the particular condition (*e.g.,* other drugs and physical therapy for rheumatoid arthritis). Such measures may allow smaller doses of corticosteroids, which are greatly to the client's advantage in decreasing adverse reactions.
- Recognize stress situations that necessitate increases in drug dosage. Clarify with the physician predictable sources of stress and the amount of drug to be taken if the stress cannot be avoided. This requires commitment and cooperation between the client and health care personnel. Close supervision is necessary, especially during the first few months of corticosteroid therapy. Common stresses include infections such as the common cold, extremes of heat or cold, surgical procedures, illness, or death of a family member. However, many stress situations are acute and unpredictable and elicit different responses from different clients.
- If diabetes mellitus results from corticosteroid therapy, teach the client as you would any other diabetic: that is, teach about drug therapy, diet, and blood glucose testing, and provide other necessary information.

Evaluation

- Interview and observe for relief of symptoms for which corticosteroids were prescribed.
- Interview and observe for accurate drug administration.
- Interview and observe for use of nondrug measures indicated for the condition being treated.
- Interview and observe for adverse drug effects on a regular basis.
- Interview regarding drug knowledge and effects to be reported to health care providers.

Principles of Therapy

RISK–BENEFIT FACTORS

1. Because corticosteroid drugs can cause serious adverse reactions, indications for their clinical use should be as clear-cut as possible. They are relatively safe for short-term treatment of self-limiting conditions, such as allergic reactions or acute exacerbations of chronic conditions. Long-term use of pharmacologic doses (more than 20 mg of hydrocortisone daily or its equivalent) produces adverse reactions. For this reason, long-term corticosteroid therapy should be reserved for life-threatening conditions or severe, disabling symptoms that do not respond to treatment with more benign drugs or other measures. Both physician and client should be convinced

that the anticipated benefits of long-term therapy are worth the risks.
2. The goal of corticosteroid therapy is usually to reduce symptoms to a tolerable level. Total suppression of symptoms is likely to require excessively large doses and produce excessive adverse effects.

DRUG SELECTION

Choice of corticosteroid drug is influenced by many factors, including the purpose for use, characteristics of specific drugs, desired route of administration, characteristics of individual clients, and expected side effects. Some guidelines for rational drug choice include the following:

1. **Adrenocortical insufficiency,** whether caused by Addison's disease, adrenalectomy, or inadequate corticotropin, requires replacement of both glucocorticoids and mineralocorticoids. Hydrocortisone and cortisone are usually the drugs of choice because they have greater mineralocorticoid activity compared with other corticosteroids. If additional mineralocorticoid activity is required, fludrocortisone is most convenient because it can be given orally.
2. **Nonendocrine disorders,** in which anti-inflammatory, antiallergic, antistress, and immunosuppressive effects are desired, can be treated by a corticosteroid drug with primarily glucocorticoid activity. Prednisone is often the glucocorticoid of choice. It has less mineralocorticoid activity than hydrocortisone and is less expensive than newer synthetic glucocorticoids.
3. **Respiratory disorders.** Beclomethasone (Vanceril), dexamethasone (Decadron), flunisolide (Aerobid), and triamcinolone (Azmacort) are corticosteroids formulated to be given by oral or nasal inhalation. Their use replaces, prevents, delays, or decreases use of systemic drugs and thereby decreases risks of serious adverse effects. Higher doses may suppress adrenocortical function.
4. **Cerebral edema** associated with brain tumors, craniotomy, or head injury. Dexamethasone (parenterally or orally) is considered the corticosteroid of choice because it is thought to penetrate the blood-brain barrier more readily and achieve higher concentrations in cerebrospinal fluids and tissues. It also has minimal sodium- and water-retaining properties. With brain tumors, the drug is more effective in metastatic lesions and glioblastomas than astrocytomas and meningiomas.
5. **Acute, life-threatening situations** require a drug that can be given parenterally, usually IV. This limits the choice of drugs because not all are available in injectable preparations. Hydrocortisone, dexamethasone, and methylprednisolone are among those that may be given parenterally.

DOSAGE FACTORS

Dosage of corticosteroid drugs is influenced by many factors, such as the specific drug to be given, the desired route of administration, the reason for use, expected adverse effects, and client characteristics. Generally, the smallest effective dose should be given for the shortest effective time. Dosage guidelines include the following:

1. Dosage must be individualized according to the severity of the disorder being treated, whether the disease is acute or chronic, and the client's response to drug therapy. If life-threatening disease is present, high doses are usually given until acute symptoms are brought under control. Then, dosage is gradually reduced until a maintenance dose is determined or the drug is discontinued. If the disease is not life-threatening, the physician may still choose to prescribe relatively high doses initially and reduce to maintenance doses or may choose to start with low doses and increase to a maintenance level.
2. Physiologic doses (about 20 mg of hydrocortisone or its equivalent daily) are given to replace or substitute for endogenous adrenocortical hormone. Pharmacologic doses (multiples of physiologic doses) are usually required for anti-inflammatory, antiallergic, antistress, and immunosuppressive effects.
3. New drugs are compared to hydrocortisone. They are more potent than hydrocortisone on a weight basis but are equipotent in anti-inflammatory effects when given in equivalent doses (see Table 24-1). Statements of equivalency with hydrocortisone are helpful in evaluating new drugs, comparing different drugs, and changing drugs or dosages. However, dosage equivalents generally apply only to drugs given orally or IV. When the drugs are given by other routes, equivalency relationships are likely to be changed.
4. Dosage for children is calculated according to severity of disease rather than weight.
5. Dosage must be reduced if hypoalbuminemia is present. Normally, corticosteroids are highly bound to serum proteins, especially albumin. With hypoalbuminemia, more drug is unbound and pharmacologically active. This increases the incidence and severity of adverse effects if dosage is not reduced.
6. For people receiving chronic corticosteroid therapy, dosage must be increased during periods of stress. Although an event that is stressful for one client may not be stressful for another, some common sources of stress for most people include surgery and anesthesia, infections, anxiety, and extremes of temperature. Some guidelines for corticosteroid dosage during stress include the following:
   a. During *minor or relatively mild illness* (viral upper respiratory infection, any febrile illness, strenuous exercise, gastroenteritis with vomiting and diarrhea, minor surgery), doubling the daily maintenance dose is usually adequate. Once the stress period is over, dosage may be reduced abruptly to the usual maintenance dose.
   b. During *major stress or severe illness*, even larger doses are necessary. For example, a client undergoing abdominal surgery may require 300 to 400 mg of hydrocortisone on the day of surgery. This dose can gradually be reduced to usual maintenance doses within about 5 days if postoperative recovery is uncomplicated. As a general rule, it is better to administer excessive doses temporarily than to risk inadequate doses and adrenal insufficiency. The client also may require sodium chloride and fluid replacement, antibiotic therapy if infection is present, and supportive measures if shock occurs.

      An acute stress situation of short duration, such as traumatic injury or invasive diagnostic tests (*e.g.*, angiograms), can usually be treated with a single dose of about 100 mg of hydrocortisone immediately after the injury or before the diagnostic test.
   c. Many chronic diseases that require long-term corticosteroid therapy are characterized by exacerbations and remissions. Dosage of corticosteroids usually must be increased during acute flare-ups of disease symptoms but can then be decreased gradually to maintenance levels.

SELECTION OF ROUTE OF ADMINISTRATION

Corticosteroid drugs can be given by several different routes to achieve local or systemic effects. When feasible, they should be given locally rather than systemically to prevent or decrease systemic toxicity. When corticosteroids must be given systemically, the oral route is preferred. Parenteral administration is indicated only for clients who are seriously ill or unable to take oral medications.

SCHEDULING GUIDELINES

Scheduling of drug administration is more important with corticosteroids than with most other drug classes. Most adverse effects occur with long-term administration of high doses. A major adverse reaction is suppression of the HPA axis and subsequent loss of adrenocortical function. Although opinions differ, the following schedules are often recommended to prevent or minimize HPA suppression:

1. **Short-term use (10 days or less) in acute situations:** Corticosteroids can be given in relatively large, divided doses for about 48 to 72 hours until the acute situation is brought under control. At

times, also, continuous IV infusions may be given. After acute symptoms subside or 48 to 72 hours have passed, the dosage is tapered so that a slightly smaller dose is given each day until the drug can be discontinued completely. Such a regimen may be useful in allergic reactions, contact dermatitis, exacerbations of chronic conditions (*e.g.,* rheumatoid arthritis, bronchial asthma), and stressful situations such as surgery.

2. **Replacement therapy in cases of chronic adrenocortical insufficiency:** Daily administration is required. The entire daily dose can be taken each morning, between 6 and 9 AM. This schedule simulates normal endogenous corticosteroid secretion.

3. **Other chronic conditions:** Alternate-day therapy (ADT) is usually preferred. ADT involves giving a double dose every other morning. This schedule allows rest periods so that adverse effects are decreased while anti-inflammatory effects continue.

    a. ADT seems to be as effective as more frequent administration in most clients with bronchial asthma, ulcerative colitis, and other conditions for which long-term corticosteroid therapy is prescribed.

    b. ADT is used only for maintenance therapy (*i.e.,* clinical signs and symptoms are controlled initially with more frequent drug administration). ADT can be started once symptoms have subsided and stabilized.

    c. ADT does not retard growth in children as do other schedules.

    d. ADT probably decreases susceptibility to infection.

    e. Intermediate-acting glucocorticoids, such as prednisone, prednisolone, and methylprednisolone, are the drugs of choice for ADT.

    f. ADT is not usually indicated in clients who have received long-term corticosteroid therapy. First, these clients already have maximal HPA suppression, so a major advantage of ADT is lost. Second, if they are transferred to ADT, recurrence of symptoms and considerable discomfort may occur on days when drugs are omitted. Clients with severe disease and very painful or disabling symptoms also may experience severe discomfort with ADT.

USE IN SPECIFIC SITUATIONS

Allergic Rhinitis

Allergic rhinitis (also called seasonal rhinitis or hay fever and perennial rhinitis) is a common problem for which corticosteroids are given by nasal spray, once or twice daily. Therapeutic effects usually occur within a few days with regular use. Systemic adverse effects are minimal with recommended doses but may occur with higher doses, including adrenocortical insufficiency from HPA suppression.

Arthritis

Corticosteroids are the most effective drugs for rapid relief of the pain, edema, and restricted mobility associated with acute episodes of joint inflammation. They are usually given on a short-term basis. When inflammation is limited to three or fewer joints, the preferred route of drug administration is by injection directly into the joint. Intra-articular injections relieve symptoms in about 2 to 8 weeks. Several formulations are available for this route; however, these drugs do not prevent disease progression and joint destruction. As a general rule, a joint should not be injected more often than three times yearly because of risks of infection and damage to intra-articular structures from the injections and from overuse when pain is relieved.

Asthma

Corticosteroids are commonly used in the treatment of asthma for anti-inflammatory and other effects. In acute asthma attacks or status asthmaticus unrelieved by an inhaled beta-adrenergic bronchodilator, high doses of systemic corticosteroids are given PO or IV along with the bronchodilator for about 5 to 10 days. Although these high doses suppress the HPA axis, the suppression only lasts for 1 to 3 days and other serious adverse effects are avoided. Thus, systemic corticosteroids are used in short courses as needed and not for long-term treatment. People who regularly use inhaled corticosteroids also need high doses of systemic drugs during acute attacks because aerosols are not effective. As soon as acute symptoms subside, dosage should be tapered to the lowest effective maintenance dose or the drug should be discontinued.

In chronic asthma, inhaled corticosteroids are drugs of first choice. This recommendation evolved from increased knowledge about the importance of inflammation in the pathophysiology of asthma and the development of aerosol corticosteroids that are effective with minimal adverse effects because there is little systemic absorption with recommended doses. Inhaled drugs may be given alone or with systemic drugs. Generally, inhaled corticosteroids can replace oral drugs when daily dosage of the oral agent has been tapered to 10 to 15 mg of prednisone or the equivalent dosage of other agents. When a client is being switched from an oral to an inhaled corticosteroid, the inhaled drug should be started during tapering of the oral drug, about 1 or 2 weeks before discontinuing or reaching the lowest anticipated dose of the oral drug. When a client requires a systemic corticosteroid, co-administration of an aerosol allows smaller doses of the systemic corticosteroid. Although the inhaled drugs can cause suppression of the HPA axis and adrenocortical function, especially at higher doses, they are much less likely to do so than systemic drugs.

In addition to their anti-inflammatory effects, corticosteroids also increase the effects of adrenergic bronchodilators that are given in asthma and other disorders to prevent or treat bronchoconstriction and bronchospasm. They perform this important function by increasing the number and responsiveness of beta-adrenergic receptors and preventing the tolerance usually associated with chronic administration of adrenergic bronchodilators. Research studies indicate increased responsiveness to beta-adrenergic bronchodilators within 2 hours and increased numbers of beta receptors within 4 hours of corticosteroid administration.

Cancer

Corticosteroids are commonly used in the treatment of lymphomas, lymphocytic leukemias, and multiple myeloma. In these disorders, corticosteroids inhibit cell reproduction and are cytotoxic to lymphocytes. In addition to their anticancer effects in hematologic malignancies, corticosteroids are beneficial in treatment of several signs and symptoms that often accompany cancer. Although the mechanisms of action are unknown and drug/dosage regimens vary widely, corticosteroids are used to treat anorexia, nausea and vomiting, cerebral edema and inflammation associated with brain metastases or radiation of the head, spinal cord compression, pain and edema related to pressure on nerves or bone metastases, graft-versus-host disease after bone marrow transplantation, and other disorders. Clients tend to feel better when taking corticosteroids although the basic disease process may be unchanged.

PREVENTION OF ACUTE ADRENOCORTICAL INSUFFICIENCY

Suppression of the hypothalamic-pituitary-adrenal (HPA) axis may occur with corticosteroid therapy and may lead to life-threatening inability to increase cortisol secretion when needed to cope with stress. It is most likely to occur with abrupt withdrawal of systemic corticosteroid drugs. The risk of significant insufficiency is high with systemic drugs given more than a few days, although the minimum dose and duration of therapy that will cause adrenal suppression are unknown. When the drugs are given for replacement therapy, adrenal insufficiency is lifelong and drug administration must be continued. When the drugs are given for purposes other than replacement and then discontinued, the HPA axis usually recovers function. However, adrenal insufficiency can persist a year or more after corticosteroid therapy is discontinued. Signs and symptoms of adrenal insufficiency are most likely to occur during physical stresses such as illness, trauma, or surgery and may include hypotension, hypoglycemia, nausea, anorexia, and mental depression.

Several strategies have been developed to minimize HPA suppression and risks of acute adrenal insufficiency. One strategy is to use local rather than systemic therapy when possible, alone or in combination with low doses of systemic drugs. Numerous preparations are available for local application, including aerosols for inhalation, formulations for topical application to the skin, eyes, and ears, and drugs for intra-articular injections. A second strategy is to give short courses of systemic therapy for acute disorders, such as acute asthma attacks, then decreasing the dose or stopping the drug within a few days. A third strategy is to gradually taper the dose, often with daily reductions. Although specific guidelines for tapering dosage have not been developed, generally higher doses and longer durations of administration require slower tapering, possibly over several weeks. The goal of tapering may be to stop the drug or to decrease the dosage to the lowest effective amount.

For people who require long-term systemic therapy (*i.e.*, are steroid-dependent), two additional strategies reduce the risk of acute adrenal insufficiency. One is ADT, which involves titrating the daily dose to the lowest effective maintenance level, then giving a double dose every other day. The other strategy is to give additional corticosteroids during physical stresses such as illness, trauma, or surgery.

USE IN CHILDREN

Corticosteroids are used for the same conditions in children as in adults. With long-term use, corticosteroids may impair growth and development by their effects on protein and bone metabolism. If stunting of growth occurs, most children have a "catch-up" spurt of growth when the drug is discontinued, so permanent stunting is unusual.

Parents and health care providers can monitor drug effects by taking weekly recordings of height and weight. ADT is less likely to impair normal growth and development than daily administration.

USE IN OLDER ADULTS

Corticosteroids are used for the same conditions in older adults as in younger ones. Older adults are especially likely to have conditions that are aggravated by the drugs (*e.g.*, congestive heart failure, hypertension, diabetes mellitus, arthritis, osteoporosis, increased susceptibility to infection, and concomitant drug therapy that increases risks of gastrointestinal ulceration and bleeding). Consequently, risk–benefit ratios of corticosteroid therapy should be carefully considered, especially for long-term therapy.

When used, lower doses are usually indicated because of decreased muscle mass, plasma volume, hepatic metabolism, and renal excretion in older adults. In addition, therapeutic and adverse responses should be monitored regularly by a health care provider (*e.g.*, blood pressure, serum electrolytes, blood glucose levels).

HOME CARE

Corticosteroids are extensively used in the home setting, by all age groups, for a wide variety of disorders, and by most routes of administration. Because of potentially serious adverse effects, especially with oral drugs, it is extremely important that these drugs be used as prescribed. A major responsibility of the home care nurse is to teach, demonstrate, supervise, monitor, or do whatever is needed to facilitate correct usage. In addition, the home care nurse needs to teach clients and caregivers interventions to minimize adverse effects of these drugs.

NURSING ACTIONS — CORTICOSTEROID DRUGS

NURSING ACTIONS	RATIONALE/EXPLANATION
1. Administer accurately **a.** Read the drug label carefully to be certain of having the correct preparation for the intended route of administration.	Many corticosteroid drugs are available in several different preparations. For example, hydrocortisone is available in formulations for intravenous (IV) or intramuscular (IM) administration, for intra-articular injection, and for topical application in creams and ointments of several different strengths. These preparations cannot be used interchangeably without causing potentially serious adverse reactions and decreasing therapeutic effects. Some drugs are available for only one use. For example, several preparations are for topical use only; beclomethasone is prepared only for oral and nasal inhalation.
b. With oral corticosteroid drugs, give with or after meals.	Opinion seems divided regarding the effectiveness of this scheduling in relation to meals. The rationale is to decrease gastric irritation and prevent development or aggravation of peptic ulcer disease. Corticosteroid drugs have long been considered ulcerogenic, but there is no valid evidence to substantiate this claim. Many physicians prescribe antacids to be given at the same time as the corticosteroid drug.
c. For IV or IM administration: (1) Follow the manufacturer's directions on the drug vial for the type and amount of diluent to add.	Instructions vary with specific preparations.
(2) Give direct IV injection over at least 1 min.	To increase safety of administration
(3) Follow the manufacturer's directions for diluting and administering by continuous IV infusions.	Instructions vary with specific preparations.
d. For oral inhalation of a corticosteroid, check the instruction leaflet that accompanies the inhaler. If the client also is receiving a bronchodilator, administer it first, then wait a few minutes before giving the corticosteroid inhalation.	Giving a bronchodilating drug by inhalation before giving the corticosteroid increases penetration of the corticosteroid into the tracheobronchial tree and increases its therapeutic effectiveness. Waiting a few minutes between the drugs decreases the likelihood of toxicity from the inhaled fluorocarbon propellants of the aerosol drugs.
2. Observe for therapeutic effects	The primary objective of corticosteroid therapy is to relieve signs and symptoms, because the drugs are not curative. Therefore, therapeutic effects depend largely on the reason for use.
a. With adrenocortical insufficiency, observe for absence or decrease of weakness, weight loss, anorexia, nausea, vomiting, hyperpigmentation, hypotension, hypoglycemia, hyponatremia, and hyperkalemia.	These signs and symptoms of impaired metabolism do not occur with adequate replacement of corticosteroids.
b. With rheumatoid arthritis, observe for decreased pain and edema in joints, greater capacity for movement, and increased ability to perform usual activities of daily living.	

NURSING ACTIONS	RATIONALE/EXPLANATION
c. With asthma and chronic obstructive pulmonary disease, observe for decrease in respiratory distress and increased tolerance of activity.	
d. With skin lesions, observe for decreasing inflammation.	
e. When the drug is given to suppress the immune response to organ transplants, therapeutic effect is the absence of signs and symptoms indicating rejection of the transplanted tissue.	
3. Observe for adverse effects	These are uncommon with replacement therapy but common with long-term administration of the pharmacologic doses used for many disease processes. Adverse reactions may affect every body tissue and organ.
a. Adrenocortical insufficiency—fainting, weakness, anorexia, nausea, vomiting, hypotension, shock, and if untreated, death	This reaction is likely to occur in clients receiving daily corticosteroid drugs who encounter stressful situations. It is caused by drug-induced suppression of the HPA axis, which makes the client unable to respond to stress by increasing adrenocortical hormone secretion.
b. Adrenocortical excess (hypercorticism or Cushing's disease)	Most adverse effects result from excessive corticosteroids.
(1) "Moon face," "buffalo hump" contour of shoulders, obese trunk, thin extremities	This appearance is caused by abnormal fat deposits in cheeks, shoulders, breasts, abdomen, and buttocks. These changes are more cosmetic than physiologically significant. However, the alterations in self-image can lead to psychological problems. These changes cannot be prevented, but they may be partially reversed if corticosteroid therapy is discontinued or reduced in dosage.
(2) Diabetes mellitus—glycosuria, hyperglycemia, polyuria, polydipsia, polyphagia, impaired healing, and other signs and symptoms	Corticosteroid drugs can cause hyperglycemia and diabetes mellitus or aggravate pre-existing diabetes mellitus by their effects on carbohydrate metabolism.
(3) Central nervous system effects—euphoria, psychological dependence, nervousness, insomnia, depression, personality and behavioral changes, aggravation of pre-existing psychiatric disorders	Some clients enjoy the drug-induced euphoria so much that they resist attempts to withdraw the drug or decrease its dosage.
(4) Musculoskeletal effects—osteoporosis, pathologic fractures, muscle weakness and atrophy, decreased linear growth in children	Demineralization of bone produces thin, weak bones that fracture easily. Fractures of vertebrae, long bones, and ribs are relatively common, especially in postmenopausal women and immobilized clients. Myopathy results from abnormal protein metabolism. Decreased growth in children results from impaired bone formation and protein metabolism.
(5) Cardiovascular, fluid, and electrolyte effects—fluid retention, edema, hypertension, congestive heart failure, hypernatremia, hypokalemia, metabolic alkalosis	These effects result largely from mineralocorticoid activity, which causes retention of sodium and water. They are more likely to occur with older corticosteroids, such as hydrocortisone and prednisone.
(6) Gastrointestinal effects—nausea, vomiting, possible peptic ulcer disease, increased appetite, obesity	
(7) Increased susceptibility to infection and delayed wound healing	Caused by suppression of normal inflammatory and immune processes and impaired protein metabolism
(8) Menstrual irregularities, acne, excessive facial hair	Caused by excessive sex hormones, primarily androgens
(9) Ocular effects—increased intraocular pressure, glaucoma, cataracts	

(continued)

NURSING ACTIONS	RATIONALE/EXPLANATION
(10) Integumentary effects—skin becomes reddened, thinner, has stretch marks, and is easily injured	

4. Observe for drug interactions
  a. Drugs that *increase* effects of corticosteroids:

(1) Adrenergics (*e.g.*, epinephrine), anticholinergics (*e.g.*, atropine), tricyclic antidepressants (*e.g.*, amitriptyline [Elavil]), antihistamines, and meperidine	Potentiation of increased intraocular pressure. The combinations are hazardous in glaucoma and should be avoided if possible.
(2) Diuretics	Excessive potassium depletion may occur because both diuretics and corticosteroids can cause hypokalemia.
(3) Estrogens	Potentiate glycosuria and anti-inflammatory effects of hydrocortisone but not those of dexamethasone, methylprednisolone, prednisolone, or prednisone
(4) Indomethacin	Increases ulcerogenic effects
(5) Salicylates	May potentiate all effects of corticosteroids by displacing the drug from plasma protein binding sites

  b. Drugs that *decrease* effects of corticosteroids:

Antihistamines, barbiturates, chloral hydrate, phenytoin, rifampin	These drugs induce microsomal enzymes in the liver and increase the rate at which corticosteroids are metabolized or deactivated.

5. Teach clients
  a. With long-term systemic corticosteroid therapy:

(1) Take the drugs as directed.	This is extremely important with these drugs. Missing a dose or two, stopping the drug, changing the amount or time of administration, or taking extra drug (except as specifically directed during stress situations) or any other alterations may result in complications. Some complications are relatively minor; several are serious, even life-threatening. When these drugs are being discontinued, the dosage is gradually reduced over several weeks. They should not be abruptly stopped.
(2) Report to the physician if unable to take a dose orally because of vomiting or some other problem.	In some circumstances, the physician may prescribe one or more injections to prevent potentially serious problems.
(3) Avoid exposure to infection when possible. Avoid crowds and people known to have an infection. Also, wash hands frequently and thoroughly.	These drugs increase the likelihood of infection, so preventive measures are necessary. Also, if infection does occur, healing is likely to be slow.
(4) Practice safety measures to avoid accidents.	To avoid falls and possible fractures due to osteoporosis; to avoid cuts or other injuries because of delayed wound healing; to avoid soft-tissue trauma because of increased tendency to bruise easily.
(5) Weigh frequently when starting corticosteroid therapy and at least weekly during long-term maintenance.	An initial weight gain is likely to occur and is usually attributed to increased appetite. Later weight gains may be caused by fluid retention.
(6) Muscle weakness and fatigue or disease symptoms may occur when drug dosage is reduced, withdrawn, or omitted (*e.g.*, the nondrug day of alternate-day therapy [ADT])	Although these symptoms may cause some discomfort, they should be tolerated if possible rather than increasing corticosteroid dose. If severe, of course, dosage or time of administration may have to be changed.
(7) Dietary changes, if indicated. Possible changes include decreasing salt and increasing potassium, calcium, protein, and vitamins D and C.	These changes may not be necessary in all clients. Limiting salt intake may be important if fluid retention or edema is a problem. The simplest way to do this is to avoid adding table

NURSING ACTIONS	RATIONALE/EXPLANATION
	salt to foods and avoid obviously salty foods, such as many snack foods and prepared sandwich meats. If more stringent restrictions seem indicated, consult a dietitian or diet manual. When sodium is retained, potassium is lost. It may be desirable for the client to increase intake of high-potassium foods, such as citrus fruits and juices or bananas. Protein, calcium, and vitamin D may help to prevent or delay osteoporosis, and vitamin C may help to prevent excessive bruising. Meat and dairy products are good sources of protein, calcium, and vitamin D; citrus fruits are good sources of vitamin C.
	Any diet teaching should be specific to the needs of the individual client and should consider food preferences and usual eating habits.
(8) Report to a health care provider:	As previously indicated, clients experiencing stress situations require larger doses of corticosteroids. It would be helpful if the physician would instruct the client on what kinds of stress situations the client can handle and for which the physician should be notified. All the other symptoms to be reported indicate adverse reactions, such as infection, sodium and fluid retention, fractures of vertebrae or ribs, and psychological problems. If these occur, they must be assessed by the physician to see if any changes in corticosteroid therapy are indicated.
(a) Stress situations	
(b) Sore throat, fever, or other signs of infection	
(c) Weight gain of 5 lb or more in a week	
(d) Swelling in ankles or elsewhere in the body	
(e) Persistent backache or chest pain	
(f) Mental depression or other mood changes	
(g) Changes in sleeping patterns	
b. With local applications of corticosteroids:	
(1) Use the drug preparation only as directed and for the purpose intended.	To increase therapeutic effects and decrease adverse reactions. As a general rule, not enough drug is absorbed to cause systemic toxicity. However, systemic toxicity can occur if excess corticosteroid is inhaled or if occlusive dressings are used over skin lesions. Local reactions may occur, especially with large doses. Most of the time, different drug preparations are used for specific purposes, such as eye drops or ear drops or application to skin lesions. These preparations must not be used interchangeably
(2) Use hand-held inhalers as follows:	
(a) Shake canister thoroughly.	
(b) Place canister between lips (both open and pursed lips have been recommended).	
(c) Exhale completely.	
(d) Activate canister while taking a slow, deep breath.	
(e) Hold breath for 10 sec or as long as possible.	
(f) Wait at least 1 min before taking additional inhalations.	
(g) Rinse mouth following inhalations to decrease the incidence of oral thrush.	
(h) Rinse mouthpiece at least once per day.	

REVIEW AND APPLICATION EXERCISES

1. What are the main characteristics and functions of cortisol?

2. What is the difference between glucocorticoid and mineralocorticoid components of corticosteroids?

3. How do glucocorticoids affect body metabolism?

4. What is meant by the HPA axis?

5. What are the mechanisms by which exogenous corticosteroids may cause adrenocortical insufficiency and excess?

6. What are adverse effects associated with chronic use of systemic corticosteroids?

7. For a client on long-term systemic corticosteroid therapy, why is it important to taper the dose and gradually discontinue the drug rather than stop it abruptly?

8. Why is alternate-day administration of a systemic corticosteroid preferred when possible?

9. What are the main differences between administering corticosteroids in adrenal insufficiency and in other disorders?

10. When a corticosteroid is given by inhalation to clients with asthma or other bronchoconstrictive disorder, what is the expected effect?

SELECTED REFERENCES

Barnes, P.J. (1995). Inhaled glucocorticoids for asthma. *New England Journal of Medicine, 332,* 868–875.

Drug facts and comparisons. (1996). St. Louis: Facts and Comparisons.

Gums, J.G. (1993). Disorders of the adrenal gland. In J.T. DiPiro, R.L. Talbert, P.E. Hayes, G.C. Yee, G.R. Matzke, & L.M. Posey (Eds.), *Pharmacotherapy: A pathophysiologic approach,* 2nd ed., pp. 1168–1182. Norwalk, CT: Appleton & Lange.

Guyton, A.C. & Hall, J.E. (1996). *Textbook of medical physiology,* 9th ed. Philadelphia: W.B. Saunders.

Kelly, H.W. & Hill, M.R. (1993). Asthma. In J.T. DiPiro, R.L. Talbert, P.E. Hayes, G.C. Yee, G.R. Matzke, & L.M. Posey (Eds.), *Pharmacotherapy: A pathophysiologic approach,* 2nd ed., pp. 408–449. Norwalk, CT: Appleton & Lange.

Porth, C.M. & Hurwitz, L.S. (1994). Alterations in endocrine control of growth and metabolism. In C.M. Porth (Ed.), *Pathophysiology: Concepts of altered health states,* 4th ed., pp. 907–926. Philadelphia: J.B. Lippincott.

Schimmer, B.P. & Parker, K.L. (1996). Adrenocorticotropic hormone; adrenocortical steroids and their synthetic analogs; inhibitors of the synthesis and actions of adrenocortical hormones. In J.G. Hardman, L.E. Limbird, P.B. Molinoff, & R.W. Ruddon (Eds.), *Goodman & Gilman's The pharmacological basis of therapeutics,* 9th ed., pp. 1459-1485. New York: McGraw-Hill.

25 Thyroid and Antithyroid Drugs

Outline

Objectives

After studying this chapter, the student will be able to:

1 Describe physiologic effects of thyroid hormone.

2 Identify effects of hypo- and hypersecretion of thyroid hormone.

3 Describe characteristics, uses and effects of thyroid drugs.

4 Describe characteristics, uses and effects of antithyroid drugs.

5 Discuss the influence of thyroid and antithyroid drugs on the metabolism of other drugs.

6 Teach clients self-care activities related to the use of thyroid and antithyroid drugs.

Key Terms

Cretinism	Myxedema
Graves' disease	Thyroiditis
Hyperthyroidism	Thyrotoxicosis
Hypothyroidism	Thyroxine

Description and Uses

The thyroid gland produces three hormones: thyroxine, triiodothyronine, and calcitonin. Thyroxine contains four atoms of iodine and is also called T_4. Triiodothyronine contains three atoms of iodine and is called T_3. Compared to thyroxine, triiodothyronine is more potent and has a more rapid onset but shorter duration of action. Despite these minor differences, the two hormones produce the same physiologic effects and have the same actions and uses. Calcitonin functions in calcium metabolism and is discussed in Chapter 26.

Production of thyroxine and triiodothyronine depends on the presence of iodine and tyrosine in the thyroid gland. Plasma iodide is derived from dietary sources and from the metabolic breakdown of thyroid hormone, which allows some iodine to be reused. The thyroid gland extracts iodide from the circulating blood, concentrates it, and secretes enzymes that change the chemically inactive iodide to free iodine atoms. Tyrosine is an amino acid derived from dietary protein. It forms the basic structure of thyroglobulin. In a series of chemical reactions, iodine atoms become attached to tyrosine to form the thyroid hormones T_3 and T_4. Once formed, the hormones are stored within the chemically inactive thyroglobulin molecule.

Thyroid hormones are released into the circulation when the thyroid gland is stimulated by thyrotropin from the anterior pituitary gland. Because the thyroglobulin molecule is too large to cross cell membranes, proteolytic enzymes break down the molecule so the active hormones can be released. After their release from thyroglobulin, the hormones become largely bound to plasma proteins. Only the small amounts left unbound are biologically active. The bound thyroid hormones are released to tissue cells very slowly. Once in the cells, the hormones combine with intracellular proteins so they are again stored. They are released slowly within the cell and used over a period of days or weeks. Once used by the cells, the thyroid hormones release the iodine atoms. Most of the iodine is reabsorbed and used to produce new thyroid hormones; the remainder is excreted in the urine.

Thyroid hormones control the rate of cellular metabolism and thereby influence the functioning of virtually every cell in the body. The heart, skeletal muscle, liver, and kidneys are especially responsive to the stimulating effects of thyroid hormones. The brain, spleen, and gonads are less responsive. Thyroid hormones are required for normal growth and development and are considered especially critical for brain and skeletal development and maturation. These hormones are thought to act mainly by controlling intra-

cellular protein synthesis. Some specific physiologic effects include:

1. Increased rate of cellular metabolism and oxygen consumption with a resultant increase in heat production
2. Increased heart rate, force of contraction, and cardiac output (increased cardiac workload)
3. Increased carbohydrate metabolism
4. Increased fat metabolism, including increased lipolytic effects of other hormones and metabolism of cholesterol to bile acids
5. Inhibition of pituitary secretion of thyrotropin

Thyroid Disorders

Thyroid disorders requiring drug therapy are goiter, hypothyroidism, and hyperthyroidism. Hypothyroidism and hyperthyroidism produce opposing effects on body tissues, depending on the levels of circulating thyroid hormone. Specific effects and clinical manifestations are listed in Table 25-1.

SIMPLE GOITER

Simple goiter is an enlargement of the thyroid gland resulting from iodine deficiency. Inadequate iodine decreases thyroid hormone production. To compensate, the anterior pituitary gland secretes more thyrotropin, which causes the thyroid to enlarge and produce more hormone. The enlarged gland may secrete enough hormone to cause disfigurement, psychological distress, dyspnea, and dysphagia. If the gland cannot secrete enough hormone despite enlargement, hypothyroidism results. Simple or endemic goiter is a common condition in some geographic areas. It is uncommon in the United States, largely because of the widespread use of iodized table salt.

Treatment of simple goiter involves giving iodine preparations and thyroid hormones to prevent further enlargement and promote regression in gland size. Large goiters may require surgical excision.

HYPOTHYROIDISM

Primary hypothyroidism occurs when disease or destruction of thyroid gland tissue causes inadequate production of thyroid hormones. Some causes of primary hypothyroidism include acute viral thyroiditis; chronic (Hashimoto's) thyroiditis, an autoimmune disorder; and treatment of hyperthyroidism with antithyroid drugs, radiation therapy, or surgery. Secondary hypothyroidism occurs when there is decreased thyrotropin from the anterior pituitary gland.

Congenital hypothyroidism (cretinism) occurs when a child is born without a thyroid gland or with a poorly

TABLE 25-1 THYROID DISORDERS AND THEIR EFFECTS ON BODY SYSTEMS

Hypothyroidism	Hyperthyroidism
Cardiovascular Effects	
Increased capillary fragility	Tachycardia
Decreased cardiac output	Increased cardiac output
Decreased blood pressure	Increased blood volume
Decreased heart rate	Increased systolic blood pressure
Cardiac enlargement	Cardiac arrhythmias
Congestive heart failure	Congestive heart failure
Anemia	
More rapid development of atherosclerosis and its complications (*e.g.*, coronary artery and peripheral vascular disease)	
Central Nervous System Effects	
Apathy and lethargy	Nervousness
Emotional dullness	Emotional instability
Slow speech, perhaps slurring and hoarseness as well	Restlessness
Hypoactive reflexes	Anxiety
Forgetfulness and mental sluggishness	Insomnia
Excessive drowsiness and sleeping	Hyperactive reflexes
Metabolic Effects	
Intolerance of cold	Intolerance of heat
Subnormal temperature	Low-grade fever
Increased serum cholesterol	Weight loss despite increased appetite
Weight gain	
Gastrointestinal Effects	
Decreased appetite	Increased appetite
Constipation	Abdominal cramps
	Diarrhea
	Nausea and vomiting
Muscular Effects	
Weakness	Weakness
Fatigue	Fatigue
Vague aches and pains	Muscle atrophy
	Tremors
Integumentary	
Dry, coarse, and thickened skin	Moist, warm, flushed skin owing to vasodilation and increased sweating
Puffy appearance of face and eyelids	
Dry and thinned hair	Hair and nails soft
Thick and hard nails	
Reproductive Effects	
Prolonged menstrual periods	Amenorrhea or oligomenorrhea
Infertility or sterility	
Decreased libido	
Miscellaneous Effects	
Increased susceptibility to infection	Dyspnea
Increased sensitivity to narcotics, barbiturates, and anesthetics owing to slowed metabolism of these drugs	Polyuria
	Hoarse, rapid speech
	Increased susceptibility to infection
	Excessive perspiration
	Localized edema around the eyeballs, which produces characteristic eye changes, including exophthalmos

functioning gland. Cretinism is uncommon in the United States but may occur with a lack of iodine in the mother's diet. Symptoms are rarely present at birth, but develop gradually during infancy and early childhood and include poor growth and development, lethargy and inactivity, feeding problems, slow pulse, subnormal temperature, and constipation. If the disorder is untreated until the child is several months old, permanent mental retardation is likely to result.

Adult hypothyroidism produces variable signs and symptoms, depending on the amount of hormone production. Initially, manifestations are mild and vague. They usually increase in incidence and severity over time as the thyroid gland gradually atrophies, and functioning glandular tissue is replaced by nonfunctioning fibrous connective tissue (see Table 25-1).

Regardless of the cause of hypothyroidism and the age at which it occurs, the specific treatment is replacement of thyroid hormone from an exogenous source. Synthetic levothyroxine is the drug of choice.

The main clinical indication for use of thyroid drugs is hypothyroidism manifested by signs and symptoms and diagnostic tests of thyroid function. They also may be used to suppress secretion of thyrotropin by the anterior pituitary gland.

HYPERTHYROIDISM

Hyperthyroidism is characterized by excessive secretion of thyroid hormone. It may be associated with Graves' disease, nodular goiter, thyroiditis, overtreatment with thyroid drugs, functioning thyroid carcinoma, and pituitary adenoma that secretes excessive thyrotropin. Hyperthyroidism usually involves an enlarged thyroid gland that has an increased number of cells and an increased rate of secretion. The hyperplastic thyroid gland may secrete 5 to 15 times the normal amount of thyroid hormone. As a result, body metabolism is greatly increased. Specific physiologic effects and clinical manifestations of hyperthyroidism are listed in Table 25-1. These effects vary, depending on the amount of circulating thyroid hormone, and they usually increase in incidence and severity with time if hyperthyroidism is not treated.

Thyroid storm or thyrotoxic crisis is a rare but severe complication characterized by extreme symptoms of hyperthyroidism, such as severe tachycardia, fever, dehydration, heart failure, and coma. It is most likely to occur in clients with hyperthyroidism that has been inadequately treated, especially when stressful situations occur (*e.g.*, trauma, infection, surgery, emotional upsets).

Treatment

Hyperthyroidism is treated by antithyroid drugs, radioactive iodine, surgery, or a combination of these methods. The drugs act by decreasing production or release of thyroid hormones. Radioactive iodine emits rays that destroy thyroid gland tissue. Subtotal thyroidectomy involves surgical excision of thyroid tissue. All these methods reduce the amount of thyroid hormones circulating in the bloodstream.

The antithyroid drugs include the thioamide derivatives (propylthiouracil and methimazole) and iodine preparations. The thioamide drugs inhibit synthesis of thyroid hormone, are inexpensive and relatively safe, and they do not damage the thyroid gland. These drugs may be used as the primary treatment (for which they may be given 6 months to 2 years) or to decrease blood levels of thyroid hormone before radioactive iodine therapy or surgery.

Radioactive iodine (RAI) is a frequently used treatment in the United States. It is generally safe, effective, inexpensive, and convenient. One disadvantage is hypothyroidism, which usually develops within a few months and requires lifelong thyroid hormone replacement therapy. Another disadvantage is the delay in therapeutic benefits. Results may not be apparent for 3 months or longer, during which time severe hyperthyroidism must be brought under control with one of the thioamide antithyroid drugs. Other iodine preparations are not used in long-term treatment of hyperthyroidism. They are indicated when a rapid clinical response is needed, as in thyroid storm and acute hyperthyroidism, or to prepare a hyperthyroid person for thyroidectomy. A thioamide drug is given to produce a euthyroid state, and an iodine preparation is given to reduce the size and vascularity of the thyroid gland to reduce the risk of excessive bleeding.

Iodine preparations inhibit the release of thyroid hormones and cause them to be stored within the gland. They reduce blood levels of thyroid hormones more quickly than thioamide drugs or radioactive iodine. Maximal effects are reached in about 10 to 15 days of continuous therapy, and this is probably the primary advantage. Several disadvantages, however, include the following:

1. They may produce goiter, hyperthyroidism, or both.
2. They cannot be used alone. Therapeutic benefits are temporary, and symptoms of hyperthyroidism may reappear and even be intensified if other treatment methods are not also used.
3. Radioactive iodine cannot be used effectively for a prolonged period in a client who has received iodine preparations. Even if the iodine preparation is discontinued, the thyroid gland is saturated with iodine and will not attract enough radioactive iodine for treatment to be effective. Also, if radioactive iodine is given later, acute hyperthyroidism is likely to result because the radioactive iodine causes the stored hormones to be released into the circulation.

4. Although giving a thioamide drug followed by an iodine preparation is standard preparation for thyroidectomy, the opposite sequence of administration is unsafe. If the iodine preparation is given first and followed by propylthiouracil or methimazole, the client is likely to experience acute hyperthyroidism because the thioamide causes release of the stored thyroid hormones.

Subtotal thyroidectomy is effective in relieving hyperthyroidism but also has several disadvantages. First, preparation for surgery requires several weeks of drug therapy. Second, there are risks involved in anesthesia and surgery and potential postoperative complications. Third, there is a high risk of eventual hypothyroidism. For these reasons, surgery is generally used for clients with large goiters or contraindications to other treatments.

Propranolol is used as an adjunctive drug in the treatment of hyperthyroidism. It relieves tachycardia, cardiac palpitations, excessive sweating, and other symptoms. Propranolol is especially helpful during the several weeks required for therapeutic results from antithyroid drugs or from radioactive iodine administration.

Individual Drugs

THYROID AGENTS (DRUGS USED IN HYPOTHYROIDISM)

Levothyroxine (Synthroid, Levothroid) is a synthetic preparation of T_4. It is more potent than thyroid, contains a uniform amount of hormone, and can be given parenterally. Compared with liothyronine, levothyroxine has a slower onset and longer duration of action. Levothyroxine is considered the drug of choice for long-term treatment of hypothyroidism.

Routes and Dosage Ranges

Adults: PO 0.05–0.1 mg/d initially, increased q1–3 wk until the desired response is obtained; usual maintenance dose is 0.1–0.2 mg/d
 Myxedema coma, IV 0.2–0.5 mg (0.1 mg/ml) in a single dose; 0.1–0.3 mg may be repeated on the second day if necessary
Older adults, clients with cardiac disorders, and clients with hypothyroidism of long duration: PO 0.0125–0.025 mg/d for 6 wk, then dose is doubled q6–8 wk until the desired response is obtained
 Myxedema coma, same as adult dosage
Children: PO no more than 0.05 mg/d initially, then increased by 0.05–0.1 mg q2 wk until the desired response is obtained; usual dosage range is 0.3–0.4 mg/d
 Myxedema coma, same as adult dosage

Liothyronine (Cytomel, Triostat) is a synthetic preparation of T_3. Compared with levothyroxine, liothyronine has a more rapid onset and a shorter duration of action. Consequently, it may be more likely to produce high concentrations in blood and tissues and cause adverse reactions. Also, it requires more frequent administration if used for long-term treatment of hypothyroidism. Only the intravenous (IV) formulation (Triostat) is used in treating myxedema coma.

Routes and Dosage Ranges

Adults: PO 25 µg/d initially, increased by 12.5–25 µg q1–2 wk until desired response is obtained
 Myxedema coma, IV 25–50 µg initially, then adjust dosage according to clinical response. Usual dosage, 65–100 µg/d, with doses at least 4 h apart and no more than 12 h apart
Older adults: PO 2.5–5 µg/d for 3–6 wk, then doubled q6 wk until the desired response is obtained
 Myxedema coma, IV 10–20 µg initially, then adjusted according to clinical response
Children: PO 5 µg/d initially, increased by 5 µg/d q3–4 d until the desired response is obtained. Doses as high as 20–80 µg may be required in cretinism
 Myxedema coma, dosage, safety and effectiveness have not been established

Liotrix (Euthroid, Thyrolar) contains levothyroxine and liothyronine in a 4:1 ratio, resembling the composition of natural thyroid hormone. Euthroid and Thyrolar are available in strengths ranging from 15 to 180 mg in thyroid equivalency.

Route and Dosage Ranges

Adults: PO 15–30 mg/d initially, increased gradually q1–2 wk until response is obtained
Older adults, clients with cardiac disorders, and clients with hypothyroidism of long duration: PO one fourth to one half the usual adult dose initially, doubled q8 wk if necessary
Children: PO same as adult dosage, increased q2 wk if necessary

ANTITHYROID AGENTS (DRUGS USED IN HYPERTHYROIDISM)

Propylthiouracil is the prototype of the thioamide antithyroid drugs. It can be used alone to treat hyperthyroidism, as part of the preoperative preparation for thyroidectomy, before or after radioactive iodine therapy, and in the treatment of thyroid storm or thyrotoxic crisis. Propylthiouracil acts by inhibiting production of thyroid hormones and peripheral conversion of T_4 to the more active T_3. It does not interfere with release of thyroid hormones previously produced and stored. Thus, therapeutic effects do not occur for several days or weeks until the stored hormones have been used. **Methimazole** (Tapazole) is similar to propylthiouracil in actions, uses, and adverse reactions, except that it lacks peripheral activity.

Propylthiouracil
Route and Dosage Ranges

Adults: PO 300–400 mg/d in divided doses q8h, until the client is euthyroid; then 100–150 mg/d in three divided doses, given for maintenance

Children >10 y: PO 150–300 mg/d in divided doses q8h; usual maintenance dose, 100–300 mg/d in two divided doses, q12h

Children 6–10 y: 50–150 mg/d in divided doses q8h Neonatal thyrotoxicosis, 10 mg/kg/d in divided doses

Methimazole
Route and Dosage Ranges

Adults: PO 15–60 mg/d initially, in divided doses q8h until the client is euthyroid; maintenance, 5–15 mg/d in two or three doses

Children: PO 0.4 mg/kg/d initially, in divided doses q8h; maintenance dose, one half initial dose

Strong iodine solution (Lugol's solution) and **saturated solution of potassium iodide** (SSKI) are iodine preparations sometimes used in short-term treatment of hyperthyroidism. The drugs inhibit release of thyroid hormones, causing them to accumulate in the thyroid gland. Lugol's solution is generally used to treat thyrotoxic crisis and to decrease the size and vascularity of the thyroid gland before thyroidectomy. SSKI is more often used as an expectorant but may be given as preparation for thyroidectomy. Iodine preparations should not be followed by propylthiouracil, methimazole, or radioactive iodine because the latter drugs cause release of stored thyroid hormone and may precipitate acute hyperthyroidism.

Strong Iodine Solution
Route and Dosage Ranges

Adults and children: PO 2–6 drops three times per day for 10 d before thyroidectomy

Potassium Iodide Solution
Route and Dosage Ranges

Adults and children: PO 5 drops three times per day for 10 d before thyroidectomy

Sodium iodide ^{131}**I** (Iodotope) is a radioactive isotope of iodine. The thyroid gland cannot differentiate between regular iodide and radioactive iodide, so it picks up the radioactive iodide from the circulating blood. As a result, small amounts of radioactive iodide can be used as a diagnostic test of thyroid function, and larger doses are used therapeutically to treat hyperthyroidism. Therapeutic doses act by emitting beta and gamma rays, which destroy thyroid tissue and thereby decrease production of thyroid hormones. It is also used to treat thyroid cancer.

Radioactive iodide is usually given in a single dose on an outpatient basis. For most clients, no special radiation precautions are necessary. If a very large dose is given, the client may be isolated for 8 days, which is the half-life of radioactive iodide. Therapeutic effects are delayed for several weeks or up to 6 months. During this time, symptoms may be controlled with thioamide drugs or propranolol. Radioactive iodide is usually given to middle-age and elderly people; it is contraindicated during pregnancy and lactation.

Routes and Dosage Ranges

Adults and children: PO, IV, dosage as calculated by a radiologist trained in nuclear medicine

Propranolol (Inderal) is an antiadrenergic, not an antithyroid, drug. It does not affect thyroid function, hormone secretion, or hormone metabolism. It is most often used to treat cardiovascular conditions, such as arrhythmias, angina pectoris, and hypertension. When given to clients with hyperthyroidism, propranolol blocks beta-adrenergic receptors in various organs and thereby controls symptoms of hyperthyroidism resulting from excessive stimulation of the sympathetic nervous system. These symptoms include tachycardia, palpitations, excessive sweating (hyperhidrosis), tremors, and nervousness. Propranolol is useful for controlling symptoms during the delayed response to thioamide drugs and radioactive iodine, before thyroidectomy, and in treating thyrotoxic crisis. When the client becomes euthyroid and hyperthyroid symptoms are controlled by definitive treatment measures, propranolol should be discontinued.

Route and Dosage Range

Adults: PO 40–160 mg/d in divided doses

Nursing Process

Assessment

- Assess for signs and symptoms of thyroid disorders (see Table 25-1). During the course of treatment with thyroid or antithyroid drugs, the client's blood level of thyroid hormone may range from low to normal to high. At either end of the continuum, signs and symptoms may be dramatic and obvious.

As blood levels change toward normal as a result of treatment, signs and symptoms become less obvious. If presenting signs and symptoms are treated too aggressively, they may change toward the opposite end of the continuum and indicate adverse drug effects. Thus, each client receiving a drug that alters thyroid function must be assessed for indicators of hypothyroidism, euthyroidism, and hyperthyroidism.

- Check laboratory reports of diagnostic test values. Commonly used tests of thyroid function and their normal values are resin T_3 uptake (RT_3U), 25% to 45%; serum T_3, 0.08 to 0.20 μg/100 ml; serum T_4, 5 to 12 μg/100 ml; serum thyroid-stimulating hormone (TSH), 0.5 to 5 μU/ml. An elevated serum TSH is the first indication of primary hypothyroidism and commonly occurs in middle-age women, even in the absence of other signs and symptoms.

Nursing Diagnoses

- Decreased Cardiac Output related to disease or drug-induced hypothyroidism
- Altered Nutrition: Less Than Body Requirements with hyperthyroidism
- Altered Nutrition: More Than Body Requirements with hypothyroidism
- Body Image Disturbance related to weight gain with hypothyroidism or weight loss and exophthalmos with hyperthyroidism
- Ineffective Individual Coping related to disease process and long-term drug therapy
- Constipation with hypothyroidism, diarrhea with hyperthyroidism
- Ineffective Thermoregulation related to changes in metabolism rate and body heat production
- Knowledge Deficit: Disease process and drug therapy

Planning/Goals

The client will:
- Achieve normal blood levels of thyroid hormone
- Receive or take drugs accurately
- Experience relief of symptoms of hypothyroidism or hyperthyroidism
- Be assisted to cope with symptoms until therapy becomes effective
- Avoid preventable adverse drug effects
- Be monitored regularly for therapeutic and adverse responses to drug therapy

Interventions

Use nondrug measures to control symptoms, increase effectiveness of drug therapy, and decrease adverse reactions. Some areas for intervention include the following:

- **Environmental temperature.** Regulate for the client's comfort, when possible. Clients with hypothyroidism are very intolerant of cold owing to their slow metabolism rate. Chilling and shivering should be prevented because of added strain on the heart. Provide blankets and warm clothing as needed. Clients with hyperthyroidism are very intolerant of heat and perspire excessively owing to their rapid metabolism rate. Provide cooling baths and lightweight clothing as needed.

- **Diet.** Despite a poor appetite, *hypothyroid* clients are often overweight. Thus, a low-calorie, weight reduction diet may be indicated. In addition, an increased intake of high-fiber foods is usually needed to prevent constipation as a result of decreased gastrointestinal secretion and motility. Despite a good appetite, *hyperthyroid* clients are often underweight because of rapid metabolism rates. They often need extra calories and nutrients to prevent tissue breakdown. These can be provided by extra meals and snacks. The client may wish to avoid highly seasoned and high-fiber foods because they may increase diarrhea.

- **Fluids.** With *hypothyroidism,* clients need an adequate intake of low-calorie fluids to prevent constipation. With *hyperthyroidism,* clients need large amounts of fluids (3000–4000 ml/d) unless contraindicated by cardiac or renal disease. The fluids are needed to eliminate heat and waste products produced by the hypermetabolic state. Much of the client's fluid loss is visible as excessive perspiration and urine output.

- **Activity.** With *hypothyroidism,* encourage activity to maintain cardiovascular, respiratory, gastrointestinal, and musculoskeletal function. With *hyperthyroidism,* encourage rest and quiet, nonstrenuous activity. Because clients differ in what they find restful, this must be determined with each one. A quiet room, reading, and soft music may be helpful. Mild sedatives are often given. The client is caught in the dilemma of needing rest because of the high metabolic rate but being unable to rest because of nervousness and excitement.

- **Skin care.** *Hypothyroid* clients are likely to have edema and dry skin. When edema is present, inspect pressure points, turn often, and avoid trauma when possible. Edema increases risks of skin breakdown and decubitus ulcer formation. Also, increased capillary fragility increases the likelihood of bruising from seemingly minor trauma. When skin is dry, use soap sparingly and lotions and other lubricants freely.

- **Eye care.** *Hyperthyroid* clients may have exophthalmos. In mild cases, use measures to protect the eye. For example, dark glasses, local lubricants, and patching of the eyes at night may be needed. Diuretic drugs and elevating the head of the bed may help reduce periorbital edema and eyeball protrusion. If the eyelids cannot close, they are sometimes taped shut to avoid corneal abrasion. In severe exophthalmos, the above measures are taken and large doses of corticosteroids are usually given.

 Teach clients:
- That the duration of drug therapy for hypothyroidism is usually lifelong and for hyperthyroidism is usually 1 y or longer
- That periodic tests of thyroid function will be needed
- That dosage adjustments will be made according to clinical response and results of thyroid function tests
- To monitor response to drug therapy by weighing themselves at least weekly and recording their pulse rate daily

Evaluation

- Interview and observe for compliance with instructions for taking medications.
- Observe for relief of symptoms.
- Check laboratory reports for normal blood levels of thyroid hormones.
- Interview and observe for adverse drug effects.
- Check appointment records for compliance with follow-up procedures.

Principles of Therapy

THYROID DRUGS

Drug Selection

Levothyroxine is considered the drug of choice for thyroid hormone replacement because of uniform potency, once-daily dosing, and low cost.

Dosage Factors

Dosage is influenced by the choice of drug, the client's age, the client's general condition, severity and duration of hypothyroidism, and clinical response to drug therapy. Specific factors include the following:

1. Dosage must be individualized to approximate the amount of thyroid hormone needed to make up the deficit in endogenous hormone production.
2. As a general rule, initial dosage is relatively small. Dosage is gradually increased at about 2-week intervals in most clients until an optimum response is obtained, and symptoms are relieved. Maintenance dosage for long-term therapy is based on the client's clinical status and periodic laboratory tests, such as measurement of serum TSH.
3. Infants requiring thyroid hormone replacement need relatively large doses. After thyroid drugs are started, the maintenance dosage is determined by periodic radioimmunoassay of serum T_4 and by periodic x-ray studies to follow bone development.
4. Clients who are elderly or have cardiovascular disease are given small initial doses. Also, increments are smaller and made at longer intervals, usually about 8 weeks. The primary reason for very cautious thyroid replacement in such clients is the high risk of adverse effects on the cardiovascular system.

Hypothyroidism and the Metabolism of Other Drugs

Changes in the rate of body metabolism affect the metabolism of various drugs. Most drugs given to a client with hypothyroidism have a prolonged effect because drug metabolism in the liver is delayed, and the glomerular filtration rate of the kidneys is decreased. Also, drug absorption from the gastrointestinal system or a parenteral injection site may be slowed. As a result, dosage of many other drugs should be reduced, including digoxin and insulin. In addition, people with hypothyroidism are especially likely to develop respiratory depression and myxedema coma with narcotic analgesics and other sedating drugs. These drugs should be avoided, but if considered necessary, they are given very cautiously and in dosages of about one third to one half the usual dose. Even then, clients must be observed very closely for respiratory depression.

Once thyroid replacement therapy is started and stabilized, the client becomes euthyroid, has a normal rate of metabolism, and can tolerate usual doses of most drugs if other influencing factors are not present. On the other hand, excessive doses of thyroid drugs may produce hyperthyroidism and a greatly increased rate of metabolism. In this instance, larger doses of most other drugs are necessary to produce the same effects. Rather than increasing dosage of other drugs, though, dosage of thyroid drugs should be reduced so the client is euthyroid again.

Duration of Replacement Therapy

Thyroid replacement therapy in the client with hypothyroidism is lifelong. Medical supervision is needed frequently during early treatment and at least annually after the client's condition has stabilized and maintenance dosage has been determined.

Adrenal Insufficiency

If adrenal insufficiency is present in a client who needs thyroid drugs, that insufficiency must be corrected by giving corticosteroid drugs before starting thyroid replacement, because thyroid hormones increase tissue metabolism and tissue demands for adrenocortical hormones. If adrenal insufficiency is not treated first, administration of thyroid hormone may cause acute adrenocortical insufficiency.

ANTITHYROID DRUGS

Dosage Factors

Dosage of the thioamide antithyroid drugs is relatively large until a euthyroid state is reached, in about 6 to 8 weeks. Then a maintenance dose, in the smallest amount that prevents recurrent symptoms of hyperthyroidism, is given for 1 year or longer. Dosage should be decreased if the thyroid gland enlarges or signs and symptoms of hypothyroidism occur.

Duration of Antithyroid Therapy

No clear-cut guidelines exist regarding duration of antithyroid drug therapy because exacerbations and remissions occur. It is usually continued until the client is euthyroid for 6 to 12 months. Then diagnostic tests to evaluate thyroid function or a trial withdrawal may be implemented to determine whether the client is likely to remain euthyroid without further drug therapy. If the drug is to be discontinued, this is usually done gradually over weeks or months.

Use in Pregnancy

Iodine preparations and thioamide antithyroid drugs are contraindicated during pregnancy because they can lead to goiter and hypothyroidism in the fetus or newborn.

Hyperthyroidism and the Metabolism of Other Drugs

Treatment of hyperthyroidism changes the rate of body metabolism, including the rate of metabolism of many drugs. During the hyperthyroid state, drug metabolism may be very rapid, and higher doses of most drugs may be necessary to achieve therapeutic results. When the client becomes euthyroid, the rate of drug metabolism is decreased. Consequently, doses of all medications should be evaluated and probably reduced to avoid severe adverse reactions.

Iodine Ingestion and Hyperthyroidism

Iodine is present in foods (especially seafood), in many medications used to treat pulmonary and other diseases (*e.g.*, Calcidrine, Organidin, Quadrinal), and in many contrast dyes used for gallbladder and other radiologic procedures. Ingestion of large amounts of iodine from these sources may result in goiter and hyperthyroidism. These conditions can develop in clients with no history of thyroid disease, but they are probably more likely in those with underlying thyroid problems.

USE IN CHILDREN

For *hypothyroidism* in children, replacement therapy is required because thyroid hormone is essential for normal growth and development. As in adults, levothy-

roxine is the drug of choice in children and dosage needs may change with growth. For congenital hypothyroidism (cretinism), drug therapy should be started within 6 weeks of birth and continued for life. Initially, the recommended dose is 10 to 15 µg/kg/d. Then, maintenance doses for long-term therapy vary with the child's age and weight, generally decreasing over time to a typical adult dose at age of 11 to 20 years. Recording height and weight at regular intervals and comparing them with growth charts is one way to monitor drug effects on growth. Adverse drug effects are similar to those seen in adults, and children should be monitored closely.

For *hyperthyroidism* in children, a thioamide antithyroid drug (propylthiouracil or methimazole) is used. Potential risks of adverse effects are similar to those in adults. Because radioactive iodine may cause cancer and chromosome damage in children, it should be used only for hyperthyroidism that cannot be controlled by other antithyroid drugs or surgery.

USE IN OLDER ADULTS

Signs and symptoms of thyroid disorders may mimic those of other disorders that often occur in older adults (*e.g.*, congestive heart failure). Therefore, a thorough physical examination and diagnostic tests of thyroid function are necessary before starting any type of treatment.

For *hypothyroidism*, levothyroxine is usually given. Thyroid replacement hormone increases the workload of the heart and may cause serious adverse effects in older adults, especially those with cardiovascular disease. Cardiac effects also may be increased in clients receiving bronchodilators or other cardiac stimulants. To decrease adverse effects, the drugs should be given in small initial doses (*e.g.*, 25 µg daily) and increased by 25 µg daily at monthly intervals until euthyroidism is attained. Then, a client may be maintained on that dose of levothyroxine for a lifetime or the dose may need to be reduced as the client gets older. Periodic measurements of serum TSH levels are indicated to monitor drug therapy, and doses can be adjusted when indicated.

Blood pressure and pulse should be monitored regularly. As a general rule, do not give the drug if the resting heart rate is more than 100 beats per minute.

For *hyperthyroidism*, propylthiouracil or methimazole may be used, but radioactive iodine is often preferred because it is associated with fewer adverse effects than other antithyroid drugs or surgery. Clients should be monitored closely for hypothyroidism, which usually develops within a year after receiving treatment for hyperthyroidism.

NURSING ACTIONS · HYPOTHALAMIC AND PITUITARY HORMONES

NURSING ACTIONS	RATIONALE/EXPLANATION
1. Administer accurately **a.** With thyroid drugs:	
(1) Administer in a single daily dose, usually before breakfast.	This allows peak drug activity during daytime hours and is less likely to interfere with sleep.
(2) Check the pulse rate before giving the drug. If the rate is over 100 per minute or if any changes in cardiac rhythm are noted, consult the physician before giving the dose.	Tachycardia or other cardiac arrhythmias may indicate adverse cardiac effects. Dosage may need to be reduced or the drug stopped temporarily.
(3) Do not switch among various brands or generic forms of the drug.	Differences in bioavailability have been identified among available products. Changes in preparations may alter dosage and therefore symptom control.
b. With antithyroid and iodine drugs:	
(1) Administer q8h.	All these drugs have rather short half-lives and must be given frequently and regularly to maintain therapeutic blood levels. In addition, if iodine preparations are not given every 8 h, symptoms of hyperthyroidism may recur.
(2) Dilute iodine solutions in a full glass of fruit juice or milk, if possible, and have the client drink the medication through a straw.	Dilution of the drug reduces gastric irritation and masks the unpleasant taste. Using a straw prevents staining the teeth.
2. Observe for therapeutic effects **a.** With thyroid drugs, observe for:	
(1) Increased energy and activity level, less lethargy and fatigue	Therapeutic effects result from a return to normal metabolic activities and relief of the symptoms of hypothyroidism. Therapeutic effects may be evident as early as 2 or 3 d after drug therapy is started or delayed up to about 2 wk. All signs and symptoms of myxedema should disappear in about 3 to 12 wk.
(2) Increased alertness and interest in surroundings	
(3) Increased appetite	
(4) Increased pulse rate and temperature	
(5) Decreased constipation	
(6) Reversal of coarseness and other changes in skin and hair	
(7) With cretinism, increased growth rate (record height periodically)	
(8) With myxedema, diuresis, weight loss, and decreased edema	
(9) Increased serum T_4	
(10) Decreased serum cholesterol and possibly decreased creatine phosphokinase, lactic dehydrogenase, and aspartate aminotransferase	These tests are often elevated with myxedema and may return to normal when thyroid replacement therapy is begun.
b. With antithyroid and iodine drugs, observe for:	
(1) Slower pulse rate	With propylthiouracil and methimazole, some therapeutic effects are apparent in 1 or 2 wk, but euthyroidism may not occur for 6 or 8 wk.
(2) Slower speech	

Nursing Actions	*Rationale/Explanation*
(3) More normal activity level (slowing of hyperactivity)	With iodine solutions, therapeutic effects may be apparent within 24 h. Maximal effects occur in about 10 to 15 d. However, therapeutic effects may not be sustained. Symptoms may reappear if the drug is given longer than a few weeks, and they may be more severe than initially.
(4) Decreased nervousness	
(5) Decreased tremors	
(6) Improved ability to sleep and rest	
(7) Weight gain	
3. Observe for adverse effects	
a. With thyroid drugs, observe for tachycardia and other cardiac arrhythmias, angina pectoris, myocardial infarction, congestive heart failure, nervousness, hyperactivity, insomnia, diarrhea, abdominal cramps, nausea and vomiting, weight loss, fever, intolerance to heat.	Most adverse reactions stem from excessive doses, and signs and symptoms produced are the same as those occurring with hyperthyroidism. Excessive thyroid hormones make the heart work very hard and fast in attempting to meet tissue demands for oxygenated blood and nutrients. Symptoms of myocardial ischemia occur when the myocardium does not get an adequate supply of oxygenated blood. Symptoms of congestive heart failure occur when the increased cardiac workload is prolonged. Cardiovascular problems are more likely to occur in clients who are elderly or who already have heart disease.
b. With propylthiouracil and methimazole, observe for:	
(1) Hypothyroidism—bradycardia, congestive heart failure, anemia, coronary artery and peripheral vascular disease, slow speech and movements, emotional and mental dullness, excessive sleeping, weight gain, constipation, skin changes, and others	
(2) Blood disorders—leukopenia, agranulocytosis, hypoprothrombinemia	Leukopenia may be difficult to evaluate because it may occur with hyperthyroidism and with antithyroid drugs. Agranulocytosis occurs rarely but is the most severe adverse reaction; the earliest symptoms are likely to be sore throat and fever. If these occur, report them to the physician immediately.
(3) Integumentary system—skin rash, pruritus, alopecia	
(4) CNS—headache, dizziness, loss of sense of taste, drowsiness, paresthesias	
(5) Gastrointestinal system—nausea, vomiting, abdominal discomfort, gastric irritation, cholestatic hepatitis	
(6) Other—lymphadenopathy, edema, joint pain, drug fever	
c. With iodine preparations, observe for:	Adverse effects are uncommon with short-term use.
(1) Iodism—metallic taste, burning in mouth, soreness of gums, excessive salivation, gastric or respiratory irritation, rhinitis, headache, redness of conjunctiva, edema of eyelids	
(2) Hypersensitivity—acneiform skin rash, pruritus, fever, jaundice, angioedema, serum sickness	Allergic reactions rarely occur.
(3) Goiter with hypothyroidism	Uncommon but may occur in adults and newborns whose mothers have taken iodides for long periods

(continued)

NURSING ACTIONS	RATIONALE/EXPLANATION
4. Observe for drug interactions **a.** Drugs that *increase* effects of the thyroid hormones:	
(1) Antidepressants (tricyclic), epinephrine, levarterenol	These drugs primarily increase catecholamines. When combined with thyroid hormones, excessive cardiovascular stimulation may occur and cause myocardial ischemia, cardiac arrhythmias, hypertension, and other adverse cardiovascular effects.
(2) Clofibrate, phenobarbital, and phenytoin	Potentiate thyroid drugs by displacement from plasma protein-binding sites or by slowing liver metabolism
b. Drugs that *decrease* effects of thyroid hormones:	
(1) Antihypertensives	These agents decrease the cardiovascular effects of catecholamines (epinephrine and norepinephrine) and thyroid hormone so angina pectoris is less likely to occur.
(2) Cholestyramine resin (Questran)	This drug decreases gastrointestinal absorption of thyroid hormones. Cholestyramine binds T_4 and T_3 almost irreversibly. If it is necessary to give these drugs concurrently, give the resin at least 4 or 5 h before or after giving the thyroid drug.
(3) Estrogens, including oral contraceptives containing estrogens	Estrogens inhibit thyroid hormones by increasing thyroxine-binding globulin. This increases the amount of bound, inactive thyroid hormones in clients with hypothyroidism. This decreased effect does not occur in clients with adequate thyroid hormone secretion because the increased binding is offset by increased T_4 production. Women taking oral contraceptives may need larger doses of thyroid hormone replacement than would otherwise be needed.
(4) Propranolol (Inderal)	This drug decreases cardiac effects of thyroid hormones. It is used in hyperthyroidism to reduce tachycardia and other symptoms of excessive cardiovascular stimulation.
c. Drugs that *increase* effects of antithyroid drugs:	
(1) Chlorpromazine, sulfonamides, oral antidiabetic drugs, xanthines	Increased risk of goiter
(2) Lithium	Acts synergistically to produce hypothyroidism
5. Teach clients **a.** Take thyroid and antithyroid drugs as directed.	Thyroid replacement hormones must be continued throughout life. Thioamide antithyroid drugs must be taken for 1 y or longer.
b. Report adverse effects (hyperthyroidism, hypothyroidism, iodism, and others).	Drug dosage may need to be reduced or the drug discontinued.
c. Avoid over-the-counter drugs or consult with physician before taking them.	Many preparations contain iodide, which can increase the likelihood of goiter with thioamides and the risk of adverse reactions from excessive doses of iodide. For example, cough syrups, some asthma medications, and some multivitamins contain iodide.
d. Ask the physician if it is necessary to avoid or restrict amounts of seafood or iodized salt.	These sources of iodide may need to be reduced or omitted during antithyroid drug therapy.

**REVIEW AND
APPLICATION EXERCISES**

1. Where is TSH produced, and what is its function?

2. What is the role of thyroid hormones in maintaining body functions?

3. What signs and symptoms are associated with hypothyroidism?

4. In primary hypothyroidism, are blood levels of TSH increased or decreased?

5. What is the drug of first choice for treating hypothyroidism?

6. What are adverse effects of drug therapy for hypothyroidism?

7. What signs and symptoms are associated with hyperthyroidism?

8. Which drugs reduce blood levels of thyroid hormone in hyperthyroidism, and how do they act?

9. What are adverse effects of drug therapy for hyperthyroidism?

10. When propranolol is used in the treatment of hyperthyroidism, what are its expected effects?

11. What is the effect of thyroid disorders on metabolism of other drugs?

SELECTED REFERENCES

Drug facts and comparisons. (1996). St. Louis: Facts and Comparisons.

Guyton, A.C. & Hall, J.E. (1996). *Textbook of medical physiology,* 9th ed. Philadelphia: W.B. Saunders.

Porth, C.M. & Hurwitz, L.S. (1994). Alterations in endocrine control of growth and metabolism. In C.M. Porth (Ed.), *Pathophysiology: Concepts of altered health states,* 4th ed., pp. 907–926. Philadelphia: J.B. Lippincott.

Reasner, C.A. II & Talbert R.L. (1993). Thyroid disorders. In J.T. DiPiro, R.L. Talbert, P.E. Hayes, G.C. Yee, G.R. Matzke, & L.M. Posey (Eds.), *Pharmacotherapy: A pathophysiologic approach,* 2nd ed., pp. 1146–1167. Norwalk, CT: Appleton & Lange.

Singer, P.A., Cooper, D.S., Levy, E.G., et al. (1995). Treatment guidelines for patients with hyperthyroidism and hypothyroidism. *Journal of the American Medical Association, 273,* 808–812.

26 Hormones That Regulate Calcium and Phosphorus Metabolism

Outline

Objectives

After studying this chapter, the student will be able to:

1 Describe the roles of parathyroid hormone, calcitonin and vitamin D in regulating calcium metabolism.

2 Identify populations at risk of developing hypocalcemia.

3 Discuss prevention and treatment of hypocalcemia.

4 Identify clients at risk of developing hypercalcemia.

5 Discuss recognition and management of hypercalcemia as a medical emergency.

Key Terms

Calciferol	**Hypocalcemia**
Calcitonin	**Tetany**
Hypercalcemia	

Description

Calcium and phosphorus metabolism is regulated primarily by three hormones: parathyroid hormone, calcitonin, and vitamin D (calciferol). These hormones are interrelated in a complex homeostatic mechanism of which the main goal is to maintain normal serum levels of calcium.

PARATHYROID HORMONE

Parathyroid hormone is secreted by the parathyroid glands located behind the thyroid gland. The primary function of parathyroid hormone is to maintain normal calcium levels in the serum or extracellular fluid. Parathyroid hormone secretion is stimulated by low serum calcium levels and inhibited by normal or high levels. Thus, secretion is controlled by a negative feedback system, as are most other hormonal secretions. Because phosphate is closely related to calcium in body functions, parathyroid hormone also regulates phosphate metabolism. As a general rule, when serum calcium levels go up, serum phosphate levels go down, and vice versa. Thus, an inverse relationship between calcium and phosphate is maintained.

When the serum calcium level falls below the normal range, parathyroid hormone raises the level by acting on bone, intestines, and kidneys. The effect of parathyroid hormone on bone is to increase bone breakdown or resorption, thereby causing calcium to move from bone into the serum. The effect on intestines is to increase absorption of calcium ingested in food, and the effect on the kidneys is to increase reabsorption of calcium in the renal tubules (thereby decreasing urinary excretion). The opposite effects occur with phosphate (*i.e.*, parathyroid hormone decreases serum phosphate and increases urinary phosphate excretion).

Disorders of parathyroid function are related to deficient production of parathyroid hormone (hypoparathyroidism) or excessive production (hyperparathyroidism). Hypoparathyroidism is most often caused by removal of or damage to the parathyroid glands during neck surgery. There are normally four parathyroid glands. Removal of two causes little, if any, change in normal function. If even a small amount of parathyroid tissue remains, a transient hypoparathyroidism may occur, but the tissue usually enlarges and secretes sufficient parathyroid hormone to meet body requirements. Hyperparathyroidism is most often caused by a tumor or hyperplasia of one of the glands. It also may result from ectopic secretion of parathyroid hormone by malignant tumors (*e.g.*, carcinomas of the lung, pancreas, kidney, ovary, prostate gland, or bladder).

Clinical manifestations and treatment of hypoparathyroidism are the same as those of hypocalcemia, which is discussed later in this chapter. Treatment of hypocalcemia includes giving a calcium preparation and perhaps vitamin D. Clinical manifestations of hyperparathyroidism are those of hypercalcemia, also discussed later in this chapter. When hypercalcemia is caused by a tumor of parathyroid tissue, the usual treatment of choice is surgical excision. When it is caused by malignant tumor, treatment of the tumor with surgery, irradiation, or chemotherapy may reduce production of parathyroid hormone.

CALCITONIN

Calcitonin is a hormone secreted by the thyroid gland. Its secretion is controlled by the concentration of ionized calcium in the blood flowing through the thyroid gland. When the serum level of ionized calcium is increased, secretion of calcitonin is increased. Calcitonin lowers serum calcium levels primarily by decreasing movement of calcium from bone to serum. Calcitonin also increases renal excretion of calcium, phosphate, sodium, and chloride, but its primary function is to lower serum calcium in the presence of hypercalcemia. Its action is rapid but of short duration. Thus, it has little effect on long-term calcium metabolism. Synthetic preparations of calcitonin are available for clinical use in the treatment of hypercalcemia and Paget's disease.

VITAMIN D (CALCIFEROL)

Vitamin D is a fat-soluble vitamin that includes both ergocalciferol (obtained from foods) and cholecalciferol (formed by exposure of skin to sunlight). It functions as a hormone and plays an important role in calcium metabolism. The main action of vitamin D is to raise serum calcium levels by increasing intestinal absorption of dietary calcium and mobilizing calcium from bone. Vitamin D is not physiologically active in the body. It must be converted to an active metabolite (1,25-dihydroxyvitamin D or calcitriol) by a series of reactions in the liver and kidneys. Parathyroid hormone and adequate renal function are required to produce the active metabolite.

The recommended intake of vitamin D is 10 μg (400 units) daily from infancy through 24 years and during pregnancy and lactation. For adults older than 24 years, 5 μg (200 units) are recommended. Milk that has been fortified with vitamin D is the best food source. Exposure of skin to sunlight is also needed to supply adequate amounts of vitamin D.

Deficiency of vitamin D causes inadequate absorption of calcium and phosphorus. This, in turn, leads to low levels of serum calcium and stimulation of parathyroid hormone secretion, which raises serum calcium levels by moving calcium from bone into serum. In children, this sequence of events produces inadequate mineralization of bone (rickets), a condition now rare in the United States. In adults, vitamin D deficiency causes osteomalacia, a condition characterized by decreased bone density and strength. Osteomalacia is more likely to occur during times of increased need for calcium, such as pregnancy and lactation.

Clinical indications for use of vitamin D supplements include prevention and treatment of rickets and osteomalacia, treatment of hypoparathyroidism, and treatment of chronic hypocalcemia when calcium supplements fail to maintain normal serum calcium levels. The major adverse reaction resulting from high dosage or prolonged administration is hypervitaminosis D. This condition of excessive accumulation of vitamin D produces signs and symptoms of hypercalcemia. The first step in treatment is to stop the administration of vitamin D. Other treatment measures are the same as for hypercalcemia from other causes and are described later in this chapter.

CALCIUM AND PHOSPHORUS

Calcium and phosphorus are discussed together because they are closely related physiologically. These mineral nutrients are found in many of the same foods, from which they are absorbed together. They are regulated by parathyroid hormone and excreted through the kidneys. They are both required, as calcium phosphate, in formation and maintenance of bones and teeth.

Calcium

Calcium is the most abundant cation in the body. About 99% of calcium is located in the bones and teeth; the rest is in the extracellular fluid and soft tissues. There is constant shifting of calcium among body compartments. This is part of the homeostatic mechanism that acts to maintain serum calcium levels at about 8.5 to 10 mg/100 ml.

About half of serum calcium is bound, mostly to serum proteins, and is physiologically inactive. The other half of the total serum calcium is ionized and physiologically active. This seemingly small amount of calcium performs vital functions. Small fluctuations in the amount of ionized calcium have profound effects on body organs. Physiologic functions of calcium include the following:

1. Participating in many metabolic processes. Ionized calcium can leave the vascular compartment and enter cells, where it participates in intracellular functions and is important in the regulation of:
   a. Cell membrane permeability and function
   b. Nerve cell excitability and transmission of impulses (e.g., it is important in nerve cell release of neurotransmitters).
   c. Contraction of cardiac, skeletal, and smooth muscle, including the electrophysiologic slow calcium channel response in cardiac and smooth muscle
   d. Blood coagulation and platelet adhesion processes
   e. Hormone secretion
   f. Enzyme activity
2. Building and maintaining bones and teeth. Bone calcium is mainly composed of calcium phosphate and calcium carbonate. In addition to these bound forms, a small amount of calcium is available for exchange with serum. This acts as a reserve supply of calcium. Calcium is constantly shifting between bone and serum as bone is formed and broken down. Calcium is taken from the serum and used in the formation of new bone by osteoblast cells; it is transferred from bone to the serum when bone is broken down by osteoclast cells. The latter process is called bone resorption. When serum calcium levels become low, calcium moves into serum at the expense of bone calcium.

The calcium requirement of normal adults is about 1000 mg daily. Increased daily amounts are needed by growing children (1200 mg), pregnant or lactating women (1200 mg), and postmenopausal women who do not take replacement estrogens (1500 mg to prevent osteoporosis).

The best source of calcium is milk or milk products. Three 8-oz glasses of milk daily contain approximately the amount needed by healthy adults. Calcium in milk is readily used by the body because milk also contains lactose and vitamin D, both of which are involved in calcium absorption. Other sources of calcium include vegetables (e.g., broccoli, spinach, kale, mustard greens) and seafood (e.g., clams, oysters).

About 30% to 50% of dietary calcium is absorbed from the small intestine; the rest is lost in feces. Some factors that aid calcium absorption include the presence of vitamin D, increased acidity of gastric secretions, the presence of lactose, moderate amounts of fat, high protein intake, and a physiologic need. Factors that inhibit calcium absorption include the following:

Vitamin D deficiency
High-fat diet, which leads to formation of insoluble calcium salts in the intestine
The presence of oxalic acid (from beet greens, chard), which combines with calcium to form insoluble calcium oxalate in the intestine
Alkalinity of intestinal secretions, which leads to formation of insoluble calcium phosphate
Diarrhea or other conditions of rapid intestinal motility, which do not allow sufficient time for absorption
Immobilization
Mental or emotional stress

Calcium is lost from the body in feces, urine, and sweat. In lactating women, relatively large amounts are lost in breast milk.

Phosphorus

1. Phosphorus is one of the most important elements in normal body function. Most phosphorus is combined with calcium in bones and teeth as calcium phosphate (about 80%). The remainder is distributed in every body cell and in extracellular fluid. It is combined with carbohydrates, lipids, proteins, and various other compounds.
2. Most phosphorus is located intracellularly (as the phosphate ion), where it performs many metabolic functions:
   a. It is an essential component of deoxyribonucleic acid, ribonucleic acid, and other nucleic acids in body cells. Thus, it is required for cell reproduction and body growth.
   b. It combines with fatty acids to form phospholipids, which are components of all cell membranes in the body. This reaction also prevents excessive amounts of free fatty acids.
   c. It forms a phosphate buffer system, which helps to maintain acid–base balance. When excess hydrogen ions are present in kidney tubules, phosphate combines with them and allows their excretion in urine. At the same time, bicarbonate is retained by the kidneys and contributes to alkalinity of body fluids. Although there are other buffering systems in the body, failure of the phosphate system leads to metabolic acidosis (retained hydrogen ions or acid and lost bicarbonate ions or base).
   d. It is necessary for cell use of glucose and production of energy.
   e. It is necessary for proper function of several B vitamins (i.e., the vitamins function as coenzymes in various chemical reactions only when combined with phosphate).
3. Daily requirements for phosphorus are about 800 mg for normal adults and about 1200 mg for growing children and pregnant or lactating women. Phosphorus is widely available in foods. Good sources are milk and dairy products, meat, poultry, fish, eggs, and nuts. There is little risk of phosphorus deficiency with an adequate intake of calcium and protein.

About 70% of dietary phosphorus is absorbed from the gastrointestinal (GI) tract. The most efficient absorption occurs when calcium and phosphorus are ingested in approximately equal amounts. Because this equal ratio is present in milk, milk is probably the best source of phosphorus. Generally, factors that increase or decrease calcium absorption act the same way on phosphorus absorption. Vitamin D enhances, but is not essential for, phosphorus absorption. Large amounts of calcium or aluminum in the GI tract may combine with phosphate to form insoluble compounds and thereby decrease absorption of phosphorus.

Phosphorus is lost from the body primarily in urine. In people with acute or chronic renal failure, phosphorus intake is restricted because excretion is impaired.

Hypocalcemia

Hypocalcemia may result from several causes, including inadequate dietary intake of calcium and vitamin D, inadequate absorption of calcium and vitamin D with diarrhea or malabsorption syndromes, hypoparathyroidism, and impaired renal function. Hypocalcemia associated with renal failure is caused by two mechanisms. First, inability to excrete phosphate in urine leads to accumulation of phosphate in the blood (hyperphosphatemia). Because phosphate levels are inversely related to calcium levels, hyperphosphatemia induces hypocalcemia. Second, when kidney function is impaired, vitamin D conversion to its active metabolite is impaired. This results in decreased intestinal absorption of calcium.

Clinical manifestations of hypocalcemia are characterized by increased neuromuscular irritability, which may progress to tetany. Tetany is characterized by numbness and tingling of the lips, fingers, and toes; twitching of facial muscles; spasms of skeletal muscle; carpopedal spasm; laryngospasm; and convulsions. In young children, hypocalcemia may be manifested by convulsions rather than tetany and erroneously diagnosed as epilepsy. This may be a serious error because anticonvulsant drugs used for epilepsy may further decrease serum calcium levels.

INDIVIDUAL DRUGS USED IN HYPOCALCEMIA

The drugs used to treat hypocalcemia are calcium and vitamin D preparations (Table 26-1). Several calcium salts may be used intravenously for acute hypocalcemia and orally for less severe or chronic hypocalcemia. These preparations differ mainly in the amounts of calcium they contain and the routes by which they may be given. Vitamin D is used in chronic hypocalcemia if calcium preparations alone cannot maintain serum calcium levels within normal range.

Nursing Process (Hypocalcemia)

Assessment

- Assess for conditions in which hypocalcemia is likely to occur (e.g., inadequate intake or absorption of calcium and vitamin D).

TABLE 26-1 DRUGS USED IN HYPOCALCEMIA

Generic/Trade Name	Routes and Dosage Ranges	
	Adults	*Children*
Calcium Preparations		
Calcium carbonate precipitated (40% calcium) (Os-Cal 500)	PO 1–1.5 g three times daily with meals (maximal daily dose, 8 g)	
Calcium chloride (10 ml of 10% solution contains 273 mg [13.6 mEq] of calcium)	IV 500 mg–1 g (5–10 ml of 10% solution) every 1–3 d, depending on clinical response or serum calcium measurements.	IV 0.2 ml/kg, up to 1–10 ml/d
Calcium citrate (21% calcium) (Citracal)	1–2 tablets (200 mg calcium per tablet) two to four times daily	
Calcium glubionate (6% calcium) (Neo-Calglucon)	PO 15 ml three times daily Pregnancy or lactation, PO 15 ml four times daily	PO 10 ml three times daily
Calcium gluceptate (8% calcium)	IV 5–20 ml IM 2–5 ml	IM 2–5 ml
Calcium gluconate (9% calcium)	PO 1–2 g three or four times daily IV 5–20 ml of 10% solution	PO, IV 500 mg/kg/d in divided doses
Calcium lactate (13% calcium)	PO 1–3 g three times daily with meals	PO 500 mg/kg/d in divided doses
Calcium phosphate dibasic (30% calcium) (Dical-D)	PO 0.5–1.5 g two or three times daily with meals	Dosage not established
Calcium phosphate tribasic (39% calcium) (Posture)	1–2 tablets (600 mg calcium per tablet) two to four times daily	
Vitamin D Preparations		
Calcifediol (Calderol)	PO 50–100 μg daily	Dosage not established
Calcitriol (Rocaltrol)	PO 0.25 μg daily initially, then adjusted according to serum calcium levels (usual daily maintenance dose, 0.5–1 μg)	
Cholecalciferol (Delta-D)	PO 400–1000 IU daily	Dosage not established
Dihydrotachysterol (Hytakerol)	PO 0.8–2.4 mg daily, then decreased for maintenance according to serum calcium levels (usual daily maintenance dose, 0.2–1.0 mg)	
Ergocalciferol (vitamin D) (Drisdol)	PO 50,000–200,000 units daily initially (average daily maintenance dose, 25,000–100,000 units)	

- Assess dietary intake of dairy products and other calcium-containing foods.
- Observe for the previously described clinical manifestations.
- Check serum calcium reports for decreased values. Although laboratories differ slightly in normal values, the total serum calcium level is about 8.8 to 10.3 mg/100 ml (SI units 2.2–2.6 mmol/L). About half of the total serum calcium (*e.g.*, 4–5 mg/100 ml) should be free ionized calcium, the physiologically active form. To interpret serum calcium levels accurately, serum albumin levels and acid–base status must be considered. Low serum albumin decreases the total serum level of calcium by decreasing the amount of calcium that is bound to protein. However, the unbound, ionized concentration is normal. Metabolic and respiratory alkalosis increase binding of calcium to serum proteins, thereby maintaining normal total serum calcium but decreasing the ionized values. Conversely, metabolic and respiratory acidosis decrease binding and therefore increase the concentration of ionized calcium.
- Check once daily for *Chvostek's sign:* Tap the facial nerve just below the temple, in front of the ear. If facial muscles twitch, hyperirritability of the nerve and potential tetany are indicated.
- Check for *Trousseau's sign:* Constrict blood circulation in an arm (usually with a blood-pressure cuff) for 3 to 5 min. This produces ischemia and increased irritability of peripheral nerves, which causes spasms of the lower arm and hand muscles (carpal spasm) if tetany is present.

Nursing Diagnoses

- Altered Nutrition: Less Than Body Requirements with hypocalcemia
- Knowledge Deficit: Recommended daily amounts and dietary sources of calcium and vitamin D
- Knowledge Deficit: Rational use of vitamin and mineral supplements
- Risk for Injury: Tetany, sedation, seizures from hypocalcemia
- Risk for Injury: Hypercalcemia related to overuse of supplements
- Constipation with oral calcium supplements

Planning/Goals

The client will:

- Achieve and maintain normal serum levels of calcium
- Increase dietary intake of calcium-containing foods
- Use calcium or vitamin D supplements with the approval and supervision of a health care provider
- Avoid hypercalcemia from overuse of supplements

Interventions

Prevent hypocalcemia when possible by assisting clients to maintain an adequate dietary intake of calcium. With an adequate protein and calcium intake, enough phosphorus will also be obtained.

- The best dietary source is milk and other dairy products, including yogurt.
- Unless contraindicated by the client's condition, recommend that adults drink at least two 8-oz glasses of milk daily. This will furnish about half the daily calcium requirement; the remainder will probably be obtained from other foods.
- Children need about four glasses of milk or an equivalent amount of calcium in milk and other foods to support normal growth and development.
- Pregnant and lactating women also need about four glasses of milk or their equivalents to meet increased needs. Vitamin and mineral supplements are often prescribed during these periods. However, some supplements contain only 250 mg of a calcium salt (equivalent to 8 oz of milk). This amount does not go very far in meeting a requirement of about 1200 mg.
- Postmenopausal women who take estrogens need the usual adult amount (1000 mg). Those who do not take estrogens need about 1500 mg to prevent or minimize osteoporosis.
- For clients who avoid or minimize their intake of dairy products because of the calories, identify low-calorie sources, such as skim milk and low-fat yogurt.

 Teach clients:

- Not to take calcium or vitamin D supplements unless recommended by a health care provider. They are rarely needed if dietary intake is adequate. Taking more than needed to maintain normal body function serves no beneficial purpose. In addition, excessive amounts are potentially more harmful than a minor deficiency.
- If a supplement is recommended, an inexpensive, over-the-counter antacid called Tums contains 200 mg per tablet. Avoid supplements containing bone meal; they may contain lead and other contaminants that are toxic to the human body.

- Exercise, especially if vigorous and weight-bearing, helps to promote and maintain strong bone. Inactivity promotes bone weakening and loss.

Evaluation

- Check laboratory reports for normal serum calcium levels.
- Interview and observe for relief of symptoms of hypocalcemia.
- Interview and observe intake of calcium-containing foods.
- Question about normal calcium requirements and how to meet them.

Principles of Therapy: Drugs Used in Hypocalcemia

1. If hypocalcemia is caused by diarrhea or malabsorption, treatment of the underlying condition will decrease loss of calcium from the body and increase absorption.
2. In severe, acute hypocalcemia, IV calcium gluconate or calcium chloride is given. For less acute situations or for long-term treatment of chronic hypocalcemia, oral calcium supplements are preferred. Vitamin D is given also if a calcium preparation alone cannot maintain serum calcium levels within a normal range.
3. When vitamin D is given to treat hypocalcemia, dosage is determined by frequent measurement of serum calcium levels. Usually, higher doses are given initially, then decreased to smaller doses for maintenance therapy.

CALCIUM–VITAMIN D COMBINATIONS

Calcium salts and vitamin D are combined in a number of commercial preparations. These are promoted as dietary supplements for children and for women during pregnancy and lactation. There is no evidence that these fixed amounts of calcium and vitamin D meet the dietary needs of most people. Therefore, calcium and vitamin D should be prescribed individually. Also, these mixtures are not indicated for maintenance therapy in chronic hypocalcemia.

DRUG INTERACTIONS

1. Calcium preparations and digoxin have similar effects on the myocardium. Therefore, if calcium is given to a digitalized client, the risks of digitalis toxicity and cardiac arrhythmias are increased. This combination must be used very cautiously.
2. Oral calcium preparations decrease effects of oral tetracycline drugs by combining with the antibiotic and preventing its absorption. They should not be given at the same time or within 2 to 3 hours of each other.

Use in Children

Hypocalcemia is uncommon in children. If it does develop, principles of using calcium or vitamin D supplements are the same as those in adults. Monitor closely for signs and symptoms of adverse drug effects.

Use in Older Adults

Calcium moves from bone to blood to maintain normal serum levels. In older adults, demineralization and weakening of bone (osteoporosis) increase risks of fractures, pain, skeletal deformity, and loss of self-care abilities. People at risk for developing osteoporosis include postmenopausal women; those with small stature, lean body mass, sedentary lifestyles, and long-term deficiencies in calcium intake; and those with diseases or drugs (*e.g.*, adrenal corticosteroids) that demineralize bone. In addition, absorption of calcium from the intestine is impaired in older adults, possibly aggravated by inadequate activation of vitamin D.

Sex hormones seem to play a role in osteoporosis. This is most evident in postmenopausal women, who comprise the group most likely to develop the disorder. Older men are also at risk; however, osteoporosis is likely to develop less often, at a later age, and to be less extensive than in older women. Thus, older adults need to continue their dietary intake of dairy products and other calcium-containing foods. Estrogen replacement drugs and calcium supplements are recommended for postmenopausal women, to prevent or treat osteoporosis. Overuse of supplements should be avoided because it may cause hypercalcemia.

NURSING ACTIONS — DRUGS USED IN HYPOCALCEMIA

Nursing Actions	*Rationale/Explanation*
1. Administer accurately **a.** Give oral calcium preparations 30 min before meals or at bedtime.	To increase absorption
b. With IV calcium preparations, inject slowly, over at least 2 min, check pulse and blood pressure closely, and preferably monitor the electrocardiogram (ECG).	Arrhythmias and hypotension may occur. Hypercalcemia is indicated on the ECG by a prolonged QT interval associated with an inverted T wave.
c. Do not mix IV calcium preparations with any other drug in the same syringe.	Calcium reacts with some other drugs and forms a precipitate.
2. Observe for therapeutic effects **a.** Relief of symptoms of neuromuscular irritability and tetany, such as decreased muscle spasms and decreased paresthesias	
b. Serum calcium levels within normal range (8.5–10 mg/100 ml)	
c. Absence of Chvostek's and Trousseau's signs	
3. Observe for adverse effects **a.** Hypercalcemia: (1) Gastrointestinal effects—anorexia, nausea, vomiting, abdominal pain, constipation (2) Central nervous system (CNS) effects—apathy, poor memory, depression, drowsiness, disorientation, coma (3) Other effects—weakness and decreased tone in skeletal and smooth muscles, dysphagia, polyuria, polydipsia, cardiac arrhythmias (4) Increased serum calcium	
b. Hypervitaminosis D—produces hypercalcemia and the clinical manifestations listed above	This is most likely to occur with chronic ingestion of 50,000 or more units of vitamin D daily. In children, accidental ingestion may lead to acute toxicity.

(continued)

NURSING ACTIONS	RATIONALE/EXPLANATION
4. Observe for drug interactions **a.** Drugs that *increase* effects of calcium:	
(1) Vitamin D	Increases intestinal absorption of calcium from both dietary and supplemental drug sources
b. Drugs that *decrease* effects of calcium:	
(1) Adrenocorticosteroids (prednisone, others), calcitonin, plicamycin, and phosphates	These drugs lower serum calcium levels by various mechanisms. They are used in the treatment of hypercalcemia and are discussed further in the next section of this chapter.
(2) Antacids	Oral calcium preparations are more soluble and better absorbed in an acid medium. Antacids decrease acidity of gastric secretions and therefore may decrease absorption of calcium.
(3) Laxatives	These drugs decrease absorption of calcium from the intestinal tract by increasing motility. This allows less time for calcium absorption.
c. Drugs that *increase* effects of vitamin D: Thiazide diuretics	Thiazide diuretics administered to hypoparathyroid clients may cause hypercalcemia (potentiate vitamin D effects).
d. Drugs that *decrease* effects of vitamin D:	
(1) Anticonvulsants (*e.g.*, phenytoin [Dilantin], primidone [Mysoline], phenobarbital)	These drugs accelerate and change the metabolism of vitamin D in the liver. As a result, vitamin D deficiency, hypocalcemia, and rickets or osteomalacia are likely to develop in clients receiving anticonvulsant drugs for seizure disorders. These problems can be prevented by increasing intake of vitamin D.
(2) Cholestyramine resin (Questran)	May decrease intestinal absorption of calcitriol (Rocaltrol)
(3) Mineral oil	Mineral oil is a fat and therefore combines with fat-soluble vitamins, such as vitamin D, and prevents their absorption from the gastrointestinal tract.
5. Teach clients **a.** If calcium or vitamin D is prescribed, take as directed.	To obtain the greatest therapeutic effect with the least likelihood of adverse effects from overdosage
b. With chronic hypocalcemia, increase dietary intake of calcium and vitamin D with milk and other dairy products. Note that foods that contain oxalic acid (*e.g.*, spinach, rhubarb) and phytic acid (*e.g.*, bran) may decrease absorption of calcium.	
c. Report signs and symptoms of hypercalcemia.	See 3(a) above.

Hypercalcemia

Hypercalcemia occurs with hyperparathyroidism, excessive ingestion of vitamin D, malignant neoplasms, prolonged immobilization, adrenocortical insufficiency, and ingestion of thiazide diuretics, estrogens, and lithium. In hospitalized clients, cancer is a common cause of hypercalcemia, especially carcinomas (of the breast, lung, head and neck, or kidney) and multiple myeloma. Cancer stimulates bone resorption or breakdown, which increases serum calcium levels. In-

creased urine output leads to fluid volume deficit. This leads, in turn, to increased reabsorption of calcium in renal tubules and decreased renal excretion of calcium. Decreased renal excretion potentiates hypercalcemia.

Clinical manifestations are caused by the decreased ability of nerves to respond to stimuli and the decreased ability of muscles to contract and relax. Hypercalcemia has a depressant effect on nerve and muscle function.

GI problems with hypercalcemia include anorexia, nausea, vomiting, constipation, and abdominal pain. Central nervous system (CNS) problems include apathy, depression, poor memory, headache, and drowsiness. Severe hypercalcemia may produce lethargy, syncope, disorientation, hallucinations, coma, and death. Other signs and symptoms include weakness and decreased tone in skeletal and smooth muscle, dysphagia, polyuria, polyphagia, and cardiac arrhythmias. In addition, calcium may be deposited in various tissues, such as the conjunctiva, cornea, and kidneys. Calcium deposits in the kidneys (renal calculi) may lead to irreversible damage and impairment of function.

Individual Drugs Used in Hypercalcemia

The agents used in hypercalcemia belong to several therapeutic classes and act by different mechanisms to lower serum calcium levels.

Calcitonin-salmon (Calcimar, Miacalcin) is used in the treatment of hypercalcemia, Paget's disease, and postmenopausal osteoporosis. In hypercalcemia, calcitonin lowers serum calcium levels by inhibiting bone resorption (i.e., movement of calcium from bone to serum). It is most likely to be effective in hypercalcemia caused by hyperparathyroidism, prolonged immobilization, or certain malignant neoplasms. In acute hypercalcemia, calcitonin may be used along with other measures to lower serum calcium levels rapidly. A single injection of calcitonin decreases serum calcium levels in about 2 hours; effects last about 6 to 8 hours. The amount of the decrease is unpredictable and varies extensively among clients. In chronic hypercalcemia, it may lose its effectiveness after several weeks.

Paget's disease is a disorder characterized by an abnormal and rapid rate of bone formation and breakdown. Calcitonin slows the rate of bone turnover, improves bone lesions on radiologic examination, and relieves bone pain. In postmenopausal osteoporosis, calcitonin prevents further bone loss and increases bone mass in the presence of adequate calcium and vitamin D. Calcitonin is available as a nasal spray for treatment of osteoporosis.

Calcitonin-human (Cibacalcin) is a synthetic preparation with the same number and sequence of amino acids as human calcitonin. It is approved for use in Paget's disease. Compared to calcitonin-salmon, calcitonin-human is more likely to cause nausea and facial flushing and less likely to cause antibody formation and allergic reactions.

Calcitonin-Salmon
Routes and Dosage Ranges

Adults: Hypercalcemia, SC, IM 4 IU/kg q12h; can be increased after 1 or 2 d to 8 IU/kg q12h; maximum dose, 8 IU/kg q6h
Paget's disease, SC, IM 50–100 IU/d
Postmenopausal osteoporosis, SC, IM 100 IU/d (along with supplemental calcium [1500 mg]

and vitamin D [400 units] daily); nasal spray (Miacalcin) 200 IU daily

Calcitonin-human
Route and Dosage Range

Adults: Paget's disease, SC 0.5 mg/d

Alendronate (Fosamax), **etidronate** (Didronel) and **pamidronate** (Aredia) are chemically related substances that inhibit calcium resorption from bone. Alendronate is used to treat osteoporosis and Paget's disease. Oral etidronate is used in the symptomatic treatment of Paget's disease and heterotopic ossification (growth of bone in abnormal locations) associated with spinal cord injury or total hip replacement. Intravenous etidronate and pamidronate are used in the treatment of malignancy-associated hypercalcemia. Etidronate is excreted by the kidneys, and dosage must be reduced in the presence of renal insufficiency.

Alendronate
Routes and Dosage Ranges

Adults: Osteoporosis in postmenopausal women, PO 10 mg once daily, with 6–8 oz of plain water, at least 30 min before the first food, beverage, or medication of the day
Paget's disease, PO 40 mg daily for 6 months. The course of therapy may be repeated if necessary.

Etidronate
Routes and Dosage Ranges

Adults: Paget's disease, PO 5 mg/kg/d for up to 6 months. The course of therapy may be repeated if symptoms recur.
Heterotopic ossification caused by spinal cord injury, PO 20 mg/kg/d for 2 wk, then 10 mg/kg/d for 10 wk
Heterotopic ossification associated with total hip replacement, PO 20 mg/kg/d for 1 month preoperatively and continued for 3 months postoperatively
Hypercalcemia of malignancy, IV 7.5 mg/kg/d, diluted in at least 250 ml of 0.9% sodium chloride solution and infused over at least 2 h daily for 3 successive days

Pamidronate
Route and Dosage Ranges

Adults: Hypercalcemia, IV 60–90 mg, reconstituted according to manufacturer's directions, diluted in 1000 ml of 0.9% or 0.45% sodium chloride solution and infused over 24 h

Furosemide (Lasix) is a potent diuretic that increases calcium excretion in urine by preventing its reabsorption in renal tubules. Furosemide can be given

IV for rapid effects in hypercalcemic crises or orally for nonemergency situations. (See Chap. 56 for further discussion of diuretic drug therapy.)

Route and Dosage Ranges

Adults: IV 80–100 mg q2h until a diuretic response is obtained or other treatment measures are initiated
Children: IV 20–40 mg q4h until a diuretic response is obtained or other treatment measures are initiated

Gallium (Ganite), like calcitonin, alendronate, etidronate, and pamidronate, inhibits calcium resorption from bone. It is used to treat hypercalcemia of malignancy that does not respond to hydration. It is excreted mainly by the kidneys and contraindicated in severe renal impairment (serum creatinine above 2.5 mg/100 ml).

Route and Dosage Ranges

Adults: IV 200 mg/m², diluted in 1000 ml of 0.9% sodium chloride or 5% dextrose injection and infused over 24 h daily for 5 consecutive days

Hydrocortisone (Solu-Cortef and others) and **prednisone** (Deltasone and others) are adrenal corticosteroid drugs that may be used to treat hypercalcemia. Because all the glucocorticoids have similar effects, others may be used. In the treatment of hypercalcemia, corticosteroid drugs antagonize effects of vitamin D and therefore decrease intestinal absorption of calcium. They are probably most useful in treating hypercalcemia resulting from excess vitamin D, sarcoidosis, and renal insufficiency. They also may be useful in treating hypercalcemia due to malignant neoplasms (*e.g.*, multiple myeloma, leukemia, lymphomas) by decreasing bone resorption. High doses or prolonged administration of corticosteroids leads to serious adverse reactions. (See Chap. 24 for further discussion of corticosteroid drug therapy.)

Hydrocortisone
Route and Dosage Range

Adults: IM, IV 100–500 mg/d

Prednisone
Route and Dosage Range

Adults: PO 40–60 mg/d initially, then gradually reduced

Plicamycin (Mithracin) lowers serum calcium levels by blocking calcium resorption from bone. It is used to treat malignancy-associated hypercalcemia that does not respond to hydration and diuretics. Calcium levels start to decline within 12 hours after a dose and reach their lowest levels in 2 to 4 days.

Route and Dosage Range

Adults: IV 25 µg/kg/d for 3 or 4 d, repeated at intervals of 1 wk or more if necessary

Phosphate salts (Neutra-Phos) inhibit intestinal absorption of calcium and increase deposition of calcium in bone. They are effective in the treatment of hypercalcemia of any etiology. A potential adverse reaction to phosphates is calcification of soft tissues due to deposition of calcium phosphate. This can lead to severe impairment of function in the kidneys and other organs. Phosphates should be given only when hypercalcemia is accompanied by hypophosphatemia. Neutra-Phos is a combination of sodium phosphate and potassium phosphate.

Route and Dosage Range

Adults: PO 1–2 tablets three or four times daily, or contents of 1 capsule mixed with 75 ml of water four times daily

0.9% Sodium chloride injection (normal saline) is an IV solution containing water, sodium, and chloride. It is included here because it is the treatment of choice for hypercalcemia and, along with furosemide, is usually effective. The sodium contained in the solution inhibits the reabsorption of calcium in renal tubules and thereby increases urinary excretion of calcium. The solution also relieves the dehydration caused by vomiting and polyuria, and it dilutes the calcium concentration of serum and urine. Saline, 4 to 6 L/d, is given first to hydrate the client, and then furosemide is given.

Nursing Process (Hypercalcemia)

Assessment
- Assess dietary intake of calcium and vitamin D.
- Assess for conditions in which hypercalcemia is likely to occur (*e.g.*, cancer, prolonged immobilization).
- Observe for signs and symptoms of hypercalcemia in clients at risk. Electrocardiogram changes indicative of hypercalcemia include a shortened QT interval and an inverted T wave.
- Assess laboratory reports of serum calcium levels for increases (above 10 mg/100 ml total, above 5 mg/100 ml ionized calcium, approximately). To determine whether an increase is significant, consider serum albumin and acid–base balance as described earlier in this chapter.
- If Paget's disease is suspected, assess for an elevated serum alkaline phosphatase and abnormal bone scan reports.

Nursing Diagnoses
- Altered Thought Processes: Confusion with hypercalcemia
- Altered Nutrition: More Than Body Requirements with hypercalcemia
- Knowledge Deficit: Disease process and drug therapy for hypercalcemia

- Fluid Volume Excess related to large amounts of 0.9% sodium chloride solution used to lower serum calcium levels
- Anxiety related to disease process and treatment
- Risk for Injury: Hypocalcemia from aggressive treatment of hypercalcemia

Planning/Goals

The client will:

- Achieve normal serum calcium levels
- Comply with instructions for safe drug usage
- Be monitored closely for therapeutic and adverse effects of drugs used to treat hypercalcemia
- Be assisted in reducing dietary calcium intake
- Comply with procedures for follow-up treatment of chronic hypercalcemia
- Avoid preventable adverse effects of treatment for acute hypercalcemia

Interventions

Prevent or minimize effects of hypercalcemia by assisting clients to decrease dietary calcium intake and prevent precipitation of calcium in the kidneys (formation of renal calculi).

- The most effective measure to decrease dietary calcium is to avoid milk and milk products.
- Antacids containing calcium (*e.g.*, Tums) also should be avoided.
- Measures to decrease formation of renal calculi include forcing fluids to about 3000 to 4000 ml/d and preventing urinary tract infections.

Teach clients:

- Expected results of treatment for hypercalcemia
- Nondrug measures to decrease risk of recurrence
- Correct drug administration, including injection techniques if indicated
- To report signs and symptoms of either hypercalcemia or hypocalcemia to a health care provider

Evaluation

- Check laboratory reports of serum calcium levels for normal values.
- Interview and observe for decreased intake of dairy products and other calcium-containing foods.
- Interview and observe for accurate drug usage and compliance with follow-up procedures.
- Interview and observe for therapeutic and adverse drug effects.

Principles of Therapy: Drugs Used in Hypercalcemia

Treatment of hypercalcemia depends largely on its cause and severity.

1. When hypercalcemia is caused by an adenoma of a parathyroid gland, surgical excision is indicated.

When it is caused by malignancy, excision or treatment is likely to decrease serum calcium levels. When it is caused by excessive intake of vitamin D, the vitamin D preparation should be stopped immediately.

Clients at risk for hypercalcemia should be monitored for early signs and symptoms so treatment can be started before severe hypercalcemia develops.

2. Acute hypercalcemia is a medical emergency and requires immediate treatment. The priority is fluid replacement and rehydration. This need can be met by intravenous (IV) saline infusion (0.9% or 0.45% NaCl), 4000 ml/d or more if kidney function is adequate. At the same time, calcium intake is limited. After rehydration, a diuretic, such as furosemide, is usually given IV to increase renal excretion of calcium and to prevent fluid overload. Because sodium, potassium, and water are also lost in the urine, these must be replaced in the IV fluids.

   With mild hypercalcemia, most clients respond to the above treatment, and further drug therapy is not needed. With moderate to severe hypercalcemia of malignancy, etidronate, gallium, or pamidronate may be given. Phosphates should not be used unless hypophosphatemia is present. They are also contraindicated in clients with persistent urinary tract infections and an alkaline urine because calcium phosphate kidney stones are likely to form in such cases.

3. Chronic hypercalcemia requires treatment of the underlying disease process and measures to control serum calcium levels (*e.g.*, a low-calcium diet, high fluid intake, and mobilization to help retain calcium in bone). Oral phosphate administration may help if other measures are ineffective.

4. Serum calcium levels should be measured to monitor effects of therapy. In acute hypercalcemia, measure them frequently.

5. For clients with severely impaired renal function who develop hypercalcemia, hemodialysis or peritoneal dialysis with a calcium-free solution is effective and safe.

USE IN CHILDREN

Guidelines for treating hypercalcemia in children are essentially the same as those for adults, with drug dosages adjusted. Safety, effectiveness, and dosages of etidronate, gallium, and pamidronate have not been established.

USE IN OLDER ADULTS

Older adults are likely to have chronic cardiovascular and other disorders that may be aggravated by hypercalcemia and its treatment. During infusion of 0.9% sodium chloride (usually 150–200 ml/h) for acute hypercalcemia, observe older adults closely for signs of congestive heart failure, pulmonary edema, and hypertension.

DRUGS USED IN HYPERCALCEMIA

NURSING ACTIONS	RATIONALE/EXPLANATION
1. Administer accurately	
a. With calcitonin, give at bedtime.	To decrease nausea and discomfort from flushing
b. With oral etidronate, give as a single dose or in divided doses. Avoid administration within 2 h of ingesting dairy products, antacids, or vitamin or mineral supplements. With IV etidronate, gallium, and pamidronate, follow manufacturers' instructions.	If gastrointestinal (GI) symptoms occur with the single dose, divided doses may relieve them. Substances containing calcium or other metals decrease absorption of etidronate. The drugs require reconstitution and diluting with IV fluids.
c. With furosemide, give IV or orally.	
d. With hydrocortisone:	
(1) Give intravenously (IV) or intramuscularly (IM).	In acute hypercalcemia, IV administration (by bolus injection or by addition to 5% dextrose in water or NaCl injection, given as an IV infusion over several hours) is preferred.
(2) Be sure to have the appropriate drug preparation for the ordered route.	Several commercial preparations of hydrocortisone are available. Some are given IV, some IM, and some by either route. Do not assume that any preparation can be given by both routes of administration.
(3) Decrease dosage gradually—do not discontinue abruptly.	Abrupt discontinuation can lead to acute adrenal insufficiency.
e. With plicamycin, give IV for a limited number of doses. See package insert for specific instructions.	
f. With phosphate salts, mix powder forms with water for oral administration. See package inserts for specific instructions.	
2. Observe for therapeutic effects	
a. Decreased serum calcium level	Calcitonin lowers serum calcium levels in approximately 2 h after injection, and effects last 6 to 8 h. Corticosteroids require 10 to 14 d to lower serum calcium. Plicamycin lowers serum calcium levels within 24 to 48 h, but effects last only 3 to 4 d.
b. Decreased signs and symptoms of hypercalcemia	
c. Decreased signs and symptoms of Paget's disease	Decreased serum alkaline phosphatase and radiologic improvement of bone lesions may require several months. Neurologic improvement may require 1 year or more.
3. Observe for adverse effects	
a. Hypocalcemia	Hypocalcemia may result from vigorous treatment of hypercalcemia, especially with etidronate, gallium, and pamidronate. This can be minimized by monitoring serum calcium levels frequently and adjusting drug dosages and other treatments.
b. With calcitonin, observe for nausea, vomiting, tissue irritation at injection sites, and allergic reactions.	Adverse reactions are usually mild and transient.
c. With etidronate and pamidronate, observe for anorexia, nausea, diarrhea, bone pain, fever, and fluid overload.	Adverse effects are more frequent and more severe at higher doses.

(continued)

NURSING ACTIONS	RATIONALE/EXPLANATION
d. With furosemide, observe for dehydration, hypokalemia, hypomagnesemia, and other fluid and electrolyte imbalances.	As furosemide exerts its therapeutic effect of removing excess calcium from the body by increased urine output, water and other electrolytes are lost as well. Adverse reactions can be prevented by avoiding overdosage of furosemide and by careful replacement of the water and electrolytes lost in the urine. Frequent measurements of serum electrolytes help determine amounts of replacement fluids and electrolytes needed.
e. With gallium, observe for renal impairment, as indicated by increasing blood urea nitrogen and serum creatinine levels.	Nephrotoxicity reportedly develops in approximately 12% of recipients.
f. With hydrocortisone and prednisone, see Chapter 24.	Adrenal corticosteroids may cause many adverse reactions, especially with high doses or prolonged administration.
g. With plicamycin, observe for bone marrow depression, nausea, vomiting, and impaired liver function.	These adverse reactions may occur but are much less likely with the small doses used for hypercalcemia than with the large doses used for malignant neoplasms.
h. With phosphates, observe for nausea, vomiting, and diarrhea.	
4. Observe for drug interactions	
a. With calcitonin, testosterone and other androgens *increase* effects; parathyroid hormone *decreases* effects.	Androgens and calcitonin have additive effects on calcium retention and inhibition of bone resorption (movement of calcium from bone to serum). Parathyroid hormone antagonizes or opposes calcitonin. Parathyroid hormone *increases* serum calcium concentration, whereas calcitonin *decreases* it.
b. With gallium, aminoglycoside antibiotics (*e.g.*, gentamicin), amphotericin B, and other nephrotoxic drugs increase nephrotoxic effects.	
c. With hydrocortisone and prednisone, see Chapter 24.	
d. With plicamycin, antineoplastic drugs that cause bone marrow depression (see Chapter 64) increase effects.	
e. With phosphate salts, avoid concomitant use of antacids containing aluminum and magnesium.	Aluminum and magnesium may combine with phosphate and thereby prevent its absorption and therapeutic effect.
5. Teach clients	
a. Maintain a low-calcium diet by limiting intake of dairy products.	One serving of milk, cheese, or other dairy product plus fruits and vegetables furnish a daily calcium intake of about 400 mg.
b. Drink 3 to 4 quarts of fluid daily if able.	To keep the urine dilute. This helps to prevent formation of kidney stones and urinary tract infections.
c. Report any signs of cystitis, such as burning or discomfort with urination.	Infections in the urinary tract can increase kidney stone formation. If they occur, early treatment is needed.

REVIEW AND APPLICATION EXERCISES

1. What are major physiologic functions of calcium?

2. What is the normal serum level of calcium?

3. What are some nursing interventions to prevent hypocalcemia?

4. What signs and symptoms may indicate hypocalcemia?

5. How is hypocalcemia treated?

6. What signs and symptoms may indicate hypercalcemia?

7. How is hypercalcemia treated?

SELECTED REFERENCES

Davis, J.R. & Sherer, K. (1994). *Applied nutrition and diet therapy for nurses,* 2nd ed. Philadelphia: W.B. Saunders.

Drug facts and comparisons. (1996). St. Louis: Facts and Comparisons.

Porth, C.M. (1994). *Pathophysiology: Concepts of altered health states,* 4th ed., pp. 591–627. Philadelphia: J.B. Lippincott.

Schultz, N.J. (1993). Body electrolyte homeostasis. In J.T. DiPiro, R.L. Talbert, P.E. Hayes, G.C. Yee, G.R. Matzke, & L.M. Posey (Eds.), *Pharmacotherapy: A pathophysiologic approach,* 2nd ed., pp. 764–796. Norwalk, CT: Appleton & Lange

Antidiabetic Drugs

Objectives

After studying this chapter, the student will be able to:

1 Describe major effects of endogenous insulin on body tissues.

2 Discuss Regular, NPH and Lente insulins in terms of mechanism of action, indications for use, route of administration, and duration of action.

3 Differentiate between human insulin and animal insulin.

4 Discuss the relationships among diet, exercise, and drug therapy in controlling diabetes.

5 Recognize normal, hypoglycemic and hyperglycemic levels of blood glucose.

6 Differentiate types of oral antidiabetic agents in terms of mechanisms of action, indications for use, adverse effects, client teaching, and nursing process implications.

7 Explain the benefits of maintaining glycemic control in preventing complications of diabetes.

8 State reasons for combinations of insulin and oral agents or two types of oral agents.

9 Teach clients how to recognize and treat hypoglycemic reactions.

10 Collaborate with nurse diabetes educators, dietitians, and others in teaching self-care activities to clients with diabetes.

(continued)

Key Terms

Diabetogenic	**Lactic acidosis**
Glucagon	**Ketoacidosis**
Hyperglycemia	**Neuropathy**
Hypoglycemia	**Polydipsia**
Insulin	**Polyphagia**
Insulin resistance	**Polyuria**

There are two types of antidiabetic drugs: insulin and oral agents. Because these drugs are used to lower blood glucose, they are also called hypoglycemic or antihyperglycemic agents. Diabetes mellitus is a common, complex disorder. To understand clinical usage of antidiabetic drugs, it is necessary to understand the characteristics of endogenous insulin, diabetes mellitus, and the drugs.

Endogenous Insulin

Insulin is a protein hormone (51 amino acids in two linked chains) secreted by beta cells in the pancreas. The average adult pancreas secretes a basal amount of 1 to 2 units/h and additional amounts (about 4 to 6 units/h) after meals or when the blood sugar level exceeds 100 mg/100 ml, with an average daily secretion of about 40 to 60 units. In a fasting state, serum insulin levels are low and stored glucose and amino acids are used for energy needs of tissues that require glucose. After a meal, serum insulin levels increase in a few minutes, peak in about 30 minutes, and decrease to baseline levels in about 3 hours.

Secreted insulin is released into the portal circulation and transported to the liver where about half is utilized or degraded and only the remaining half reaches the systemic circulation. Once in the systemic circulation, insulin circulates mainly in an unbound form and is transported to most body cells.

At the cellular level (Figure 27-1), insulin binds with and activates receptors on the cell membranes of about 80% of body cells. Liver, muscle and adipose cells have many insulin receptors and are primary tissues for insulin action. After insulin-receptor binding occurs, cell membranes become highly permeable to glucose and allow rapid entry of glucose into the cells. The cell membranes also become more permeable to amino acids, fatty acids, and electrolytes such as potassium, magnesium, and phosphate ions. Cellular metabolism is altered by the movement of these substances into the cells, activation of some enzymes and inactivation of others, movement of proteins between cellular compartments, changes in the amounts of proteins produced, and perhaps other mechanisms. Overall, the

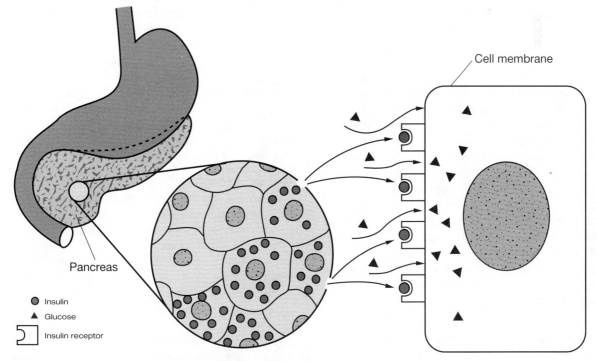

Figure 27-1
Normal glucose metabolism. Once insulin binds with receptors on the cell membrane, glucose can move into the cell, promoting cellular metabolism and energy production.

changes in cellular metabolism stimulate anabolic effects (*e.g.*, utilization and storage of glucose, amino acids and fatty acids) and inhibit catabolic processes (*e.g.*, breakdown of glycogen, fat, and protein). After binding to insulin and entering the cell, receptors may be degraded or recycled back to the cell surface.

Insulin is cleared from circulating blood in about 10 to 15 minutes because of rapid binding to peripheral tissues or metabolic breakdown. The insulin that does not combine with receptors is metabolized in the liver, kidneys, plasma, and muscles. In the kidneys, insulin is filtered by the glomeruli and reabsorbed by the tubules, which also degrade it. Severe renal impairment slows the clearance of insulin from the blood.

Physiologically, insulin plays a major role in metabolism of carbohydrate, fat, and protein (Box 27-1). These foodstuffs are broken down into molecules of glucose, lipids, and amino acids, respectively. These molecules enter the cells and are converted to energy for cellular activities. The energy can be used immediately or converted to storage forms for later use. When carrying out its metabolic functions, the overall effect of insulin is to lower blood glucose levels, primarily by the following mechanisms:

1. In the liver, insulin acts to *decrease* breakdown of glycogen (glycogenolysis), formation of new glucose from fatty acids and amino acids (gluconeogenesis), and formation of ketone bodies (ketogenesis). At the same time, it acts to *increase* synthesis and storage of glycogen and fatty acids.
2. In adipose tissue, insulin acts to *decrease* breakdown of fat (lipolysis) and to *increase* production of glycerol and fatty acids.
3. In muscle tissue, insulin acts to *decrease* protein breakdown and amino acid output and to *increase* amino acid uptake, protein synthesis, and glycogen synthesis.

REGULATION OF INSULIN SECRETION

Insulin is the only hormone known to decrease blood sugar; however, several hormones increase blood sugar. Insulin secretion is a complex process with a

---

BOX 27-1. EFFECTS OF INSULIN ON METABOLISM

Carbohydrate Metabolism
- Insulin increases glucose transport into most body cells. Complete lack of insulin allows transport of about one fourth the normal amount of glucose. Insulin facilitates glucose transport into skeletal muscle, adipose tissue, the heart, and some smooth muscle organs, such as the uterus; it must be present for muscle and fat tissues to utilize glucose for energy. It does not increase glucose transport into brain cells, red blood cells, intestinal mucosal cells, or tubular epithelial cells of the kidney.
- Insulin regulates glucose metabolism and homeostasis. The main goal of glucose metabolism is to produce energy for cellular functions. If excess glucose is present after this need is met, it is converted to glycogen and stored for future energy needs or converted to fat and stored. The excess glucose transported to liver cells is converted to fat only after glycogen stores are saturated. When insulin is absent or blood glucose levels are low, these stored forms of glucose can be reconverted. The liver is especially important in restoring blood sugar levels by breaking down glycogen or by forming new glucose.

Fat Metabolism
- Insulin promotes transport of glucose into fat cells. Once inside the cell, glucose is broken down. One of the breakdown products is alpha-glycerophosphate, which

combines with fatty acids to form triglycerides. This is the mechanism by which insulin promotes fat storage.
- When insulin is lacking, fat is not stored in the fat cells. Instead, it is released into the bloodstream in the form of free fatty acids. Blood concentrations of other lipids (triglycerides, cholesterol, phospholipids) are also increased. The high blood lipid concentration probably accounts for the atherosclerosis that tends to develop early and progress more rapidly in people with diabetes mellitus. Also, when more fatty acids are released than the body can use as fuel, some fatty acids are converted into ketone bodies. Excessive amounts of ketones produce acidosis and coma.

Protein Metabolism
- Insulin increases the total amount of body protein by increasing transport of amino acids into cells and synthesis of protein within the cells. The basic mechanism of these effects is unknown.
- Insulin potentiates the effects of growth hormone.
- Lack of insulin causes protein depletion and breakdown into amino acids. These amino acids are released into the bloodstream and transported to the liver for energy or gluconeogenesis. These proteins are not replaced by synthesis of new proteins. The overall consequences of protein wasting include abnormal functioning of many body organs, severe weakness, and weight loss.

major function of providing adequate glucose in the blood for cellular metabolism and energy needs, during both fasting and feeding. The process involves coordination of numerous factors, including various nutrients, gastrointestinal (GI) and pancreatic hormones, and the autonomic nervous system.

Factors that stimulate insulin secretion include glucose, amino acids, fatty acids, ketone bodies, and stimulation of beta$_2$-adrenergic receptors or vagal nerves. Glucose is the major stimulus to insulin secretion in humans. Oral glucose is more effective than intravenous (IV) glucose in stimulating insulin secretion because glucose or food in the digestive tract induces the release of GI hormones (*e.g.*, gastrin, secretin, cholecystokinin, gastric inhibitory peptide) and stimulates vagal activity. Other hormones that raise blood glucose levels and stimulate insulin secretion include glucagon, growth hormone, cortisol and, to a lesser extent, progesterone and estrogen. Excessive, prolonged, endogenous secretion or administration of pharmacologic preparations of these hormones can exhaust the ability of pancreatic beta cells to produce insulin and thereby cause diabetes mellitus.

Factors that inhibit insulin secretion include stimulation of pancreatic alpha$_2$-adrenergic receptors and stress conditions such as hypoxia, hypothermia, surgery or severe burns.

Diabetes Mellitus

CHARACTERISTICS

Diabetes mellitus is a chronic systemic disease characterized by metabolic and vascular abnormalities. Metabolic problems occur early in the disease process and are related to changes in the metabolism of carbohydrate, fat, and protein. One of the primary clinical manifestations of disordered metabolism is hyperglycemia. Vascular problems include development and progression of atherosclerosis throughout the body and changes in small blood vessels, which especially affect the retina and kidney. Clinical manifestations of vascular disorders may include hypertension, myocardial infarction, stroke, retinopathy, blindness, nephropathy, and peripheral vascular disease.

CLASSIFICATIONS

The two major classifications of diabetes mellitus are type I and type II. Although both types are characterized by hyperglycemia, they differ significantly in onset, course, treatment, and pathologic changes. Secondary diabetes may be induced by certain disease processes, certain drugs, and pregnancy.

Type I

Type I, or insulin-dependent, diabetes mellitus (IDDM) is thought to be a genetic, autoimmune disorder characterized by the production of antibodies against pancreatic beta cells and the body's own insulin. The anti-beta cell antibodies produce an inflammatory reaction in the beta cell area that gradually destroys the cells and reduces insulin secretion. When about 10% to 20% of functioning beta cells remain, hyperglycemia and other symptoms of diabetes develop. Eventually, all the beta cells are destroyed, and no insulin is produced. The anti-insulin antibodies destroy or decrease the effectiveness of insulin.

Type I diabetes may occur at any age but usually starts before 20 years of age. It generally has a sudden onset; produces more severe symptoms; is more difficult to control; produces a high incidence of complications, such as diabetic ketoacidosis (DKA) and renal failure; and requires administration of exogenous insulin. Only about 10% of diabetics have type I diabetes.

Type II

Type II, or non–insulin-dependent, diabetes mellitus (NIDDM), is characterized by hyperglycemia and peripheral tissue resistance to insulin. The hyperglycemia results from increased production of glucose by the liver and decreased uptake of glucose in muscle and fat. Pancreatic beta cells have an impaired response to the hyperglycemia, thereby causing an insulin deficiency. In addition, the liver and peripheral tissues have an impaired response to the biologic action of insulin (insulin resistance). Insulin resistance has been attributed to abnormalities in insulin receptors, but studies indicate that most people with NIDDM have insulin receptors that are normal in number, activity, and binding capacity. Postreceptor, intracellular mechanisms may be responsible. Opinions differ about the relative importance of insulin deficiency and insulin resistance in the pathophysiology of NIDDM.

Type II diabetes may occur at any age but usually starts after 40 years of age. It usually has a gradual onset, produces less severe symptoms initially, is easier to control, causes less DKA and renal failure but more myocardial infarctions and strokes, and does not necessarily require exogenous insulin, because endogenous insulin is still produced by pancreatic beta cells. Insulin may be present but unable to act effectively to lower blood sugar. Approximately 90% of diabetics have type II diabetes; 20% to 30% of them require exogenous insulin.

ETIOLOGY

IDDM is an autoimmune disease of the pancreatic beta cell, with destruction of the cells occurring over several years and subsequent insulin deficiency. The cause of the autoimmune attack on beta cells is unclear but is thought to involve a genetic predisposition and one or more environmental triggers such as a viral infection. Other possible triggers include exposure to cow's milk during the first 3 to 4 months of life (antibodies to milk protein are found in most children with newly diagnosed IDDM); sex hormones (increased during puberty and pregnancy); and possibly insulin itself (antibodies to insulin are found in the blood). The clinical onset of IDDM may be sudden, but the damage to pancreatic beta cells occurs slowly. Overt IDDM may occur at any time during this progressive loss of beta cells if acute illness or stress increases the body's demand for insulin beyond the capacity of the remaining beta cells to secrete insulin.

NIDDM is a heterogenous disease, and etiology probably involves multiple factors such as a genetic predisposition (possibly involving a variety of genes) and environmental factors. Obesity is considered to be a major cause of type II diabetes. With obesity and chronic ingestion of excess calories, more insulin is required. The increased need leads to prolonged stimulation and eventual "fatigue" of pancreatic beta cells. As a result, the cells become less responsive to elevated blood sugar levels and less able to produce enough insulin to meet metabolic needs.

Disease-induced diabetes mellitus can result from any condition that damages or removes pancreatic beta cells. In addition to the autoimmune process described previously, such conditions include cancer, pancreatitis, surgical excision of pancreatic tissue, and viral infections.

Hormone-induced diabetes may result from excessive amounts of some hormones, whether from endogenous oversecretion or from excessive administration of exogenous hormones. These include adrenal corticosteroids, growth hormone, glucagon, and thyroid hormone.

Gestational diabetes is a type of glucose intolerance that develops during pregnancy. It occurs in about 2% of pregnancies and requires insulin therapy to decrease risks of birth defects. It usually subsides after delivery, but as many as 30% of these women are estimated to develop type II diabetes within 10 to 15 years.

SIGNS AND SYMPTOMS

Most signs and symptoms of diabetes mellitus stem from a relative or absolute lack of insulin and the subsequent metabolic abnormalities. The incidence and severity of clinical manifestations are correlated with the amount of effective insulin. In type I diabetes, insulin secretion is absent or severely impaired. Clinical signs and symptoms may be precipitated by infection, rapid growth, pregnancy, or other factors that increase demand for insulin. In type II diabetes, insulin is secreted but is inadequate or ineffective, especially when insulin demand is increased by obesity, pregnancy, aging, or other factors. In many people, signs and symptoms occur with obesity and subside with normal weight.

Most early manifestations result from disordered carbohydrate metabolism, which causes excess glucose to accumulate in the blood (hyperglycemia). Hyperglycemia produces glucosuria, which, in turn, produces polydipsia, polyuria, dehydration, and polyphagia.

Glucosuria usually appears when the blood glucose level is about twice the normal value and the kidneys receive more glucose than can be reabsorbed. However, renal threshold varies, and the amount of glucose lost in the urine does not accurately reflect blood glucose. In very young people, glucose tends to appear in urine at much lower or even normal blood glucose levels. In older people, the ability of the kidneys to excrete excess glucose from the blood is decreased. Therefore, some older people can have rather high blood glucose levels with little or no glucose appearing in the urine.

When large amounts of glucose are present, water is pulled into the renal tubule. This results in a greatly increased urine output (polyuria). The excessive loss of fluid in urine (osmotic diuresis) leads to increased thirst (polydipsia) and, if fluid intake is inadequate, to fluid volume deficit (dehydration). Dehydration also occurs because high blood glucose levels increase osmotic pressure in the bloodstream, and fluid is pulled out of the cells in the body's attempt to regain homeostasis.

Polyphagia (increased appetite) occurs because the body cannot use ingested foods. Many people with diabetes lose weight because of abnormal metabolism.

COMPLICATIONS

Complications of diabetes mellitus are common and potentially disabling or life-threatening (Box 27-2). They are attributed to insulin deficiency and the resultant metabolic abnormalities. These metabolic abnormalities, especially those associated with hyperglycemia, can cause early, acute complications, such as DKA or nonketotic hyperosmolar coma. Eventually, metabolic abnormalities lead to changes in structure and function of blood vessels and other body tissues. Complications can be decreased or delayed by controlling hyperglycemia and normalizing metabolic processes.

BOX 27-2. COMPLICATIONS OF DIABETES MELLITUS

Diabetic ketoacidosis (DKA)

This acute, life-threatening complication of diabetes occurs with severe insulin deficiency. In the absence of insulin, glucose cannot be used by body cells for energy, and fat is mobilized from adipose tissue to furnish a fuel source. The mobilized fat circulates in the bloodstream, from which it is extracted by the liver and broken down into glycerol and fatty acids. The fatty acids are further changed in the liver to ketone bodies (acetoacetic acid, acetone, beta-hydroxybutyric acid), which then enter the bloodstream and are circulated to body cells for metabolic conversion to energy, carbon dioxide, and water.

Owing to these metabolic abnormalities, clinical signs and symptoms develop rather rapidly because ketone bodies tend to be produced more rapidly than body cells can use them. They accumulate and produce acidemia (a drop in blood pH and an increase in blood hydrogen ions). The body attempts to buffer the acidic hydrogen ions by exchanging them for intracellular potassium ions. Hydrogen ions enter body cells, and potassium ions leave the cells to be excreted in the urine. Another attempt to remove excess acid involves the lungs. Deep, labored respirations, called Kussmaul respirations, eliminate more carbon dioxide and prevent formation of carbonic acid. A third attempt to regain homeostasis involves the kidneys, which excrete some of the ketones, thereby producing acetone in the urine.

DKA worsens as the compensatory mechanisms fail. Clinical signs and symptoms vary and become progressively more severe. Early ones include blurred vision, anorexia, nausea and vomiting, thirst, and polyuria. Later ones include drowsiness, which progresses to stupor and coma, Kussmaul breathing, dehydration and other signs of fluid and electrolyte imbalances, and decreased blood pressure, increased pulse, and other signs of shock.

Hyperglycemic Hyperosmolar Nonketotic Coma

This is another type of diabetic coma that is potentially life threatening. It is relatively rare and carries a high mortality rate. The term *hyperosmolar* refers to an excessive amount of glucose, electrolytes, and other solutes in the blood in relation to the amount of water.

Like DKA, hyperosmolar coma is characterized by hyperglycemia, which leads to osmotic diuresis and resultant thirst, polyuria, dehydration, and electrolyte losses, as well as neurologic signs ranging from drowsiness to stupor to coma. Additional clinical problems may include hypovolemic shock, thrombosis, renal problems, or stroke. In contrast to DKA, hyperosmolar coma occurs in people with previously unknown or mild diabetes, usually following an illness; occurs in hyperglycemic conditions other than diabetes (*e.g.*, severe burns, corticosteroid drug therapy); and does not cause ketosis.

Cardiovascular Complications

Persons with diabetes develop generalized atherosclerosis that occurs at an earlier age, progresses more rapidly, and becomes more severe than in persons who do not have diabetes. Changes occur in large and small blood vessels. Reasons for vascular changes are unclear, but the sequence of events is thought to involve damage to the endothelial lining, followed by platelet aggregation, lipid deposition, plaque formation, and thrombosis in the damaged area.

Vascular disease is a leading cause of death in people with diabetes. It is also a leading cause of morbidity, because people with diabetes are more likely to have myocardial infarction, peripheral arterial insufficiency, kidney failure, and blindness than nondiabetics. Other vascular complications include angina pectoris, congestive heart failure, hypertension, and cerebral thrombosis (stroke).

Nephropathy

The several types of kidney lesions in diabetes mellitus are collectively called *diabetic nephropathy*. One such lesion is diffuse glomerulosclerosis, which is found in about 90% of people who have had diabetes for more than 10 years. Another lesion is called *nodular glomerulosclerosis*, or Kimmelstiel-Wilson syndrome. It occurs in 10% to 25% of diabetics. A third lesion is acute or chronic pyelonephritis. Although pyelonephritis also occurs in nondiabetics, it is usually more severe in diabetics. A fourth lesion involves atherosclerosis and arteriosclerosis of renal arteries as a manifestation of generalized atherosclerosis. These disorders all produce abnormal renal function and may cause renal failure.

As with most other complications, nephropathy can be decreased and delayed by normalizing blood glucose levels. In addition, administration of angiotensin-converting enzyme (ACE) inhibitors (*e.g.*, captopril, enalapril, others) has protective effects on the kidney with both type I and type II diabetes and in both normotensive and hypertensive persons. Although ACE inhibitors are also used in the treatment of hypertension, their ability to delay nephropathy seems to be independent of antihypertensive effects. Additional measures to preserve renal function include effective treatment of hypertension, limited intake of dietary protein, prompt treatment of urinary tract infections, and avoidance of nephrotoxic drugs when possible.

Retinopathy

This is the most common and most serious ocular complication of diabetes, although cataract formation and glaucoma may develop at an earlier age in the diabetic. Diabetic retinopathy is related to the duration of diabetes.

(continued)

BOX 27-2. (CONTINUED)

About 50% of diabetics have some degree of retinopathy after 10 years, about 80% to 90% after 20 years. Retinopathy results from vascular changes, and the severity is correlated with the degree of generalized vascular disease. Hemorrhage, edema, and exudates may be seen through the ophthalmoscope. Retinal detachment may occur.

Neuropathy

Several nonspecific neurologic disorders are often associated with diabetes mellitus. The degenerative changes in nerves that produce neuropathy are attributed to sorbitol, an alcohol produced by glucose metabolism, and nerve fiber ischemia from vascular disorders.

In the extremities, neuropathy causes discomfort and impairment of sensory and motor functions. Injuries often result, usually in the feet, and even minor injuries may eventually necessitate leg amputation. In the cardiovascular system, silent myocardial infarction, postural hypotension, and impaired response to sympathetic or parasympathetic stimulation may occur. Another autonomic manifestation is the absence of warning signs of hypoglycemia. In the gastrointestinal system, neuropathy may cause disturbances of motility (*e.g.*, gastroparesis) and changes in bowel function. In the genitourinary system, bladder atony may cause urine retention and urinary tract infections. Impotence and retrograde ejaculation may occur in men.

Other Complications

Arthropathy and osteolysis may develop, probably from trauma and decreased ability to perceive pain. Diabetics are more susceptible to infections, especially tuberculosis, pneumonia, and urinary tract and skin infections. When infections occur, they tend to progress more rapidly and become more severe. Infections are attributed to impairment of phagocytosis and other defense mechanisms. Women with diabetes are more likely to develop toxemia and other complications of pregnancy. Babies born to diabetic mothers are more likely to be premature or stillborn.

Hypoglycemic Drugs

Individual insulins and oral antidiabetic drugs are listed in Tables 27-1 and 27-2, respectively.

INSULIN

1. Available insulin preparations are combinations of beef and pork insulins, single-component pork insulin, and human insulin. Early products contained proinsulin and other protein contaminants that caused a relatively high incidence of allergic reactions and insulin antibody formation. Newer products are highly purified and less likely to be antigenic. Beef insulin differs from human insulin by three amino acids and is more antigenic than pork insulin. Pork insulin differs from human insulin by one amino acid. Human insulin is produced in the laboratory with recombinant deoxyribonucleic acid techniques using strains of *Escherichia coli* or yeast or by modifying pork insulin to replace the single different amino acid. Human insulin has the same number and sequence of amino acids as endogenous insulin. It is not derived from the human pancreas.

    In addition to the above preparations, a new kind of insulin called an insulin analog was developed to improve the absorption and/or action of insulin. Insulin lispro (Humalog) is identical to human insulin except for the substitution of two amino acids (lysine and proline). Insulin lispro is absorbed much more rapidly and has a shorter half-life after subcutaneous (SC) injection than regular human insulin. As a result, it is similar to physiologic insulin secretion after eating a meal, more effective at blunting postprandial hyperglycemia, and less likely to cause hypoglycemia before the next meal. Injection just before a meal produces hypoglycemic effects similar to those of an injection of conventional regular insulin given 30 minutes before a meal. Insulin analogs are expected to be widely used, and numerous others are being investigated.

2. Insulin cannot be given orally because it is a protein that is destroyed by proteolytic enzymes in the GI tract. It is given only by the parenteral route, most often SC. When exogenous insulin is given SC, its action differs from that of endogenous insulin. One difference is that the rise and fall of serum insulin levels occur more slowly than the physiologic pattern of rapid rise and fall in response to food intake. Another difference is that the injected insulin diffuses into the peripheral circulation instead of being released into the portal circulation. The effect of secreted insulin on hepatic metabolism is eliminated.

3. Insulin preparations differ primarily in onset and duration of action. They are usually categorized as short-, intermediate-, or long-acting insulins. Short-acting insulins have a rapid onset and a short duration of action. Intermediate- and long-acting insulins are modified by adding protamine (a large, insolu-

TABLE 27-1 INSULIN

Generic/Trade Name	Characteristics	Routes and Dosage Ranges	Action (h)		
			Onset	Peak	Duration
Short-Acting Insulins					
Insulin injection (Insulin, Regular Iletin I Purified preparations: Regular Iletin II [beef or pork], Actrapid (pork). Human insulin: Humulin R, Novolin R)	1. A clear liquid solution with the appearance of water 2. The hypoglycemic drug of choice for diabetics experiencing acute or emergency situations, diabetic ketoacidosis, hyperosmolar nonketotic coma, severe infections or other illnesses, major surgery, and pregnancy 3. The only insulin preparation that can be given IV 4. Rarely used alone for long-term maintenance but may be combined with an intermediate-acting insulin (*e.g.,* NPH) for this purpose	SC, dosage individualized according to blood glucose levels. For sliding scale, 5–20 units before meals and bedtime, depending on blood glucose levels IV, dosage individualized. For ketoacidosis, regular insulin may be given by direct injection, intermittent infusion, or continuous infusion. One regimen involves an initial bolus injection of 10–20 units followed by a continuous low-dose infusion of 2–10 units/h, based on hourly blood and urine glucose levels	½–1	2–3	5–7
Prompt insulin zinc suspension (Semilente Insulin, Semilente Iletin I Purified preparation: Semitard [pork])	1. Modified by chemical combination with zinc to produce small crystals, which are rapidly absorbed 2. Rarely used alone; most often used in combination with intermediate (Lente) or long-acting (Ultralente) insulins 3. A suspension that is milky or cloudy when mixed thoroughly in the drug vial 4. Given *only* SC 5. Not recommended in emergencies	SC, dosage individualized. Initially, 10–20 units once or twice daily may be given.	½–1½	4–6	12–16
Intermediate Acting Insulins					
Isophane insulin suspension (NPH Iletin I, NPH Insulin Purified preparations: Iletin II [beef or pork], NPH purified pork Human insulin: Humulin N, Novolin N)	1. Commonly used for long-term administration 2. Modified by addition of protamine (a protein) and zinc 3. A suspension with a cloudy appearance when correctly mixed in the drug vial 4. Given *only* SC 5. Not recommended for use in acute situations 6. Hypoglycemic reactions are more likely to occur during mid-to-late afternoon	SC, dosage individualized. Initially, 7–26 units may be given once or twice daily.	1–1½	8–12	18–24
Insulin zinc suspension (Lente insulin Lente Iletin I	1. Modified by addition of zinc 2. A mixture of 30% Semilente and 70% Ultralente. The	SC, dosage individualized. Initially, 7–26 units may be given once or twice daily.	1–2	8–12	18–24

(continued)

TABLE 27-1	INSULIN (Continued)				
Generic/Trade Name	Characteristics	Routes and Dosage Ranges	Onset	Peak	Duration
Purified preparations: Lente Iletin II [beef or pork], Lente purified pork Human insulin: Novolin L)	small crystals of Semilente are rapidly absorbed, and the large crystals of Ultralente are slowly absorbed 3. May be used interchangeably with NPH insulin 4. A suspension with a cloudy appearance when correctly mixed in the drug vial 5. Given *only* SC				
Long-Acting Insulin					
Extended insulin zinc suspension (Ultralente Purified preparation: Ultratard [beef])	1. Modified by addition of zinc and formation of large crystals, which are slowly absorbed 2. Hypoglycemic reactions are frequent and likely to occur during sleep. 3. Rarely used alone; may be combined with Lente or Semilente	SC, dosage individualized. Initially, 7–26 units may be given once daily	4–8	10–30	36 plus
Insulin Mixtures					
NPH 70% **Regular 30%** (Humulin 70/30, Novolin 70/30)	1. Stable mixture 2. Onset, peak, and duration of action same as individual components	SC, dosage individualized			
NPH 50% **Regular 50%** (Humulin 50/50)	See Humulin 70/30, above	SC, dosage individualized			
Insulin Analog					
Insulin lispro (Humalog)	1. A synthetic insulin of recombinant DNA origin, created by reversing two amino acids 2. Has a faster onset and a shorter duration of action than human regular insulin 3. Intended for use with a longer-acting insulin	SC, dosage individualized, 15 min before meals			

ble protein), zinc, or both to slow absorption and prolong drug action.

4. U-100 is the main insulin concentration in the United States. This means that it contains 100 units of insulin per milliliter of solution. U-100 insulin can be accurately measured only in a syringe designed for use with U-100 insulin. In addition, stable mixtures of 70% NPH and 30% regular insulin (*e.g.,* Humulin 70/30) or 50% each (Humulin 50/50) are available. The mixtures are more convenient and may be more accurately measured when both an intermediate- and a short-acting insulin are needed.

5. Insulin absorption is delayed or decreased when it is injected into SC tissue with lipodystrophy or other lesions, when circulatory problems (*e.g.,* edema or hypotension) are present, by insulin-binding antibodies

TABLE 27-2 ORAL DRUGS FOR DIABETES MELLITUS

Generic/Trade Name	Characteristics	Routes and Dosage Ranges
Sulfonylureas		
First generation		
Acetohexamide (Dymelor)	Duration of action intermediate (12–24 h) Has uricosuric effects, therefore useful in patients with gout	PO, dosage individualized. Usual range, 250 mg– 1.5 g; maximal daily dose, 1.5 g. Dosages of 1 g or less daily can be given in a single dose. Dosage of 1.5 g daily should be given in two divided doses, before morning and evening meals.
Chlorpropamide (Diabinese)	Long-acting (up to 72 h) When chlorpropamide therapy is started, therapeutic effects may not be evident for 1–2 wk. When the drug is discontinued, several weeks are required for complete elimination of the drug from the body.	PO, dosage individualized. Initially, 100–250 mg daily in a single dose. Dosage may be increased or decreased by 50–125 mg at weekly intervals. Usual maintenance dose is 100–500 mg daily. Avoid doses greater than 750 mg daily.
Tolazamide (Tolinase)	Intermediate-acting (10–14 h) Does not have antidiuretic effects, thus useful in patients with congestive heart failure, hepatic cirrhosis, or other conditions characterized by fluid retention and edema	PO, dosage individualized. Initially, 100–250 mg daily is given in a single dose. Dosage may be adjusted every 4–6 d, as needed. If 500 mg or more is required daily, two divided doses are given.
Tolbutamide (Orinase)	Short-acting agent (6–12 h)	PO, dosage individualized. Initially, 500 mg is given in divided doses, twice daily. Maintenance dose is 250 mg–3 g daily, in divided doses.
Second generation		
Glimepiride (Amaryl)	Newer agent that seems to offer no significant advantage over glipizide and glyburide.	PO, initially 1–2 mg once daily, with breakfast or first main meal. Maximum starting dose 2 mg or less. Maintenance dose 1–4 mg once daily. After a dose of 2 mg is reached, increase dose in increments of 2 mg or less at 1- to 2-week intervals, based on blood glucose levels. Maximum recommended dose, 8 mg once daily. In combination with insulin, PO 8 mg once daily with the first main meal.
Glipizide (Glucotrol)	Onset of action about 1–1.5 h; duration 10–16 h	PO, initially 5 mg daily in a single dose, 30 min before breakfast. Maximum dose, 40 mg daily. In elderly, may start with 2.5 mg daily
Glyburide (DiaBeta, Micronase, Glynase Pres Tab)	Onset of action about 2–4 h; duration 24 h. Glynase is better absorbed, acts faster (onset about 1 h; duration 24 h), and is given in smaller doses than other forms of glyburide	PO, initially 2.5–5 mg daily in a single dose, with breakfast. Maximum dose, 20 mg daily. Glynase PO initially 1.5–3 mg daily with breakfast. Maximum dose, 12 mg daily.
Alpha-glucosidase inhibitors		
Acarbose (Precose)	Delays digestion of carbohydrate foods when acarbose and food are present in GI tract at the same time	PO, initially 25 mg, three times daily with first bite of main meals; increase at 4- to 8-week intervals to a maximum dose of 50 mg three times daily (for patients weighing under 60 kg) if necessary, depending on 1-h postprandial blood glucose levels and tolerance. Clients weighing more than 60 kg may need doses up to 100 mg three times daily (the maximum dose).

(continued)

TABLE 27-2	ORAL DRUGS FOR DIABETES MELLITUS (Continued)	
Generic/Trade Name	**Characteristics**	**Routes and Dosage Ranges**
Miglitol (Glyset)	Delays digestion of carbohydrates in the GI tract	PO, initially 25 mg three times daily with the first bite of each main meal, gradually increased if necessary. Maximum dose, 100 mg three times daily
Biguanide **Metformin** (Glucophage)	Older adults are at higher risk of developing lactic acidosis, a rare but potentially fatal reaction. Thus, smaller doses and monitoring of renal function are recommended.	PO, initially 500 mg twice daily, with morning and evening meals; increase dose in increments of 500 mg/d every 2–3 weeks if necessary, up to a maximum of 3000 mg daily, based on patient tolerance and blood glucose levels. In elderly patients, do not increase to maximum dose.
Insulin-enhancing agent **Troglitazone** (Rezulin)	Increases effects of circulating insulin Causes few adverse effects; does not cause hypoglycemia	PO 400 mg once daily in the morning

(which develop after 2 or 3 months of insulin administration), and by injecting cold (*i.e.*, refrigerated) insulin.

6. Temperature extremes can cause loss of potency. Insulin retains potency up to 36 months under refrigeration and about 18 to 24 months at room temperature. At high temperatures (about 100°F or 37.8°C), insulin loses potency in about 2 months. If frozen, insulin remains potent but tends to clump or precipitate. This prevents withdrawal of an accurate dose, and the vial should be discarded.

ORAL HYPOGLYCEMIC DRUGS

There are four types of oral antidiabetic agents. The oldest and largest group is the sulfonylureas. Newer drugs include two alpha-glucosidase inhibitors, a biguanide, and an insulin-enhancing agent.

Sulfonylureas

The sulfonylureas are chemically related to sulfonamide antibacterial drugs; are well absorbed with oral administration; have the same mechanisms of action, indications for use, and contraindications; are more than 90% bound to plasma proteins; produce hypoglycemia as a major adverse effect; are metabolized in the liver; and metabolites are excreted primarily by the kidneys (except for glyburide, which is excreted about 50% in urine and 50% in bile). The drugs vary in duration of action. Although generally well absorbed, food and hyperglycemia can reduce absorption. Hyperglycemia can slow the absorption of many drugs because it inhibits gastric and intestinal motility.

The four older agents are called first-generation sulfonylureas. Metabolism of acetohexamide (Dymelor) and chlorpropamide (Diabinese) produces active metabolites that contribute to their duration of action. Metabolism of tolazamide (Tolinase) and tolbutamide (Orinase) produces inactive metabolites.

Glipizide (Glucotrol), glyburide (DiaBeta, Micronase), and glimepiride (Amaryl) are called second-generation sulfonylureas. They are similar in therapeutic and adverse effects. Compared to first-generation drugs, they are more potent (*i.e.*, have greater hypoglycemic effects per milligram) and produce similar hypoglycemia but are less likely to cause other adverse effects. They are metabolized to inactive compounds, which may be advantageous in clients with impaired renal function. Glimepiride is the only sulfonylurea that is FDA-approved for combination therapy with insulin, although others would presumably produce the same effects.

In addition to their hypoglycemic actions, oral sulfonylureas have other pharmacologic activities. For example, acetohexamide, tolazamide, glyburide, and glipizide have mild diuretic effects; acetohexamide has uricosuric effects; and chlorpropamide may potentiate the action of antidiuretic hormone.

Alpha-glucosidase Inhibitors

Acarbose (Precose) and miglitol (Glyset) inhibit alpha-glucosidase enzymes (*e.g.*, sucrase, maltase, amylase) in the GI tract and thereby delay digestion of complex carbohydrates into glucose and other simple sugars. As a result, glucose absorption is delayed and there is a smaller increase in blood glucose levels following a meal.

Acarbose and miglitol are metabolized within the GI tract, by digestive enzymes and intestinal bacteria. Some of the metabolites are absorbed systemically and excreted in urine; plasma concentrations are increased in the presence of renal impairment. These drugs are used to treat NIDDM when hyperglycemia is not controlled by diet alone. One of the drugs may be given alone or combined with a sulfonylurea.

Biguanide

Metformin (Glucophage) increases the use of glucose by muscle and fat cells, decreases hepatic glucose production, and decreases intestinal absorption of glucose. It is preferably called an antihyperglycemic rather than a hypoglycemic agent because it does not cause hypoglycemia, even in large doses, when used alone. It has no effect on pancreatic insulin secretion and no significant effects on secretion of other hormones involved in blood glucose regulation (*e.g.*, glucagon, cortisol, growth hormone, somatostatin).

Metformin is absorbed from the small intestine. It circulates without binding to plasma proteins and has a serum half-life of 1.3 to 4.5 hours. It is not metabolized in the liver but is excreted unchanged in the urine. Metformin is used to treat NIDDM when hyperglycemia is not controlled with diet alone or with diet and a sulfonylurea. Metformin may be given alone or in combination with a sulfonylurea.

Insulin-Enhancing Agent

Troglitazone (Rezulin) is the first thiazolidinedione, a new category of oral antidiabetic agents. It decreases insulin resistance by increasing uptake of glucose by skeletal muscles and by decreasing production of glucose by the liver. Overall, the drug increases the effectiveness of circulating insulin; it does not stimulate insulin secretion.

MECHANISMS OF ACTION

Exogenous insulin has the same mechanism of action as the endogenous hormone. Oral sulfonylureas lower blood glucose mainly by increasing secretion of insulin. They may also increase peripheral use of glucose, decrease production of glucose in the liver, increase the number of insulin receptors, or alter postreceptor actions to increase tissue responsiveness to insulin. Because the drugs stimulate pancreatic beta cells to produce and release more insulin, they are effective only when functioning pancreatic beta cells are present. Acarbose and miglitol prevent absorption of carbohydrates from the intestine; metformin decreases absorption and production of glucose and stimulates tissue uptake of glucose; and troglitazone decreases insulin

resistance. Thus, the nonsulfonylurea agents decrease hyperglycemia by a varitey of mechanisms. They do not increase insulin secretion.

INDICATIONS FOR USE

The primary clinical indication for insulin is treatment of diabetes mellitus. Because diabetes is characterized by a relative or absolute lack of the natural pancreatic hormone, insulin from a source outside the body is needed as a substitute or replacement. Insulin is the only effective treatment for type I diabetes (IDDM), because little, if any, endogenous insulin is produced and metabolism is severely impaired. Insulin is required for 20% to 30% of type II diabetics (NIDDM) who cannot control their disease with diet, weight control, and oral agents. It may be needed for anyone with diabetes during times of stress, such as illness, infection or surgery. Insulin also is used to control diabetes induced by chronic pancreatitis, surgical excision of pancreatic tissue, hormones and other drugs, and pregnancy (gestational diabetes). In nondiabetics, insulin is used to prevent or treat hyperglycemia induced by IV hyperalimentation solutions and to treat hyperkalemia. In hyperkalemia, an IV infusion of insulin and dextrose solution causes potassium to move from the blood into the cell; it does not eliminate potassium from the body.

Oral hypoglycemic agents are indicated for clients with symptomatic type II diabetes that cannot be controlled by diet or weight loss. In addition, when hyperglycemia is not controlled by diet and a single drug, a sulfonylurea may be given along with acarbose, miglitol, or metformin. In some instances, an oral agent is given along with insulin in type II diabetes.

CONTRAINDICATIONS FOR USE

The only clear-cut contraindication to the use of insulin is hypoglycemia (because of the risk of brain damage). Beef or pork insulin is contraindicated in clients allergic to the animal proteins.

Oral sulfonylureas are contraindicated in clients with hypersensitivity to them, with severe renal or hepatic impairment, and during pregnancy. They are unlikely to be effective during periods of stress, such as major surgery, severe illness, or infection. Insulin is usually required in these circumstances.

Acarbose and miglitol are contraindicated in clients with hypersensitivity; DKA; hepatic cirrhosis; inflammatory and other intestinal disorders; and severe renal impairment.

Metformin is contraindicated in clients with diabetes complicated by fever, severe infections, severe trauma, major surgery, acidosis, or pregnancy (insulin is indicated in these conditions). It is also contraindicated with serious hepatic or renal impairment, cardiac or respiratory insufficiency, hypoxia from any cause, or a history of lactic acidosis because these conditions may increase production of lactate and risk of potentially fatal lactic acidosis.

Nursing Process

Assessment

Assess the client's knowledge, attitude, and condition in relation to diabetes, the prescribed treatment plan, and complications. Assessment data should include past manifestations of the disease process and the client's response to them, present status, and potential problem areas.

- *Historic data* include age at onset of diabetes, prescribed control measures and their effectiveness, the ease or difficulty of complying with the prescribed treatment, occurrence of complications such as ketoacidosis, and whether other disease processes have interfered with diabetes control.
- *Assess the client's current status,* including subjective and objective information related to the following areas:
  - **Diet.** Ask how many calories are prescribed, how they are calculated (food exchanges, weighing portions, or other), who prepares the food, what factors help in following the diet, what factors interfere with following the diet, the present weight and whether there has been a recent increase or decrease in weight. Also, list specific foods eaten at home during a 1- to 3-day period. This information assists in evaluating the nutritional adequacy of the diet actually taken and the client's adherence to the prescribed diet.
  - **Activity.** Ask the client to describe usual activities of daily living, including those related to work, home, and recreation. Does the client have a regular exercise program?
  - **Medication.** If the client takes insulin, ask what kind, how much, who administers it, usual time of administration, sites used for injections, if a hypoglycemic reaction to insulin has ever been experienced, and if so, how it was handled. This information helps to assess knowledge, usual practices, and teaching needs. If the client takes an oral antidiabetic drug, ask the name, the prescribed dosage and time, and the dosage and time actually taken.
  - **Monitoring methods.** Blood testing for glucose and urine testing for ketones (*e.g.,* when ill and unable to eat) are the two main methods of monitoring disease control and response to treatment. Try to determine the method used, the frequency of testing, and the pattern of results. If possible, observe the client performing and interpreting an actual test to assess accuracy.
  - **Skin and mucous membranes.** Inspect for signs of infection and any other lesions. Infections are relatively common in axillary and groin areas, because these are areas with large numbers of microorganisms. Periodontal disease, also called pyrrhea, is relatively common and may be manifested by inflammation and bleeding of the gums. Women with diabetes are susceptible to monilial vaginitis and infections underneath the breasts. Check the sites of insulin injection for atrophy (dimpling or indentation), hypertrophy (nodules or lumps), and fibrosis (hardened areas). Check the lower leg for brown spots; these are caused by small hemorrhages into the skin and may indicate widespread changes in the blood vessels.

Problems are especially likely to develop in the feet from infection, trauma, pressure, vascular insufficiency, and neuropathy. Therefore, inspect the feet for calluses, ulcers, and signs of infection. When such problems develop, sensory impairment from neuropathy may delay detection, and impaired circulation may delay healing. Check pedal pulses, color, and temperature in both feet to assist in evaluating the adequacy of arterial blood flow to the feet.

- **Eyes.** Ask if the client has experienced any changes in visual acuity or blurring of vision and if eyes are examined regularly. Diabetics are prone to develop retinopathy, cataracts, and possibly glaucoma.
- **Cardiovascular system.** Clients with diabetes have a high incidence of atherosclerosis, which makes them susceptible to cardiovascular problems (*e.g.,* hypertension, angina pectoris, myocardial infarction, and peripheral vascular disease). Therefore, check blood pressure, ask if chest pains ever occur, and ask about pain in the legs with exercise (intermittent claudication).
- **Genitourinary system.** People with diabetes often have kidney and bladder problems. Assess for signs of urinary tract infection, such as burning on urination; albumin, white blood cells, or blood in urine; edema; increased urination at night; difficulty voiding; generalized itching; easy bleeding and bruising; fatigue; and muscular weakness. Impotence may develop in male diabetics and is probably caused by neuropathy.
- Assess blood sugar reports for increases or decreases. Two or more fasting blood glucose levels above 140 mg/100 ml are diagnostic of diabetes mellitus. Also, 2-hour postprandial blood sugars above 140 mg/100 ml for people younger than 50 years and above 180 mg for people over 60 are significant. Decreased blood sugar levels are especially dangerous at 40 mg/100 ml or below.
- Assess the glycosylated hemoglobin (also called glycohemoglobin and hemoglobin A_{1c}) level when available. This test indicates glucose bound to hemoglobin in red blood cells when the red blood cell is exposed to high levels of blood glucose. The binding is irreversible and lasts for the life span of the red blood cell (about 120 days). The test reflects the average blood sugar for about 2 to 3 months before the test is done and indicates whether blood sugar is being controlled within desirable ranges.

Test results are not affected by several factors that alter blood sugar levels, such as time of day, food intake, exercise, recently administered antidiabetic drugs, emotional stress, or patient cooperation. The test is especially useful with children, labile diabetics, and those who have abnormal renal thresholds for glucose, who do not test blood glucose regularly, or who change their usual habits before a scheduled appointment with a health care provider so that their blood sugar control appears better that it actually is.

Nursing Diagnoses

- Altered Tissue Perfusion related to atherosclerosis and vascular impairment
- Sensory/Perceptual Alterations related to impaired vision
- Sensory/Perceptual Alterations related to neuropathy, especially in the legs
- Ineffective Individual Coping related to chronic illness and required treatment

- Anxiety: Managing a chronic illness, finger sticks, insulin injections
- Risk for Injury: Trauma, infection, hypoglycemia, hyperglycemia
- Noncompliance related to inability or unwillingness to manage the disease process and required treatment
- Knowledge Deficit: Disease process and management
- Knowledge Deficit: Administration and effects of antidiabetic drugs
- Knowledge Deficit: Interrelationships among diet, exercise, and antidiabetic drugs
- Knowledge Deficit: Management of hypoglycemia, "sick days," and other complications

Planning/Goals

The client will:

- Learn self-care activities at an individualized pace
- Manage drug therapy to prevent or minimize hypoglycemia and other adverse effects
- Develop a consistent pattern of diet and exercise
- Use available resources to learn about the disease process and how to manage it
- Administer antidiabetic drugs accurately
- Self-monitor blood glucose and urine ketones appropriately
- Keep appointments for follow-up and monitoring procedures by a health care provider

Interventions

Use nondrug measures to improve control of diabetes and to help prevent complications.

- Assist the client in maintaining the prescribed diet. Specific measures vary but may include teaching the client and family about the importance of diet, referring the client to a dietitian, and helping the client identify and modify factors that decrease compliance with the diet. If the client is obese, assist in developing a program to lose weight and then maintain weight at a more nearly normal level.
- Assist the client to develop and maintain a regular exercise program.
- Perform and interpret blood tests for glucose accurately, and teach clients and family members to do so. Self-monitoring of blood glucose levels allows the client to see the effects of diet, exercise, and hypoglycemic medications on blood glucose levels and may promote compliance.

    Several products are available for home glucose monitoring. All involve obtaining a drop of capillary blood from a finger with a sterile lancet. The blood is placed on a semipermeable membrane that contains a reagent. The amount of blood glucose, in milligrams per 100 ml, can be read visually or with various machines (*e.g.*, Accu-Chek Glucometer). The latter method is more accurate but less convenient and more expensive than visual reading.
- Test urine for ketones when the client is sick, when blood glucose levels are above 240 mg/100 ml, and when episodes of nocturnal hypoglycemia are suspected. Also teach clients and family members to test urine when indicated.
- Promote early recognition and treatment of problems by observing for signs and symptoms of urinary tract infection, peripheral vascular disease, vision changes, ketoacidosis, hypoglycemia, and others. Teach clients and families to observe for these conditions and report their occurrence.

- Discuss the importance of regular visits to the physician, clinic, or other facility for blood sugar measurements, weights, blood pressure measurements, and eye examinations.
- Perform and teach correct foot care. Have the client observe the following safeguards: Avoid going barefoot to prevent trauma to the feet; wear correctly fitted shoes; wash the feet daily with warm water, dry well, inspect for any lesions or pressure areas, and apply lanolin if the skin is dry; wear cotton or wool socks, because they are more absorbent than synthetic materials, such as nylon; cut toenails straight across and only after the feet have been soaked in warm water and washed thoroughly. Teach the client to avoid use of hot-water bottles or electric heating pads, cutting toenails if vision is impaired, use of strong antiseptics on the feet, and cutting corns or calluses. Also teach the client to report any lesions on the feet to the physician.

Teach clients:

- The nature and characteristics of diabetes mellitus and proposed control measures. Few diseases require as much adaptation in activities of daily living as diabetes mellitus. The client must be well informed to control the disease, minimize complications, and achieve an optimal quality of life.
- Signs and symptoms of hyperglycemia: increased blood glucose and excessive thirst, hunger, and urine output. Persistent hyperglycemia may indicate a need to change some aspect of the treatment program, such as diet or medication.
- Symptoms of hypoglycemia: sweating, nervousness, hunger, weakness, tremors, and mental confusion. Hypoglycemia may indicate too much medication or exercise or too little food. If it occurs, take about 4 oz of orange juice, two lumps of sugar, or a few bites of candy. Repeat in 10 to 15 minutes if necessary. Avoid taking so much sugar that hyperglycemia occurs.
- The importance of diet, weight control, and exercise in control of diabetes. Maintaining normal weight and avoiding excessive caloric intake decrease the need for medication, decrease the workload of the pancreas, and help the body use insulin more efficiently. Exercise improves use of insulin and helps to promote more normal blood glucose levels.
- Measures to delay, prevent, or decrease severity of complications. These measures are wide ranging and include regular medical supervision, preferably by a diabetologist, regular vision and glaucoma testing, and special foot care. The goal of such measures is to prevent complications. If they cannot be prevented, early recognition and treatment may minimize their severity.
- Take only drugs prescribed by a physician who knows the client has diabetes. Avoid other prescriptions and over-the-counter drugs unless these are discussed with the physician treating the patient, because adverse reactions and interactions may occur. For example, nasal decongestants (alone or in multi-ingredient cold remedies) and asthma medications may cause tachycardia and nervousness, which may be interpreted as hypoglycemia. In addition, liquid cold remedies and cough syrups may contain sugar and raise blood glucose levels. Aspirin and other salicylates in over-the-counter preparations for pain may increase the likelihood of hypoglycemia.

- Test blood regularly for glucose. A frequently recommended schedule is before meals and at bedtime. The optimal frequency of blood glucose monitoring has not been established.

Evaluation

- Check blood sugar reports regularly for normal or abnormal values.
- Check glycosylated hemoglobin reports when available.
- Interview and observe for therapeutic and adverse responses to antidiabetic drugs.
- Interview and observe for compliance with prescribed treatment.
- Interview clients and family members about the frequency and length of hospitalizations for diabetes mellitus.

Principles of Therapy

TREATMENT REGIMENS

When possible, it is desirable to have an interdisciplinary diabetes care team (e.g., physician, nurse diabetes educator, dietitian, and perhaps others) work with the client to design, monitor, and revise an individualized treatment plan. This is especially important for clients with newly diagnosed diabetes mellitus, to assist them in learning to manage their disease and make appropriate lifestyle changes.

For most clients, the goal of treatment is to maintain blood glucose at normal or near-normal levels. There is strong evidence in clients with type I and increasing evidence in clients with type II diabetes that strict control of blood sugar decreases complications of diabetes. The treatment regimen chosen for a particular client depends on the type of diabetes, the client's age and general condition, and the client's ability and willingness to comply with the prescribed therapy.

In type I diabetes, the only effective treatment measures are insulin, diet, and exercise. In type II diabetes, the initial treatment of choice is diet therapy and weight control. If this regimen is ineffective, oral agents or insulin may be added.

GUIDELINES FOR INSULIN THERAPY

Choice of Preparation

When insulin therapy is indicated, the physician may choose from several preparations that vary in composition, onset and duration of action, and other characteristics. Some factors to be considered include the following:

1. Human insulin is preferred for newly diagnosed type I diabetes, gestational diabetes, poorly controlled diabetes, and diabetics undergoing surgery or experiencing illness that requires short-term insulin therapy. Human insulin is less likely to cause allergic reactions and insulin-antibody formation.
2. Isophane insulin (NPH) or insulin zinc suspension (Lente) is often used for long-term insulin therapy. NPH is more commonly used.
3. Regular insulin (insulin injection) is the only preparation that has a rapid onset of action and can be given IV. Therefore, it is the insulin of choice during acute situations, such as DKA, severe infection or other illness, and surgical procedures.
4. For many clients, a combination of regular insulin and an intermediate-acting insulin, most often NPH, provides more consistent control of blood glucose levels. Although several regimens are used, a common one is a mixture of regular and intermediate insulins, administered before the morning and evening meals. A commercial mixture is more convenient and probably more accurate than a mixture prepared by a client or caregiver, if the proportions of insulins are appropriate for the client.
5. For clients with local or systemic manifestations of insulin allergy, the insulin of choice is either human insulin or purified pork insulin.

Dosage Factors

Dosage of insulin must be individualized according to blood glucose levels. The goal is to alleviate symptoms of hyperglycemia and reestablish metabolic and fluid balance without causing hypoglycemia. An initial dose of approximately 0.5 to 1 unit/kg/d may be started and then adjusted to maintain blood glucose levels (tested before meals and at bedtime) of 80 to 140 mg/100 ml. However, many factors influence blood glucose response to exogenous insulin and therefore influence insulin requirements.

1. Factors that increase insulin requirements include weight gain, increased caloric intake, pregnancy, decreased activity, acute infections, hyperadrenocorticism (Cushing's disease), primary hyperparathyroidism, acromegaly, hypokalemia, and drugs such as adrenocorticosteroids, thyroid, epinephrine, and thiazide diuretics. Clients who are obese may require about 2 units/kg/d because of resistance to insulin in peripheral tissues.
2. Factors that decrease insulin requirements include weight reduction; decreased caloric intake; increased physical activity; development of renal insufficiency; stopping administration of adrenocorticosteroids, thyroid, epinephrine, and diuretics; hypothyroidism; hypopituitarism; recovery from hyperthyroidism; recovery from acute infections; and the "honeymoon period," which sometimes occurs with type I diabetes.

People who need less than 0.5 unit/kg/d may produce some endogenous insulin or their tissues may be more responsive to insulin because of exercise and good physical conditioning. Renal insufficiency decreases dosage requirements because less insulin is metabolized in the kidneys than with normal renal function. The honeymoon period, characterized by recovery of islet cell function and temporary production of insulin, may occur after diabetes is first diagnosed. Insulin requirements may decrease rapidly, and if the dosage is not decreased, severe hypoglycemic reactions may result.

3. In acute situations, dosage of regular insulin needs frequent adjustments based on measurements of blood glucose. If insulin is given IV in a continuous infusion, about 20% to 30% of the added insulin becomes bound to the container of IV fluids and to the plastic infusion set. It is recommended that 10 to 50 ml of the solution be discarded to saturate binding sites.

4. Dosage of insulin for long-term therapy is determined by blood glucose levels at various times of the day and adjusted when indicated (*e.g.*, because of illness or changes in physical activity). Titrating insulin dosage may be difficult and time consuming; it requires cooperation and collaboration between clients and health care providers.

5. Insulin pumps have advantages and disadvantages and are used by relatively few people. These devices allow continuous SC administration of regular insulin. A basal amount of insulin is injected (*e.g.*, 1 unit/h or a calculated fraction of the dose used previously) continuously, with bolus injections before meals. This method of insulin administration maintains more normal blood glucose levels and avoids wide fluctuations. Candidates for insulin pumps include clients with diabetes that is poorly controlled with other methods and those who are able and willing to care for the devices properly.

Timing of Insulin Administration

Many clients who take insulin seem to need at least two injections daily to control hyperglycemia. A common regimen is one half to two thirds of the total daily dose in the morning, before breakfast, and the remaining one half or one third before the evening meal or at bedtime.

Selection of Subcutaneous Sites for Insulin Injections

Several factors affect insulin absorption from injection sites, including the site location, environmental temperature, and exercise or massage. Research studies indicate that insulin is absorbed fastest from the ab-

domen, then the deltoid, thigh, and hip. Because of these differences, many clinicians recommend rotating injection sites *within* areas (*e.g.*, using several sites in the abdomen before moving to another area) on a daily basis. This technique decreases rotations *between* areas and promotes more consistent blood glucose levels. In relation to temperature, insulin is absorbed more rapidly in warmer sites and environments. In relation to exercise, persons who exercise should avoid injecting insulin into SC tissue near the muscles to be used. The increased blood flow that accompanies exercise promotes rapid absorption and may lead to hypoglycemia.

Timing of Food Intake

Clients receiving insulin need food at the peak action time of the insulin preparation being used and at bedtime. The food is usually taken as a between-meal and a bedtime snack. These snacks help prevent hypoglycemic reactions between meals and at night. When hypoglycemia occurs during sleep, recognition and treatment may be delayed. This delay may allow the reaction to become more severe.

Diabetic Ketoacidosis

Insulin therapy is a major component of any treatment program for DKA. Clients with DKA have a deficiency in the total amount of insulin in the body and a resistance to the action of the insulin that is available, probably owing to acidosis, hyperosmolality, infection, and other factors. To be effective, insulin therapy must be individualized according to frequent measurements of blood glucose. Low doses, given by continuous IV infusion, are preferred in most circumstances.

Other measures that usually must accompany insulin to treat DKA effectively include identification and treatment of conditions that precipitate DKA, administration of IV fluids to correct hyperosmolality and dehydration, administration of potassium supplements to maintain normal serum potassium levels, and administration of sodium bicarbonate to correct metabolic acidosis.

Although other conditions may predispose diabetics to the development of DKA, infection is one of the most common and important. If no obvious source of infection is identified, cultures of blood, urine, and throat swabs are recommended. When infection is identified, antibacterial drug therapy may be indicated.

IV fluids, possibly the most important first step in treating DKA, usually consist of 0.9% sodium chloride, an isotonic solution. Hypotonic solutions are usually avoided because they allow intracellular fluid shifts and may cause cerebral, pulmonary, and peripheral edema.

Although serum potassium levels may be normal at first, they fall rapidly after insulin and IV fluid therapy are begun. Decreased serum potassium levels are caused by expansion of extracellular fluid volume, movement of potassium into cells, and continued loss of potassium in the urine as long as hyperglycemia persists. For these reasons, potassium supplements are usually added to IV fluids. Because both hypokalemia and hyperkalemia can cause serious cardiovascular disturbances, dosage of potassium supplements must be based on frequent measurements of serum potassium levels. Also, continuous or frequent electrocardiogram monitoring is recommended.

Severe acidosis can cause serious cardiovascular disturbances. Specifically, these disturbances usually stem from peripheral vasodilation and decreased cardiac output with hypotension and shock. Acidosis generally can be corrected by giving fluids and insulin.

Sodium bicarbonate may be given if the pH is less than 7.2. If used, sodium bicarbonate should be given slowly and cautiously. Rapid alkalinization can cause potassium to move into body cells faster than it can be replaced IV. The result may be severe hypokalemia and cardiac arrhythmias. Also, giving excessive amounts of sodium bicarbonate can produce alkalosis.

Treatment of the Unconscious Client

When a person with diabetes becomes unconscious and it cannot be determined whether the unconsciousness is caused by DKA or by hypoglycemia from insulin (*i.e.*, by measuring blood glucose levels), treat the client for hypoglycemia. If hypoglycemia is the cause of unconsciousness, giving some form of glucose may avert brain damage, which results from severe, prolonged hypoglycemia. If DKA is the cause of unconsciousness, giving glucose will not harm the client. Sudden unconsciousness in the insulin-dependent diabetic is most likely to result from an insulin reaction; DKA usually develops gradually over several days or even weeks.

Hyperosmolar Nonketoacidotic Diabetic Coma

Treatment of hyperosmolar nonketoacidotic diabetic coma is similar to that of DKA in that insulin, IV fluids, and potassium supplements are major components. Regular insulin is given by continuous IV infusion, and dosage is individualized according to frequent measurements of blood glucose levels. IV fluids are given to correct the profound dehydration and hyperosmolality, and potassium is given IV to replace the large amounts lost in urine during a hyperglycemic state.

Insulin Therapy During the Perioperative Period

Clients with diabetes who undergo major surgery have increased risks of both surgical and diabetic complications. Risks associated with surgery and anesthesia are greater if diabetes is not well controlled and complications of diabetes (*e.g.*, hypertension, nephropathy, vascular damage) are already evident. Hyperglycemia and poor metabolic control are associated with increased susceptibility to infection, poor wound healing, and fluid and electrolyte imbalances. Risks of diabetic complications are increased because the stress of surgery increases insulin requirements and may precipitate ketosis or DKA. Metabolic responses to stress include increased secretion of catecholamines, cortisol, glucagon, and growth hormone, all of which increase blood sugar levels. In addition to hyperglycemia, protein breakdown, lipolysis, ketogenesis, and insulin resistance occur. The risk of hypoglycemia is also increased.

The goals of diabetes management are to avoid hypoglycemia, severe hyperglycemia, ketoacidosis, and fluid and electrolye imbalances. Generally, mild hyperglycemia (*e.g.*, blood glucose levels between 150 and 250 mg/100 ml) is considered safer for the client than hypoglycemia, which may go unrecognized during anesthesia and surgery. Because surgery is a stressful event that increases blood glucose levels and the body's need for insulin, insulin therapy is usually required.

The goal of insulin therapy is to avoid ketosis from inadequate insulin and hypoglycemia from excessive insulin. Specific actions to reach this goal depend largely on the severity of diabetes and the type of surgical procedure. Diabetes should be well controlled before any type of surgery. Minor procedures usually require little change in the usual treatment program; major operations usually require a different medication regimen.

As a general rule, regular, short-acting insulin is used in all patients with diabetes who have major surgery or any surgery requiring general anesthesia. For clients who have been insulin dependent and using an intermediate-acting insulin, a different regimen using regular insulin in doses approximating the usual daily requirement is needed. For clients who usually manage their diabetes with diet alone or with diet and oral hypoglycemic medications, insulin therapy is started. Small doses are usually required.

Preoperatively, for elective major surgery, clients should be scheduled early in the day to avoid prolonged fasting. In addition, most authorities recommend omitting usual doses of insulin on the day of surgery and oral antidiabetic medications for 1 or 2 days before surgery. While the patient is receiving nothing by mouth, preoperatively and intraoperatively, IV insulin is usually given. Along with the insulin, clients need adequate sources of carbohydrate. This is usually supplied by IV solutions of 5% or 10% dextrose solutions.

Postoperatively, IV insulin and dextrose may be continued until the patient is able to eat and drink. Regular insulin also can be given SC every 4 to 6 hours, with frequent blood glucose measurements. Oral fluids and foods that contain carbohydrate should be resumed as soon as possible. When meals are fully tolerated, the preoperative insulin or oral medication regimen can be resumed. Additional regular insulin can be given for elevated blood glucose and ketones, if indicated.

ORAL ANTIDIABETIC DRUGS

Sulfonylureas

1. Sulfonylureas are not effective in all clients with type II diabetes mellitus. Even when carefully selected, many clients experience primary or secondary treatment failure. Primary failure involves a lack of initial response to the drugs. Secondary failure means that a therapeutic response occurs when the drugs are first given, but the drugs eventually become ineffective. The reasons for secondary failure are unclear but may include decreased compliance with diet instructions, failure to take the drugs as prescribed, or decreased ability of the pancreatic beta cells to produce more insulin in response to the drugs.
2. All the sulfonylureas must be used cautiously in clients with impaired renal or hepatic function.
3. Dosage of sulfonylureas is usually started at lower amounts and increased gradually until the fasting blood glucose level is 110 mg/100 ml or less. The lowest dose that will achieve normal levels of both fasting and postprandial blood sugars is recommended.
4. Sulfonylureas are not recommended for use during pregnancy because some of these drugs cross the placenta and may cause hypoglycemia and even fetal death. Also, an increased risk of congenital anomalies is possible. A third reason is the risk that women with gestational diabetes will develop overt diabetes because the drugs stimulate an already overstimulated pancreas.

Alpha-glucosidase Inhibitors

1. The important differences between acarbose and miglitol and other oral antidiabetic drugs are that the alpha-glucosidase inhibitors do not alter insulin secretion and do not cause hypoglycemia.

2. Acarbose and miglitol should be taken at the beginning of a meal so they will be present in the GI tract with food and able to block digestion of carbohydrates.
3. Clients taking acarbose and miglitol should continue their diet, exercise, and blood glucose testing routines. During initiation and dosage titration, the client's response can be monitored by measuring 1-hour postprandial blood glucose levels. During long-term therapy, measurement of glycosylated hemoglobin is recommended about every 3 months to evaluate glycemic control. The goal of treatment is to lower the postprandial blood glucose and the glycosylated hemoglobin levels to normal or near normal.

Biguanide

1. Renal function should be assessed before starting metformin therapy and at least annually during long-term therapy. The drug should not be given initially if renal impairment is present; it should be stopped if renal impairment occurs during treatment.
2. As with other antidiabetic drugs, clients taking metformin should continue their diet, exercise, and blood glucose testing regimens. During initiation and dosage titration, the client's response can be monitored by measuring blood glucose levels. During long-term therapy, measurement of glycosylated hemoglobin is recommended about every 3 months to evaluate glycemic control. The goal of treatment is to lower the fasting blood glucose and the glycosylated hemoglobin levels to normal or near normal.
3. Parenteral radiographic contrast media containing iodine (*e.g.*, Cholografin, Hypaque, Omnipaque) may cause renal failure, and they have been associated with lactic acidosis in patients receiving metformin. Metformin should be discontinued at least 48 hours before diagnostic tests are performed with these materials. In addition, metformin should not be resumed for at least 48 hours after the tests are done and until tests indicate renal function is normal.

COMBINATION DRUG THERAPY FOR NIDDM

Combination drug therapy is an increasing trend in NIDDM that is not controlled by diet or by diet and single-drug therapy. Various combinations are being used, with evidence of increased effectiveness in metabolic control. One combination is insulin plus a sulfonylurea. Advantages indicated by several studies include lower fasting blood glucose levels; decreased glycosylated hemoglobin levels; increased secretion of endogenous insulin; smaller daily doses of insulin; and no significant change in body weight. The role of insulin analogs such as insulin lispro (Humalog) in combination drug therapy is not clear.

Oral agents are also being combined, such as acarbose plus a sulfonylurea or metformin plus a sulfonylurea. These combinations have been investigated in clinical trials, and acarbose and metformin are FDA-approved for use with sulfonylureas. However, clinical experience with the combinations is limited, and optimal therapy is still being defined.

HYPOGLYCEMIA: CHARACTERISTICS AND TREATMENT

Hypoglycemia may occur with insulin, oral sulfonylureas, or metformin. When suspected, the blood glucose level should be measured if at all possible, although signs and symptoms and the plasma glucose level at which they occur vary from person to person. Hypoglycemia is usually defined as a blood glucose below 60 to 70 mg/dl and is especially dangerous about 40 mg/dl or below. Central nervous system (CNS) effects of hypoglycemia may lead to accidental injury or permanent brain damage; cardiovascular effects may lead to cardiac arrhythmias or myocardial infarction. Severe hypoglycemia is especially likely to occur in clients receiving intensive insulin therapy (i.e., continuous SC infusion or three or more injections daily). Other causes include omitting or delaying meals; an excessive or incorrect dose of insulin or an oral agent; altered sensitivity to insulin; decreased clearance of insulin or an oral agent (e.g., with renal insufficiency); decreased glucose intake; decreased production of glucose in the liver; giving an insulin injection IM or IV rather than SC; drug interactions that decrease blood glucose levels; increased physical exertion; and ethanol ingestion.

Normally, when hypoglycemia occurs, several hormones (glucagon, epinephrine, growth hormone and cortisol) work to restore and maintain blood glucose levels. Glucagon and epinephrine, the dominant counterregulatory hormones, act rapidly because they are activated as soon as blood glucose levels start declining. Growth hormone and cortisol act more slowly, about 2 hours after hypoglycemia occurs. The person with diabetes who develops hypoglycemia may have impaired secretion of these counterregulatory hormones. Such impairment is especially likely in patients with IDDM. Decreased secretion of glucagon is often evident in patients who have had diabetes for 5 years or longer. Decreased secretion of epinephrine also occurs in persons who have been treated with insulin for several years. Decreased epinephrine decreases tachycar-

dia, a common sign of hypoglycemia, and may delay recognition and treatment.

When hypoglycemic reactions occur with insulin, sulfonylureas, or metformin, treatment consists of the immediate administration of a rapidly absorbed carbohydrate. If the client is awake and can swallow, the carbohydrate is given orally. About 10 to 15 g of carbohydrate are usually sufficient and can be furnished by a variety of foods and fluids (e.g., two sugar cubes; 1 to 2 teaspoons of sugar, syrup, honey, or jelly; two or three small pieces of candy; five or six Lifesavers candies; 4 oz of fruit juice, such as orange, apple, or grape; 4 oz of ginger ale; coffee or tea with 2 teaspoons of sugar added). Concentrated glucose products available include gel formulations (e.g., Glutose, Insta-Glucose, Monojel) and chewable tablets (e.g., B-D Glucose). All these products must be swallowed to be effective. Symptoms usually subside within 15 to 20 minutes. If they do not subside, the patient should take another 10 to 15 g of oral carbohydrate. Once hypoglycemia is relieved, the person should have a snack or a meal. Slowly absorbed carbohydrate and protein foods, such as milk, cheese, and bread, are needed to replace glycogen stores in the liver and to prevent secondary hypoglycemia from rapid use of the carbohydrates given earlier. *If acarbose or miglitol has been taken with a sulfonylurea or metformin and a hypoglycemic reaction occurs, glucose (oral or IV) or glucagon must be given for treatment. Sucrose (table sugar) and other oral carbohydrates will not relieve hypoglycemia because the presence of acarbose or miglitol prevents their digestion and absorption from the GI tract.*

If the client cannot swallow or is unconscious, carbohydrate cannot be given orally because of the risks of aspiration. Therefore, the treatment choices involve parenteral glucose or glucagon. If the client is in a health care facility where medical help is readily available, IV glucose in a 25% or 50% concentrated solution is the treatment of choice. It acts rapidly to raise blood glucose levels and arouse the client. If the client is at home or elsewhere, glucagon may be given if available and there is someone to inject it. A family member may be taught to give glucagon SC or IM. It can also be given IV. The usual adult dose is 0.5 to 1 mg. Glucagon is a pancreatic hormone that increases blood sugar by converting liver glycogen to glucose. It is effective only when liver glycogen is present. Some clients cannot respond to glucagon because glycogen stores are depleted by such conditions as starvation, adrenal insufficiency, or chronic hypoglycemia. The hyperglycemic effect of glucagon occurs more slowly than that of IV glucose and is of relatively brief duration. If the client does not respond to one or two doses of glucagon within 20 minutes, IV glucose is indicated.

Although the main goal of treatment is to relieve hypoglycemia and restore the brain's supply of glucose, a secondary goal is to avoid overtreatment and excessive hyperglycemia. Caution is needed in the treatment of hypoglycemia. The client having a hypoglycemic reaction should not use it as an excuse to eat large amounts of food in addition to or instead of the prescribed diet. Health care personnel caring for the client should avoid giving excessive amounts of glucose. Repeated episodes of hypoglycemia mean that the therapeutic regimen and client compliance must be reevaluated.

USE IN CHILDREN

Insulin is the only drug indicated for use in type I diabetes. Because children with diabetes cannot produce insulin, insulin is required as replacement therapy. Several factors influence diabetes management and insulin therapy in children, including the following:

1. Effective management of IDDM requires a rather rigid schedule of meals, snacks, blood glucose monitoring, insulin injections and dose adjustments, and exercise. Such a schedule is difficult to implement in children, but extrememly important in promoting normal growth and development. A major factor in optimal treatment is a supportive family in which at least one member is thoroughly educated about IDDM. Less-than-optimal treatment can lead to stunted growth, delayed puberty, and early development of complications such as retinopathy, nephropathy, or neuropathy.

2. Infections and other illnesses in children with IDDM may cause wide fluctuations in blood glucose levels and interfere with metabolic control. For example, some infections cause hypoglycemia; others, especially chronic infections, are likely to cause hyperglycemia and insulin resistance and may precipitate ketoacidosis. As a result, insulin requirements may vary widely during illness episodes and should be based on blood glucose and urine ketone levels. Young children often develop hypoglycemia, partly because of anorexia and smaller glycogen reserves.

3. During illness, children with IDDM are highly susceptible to dehydration, and an adequate fluid intake is very important. Many clinicians recommend sugar-containing liquids (*e.g.*, regular sodas, clear juices, regular gelatin desserts) if blood glucose values are lower than 250 mg/dl. When blood glucose values are greater than 250 mg/dl, diet soda, unsweetened tea, and other fluids without sugar should be given.

4. For infants and toddlers who weigh less than 10 kg or require less than 5 units of insulin per day, a di-

luted insulin can be used because such small doses are hard to measure in a U-100 syringe. The most common dilution is U-10, and a diluent is available from most insulin manufacturers. Vials of diluted insulin should be clearly labeled and discarded after 1 month.

5. Rotation of injection sites is important in infants and young children because of the relatively small areas for injection at each anatomic site and to prevent lipodystrophy.

6. Young children usually adjust to injections and blood glucose monitoring better when the parents express less anxiety about these vital procedures.

7. Avoiding hypoglycemia is a major goal in infants and young children because of potentially damaging effects on growth and development. For example, the brain and spinal cord do not develop normally without an available source of glucose. Animal studies indicate that prolonged hypoglycemia results in decreased brain weight, numbers of neurons, and protein content. Myelinization of nerve cells is also decreased. Because complex motor and intellectual functions require an intact CNS, frequent, severe, or prolonged hypoglycemia can be a serious problem in infants, toddlers, and preschoolers. In addition, recognition of hypoglycemia may be delayed because signs and symptoms are not very specific and the children may be unable to communicate signs and symptoms to parents or caregivers. Because of these difficulties, most pediatric diabetologists recommend maintaining blood glucose levels between 100 and 200 mg/dl to prevent hypoglycemia. In addition, *the bedtime snack and blood glucose measurement should never be skipped.*

8. Signs and symptoms of hypoglycemia in older children are similar to those in adults (*e.g.*, hunger, sweating, tachycardia). In young children, hypoglycemia may be manifested by changes in behavior, including severe hunger, irritability, and lethargy. In addition, mental functioning may be impaired in all age groups, even with mild hypoglycemia. Any time hypoglycemia is suspected, blood glucose should be tested.

9. Adolescents with IDDM may resist adhering to their prescribed treatment regimens, and effective management may be especially difficult during this developmental period. In one study of 59 adolescents and young adults with IDDM (Dunning, 1995), results indicated that 66% sometimes delayed or omitted insulin to fit in socially (by eating more, sleeping in, or drinking alcohol) and 38% (mostly females) decreased their prescribed insulin dose to control their weight. Omitting or decreasing insulin dosage may lead to repeated episodes of ketoacidosis.

USE IN OLDER ADULTS

General precautions for safe and effective use of antidiabetic drugs apply to older adults, including close monitoring of blood glucose levels. In addition, older adults may have impaired vision or other problems that decrease their ability to perform needed tasks (*e.g.*, self-administration of insulin, monitoring blood glucose levels, managing diet and exercise). They also may have other disorders and may take other drugs that complicate management of diabetes. For example, thiazide diuretics, corticosteroids, estrogens, and other drugs may cause hyperglycemia, thereby increasing dosage requirements for antidiabetic drugs.

With oral sulfonylureas, drugs with a short duration of action and inactive metabolites are considered safer, especially with impaired liver or kidney function. Chlorpropamide is not recommended because of its long duration of action.

Older adults may experience an exaggerated response to oral agents. This may be averted by starting with a low dose, then increasing or decreasing the dose according to blood glucose levels and clinical response. If hypoglycemic reactions occur, dosage may need to be reduced.

There has been little research and clinical experience with newer antidiabetic drugs in older adults. The insulin analog (Humalog) appears to have some advantages over conventional insulin, but its role is undefined. Glimepiride is similar to other second-generation sulfonylureas. Acarbose, miglitol, and metformin may not be as useful in older adults as in younger ones because of the high prevalence of impaired renal function. These drugs are relatively contraindicated in clients with renal insufficiency because they have a longer half-life and may accumulate. With metformin, dosage should be based on periodic tests of renal function and the drug should be stopped if renal impairment occurs (*i.e.*, serum creatinine increases) or if serum lactate increases. In addition, dosage should not be titrated to the maximum amount recommended for younger adults.

HOME CARE

Most diabetes care is delivered in ambulatory care settings or in the home. Hospitalization generally occurs only for complications, and clients are quickly discharged if possible. Any client with diabetes is likely to need home care sometime during the course of the disease. The home care nurse has an important role to play in assisting clients of multiple age groups to learn self-care and assisting caregivers to support client efforts or actively participate in diabetes management. Some aspects of this role include mobilizing and coordinating health care providers and community resources, teaching and supporting clients and caregivers, monitoring the client's health status and progress in disease management, and preventing or solving problems.

The person with diabetes has a tremendous amount of information to learn about living with this disease on a day-to-day basis. For most clients, the goal of diabetes education is self-care in terms of diet, exercise, medication administration, blood glucose monitoring, and prevention and recognition of complications. For some clients, a parent or caregiver may assume most of the responsibility for diabetes management. Because of the amount and complexity of information, a multidisciplinary health care team that includes a nurse diabetes educator is preferred in home care as in other settings. The role of the home care nurse may include initial teaching and/or reinforcement and follow-up of teaching done by others.

One important topic to include in home care teaching is management of sick days. Illness that would be minor in persons without diabetes may become a major illness or medical emergency in persons with diabetes. Everyone involved should be vigilant about recognizing and seeking prompt treatment for any illness. The main goal during any illness is to prevent complications such as severe hyperglycemia, dehydration, and DKA. This goal is best achieved by a well-informed and motivated patient. If the patient is unable to provide self-care because of the illness, a family member or other caregiver is needed.

Illness can affect diabetes control in several ways. First, illness causes a stress response. Part of the stress response is increased secretion of glucagon, epinephrine, growth hormone, and cortisol, hormones that raise blood glucose levels (by stimulating gluconeogenesis and inhibiting insulin action) and cause ketosis (by stimulating lipolysis and ketogenesis). Second, if the illness makes a person unable or unwilling to eat, hypoglycemia can occur. Third, if the illness affects GI function (*e.g.*, causes vomiting or diarrhea), the person may be unable to drink enough fluids to prevent dehydration and electrolyte imbalance. In addition, hyperglycemia induces an osmotic diuresis that increases dehydration and electrolyte imbalances.

Because of the potentially serious effects of other illnesses on diabetes management, patients with diabetes should be taught how to adjust their usual regimens to maintain metabolic balance and prevent severe complications. It is desirable for a health care provider to discuss specific, individualized guidelines with each patient and update them regularly. Some general guidelines for client and/or caregiver include the following:

1. Monitor blood glucose at least four times daily; test urine for ketones when the blood glucose level exceeds 240 mg/dl. Teach at least one person other than the client when and how to do the tests, in case the client is unable to do them.
2. Continue to take the usual dose of insulin or oral antidiabetic agent. Additional insulin also may be needed, especially if ketosis develops. Ketones in the urine indicate insulin deficiency or insulin resistance, and an additional insulin dose is usually needed.
3. If a client is unable or unwilling to eat solid food, provide easily digested liquids or semiliquid foods. About 15 g of carbohydrate every 1 to 2 hours are usually enough and can be provided by ½ cup of apple juice, applesauce, cola, cranberry juice, eggnog, Cream of Wheat cereal, custard, vanilla ice cream, regular gelatin, or frozen yogurt.
4. Drink 8 to 12 oz of fluid every hour, including water, tea, broth, diet soda, or a carbohydrate-containing fluid.
5. Notify the physician who manages the diabetes if the client:
   a. has an elevated before-meal blood glucose (>250 mg/dl);
   b. is unable to eat normally for more than 24 hours;
   c. develops fever above 100°F;
   d. has vomiting or diarrhea longer than about 6 hours;
   e. has ketonuria or symptoms of ketoacidosis;
   f. develops other severe symptoms such as difficulty in breathing, chest pain, severe abdominal pain, or severe dehydration.

Clients and caregivers may also need teaching about home management of hypoglycemic reactions. If the client is conscious and able to swallow, a rapidly absorbed source of oral glucose is needed, as described previously. If the client is unconscious, injection of glucagon is the treatment of choice. For clients who take insulin, glucagon should be available in the home and a caregiver should know how to give it. Preparing and administering glucagon is a simple procedure and can be taught in a few minutes. The person receiving glucagon should be placed in a side-lying position, to prevent aspiration if the medication causes vomiting. In addition, the person should be fed immediately upon regaining consciousness, because glucagon has a short duration of action.

ANTIDIABETIC DRUGS

NURSING ACTIONS	RATIONALE/EXPLANATION
1. Administer accurately	
a. With insulin:	
(1) Store the insulin vial in current use and administer insulin at room temperature. Refrigerate extra vials.	Cold insulin is more likely to cause lipodystrophy, local sensitivity reactions, discomfort, and delayed absorption. Insulin preparations are stable for months at room temperature if temperature extremes are avoided.
(2) Avoid freezing temperatures (32°F) or high temperatures (95°F or above).	Extremes of temperature decrease insulin potency and cause clumping of the suspended particles of modified insulins (all except regular insulin). This clumping phenomenon causes inaccurate dosage even if the volume is accurately measured.
(3) Use only an insulin syringe calibrated to measure U-100 insulin.	For accurate measurement of the prescribed dose.
(4) With modified insulin preparations, which includes all except regular, short-acting insulin, invert and rotate the vial before withdrawing the insulin. Do not shake the vial.	These insulin preparations are suspensions, and the components separate on standing. Unless the particles are resuspended in the solution and distributed evenly, dosage will be inaccurate. Shaking the vial causes air bubbles, which enter the syringe and interfere with accurate measurement of the prescribed dose.
(5) When a mixture of two insulins is prescribed, such as regular and NPH, prepare in the following sequence:	It is important that the two insulins be drawn up in the same sequence every time. Most authorities recommend that regu-

(continued)

NURSING ACTIONS	*RATIONALE/EXPLANATION*
(a) Draw into the insulin syringe the amount of air equal to the total amount of both insulins. (b) Draw up the regular insulin first. Inject the equivalent portion of air, and aspirate the ordered dose. (c) With the NPH vial, insert the remaining air (avoid injecting regular insulin into the NPH vial), and aspirate the ordered dose. (d) Expel air bubbles, if present, and verify that the correct dosage is in the syringe.	lar insulin *always* be drawn up first. This avoids contamination of the regular insulin with the NPH. Because regular insulin combines with excess protamine in NPH, the concentration of regular insulin is changed when they are mixed. Following the same sequence also leaves the same type of insulin in the needle and syringe (dead space) every time. Although dead space is not usually considered a significant factor with available insulin syringes, it may be with small doses.
(e) Administer the combined insulins *consistently* within 15 min of mixing or after a longer period; that is, do not give one dose within 15 min of mixing and another 2 h or days after mixing.	As stated previously, regular insulin combines with excess protamine when combined with NPH insulin. This reaction, which occurs within 15 min of mixing, alters the amount of regular insulin present. After about 15 min, the mixture is stable for about 1 month at room temperature and 3 months when refrigerated. Thus, to administer the same dose consistently, the mixture must be given at about the same time interval after mixing. NPH and regular insulins are most often combined. The Lente insulins mix well with each other. However, if a Lente insulin is mixed with regular insulin, they interact up to 24 h. If administered during this time, the dose of each insulin is unknown and variable. After 24 h, the mixture is stable for 1 month at room temperature and 3 months when refrigerated.
(6) Rotate injection sites systematically, and use all available sites. These include the thighs, abdomen, upper back, upper arms, and buttocks unless some of these locations are contraindicated.	Frequent injection in the same site can cause tissue fibrosis, erratic absorption, and deposits of unabsorbed insulin. Also, if insulin is usually injected into fibrotic tissue where absorption is slow, injection into healthy tissue may result in hypoglycemia because of more rapid absorption. Further, deposits of unabsorbed insulin may initially lead to hyperglycemia. If dosage is increased to control the apparent hyperglycemia, hypoglycemia may occur. In addition, a sudden increase in physical activity is likely to increase subcutaneous blood circulation, causing rapid absorption of insulin.
(7) Rotate sites within the same anatomic area (*e.g.*, abdomen) until all sites are used. Avoid random rotation between the abdomen and thigh or arm, for example.	Rates of absorption differ among anatomic sites, and random rotation increases risks of hypoglycemic reactions. Some authorities recommend giving all insulin injections in the abdomen.
(8) Inject insulin at a 90-degree angle into a subcutaneous pocket created by raising subcutaneous tissue away from muscle tissue. Avoid intramuscular injection.	Injection into a subcutaneous pocket is thought to produce less tissue irritation and better absorption than injection into subcutaneous tissue. Intramuscular injection should not be used because of rapid absorption.
b. With oral sulfonylureas: Give a single daily dose about 30 min before breakfast; give a second daily dose about 30 min before the evening meal.	To promote absorption and effective plasma levels. Most of these drugs are given once or twice daily.
c. With acarbose and miglitol: Give at the beginning of each main meal, three times daily.	These drugs must be in the GI tract when carbohydrate foods are ingested.
d. With metformin: Give two daily doses with morning and evening meals; give three daily doses with meals.	Giving with food decreases GI upset
e. With troglitazone: Give once daily, in the morning	

NURSING ACTIONS	RATIONALE/EXPLANATION
2. Observe for therapeutic effects	
a. Improved blood glucose levels (fasting, preprandial, and postprandial) and glycosylated hemoglobin levels	The general goal of antidiabetic drug therapy is normal or near-normal blood glucose levels. However, specific targeted levels for individuals vary, depending on intensity of treatment, risks of hypoglycemia, and other factors. Improved metabolic control can prevent or delay complications.
b. Absent or decreased ketones in urine (N = none)	In diabetes, ketonuria indicates insulin deficiency and impending DKA if preventive measures are not taken. Thus, always report the presence of ketones. In addition, when adequate insulin is given, ketonuria decreases. Ketonuria does not often occur with NIDDM.
c. Absent or decreased pruritus, polyuria, polydipsia, polyphagia, and fatigue	These signs and symptoms occur in the presence of hyperglycemia. When blood sugar levels are lowered with antidiabetic drugs, they tend to subside.
d. Decreased complications of diabetes	
3. Observe for adverse effects	
a. With insulin and oral sulfonylureas:	
(1) Hypoglycemia	Hypoglycemia is more likely to occur with insulin than with oral agents and at peak action times of the insulin being used (*e.g.*, 2–3 h after injection of regular insulin; 8–12 h after injection of NPH or Lente insulins).
(a) SNS activation–tachycardia, palpitations, nervousness, weakness, hunger, perspiration	The sympathetic nervous system is activated as part of the stress response to low blood glucose levels. Epinephrine and other hormones act to raise blood glucose levels.
(b) CNS impairment–mental confusion, incoherent speech, blurred vision, double vision, headache, convulsions, coma	There is an inadequate supply of glucose for normal brain function.
b. With insulin	
(1) Local insulin allergy–erythema, induration, itching at injection sites	Allergic reactions are less common with increased use of human insulin and decreased use of animal insulins.
(2) Systemic allergic reactions–skin rash, dyspnea, tachycardia, hypotension, angioedema, anaphylaxis	Infrequent; anaphylaxis is rare. If a severe systemic reaction occurs, skin testing and desensitization are usually required even if patients are switched from animal to human insulin.
(3) Lipodystrophy–atrophy and "dimpling" at injection site; hypertrophy at injection site	These changes in subcutaneous fat occur from too-frequent injections into the same site. They are less likely to occur with human insulin.
c. With oral sulfonylureas	
(1) Hypoglycemia–see above	Hypoglycemia occurs less commonly with oral agents than with insulin. It is more likely to occur in patients who are elderly, debilitated, or who have impaired renal and hepatic function.
(2) Allergic skin reactions–skin rash, urticaria, erythema, pruritus	These reactions may subside with continued use of the drug. If they do not subside, the drug should be discontinued.
(3) GI upset–nausea, heartburn	These are the most commonly reported adverse effects. If severe, reducing drug dosage usually relieves.
(4) Miscellaneous–fluid retention and hyponatremia; facial flushing if alcohol is ingested; hematologic disorders (hemolytic or aplastic anemia, leukopenia, thrombocytopenia, others)	These are less common adverse effects.

(continued)

NURSING ACTIONS	RATIONALE/EXPLANATION
d. With acarbose and miglitol	
GI symptoms—flatulence, diarrhea, abdominal pain	These are commonly reported. They are caused by the presence of undigested carbohydrate in the lower GI tract and usually subside with continued therapy.
e. With metformin	
(1) GI effects—anorexia, nausea, vomiting, diarrhea, abdominal discomfort, decreased intestinal absorption of folate and vitamin B$_{12}$	GI symptoms are the most frequently reported adverse effects. They may be minimized by increasing drug dosage slowly and taking the drug with meals.
(2) Hypoglycemia	Hypoglycemia is uncommon when metformin is taken as the sole antidiabetic drug but may occur if taken with a sulfonylurea. It also occurs if taken with alcohol.
(3) Allergic skin reactions—eczema, pruritus, erythema, urticaria	
(4) Lactic acidosis—drowsiness, malaise, respiratory distress, bradycardia and hypotension (if severe), blood lactate levels above 5 mmol/l, blood pH below 7.35	A rare but serious adverse effect (about 50% fatal). Most likely with renal or hepatic impairment, advanced age, or hypoxia. This is a medical emergency that requires hospitalization for treatment. Hemodialysis is effective in correcting acidosis and removing metformin.
	Lactic acidosis may be prevented by monitoring plasma lactate levels and stopping the drug if they exceed 3 mmol/l. Other reasons to stop the drug include patients experiencing decreased renal or hepatic function, a prolonged fast, or a very low calorie diet. The drug should be stopped immediately if a patient has a myocardial infarction or septicemia.
f. With troglitazone	
(1) GI symptoms—nausea, vomiting, diarrhea	Few adverse effects have been reported; those reported have been mild.
(2) Edema	
(3) Dizziness	
4. Observe for drug interactions	
a. Drugs that *increase* effects of insulin:	
(1) Oral sulfonylurea hypoglycemic agents	These agents are increasingly being used with insulin in the treatment of some patients with NIDDM. The risks of hypoglycemia are probably greater with the combination but depend on the dosage of each drug and other factors that affect blood glucose levels.
(2) Alcohol	Increased hypoglycemia. Ethanol inhibits gluconeogenesis (in persons with or without diabetes).
(3) Beta-adrenergic blocking agents (*e.g.*, propranolol, others)	These drugs increase hypoglycemia by inhibiting the effects of catecholamines on gluconeogenesis and glycogenolysis (effects that normally raise blood glucose levels in response to hypoglycemia). They also may mask signs and symptoms of hypoglycemia (*e.g.*, tachycardia, tremors) that normally occur with a hypoglycemia-induced activation of the sympathetic nervous system.
(4) Monoamine oxidase (MAO) inhibitors	These drugs may significantly potentiate and prolong insulin-induced hypoglycemia. Such a combination is hazardous and should be used very cautiously, if at all.

NURSING ACTIONS	RATIONALE/EXPLANATION
(5) Salicylates	Salicylates increase risks of hypoglycemia by increasing insulin secretion.
b. Drugs that *decrease* effects of insulin:	These drugs are often called *diabetogenic* because of their tendencies to raise blood sugar levels.
(1) Corticosteroids (*e.g.,* hydrocortisone)	Antagonize hypoglycemic effects, produce hyperglycemia
(2) Diuretics (especially thiazide diuretics, such as hydrochlorothiazide)	These drugs antagonize hypoglycemic effects of insulin and may cause hyperglycemia.
(3) Epinephrine	This adrenergic drug tends to raise blood glucose levels and thereby antagonize hypoglycemic effects of insulin.
(4) Glucagon	In small doses, glucagon is used to counteract hypoglycemia induced by insulin. Glucagon raises blood glucose levels by converting liver glycogen to glucose.
(5) Oral contraceptives	Tend to raise blood glucose levels and thereby antagonize insulin effects. Insulin dosage may need to be increased.
(6) Phenytoin (Dilantin)	Inhibits insulin secretion and may cause severe hyperglycemia.
(7) Propranolol (Inderal)	May inhibit insulin release
(8) Thyroid preparations (*e.g.,* levothyroxine [Synthroid])	May cause hyperglycemia
c. Drugs that *increase* effects of oral sulfonylureas:	
(1) Acarbose, miglitol, and metformin	Either of these newer drugs may be used concomitantly with a sulfonylurea to improve glycemic control in patients with NIDDM. There is an increased risk of hypoglycemia with the combination.
(2) Acidifying agents (*e.g.,* ascorbic acid) and probenecid (Benemid)	Increase effects by slowing the rate of urinary excretion.
(3) Alcohol	Additive hypoglycemia. If alcohol use is chronic and heavy, oral hypoglycemic agents may be metabolized more rapidly and *hyperglycemia* may occur.
(4) Allopurinol (Zyloprim), cyclophosphamide (Cytoxan), MAO inhibitors, sulfinpyrazone (Anturane); tetracyclines	Increase hypoglycemia, mechanisms unclear
(5) Anticoagulants, oral	Increase hypoglycemia by slowing metabolism of oral antidiabetic agents and possibly by decreasing their urinary excretion.
(6) Insulin	Additive hypoglycemia
(7) Salicylates (*e.g.,* aspirin) and sulfonamides	Increase hypoglycemia by displacing oral antidiabetic agents from protein-binding sites
d. Drugs that *decrease* effects of oral sulfonylureas:	
(1) Alcohol	Heavy, chronic intake of alcohol induces metabolizing enzymes in the liver. This increases the rate of metabolism of oral antidiabetic drugs, shortens their half-lives, and may produce hyperglycemia.
(2) Beta-blocking agents	Decrease hypoglycemic effects, possibly by decreasing release of insulin in the pancreas
(3) Corticosteroids, diuretics, epinephrine, estrogens, and oral contraceptives	These drugs have hyperglycemic effects.

(continued)

Nursing Actions	*Rationale/Explanation*
(4) Glucagon	Raises blood glucose levels. It is used to treat severe hypoglycemia induced by insulin or oral antidiabetic agents.
(5) Nicotinic acid	Large doses have a hyperglycemic effect.
(6) Phenytoin (Dilantin)	Inhibits insulin secretion and has hyperglycemic effects
(7) Rifampin	Increases the rate of metabolism of oral antidiabetic agents by inducing liver-metabolizing enzymes
(8) Thyroid preparations	Antagonize the hypoglycemic effects of oral antidiabetic drugs
e. Drugs that *decrease* effects of acarbose and miglitol	
(1) Digestive enzymes	Decrease effects and should not be used concomitantly with acarbose
(2) Intestinal adsorbents (*e.g.,* charcoal)	Decrease effects and should not be used concomitantly with acarbose
f. Drugs that *increase* effects of metformin	
(1) Alcohol	Increases risk of hypoglycemia and lactic acidosis. Patients should avoid acute and chronic ingestion of excessive alcohol.
(2) Cimetidine	Increases risk of hypoglycemia. Cimetidine interferes with metabolism and increases blood levels of metformin.
(3) Furosemide	Increases blood levels of metformin
(4) Nifedipine	Apparently increases absorption of metformin
(5) Sulfonylurea hypoglycemic agents	The combination of these drugs is used therapeutically to improve control of hyperglycemia in NIDDM, but it also increases risk of hypoglycemia.
5. Teach clients	
a. With insulin-dependent diabetics teach:	
(1) Characteristics of the prescribed insulin preparations, including the expected time of peak insulin activity	The client may be able to eat at the time of peak insulin activity and reduce the likelihood of hypoglycemia. If hypoglycemia does occur, it is important that it be recognized as early as possible so some kind of fast-acting carbohydrate can be taken.
(2) Correct techniques for self-administration of insulin:	
(a) Use sterile technique.	
(b) Draw up insulin in a good light.	
(c) Use appropriate needle and syringe.	
(d) If it is necessary to mix two insulin preparations, draw them up as specified in 1a(5), above.	For accurate dosage
(e) Inject at a 90-degree angle.	To prevent local reactions
(f) Rotate injection sites.	To prevent fibrosis, loss, or enlargement of subcutaneous tissue. If these changes occur, unpredictable absorption of the insulin may lead to unstable blood sugar levels and hyperglycemia or hypoglycemia.
(g) Aspirate.	To avoid inadvertent injection into a blood vessel. Some authorities do not believe aspiration is necessary.
(h) Change insulin dosage only if instructed to do so and the circumstances are specified.	

NURSING ACTIONS	RATIONALE/EXPLANATION
(i) Keep several days' supply of insulin, syringes, and needles on hand.	To allow for weather or other conditions that might prevent replacement of insulin or other supplies when needed.
(j) Carry sugar or candy.	For immediate use if a hypoglycemic reaction occurs
(k) If illness occurs, take the usual daily dose of insulin; do not omit insulin. Check blood glucose levels frequently. Test urine for ketones; if unable to test own urine, have someone else do it. Rest, keep warm, do not exercise, keep someone with you if possible, and drink some fluids every hour if able—broth and clear soups help.	Diabetics who cannot eat because of nausea, vomiting, or other difficulty commonly omit their insulin. Such a practice increases the likelihood of DKA. Insulin requirements are often increased during illness, probably owing to stress, decreased activity, and other factors. The Joslin Diabetes Foundation recommends keeping a bottle of regular, short-acting insulin on hand even if it is not used ordinarily. The client's physician should be consulted regarding this, and the circumstances in which any supplemental insulin should be taken.
(l) Reduce insulin dosage or eat extra food if you expect to exercise more than usual.	Specific recommendations should be individualized and worked out with the physician in relation to the type of exercise.
b. With oral hypoglycemic agents, teach:	
(1) Signs and symptoms of hypoglycemia	Hypoglycemic reactions may occur with oral antidiabetic drugs, although they are less common than with insulin.
(2) Do not skip meals and snacks.	This increases the risk of hypoglycemic reactions.
(3) More food may be needed if vigorous exercise is undertaken.	Exercise decreases the need for insulin. Thus, smaller doses of the oral drugs or larger amounts of food are needed. Specific recommendations from the physician will consider the type of exercise.

REVIEW AND APPLICATION EXERCISES

1. What is the function of insulin in normal cellular metabolism?

2. What is the effect of insulin on blood glucose levels?

3. What are the effects of cortisol, epinephrine, glucagon, and growth hormone on blood glucose levels?

4. What are the major differences between type I and type II diabetes?

5. What are sources of exogenous insulin drug preparations?

6. What are advantages and disadvantages of human insulin preparations?

7. What is the rationale for maintaining near-normal blood glucose levels?

8. What is the major risk of maintaining near-normal blood glucose levels?

9. At what blood glucose range is brain damage most likely to occur?

10. Compare regular, NPH, and Lente insulins in terms of onset, peak, and duration of action.

11. In a diabetic client with typical signs and symptoms, distinguish between manifestations of hyperglycemia and hypoglycemia.

12. Contrast insulin and oral hypoglycemic agents in terms of mechanism of action, route of administration, indications for use, contraindications for use, and adverse effects.

13. For an adult client newly diagnosed with type II diabetes, state interventions to assist the client in learning self-care.

14. How could the nurse accurately respond to a child with diabetes mellitus who asks why he cannot take pills like his grandmother does?

15. Prepare a teaching plan for a client starting insulin therapy and for a client starting an oral hypoglycemic drug.

SELECTED REFERENCES

AADE position statement: Individualization of diabetes education and management. (1995). *The Diabetes Educator, 21*(2), 105.

Bloomgarden, Z.T. (1996). American Diabetes Association Postgraduate course, 1996: Treatment and prevention of diabetes. *Diabetes Care, 19*(7), 784–786.

Campbell, S., & Mooradian, A.D. (1993). Diabetes mellitus. In R. Bressler & M.D. Katz (Eds.), *Geriatric pharmacology*, pp. 409–425. New York: McGraw-Hill.

Cirone, N. (1996). Diabetes in the elderly, Part I. Unmasking a hidden disorder. *Nursing 96, 26*(3), 34–39.

Cirone, N. & Schwartz, N. (1996). Diabetes in the elderly, Part II. Finding the balance for drug therapy. *Nursing 96, 26*(3), 40–45.

Clark, C.M., Jr. & Lee, D.A. (1995). Prevention and treatment of the complications of diabetes mellitus. *New England Journal of Medicine, 332*, 1207–1210.

Cox, D.J., Gonder-Frederick, L.A., Schroeder, D.B., Cryer, P.E., & Clarke, W.L. (1993). Disruptive effects of acute hypoglycemia on speed of cognitive and motor performance. *Diabetes Care, 16*(10), 1391–1393.

Cziraky, M.J., Mehra, I.V., Wilson, M.D., & Bakris, G.L. (1996). Current issues in treating the hypertensive patient with diabetes: Focus on diabetic nephropathy. *The Annals of Pharmacotherapy, 30*, 791–798.

Davis, S.N. & Granner, D.K. (1996). Insulin, oral hypoglycemic agents, and the pharmacology of the endocrine pancreas. In J.G. Hardman, L.E. Limbird, P.B. Molinoff, & R.W. Ruddon (Eds.), *Goodman & Gilman's The pharmacological basis of therapeutics*, 9th ed., pp. 1487–1517. New York: McGraw-Hill.

The Diabetes Control and Complications Trial Research Group. (1993). The effect of intensive treatment of diabetes on the development and progression of long-term complications in insulin-dependent diabetes mellitus. *New England Journal of Medicine, 14*, 977–986.

Drug facts and comparisons. (1996). St Louis: Facts and Comparisons.

Dunning, P.L. (1995). Young adult perspective of insulin-dependent diabetes. *The Diabetes Educator, 21*(1), 58–65.

Guyton, A.C. & Hall, J.E. (1996). *Textbook of medical physiology*, 9th ed. Philadelphia: W.B. Saunders.

Henry, R.R. (1996). Glucose control and insulin resistance in non-insulin-dependent diabetes mellitus. *Annals of Internal Medicine, 124*(1, part 2), 97–103.

Henry, R.R. & Genuth, S. (1996). Forum one: Current recommendations about intensification of metabolic control in non-insulin-dependent diabetes mellitus. *Annals of Internal Medicine, 124*(1, part 2), 175–177.

Hernandez, C.A. (1995). The experience of living with insulin-dependent diabetes: Lessons for the diabetes educator. *The Diabetes Educator, 21*(1), 33–37.

Kupecz, D. (1995). Metformin: An antihyperglycemic drug for non-insulin dependent diabetes mellitus. *Nurse Practitioner, 20*(7), 70–72.

Mason, B.J., Matsuyama, J.R., & Jue, S.G. (1995). Assessment of sulfonylurea adherence and metabolic control. *The Diabetes Educator, 21*, 52–57.

Melkus, G.D. (1993). Type II non-insulin-dependent diabetes mellitus. *Nursing Clinics of North America, 28*(1), 25–33.

Pandit, M.K., Burke, J., Gustafson, A.B., Minocha, A., & Peiris, A.N. (1993). Drug-induced disorders of glucose tolerance. *Annals of Internal Medicine, 118*, 529–537.

Porth, C.M. & Hurwitz, L.S. (1994). Diabetes mellitus. In C.M. Porth (Ed.), *Pathophysiology: Concepts of altered health states*, 4th ed., pp. 927–948. Philadelphia: J.B. Lippincott.

White, J.R., Jr. & Campbell, R.K. (1996). Pharmacologic therapies in the management of diabetes mellitus. In D. Haire-Joshu, *Management of diabetes mellitus: Perspectives of care across the life span*, 2nd ed., pp. 202–233. St. Louis: Mosby-Year Book.

Estrogens, Progestins, and Oral Contraceptives

Objectives

After studying this chapter, the student will be able to:

1 Discuss effects of endogenous estrogens and progestins.

2 Describe advantages and disadvantages of postmenopausal hormone replacement therapy (HRT).

3 Describe adverse effects associated with estrogens, progestins, and oral contraceptives.

4 Apply nursing process with clients taking estrogens, progestins, and oral contraceptives.

Key Terms

Contraception

Menopause

Menstrual cycle

Menstrual disorders

Osteoporosis

Ovulation

Thromboembolic disorders

Estrogens and progestins are female sex hormones produced primarily by the ovaries and secondarily by the adrenal cortices in nonpregnant women. In pregnant women, large amounts of estrogens are produced by the placenta.

Like other steroid hormones, estrogens and progestins are synthesized from cholesterol. The ovaries and adrenal glands can manufacture cholesterol or extract it from the blood. Through a series of chemical reactions, cholesterol is converted to progesterone, then to the androgens, testosterone and androstenedione. These male sex hormones are used by the ovaries to produce estrogens. After formation, the hormones are secreted into the bloodstream in response to stimulation by the anterior pituitary gonadotropic hormones, follicle-stimulating hormone (FSH), and luteinizing hormone (LH). In the bloodstream, the hormones combine with serum proteins and are transported to target tissues where they enter body cells. They cross cell membranes easily because of their steroid molecular structure and lipid solubility. Once inside the cells, they stimulate cellular protein synthesis.

Estrogens

Three estrogens (estradiol, estrone, and estriol) are secreted in significant amounts. Estradiol is considered the major estrogen because it usually exerts more estrogenic activity than the other two combined. The main function of the estrogens is to promote growth in tissues related to reproduction and sexual characteristics in the female. More specific effects of estrogens on body tissues include the following:

1. **Breasts.** Estrogens stimulate growth of breast tissue at puberty by causing deposition of fat, formation of connective tissue, and construction of ducts. These ducts become part of the milk-producing apparatus after additional stimulation by progesterone.
2. **Sexual organs.** At puberty, estrogen secretion increases greatly and produces enlargement and other changes in the sexual organs. The fallopian tubes, uterus, vagina, and external genitalia increase in size. The endometrial lining of the uterus proliferates and develops glands that will later nourish the implanted ovum when pregnancy occurs. The epithelial lining of the vagina becomes more resistant to trauma and infection.
3. **Skeleton.** Estrogen stimulates skeletal growth so that, beginning at puberty, height increases rapidly for several years. Estrogen then causes the epiphyses to unite with the shafts of the long bones, and linear growth is halted. This effect of estrogen is stronger than the similar effect of testosterone in the male. Consequently, females stop growing in height sev-

eral years earlier than males and on the average are shorter than males. Estrogen also conserves calcium and phosphorus. This action promotes bone formation and decreases bone resorption. An additional skeletal effect of estrogen is to broaden the pelvis in preparation for childbirth.

4. **Skin and subcutaneous tissue.** Estrogen increases vascularity in the skin. This leads to greater skin warmth and likelihood of bleeding in women. Estrogen also causes deposition of fat in subcutaneous tissue, especially in the breasts, thighs, and buttocks, which produces the characteristic female figure.
5. **Anterior pituitary gland.** Estrogens decrease pituitary secretion of FSH and increase secretion of LH when blood levels are sufficiently high. Thus, they control their own secretion, in part, by feedback mechanisms to the anterior pituitary gland.
6. **Metabolism.** Estrogens affect the metabolic processes of both reproductive and nonreproductive tissues and estrogen receptors are found in female reproductive organs, breast tissue, bone, the brain, liver, heart, and blood vessels. They are also found in various tissues in men. Metabolic effects include protein anabolism, increased bone growth and epiphyseal closure in young girls, decreased bone resorption in postmenopausal women, and increased sodium and water retention, serum triglycerides, and high-density lipoproteins (HDL or "good" cholesterol because of cardioprotective effects). Low-density lipoproteins (LDL or "bad" cholesterol because of cardiotoxic effects) are decreased. In addition to effects on serum lipids, estrogens increase the amount of cholesterol in bile and thereby increase gallstone formation.
7. **Blood coagulation.** Estrogen enhances coagulation by increasing blood levels of several clotting factors, including prothrombin and factors VII, IX, and X and probably increases platelet aggregation.

In nonpregnant women, between puberty and menopause, estrogens are secreted in a monthly cycle called the menstrual cycle. During the first half of the cycle, before ovulation, estrogens are secreted in progressively larger amounts. During the second half of the cycle, estrogens and progesterone are secreted in increasing amounts until about 2 days before the onset of menstruation. At that time, secretion of both hormones decreases abruptly. When the endometrial lining of the uterus loses its hormonal stimulation, it is discharged vaginally as menstrual flow.

During pregnancy, the placenta produces large amounts of estrogen, mainly estriol. The increased estrogen causes enlargement of the uterus and breasts, growth of glandular tissue in the breasts, and relaxation of ligaments and joints in the pelvis. All these changes are necessary for growth and birth of the fetus.

Finally, estrogens are inactivated in the liver. They are conjugated with glucuronic acid or sulfuric acid, which makes them water soluble and readily excreted through the kidneys. About 80% of the conjugates are excreted in urine, with the remainder excreted in bile. Impaired liver function increases estrogen activity and may produce signs and symptoms of estrogen excess in males and females.

Progesterone

Progesterone is a progestin concerned almost entirely with reproduction. In the nonpregnant woman, progesterone is secreted by the corpus luteum during the last half of the menstrual cycle, after ovulation. This hormone continues the changes in the endometrial lining of the uterus begun by estrogens during the first half of the menstrual cycle. These changes provide for implantation and nourishment of a fertilized ovum. When fertilization does not take place, the levels of estrogen and progesterone decrease, and menstruation occurs.

If the ovum is fertilized, progesterone acts to maintain the pregnancy. The corpus luteum produces progesterone during the first few weeks of gestation. Then, the placenta produces the progesterone needed to maintain the endometrial lining of the uterus. In addition to its effects on the uterus, progesterone prepares the breasts for lactation by promoting development of milk-producing cells. Milk is not secreted, however, until the cells are further stimulated by prolactin from the anterior pituitary gland. Progesterone also may help maintain pregnancy by decreasing uterine contractility. This, in turn, decreases the risk of spontaneous abortion.

Progesterone generally has opposite effects on lipid metabolism compared with estrogen. That is, progestins decrease HDL and increase LDL, both of which increase risks of cardiovascular disease. Physiologic progesterone increases insulin levels but does not usually impair glucose tolerance. However, long-term administration of potent synthetic progestins such as norgestrel may decrease glucose tolerance and make diabetes mellitus more difficult to control. Like estrogen, progesterone is metabolized in the liver.

Estrogens and Progestins Used as Drugs

1. When estrogens and progestins are given from exogenous sources as drugs for therapeutic purposes, they produce the same effects as endogenous (naturally occurring) hormones.

2. Several preparations of estrogens and progestins are available for various purposes and routes of administration:
    a. *Naturally occurring, nonconjugated estrogens* (estradiol, estrone) *and natural progesterone* are given intramuscularly because they are rapidly metabolized if given orally. Some crystalline suspensions of estrogens and oil solutions of both estrogens and progesterone prolong drug action by slowing absorption.
    b. *Conjugated estrogens* (Premarin) and some synthetic derivatives of natural estrogens (*e.g.*, ethinyl estradiol) and natural progesterone (*e.g.*, norethindrone) are chemically modified to be effective with oral administration.
    c. *Nonsteroidal, synthetic preparations* are usually given orally or topically. They are chemically altered to slow their metabolism in the liver. They are also less bound to serum proteins than the naturally occurring hormones.

3. Most oral contraceptives consist of a synthetic estrogen (*e.g.*, ethinyl estradiol) and a synthetic progestin (*e.g.*, norethindrone). Monophasic contraceptives contain fixed amounts of both components. Biphasics and triphasics contain either fixed amounts of estrogen and varied amounts of progestins or varied amounts of both estrogens and progestins. Biphasic and triphasic preparations mimic normal variations of hormone secretion, decrease the total dosage of hormones, and may decrease adverse effects.

    These contraceptives are dispensed in containers with color-coded tablets that must be taken in the correct sequence. Dispensers with 28 tablets contain seven inactive or placebo tablets of a third color. A few contraceptive products contain a progestin only. These are somewhat less effective in preventing pregnancy and are more likely to cause vaginal bleeding irregularities, which makes them less acceptable to many women.

Mechanism of Action

The precise mechanism by which estrogens and progestins produce their effects is unknown. Estrogens circulate briefly in the bloodstream before reaching target cells, where they enter the cells and combine with receptor proteins in cell cytoplasm. The estrogen-receptor complex then interacts with deoxyribonucleic acid (DNA) to produce ribonucleic acid and new DNA. These substances stimulate cell reproduction and production of various proteins. Progestins also diffuse freely into cells, where they bind to progesterone receptors.

Oral contraceptives act by several mechanisms. First, they inhibit hypothalamic secretion of gonadotropin-releasing hormone, which inhibits pituitary secretion of FSH and LH. When these gonadotropic hormones are absent, ovulation and therefore conception cannot occur. Second, the drugs produce cervical mucus that resists penetration of spermatozoa into the upper reproductive tract. Third, the drugs interfere with endometrial maturation and reception of ova that are released and fertilized. These overlapping mechanisms make the drugs highly effective in preventing pregnancy.

INDICATIONS FOR USE

Estrogen

1. **As replacement therapy in deficiency states.** Deficiency states usually result from hypofunction of the pituitary gland or the ovaries and may occur anytime during the life cycle. For example, in the adolescent girl with delayed sexual development, estrogen can be given to produce the changes that normally occur at puberty. In the woman of reproductive age (about age 12 to 45), estrogens are sometimes used in menstrual disorders, including amenorrhea and abnormal uterine bleeding due to estrogen deficiency.

2. **As a component in birth control pills.** Estrogens, usually combined with a progestin, are used widely in the 12- to 45-year age group to control fertility. If pregnancy does occur, estrogens are contraindicated because their use during pregnancy has been associated with the occurrence of vaginal cancer in female offspring and possible harmful effects on male offspring.

3. **During menopause.** Estrogens are given to relieve atrophic vaginitis and vasomotor instability, which produces "hot flashes," and to prevent osteoporosis. They also may prevent or delay coronary atherosclerosis and subsequent myocardial infarction. When estrogen is given to women with a uterus, a progestin is also given to prevent endometrial cancer.

4. **Other clinical uses.** Estrogen is used to treat metastatic breast cancer in women more than 5 years postmenopause, metastatic prostate cancer in men, acne and hirsutism in women with excessive male sex hormone secretion, and excessive height in young girls.

Progestins

Progestins are most often used for contraception, alone or with estradiol or mestranol in oral contraceptive pills, and for hormone replacement therapy (HRT) in postmenopausal women, with an estrogen preparation. In HRT, the purpose of a progestin is to prevent endometrial cancer. Progestins also are used to suppress ovarian function in dysmenorrhea, endometriosis, and uterine bleeding. These uses of oral progestins are

extensions of the physiologic actions of progesterone on the neuroendocrine control of ovarian function and on the endometrium.

Hormonal Contraceptives

The primary clinical indication for the use of hormonal contraceptives is to control fertility and prevent pregnancy. Several products are used as postcoital contraceptives following unprotected sexual intercourse. These preparations also are used to treat various menstrual disorders, such as amenorrhea and dysmenorrhea.

CONTRAINDICATIONS FOR USE

Because of their widespread effects on body tissues and reported adverse reactions, estrogens, progestins, and oral contraceptives are contraindicated in:

1. Known or suspected pregnancy, because damage to the fetus may result
2. Presence of thromboembolic disorders, such as thrombophlebitis, deep vein thrombosis, or pulmonary embolism
3. Known or suspected cancers of breast or genital tissues, because the drugs may stimulate tumor growth. An exception is use of estrogens for treatment of metastatic breast cancer in women at least 5 years postmenopause.
4. Undiagnosed vaginal or uterine bleeding
5. Fibroid tumors of the uterus
6. Active liver disease or impaired liver function
7. History of cerebrovascular disease, coronary artery disease, thrombophlebitis, hypertension, or conditions predisposing to these disease processes
8. Women older than age 35 who smoke cigarettes. These women have a greater risk of thromboembolic disorders if they take oral contraceptives, possibly because of increased platelet aggregation with estrogen ingestion and cigarette smoking. In addition, estrogen increases hepatic production of blood clotting factors.
9. Family history of breast or reproductive system cancer

Individual Estrogens, Progestins, and Oral Contraceptives

Table 28-1 lists the clinical indications, routes of administration, and dosages of estrogens. Table 28-2 provides the clinical indications, routes of administration, and dosages of progestins. Oral contraceptive agents are listed in Table 28-3.

TABLE 28-1 ESTROGENS

Generic/Trade Name	Routes and Dosage Ranges for Various Indications							
	Menopausal Symptoms	Female Hypogonadism	Prevention of Osteoporosis	Postcoital Contraception	Breast Cancer	Prostate Cancer	Other
Chlorotrianisene (Tace)	PO 12–25 mg daily for 21 d, followed by 7 d without the drug	PO 12–25 mg daily for 21 d				PO 12–25 mg daily	
Conjugated estrogens (Premarin)	PO 0.3–1.25 mg daily for 21 d followed by 7 d without the drug	PO 2.5–7.5 mg daily in divided doses, cyclically, 20 d on, 10 d off the drug	PO 0.625 mg daily for 21 d, then 7 d without the drug		PO 10 mg tid for at least 3 months	PO 1.25–2.5 mg three times daily	Dysfunctional uterine bleeding: IM or IV for emergency use, 25 mg, repeated in 6–12 h if necessary. Atrophic vaginitis: topically, 2.4 g of vaginal cream inserted daily
Dienestrol (DV)							Atrophic or senile vaginitis: topically, vaginal cream applied two or three times daily for about 2 wk, then reduced to three times weekly
Diethylstilbestrol (Stilbestrol)	PO 0.2–0.5 mg daily for 21 d, followed by 7 d without the drug	PO 0.2–0 5 mg daily for 21 d, followed by 7 d without the drug		PO 25 mg twice daily for 5 d	PO 15 mg daily	PO 1–3 mg daily	
Diethylstilbestrol diphosphate (Stilphostrol)						PO 50–200 mg three times daily, IV 0.5 g first day, 1 g daily for next 5 d. Maintenance, 0.25–0.5 g one or two times weekly	
Esterified estrogens (Estratab)	PO 0.3–1.25 mg daily for 21 d, then 7 d without the drug	PO 2.5–7.5 mg daily, in divided doses, for 21 d, then 7 d without the drug			PO 10 mg three times daily for at least 3 months	PO 1.25–2.5 mg one to three times daily	

(continued)

355

TABLE 28-1 ESTROGENS (Continued)

Generic/Trade Name	Routes and Dosage Ranges for Various Indications						
	Menopausal Symptoms	Female Hypogonadism	Prevention of Osteoporosis	Postcoital Contraception	Breast Cancer	Prostate Cancer	Other
Estradiol (Estrace)	PO 1–2 mg daily for 3 wk, then 1 wk off or daily Monday through Friday, none on Saturday or Sunday		PO 0.5 mg daily for 23 d and no drug for 5 d each month		PO 10 mg three times daily for at least 3 months	PO 1–2 mg three times daily for at least 3 months	
Estradiol cypionate (Depo-Estradiol)	IM 1–5 mg q3–4 wk	IM 1.5–2 mg at monthly intervals					
Estradiol transdermal system (Estraderm)	Topically to skin, 1 patch one or two times weekly for 3 wk followed by 1 wk off (cyclically)	Same as for menopause	0.05 mg daily				
Estradiol valerate (Delestrogen)	IM 10–20 mg q4 wk	IM 10–20 mg q4 wk				IM 30 mg q1–2 wk	
Estrone (Theelin)	IM 0.1–0.5 mg weekly in single or divided doses	IM 0.1–2 mg weekly		PO 5 mg three times daily for 5 d		IM 2–4 mg q3–4 d	Dysfunctional uterine bleeding: IM 2–4 mg daily for several days until bleeding is controlled, followed by progestin for 1 wk Ovarian failure: same dosage as for female hypogonadism Atrophic vaginitis: topically, 1–2 g vaginal cream daily
Estropipate (Ogen)	PO 0.625–5 mg daily, cyclically	PO 1.25–7.5 mg daily for 3 wk, followed by an 8- to 10-d rest period. Repeat as needed.	PO 0.625 mg daily 25 d, no drug 6 d each month				
Ethinyl estradiol (Estinyl)	PO 0.02–0.05 mg daily, cyclically	PO 0.05 mg one to three times daily for 2 wk with addition of progestin for last 2 wk of month		PO 2.5 mg twice daily for 5 d when given alone; PO 100 μg for two doses, 12 h apart when given with norgestrel 1 mg	PO 1 mg three times daily	PO 0.15–2 mg daily	
Quinestrol (Estrovis)	PO 100 μg daily for 7 d, then 100–200 μg once weekly						Atrophic vaginitis: PO 100 μg daily for 7 d, then 100–200 μg weekly

TABLE 28-2	PROGESTINS			
	Routes and Dosage Ranges for Various Indications			
Generic/Trade Name	*Menstrual Disorders*	*Endometriosis*	*Endometrial Cancer*	*Other*
Hydroxyprogesterone caproate (Hylutin)	Amenorrhea, dysfunctional uterine bleeding: IM 375 mg. If no bleeding after 21 d, begin cyclic therapy with estradiol and repeat q4 wk for 4 cycles			Uterine adenocarcinoma: IM 1 g or more initially; repeat one or more times each week (maximum, 7 g/wk). Stop when relapse occurs or after 12 wk with no response. Test for endogenous estrogen production: IM 250 mg, repeated in 4 wk. Bleeding 7–14 d after injection indicates endogenous estrogen.
Medroxyprogesterone acetate (Depo-Provera, Provera)	Dysfunctional uterine bleeding: PO 5–10 mg daily for 5–10 d beginning on 16th or 21st day of cycle		IM 400–1000 mg weekly until improvement, then 400 mg monthly	
Megestrol acetate (Megace)	Amenorrhea: PO 5–10 mg daily for 5–10 d		PO 40–320 mg daily in four divided doses for at least 2 months	Breast cancer: PO 160 mg daily in four divided doses for at least 2 months
Norethindrone acetate (Aygestin)	Amenorrhea, dysfunctional uterine bleeding: PO 2.5–10 mg daily, starting on 5th day of menstrual cycle and ending on 25th day	PO 5 mg daily for 2 wk, increased by 2.5 mg daily every 2 wk to dose of 15 mg. Then give 10–15 mg daily for maintenance.		Contraception: (See Table 28-3.)
Progesterone	Amenorrhea, dysfunctional uterine bleeding: IM 5–10 mg for 6–8 consecutive days			

Nursing Process

Assessment

Before drug therapy is started, clients need a thorough history and physical examination, including measurements of blood pressure, serum cholesterol, and triglycerides. These parameters must be monitored periodically as long as the drugs are taken.

- Assess for conditions in which estrogens and progestins are used (*e.g.,* menstrual disorders, menopausal symptoms).
- Assess for conditions that increase risks of adverse effects or are contraindications for hormonal therapy (*e.g.,* thromboembolic disorders, pregnancy).

- Record blood pressure with each outpatient contact or regularly with hospitalized clients. Increases are likely because of estrogen-induced increases in angiotensinogen, a precursor to the strong pressor substance, angiotensin. Sodium and water retention also occur.
- Check laboratory reports of cholesterol and triglyceride levels when available.
- Assess diet and presence of cigarette smoking. A high-fat diet increases the risks of gallbladder disease and perhaps other problems; cigarette smoking clearly increases risks of cardiovascular disease in women over 35 who take oral contraceptives.
- Assess the client's willingness to comply with instructions about drug therapy and follow-up procedures.

TABLE 28-3 ORAL AND OTHER CONTRACEPTIVES

Trade Name	Phase	Estrogen (µg)	Progestin (mg)
Monophasics			
Brevicon		Ethinyl estradiol 35	Norethindrone 0.5
Demulen 1/35		Ethinyl estradiol 35	Ethynodiol diacetate 1
Demulen 1/50		Ethinyl estradiol 50	Ethynodiol diacetate 1
Desogen		Ethinyl estradiol 30	Desogestrel 0.15
Genora 0.5/35		Ethinyl estradiol 35	Norethindrone 0.5
Genora 1/35		Ethinyl estradiol 35	Norethindrone 1
Genora 1/50		Mestranol 50	Levonorgestrel 0.15
Levlen		Ethinyl estradiol 30	Norethindrone acetate 1
Loestrin 21 1/20		Ethinyl estradiol 20	Norethindrone acetate 1.5
Loestrin 21 1.5/30		Ethinyl estradiol 30	Norethindrone acetate 1
Loestrin Fe 1/20		Ethinyl estradiol 20	Norethindrone acetate 1.5
Loestrin Fe 1.5/30		Ethinyl estradiol 30	Norgestrel 0.3
Lo/Ovral		Ethinyl estradiol 30	Norethindrone 0.5
Modicon		Ethinyl estradiol 35	Norethindrone 1
N.E.E. 1/35		Ethinyl estradiol 35	Norethindrone 0.5
Nelova 0.5/35E		Ethinyl estradiol 35	Norethindrone 1
Nelova 1/35E		Ethinyl estradiol 35	Norethindrone 1
Nelova 1/50M		Mestranol 50	Norethindrone 1
Norcept-E 1/35		Ethinyl estradiol 35	Levonorgestrel 0.15
Nordette		Ethinyl estradiol 30	Norethindrone 1
Norethin 1/35E		Ethinyl estradiol 35	Norethindrone 1
Norethin 1/50		Mestranol 50	Norethindrone 1
Norinyl 1 + 35		Ethinyl estradiol 35	Norethindrone 1
Norinyl 1 + 50		Mestranol 50	Norethindrone acetate 1
Ortho-Cept		Ethinyl estradiol 30	Desogestrel 0.15
Ortho-Cyclen		Ethinyl estradiol 35	Norgestimate 0.25
Ortho-Novum 1/35		Ethinyl estradiol 35	Norethindrone 1
Ortho-Novum 1/50		Mestranol 50	Norethindrone 0.4
Ovcon-35		Ethinyl estradiol 35	Norethindrone 1
Ovcon-50		Ethinyl estradiol 50	Norgestrel 0.5
Ovral		Ethinyl estradiol 50	
Biphasics			
Jenest-28	I: 10 d	Ethinyl estradiol 35	Norethindrone 0.5
	II: 11 d	Ethinyl estradiol 35	Norethindrone 1
Nelova 10/11	I: 10 d	Ethinyl estradiol 35	Norethindrone 0.5
	II: 11 d	Ethinyl estradiol 35	Norethindrone 1
Ortho-Novum 10/11	I: 10 d	Ethinyl estradiol 35	Norethindrone 0.5
	II: 11 d	Ethinyl estradiol 35	Norethindrone 1
Triphasics			
Ortho-Novum 7/7/7	I: 7 d	Ethinyl estradiol 35	Norethindrone 0.5
	II: 7 d	Ethinyl estradiol 35	Norethindrone 0.75
	III: 7 d	Ethinyl estradiol 35	Norethindrone 1
Ortho Tri-Cyclen	I: 7 d	Ethinyl estradiol 35	Norgestimate 0.18
	II: 9 d	Ethinyl estradiol 35	Norgestimate 0.215
	III: 5 d	Ethinyl estradiol 35	Norgestimate 0.25
Tri-Levlen	I: 6 d	Ethinyl estradiol 30	Levonorgestrel 0.05
	II: 5 d	Ethinyl estradiol 40	Levonorgestrel 0.75
	III: 10 d	Ethinyl estradiol 30	Levonorgestrel 0.125
Tri-Norinyl	I: 7 d	Ethinyl estradiol 35	Norethindrone 0.5
	II: 9 d	Ethinyl estradiol 35	Norethindrone 1
	III: 5 d	Ethinyl estradiol 35	Norethindrone 0.5

| TABLE 28-3 | ORAL AND OTHER CONTRACEPTIVES (Continued) |

Trade Name	Phase	Estrogen (μg)	Progestin (mg)
Triphasil	I: 6 d	Ethinyl estradiol 30	Levonorgestrel 0.05
	II: 5 d	Ethinyl estradiol 40	Levonorgestrel 0.075
	III: 10 d	Ethinyl estradiol 30	Levonorgestrel 0.125
Progestin-Only Products			
Depo-Provera			Medroxyprogesterone 1.50
Micronor			Norethindrone 0.35
Norplant subdermal system			Levonorgestrel 216
Nor-QD			Norethindrone 0.35
Ovrette			Norgestrel 0.075
Progestasert intrauterine			Progesterone 38

- Assess for signs and symptoms of thromboembolic disorders regularly. These are most likely to occur in women over age 35 who take oral contraceptives and women or men who take large doses for cancer; they have not been associated with postmenopausal estrogen replacement therapy.

Nursing Diagnoses

- Body Image Disturbance in females, related to effects of hormone deficiency states
- Body Image Disturbance in males, related to feminizing effects and impotence from female hormones
- Altered Tissue Perfusion related to thromboembolic effects of drugs
- Fluid Volume Excess related to sodium and water retention
- Knowledge Deficit: Effects of hormonal therapy
- Risk for Injury related to increased risks of hypertension and gallbladder disease

Planning/Goals

The client will:
- Be assisted to cope with self-concept and body image changes
- Receive or take the drugs accurately
- Experience relief of symptoms for which the drugs are given
- Avoid preventable adverse drug effects
- Keep appointments for monitoring of drug effects

Interventions

- Assist female clients of childbearing age to choose an appropriate contraceptive method. If the choice is an estrogen-progestin combination, help the client take it accurately.
- Help postmenopausal women plan for adequate calcium and vitamin D in the diet.

Teach clients:
- Medical supervision, usually every 6 to 12 months, is necessary to check blood pressure, breasts, pelvis, and other areas for possible adverse reactions when these drugs are taken for long periods.

- Women with diabetes should report increased blood glucose levels.
- Women who take oral contraceptives should not smoke cigarettes. Cigarette smoking increases risks of thromboembolic disorders.
- Men who receive estrogens should know that feminizing effects and impotence are temporary and subside when drug therapy is discontinued.

Evaluation

- Interview and observe for compliance with instructions for taking the drugs.
- Interview and observe for therapeutic and adverse drug effects.

Principles of Therapy

NEED FOR CONTINUOUS SUPERVISION

Because estrogens, progestins, and oral contraceptives are usually taken for several months or years and may cause adverse reactions, clients taking these drugs need continued medical supervision. Before the drugs are given, a complete medical history; a physical examination, including breast and pelvic examinations and a Pap smear; urinalysis; and weight and blood pressure measurements are recommended. These examinations should be repeated periodically, at least annually, as long as the client is taking these drugs.

DRUG SELECTION FACTORS

Choice of preparation depends on the reason for use, desired route of administration, and duration of action. Conjugated estrogen (*e.g.,* Premarin) is a commonly used oral estrogen and medroxyprogesterone (*e.g.,* Provera) is a commonly used oral progestin.

The choice of combination oral contraceptives may be determined by the progestin component. Some progestins are more likely to cause weight gain, acne, and changes in blood lipids that increase risks of myocardial infarction or stroke. These adverse effects are attributed mainly to the androgenic activity of the progestin, and some progestins have more androgenic effects than others. Progestins with the least androgenic activity are desogestrel and norgestimate; those with intermediate activity include norethindrone and ethynodiol diacetate; and norgestrel has the highest androgenic effects. In addition, there are long-acting progestin contraceptive preparations such as IM depot medroxyprogesterone (Depo-Provera) that lasts about 3 months per injection, intrauterine progesterone that lasts 1 year, and levonorgestrel subcutaneous implants (Norplant) that last 5 years.

For postcoital contraception, several drugs are used, including a combination of ethinyl estradiol and norgestrel, ethinyl estradiol alone, conjugated estrogens, estrone, or diethylstilbestrol. Such usage is recommended for females who are victims of rape or incest or whose physical or mental health is threatened by pregnancy. To be effective, the drug should be started within 24 hours if possible and no later than 72 hours after exposure. The mechanism of action is unclear, but the drugs are thought to interfere with tubal transport or endometrial implantation of the ovum.

DOSAGE FACTORS

Although dosage needs vary with clients and the conditions for which the drugs are prescribed, a general rule is to use the smallest effective dose for the shortest effective time. Estrogens are usually given cyclically. In one regimen, the drug is taken for 3 weeks, then omitted for 1 week; in another, it is omitted the first 5 days of each month. These regimens more closely resemble normal secretion of estrogen and avoid prolonged stimulation of body tissues. A progestin may be added for 10 days each month.

USE IN SPECIFIC SITUATIONS

Menopause and Postmenopause

In treatment of women during menopause, hormonal replacement therapy (HRT) prevents vasomotor instability ("hot flashes") and other menopausal symptoms resulting from estrogen deficiency; during postmenopausal years, HRT prevents osteoporosis and decreases risks of myocardial infarction or stroke. Osteoporosis involves thin, weak bones that fracture easily, including the vertebrae and hips. Estrogens are more effective in preventing bone loss than restoring bone after loss has occurred. Thus, therapy should be initiated soon after menopause and continued indefinitely. Bone loss

resumes when treatment is discontinued. Treatment is more effective if the client consumes adequate calcium in the diet and participates in weight-bearing exercises. In relation to cardiovascular disease, evidence indicates that current doses do not increase the risk of hypertension, myocardial infarction, stroke or venous thrombosis except in women with other risk factors, such as those older than 35 years who smoke. In women who do not smoke, estrogens actually have protective effects, which are attributed to increases in HDL cholesterol and decreases in LDL cholesterol. When a progestin is added, cardiovascular protective effects may be decreased or lost because progestins have opposite effects on blood lipids.

A commonly prescribed regimen is a conjugated estrogen, such as Premarin, 0.625 mg to 1.25 mg daily for 25 days of each month, with a progestin, such as Provera, 10 mg daily for 10 days of each month, on days 15 to 25 of the cycle. The main function of the progestin is to decrease the risk of endometrial cancer; thus, some authorities do not prescribe progestin for the hysterectomized woman. Estradiol is also available as a transdermal patch (Estradrem), which releases the drug slowly, provides more consistent blood levels than oral formulations, and is applied weekly.

Contraception

Estrogen and progestin contraceptive preparations are nearly 100% effective in preventing pregnancy. Some guidelines for using these preparations include the following:

1. Numerous oral contraceptive (OC) preparations are available, with different components and different doses of components, so that a preparation can be chosen to meet individual needs. In many cases, the initial OC of choice contains an estrogen and a progestin. The estrogen dose in most OCs is 30 to 35 µg. Smaller amounts (*e.g.*, 20 µg) may be adequate for small or underweight women; larger amounts (*e.g.*, 50 µg) may be needed for large or overweight women. When estrogen is contraindicated, a progestin-only OC may be used.
2. Currently available products contain relatively small amounts of estrogen and cause fewer adverse effects than earlier products. Despite the decreased estrogen dosage, oral contraceptives may still be safest when given to nonsmoking women under 35 years of age who do not have a history of thromboembolic problems, diabetes mellitus, hypertension, or migraine.
3. Assess each client's need and desire for oral contraceptives, as well as her willingness to comply with the prescribed regimen. Assessment information includes the client's knowledge about oral contra-

ceptives and other methods of birth control. Compliance involves the willingness to take the drugs as prescribed, to have examinations of breasts and pelvis and blood pressure measurements every 6 to 12 months, and to stop the oral contraceptive periodically (other contraceptive methods can be used during these periods). Assessment also includes identifying clients in whom oral contraceptives are contraindicated or who are at increased risk of adverse reactions.

4. The most effective and widely used oral contraceptives are estrogen-progestin combinations (see Table 28-3). Effects of estrogen components are similar when prescribed in equipotent doses, but progestins differ in progestogenic, estrogenic, antiestrogenic, and androgenic activity. Consequently, adverse effects may differ to some extent, and a client may be able to tolerate one oral contraceptive better than another.

5. Oral contraceptives decrease effects of oral anticoagulants, insulin and oral antidiabetic agents, antihypertensive drugs, and drugs used to lower serum cholesterol. If oral contraceptives are used concurrently with these drug groups, dosage of these groups may need to be increased. If oral contraceptives are discontinued, dosage of the other drugs may need to be decreased.

Cancer

When estrogens and progestins are used in the treatment of cancer, several factors must be considered. First, the goals of treatment are palliation of symptoms and shrinkage of tumor tissue rather than cure. Second, these drugs have limited effectiveness, and careful selection of recipients is essential. Estrogens are recommended only for men with recurrent or metastatic cancer of the prostate gland and for postmenopausal women with recurrent or metastatic breast cancer. Progestins are used for metastatic cancer of the endometrium. Third, relatively large doses are needed for antineoplastic effects, and the drugs are given continuously rather than cyclically. This means that adverse reactions are more likely to occur and that most symptoms result from hormone excess.

USE IN CHILDREN

There is little information about effects of estrogens in children, and the drugs are not indicated for use. Because the drugs cause epiphyseal closure, they should be used with caution before completion of bone growth and attainment of adult height. When hormonal contraceptives are given to adolescent girls, the smallest effective doses should be used, as in other populations.

USE IN OLDER ADULTS

Estrogens alone or estrogens and progestins are commonly used in postmenopausal women, whether menopause is physiologic or surgically induced by excision of both ovaries. Progestins reduce the risk of endometrial cancer in women who have not had hysterectomies. In men who receive estrogens for metastatic cancer of the prostate gland, feminizing effects may occur in older men as in younger ones.

 ## HOME CARE

Estrogens, progestins, and oral contraceptives are usually self-administered at home. The home care nurse may encounter patients or family members taking one of the drugs when visiting the home for another purpose. Teaching or assisting clients to take the drugs as prescribed may be needed. In addition, clients may need encouragement to keep appointments for follow-up supervision and monitoring of blood pressure and so forth. When visiting families that include adolescent girls or young women, the nurse may need to teach about birth control or preventing osteoporosis by improving diet and exercise patterns.

 ESTROGENS, PROGESTINS, AND ORAL CONTRACEPTIVES

NURSING ACTIONS	*RATIONALE/EXPLANATION*
1. Administer accurately	
a. Give oral estrogens, progestins, and contraceptive preparations after meals or at bedtime.	To decrease nausea, a common adverse reaction
b. With aqueous suspensions to be given IM, roll the vial between the hands several times.	To be sure that drug particles are evenly distributed through the liquid vehicle
c. Give oil preparations deeply into a large muscle mass, preferably gluteal muscles.	

(continued)

Nursing Actions	*Rationale/Explanation*
2. Observe for therapeutic effects	Therapeutic effects vary, depending on the reason for use.
a. With estrogens:	
(1) When given for menopausal symptoms, observe for decrease in "hot flashes" and vaginal problems.	
(2) When given for amenorrhea, observe for menstruation.	
(3) When given for female hypogonadism, observe for menstruation, breast enlargement, axillary and pubic hair, and other secondary sexual characteristics.	
(4) When used in cancer of the breast or prostate gland, observe for relief of symptoms.	
b. With progestins:	
(1) When given for menstrual disorders, such as abnormal uterine bleeding, amenorrhea, dysmenorrhea, premenstrual discomfort, and endometriosis, observe for relief of symptoms.	
3. Observe for adverse effects	
a. With estrogens	
(1) Menstrual disorders—breakthrough bleeding, dysmenorrhea, amenorrhea, exacerbation of endometriosis	Estrogen drugs may alter hormonal balance
(2) Gastrointestinal system—nausea, vomiting, abdominal cramps, bloating, cholestatic jaundice, colitis, acute pancreatitis	Nausea commonly occurs but usually subsides within 1 to 2 wk of continued therapy. When high doses of estrogens are used as postcoital contraceptives, nausea and vomiting may be severe enough to require administration of antiemetic drugs.
(3) Cardiovascular system—thromboembolic conditions such as thrombophlebitis, pulmonary embolism, cerebral thrombosis, and coronary thrombosis; edema and weight gain	Thromboembolic disorders were associated with earlier oral contraceptive pills which contained larger amounts of estrogen than those currently used. The only population groups now considered at high risk for thromboembolic disorders are women older than 35 y who take oral contraceptives, even low-estrogen preparations, and men or women who receive large doses of estrogens for treatment of cancer. Edema and weight gain are caused by fluid retention.
(4) Central nervous system—headache, migraine, dizziness, mental depression, convulsions	Estrogens may cause or aggravate migraine in some women; the mechanism is unknown.
(5) Cancer—endometrial and possibly breast cancer	When estrogens are used alone in postmenopausal women, they cause endometrial hyperplasia and may cause endometrial cancer. This effect can be prevented by also giving a progestin, which opposes the effects of estrogen on the endometrium. Opinions differ regarding estrogens as a cause of breast cancer. Most studies indicate little risk; a few indicate some risk, especially with high doses for prolonged periods (*i.e.*, 10 y or longer.
b. With progestins	
(1) Menstrual disorders—breakthrough bleeding	Irregular vaginal bleeding is a common adverse effect that decreases during the first year of use. This is a major reason that some women do not want to take progestin-only contraceptives.

NURSING ACTIONS	RATIONALE/EXPLANATION
(2) Cardiovascular system—decreased HDL and increased LDL cholesterol	These adverse effects on plasma lipids potentially increase the risks of cardiovascular disease. Long-term effects of progestins on thrombosis and other cardiovascular disorders are unclear, because these drugs have not been investigated as much as combined estrogen-progestin oral contraceptives.
(3) Gastrointestinal system—nausea, increased or decreased weight	Nausea may be decreased by taking with food.
(4) Endocrine system—impaired glucose tolerance	Impaired glucose tolerance may occur, especially in people with diabetes mellitus.
(5) Central nervous system—drowsiness, insomnia, mental depression	
(6) Miscellaneous effects—edema, weight gain	
c. Combined estrogen and progestin oral contraceptives	
(1) Gastrointestinal effects—nausea, others	Nausea can be minimized by taking the drugs with food or at bedtime.
(2) Cardiovascular effects—thromboembolism, myocardial infarction, stroke, hypertension	These effects occurred with earlier oral contraceptives, which contained larger amounts of estrogen than those currently used and are much less common in most people who take low-dose preparations. However, for women over 35 who smoke, there is an increased risk of myocardial infarction and other cardiovascular disorders even with low-dose pills.
(3) Gallbladder disease—cholelithiasis and cholecystitis	Women who use oral contraceptives are two to three times as likely to develop gallstones as nonusers. This is attributed to increased concentration of cholesterol in bile acids, which leads to decreased solubility and increased precipitation of stones.
(4) Miscellaneous—edema, weight gain, headache	
4. Observe for drug interactions	
a. Drugs that *decrease* effects of estrogens, progestins, and oral contraceptives:	
(1) Anticonvulsants, barbiturates, rifampin	Decrease effects by inducing enzymes that accelerate metabolism of estrogens and progestins
(2) Antimicrobials—ampicillin, chloramphenicol, neomycin, nitrofurantoin, penicillin V, sulfonamides, tetracyclines	By disrupting the normal bacterial flora of the gastrointestinal tract, antimicrobial drugs may decrease or eliminate enterohepatic circulation of estrogens and their conjugates. This action may decrease effectiveness of the contraceptive or cause breakthrough bleeding.
5. Teach clients	
a. Take estrogens, progestins, or oral contraceptives with meals or food or at bedtime.	To decrease nausea, a common adverse reaction
b. If cyclic therapy is prescribed, take the drug for 3 wk and then omit it for 1 wk. Explain that menstruation occurs but pregnancy does not because ovulation has been prevented. With oral contraceptives, consult the physician about what to do if one or more daily doses are omitted for any reason. Another method of contraception may be needed temporarily because ovulation may have occurred.	

(continued)

NURSING ACTIONS	RATIONALE/EXPLANATION
c. Teach women receiving vaginal suppositories of estrogen how to insert them correctly.	
d. Teach women using transdermal estrogen (*e.g.*, Estraderm) to apply it to clean, dry skin, preferably the abdomen; to press tightly about 10 sec to get a good seal; and to rotate sites so that at least 1 wk passes between applications to a site.	To maintain placement and therapeutic effects
e. When an estrogen or oral contraceptive is used as a postcoital contraceptive, teach clients to take the drug despite the nausea that often occurs.	This drug must be taken as prescribed to be effective in preventing pregnancy.
f. Clients should weigh themselves at least weekly and report sudden weight gain.	Fluid retention and edema may occur and produce weight gain.
g. Clients should report any unusual vaginal bleeding.	This may be caused by excessive amounts of estrogen.
h. Clients should observe for and report adverse reactions, such as calf tenderness, redness, or swelling, which are signs of thrombophlebitis.	

REVIEW AND APPLICATION EXERCISES

1. What are reproductive and nonreproductive functions of estrogens?

2. What are the functions of progestins?

3. What is considered the major mechanism of action of oral contraceptives?

4. What are adverse effects of oral contraceptives, and how can they be prevented or minimized?

5. What are the advantages and disadvantages of postmenopausal estrogen replacement therapy?

SELECTED REFERENCES

Drug facts and comparisons. (1996). St. Louis: Facts and Comparisons.

Guyton, A.C. & Hall, J.E. (1996). *Textbook of medical physiology*, 9th ed. Philadelphia: W.B. Saunders.

Moore, A.O., Mullins, P.M., & Pugh, M.C. (1993). Hormonal replacement therapy. In J.T. DiPiro, R.L. Talbert, P.E. Hayes, G.C. Yee, G.R. Matzke, & L.M. Posey (Eds.), *Pharmacotherapy: A pathophysiologic approach*, 2nd ed., pp. 1241–1250. Norwalk, CT: Appleton & Lange.

Three-month contraceptive injection approved. (1993). *FDA Medical Bulletin*, 23(1), 6.

Williams, C.L. & Stancel, G.M. (1996). Estrogens and progestins. In J.G. Hardman, L.E. Limbird, P.B. Molinoff, and R.W. Ruddon (Eds.), *Goodman and Gilman's The pharmacological basis of therapeutics*, 9th ed., pp. 1411–1440. New York: McGraw-Hill.

29 Androgens and Anabolic Steroids

Outline

Androgens

Anabolic Steroids

Testosterone

Abuse of Androgenic and Anabolic Steroid Drugs

Characteristics of Androgenic and Anabolic Steroid Drugs
mechanism of action
indications for use
contraindications for use

Nursing Process
assessment
nursing diagnoses
planning/goals
interventions
evaluation

Principles of Therapy
use in children
use in older adults

Objectives

After studying this chapter, the student will be able to:

1 Discuss effects of endogenous androgens.

2 Discuss uses and effects of exogenous androgens and anabolic steroids.

3 Discuss the rationale for using danazol to treat women with endometriosis or fibrocystic breast disease

4 Describe potential consequences of abusing anabolic steroids.

Key Terms

Anabolism	**Jaundice**
Buccal	**Masculinizing**
Epiphyseal closure	**Steroid hormone**
Hirsutism	

Androgens

Androgens are male sex hormones secreted by the testes in men, the ovaries in women, and the adrenal cortices of both sexes. Like the female sex hormones, the naturally occurring male sex hormones are steroids synthesized from cholesterol. The sex organs and adrenal glands can produce cholesterol or remove it from the blood. Cholesterol then undergoes a series of conversions to progesterone, androgenic prehormones, and finally testosterone. The androgens produced by the ovaries have little androgenic activity and are used mainly as precursor substances for the production of naturally occurring estrogens. The adrenal glands produce about five androgens, including androstenedione and dehydroepiandrosterone, but these ordinarily have little masculinizing effect.

Anabolic Steroids

Anabolic steroids are synthetic drugs with increased anabolic activity and decreased androgenic activity when compared with testosterone. They were developed during attempts to modify testosterone so that its tissue-building and growth-stimulating effects could be retained while its masculinizing effects could be eliminated or reduced.

Testosterone

Testosterone is normally the only important male sex hormone. It is secreted by the Leydig's cells in the testes in response to stimulation by luteinizing hormone (LH) or interstitial cell-stimulating hormone (ICSH) from the anterior pituitary gland. The main functions of testosterone are related to the development of male sexual characteristics, reproduction, and metabolism. Specific effects of testosterone on body tissues include the following:

1. **Fetal development.** Large amounts of chorionic gonadotropin are produced by the placenta during pregnancy. Chorionic gonadotropin is similar to LH from the anterior pituitary gland. It promotes development of the interstitial or Leydig's cells in fetal testes, which then secrete testosterone. Testosterone production begins about the second month of fetal life. When present, testosterone promotes development of male sexual characteristics, such as the penis, scrotum, prostate gland, seminal vesicles, and seminiferous tubules and suppresses development of female sexual characteristics. In the absence

of testosterone, the fetus develops female sexual characteristics.

Testosterone also provides the stimulus for the descent of the testes into the scrotum. This normally occurs after the seventh month of pregnancy, when the fetal testes are secreting relatively large amounts of testosterone. If the testes do not descend before birth, administration of testosterone or gonadotropic hormone, which stimulates testosterone secretion, will produce descent in most cases.

2. **Adult development.** Little testosterone is secreted in male children until approximately age 11 to 13 years. At the onset of puberty, testosterone secretion increases rapidly and remains at a relatively high level until about 50 years of age, after which it gradually declines.

   a. The testosterone secreted at puberty acts as a growth hormone to produce enlargement of the penis, testes, and scrotum until about 20 years of age. The prostate gland, seminal vesicles, seminiferous tubules, and vas deferens also increase in size and functional ability. Under the combined influence of testosterone and follicle-stimulating hormone (FSH) from the anterior pituitary gland, sperm production is initiated and maintained throughout the man's reproductive life.

   b. **Skin.** Testosterone increases skin thickness and activity of the sebaceous glands. Acne in the adolescent male is attributed to the increased production of testosterone.

   c. **Voice.** The larynx enlarges and deepens the voice of the adult male.

   d. **Hair.** Testosterone produces the distribution of hair growth on the face, limbs, and trunk typical of the adult male. In men with a genetic trait toward baldness, large amounts of testosterone cause alopecia (baldness) of the scalp.

   e. **Skeletal muscles.** Testosterone is largely responsible for the larger, more powerful muscles of men. This characteristic is caused by the effects of testosterone on protein metabolism. Testosterone helps the body retain nitrogen, form new amino acids, and build new muscle protein. At the same time, it slows the loss of nitrogen and amino acids formed by the constant breakdown of body tissues. Overall, testosterone increases protein anabolism (buildup) and decreases protein catabolism (breakdown).

   f. **Bone.** Testosterone makes bones thicker and longer. After puberty, more protein and calcium are deposited and retained in bone matrix. This causes a rapid rate of bone growth. The height of a male adolescent increases rapidly for a time, then stops as epiphyseal closure occurs. This happens when the cartilage at the end of the long bones in the arms and legs becomes bone. Further lengthening of the bones is then prevented.

g. **Anterior pituitary function.** High blood levels of testosterone decrease secretion of FSH and of LH or ICSH from the anterior pituitary gland. This, in turn, decreases testosterone production.

After testosterone is secreted by the testes, most of it binds reversibly to plasma proteins. It then circulates in the bloodstream for a half hour or less before it becomes attached to tissues or is broken down into inactive products. The portion that is attached to tissues enters the cells and is changed to dihydrotestosterone. The dihydrotestosterone binds with receptors within the cell and stimulates increased production of protein by the cell. The portion that does not become attached to tissues is converted into androsterone and dehydroepiandrosterone by the liver. These are conjugated with glucuronic or sulfuric acid and excreted in the bile or urine.

Abuse of Androgenic and Anabolic Steroid Drugs

These drugs, especially the anabolic steroids, are widely abused in attempts to enhance muscle development, muscle strength, and athletic performance. Athletes are considered a high-risk group, because some start taking the drugs in their early teen years and continue for years. Abusers usually take massive doses and often take several drugs or combine injectable and oral drugs for maximum effects. The large doses produce potentially serious adverse effects in several body tissues:

- Liver disorders include benign and malignant neoplasms, cholestatic hepatitis and jaundice, and peliosis hepatis, a disorder in which blood-filled cysts develop in the liver and may lead to hemorrhage or liver failure.
- Central nervous system disorders include aggression, hostility, combativeness, and dependence characterized by preoccupation with drug use, inability to stop taking the drugs, and withdrawal symptoms similar to those that occur with alcohol, cocaine, and narcotics.
- Reproductive system disorders include testicular atrophy, low sperm counts, and impotence in men. They include menstrual irregularities, baldness, hirsutism, and deepening of the voice in women.
- Metabolic disorders include increased serum cholesterol, with increased risk of cardiovascular disease and retention of fluids, with edema and other imbalances. Fluid and electrolyte retention contribute to the increased weight associated with drug use.
- Dermatologic disorders include moderate to severe acne in both sexes, depending on drug dosage.

Many of these adverse effects persist several months after the drugs are stopped and may be irreversible.

Because of their abuse potential, the drugs were legally designated as Schedule III controlled substances in 1991. Although nonprescription sales of the drugs are illegal, they are readily available.

Characteristics of Androgenic and Anabolic Steroid Drugs

Individual androgens and anabolic steroids are listed in Table 29-1.

1. When male sex hormones or androgens are given from exogenous sources for therapeutic purposes, they produce the same effects as the naturally occurring hormones.
2. Male sex hormones given to women antagonize or reduce the effects of female sex hormones. Thus, administration of testosterone to women can suppress menstruation and cause atrophy of the endometrial lining of the uterus.
3. Most exogenous androgens are given intramuscularly or orally. Naturally occurring androgens are given by injection because they are rapidly metabolized by the liver if given orally. Some esters of testosterone have been modified to slow the rate of metabolism and thus prolong action. Testosterone transdermal systems are also available.
4. All synthetic anabolic steroids are weak androgens. Consequently, giving these drugs for anabolic effects also produces masculinizing effects. This characteristic limits the clinical usefulness of these drugs in women and children. Profound changes in growth and sexual development may occur if these drugs are given to young children.

MECHANISM OF ACTION

Androgenic and anabolic drugs penetrate the cell membrane and bind to receptor proteins in the cell cytoplasm. The steroid-receptor complex is then transported to the nucleus where it activates ribonucleic and deoxyribonucleic acid production and stimulates cellular synthesis of protein. Production of protein increases in body cells, especially those associated with male sexual characteristics.

| TABLE 29-1 | ANDROGENS AND ANABOLIC STEROIDS |

Generic/Trade Name	Routes and Dosage Ranges for Various Indications		
	Hypogonadism	*Breast Cancer*	*Other*
Androgens			
Testosterone aqueous (Histerone, others)	IM 25–50 mg two to three times weekly PO 10–40 mg daily Buccal tablets 5–20 mg daily	IM 50–100 mg three times weekly	Cryptorchidism: PO 30 mg daily; buccal tablets, 15 mg daily
Testosterone cypionate (Depo-Testosterone)	IM 50–200 mg every 2–4 wk	IM 200–400 mg every 2–4 wk	
Testosterone enanthate (Delatestryl)	IM 50–200 mg every 2–4 wk	IM 50–100 mg three times weekly	
Testosterone transdermal systems (Androderm, Testoderm)	Apply two Androderm systems (dose of 5 mg) nightly to back, abdomen, upper arm or thigh; apply Testoderm (one 6-mg system) to scrotal sac daily		
Testolactone (Teslac)	PO 5–20 mg daily daily	PO 250 mg four times	
Fluoxymesterone (Halotestin)		PO 10–40 mg daily in divided doses	
Methyltestosterone (Oreton methyl)		PO 200 mg daily in divided doses Buccal tablets 100 mg daily	Cryptorchidism: PO 30 mg daily; buccal tablets, 15 mg daily
Danazol (Danocrine)			Endometriosis: PO 800 mg daily in two divided doses for 3–9 months Fibrocystic breast disease: PO 100–400 mg daily in two divided doses for 3–6 months Hereditary angioedema prophylaxis: PO 200 mg two to three times daily initially, reduce for maintenance
Anabolic Steroids			
Nandrolone decanoate (Deca-Durabolin)			Anemia of renal disease: IM Women: 50–100 mg weekly Men: 100–200 mg weekly Children (2–13 years): 25–50 mg every 3–4 wk
Nandrolone phenpropionate (Durabolin)		IM 50–100 mg weekly	
Oxandrolone (Oxandrin)			Tissue building; osteoporosis: Adults: PO 5–10 mg daily in divided doses (up to 20 mg daily) for 2–4 weeks. Repeat after a rest period, if desired. Do not use longer than 3 months. Children: PO 0.1 mg/kg/d
Oxymetholone (Anadrol-50)			Anemia: PO 1–5 mg/kg/d
Stanazolol (Winstrol)			Hereditary angioedema prophylaxis: PO 2 mg three times daily initially; maintenance dose, 2 mg daily

INDICATIONS FOR USE

With male sex hormones, the most clear-cut indication for use is to treat androgen deficiency states (*e.g.*, hypogonadism, cryptorchidism, impotence, oligospermia) in boys and men. Hypogonadism may result from hypothalamic-pituitary or testicular dysfunction. In prepubertal boys, administration of the drugs stimulates the development of masculine characteristics. In postpubertal men who become androgen deficient, the hormones reestablish and maintain masculine characteristics and functions.

In women, male sex hormones are most often used in the palliative treatment of metastatic breast cancer. These women are usually premenopausal or menopausal and have breast tumors in which growth is stimulated by estrogen, the major female sex hormone. The male sex hormones inhibit the stimulating effects of estrogen. In addition, danazol (Danocrine) may be used to prevent or treat endometriosis, fibrocystic breast disease, or hereditary angioedema.

Anabolic steroids are occasionally used to treat tissue wasting (*e.g.*, catabolic states associated with severe illnesses, burns, trauma, and long-term use of adrenal corticosteroids), some types of anemia, hereditary angioedema, or metastatic breast cancer in women. These drugs are more often abused for body-building purposes than used for therapeutic effects.

CONTRAINDICATIONS FOR USE

Androgens and anabolic steroids are contraindicated during pregnancy (because of possible masculinizing effects on a female fetus), in clients with pre-existing liver disease, and in men with prostate gland disorders. Men with enlarged prostates may develop additional enlargement, and men with prostatic cancer may experience tumor growth. Although not contraindicated in children, these drugs must be used very cautiously and with x-rays approximately every 6 months to evaluate bone growth.

Nursing Process

Assessment

Before drug therapy is started, clients need a thorough history and physical examination. Periodic monitoring of the client's condition is needed throughout drug therapy.
- Assess for conditions in which androgens and anabolic steroids are used (*e.g.*, deficiency states, debilitating illness).
- Assess for conditions that increase risks of adverse effects or are contraindications (*e.g.*, pregnancy, liver disease, prostatic hypertrophy).
- Check laboratory reports of liver function tests (the drugs may cause cholestatic jaundice and liver damage), serum electrolytes (the drugs may cause sodium and water reten-

tion), and serum lipids (the drugs may increase levels and aggravate atherosclerosis).
- Assess weight and blood pressure regularly. These may be elevated by retention of sodium and water with resultant edema, especially in clients with congestive heart failure.
- For children, check x-ray reports of bone growth status initially and about every 6 months while the drugs are being taken.
- Assess the client's attitude toward taking male sex hormones.
- Assess the client's willingness to comply with instructions for taking the drugs and follow-up procedures.

Nursing Diagnoses

- Body Image Disturbance in females related to masculinizing effects and menstrual irregularities
- Sexual Dysfunction in males related to impotence and changes in libido
- Ineffective Individual Coping related to use of androgens and anabolic steroids for nonmedical purposes
- Knowledge Deficit: Physiologic and psychological consequences of overuse and abuse of the drugs to enhance athletic performance
- Noncompliance: Overuse
- Fluid Volume Excess related to sodium and water retention
- Risk for Injury: Liver disease and other serious adverse drug effects
- Risk for Violence: Directed at Others related to feelings of aggression and hostility in those who take large doses

Planning/Goals

The client will:
- Use the drugs for medical purposes only
- Receive or take the drugs as prescribed
- Avoid overuse and abuse of drugs for "body building"
- Be counseled regarding effects of overuse and abuse if identified as being at risk (*e.g.*, athletes, especially weight lifters and football players)
- Avoid preventable adverse drug effects
- Comply with monitoring and follow-up procedures

Interventions

- Assist clients to use the drug correctly.
- Assist clients to reduce sodium intake if edema develops.
- Assist clients with severe injuries or burns to increase intake of protein, calories, and other nutrients.
- Record weight and blood pressure at regular intervals.
- Participate in school or community programs to inform children, parents, coaches, athletic trainers, and others of the risks of inappropriate use of androgens and anabolic steroids.

 Teach clients:
- Take the drugs only if prescribed and as prescribed. Usage by athletes for body building is inappropriate and, if not prescribed by a licensed physician, illegal.
- Continue medical supervision as long as the drugs are being taken.
- Weigh yourself once or twice weekly, and record the amount.

Evaluation

- Interview and observe for compliance with instructions for taking prescribed drugs.
- Interview and observe for therapeutic and adverse drug effects.
- Question athletes about illegal use of the drugs.
- Observe athletes for increased weight and behavioral changes that may indicate drug abuse.

Principles of Therapy

1. When androgen or anabolic steroids are used in the treatment of metastatic breast cancer or refractory anemia, the required dosage may be two to three times the amount needed for androgen replacement therapy. These high dosages increase the incidence of adverse reactions.
2. When these drugs are given to women and prepubertal males, good skin care is indicated to decrease the incidence and severity of acne.
3. Drug therapy with androgens and anabolic steroids may be short or long term, depending on the condition in question, the client's response to treatment, and the incidence of adverse reactions. If feasible, intermittent rather than continuous therapy is recommended.
4. Androgens generally potentiate oral anticoagulants, oral antidiabetic agents, and insulin. Dosage of these drugs may need to be decreased during concurrent therapy with androgens or anabolic drugs.

USE IN CHILDREN

The main indication for use of androgens in children is for boys with established deficiency states. Because the drugs cause epiphyseal closure, hands and wrists should be x-rayed every 6 months to detect bone maturation and prevent loss of adult height. Stimulation of skeletal growth continues for about 6 months after drug therapy is stopped. If premature puberty occurs (precocious sexual development, enlarged penis), the drug should be stopped. The drugs may cause or aggravate acne. Scrupulous hygiene and other antiacne treatment may be needed, especially in adolescent boys.

Long-term use of danazol or stanazolol to prevent attacks of hereditary angioedema is not recommended in children because such attacks are infrequent and adverse drug effects are likely to occur.

USE IN OLDER ADULTS

The main indication for use of androgens is a deficiency state in men. Older adults often have hypertension and other cardiovascular disorders that may be aggravated by the sodium and water retention associated with androgens and anabolic steroids. In men, the drugs may increase prostate size and interfere with urination, increase risk of prostatic cancer, and cause excessive sexual stimulation and priapism.

The main reason for use of the drugs in older women is treatment of metastatic breast cancer. Masculinizing effects may occur.

ANDROGENS AND ANABOLIC STEROIDS

NURSING ACTIONS	RATIONALE/EXPLANATION
1. Administer accurately **a.** Give IM preparations of testosterone, other androgens and anabolic steroids deeply, preferably in the gluteal muscle.	
b. Give oral preparations before or with meals, in divided doses.	To decrease gastrointestinal disturbances
c. For buccal preparations:	
(1) Give in divided doses.	
(2) Place the tablet between the cheek and gum.	Buccal preparations must be absorbed through the mucous membranes.
(3) Instruct the client not to swallow the tablet and not to drink, chew, or smoke until the tablet is completely absorbed.	
(4) Maintain oral hygiene.	To decrease irritation and risk of infection

NURSING ACTIONS	RATIONALE/EXPLANATION
d. With transdermal systems:	Correct site selection and application are necessary for therapeutic effects. Scrotal skin is more permeable to testosterone than other skin areas.
(1) Apply 2 Androderm systems nightly to clean, dry skin on back, abdomen, upper arm, or thigh. Do *not* apply to scrotum. Rotate sites, with 7 days between applications to a site. Press firmly into place for adherence.	
(2) Apply 1 Testoderm system to clean, dry scrotal skin (shaved, for best adherence) once daily.	
2. Observe for therapeutic effects	
a. When the drug is given for hypogonadism, observe for masculinizing effects, such as growth of sexual organs, deepening of voice, growth of body hair, and acne.	
b. When the drug is given for anabolic effects, observe for increased appetite, euphoria, or statements of feeling better.	
c. When the drug is given for cancer, observe for decreased pain and increased reports of feeling better.	
d. When the drug is given for anemia, observe complete blood count reports for increased red blood cells, hematocrit, and hemoglobin.	
3. Observe for adverse reactions	
a. Virilism or masculinizing effects:	
(1) In adult men with adequate secretion of testosterone—priapism, increased sexual desire, reduced sperm count, and prostate enlargement	
(2) In prepubertal boys—premature development of sex organs and secondary sexual characteristics, such as enlargement of the penis, priapism, pubic hair	
(3) In women—masculinizing effects include hirsutism, deepening of the voice, menstrual irregularities	
b. Jaundice—dark urine, yellow skin and sclera, itching	
c. Edema	More likely in clients who are elderly or who have heart or kidney disease
d. Hypercalcemia	More likely in women with advanced breast cancer
e. Difficulty voiding due to prostate enlargement	More likely in middle-age or elderly men
f. Inadequate growth in height of children	
4. Observe for drug interactions	
a. Drugs that *decrease* effects of androgens and anabolic agents:	
(1) Aminopyrine	Increases the rate of metabolism
(2) Antihistamines	Increase enzyme induction
(3) Barbiturates	Increase enzyme induction and rate of metabolism
(4) Calcitonin	Decreases calcium retention and thus antagonizes calcium-retaining effects of androgens

(continued)

NURSING ACTIONS	RATIONALE/EXPLANATION
(5) Chlorcyclizine (Perazil)	Increases metabolism
(6) Estrogens	Antagonize the anticancer effects of androgens
5. Teach clients **a.** Correct use of buccal tablets and transdermal systems	
b. Report adverse reactions, such as jaundice, edema, masculinizing effects.	
c. Weigh weekly, and report gains.	May indicate fluid retention and edema or a therapeutic effect of anabolic drugs
d. Practice frequent and thorough skin cleansing.	To decrease acne, which is most likely to occur in women and children
e. With anabolic drugs, eat a well-balanced diet.	Adequate protein and calories are necessary for full anabolic effects. Folic acid is necessary when these drugs are given for anemia.

REVIEW AND APPLICATION EXERCISES

1. How does testosterone promote development of male sexual characteristics?

2. What is the major clinical indication for therapeutic use of testosterone and related androgens?

3. What is the difference between androgenic activity and anabolic activity?

4. What are the adverse effects of using large doses of anabolic steroids in body-building efforts?

5. If your 14-year-old brother said some friends were telling him to take drugs to increase muscle development and athletic ability, how would you reply? Justify your answer.

SELECTED REFERENCES

Drug facts and comparisons. (1996). St. Louis: Facts and Comparisons.

Guyton, A.C. & Hall, J.E. (1996). *Textbook of medical physiology,* 9th ed. Philadelphia: W.B. Saunders.

Su, T.P., Pagliaro, M., Schmidt, P.J., Pickar, D., Wolkowitz, O., & Rubinow, D.R. (1993). Neuropsychiatric effects of anabolic steroids in male normal volunteers. *Journal of the American Medical Association, 269,* 2760–2764.

Wilson, J.D. (1996). Androgens. In J.G. Hardman, L.E. Limbird, P.B. Molinoff, R.W. Ruddon (Eds.), *Goodman & Gilman's The pharmacological basis of therapeutics,* 9th ed., pp. 1441–1455. New York: McGraw-Hill.

Section V

Nutrients, Fluids, and Electrolytes

Nutritional Products, Anorexiants, and Digestants

Outline

Objectives

After studying this chapter, the student will be able to:

1 Discuss the importance of water, carbohydrates, proteins, and fats in maintaining health.

2 Identify clients at risk of developing fluid disorders.

3 Identify clients at risk of developing undernutrition.

4 Discuss nutrients needed to promote tissue healing and recovery from illness.

5 Discuss common disorders and drugs that interfere with nutrition.

6 Describe nursing interventions to maintain fluid balance.

7 Describe nursing interventions to increase calorie-protein intake in undernourished clients.

8 Review health consequences of obesity.

9 Discuss nursing interventions to assist obese clients in weight management.

Key Terms

Anorexiants	**Parenteral nutrition**
Enteral nutrition	**Sedentary**
Malabsorption	**Undernutrition**
Obesity	

Nutritional Products

Water, carbohydrates, proteins, fats, vitamins, and minerals are required for human nutrition, to promote or maintain health, to prevent illness, and to promote recovery from illness. The first four nutrients are discussed in this chapter; vitamins and minerals are discussed in the following chapters.

Water, carbohydrates, proteins, and fats are necessary for life. Water is second only to oxygen in importance, because a person can live only a few days without water intake. Proteins are basic anatomic and physiologic components of all body cells and tissues. Carbohydrates and fats serve primarily as sources of energy for cell metabolism.

Energy is measured in terms of kilocalories (kcal) per gram of food oxidized in the body. Carbohydrates are oxidized first and provide an immediate source of energy; fats are used second and provide a long-term or reserve supply of energy; and proteins are used last. Undernutrition, starvation, and death occur within a few weeks when there is no intake of carbohydrates, proteins, and fats. Table 30-1 lists more specific characteristics of water, carbohydrates, proteins, and fats in relation to normal nutrition.

When inadequate or excessive amounts of these nutrients are ingested, nutritional disorders result. These disorders include water deficit (also called dehydration or fluid volume deficit), water excess (also called water intoxication or fluid volume excess), undernutrition, and obesity. Causes and clinical manifestations of water imbalances are listed in Table 30-2; protein–calorie imbalances are described in Table 30-3.

Numerous products are available to supplement or substitute for dietary intake in clients who cannot ingest, digest, absorb, or use nutrients. For example, liquid formulas are available for oral or tube feedings. Many liquid formulas are nutritionally complete, except for water, when given in sufficient quantities. Others are nutritionally incomplete but useful in certain circumstances. Additional water is given to meet fluid needs. A variety of intravenous (IV) fluids is also available. Most IV fluids are nutritionally incomplete and are designed for short-term use when oral or tube feedings are contraindicated. They are most useful in meeting fluid and electrolyte needs.

When nutrients must be provided parenterally for more than a few days, a special nutritional formula can be given. Parenteral nutritional formulas can be designed to meet all nutritional needs or to supplement other feeding methods. Fat emulsions also are administered to supply additional calories and essential fatty acids. For nutritional deficiencies due to malabsorption of carbohydrates, protein, and fat, pancreatic enzymes may be given to aid digestion.

Anorexiants

In nutritional excesses or obesity, anorexiant drugs are sometimes given to decrease appetite (Table 30-4). Amphetamines (see Chap. 16) have been used for this purpose, but they have a high potential for abuse and dependence. Other anorexiant drugs are similar to amphetamines but are promoted for use only in appetite control. These drugs should be part of a weight-reduction program that also includes calorie restriction, exercise, medical supervision, and psychological support. These drugs may lead to abuse and dependence of the amphetamine type, and their use is regulated by the Controlled Substances Act. Anorexiant drugs are contraindicated in cardiovascular disease, hyperthyroidism, glaucoma, and agitated psychological disturbances.

Phenylpropanolamine is an adrenergic drug commonly used as a nasal decongestant in over-the-counter cold remedies. It is also the active ingredient in over-the-counter appetite suppressants (*e.g.*, Dexatrim, Acutrim). Effectiveness of the drug in weight reduction is limited, and its use has been associated with psychosis, hypertension, stroke, renal failure, cardiac arrhythmias, and death. These adverse effects have occurred with recommended doses but are especially likely with overdoses or concomitant use of other stimulants, such as caffeine.

Individual Nutritional Products for Oral or Tube Feeding

NUTRITIONALLY COMPLETE LIQUID FORMULAS FOR GENERAL USE

Ensure (orally [PO] or TF 2000 ml), **Isocal** (PO or TF 2000 ml), **Osmolite** (TF 2000 ml), and **Sustacal** (PO or TF 1080 ml) are examples of formulas that provide recommended dietary allowances (RDAs) for protein, vitamins, and minerals. Most of the formulas provide 1 calorie per milliliter.

When given in the designated amounts, these formulas meet basic nutritional needs for adults. However, amounts should be individualized according to (*text continues on page 380*)

TABLE 30-1   WATER, CARBOHYDRATES, PROTEINS, AND FATS

Characteristics	Functions	Requirements	Normal Sources	Normal Losses
Water 1. Major chemical constituent of the body 2. Intracellular fluid includes the water inside body cells. 3. Extracellular fluid includes the water or liquid portion of blood, lymph, spinal fluid, saliva, gastrointestinal secretions, bile, sweat, urine, and the tissue fluid that surrounds body cells.	1. Serves as a solvent or medium in which all cell metabolism occurs 2. Maintains blood volume 3. Transports nutrients to body cells 4. Assists in maintaining electrolyte balance in blood and cells 5. Assists in maintaining body temperature	Approximately 2000–3000 ml daily, depending on activity, environmental temperature, and other factors	1. Drinking water and other beverages (about 1200 ml/d) 2. Water in foods (about 1000 ml/d) 3. Water produced by oxidation of foods in the body (about 300 ml/d)	1. Urine (about 1500 ml/d) 2. Insensible losses from skin and lungs (about 900 ml/d) 3. Feces (about 100 ml/d)
Carbohydrates 1. Chemical substances composed of carbon, hydrogen, and oxygen 2. The major source of energy for body activities. When oxidized in the body, carbohydrates furnish 4 kcal of energy per gram. 3. They must be broken down into glucose, galactose, or fructose before they can be absorbed. The simple sugars can then be used for energy or stored as glycogen	1. Provide glucose, which is necessary for normal cellular metabolism 2. Conserve body proteins for tissue building and repair by preventing use of proteins for energy 3. Promote normal fat metabolism 4. Promote normal function of nerve cells. Glucose is the only source of energy that can be used by the brain. 5. Promote growth of normal intestinal bacteria by providing lactose. These bacteria synthesize certain vitamins, mainly vitamin K. 6. Promote normal bowel elimination by stimulating peristalsis, absorbing water and increasing the bulk of intestinal contents. This function is fulfilled by complex or indigestible carbohydrates.	Approximately 2000 kcal daily for the average adult female (58 kg or 127 lb) and 2700 kcal for the average adult male (70 kg or 154 lb). Requirements vary, depending on age, size, activity, and other factors. They increase in pregnancy and lactation; rapid growth periods of infancy, early childhood, and adolescence; periods of strenuous activity; and disorders such as fever, hyperthyroidism, severe burns, trauma, or surgery. They decrease with sedentary activities and in elderly people.	Grains, fruits, and vegetables are good sources of carbohydrates and other essential nutrients. Candy and carbonated beverages contain kilocalories but lack other nutrients. Glycogen is a reserve supply of glucose that can be mobilized to meet energy needs. The amount available is relatively small—approximately 110 g in the liver and 225 g in muscle. For some people, this amount would not meet requirements for 24 h during a fasting state.	Waste products from carbohydrate metabolism are mainly carbon dioxide and water. Carbon dioxide is mainly excreted through the lungs, and water may be excreted in urine or used for other metabolic processes.

(continued)

377

TABLE 30-1 WATER, CARBOHYDRATES, PROTEINS, AND FATS (Continued)

Characteristics	Functions	Requirements	Normal Sources	Normal Losses
Proteins				
1. Chemical substances composed of carbon, hydrogen, water, nitrogen, phosphorus. When broken down in the body, proteins yield 4 kcal of energy per gram. They are used for energy only when intake of carbohydrates and fats is inadequate. 2. Most proteins are found in muscle tissue; others are found in soft tissues, bones, teeth, and blood and other body fluids.	1. Furnish amino acids for growth of new tissue and repair of damaged or worn-out tissue. Amino acids are the basic constituents or building blocks of all body cells. 2. Serve as components of numerous body fluids and secretions, including enzymes, many hormones, milk, mucus, and sperm. (Sweat, bile, and urine are normally protein free.) 3. Assist in maintaining normal osmotic pressure in the blood. Albumin is especially important in fulfilling this function. 4. Transport various substances in the blood. Lipid-carrying plasma proteins transport fat-soluble vitamins, cholesterol, triglycerides, and phospholipids. Transferrin carries iron, and another protein carries calcium. Albumin transports free fatty acids, bilirubin, and many drugs.	Approximately 0.8 g/kg of body weight daily This amount maintains normal nitrogen balance and tissue growth and repair. An average adult female (58 kg) requires about 46 g; an average adult male (70 kg) requires about 56 g. Requirements increase during growth periods of children, pregnancy and lactation, fever, burn injuries, surgery, hyperthyroidism, and stress. Older adults need the same amount of protein (0.8 g/kg) as younger adults.	Animal foods, such as meat, fish, poultry, milk, eggs, and cheese, provide "complete" proteins, which contain all the essential amino acids. Proteins from beans, breads, and cereals are incomplete, but they can be combined in ways that provide adequate intake.	Nitrogenous waste products, ammonia, urea, and uric acid are excreted in the urine.

5. Provide immunoglobulins or antibodies, which are important in resistance to disease

Fats (lipids)

1. Several different chemical substances of which the major ones are triglycerides, phospholipids, and cholesterol. More than 98% of natural fats are triglycerides.
2. Second choice as energy source, after carbohydrates. They furnish 9 kcal of energy per gram.
3. Excess dietary fats are stored, excess carbohydrates and proteins are converted to fat and stored in adipose tissue

1. Provide energy for body metabolism
2. Conserve proteins for tissue synthesis by preventing use of proteins for energy
3. Protect organs from injury
4. Conserve body heat and help maintain normal body temperature
5. Conserve thiamine, a vitamin that is required for carbohydrate metabolism but not fat metabolism
6. Promote intestinal absorption of fat-soluble vitamins
7. Increase palatability of foods
8. Slow gastric emptying, thereby increasing and prolonging satiety
9. Promote normal growth and development
10. Serve as essential components of cells and cell membranes
11. Protect against entry of foreign substances and loss of water through the skin

Approximately 50–130 g daily (900–1200 kilocalories in a 3000-kcal diet). Requirements depend on weight, size, amount of carbohydrate ingested, physical activity, and other factors

High amounts of fat are contained in meat, egg yolk, cheese, butter, whole milk, salad dressings, cream, and ice cream.
In addition to food sources, triglycerides and cholesterol are formed in the liver. Cholesterol in foods is only about 50% absorbed.

Fats are excreted in sweat, bile, and feces or are oxidized to carbon dioxide and water, which are excreted.

TABLE 30-2	WATER IMBALANCES

Water Deficit

Causes	*Signs and Symptoms*
1. Inadequate fluid intake, most likely to occur in people who are comatose, unable to swallow, or otherwise incapacitated 2. Excessive fluid loss due to vomiting, diarrhea, fever, diuretic drug therapy, high environmental temperatures, strenuous physical activity, or excessive sweating 3. A combination of 1 and 2	1. Thirst 2. Oliguria and concentrated urine 3. Weakness 4. Dry tongue and oral mucous membranes 5. Flushed skin 6. Weight loss 7. Fever 8. Increased hematocrit 9. Mental disturbances ranging from mild confusion to delirium, convulsions, and coma 10. Hypovolemic shock if the deficiency is severe or develops rapidly

Water Excess

Causes	*Signs and Symptoms*
1. Excessive intake, most likely to occur with excessive amounts or rapid infusion of IV fluids 2. Impaired excretion of fluids due to endocrine, renal, cardiovascular, or central nervous system disorders	1. Drowsiness 2. Weakness and lethargy 3. Weight gain 4. Edema 5. Low serum sodium and hematocrit 6. Disorientation 7. Circulatory overload and pulmonary edema if water excess is severe or develops rapidly

nutritional needs and whether the formula is being used to supplement or substitute for other sources of food and fluids. **PediaSure** is a nutritionally complete formula for enteral use in children 1 to 6 years old.

NUTRITIONAL AGENTS FOR SPECIFIC USES (DEFINED FORMULA OR ELEMENTAL DIETS)

Lofenalac is a low-phenylalanine preparation used only in infants and children with phenylketonuria, a metabolic disorder in which phenylalanine cannot be metabolized normally. Lofenalac is inadequate for complete nutrition and growth, although it meets Food & Drug Administration (FDA) requirements for infant formulas. For growth needs, it is recommended that about 85% of the child's protein needs be supplied with Lofenalac and the remaining 10% to 15% be supplied with foods containing phenylalanine, which is an essential amino acid.

Nursoy, ProSobee, Isomil, and **Soyalac** are hypoallergenic, milk-free formulas. They derive their protein from soybean products rather than milk. They provide 20 calories/oz when mixed or diluted as directed and provide all other essential nutrients for normal growth and development. They are used as milk substitutes for clients who are allergic to milk (most often infants).

Nutramigen is a nutritionally complete hypoallergenic formula containing predigested protein. It is used for infants and children who are allergic to ordinary food proteins or who have diarrhea or other gastrointestinal (GI) problems.

Portagen is a nutritionally complete formula that contains medium-chain triglycerides, an easily digested form of fat. It is used primarily in clients with fat malabsorption problems. It may be used as the complete diet, as a beverage with meals, or as an addition to various recipes. It may induce coma in clients with severe hepatic cirrhosis.

Precision diets are nutritionally complete, low-residue formulas for oral or tube feedings. The **high-nitrogen diet** provides 125 g of protein or 20 g of nitrogen, 3000 kcal, and recommended amounts of essential vitamins and minerals in ten 3-oz servings. The **low-residue** formula contains 45 g of protein or 7.2 g of nitrogen (a maintenance amount of protein), 1900 kcal, and essential vitamins and minerals in six 3-oz servings. The **isotonic** diet contains

TABLE 30-3	CARBOHYDRATE, PROTEIN, AND FAT IMBALANCES

Protein-Calorie Deficit	
Causes	*Signs and Symptoms*
1. Inadequate intake of protein, carbohydrate, and fat 2. Impaired ability to digest, absorb, or use nutrients 3. Excessive losses	1. Weight loss with eventual loss of subcutaneous fat and muscle mass 2. Increased susceptibility to infection 3. Weakness and fatigability 4. Dry, scaly skin 5. Impaired healing 6. Impaired growth and development in children 7. Edema 8. Decreased hemoglobin 9. Acidosis 10. Disordered brain function 11. Coma 12. Starvation

Protein-Calorie Excess	
Causes	*Signs and Symptoms*
1. Excessive intake, especially of carbohydrates and fats	1. Weight gain 2. Obesity

the same amounts of protein, vitamins, and minerals as the low-residue formula but is isotonic rather than hypertonic and provides 1500 kcal in six 2-oz servings.

These preparations are ingested or given by tube slowly over 4 hours. The carbohydrate content may produce hyperglycemia; therefore, they should not be used in clients with diabetes mellitus. These formulas can be given to children if the amount is calculated to provide recommended amounts of nutrients for the particular age group.

Pregestimil is an infant formula that contains easily digested protein, fat, and carbohydrate. It is used in infants with diarrhea, dietary intolerances, or malabsorption syndromes.

Pulmocare and **Nutrivent** may be used for clients with chronic obstructive pulmonary disease or respiratory insufficiency. Clients with impaired breathing have difficulty eliminating sufficient quantities of carbon dioxide, a waste product of carbohydrate metabolism. When carbon dioxide accumulates in the body, it may produce respiratory acidosis and respiratory failure. These products are high in fat and low in carbohydrates because fat metabolism produces less carbon dioxide than carbohydrate metabolism.

TraumaCal, a high-protein formula with easily assimilated amino acids and other nutrients, was developed for clients with severe trauma or burn injuries to help meet nutritional needs and promote healing. It contains 1.5 calories/ml.

Vivonex is a nutritionally complete diet that contains crystalline amino acids as its protein or nitrogen source. It can be used for oral or tube feedings. It requires virtually no digestion and leaves virtually no fecal residue, so it is especially useful in GI disorders. The amount, concentration, and rate of administration can be adjusted to meet nutritional needs and tolerance in adults and children.

NUTRITIONALLY INCOMPLETE SUPPLEMENTS

Amin-Aid is used as a source of protein for clients with acute and chronic renal insufficiency in whom dietary protein must be restricted. Amin-Aid supplies amino acids, carbohydrates, and a few electrolytes.

Casec is an oral protein supplement for use in infants, children, or adults.

Citrotein is an oral dietary supplement that provides protein, vitamins, and minerals. It is especially useful when appetite and food intake are decreased or during rapid growth periods when intake does not meet nutritional needs.

Gevral Protein is an oral supplement used to increase intake of protein, vitamins, and minerals. The powder can be mixed with water, milk, or other cold liquids, added to cereals, or mixed into desserts.

Lipomul (corn oil) and **Microlipid** (safflower oil) are fat supplements containing unsaturated fats.

Lonalac, an oral supplement, is used as a milk substitute in sodium-restricted diets or to increase protein intake when sodium must be restricted.

TABLE 30-4 **ANOREXIANTS**

Generic/ Trade Name	Route and Dosage Range (Adults)	Status Under Controlled Substances Act	Remarks
Benzphetamine (Didrex)	PO 25–50 mg one to three times daily	Schedule III	Dosages not established for children under 12 years of age
Dexfenfluramine (Redux)	PO 15 mg twice daily with meals	Schedule IV	May cause pulmonary hypertension, most likely with use longer than 3 months
Diethylpropion (Tenuate)	PO 25 mg three times daily	Schedule IV	
Fenfluramine (Pondimin)	PO 20–40 mg three times daily: maximal daily dose, 120 mg	Schedule IV	Fenfluramine generally has the same actions, uses, and characteristics as the other non-amphetamine anorexiant drugs. An important difference, however, is that fenfluramine depresses, rather than stimulates, the central nervous system.
Mazindol (Sanorex)	PO 1 mg three times daily	Schedule III	
Phendimetrazine (Plegine)	PO 35 mg two or three times daily or 105 mg once daily	Schedule III	
Phentermine hydrochloride (Fastin)	PO 8.0 mg three times daily or 15–37 mg daily in the morning	Schedule IV	
Phentermine resin (Ionamin)	PO 15–30 mg once daily	Schedule IV	

MCT Oil is a preparation of medium-chain triglycerides derived from coconut oil. MCT Oil is more easily digested than fats contained in most foods, which are mainly long-chain triglycerides. The medium-chain triglycerides are water soluble, are absorbed into the portal vein rather than lymphatic channels, and do not require the presence of bile salts for absorption. Thus, they are useful in children or adults with fat malabsorption syndromes. Although they are useful as a caloric substitute for dietary fat (1 tablespoon provides 115 kcal), they do not promote absorption of fat-soluble vitamins or provide essential fatty acids as the long-chain triglycerides do. MCT Oil can be mixed with fruit juices, used with salads or vegetables, or used in cooking and baking. Limited amounts of this product should be used in clients with severe hepatic cirrhosis because of the risk of precipitating encephalopathy and coma.

Polycose is an oral supplement used to increase caloric intake. Derived from carbohydrate, Polycose may be used by clients on protein-, electrolyte-, or fat-restricted diets. Available in liquid and powder, Polycose may be mixed with water or other beverages and with foods. Amounts taken should be determined by taste, calories needed, and tolerance.

COMPLETE INFANT FORMULAS

Enfamil, Similac, and **SMA** are commonly used complete nutritional formulas for full-term infants. Either may be used alone for bottle-fed infants or as a supplement for breast-fed infants. These preparations are quite similar to human breast milk. Their only deficiency is in iron, which may be given separately or in a formula preparation containing iron. **Enfamil Premature, Special Care Similac,** and **Preemie SMA** are formulations for preterm infants because their nutritional needs differ from those of full-term infants.

Intravenous Fluids

Dextrose injection is available in preparations containing 2.5%, 5%, 10%, 20%, 25%, 30%, 40%, 50%, 60%, and 70% dextrose. The most frequently used concentration is 5% dextrose in water or sodium chloride injection. A concentration of 5% dextrose in water is approximately isotonic with blood. It provides water and 170 kcal/l. The dextrose is rapidly used, leaving "free" water for excreting waste products, maintaining renal function, and maintaining urine output. The 10% dextrose solution provides double the amount of calories in the same volume of fluid but is hypertonic and therefore may cause phlebitis. Except for 25% or 50% solutions sometimes used to treat hypoglycemia, the higher concentrations are used primarily to provide calories in parenteral nutrition. They are hypertonic and must be given through a central or subclavian catheter.

Dextrose and sodium chloride injection is available in various concentrations. The most frequently used are 5% dextrose in 0.225% or 0.45% sodium chloride (also called $D_5\frac{1}{4}$ and $D_5\frac{1}{2}$ normal saline, respectively). These provide about 170 kcal/l, water, sodium, and chloride. They are frequently used for maintenance therapy, usually with added potassium chloride, in clients who cannot eat or drink. They also are used for replacement therapy when large amounts of fluid are lost, for keeping IV lines open, and for administering medications.

Crystalline amino acid solutions (Aminosyn, Freamine) contain essential and nonessential amino acids. These solutions are most often used with concentrated dextrose injection in parenteral nutrition.

Fat emulsions (Intralipid, Liposyn) provide concentrated calories and essential fatty acids. The emulsion is usually given as part of parenteral nutrition. More calories can be supplied with a fat emulsion than with dextrose-protein solutions alone. It is available in 10% and 20% emulsions; 500 ml of 10% emulsion provides 550 calories.

Pancreatic Enzymes

Pancreatin is an oral preparation of pancreatic enzymes used to aid digestion and absorption of dietary carbohydrate, protein, and fat in conditions characterized by pancreatic enzyme deficiency. These conditions include cystic fibrosis, chronic pancreatitis, pancreatectomy, and pancreatic obstruction. **Pancrelipase** (Viokase) is essentially the same as pancreatin except that it may be more effective in steatorrhea (excess fat in the feces).

Pancreatin
Route and Dosage Ranges

Adults: PO 1 or 2 capsules or tablets with meals or snacks

Children: PO 1 or 2 capsules or tablets with each meal initially, increased in amount or frequency if necessary and if adverse effects do not occur

Pancrelipase
Route and Dosage Ranges

Adults: PO 1 to 3 capsules or tablets before or with meals or snacks; or 1 or 2 packets of powder with meals or snacks

Nursing Process

Assessment

Assess each client for current or potential nutritional disorders. Some specific assessment factors include the following:
- What are usual drinking and eating patterns? Does fluid intake seem adequate? Does food intake seem adequate in terms of normal nutrition? Is the client financially able to purchase sufficient food? What are fluid and food likes and dislikes?
- Does the client know the basic foods for normal nutrition? Does the client view nutrition as important in maintaining health?
- Does the client appear overweight or underweight? How does current weight compare with the ideal weight for age and height?
- Does the client have symptoms, disease processes, treatment measures, medications, or diagnostic tests that are likely to interfere with nutrition? For example, many illnesses and oral medications cause anorexia, nausea, vomiting, and diarrhea.
- Are any conditions present that increase or decrease nutritional requirements?
- Check available reports of laboratory tests, such as serum proteins, complete blood count, and blood glucose. Nutritional disorders, as well as many other disorders, may cause abnormal values.

Nursing Diagnoses

- Altered Nutrition: Less Than Body Requirements related to inadequate intake
- Altered Nutrition: Less Than Body Requirements related to impaired ability to digest and absorb nutrients
- Altered Nutrition: More Than Body Requirements related to excessive intake
- Fluid Volume Deficit related to inadequate intake
- Fluid Volume Excess related to excessive intake
- Diarrhea related to enteral nutrition
- Altered Growth and Development related to nutrient deficiency
- Altered Protection related to nutrient deficiency
- Self-Care Deficit: Feeding
- Body Image Disturbance related to excessive weight loss or weight gain
- Knowledge Deficit: Normal nutrition
- Knowledge Deficit: Nutritional needs during illness
- Risk for Infection related to microbial contamination of enteral formulas
- Risk for Infection related to impaired tissue integrity with parenteral therapy

Planning/Goals

The client will:
- Improve nutritional status in relation to body needs
- Maintain fluid and electrolyte balance
- Avoid complications of enteral nutrition, including aspiration, diarrhea, fluid volume deficit or excess, and infection
- Avoid complications of parenteral nutrition, including fluid volume deficit or excess and infection
- Identify the types and amounts of foods to meet nutritional needs
- Avoid overuse and abuse of anorexiant drugs

Interventions

Implement measures to prevent nutritional disorders by promoting a well-balanced diet for all clients. Depending on the client's condition, diet orders, food preferences, knowledge and attitudes about nutrition, and other factors, specific activities may include the following:

- Provide food and fluid the client is willing and able to take, at preferred times when possible.
- Assist the client to a sitting position, cut meat, open containers, feed the client, and perform other actions if indicated.
- Treat symptoms or disorders that are likely to interfere with nutrition, such as pain, nausea, vomiting, or diarrhea.
- Consult with the physician or dietitian when needed, especially when special diets are ordered. Compliance is improved when the ordered diet differs as little as possible from the usual diet. Also, preferred foods often may be substituted for disliked ones.
- Promote exercise and activity. For the undernourished client, this may increase appetite, improve digestion, and aid bowel elimination. Exercise may decrease appetite and distract the overweight or obese client from hunger.
- Minimize the use of sedative-type drugs when appropriate. Although no one should be denied pain relief, strong analgesics and other sedatives may cause drowsiness and decreased desire or ability to eat and drink.
- Weigh clients at regular intervals.
- Use available resources to individualize nutritional care according to the client's clinical status and needs. For example, in hospitalized clients who are able to eat, consult a nutritionist about providing foods the client is able and willing to take. In hospitalized or outpatient clients who need a nutritional supplement, consult a nutritionist about choices, amounts, and costs.
- For clients receiving parenteral nutrition, monitor weight, fluid intake, urine output, vital signs, blood glucose, serum electrolytes, and other laboratory tests (*e.g.,* complete blood count, serum proteins) daily or weekly, according to the client's status and whether hospitalized or at home.

 Teach clients:

- The importance of nutrition in promoting health and recovery from illness
- The kinds and amounts of food and fluids needed for normal nutrition
- Ways of adapting restricted diets to increase their acceptability
- Benefits to be gained from nutritional agents, whether given orally, intravenously, or by tube feeding
- Benefits and techniques of weight control
- That anorexiant drugs should be combined with restricted calorie intake and increased exercise

Evaluation

- Observe the undernourished client for quantity and quality of nutrient intake, weight gain, and improvement in laboratory tests of nutritional status (*e.g.,* serum proteins, blood sugar, electrolytes).
- Observe the obese client for food intake, weight loss, and appropriate use of exercise or anorexiant drugs.
- Observe children for quantity and quality of food intake and appropriate increases in height and weight.
- Interview and observe for signs and symptoms of complications of enteral and parenteral nutrition.

Principles of Therapy

MANAGING FLUID DISORDERS

Fluid Deficiency

Treatment of fluid deficiency is aimed toward increasing intake or decreasing loss, depending on causative factors. The safest and most effective way of replacing body fluids is to give oral fluids when possible. Water is probably best, at least initially. Fluids containing large amounts of carbohydrate, fat, or protein are hypertonic and may increase fluid volume deficit if taken without sufficient water. If the client cannot take oral food or fluids for a few days or can take only limited amounts, IV fluids can be used to provide complete or supplemental amounts of fluids. Frequently used solutions include 5% dextrose in water or sodium chloride.

To meet fluid needs over a longer period, a nasogastric or other GI tube may be used to administer fluids. Fluid needs must be assessed carefully for the client receiving food and fluid only by tube. Additional water is needed after or between tube feedings. Another way of meeting long-term fluid needs when the GI tract cannot be used is parenteral nutrition. These IV solutions provide other nutrients as well as fluids.

Optimal amounts of fluid may vary greatly. For most clients, 2000 to 3000 ml daily is adequate. A person with severe heart failure or oliguric kidney disease needs smaller amounts, but someone with fever or extra losses (*e.g.,* vomiting, diarrhea) needs more.

Fluid Excess

Treatment of fluid excess is aimed toward decreasing intake and increasing loss. In acute circulatory overload or pulmonary edema, the usual treatment is to stop fluid intake (if the client is receiving IV fluids, slow the rate but keep the vein open for medication) and administer diuretics. Because fluid excess may be a life-threatening emergency, prevention is better than treatment.

MANAGING UNDERNUTRITION

Undernutrition impairs the function of essentially every body organ, impairs wound healing, and increases risks of infection. The goal of treatment is to provide an adequate quantity and quality of nutrients to meet tissue needs. Requirements for nutrients vary with age, level of activity, level of health or illness, and other factors that must be considered when designing appropriate therapy.

Oral Feedings

The safest and most effective way of increasing nutritional intake is by oral feedings when feasible. High-protein, high-calorie foods can be included in many diets and given as between-meal or bedtime snacks. If the client cannot ingest enough food and fluid, many of the commercial nutritional preparations can be given as between-meal supplements to increase intake of protein and calories. These preparations vary in taste and acceptability. Measures to improve taste may include chilling, serving over ice, or mixing with fruit juice or another beverage. Specific methods depend on the client's taste preferences and the available formulas. Refer to instructions, usually on the labels, for appropriate diluting and mixing of beverages.

Enteral (Tube) Feedings

When oral feeding is contraindicated but the GI tract is functioning, tube feeding has several advantages over IV fluids, especially for long-term use. First, tube feeding is usually safer, more convenient, and more economical. Second, it helps to prevent GI atrophy, maintain GI function, and maintain immune system function. Third, several tubes and placement sites are available. For example, a nasogastric tube may be used for about 4 weeks. For long-term feedings, a gastrostomy tube may be placed percutaneously (called percutaneous endoscopic gastrostomy tubes or PEG) or surgically. Nasointestinal tubes are recommended for clients at risk of aspiration from gastric feedings or with gastric disorders. Except for gastrostomy tubes, the tubes should be soft and small bore to decrease trauma.

When tube feedings are the client's only source of nutrients, they should be nutritionally complete and given in amounts calculated to provide adequate water, protein, calories, vitamins, and minerals. Although tube-feeding formulas vary in osmolality and volume needed for adequate intake of nutrients, any of the complete formulas can be used effectively. Other guidelines include the following:

1. Once the kind and amount of formula are chosen, the method of feeding is selected. For feedings that enter the stomach, an intermittent schedule of administration every 4 to 6 hours, over 30 to 60 minutes, is usually recommended. For feedings that enter the duodenum or jejunum, a continuous drip method is required because the small bowel cannot tolerate the larger volumes of intermittent feedings. Continuous feedings require an infusion pump for accurate control of the flow rate. When used at home, enteral feedings are often given overnight, to allow daytime oral feedings and more activity if feasible for the client.

2. A common practice has been to initiate feedings with small amounts of diluted solution (*i.e.,* half strength), then increase to larger amounts and full strength. The rationale is to decrease the diarrhea and dehydration that may ensue when hypertonic solutions are given, and water is drawn into the GI tract. Some authorities question the value of this regimen and prefer starting with small amounts of full-strength formulas. Isocal and Osmolite are isotonic and should be given full strength. Most formulas provide 1 kcal/ml so that caloric intake can be quickly calculated. Water can be given with, after, or between regular feedings and with medications, according to the client's fluid needs.

3. Other than problems resulting from hypertonic solutions and inadequate fluid intake (diarrhea, fluid volume deficit, hypernatremia), a major complication of tube feeding is aspiration of the formula into the lungs. This is more likely to occur with unconscious clients. It can be prevented by correctly positioning clients, verifying tube placement (before every intermittent feeding and about every 4 hours with continuous feedings), and giving feedings slowly.

Parenteral Feedings

Parenteral feedings are indicated when the GI tract is nonfunctioning; when enteral feedings would aggravate conditions such as inflammatory bowel diseases or pancreatitis; and when nutritional needs cannot be met by enteral feedings. For short-term use (about 3 to 5 days) of IV fluids, the goal is to provide adequate amounts of fluids and electrolytes and enough carbohydrate to minimize oxidation of body protein and fat for energy. Choice of specific solution depends on individual needs but should contain at least 5% dextrose. A frequently used solution is 5% dextrose in 0.22% sodium chloride, 2000 to 3000 ml/24 hours. Potassium chloride is often added, and vitamins may be added. These solutions are nutritionally inadequate.

Parenteral Nutrition

For long-term IV feedings (weeks to months), the goal is to provide all nutrients required for normal body functioning, including tissue growth. This goal can be met with parenteral nutrition. Basic nutritional solutions provide water, carbohydrate, protein, vitamins, and minerals. Originally, calories were supplied primarily by 25% to 50% glucose. This resulted in a hypertonic solution that had to be given in a central vein so it could be diluted rapidly. Although effective, central parenteral nutrition requires special techniques to increase safety and decrease complications. For example, a physician must insert the central IV catheter, and placement must be verified by a chest x-ray. Complications include air embolism and pneumothorax. Peripheral parenteral nutrition (PPN) was then developed. PPN, which contains 5% or 10% dextrose, can be given alone or in combination with oral or enteral feedings to increase nutrient intake.

IV fat emulsions provide additional calories and essential fatty acids. These solutions are isotonic and may be given centrally or peripherally. When given peripherally, they are coinfused with the PPN solution. The fat emulsion is thought to protect the vein and decrease or delay phlebitis.

Home administration of central parenteral nutrition and PPN is increasing. Guidelines for both methods include the following:

1. Administer with an infusion pump to control the flow rate accurately. The solution must be given at a consistent rate so nutrients can be used and complications prevented. The initial flow rate is usually 50 ml/h; flow rate is then increased as tolerated to meet nutritional requirements (about 1500 to 3000 ml/d). With home administration, the entire daily amount may be infused overnight.
2. To prevent infection, several measures are indicated. First, the IV catheter must be inserted with aseptic technique. Second, all solutions must be prepared aseptically in a pharmacy under a laminar flow hood. Third, use an 0.45- to 0.22-μm inline filter. Fourth, change solution containers and tubing every 24 hours. Fifth, change the dressing at the venipuncture site every 48 hours. Most hospitals and home health agencies have established protocols regarding dressing changes. These usually include cleansing around the catheter with povidone-iodine solution (Betadine), applying povidone-iodine ointment, and reapplying an occlusive dressing. Sterile technique is used throughout.
3. "Piggyback" fat emulsions into the IV line beyond the filter.

MANAGING OVERWEIGHT OR OBESITY

1. For effective weight loss and continued weight control, the main elements are decreasing caloric intake and increasing exercise (caloric output). This largely depends on the client's motivation and self-discipline in changing eating habits. This is very difficult for most people to do.
2. Many reduction diets and regimens have been proposed. Among the more successful programs are groups that meet regularly and offer psychological support and diet plans. Among the more radical treatments are surgical procedures that limit the amount of food and fluid that can be ingested.

3. Drug therapy is assuming an increasingly important role in the treatment of obesity. Recent studies indicate the drugs are effective as long as they are taken, but weight gain recurs when the drugs are stopped. Some clinicians are prescribing a combination of fenfluramine and phentermine for a year or longer. Dexfenfluramine (Redux) was the first anti-obesity drug approved by the FDA for many years. It decreases reuptake of serotonin in the brain. This action increases the amount of serotonin in brain centers that control hunger and decreases appetite. Although used up to a year in a clinical trial, most clinicians do not recommend its use longer than 3 months because of a potentially fatal adverse effect of pulmonary hypertension.
4. The role of the nurse may involve counseling about benefits to be gained from weight loss, the undesirability and hazards of "fad" diets, and specific ways of decreasing caloric intake, such as low-calorie snacks, participating in noneating activities, and not buying favorite high-calorie foods. Any program for weight control must be individualized, and continued support must be available.

NUTRITIONAL SUPPORT FOR CHILDREN

Children generally need increased amounts of water, protein, carbohydrate, and fat in proportion to their size to support growth and increased physical activity. However, reports of childhood obesity and inadequate exercise abound. Therefore, the goal of nutritional support is to meet needs without promoting obesity.

With tube feedings, to prevent nausea and regurgitation, the recommended rate of administration is no more than 5 ml every 5 to 10 minutes for premature and small infants and 10 ml/min for older infants and children. Preparation of formulas, positioning of children, and administration are the same as for adults to prevent aspiration, diarrhea, and infection.

Parenteral nutrition may be indicated in infants and children who cannot eat or be fed enterally. With newborns, especially preterm and low–birth-weight infants, parenteral nutrition is needed within about 3 days of birth because they have little nutritional reserve. However, lipid emulsions should be given very cautiously in preterm infants because deaths have been attributed to increased serum levels of lipids and free fatty acids. With other infants and children, parenteral nutrition may be used during medical illnesses or perioperative conditions to improve or maintain nutritional status. Overall, benefits include weight gain, increased height, increased liver synthesis of plasma proteins, and improved healing and recovery.

NUTRITIONAL SUPPORT FOR OLDER ADULTS

Older adults are at risk of developing deficits and excesses in fluid volume. Inadequate intake is common and may result from numerous causes (*e.g.,* impaired thirst mechanism, impaired ability to obtain and drink fluids, inadequate water with hyperosmolar tube feedings). Increased losses also occur with diuretic drugs, which are commonly prescribed for older adults. Fluid volume excess is most likely to occur with large amounts or rapid administration of IV fluids, especially in older adults with impaired cardiovascular function.

Older adults also are at risk of undernutrition and overnutrition in terms of protein, carbohydrate, and fat intake. Inadequate intake may result from the inability to obtain and prepare food, as well as disease processes that interfere with the ability to digest and use nutrients. When alternative feeding methods (tube feedings, IV fluids) are used, careful assessment of nutritional status is required to avoid deficits or excesses. Excessive intake may result from continuing usual eating patterns while exercising less. Caloric needs are usually decreased in older adults, primarily because of slowed metabolism and decreased physical activity. With the high incidence of atherosclerosis and cardiovascular disease in older adults, it is especially important that fat intake be reduced.

HOME CARE

The home care nurse is likely to be involved with nutritional matters in almost any home care setting. Because nutrition is so important to health, the home care nurse should take advantage of any opportunity for health promotion in this area. Health promotion may involve assessing the nutritional status of all members of the household, especially children, elderly adults, and those with obvious deficiencies or excesses, and providing counseling or other assistance to improve nutritional status. For clients receiving tube feedings at home, the home care nurse may teach about the goals of treatment, administration, preparation or storage of solutions, equipment (*e.g.,* obtaining, cleaning), and monitoring responses (*e.g.,* weight, urine output).

For clients receiving parenteral nutrition at home, solutions, infusion pumps, and other equipment are often obtained from a pharmacy, home health agency, or independent company. The home care nurse may not be involved in the initial setup but is likely to participate in ongoing client care, monitoring of client responses, and supporting caregivers. In addition, the home care nurse may need to coordinate activities among physicians, IV therapy personnel, and other health care providers.

| NURSING ACTIONS | NUTRITIONAL PRODUCTS AND ANOREXIANTS |

NURSING ACTIONS	RATIONALE/EXPLANATION
1. Administer accurately **a.** For oral supplemental feedings:	
(1) Give at the preferred time and temperature, when possible.	To increase the likelihood the feeding will be taken. Chilling the formula may increase palatability.
(2) Mix powders or concentrated liquid preparations in preferred beverages if not contraindicated.	Some can be mixed with fruit juice, milk, tea, or coffee, which may improve taste and acceptability.
(3) Provide flavoring packets when available and preferred by the client.	To improve taste and add variety.
b. For IV feedings:	
(1) Administer fluids at the prescribed flow rate. Use an infusion control device for hyperalimentation solutions.	To administer sufficient fluids without a rapid flow rate. Rapid flow rates or large amounts of IV fluids can cause circulatory overload and pulmonary edema. In addition, hyperglycemia and osmotic diuresis may occur with hyperalimentation solutions.
(2) With IV fat emulsions, connect to the primary IV line beyond the filter; start slowly (0.5–1 ml/min) for about 30 minutes. If no adverse effects occur, increase rate to a maximum of 125 ml/h for the 10% solution or 60 ml/h for a 20% solution.	Lipid emulsions should not be filtered.

(continued)

NURSING ACTIONS	RATIONALE/EXPLANATION
(3) Use sterile technique when changing containers, tubings, or dressings.	To prevent infection
(4) When adding drugs, use sterile technique, and add only those drugs known to be compatible with the IV solution.	To avoid physical or chemical incompatibility
(5) Do not administer antibiotics or other drugs through central venous catheters.	To avoid incompatibilities and possible precipitation or inactivation of the drug or fluid components
c. For tube feedings:	
(1) Have the client sitting, if possible.	To decrease risks of aspirating formula into lungs
(2) Check tube placement before each feeding by aspirating stomach contents or instilling air into the tube while listening over the stomach with a stethoscope.	To prevent aspiration or accidental instillation of feedings into lungs
(3) Give the solution at room temperature.	Cold formulas may cause abdominal cramping.
(4) If giving by intermittent instillation, do not give more than 500 ml per feeding, including water for rinsing the tube.	To avoid gastric distention, possible vomiting, and aspiration into lungs
(5) Give by gravity flow (over 30–60 minutes) or infusion pump.	Rapid administration may cause nausea, vomiting, and other symptoms.
(6) With continuous feedings, change containers and tubing daily. With intermittent bolus feedings, rinse all equipment after each use, and change at least every 24 hours.	Most tube feeding formulas are milk based and provide a good culture medium for bacterial growth. Clean technique, not sterile technique, is required.
(7) Give an adequate amount of water, based on assessment of fluid needs. This may be done by mixing water with the tube feeding formula, giving it after the tube feeding, or giving it between feedings.	To avoid dehydration and promote fluid balance. Most clients receiving 1500 to 2000 ml of tube feeding formula daily will need 1000 ml or more of water daily.
(8) Rinse nasogastric tubes with at least 50 to 100 ml water after each bolus feeding or administration of medications through the tube.	To keep the tube patent and functioning. This water is included in calculation of fluid intake.
(9) When medications are ordered by tube, liquid preparations are preferred over crushed tablets or powders emptied from capsules.	Tablets or powders may stick in the tube lumen. This may mean the full dose of the medication does not reach the stomach. Also, the tube is likely to become obstructed.
d. With pancreatic enzymes, give with meals or food.	To obtain therapeutic effects, these agents must be in the small intestine when food is present.
e. With anorexiant drugs:	
(1) Give single-dose drugs in the early morning.	For maximum appetite-suppressant effects during the day
(2) Give multiple-dose preparations 30 to 60 minutes before meals and the last dose of the day about 6 hours before bedtime.	For maximum appetite-suppressant effects at mealtime and to avoid interference with sleep from the drug's stimulating effects on the central nervous system (CNS)
2. Observe for therapeutic effects **a.** With water and other fluids, observe for fluid balance (amber-colored urine, about 1500 ml daily; moist mucous membranes in the oral cavity; adequate skin turgor).	
b. With nutritional formulas given orally or by tube feeding, observe for weight gain and increased serum albumin. For infants and children receiving milk substitutes, observe for decreased diarrhea and weight gain.	Therapeutic effects depend on the reason for use (*i.e.*, prevention or treatment of undernutrition).

NURSING ACTIONS	RATIONALE/EXPLANATION
c. With parenteral hyperalimentation, observe for weight maintenance or gain and normal serum levels of glucose, electrolytes, and protein.	These are indications of improved metabolism, nitrogen balance, and nutritional status. When parenteral hyperalimentation is used for gastrointestinal malabsorption syndromes, diarrhea and other symptoms are usually relieved when oral feedings are stopped.
d. With pancreatic enzymes, observe for decreased diarrhea and steatorrhea.	The pancreatic enzymes function the same way as endogenous enzymes to aid digestion of carbohydrate, protein, and fat.
e. With anorexiant drugs, observe for decreased caloric intake and weight loss.	The recommended rate of weight loss is about 2 to 3 lb weekly.
3. Observe for adverse effects a. With fluids, observe for peripheral edema, circulatory overload, and pulmonary edema (severe dyspnea, crackles).	Fluid excess is most likely to occur with rapid administration or large amounts of IV fluids, especially in people who are elderly or have congestive heart failure.
b. With commercial nutritional formulas (except Osmolite and Isocal), observe for hypotension, tachycardia, increased urine output, dehydration, nausea, vomiting, or diarrhea.	These adverse reactions are usually attributed to the hyperosmolality or hypertonicity of the preparations. They can be prevented or minimized by starting with small amounts of formula, given slowly.
c. With parenteral hyperalimentation, observe for elevated blood and urine glucose levels, signs of infection (fever, inflammation at the venipuncture site), concentrated urine of high specific gravity (1.035 or above), hypertension, dyspnea.	These signs and symptoms indicate complications of therapy. Except for infection, they are likely to occur when the solution is given in a concentration or at a rate that delivers more glucose than can be used. This produces hyperglycemia, which in turn causes excessive amounts of fluid to be excreted in the urine (osmotic diuresis). Hyperglycemic, hyperosmolar, nonketotic coma also may occur.
d. With IV fat emulsions, observe for signs of fat embolism (dyspnea, fever, chills, pain in the chest and back), phlebitis from vein irritation, and sepsis from contamination. Hyperlipidemia and hepatomegaly also may occur.	Thrombophlebitis and sepsis are the most frequent adverse effects.
e. With anorexiant drugs, observe for:	
(1) Nervousness, insomnia, hyperactivity	These adverse effects are caused by excessive stimulation of the CNS. They are more likely to occur with large doses or too frequent administration.
(2) Hypertension	Anorexiant drugs stimulate the sympathetic nervous system and may cause or aggravate hypertension.
(3) Development of tolerance to appetite-suppressant effects	This usually occurs within 4 to 6 weeks and is an indication for discontinuing drug administration. Continued administration does not maintain appetite-suppressant effects but increases incidence of adverse effects. In addition, taking large doses of the drug does not restore appetite-suppressant effects.
(4) Signs of psychological drug dependence	More likely with large doses or long-term use
(5) With fenfluramine, observe for drowsiness during use and mental depression when the drug is discontinued.	Fenfluramine causes CNS depression rather than the stimulation that occurs with other anorexiant drugs.

(continued)

NURSING ACTIONS | *RATIONALE/EXPLANATION*

4. Observe for drug interactions with anorexiants
  a. Drugs that *increase* effects:

    (1) Alkalinizing agents (*e.g.,* sodium bicarbonate)

                Potentiate anorexiants by increasing gastrointestinal absorption and decreasing urinary excretion

    (2) Antidepressants, tricyclic

                May increase hypertensive effects of anorexiants

    (3) Monoamine oxidase (MAO) inhibitors

                Increase hypertensive effects. Anorexiants should not be given within 2 weeks of MAO inhibitors because of possible hypertensive crisis.

    (4) Other CNS stimulants

                Additive stimulant effects

    (5) Other sympathomimetic drugs (*e.g.,* epinephrine, isoproterenol)

                Additive hypertensive and other cardiovascular effects

  b. Drugs that *decrease* effects:

    (1) Acidifying agents (*e.g.,* ascorbic acid)

                Decrease gastrointestinal absorption and increase urinary excretion

    (2) Antihypertensive drugs

                Anorexiants have blood pressure-raising effects that antagonize blood pressure-lowering effects of drugs used for hypertension

    (3) CNS depressants (*e.g.,* alcohol, chlorpromazine)

                  Antagonize or decrease effects

5. Teach clients
  a. Most intravenous fluids are nutritionally inadequate and useful only for short-term treatment. Thus, return to oral feedings is desirable as soon as tolerated after surgery or illness.

  b. Take pancreatic enzymes with food.

                To obtain the therapeutic benefit of increased digestion and absorption of foods

  c. Take anorexiants in the dosage and for the length of time prescribed.

                Excessive dosage will cause potentially serious adverse reactions. These drugs lose their appetite-deppressant effects in 4 to 6 weeks. Prolonged use may lead to psychological dependence.

REVIEW AND APPLICATION EXERCISES

1. How does an adequate fluid balance help to maintain normal body functioning?

2. Differentiate clients who are at high risk of developing fluid imbalances.

3. When assessing a client's fluid balance, what signs and symptoms indicate fluid volume deficit or excess?

4. What are pharmacologic and nonpharmacologic interventions to restore fluid balance when an imbalance occurs?

5. For clients who are unable to ingest food, which nutrients can be provided with IV nutritional formulas?

6. How do peripheral IV nutritional formulas differ from those that must be given with a "deep line"?

7. What is the role of lipid emulsions in parenteral nutrition?

8. In an infant receiving parenteral nutrition, what is the best way to assess the adequacy of nutritional status?

9. In an outpatient or home care client with a protein-calorie deficit and various commercial nutritional supplements or replacement formulas:
    Analyze the types and amounts of nutrients provided.
    Choose a supplement to recommend to the client or caregiver.

Designate the amount to be taken daily for optimum nutritional status.

Suggest ways to increase palatability and client ingestion of the nutrients.

10. With an obese client who requests anorexiant drugs to assist with weight loss, discuss the advantages and disadvantages of drug therapy versus nonpharmacologic weight loss measures.

SELECTED REFERENCES

Chessman, K.H., & Anderson, J.D. (1997). Pediatric and geriatric nutrition support. In J.T. DiPiro, R.L. Talbert, G.C. Yee, G.R. Matzke, B.G. Wells, & L.M. Posey (Eds.), *Pharmacotherapy: A pathophysiologic approach*, 3rd ed., pp. 2787–2804. Stamford, CT: Appleton & Lange.

Corman, L.C. (1993). The role of nutrition in sickness and in health. *Medical Clinics of North America, 77*(4), 711–724.

Darby, M.K., & Loughead, J.L. (1996). Neonatal nutritional requirements and formula composition: A review. *Journal of Obstetrics, Gynecology, and Neonatal Nursing, 25*(3), 209–217.

Davis, J.R., & Sherer, K. (1994). *Applied nutrition and diet therapy for nurses*, 2nd ed. Philadelphia: W.B. Saunders.

Drug facts and comparisons. (Updated monthly). St. Louis: Facts and Comparisons.

Janson, D.D. (1997). Enteral nutrition. In J.T. DiPiro, R.L. Talbert, G.C. Yee, G.R. Matzke, B.G. Wells, & L.M. Posey (Eds.), *Pharmacotherapy: A pathophysiologic approach*, 3rd ed., pp. 2759–2785. Stamford, CT: Appleton & Lange.

Mattox, T.W. (1997). Parenteral nutrition. In J.T. DiPiro, R.L. Talbert, G.C. Yee, G.R. Matzke, B.G. Wells, & L.M. Posey (Eds.), *Pharmacotherapy: A pathophysiologic approach*, 3rd ed., pp. 2735–2758). Stamford, CT: Appleton & Lange.

Morrissey, N.A. (1996). Gastrointestinal intubation and special nutritional management. In S.C. Smeltzer & B.G. Bare, *Brunner and Suddarth's textbook of medical-surgical nursing*, 8th ed., pp. 859–883. Philadelphia: Lippincott-Raven.

Pleuss, J. (1994). Alterations in nutritional status. In C.M. Porth (Ed.), *Pathophysiology: Concepts of altered health states*, 3rd ed., pp. 873–895. Philadelphia: J.B. Lippincott.

Stenson, W.F. & Eisenberg, P. (1997). Parenteral and enteral nutrition. In W.N. Kelley (Ed.), *Textbook of internal medicine*, 3rd ed., pp. 890–902. Philadelphia: Lippincott-Raven.

Stunkard, A.J. & Wadden, T.A. (1997). Obesity. In W.N. Kelley (Ed.), *Textbook of internal medicine*, 3rd ed., pp. 192–198. Philadelphia: Lippincott-Raven.

Wallace, J.I. & Schwartz, R.S. (1997). Geriatric clinical nutrition including malnutrition and cachexia. In W.N. Kelley (Ed.), *Textbook of internal medicine*, 3rd ed., pp. 2554–2560. Philadelphia: Lippincott-Raven.

Williams, L., Davis, J.A., & Lowenthal, D.T. (1993). The influence of food on the absorption and metabolism of drugs. *Medical Clinics of North America, 77*(4), 815–829.

Vitamins

Objectives

After studying this chapter, the student will be able to:

1 Review functions and food sources of essential vitamins.

2 Differentiate between maintenance and therapeutic doses of vitamins.

3 Identify clients at risk of developing vitamin deficiency or excess.

4 Delineate circumstances in which therapeutic vitamins are likely to be needed.

5 Describe adverse effects associated with overdose of fat-soluble and selected water-soluble vitamins.

6 Discuss the rationale for administering vitamin K to newborns.

Key Terms

Coenzyme

Fat-soluble vitamins

Megadose

Megaloblastic anemia

Pernicious anemia

Vitamin deficiencies

Vitamin excesses

Water-soluble vitamins

Description and Uses

Vitamins are a group of substances necessary for normal body metabolism of fat, carbohydrate, and protein. They act mainly as coenzymes to help convert carbohydrate and fat into energy and form bones and tissues. These compounds vary greatly in chemical structure and function. They are effective in small amounts and are normally obtained from foods. Vitamins are usually classified as fat soluble (A, D, E, K) and water soluble (B complex, C). Fat-soluble vitamins are absorbed from the intestine with dietary fat, and absorption requires the presence of bile salts and pancreatic lipase. These vitamins are relatively stable in cooking. Water-soluble vitamins are readily absorbed but are also readily lost by improper cooking and storage. Vitamin D is discussed in Chapter 26 because of its major role in bone metabolism.

Table 31-1 summarizes the characteristics, functions, food sources, and recommended amounts of vitamins. The recommended dietary allowances (RDAs) were established by the Food and Nutrition Board of the National Academy of Sciences for daily intake by healthy adults and children and are periodically revised according to newer information. When inadequate amounts of vitamins are ingested, vitamin deficiencies result. Deficiency states are uncommon in people who can eat and are generally healthy. They are more likely to occur with disease processes that interfere with absorption or use of vitamins. When excessive amounts of fat-soluble vitamins are taken, excess states may occur because fat-soluble vitamins accumulate in the body. Excess states do not occur with dietary intake of water-soluble vitamins because these vitamins are rapidly excreted in the urine. Causes and clinical manifestations of vitamin disorders are listed in Table 31-2.

TABLE 31-1 VITAMINS AS NUTRIENTS

	Characteristics	Functions	Recommended Dietary Allowances (RDAs)	Dietary Sources
Fat-Soluble Vitamins				
Vitamin A (Retinol)	1. Obtained from animal foods and plant foods that contain carotenoids (precursors of vitamin A) 2. About one third of carotenoids are absorbed, and they become active in body functioning only after conversion to retinol in the wall of the small intestine. 3. Retinol, another name for preformed vitamin A, is the physiologically active form. 4. Vitamin A activity is expressed in retinol equivalents (RE), which include both preformed vitamin A and carotenoids. 1 RE = 1 µg retinol or 6 µg beta-carotene.	Required for normal vision, growth, bone development, skin, and mucous membrane	Women: 800 RE (4000 IU) Men: 1000 RE (5000 IU) Pregnant women: 1000 RE (5000 IU) Lactating women: 1200 RE (6000 IU) Children 1–10 years: 400–700 RE (2000–3500 IU); 11 years and older: same as adults	Preformed vitamin A—meat, butter and fortified margarine, egg yolk, whole milk, cheese made from whole milk Carotenoids—turnip and collard greens, carrots, sweet potatoes, squash, apricots, peaches, cantaloupe
Vitamin E	1. A group of substances called tocopherols, of which alpha-tocopherol is most biologically active	It is thought to act as an antioxidant in preventing destruction of certain fats, including the lipid	Women: 8 mg alpha TE Men: 10 mg alpha TE Children up to 10 years: 3–7 mg alpha	Cereals, green vegetables, egg yolk, milk fat, butter, meat, vegetable oils

(continued)

| TABLE 31-1 | VITAMINS AS NUTRIENTS (Continued) |

	Characteristics	Functions	Recommended Dietary Allowances (RDAs)	Dietary Sources
	2. Vitamin E activity is expressed in milligrams of alpha-tocopherol equivalents (alpha TE).	portion of cell membranes. It also may increase absorption, hepatic storage, and use of vitamin A.	TE; 11 years and older, same as adults	
Vitamin K	1. Occurs naturally in two forms: phytonadione (K$_1$), found in plant foods, and menaquinone (K$_2$), synthesized in the intestine by bacteria 2. Absorbed mainly from the upper intestine in the presence of bile and dietary fats	Essential for normal blood clotting. Activates precursor proteins, found in the liver, into clotting factors: prothrombin (factor II), proconvertin (factor VII), plasma thromboplastin component (factor IX), and Stuart factor (factor X)	1 μg/kg	Green leafy vegetables (spinach, kale, cabbage, lettuce), cauliflower, tomatoes, wheat bran, cheese, egg yolk, liver
Vitamin D	See Chapter 26.			
Water-Soluble Vitamins				
B-Complex Vitamins **Biotin**	Must be obtained from dietary intake. There is also some synthesis by intestinal bacteria, and a portion is absorbed.	Essential in fat and carbohydrate metabolism	Not established; provisionally set at 30–100 μg	Meat, especially liver, egg yolk, nuts, cereals; most vegetables
Cyanocobalamin (vitamin B$_{12}$)	In addition to food sources, some is also obtained from tissue storage in the liver and from recovery of cyanocobalamin secreted in bile and reabsorbed in the small intestine.	Essential for normal metabolism of all body cells (especially those of the bone marrow, nervous tissue, and gastrointestinal tract); normal red blood cells; growth; and metabolism of carbohydrate, protein, and fat	Adults: 2 μg Children: 0.7–1.4 μg Infants: 0.3–0.5 μg	Meat, especially liver, eggs, fish, cheese
Folic acid (folate)	1. Obtained from foods and the enterohepatic cycle. The latter provides an endogenous source, because folate is excreted in bile, reabsorbed in the small bowel, and reused. 2. May be lost from vegetables stored at room temperature or cooked at high temperatures.	Essential for normal metabolism of all body cells, for normal red blood cells, and for growth	Women: 180 μg Men: 200 μg Pregnant women or sexually active women of child-bearing age: 400 μg Lactating women: 260–280 μg Children, 1–10 years: 50–100 μg; 11–14 years, 150 μg Infants: 25–35 μg	Liver, kidney beans, fresh green vegetables (spinach, broccoli, asparagus)

TABLE 31-1   **VITAMINS AS NUTRIENTS** (Continued)

	Characteristics	Functions	Recommended Dietary Allowances (RDAs)	Dietary Sources
Niacin (vitamin B$_3$)	1. Obtained from food and endogenous synthesis from tryptophan. 2. Niacin activity is expressed in niacin equivalents (NE): 1 mg of niacin or 60 mg tryptophan = 1 NE.	Essential for glycolysis, fat synthesis, and tissue respiration. It functions as a coenzyme in many metabolic processes (after conversion to nicotinamide, the physiologically active form).	Women: 15 NE Men: 20 NE Pregnant women: 17 NE Lactating women: 20 NE Children, 1–10 years: 9–13 NE Males, 11–14 years: 17 NE; females, 11–14 years, 15 NE Infants: 5–6 NE	Meat, poultry, fish, peanuts
Pantothenic acid (vitamin B$_5$)		A component of coenzyme A and essential for cellular metabolism (intermediary metabolism of carbohydrate, fat, and protein; release of energy from carbohydrate; fatty acid metabolism; synthesis of cholesterol, steroid hormones, phospholipids, and porphyrin)	Not established. Estimated at 4–7 mg.	Eggs, liver, salmon, yeast, cauliflower, broccoli, lean beef, potatoes, tomatoes
Pyridoxine (vitamin B$_6$)	Occurs in three forms (pyridoxal, pyridoxine, and pyridoxamine), all of which are converted in the body to pyridoxal phosphate, the physiologically active form.	1. Serves as a coenzyme in many metabolic processes 2. Functions in metabolism of carbohydrate, protein, and fat 3. Required for formation of tryptophan and conversion of tryptophan to niacin 4. As part of the enzyme phosphorylase, helps release glycogen from the liver and muscle tissue 5. Functions in metabolism of the central nervous system 6. Helps maintain cellular immunity	Women: 1.6 mg Men: 2 mg Pregnant women: 2.2 mg Lactating women: 2.1 mg Children, 1–10 years: 1–1.4 mg Males, 11–14 years, 1.7 mg; females 11–14 years, 1.4 mg Infants: 0.3–0.6 mg	Yeast, wheat germ, liver and other glandular meats, whole grain cereals, potatoes, legumes
Riboflavin (vitamin B$_2$)		1. Serves as a coenzyme in metabolism	Women: 1.3 mg Men: 1.7 mg	Milk, cheddar and cottage cheese,

(continued)

			Recommended Dietary Allowances (RDAs)	Dietary Sources

TABLE 31-1   VITAMINS AS NUTRIENTS (Continued)

	Characteristics	Functions	Recommended Dietary Allowances (RDAs)	Dietary Sources
		2. Necessary for growth 3. May function in production of corticosteroids and red blood cells and gluconeogenesis	Pregnant women: 1.6 mg Lactating women: 1.7 mg Children, 1–10 years: 0.8–1.2 mg Males, 11–14 years: 1.5 mg; females, 11–14 years, 1.3 mg Infants: 0.4–0.5 mg	meat, eggs, green leafy vegetables
Thiamine (vitamin B₁)		A coenzyme in carbohydrate metabolism and essential for energy production	Women: 1.1 mg Men: 1.5 mg Pregnant women: 1.5 mg Lactating women: 1.6 mg Children, 1–10 years: 0.7–1 mg Males, 11–14 years, 1.3 mg; females, 11–14 years, 1.1 mg Infants: 0.3–0.4 mg	Meat, poultry, fish, egg yolk, dried beans, whole grain cereal products, peanuts
Vitamin C				
Vitamin C (ascorbic acid)	1. Dietary vitamin C is well absorbed from the intestinal tract and distributed widely in body tissues. 2. Not stored in body to a significant extent. Once tissues are saturated with about 1500 mg, any excess is excreted in the urine.	1. Essential for collagen formation (collagen is a fibrous protein in connective tissue throughout the body, including skin, ligaments, cartilage, bone, and teeth) 2. Required for wound healing and tissue repair, metabolism of iron and folic acid, synthesis of fats and proteins, preservation of blood vessel integrity, and resistance to infection	Adults: 60 mg Pregnant women: 70 mg Lactating women: 90–95 mg Children, infancy–14 years: 30–50 mg; 15 years and older, 60 mg	Fruits and vegetables, especially citrus fruits and juices

PRESCRIPTION VITAMINS

Vitamins prescribed by health care providers to prevent or treat deficiencies exert the same physiologic effects as those obtained from foods. Synthetic vitamins have the same structure and function as natural vitamins derived from plant and animal sources. There is no evidence that natural vitamins are superior to synthetic vitamins. Natural vitamins are usually much more expensive.

NONPRESCRIPTION VITAMINS

There are many commercially available vitamin preparations; some contain a single vitamin, and some contain multiple vitamins. The only clear-cut indications for use of these products are prevention and treatment of vitamin deficiencies. Because vitamins are essential nutrients, some people believe that large doses (megadoses)

(*text continues on page 401*)

TABLE 31-2   VITAMIN IMBALANCES

	Deficiency States		Excess States	
	Causes	*Signs and Symptoms*	*Causes*	*Signs and Symptoms*

Fat-Soluble Vitamins

Vitamin A

Deficiency States — Causes: Rarely caused by inadequate dietary intake in the United States; usually occurs with disease processes that interfere with intake, absorption, or use. Absorption is decreased with a lack of dietary fat or bile salts (from biliary tract obstruction), inflammatory gastrointestinal (GI) conditions, and other conditions characterized by malabsorption and diarrhea. Hepatitis or hepatic cirrhosis may prevent liver storage of vitamin A.

Deficiency States — Signs and Symptoms: Night blindness Xerophthalmia, which may progress to corneal ulceration and blindness Changes in skin and mucous membranes that lead to skin lesions and infections, respiratory tract infections, and urinary calculi

Excess States — Causes: Excessive intake of vitamin A, which is unlikely with dietary intake but can occur with overuse of vitamin A supplements

Excess States — Signs and Symptoms: Anorexia Vomiting Irritability Headache Skin changes (dryness, itching, desquamation, dermatitis) Later manifestations may include fatigue, pain in muscles, bones, and joints, gingivitis, enlargement of spleen and liver, altered liver function, increased intracranial pressure, and other neurologic signs. Congenital abnormalities may occur in newborns whose mothers took excessive vitamin A during pregnancy. Acute toxicity, with increased intracranial pressure, bulging fontanels, and vomiting, may occur in infants who are given vitamin A. Plasma retinol levels above 100 μg/dl

Vitamin E

Deficiency States — Causes: Deficiency is rare.

Excess States — Causes: Excessive intake of vitamin E, which is rare with dietary intake but can occur with overuse of vitamin E supplements

Excess States — Signs and Symptoms: Fatigue, nausea, headache, blurred vision, diarrhea

Vitamin K

Deficiency States — Causes: Inadequate intake, absorption, or use. Rarely caused by inadequate intake after infancy. Occurs commonly in newborns owing to lack of dietary intake of vitamin K and lack of intestinal synthesis of the vitamin during the first week of life. After infancy, defi-

Deficiency States — Signs and Symptoms: Abnormal bleeding (melena, hematemesis, hematuria, epistaxis, petechiae, ecchymoses, hypovolemic shock)

Excess States — Causes: Unlikely to occur from dietary intake; may occur when vitamin K is given as an antidote for oral anticoagulants

Excess States — Signs and Symptoms: Clinical manifestations rarely occur. However, when vitamin K is given to someone who is receiving warfarin (Coumadin), the client can be made "warfarin-resistant" for 2–3 wk.

(continued)

TABLE 31-2	VITAMIN IMBALANCES (CONTINUED)			
	Deficiency States		**Excess States**	
	Causes	*Signs and Symptoms*	*Causes*	*Signs and Symptoms*
	ciency usually results from diseases that interfere with absorption (biliary tract and GI disorders) or use (hepatic cirrhosis and hepatitis). In alcoholics, deficiency commonly occurs and probably results from decreased intake and impaired use. Drug-induced deficiency occurs with oral coumarin anticoagulants and some other drugs that act as vitamin K antagonists. Also, antibiotics reduce bacterial synthesis of vitamin K in the intestine, but this is a rare cause of deficiency.			
Vitamin D	See Chapter 26.			
Water-Soluble Vitamins			Megadoses of pharmaceutical vitamin supplements	Signs and symptoms of excess states not established for most water-soluble vitamins
Biotin	Inadequate intake or impaired absorption. Biotin deficiency is rare.	Anorexia Nausea Depression Muscle pain Dermatitis		
Cyanocobalamin (vitamin B$_{12}$)	Usually impaired absorption from a lack of hydrochloric acid or intrinsic factor in the stomach	Megaloblastic or pernicious anemia: 1. Decreased numbers of red blood cells (RBC) 2. Abnormally large, immature RBC 3. Fatigue 4. Dyspnea 5. With severe deficiency, leukopenia, thrombocytopenia, cardiac arrhythmias, heart failure, or infections may occur.		

		Neurologic signs and symptoms: 1. Paresthesias in hands and feet 2. Unsteady gait 3. Depressed deep-tendon reflexes 4. With severe deficiency, loss of memory, confusion, delusions, hallucinations, and psychosis may occur. Nerve damage may be irreversible.	
Folic acid	Inadequate diet Impaired absorption (intestinal disorders) Greatly increased requirements (pregnancy, lactation, hemolytic anemias) Ingestion of folate antagonist drugs (*e.g.,* methotrexate) Alcoholism is a common cause. It interferes with intake and absorption.	Megaloblastic anemia that cannot be distinguished from the anemia produced by B_{12} deficiency Impaired growth in children Glossitis GI problems (folic acid deficiency does not produce neurologic signs and symptoms as B_{12} deficiency does)	
Niacin (vitamin B_3)	Inadequate diet or impaired absorption	Pellagra: 1. Erythematous skin lesions 2. GI problems (stomatitis, glossitis, enteritis, diarrhea) 3. CNS problems (headache, dizziness, insomnia, depression, memory loss) 4. With severe deficiency, delusions, hallucinations, and impairment of peripheral motor and sensory nerves may occur.	Large doses (2–6 g daily) used to treat hyperlipidemia Flushing, pruritus, hyperglycemia, hyperuricemia, increased liver enzymes
Pantothenic acid (vitamin B_5)	No deficiency state established		
Pyridoxine (vitamin B_6)	Inadequate intake or impaired absorption	1. Skin and mucous membrane lesions (seborrheic dermatitis, intertrigo, glossitis, stomatitis) 2. Neurologic problems (convulsions, peripheral neuritis, mental depression)	

(continued)

TABLE 31-2   VITAMIN IMBALANCES (CONTINUED)

	Deficiency States		Excess States	
	Causes	Signs and Symptoms	Causes	Signs and Symptoms
Riboflavin (vitamin B$_2$)	Inadequate intake or impaired absorption. Uncommon and usually occurs with deficiencies of other B-complex vitamins	Glossitis and stomatitis Seborrheic dermatitis Eye disorders (burning, itching, lacrimation, photophobia, vascularization of the cornea)		
Thiamine (vitamin B$_1$)	Inadequate diet, especially among pregnant women and infants; impaired absorption due to GI disorders Alcoholism	Mild deficiency—fatigue, anorexia, retarded growth, mental depression, irritability, apathy, lethargy Severe deficiency (beriberi)—peripheral neuritis, personality disturbances, heart failure, edema, Wernicke–Korsakoff syndrome in alcoholics		
Vitamin C (ascorbic acid)	Inadequate dietary intake (most likely in infants, older adults, indigent people, and alcoholics) Increased requirements (people who smoke cigarettes, take oral contraceptives, or have acute or chronic illness) Megadoses that are abruptly discontinued may cause a rebound deficiency. Deficiency also may occur in infants whose mothers took megadoses during pregnancy.	1. Mild deficiency—irritability, malaise, arthralgia, increased tendency to bleed 2. Severe deficiency—scurvy and adverse effects on most body tissues (gingivitis; bleeding of gums, skin, joints, and other areas; disturbances of bone growth; anemia; and loosening of teeth). If not treated, coma and death may occur.	Megadoses may produce excessive amounts of oxalate in the urine.	Renal calculi

promote health and provide other beneficial effects. There is no evidence that amounts beyond those needed for normal body functioning serve any beneficial effects; excessive intake of vitamins causes harmful effects. Thus, "megavitamins" should never be self-prescribed.

Many multivitamin preparations do not require a physician's prescription. These preparations vary widely in number, type, and amount of specific ingredients. Although useful in certain situations, they cannot be used interchangeably or indiscriminately with safety. More specific characteristics include the following:

1. Preparations promoted for use as dietary supplements may contain 50% of the amounts recommended for daily intake. In healthy people who eat a well-balanced diet, nutrient needs may be greatly exceeded.

2. Preparations for therapeutic use may contain 300% to 500% of the amounts recommended for daily intake in normal circumstances. These should not contain more than recommended amounts of vitamin D, folic acid, and vitamin A.

3. Multivitamin preparations often contain minerals as well, usually in amounts much smaller than those recommended for daily intake.

Individual vitamin preparations are listed in Table 31-3.

TABLE 31-3 VITAMIN DRUG PREPARATIONS

Generic/Trade Name	Routes and Dosage Ranges
Fat-Soluble Vitamins	
Vitamin A (Aquasol A)	Adults with severe deficiency: PO 100,000–500,000 U daily for 3 d, then 50,000 U daily for 2 wk, then 10,000–20,000 U daily for another 2 mo. IM 50,000–100,000 U daily for 3 d, then 50,000 U daily for 2 wk
	Children over 8 years with severe deficiency: PO, IM, same as adults
	Infants and children under 8 years: 10,000–15,000 U daily for 10 d
Vitamin E (Aquasol E)	Adults: PO, IM 60–100 U daily
	Children: PO, IM 25–60 U daily
Vitamin K	Adults and children: PO, IM 5–15 mg daily
Menadione sodium diphosphate (Synkayvite)	Adults: PO 5–10 mg daily; SC, IM, IV 5–15 mg daily
	Children: PO, SC, IM, IV 5–10 mg daily
Phytonadione (Mephyton, Aqua-Mephyton)	Adults and children: PO, SC, IM 2.5–25 mg daily
	Newborns: IV, IM 0.5–2 mg immediately after birth to *prevent* hemorrhagic disease of neonates; 1–2 mg daily to *treat* hemorrhagic disease
Water-Soluble Vitamins	
B-Complex Vitamins	
Calcium pantothenate (B$_5$)	Adults: PO 10–20 mg daily
Cyanocobalamin (B$_{12}$) (Rubramin)	Adults and children: PO 10–250 µg daily for 1 mo in an oral therapeutic multivitamin preparation when deficiency is due to increased requirements and gastrointestinal absorption is normal
	IM, SC, IV 30 µg daily for 5–10 d, then 100–200 µg monthly
Folic acid (Folvite)	Adults and children: PO, SC, IM, IV up to 1 mg daily until symptoms decrease and blood tests are normal, then maintenance dose of 0.1–0.25 mg daily
Niacin (nicotinic acid), **niacinamide** (nicotinamide)	Deficiency, PO, IM, IV 50–100 mg daily
	Pellagra, 500 mg daily
	Hyperlipidemia, 2–6 g daily
Pyridoxine (B$_6$)	Deficiency, PO, IM, IV 10–20 mg daily for 3 wk, then 2–5 mg daily
	Anemia, peripheral neuritis, 100–200 mg daily
	Pyridoxine dependency syndrome, up to 600 mg daily
Riboflavin	PO 5–25 mg daily
Thiamine (B$_1$)	PO 10–30 mg daily; IM 10–20 mg three times daily for 2 wk, supplemented with 5–10 mg orally; IV 100–200 mg
Vitamin C	
Vitamin C (ascorbic acid)	Deficiency, PO, IM, IV 100–500 mg daily
	Scurvy, 300–1000 mg daily for at least 2 wk
	Infants receiving formula, 35–50 mg daily for first few weeks of life
	Urinary acidification, 4–12 g daily in divided doses every 4 h
	Prophylaxis, 50–100 mg daily

Nursing Process

Assessment

Assess each client for current or potential vitamin disorders during an overall assessment of nutritional status. Specific assessment factors related to vitamins include the following:

- Deficiency states are more common than excess states.
- People with other nutritional deficiencies are likely to have vitamin deficiencies as well.
- Deficiencies of water-soluble vitamins (B complex and C) are more common than those of fat-soluble vitamins.
- Vitamin deficiencies are usually multiple, and signs and symptoms often overlap, especially with B-complex deficiency states.
- Vitamin requirements are generally increased during infancy, pregnancy, lactation, fever, hyperthyroidism, and probably most illnesses. Thus, a vitamin intake that is normally adequate may become inadequate in certain circumstances.
- Vitamin deficiencies are likely to occur in people who are poor, elderly, chronically or severely ill, or alcoholic.
- Vitamin excess states are uncommonly caused by excessive dietary intake but may occur with use of vitamin drug preparations, especially if megadoses are taken.

Nursing Diagnoses

- Altered Nutrition: Less Than Body Requirements related to vitamin deficiency
- Altered Nutrition: More Than Body Requirements related to vitamin excess with overuse of supplements
- Risk for Injury related to vitamin deficiency or overdose
- Knowledge Deficit: Importance of adequate vitamin intake in normal body functioning
- Knowledge Deficit: Dietary sources of various vitamins
- Knowledge Deficit: Adverse effects of self-prescribed megadoses of vitamins

Planning/Goals

The client will:
- Ingest appropriate amounts and sources of dietary vitamins
- Avoid megadoses of vitamin supplements
- Avoid symptoms of vitamin deficiency or overdose

Interventions

Implement measures to prevent vitamin disorders; the safest and most effective way to prevent vitamin deficiencies is by increasing dietary intake of vitamins:

- A well-balanced, varied diet that is adequate in proteins and calories is adequate in vitamins for most people. Exceptions are those who have increased requirements or conditions that interfere with absorption or use of vitamins.
- Water-soluble vitamins are often destroyed by cooking or discarded in cooking water. Eating raw fruits and vegetables prevents loss of vitamins during cooking. When fruits and vegetables are cooked, vitamin losses can be minimized by using small amounts of water, steaming or pressure cooking for the shortest effective time, and keeping cooking utensils covered.

  In addition to cooking losses, vitamin C is lost with exposure of foods to air. Consequently, fruits and vegetables, including juices, should be kept covered during storage.

- When vitamin deficiency stems from inadequate dietary intake, correcting the diet is preferred over administering supplemental vitamins when feasible. For vitamin A deficiency, increasing daily intake of plant and animal sources may be sufficient. For vitamin C deficiency, citrus juices can be used therapeutically. Because about 4 oz of orange juice daily meets requirements, larger amounts can relieve deficiency. When folic acid deficiency anemia stems from dietary lack, one fresh, uncooked fruit or vegetable or one glass of fruit juice added to the daily diet will probably correct the deficiency (except during pregnancy, when folate requirements are increased).
- Even when vitamin supplements are considered necessary, dietary sources should be increased for immediate and long-term benefit.
- Clients receiving only intravenous (IV) fluids or a clear liquid diet for more than 2 or 3 days probably need replacement vitamins.

  When requirements are increased or absorption is decreased, vitamins may be needed as dietary supplements to prevent deficiencies. Vitamin preparations must be chosen carefully because they differ widely in the specific vitamins contained and in the amounts of each. Their use should be based on recommended amounts after assessing eating habits and the usual dietary supply of vitamins.

  Some oral multivitamin preparations considered appropriate for supplemental use are Adeflor, Poly-Vi-Flor, Poly-Vi-Sol, Tri-Vi-Flor, Tri-Vi-Sol, and Vi-Daylin for children and Dayalets for adults. These contain less than 150% of the RDA for all ingredients. Preparations containing fluoride require a prescription.

 Teach clients:

- That the safest and most effective way to obtain needed vitamins is to eat a varied, well-balanced diet
- Which foods are good sources of vitamins, and ways to cook and store them to preserve vitamin content. Emphasize the need for adequate folic acid intake for sexually active females of childbearing potential, to prevent severe deformities (neural tube defects) in infants.
- To avoid excessive intake of any vitamin preparation. Excessive amounts do not promote health, strength, or youth. Instead, they may cause serious adverse reactions.

  With fat-soluble vitamins, the dangers of overdosage have long been known. With water-soluble vitamins, overdosage has been considered wasteful and expensive but not dangerous because these vitamins are rapidly excreted in the urine. However, evidence indicates that prolonged intake of excessive amounts of certain water-soluble vitamins can cause serious adverse effects. For example, large amounts of niacin (used to treat hyperlipidemia) may cause gastrointestinal (GI) problems, flushing, skin rashes, and pruritus and may exacerbate asthma, uricosuria, and gouty arthritis. Long-term ingestion of high doses of pyridoxine has been associated with peripheral neuropathies characterized by decreased sensation in limbs, perioral numbness, and ataxia. These symptoms improved after pyridoxine was withdrawn but were not completely eliminated. Large amounts of vitamin C (1 g or more) may cause diarrhea, uricosuria, and oxalate kidney stones. They also increase estrogen levels, decrease activity of oral anticoagulants, and, when taken by pregnant women, have caused scurvy in infants when they no longer received the large amounts to which they were exposed in utero.

Evaluation

- Interview about and observe the amount and type of food intake.
- Interview about and observe for signs of vitamin deficiency or overdose.

Principles of Therapy

MANAGING VITAMIN DISORDERS

Vitamin disorders should be recognized as early as possible and appropriate treatment initiated. Early recognition and treatment can prevent a mild deficiency or excess from becoming severe. Some guidelines include the following:

1. **Vitamin deficiency.** For deficiency states, oral vitamin preparations are preferred when possible. They are usually effective (except in malabsorption syndromes), safe, convenient to administer, and relatively inexpensive. If the deficiency involves only a single vitamin, then that vitamin alone is indicated. However, multiple deficiencies are common, and a multivitamin preparation may be needed. Although dosages for deficiencies are generally higher than those for dietary supplements, dosages should be titrated as nearly as possible to the amounts needed by the body.

   Multivitamin preparations for treating deficiencies contain more than 150% of the RDA. They should be used only for therapeutic purposes and for limited periods. Some oral preparations considered appropriate for therapeutic use include Abdec, Abdol, Adeflor, Betalin Complex Elixir, Multicebrin, Natalins, Surbex, Tri-Vi-Sol, and Vi-Daylin. Several of these may be used for adults or children. Other preparations are available for use during pregnancy and lactation or for parenteral use.

   When fat-soluble vitamins are given to correct deficiency, there is a risk of producing excess states. When water-soluble vitamins are given, excesses are less likely but may occur with large doses. These factors must be considered when determining vitamin dosage.

2. **Vitamin excess.** For excess states, the usual treatment is to stop administration of the vitamin preparation. There are no specific antidotes or antagonists.

Disorders of Fat-Soluble Vitamins A and K

1. With vitamin A deficiency, increase intake of foods containing vitamin A or carotene when feasible. Use a single, pure form of vitamin A rather than a multivitamin unless multiple deficiencies are present. Give doses no larger than 25,000 U daily unless a severe deficiency is present. Give orally if not contraindicated; give intramuscularly if GI absorption is severely impaired or ocular symptoms are severe. With vitamin A excess, immediately stop known sources of the vitamin.

2. With vitamin K deficiency or hypoprothrombinemia, bleeding may occur spontaneously or in response to trauma. Thus, administration of vitamin K and measures to prevent bleeding are indicated. If the deficiency is not severe, oral vitamin K may be given for a few days until serum prothrombin activity returns to a normal range. In obstructive jaundice, bile salts must be given at the same time as oral vitamin K, or vitamin K must be given parenterally. In malabsorption syndromes or diarrhea, parenteral administration is probably necessary. A single dose of vitamin K may be sufficient.

   With severe bleeding, vitamin K may be given intravenously. IV vitamin K must be given very slowly to decrease risks of hypotension and shock. Unfortunately, a therapeutic response does not occur for at least 4 hours. For more rapid control of bleeding, transfusions of plasma or whole blood are needed. When bleeding is caused by oral anticoagulant drugs, avoid overdoses of vitamin K. Oral anticoagulants are usually given for thromboembolic disorders. Giving vitamin K as an antidote to control bleeding reestablishes the risks of thrombi. Measures to prevent bleeding include avoiding trauma, injections, and drugs that may cause bleeding.

Disorders of B-complex Vitamins

1. Most deficiencies of B-complex vitamins are multiple rather than single. Also, many of these vitamins are obtained from the same foods. Treating deficiencies consists of increasing intake of foods containing B-complex vitamins or giving multivitamin preparations. Multivitamin preparations vary greatly in composition and therefore must be carefully chosen. Most preparations contain thiamine, riboflavin, niacin, pyridoxine, and cyanocobalamin. Other vitamins may be included in the formulations.

   If a single deficiency seems predominant, that vitamin may be given alone or in conjunction with a multivitamin preparation. For example, thiamine deficiency is common in alcoholic clients, partly because large amounts of thiamine are used to metabolize alcohol.

2. Some relatively rare types of anemia occur with deficiencies of certain B-complex vitamins. One type of anemia occurs with pyridoxine deficiency and is relieved by administration of pyridoxine. Megaloblastic anemias, characterized by abnormally large, immature red blood cells, occur with deficiency of folic acid or vitamin B_{12}. If megaloblastic anemia is severe, treatment is usually instituted with folic acid and vitamin B_{12}.

   a. In pernicious anemia, vitamin B_{12} must be given by intramuscular or subcutaneous injection because oral forms are not absorbed from the GI tract. Vitamin B_{12} injections are specific therapy for pernicious anemia and must be continued for life. Vitamin B_{12} is sometimes given to prevent pernicious anemia in clients who are strict vegetarians, who have had gastrectomy, or who have chronic small bowel disease. Pernicious anemia must be differentiated from other megaloblastic anemias for appropriate therapy. Pernicious anemia and other megaloblastic anemias respond to administration of folic acid. However, if folic acid alone is given to the client with pernicious anemia, hematologic abnormalities disappear but neurologic deterioration continues.

   b. In other types of megaloblastic anemias, vitamin B_{12} or folic acid is indicated. Although both of these are included in many multivitamin preparations, they usually must be given separately for therapeutic purposes. With vitamin B_{12}, doses of more than 100 µg are not useful because any excess of that amount is rapidly excreted in urine. It may be given as a single dose of 1000 µg when performing the Schilling test for pernicious anemia. With folic acid, oral administration is indicated for most clients. Daily doses in excess of 1 mg are not useful because any excess is excreted in the urine.

Disorders of Vitamin C

Treatment of vitamin C deficiency involves increased intake of vitamin C from dietary or pharmaceutical sources. Vitamin C (ascorbic acid) is available alone for oral, intramuscular, or IV administration. It is also an ingredient in most multivitamin preparations for oral or parenteral use.

USE IN CHILDREN

Children need sufficient amounts of all required vitamins to support growth and normal body functioning. In the healthy child, a varied, well-balanced diet is preferred over vitamin supplements.

If supplements are given, dosages should not exceed recommended amounts. There is a risk of overdosage by children and their parents. Because of manufacturers' marketing strategies, many supplements are available in flavors and shapes (*e.g.*, cartoon characters, animals) designed to appeal to children. Younger children may think of these supplements as "candy" and take more than recommended if they are accessible. Thus, they should be stored out of reach and dispensed by an adult. Parents may lack knowledge of nutrition or be overly concerned about the adequacy of a child's diet. Their wish to promote health may lead them to give supplements when they are not needed or to give more than recommended amounts. Parents may need information about the potential hazards of acute and chronic vitamin overdoses.

USE IN OLDER ADULTS

Vitamin requirements are the same as for younger adults. However, deficiencies are common in older adults, especially of vitamins A, D, folic acid, riboflavin, and thiamine. Numerous factors may contribute to deficiencies, including limited income, anorexia, lack of teeth or ill-fitting dentures, drugs that decrease absorption of dietary nutrients, and disease processes that interfere with the ability to obtain, prepare, or eat adequate amounts of a variety of foods.

Every older adult should be carefully assessed regarding nutritional status and use of drugs that interact with dietary nutrients. If an older adult cannot eat a varied, well-balanced diet for any reason, a vitamin supplement is probably desirable. In addition, requirements may be increased during illnesses, especially those affecting GI function. Overdoses, especially of the fat-soluble vitamins A and D, may cause toxicity and should be avoided.

 ## HOME CARE

The home care nurse needs to assess household members and the home setting for indications of vitamin deficiencies or use of megadoses. If actual or potential difficulties are found, the nurse may need to counsel household members about dietary sources of vitamins and adverse effects of excessive vitamin intake.

NURSING ACTIONS   VITAMINS

NURSING ACTIONS	RATIONALE/EXPLANATION
1. Administer accurately **a.** With fat-soluble vitamins:	
(1) Give as directed.	To increase therapeutic effects and avoid adverse reactions
(2) Do not give oral preparations at the same time as mineral oil.	Mineral oil absorbs the vitamins and thus prevents their systemic absorption.
(3) For subcutaneous or intramuscular administration of vitamin K, aspirate carefully to avoid intravenous injection, apply gentle pressure to the injection site, and inspect the site frequently. For intravenous injection, vitamin K may be given by direct injection or diluted in intravenous fluids (*e.g.*, 5% dextrose in water or saline).	Vitamin K is given to clients with hypoprothrombinemia, which causes a bleeding tendency. Thus, any injection may cause trauma and bleeding at the injection site.
(4) Administer intravenous vitamin K slowly, at a rate not to exceed 1 mg/min, whether diluted or undiluted.	Intravenous phytonadione may cause hypotension and shock from an anaphylactic type of reaction.
b. With B-complex vitamins:	
(1) Give parenteral cyanocobalamin (vitamin B_{12}) intramuscularly or deep subcutaneously.	
(2) Give oral niacin preparations, except for timed-release forms, with or after meals or at bedtime. Have the client sit or lie down for about ½ hour after administration.	To decrease anorexia, nausea, vomiting, diarrhea, and flatulence. Niacin causes vasodilation, which may result in dizziness, hypotension, and possibly injury from falls. Vasodilation occurs within a few minutes and may last 1 hour.
(3) Give intramuscular thiamine deeply into a large muscle mass. Avoid the intravenous route.	To decrease pain at the injection site. Hypotension and anaphylactic shock have occurred with rapid intravenous administration and large doses.
2. Observe for therapeutic effects (mainly decreased signs and symptoms of deficiency) **a.** With vitamin A, observe for improved vision, especially in dim light or at night, less dryness in eyes and conjunctiva (xerophthalmia), improvement in skin lesions.	Night blindness is usually relieved within a few days. Skin lesions may not completely disappear for several weeks.
b. With vitamin K, observe for decreased bleeding and more nearly normal blood coagulation tests (*e.g.*, prothrombin time).	Blood coagulation tests usually improve within 4 to 12 hours.
c. With B-complex vitamins, observe for decreased or absent stomatitis, glossitis, cheilosis, seborrheic dermatitis, neurologic problems (neuritis, convulsions, mental deterioration, psychotic symptoms), cardiovascular problems (edema, heart failure), and eye problems (itching, burning, photophobia).	Deficiencies of B-complex vitamins commonly occur together and produce many similar manifestations.
d. With vitamin B_{12} and folic acid, observe for increased appetite, strength and feeling of well-being, increased reticulocyte counts, and increased numbers of normal red blood cells, hemoglobin, and hematocrit.	Therapeutic effects may be quite rapid and dramatic. The client usually feels better within 24 to 48 hours, and normal red blood cells begin to appear. Anemia is decreased within about 2 weeks, but 4 to 8 weeks may be needed for complete blood count to return to normal.
e. With vitamin C, observe for decreased or absent malaise, irritability, and bleeding tendencies (easy bruising of skin, bleeding gums, nosebleeds, and so on).	

(continued)

NURSING ACTIONS	*RATIONALE/EXPLANATION*
3. Observe for adverse reactions **a.** With vitamin A, observe for signs of hypervitaminosis A (anorexia, vomiting, irritability, headache, skin changes [dryness, dermatitis, itching, desquamation], fatigue, pain in muscles, bones, and joints, and other clinical manifestations, and serum levels of vitamin A above 1200 U/100 ml).	Severity of manifestations depends largely on dose and duration of excess vitamin A intake. Very severe states produce additional clinical signs, including enlargement of liver and spleen, altered liver function, increased intracranial pressure, and other neurologic manifestations.
b. With vitamin K, observe for hypotension and signs of anaphylactic shock with intravenous phytonadione.	Vitamin K rarely produces adverse reactions. Giving intravenous phytonadione slowly may prevent adverse reactions.
c. With B-complex vitamins, observe for hypotension and anaphylactic shock with parenteral niacin, thiamine, cyanocobalamin, and folic acid; anorexia, nausea, vomiting and diarrhea, and postural hypotension with oral niacin.	Adverse reactions are generally rare. They are unlikely with B-complex multivitamin preparations. They are most likely to occur with large intravenous doses and rapid administration.
d. With vitamin C megadoses, observe for diarrhea and rebound deficiency if stopped abruptly.	Adverse reactions are rare with usual doses and methods of administration.
4. Observe for drug interactions **a.** Fat-soluble vitamins:	
(1) Bile salts *increase* effects.	Increase intestinal absorption
(2) Laxatives, especially mineral oil, *decrease* effects.	Mineral oil combines with fat-soluble vitamins and prevents their absorption if both are taken at the same time. Excessive or chronic laxative use decreases intestinal absorption.
(3) Antibiotics may *decrease* effects	With vitamin K, antibiotics decrease production by decreasing intestinal bacteria. With others, antibiotics may cause diarrhea and subsequent malabsorption.
b. B-complex vitamins:	
(1) Cycloserine (antituberculosis drug) *decreases* effects.	By increasing urinary excretion of vitamin B-complex
(2) Isoniazid (INH) *decreases* effect.	INH has an antipyridoxine effect. When INH is given for prevention or treatment of tuberculosis, pyridoxine is usually given also.
(3) With folic acid: alcohol, methotrexate, oral contraceptives, phenytoin, and triamterene *decrease* effects.	Alcohol alters liver function and leads to poor hepatic storage of folic acid. Methotrexate and phenytoin act as antagonists to folic acid and may cause folic acid deficiency. Oral contraceptives decrease absorption of folic acid.
5. Teach clients **a.** Avoid large doses of vitamins unless specifically prescribed by the physician.	To avoid adverse effects
b. If supplementary vitamins are taken, it is probably advisable to consult a physician.	Available preparations differ widely in amounts and types of vitamin content.
c. Take prescribed vitamins as directed and for the appropriate time.	In pernicious anemia, vitamin B_{12} injections must be taken for the remainder of life. In pregnancy and lactation, vitamins are usually taken only during this period of increased need.

REVIEW AND APPLICATION EXERCISES

1. What roles do vitamins play in normal body functioning?

2. Identify client populations who are at risk for vitamin deficiencies and excesses.

3. How would you assess a client for vitamin imbalances?

4. What are clinical indications for therapeutic use of specific vitamin drug preparations?

5. Are fat-soluble or water-soluble vitamins more toxic in overdoses and why?

6. For an outpatient or home care client who is likely to have vitamin deficiencies, what information can you provide to increase vitamin intake from food?

7. For a client who asks your advice about taking a multivitamin supplement daily, how would you reply? Justify your answer.

SELECTED REFERENCES

Chessman, K.H. & Anderson, J.D. (1997). Pediatric and geriatric nutrition support. In J.T. DiPiro, R.L. Talbert, G.C. Yee, G.R. Matzke, B.G. Wells, & L.M. Posey (Eds.), *Pharmacotherapy: A pathophysiologic approach*, 3rd ed., pp. 2787–2804. Stamford, CT: Appleton & Lange.

Corman, L.C. (1993). The role of nutrition in sickness and in health. *Medical Clinics of North America*, 77(4), 711–724.

Darby, M.K. & Loughead, J.L. (1996). Neonatal nutritional requirements and formula composition: A review. *Journal of Obstetrics, Gynecology, and Neonatal Nursing*, 25(3), 209–217.

Davis, J.R. & Sherer, K. (1994). *Applied nutrition and diet therapy for nurses*, 2nd ed. Philadelphia: W.B. Saunders.

Drug facts and comparisons. (Updated monthly). St. Louis: Facts and Comparisons.

Hillman, R.S. (1996). Hematopoietic agents: Growth factors, minerals, and vitamins. In J.G. Hardman, L.E. Limbird, P.B. Molinoff, & R.W. Ruddon (Eds.), *Goodman & Gilman's The pharmacological basis of therapeutics*, 9th ed., pp. 1311–1340. New York: McGraw-Hill.

Marcus, R. & Coulston, A.M. (1996). Water-soluble vitamins. In J.G. Hardman, L.E. Limbird, P.B. Molinoff, & R.W. Ruddon (Eds.), *Goodman & Gilman's The pharmacological basis of therapeutics*, 9th ed., pp. 1555–1572. New York: McGraw-Hill.

Marcus, R. & Coulston, A.M. (1996). Fat-soluble vitamins. In J.G. Hardman, L.E. Limbird, P.B. Molinoff, & R.W. Ruddon (Eds.), *Goodman & Gilman's The pharmacological basis of therapeutics*, 9th ed., pp. 1573–1590. New York: McGraw-Hill.

Pleuss, J. (1994). Alterations in nutritional status. In C.M. Porth (Ed.), *Pathophysiology: Concepts of altered health states*, 3rd ed., pp. 873–895. Philadelphia: J.B. Lippincott.

Stenson, W.F. & Eisenberg, P. (1997). Parenteral and enteral nutrition. In W.N. Kelley (Ed.), *Textbook of internal medicine*, 3rd ed., pp. 890–902. Philadelphia: Lippincott-Raven.

Wallace, J.I. & Schwartz, R.S. (1997). Geriatric clinical nutrition including malnutrition and cachexia. In W.N. Kelley (Ed.), *Textbook of internal medicine*, 3rd ed., pp. 2554–2560. Philadelphia: Lippincott-Raven.

Williams, L., Davis, J.A., & Lowenthal, D.T. (1993). The influence of food on the absorption and metabolism of drugs. *Medical Clinics of North America*, 77(4), 815–829.

32 Minerals and Electrolytes

Objectives

After studying this chapter, the student will be able to:

1 Discuss functions and food sources of major minerals.

2 Identify clients at risk of developing selected mineral and electrolyte imbalances.

3 Describe signs, symptoms and treatment of sodium, potassium, and magnesium imbalances.

4 Describe signs, symptoms and treatment of iron deficiency anemia.

5 Discuss the chelating agents used to remove excessive copper, iron, and lead from body tissues.

6 Apply nursing process skills to prevent, recognize, or treat mineral or electrolyte imbalances.

Key Terms

Acidosis	**Hyperkalemia**
Alkalosis	**Hypokalemia**
Chelating agents	**Micronutrients**
Electrolyte	

Description and Uses

Minerals and electrolytes are essential constituents of bone, teeth, cell membranes, and connective tissue. They are also components of many essential enzymes. In general, they function to maintain fluid, electrolyte, and acid–base balance; maintain osmotic pressure; maintain nerve and muscle function; assist in transfer of essential compounds across cell membranes; and influence the growth process.

Minerals occur in the body and foods mainly in ionic form. Ions are electrically charged particles. Metals (*e.g.,* sodium, potassium, calcium, magnesium) form positive ions or cations; nonmetals (*e.g.,* chlorine, phosphorus, sulfur) form negative ions or anions. These cations and anions combine to form salts or compounds that are physiologically inactive and electrically neutral. When placed in solution, such as a body fluid, the components separate into electrically charged particles called *electrolytes.* For example, sodium and chlorine combine to form sodium chloride (NaCl). (Table salt is composed of NaCl.) In a solution, NaCl separates into Na+ and Cl− ions. (The plus sign following Na means that Na is a cation. The minus sign following Cl means that Cl is an anion.) At any given time, the body must maintain an equal number of positive and negative charges. Therefore, the ions are constantly combining and separating to maintain electrical neutrality or electrolyte balance.

These electrolytes also maintain the acid–base balance of body fluids, which is necessary for normal body functioning. When foods are digested in the body, they produce mineral residues that react chemically as acids or bases. Acids are usually anions, such as chloride, bicarbonate, sulfate, and phosphate. Bases are usually cations, such as sodium, potassium, calcium, and magnesium. If approximately equal amounts of cations and anions are present in the mineral residue, the residue is essentially neutral, and the pH of body fluids does not require adjustment. If there is an excess of cations (base), the body must draw on its anions (acid) to combine with the cations, render them physiologically inactive, and restore the normal pH of the blood. Excess cations are excreted in the urine, mainly in combination with the anion phosphate. If there is an excess of anions (acid), usually sulfate or phosphate, they combine with hydrogen ions or other cations and are excreted in the urine.

MACRONUTRIENTS

There are 22 minerals thought to be necessary for human nutrition. Some of these (calcium, phosphorus, sodium, potassium, magnesium, chlorine, sulfur) are required in relatively large amounts and thus are sometimes called *macronutrients.* Calcium and phosphorus are discussed in Chapter 26. Sulfur is a component of cellular protein molecules, several amino acids, B vitamins, insulin, and other essential body substances. No recommended dietary allowances (RDAs) have been established; the dietary source is protein foods. The other macronutrients are described here in terms of characteristics, functions, RDAs, and food sources (Table 32-1). Imbalances of macronutrients are classified as deficiency states and excess states. Sodium imbalances (hyponatremia and hypernatremia) are described in Table 32-2, potassium imbalances (hypokalemia and hyper-

TABLE 32-1	MINERALS AND ELECTROLYTES		
Characteristics	**Functions**	**Recommended Dietary Allowances (RDAs)**	**Food Sources**
Sodium			
1. Major cation in extracellular body fluids (blood, lymph, tissue fluid) 2. Small amount in intracellular fluid 3. Large amounts of sodium in saliva, gastric secretions, bile, pancreatic and intestinal secretions	1. Assists in regulating osmotic pressure, water balance, conduction of electrical impulses in nerves and muscles, electrolyte and acid–base balance 2. Influences permeability of cell membranes and assists in movement of substances across cell membranes 3. Participates in many intracellular chemical reactions	About 2 g (estimated)	1. Present in most foods. Proteins contain relatively large amounts, vegetables and cereals contain moderate to small amounts, fruits contain little or no sodium. 2. Major source of sodium in the diet is table salt added to food in cooking, processing, or seasoning. One teaspoon contains 2.3 g of sodium. 3. Water in some areas may contain significant amounts of sodium.

(continued)

TABLE 32-1	MINERALS AND ELECTROLYTES (Continued)

Characteristics	Functions	Recommended Dietary Allowances (RDAs)	Food Sources
Potassium			
1. Major cation in intracellular body fluids 2. Present in all body fluids 3. Eliminated from the body primarily in urine. Normally functioning kidneys excrete excessive amounts of potassium, but they cannot conserve potassium when intake is low or absent. The kidneys excrete 10 mEq or more daily in the absence of intake. Potassium excretion is influenced by acid–base balance and aldosterone secretion. 4. A small amount of potassium is normally lost in feces and sweat.	1. Within cells, helps to maintain osmotic pressure, fluid and electrolyte balance, and acid–base balance 2. In extracellular fluid, functions with sodium and calcium to regulate neuromuscular excitability. Potassium is required for conduction of nerve impulses and contraction of skeletal and smooth muscle. It is especially important in activity of the myocardium. 3. Participates in carbohydrate and protein metabolism. Helps transport glucose into cells and is required for glycogen formation and storage. Required for synthesis of muscle proteins from amino acids and other components.	About 40 mEq	Present in most foods, including meat, whole-grain breads or cereals, bananas, citrus fruits, tomatoes, and broccoli
Magnesium			
1. A cation occurring primarily in intracellular fluid 2. Widely distributed in the body, about half in bone tissue and the remainder in soft tissue and body fluids 3. Most dietary magnesium is not absorbed from the gastrointestinal tract and is excreted in feces.	1. Required for conduction of nerve impulses and contraction of muscle 2. Especially important in functions of cardiac and skeletal muscles 3. Serves as a component of many enzymes 4. Essential for metabolism of carbohydrate and protein	About 300 mg for adults. Increased amounts recommended for pregnant or lactating women and children.	Present in many foods; diet adequate in other respects contains adequate magnesium. Good food sources include nuts, cereal grains, dark green vegetables, and seafoods.
Chloride			
1. Ionized form of element chlorine 2. The main anion of extracellular fluid 3. Almost all chloride is normally excreted by the kidneys.	1. Functions with sodium to help maintain osmotic pressure and water balance. 2. Forms hydrochloric acid (HCl) in gastric mucosal cells 3. Helps regulate electrolyte and acid–base balance by competing with bicarbonate ions for sodium 4. Participates in a homeostatic buffering mechanism in which chloride shifts in and out of red blood cells in exchange for bicarbonate	80–110 mEq	Most dietary chloride is ingested as sodium chloride (NaCl), and foods high in sodium are also high in chloride.

TABLE 32-2	SODIUM IMBALANCES	
Causes	**Pathophysiology**	**Signs and Symptoms**
Hyponatremia		
1. Inadequate intake. Unusual but may occur with sodium-restricted diets and diuretic drug therapy or when water only is ingested after water and sodium are lost (*e.g.*, excessive sweating) 2. Excessive losses. More common and occur with vomiting, gastrointestinal (GI) suction, diarrhea, excessive water enemas, excessive perspiration, burn wounds, and adrenal insufficiency states (*e.g.*, Addison's disease). 3. Excessive dilution of body fluids with water	1. Decreased serum sodium 2. Decreased plasma volume and cardiac output 3. Decreased blood flow to kidneys, decreased glomerular filtration rate, and decreased ability of kidneys to excrete water 4. Overhydration and swelling of brain cells (cerebral edema). Leads to impaired neurologic and muscular functions. 5. GI changes	1. Serum sodium <135 mEq/L 2. Hypotension and tachycardia 3. Oliguria and increased blood urea nitrogen (BUN) 4. Headache, dizziness, weakness, lethargy, restlessness, confusion, delirium, muscle tremors, convulsions, ataxia, aphasia 5. Anorexia, nausea, and vomiting are common; abdominal cramps and paralytic ileus may develop.
Hypernatremia		
1. Deficiency of water in proportion to the amount of sodium present. Water deficiency results from lack of intake or excessive losses (diarrhea, diuretic drugs, excessive sweating). 2. Excessive intake of sodium. An uncommon cause of hypernatremia because the thirst mechanism is normally activated, and water intake is increased. 3. Sodium retention due to hyperaldosteronism and Cushing's disease	1. Increased serum sodium 2. Hypernatremia due to water deficiency decreases fluid volume in extracellular fluid and intracellular fluid compartments (dehydration). 3. Hypernatremia due to sodium gain increases extracellular fluid volume and decreases intracellular fluid volume as water is pulled out of cells.	1. Serum sodium >145 mEq/L 2. Lethargy, disorientation, hyperactive reflexes, muscle rigidity, tremors and spasms, irritability, coma, cerebral hemorrhage, subdural hematoma 3. Hypotension 4. Fever, dry skin, and dry mucous membranes 5. Oliguria, concentrated urine with a high specific gravity, and increased BUN

kalemia) in Table 32-3, magnesium imbalances (hypomagnesemia and hypermagnesemia) in Table 32-4, and chloride imbalances (hypochloremic metabolic alkalosis and hyperchloremic metabolic acidosis) in Table 32-5. Each imbalance is described in terms of causes, pathophysiology, and clinical signs and symptoms.

MICRONUTRIENTS

The other 15 minerals are required in small amounts and are often called *micronutrients* or *trace elements*. Eight trace elements (chromium, cobalt, copper, fluoride, iodine, iron, selenium, and zinc) have relatively well-defined roles in human nutrition (Table 32-6). Because of their clinical importance, iron imbalances are discussed separately in Table 32-7. Other trace elements (manganese, molybdenum, nickel, silicon, tin, and vanadium) are present in many body tissues. Some are components of enzymes and may be necessary for normal growth, structure, and function of connective tissue. For

most of these, requirements are unknown, and states of deficiency or excess have not been identified in humans.

Several pharmacologic agents are used to prevent or treat mineral–electrolyte imbalances. Usually, neutral salts of minerals (*e.g.*, potassium chloride) are used in deficiency states, and nonmineral drug preparations are used in excess states.

Individual Agents Used in Mineral–Electrolyte and Acid–Base Imbalances

ACIDIFYING AGENT

Ammonium chloride (NH_4Cl) is a systemic acidifying agent occasionally used in the treatment of hypochloremic metabolic alkalosis. As a general rule, chloride is preferably replaced with sodium chloride or potassium chloride rather than ammonium chloride. However,

TABLE 32-3	POTASSIUM IMBALANCES	
Causes	**Pathophysiology**	**Signs and Symptoms**

Hypokalemia

1. Inadequate intake. Uncommon in clients who can eat; may occur in those unable to eat or receiving only potassium-free IV fluids for several days. 2. Excessive losses from the gastrointestinal tract (vomiting, gastric suction, diarrhea, overuse of laxatives and enemas) or urinary tract (polyuria from diuretic drugs, renal disease, excessive aldosterone) 3. Movement of potassium out of serum and into cells. This occurs with administration of insulin and glucose in treatment of diabetic ketoacidosis and in metabolic alkalosis.	1. Decreased serum potassium 2. Impaired cardiac conduction 3. Decreased strength of myocardial contraction and decreased cardiac output. Decreased response to catecholamines and other substances that normally raise blood pressure. 4. Neurologic changes due to impaired conduction of nerve impulses 5. Impaired function of skeletal, smooth, and cardiac muscle, most likely with serum potassium <2.5 mEq/L. Electrical impulses are slowed until muscle contraction cannot occur. 6. Slowed gastric emptying and decreased intestinal motility, probably caused by muscle weakness 7. Decreased ability of kidney to concentrate urine and excrete acid. Decreased glomerular filtration rate with prolonged potassium deficiency. 8. Impaired carbohydrate metabolism and decreased secretion of insulin	1. Serum potassium <3.5 mEq/L 2. Arrhythmias and electrocardiogram (ECG) changes (depressed ST segment; flattened or inverted T wave; increased amplitude of P wave; prolonged P-R interval; prolonged QRS complex with normal shape and size). Premature atrial and ventricular beats or atrioventricular block may occur, usually in people taking digitalis. Death from cardiac arrest may occur. 3. Postural hypotension 4. Confusion, memory impairment, lethargy, apathy, drowsiness, irritability, delirium 5. Muscle weakness and possibly paralysis. Weakness of leg muscles usually occurs first. Then weakness ascends to include respiratory muscles and cause respiratory insufficiency. 6. Abdominal distention, constipation, paralytic ileus 7. Polyuria, polydipsia, nocturia. Prolonged deficiency may increase serum creatinine and BUN. 8. Hyperglycemia

Hyperkalemia

1. Excess intake. Uncommon with normal kidney function. 2. Impaired excretion due to renal insufficiency, oliguria, potassium-saving diuretics, aldosterone deficiency, or adrenocortical deficiency 3. Combination of the above factors. Non-food sources of potassium include potassium supplements, salt substitutes, transfusions of old blood, and potassium salts of penicillin (penicillin G potassium contains 1.7 mEq potassium per 1 million units). 4. Movement of potassium from cells into serum with burns, crushing injuries, and acidosis	1. Increased serum potassium 2. Impaired conduction of nerve impulses and muscle contraction 3. Impaired cardiac conduction. Hyperkalemia "anesthetizes" nerve and muscle cells so electrical current cannot be built up to a sufficient level (repolarization) for an electrical impulse to be initiated and conducted.	1. Serum potassium >5 mEq/L 2. Muscle weakness, possibly paralysis and respiratory insufficiency 3. Cardiotoxicity, with arrhythmias or cardiac arrest. Cardiac effects are not usually severe until serum levels are 7 mEq/L or above. ECG changes include a high, peaked T wave, prolonged P-R interval, absence of P waves, and prolonged QRS complex.

sodium chloride may be contraindicated in an edematous client, or the alkalosis may be unresponsive to sodium or potassium chloride. Ammonium chloride is also sometimes used as a urinary acidifier to facilitate the action or excretion of other drugs.

Routes and Dosage Ranges

Adults: PO 1–3 g two or four times daily
IV 100–500 ml of a 2% solution, infused over a 3-h period; dosage depends on client's status and on serum chloride concentration.

TABLE 32-4 MAGNESIUM IMBALANCES

Causes	Pathophysiology	Signs and Symptoms
Hypomagnesemia 1. Inadequate dietary intake or prolonged administration of magnesium-free IV fluids 2. Decreased absorption, as occurs with alcoholism 3. Excessive losses with diuretic drugs, diarrhea, or diabetic acidosis	1. Decreased serum magnesium 2. Impaired conduction of nerve impulses and muscle contraction	1. Serum magnesium <1.5 mEq/L 2. Confusion, restlessness, irritability, vertigo, ataxia, seizures 3. Muscle tremors, carpopedal spasm, nystagmus, generalized spasticity 4. Tachycardia, hypotension, premature atrial and ventricular beats
Hypermagnesemia 1. Renal failure 2. Impaired renal function accompanied by excessive intake of magnesium salts in antacids or cathartics 3. Overtreatment of magnesium deficiency	1. Increased serum magnesium 2. Depressant effects on central nervous and neuromuscular systems, which block transmission of electrical impulses	1. Serum magnesium >2.5 mEq/L 2. Skeletal muscle weakness and paralysis, cardiac arrhythmias, hypotension, respiratory insufficiency, drowsiness, lethargy, coma

ALKALINIZING AGENTS

Sodium bicarbonate has long been used to treat metabolic acidosis, which occurs with severe renal disease, diabetes mellitus, circulatory impairment due to hypotension, shock or fluid volume deficit, and cardiac arrest. The drug dissociates into sodium and bicarbonate ions; the bicarbonate ions combine with free hydrogen ions to form carbonic acid. This action reduces the number of free hydrogen ions and thereby raises blood pH toward normal (7.35–7.45). However, the drug is not generally recommended now unless the acidosis is severe (*e.g.*, pH < 7.1), or clinical shock is present. Even then, usage must be based on frequent measurements of arterial blood gases and careful titration to avoid inducing alkalosis. Alkalosis makes the myocardium more sensitive to stimuli and increases the occurrence of arrhythmias. It also alters the oxyhemoglobin dissociation curve so less oxygen is released, and hypoxemia becomes even more severe. Thus, drug administration may be more harmful than helpful. In most instances, treating the underlying cause of the acidosis is safer and more effective. For example, in diabetic ketoacidosis, fluid replacement and insulin may be effective. In cardiac arrest, interventions to maintain circulation and ventilation are more effective in alleviating acidosis.

Sodium bicarbonate also is used to alkalinize the urine. Alkalinization increases solubility of uric acid and sulfonamide drugs and increases excretion of some acids (*e.g.*, salicylates, phenobarbital) when taken in overdose.

Routes and Dosage Ranges

Adults: PO 325 mg to 2 g, up to four times per day; maximum daily dose, 16 g for adults under 60 years, 8 g for adults over 60 years

IV dosage individualized according to arterial blood gases

Children: IV dosage individualized according to arterial blood gases

CATION EXCHANGE RESIN

Sodium polystyrene sulfonate (Kayexalate) is a cation exchange resin used clinically only in treatment of hyperkalemia. Given orally or rectally, the resin acts in the colon to release sodium and combine with potassium. Potassium is then eliminated from the body in the feces. Each gram of resin removes about 1 mEq of potassium. This drug is ineffective in severe, acute hyperkalemia because several hours are required to lower serum potassium levels. Thus, the resin is more likely to be used after other measures (*e.g.*, insulin and glucose infusions) have lowered dangerously high serum potassium levels. Insulin and glucose lower serum potassium levels by driving potassium into the cells. They do not remove potassium from the body.

Routes and Dosage Ranges

Adults: PO 15 g in 100–200 ml of water and 70% sorbitol, one to four times daily

Rectally (retention enema) 30–50 g in 100–200 ml of water and 70% sorbitol q6h

CHELATING AGENTS (METAL ANTAGONISTS)

Deferoxamine mesylate (Desferal) is a chelating agent for iron and is the only drug available for removing excess iron from the body. When given orally within a few hours after oral ingestion of iron preparations, deferoxamine combines with the iron in the bowel lumen and

TABLE 32-5	CHLORIDE IMBALANCES	
Causes	**Pathophysiology**	**Signs and Symptoms**
Hypochloremic Metabolic Alkalosis		
1. Excessive losses of chloride from vomiting, gastric suctioning, diuretic drug therapy, diabetic ketoacidosis, excessive perspiration, or adreno-cortical insufficiency 2. Excessive ingestion of bicarbonate or base	1. Decreased serum chloride 2. When chloride is lost, the body retains bicarbonate to maintain electroneutrality in extracellular fluids. The result is metabolic alkalosis, a relative deficiency of acid, and a relative excess of base. Hypokalemia is often present as well. 3. Hyperexcitability of the nervous system 4. Retention of carbon dioxide (acid) as a compensatory attempt to restore acid–base balance 5. Fluid loss and decreased plasma volume	1. Serum chloride <95 mEq/L; arterial blood pH >7.45 2. Paresthesias of face and extremities 3. Muscle spasms and tetany, which cannot be distinguished from the tetany produced by hypocalcemia 4. Slow, shallow respirations 5. Dehydration 6. Hypotension
Hyperchloremic Metabolic Acidosis		
1. Most often caused by dehydration 2. Deficient bicarbonate 3. Hyperparathyroidism 4. Respiratory alkalosis 5. Excessive administration of sodium chloride or ammonium chloride	1. Increased serum chloride 2. In dehydration, the kidneys reabsorb water in an attempt to relieve the fluid deficit. Large amounts of chloride are reabsorbed along with the water. The result is metabolic acidosis, a relative excess of acid, and a relative deficiency of base. 3. Central nervous system depression 4. Increased exhalation of carbon dioxide as a compensatory attempt to restore acid–base balance	1. Serum chloride >103 mEq/L; arterial blood pH <7.35 2. Lethargy, stupor, disorientation, and coma if acidosis is not treated 3. Increased rate and depth of respiration

prevents its absorption. When given parenterally, it removes iron from storage sites (*e.g.,* ferrin, hemosiderin) and combines with the iron to produce a water-soluble compound that can be excreted by the kidneys. The drug can remove about 10 to 50 mg of iron per day. The urine becomes reddish brown from the iron content.

The major indication for use of deferoxamine is acute iron intoxication. It is also used in hemochromatosis due to blood transfusions or hemosiderosis due to certain hemolytic anemias. In these chronic conditions characterized by accumulation of iron in tissues, phlebotomy may be more effective in removing iron. Deferoxamine is more likely to be used in clients who are too anemic or hypoproteinemic to tolerate the blood loss.

Routes and Dosage Ranges

Adults and children: PO 4–8 g, given within a few hours of oral ingestion of iron preparations
    IM 1 g initially, then 500 mg q4h for two doses, then 500 mg q4–12h if needed; maximum dose, 6 g/24 h

IV 1 g slowly (not to exceed 15 mg/kg/h), then 500 mg q4h for two doses, then 500 mg q4–12h if necessary; maximum dose, 6 g/24 h. This route is used only in the client in shock.

Penicillamine (Cuprimine) is a drug that chelates copper, zinc, mercury, and lead to form soluble complexes that are excreted in the urine. The main therapeutic use of penicillamine is to remove excess copper in clients with Wilson's disease (see Table 32-6). It also can be used prophylactically, before clinical manifestations occur, in clients likely to develop this hereditary condition. Penicillamine may be used to treat cystinuria, a hereditary metabolic disorder characterized by large amounts of cystine in the urine and renal calculi. It may be used in lead poisoning and severe rheumatoid arthritis that does not respond to conventional treatment measures.

Route and Dosage Ranges

Adults and older children: Wilson's disease, PO 250 mg four times per day, increased gradually, if necessary, up to 2 g/d

(*text continues on page 419*)

TABLE 32-6	SELECTED TRACE ELEMENTS		

Characteristics	Functions	Recommended Dietary Allowances (RDAs)	Food Sources
Chromium			
1. Deficiency state identified in humans and several animal species 2. Deficiency produces impaired glucose tolerance (hyperglycemia, glycosuria), impaired growth and reproduction, and decreased life span.	Aids glucose use by increasing effectiveness of insulin and facilitating transport of glucose across cell membranes	Not established	Brewer's yeast and whole wheat products
Cobalt			
1. Most body cobalt is stored in the liver; some is stored in the spleen, kidneys, and pancreas. 2. Excreted mainly in urine with smaller amounts excreted in feces and perspiration. 3. In humans, deficiency of vitamin B_{12} produces pernicious anemia. 4. Excess state not established for humans. In animals, excess cobalt produces polycythemia, bone marrow hyperplasia, and increased blood volume.	A component of vitamin B_{12}, which is required for normal function of all body cells and for maturation of red blood cells	About 1 mg in the form of vitamin B_{12}	Animal foods, including liver, muscle meats, and shellfish. Fruits, vegetables, and cereals contain no cobalt as vitamin B_{12}.
Copper			
1. Found in many body tissues including the brain, liver, heart, kidneys, bone, and muscle 2. Eliminated from the body in urine, sweat, feces, and menstrual flow 3. Human deficiency occurs with lack of food intake, malabsorption syndromes, and prolonged administration of copper-free IV hyperalimentation solutions 4. Signs and symptoms of deficiency include decreased serum levels of copper and ceruloplasmin (a plasma protein	1. A component of many enzymes 2. Essential for correct functioning of the central nervous, cardiovascular, and skeletal systems 3. Important in formation of red blood cells, apparently by regulating storage and release of iron for hemoglobin	Not established; estimated at about 2 mg	Many foods, including liver, shellfish, nuts, cereals, poultry, dried fruits

(continued)

TABLE 32-6 **SELECTED TRACE ELEMENTS** (Continued)

Characteristics	Functions	Recommended Dietary Allowances (RDAs)	Food Sources
that transports copper); decreased iron absorption; anemia from impaired erythropoiesis; leukopenia. Death can occur. In infants, three deficiency syndromes have been identified. One is characterized by anemia, a second by chronic malnutrition and diarrhea, and a third (Menke's syndrome) by retarded growth and progressive mental deterioration. 5. Copper excess (hypercupremia) may occur in women who take oral contraceptives or who are pregnant and in clients with infections or liver disease. Wilson's disease is a rare hereditary disorder characterized by accumulation of copper in vital organs (brain, liver, kidneys). Signs and symptoms vary according to affected organs.			
Fluoride			
1. Present in water, soil, plants, and animals in small amounts. Often added to community supplies of drinking water. 2. Accumulates in the body until about 50–60 years of age 3. Fluoride deficiency is indicated by dental caries and possibly a greater incidence of osteoporosis. 4. Fluoride excess results in mottling of teeth and osteosclerosis.	1. A component of tooth enamel 2. Strengthens bones, probably by promoting calcium retention in bones 3. Adequate intake before ages 50–60 years may decrease osteoporosis and fractures during later years.	Not established; average daily intake estimated at about 4 mg	Beef, canned salmon, eggs. Very little in milk, cereal grains, fruits, and vegetables. Fluoride content of foods depends on fluoride content of soil where they are grown.
Iodine			
1. Iodine deficiency causes thyroid gland enlargement and may cause hypothyroidism 2. Iodine excess (iodism) produces edema, fever,	Essential component of thyroid hormones	150 mg for adults, larger amounts for children and pregnant or lactating women	Seafood is the best source. In vegetables, iodine content varies with the amount of iodine in soil where grown. In milk and eggs, content depends on the amount present in animal feed.

TABLE 32-6 SELECTED TRACE ELEMENTS

Characteristics	Functions	Recommended Dietary Allowances (RDAs)	Food Sources
conjunctivitis, lymphadenopathy, stomatitis, vomiting, and coryza. Iodism is unlikely with dietary intake but may occur with excessive intake of drugs containing iodine.			

Iron

Characteristics	Functions	Recommended Dietary Allowances (RDAs)	Food Sources
1. Nearly three fourths of body iron is in hemoglobin in red blood cells; about one fourth is stored in the liver, bone marrow, and spleen as ferritin and hemosiderin; the remaining small amount is in myoglobin and enzymes or bound to transferrin in plasma. 2. Absorption of iron from foods varies widely and is estimated to be about 10% under normal circumstances. It is influenced by several factors: A. Factors that *increase* absorption: (1) Presence of dietary ascorbic acid (2) Acidity of gastric fluids increases solubility of dietary iron. (3) Presence of calcium. Calcium combines with phosphate, oxalate, and phytate. If this reaction does not occur, iron combines with these substances and produces nonabsorbable compounds. (4) Physiologic states that increase iron absorption include periods of increased blood	1. Essential component of hemoglobin, myoglobin, and several enzymes 2. Hemoglobin is required for transport and use of oxygen by body cells; myoglobin aids oxygen transport and use by muscle cells; enzymes are important for cellular respiration.	10 mg for men and older women 18 mg for women during childbearing years and children during periods of rapid growth	Liver and other organ meats, lean meat, shellfish, dried beans and vegetables, egg yolks, dried fruits, molasses, whole grain and enriched breads. Milk and milk products contain essentially no iron.

(continued)

TABLE 32-6	SELECTED TRACE ELEMENTS (Continued)

Characteristics	Functions	Recommended Dietary Allowances (RDAs)	Food Sources

formation, such as pregnancy and growth. Also more iron is absorbed when iron deficiency is present.
B. Factors that *decrease* absorption:
  (1) Lack of hydrochloric acid in the stomach or administration of antacids, which produces an alkaline environment
  (2) Combination of iron with phosphates, oxalates, or phytates in the intestine. This results in insoluble and nonabsorbable compounds.
  (3) Increased motility of the intestines, which decreases absorption of iron by decreasing contact time with the mucosa
  (4) Steatorrhea or any malabsorption disorder			

Selenium			
1. Has antioxidant properties similar to those of vitamin E 2. Deficiency most likely with long-term IV therapy. Signs and symptoms include myocardial abnormalities and other muscle discomfort and weakness. 3. Highly toxic in excessive amounts. Signs and symptoms include fatigue, peripheral neuropathy, nausea, diarrhea, and alopecia.	Important for function of myocardium and probably other muscles	70 µg for men; 55 µg for women, increased to 65 µg during pregnancy and 75 µg during lactation	Fish, meat, breads, and cereals

TABLE 32-6	SELECTED TRACE ELEMENTS		
Characteristics	**Functions**	**Recommended Dietary Allowances (RDAs)**	**Food Sources**
Zinc			
1. Deficiency may occur in liver cirrhosis, hepatitis, nephrosis, malabsorption syndromes, chronic infections, malignant diseases, myocardial infarction, hypothyroidism, and prolonged administration of zinc-free IV hyperalimentation solutions. Signs and symptoms are most evident in growing children and include impaired growth, hypogonadism in males, anorexia, and sensory impairment (loss of taste and smell). Also, if the client has had surgery, wound healing may be delayed. 2. Zinc excess is unlikely with dietary intake but may develop with excessive ingestion or inhalation of zinc. Ingestion may cause nausea, vomiting, and diarrhea; inhalation may cause vomiting, headache, and fever.	1. A component of many enzymes that are essential for normal metabolism (*e.g.*, carbonic anhydrase, lactic dehydrogenase, alkaline phosphatase). 2. Necessary for normal cell growth, synthesis of nucleic acids (RNA and DNA), and synthesis of carbohydrates and proteins 3. May be essential for use of vitamin A	15 mg for adolescents and adults 10 mg for preadolescents 25–30 mg for pregnant and lactating women	Animal proteins, such as meat, liver, eggs, and seafood. Wheat germ is also a good source.

Lead poisoning, PO 250–500 mg twice a day

Rheumatoid arthritis, PO 125–250 mg/d for 4 weeks, increased by 125–250 mg/d at 1- to 3-month intervals, if necessary

Usual maintenance dose, 500–750 mg/d; maximum dose, 1000–1500 mg/d

Infants over 6 months and young children: Wilson's disease, PO 250 mg/d, dissolved in fruit juice

Lead poisoning, PO 125 mg three times per day

Succimer (Chemet) is a drug that chelates lead to form water-soluble complexes that are excreted in the urine. The main therapeutic use is to treat lead poisoning in children with blood levels above 45 µg/100 ml. The most common adverse effects are gastrointestinal (GI; *e.g.*, anorexia, nausea, vomiting, diarrhea).

Route and Dosage Ranges

Children: PO 10 mg/kg or 350 mg/m^2 every 8 hours for 5 days, then every 12 hours for 14 days (total of 19 days of drug administration). For young children who cannot swallow capsules, the capsule contents can be sprinkled on soft food or given with a spoon.

IRON PREPARATIONS

Ferrous gluconate (Fergon) is an oral iron preparation that is effective in treating iron deficiency anemia. It may be less irritating to GI mucosa and therefore better tolerated than ferrous sulfate. Ferrous gluconate contains about 12% elemental iron, so each 320-mg tablet

TABLE 32-7	IRON IMBALANCES	
Causes	**Pathophysiology**	**Signs and Symptoms**
Deficiency State		
1. Inadequate intake of iron in the diet 2. Faulty absorption of iron 3. Blood loss in gastrointestinal bleeding, heavy or prolonged menstrual flow, traumatic injury, and other conditions	1. Impaired erythropoiesis 2. Inadequate hemoglobin to transport sufficient oxygen to body tissues 3. Iron deficiency increases absorption of other minerals (*e.g.*, lead, cobalt, manganese) and may produce signs of excess.	1. Anemia (decrease in red blood cells, hemoglobin, and hematocrit) 2. With gradual development of anemia, minimal symptoms occur 3. With rapid development of anemia or severe anemia, dyspnea, fatigue, tachycardia, malaise, and drowsiness occur.
Acute Excess State		
Acute iron poisoning usually occurs in small children who take several tablets of an iron preparation.	Acute toxicity	Vomiting, diarrhea, melena, abdominal pain, shock, convulsions, and metabolic acidosis. Death may occur within 24 h if treatment is not prompt.
Chronic Excess State		
Chronic iron excess (hemochromatosis) is rare but may be caused by long-term ingestion of excessive iron salts (*e.g.*, ferrous sulfate), large numbers of blood transfusions, or a rare genetic trait that promotes iron absorption.	Excess iron is deposited in the heart, pancreas, kidney, liver, and other organs. It impairs cell function and eventually destroys cells.	Cardiac arrhythmias, heart failure, diabetes mellitus, bronze pigmentation of skin, liver enlargement, arthropathy, and others

contains about 38 mg of iron. Indications for use, adverse reactions, and contraindications are the same as for ferrous sulfate.

Route and Dosage Ranges

Adults: PO 320–640 mg (40–80 mg elemental iron) three times per day

Children: PO 100–300 mg (12.5–37.5 mg elemental iron) three times per day

Infants: PO 100 mg or 30 drops of elixir initially, gradually increased to 300 mg or 5 ml of elixir daily (15–37.5 mg elemental iron) in divided doses

Ferrous sulfate (Feosol), which contains 20% elemental iron, is the prototype of oral iron preparations and the preparation of choice for prevention or treatment of iron deficiency anemia. It may be used as an iron supplement during periods of increased requirements (*e.g.*, childhood, pregnancy). Nausea and other GI symptoms may result from gastric irritation. Ferrous sulfate and other oral iron preparations discolor feces, producing a black-green color that may be mistaken for blood in the stool. Contraindications to oral iron preparations include peptic ulcer disease, inflammatory intestinal disorders, anemias other than iron deficiency anemia, multiple blood transfusions, hemochromatosis, and hemosiderosis.

Route and Dosage Ranges

Adults: PO 300 mg–1.2 g (60–240 mg elemental iron) daily in three or four divided doses

Children 6–12 years: PO 120–600 mg (24–120 mg elemental iron) daily in divided doses

Infants and children <6 years: 300 mg (60 mg elemental iron) daily in divided doses

Iron dextran injection (InFeD) is a parenteral form of iron useful in treating confirmed iron deficiency anemia when oral supplements are not feasible. One ml equals 50 mg of elemental iron. Reasons for using iron dextran injection include peptic ulcer or inflammatory bowel disease that is likely to be aggravated by oral iron preparations; the client's inability or unwillingness to take oral preparations; and a shortage of time for correcting the iron deficiency (*e.g.*, late pregnancy or preoperative status). One of the major advantages of parenteral iron is that body iron stores can be replenished rapidly. The drug is contraindicated in anemias not associated with iron deficiency and hypersensitivity to the drug (fatal anaphylactoid reactions have occurred).

Dosage is calculated for individual patients according to hemoglobin and weight (see manufacturer's literature).

MAGNESIUM PREPARATION

Magnesium oxide or **hydroxide** may be given for mild hypomagnesemia in asymptomatic patients. **Magnesium sulfate** is given parenterally for moderate to severe hypomagnesemia, convulsions associated with pregnancy (eclampsia), and prevention of hypomagnesemia in total parenteral nutrition. Therapeutic effects in these conditions are attributed to the drug's depressant effects on the central nervous system and smooth, skeletal, and cardiac muscle. Oral magnesium salts may cause diarrhea; their uses as antacids and cathartics are discussed in Chapters 60 and 61, respectively. Magnesium preparations are contraindicated in clients who have impaired renal function or who are comatose.

Routes and Dosage Ranges

Adults: Hypomagnesemia, PO magnesium oxide 250–500 mg three or four times daily, Milk of Magnesia 5 ml four times daily, or a magnesium-containing antacid 15 ml three times daily; IM 1–2 g (2–4 ml of 50% solution) once or twice daily based on serum magnesium levels
Eclampsia, IM 1–2 g (2–4 ml of 50% solution) initially, then 1 g q30 min until seizures stop
Convulsive seizures, IM 1 g (2 ml of 50% solution) repeated PRN
IV, do not exceed 150 mg/min (1.5 ml/min of a 10% solution, 3 ml/min of a 5% solution)
Older children: IM, same dosage as adults

POTASSIUM PREPARATIONS

Potassium chloride is usually the drug of choice for preventing or treating hypokalemia, because deficiencies of potassium and chloride often occur together. It is often prescribed for clients who are receiving potassium-losing diuretics (*e.g.,* hydrochlorothiazide, furosemide), those who are receiving digoxin (hypokalemia increases risks of digitalis toxicity), and those who are receiving only intravenous (IV) fluids because of surgical procedures, GI disease, or other conditions. Potassium chloride also may be used to replace chloride in hypochloremic metabolic alkalosis.

Potassium chloride can be given orally or IV. Oral preparations are recommended when feasible, but one disadvantage of oral liquid preparations is an unpleasant taste. This has led to production of various flavored powders, liquids, and effervescent tablets (*e.g.,* Kay Ciel Elixir, K-Lor, Klorvess). Tablets containing a wax matrix (*e.g.,* Slow-K) are effective and better tolerated by most clients than liquid formulations. IV preparations of potassium chloride must be diluted before administration to prevent hyperkalemia, cardiotoxicity, and severe pain at the injection site.

Potassium chloride is contraindicated in clients with renal failure and in those receiving potassium-saving diuretics, such as triamterene, spironolactone, or amiloride.

Potassium gluconate (Kaon) and **potassium bicarbonate and citrate** (K-Lyte) are oral preparations of potassium salts other than chloride. They are supposedly more palatable and therefore more likely to be taken than oral potassium chloride preparations. The major indication for their use is the occasional hypokalemia associated with hyperchloremia. If given to a client with hypokalemia and hypochloremia, these preparations do not replace chloride, and another source of chloride must be given. Adverse reactions and contraindications are the same as for potassium chloride.

Routes and Dosage Ranges

Adults: PO 15–20 mEq two to four times per day
IV (potassium chloride injection) about 40–100 mEq/24 h. Dosage must be individualized and depends on serum potassium levels and total potassium body stores. Potassium chloride (KCl) must be diluted. A generally safe dosage range is 20–60 mEq, diluted in 1000 ml of dextrose or sodium chloride IV solution and given no faster than 10–15 mEq/h or 60–120 mEq/24 h.

SODIUM PREPARATIONS

Sodium chloride injection is available in several concentrations and sizes for IV use. Concentrations are 0.45% (hypotonic solution), 0.9% (isotonic), and 3% (hypertonic). Sodium chloride is also available in combination with dextrose. Five percent dextrose in 0.22% sodium chloride and 5% dextrose in 0.45% sodium chloride are frequently used solutions for IV fluid therapy. They contain 38.5 and 77 mEq/L, respectively, of sodium and chloride. Isotonic or 0.9% sodium chloride contains 154 mEq of both sodium and chloride. This solution may be used to treat hyponatremia. The 3% solution contains 513 mEq of sodium and chloride per liter. It may be used in severe hyponatremia but is rarely necessary. Because of the high risk of circulatory overload and pulmonary edema, it must be given in small amounts (200–400 ml) and administered slowly (no faster than 100 ml/h).

Route and Dosage Range

Adults: IV 1500–3000 ml of 0.22%, 0.45% solution/24 h depending on client's fluid needs; about 50 ml/h to keep IV lines open

ZINC PREPARATION

Zinc sulfate is available in tablets containing 110, 200, or 220 mg of zinc sulfate (equivalent to 25, 47, and 50 mg of elemental zinc, respectively) and in capsules containing 220 mg of zinc sulfate (equivalent to 50 mg of elemental zinc). It is also an ingredient in several vitamin–mineral combination products. Zinc sulfate is given orally as a dietary supplement to prevent or treat zinc deficiency. In malnourished clients, it may be used to promote wound healing after surgery. There is no evidence, though, that zinc promotes wound healing or has any other beneficial effect in the absence of zinc deficiency.

Route and Dosage Range

Adults: PO 25–50 mg elemental zinc daily

MULTIPLE MINERAL– ELECTROLYTE PREPARATIONS

There are numerous commercially prepared electrolyte solutions for IV use. One group provides *maintenance* amounts of fluids and electrolytes when oral intake of food and fluids is restricted or contraindicated. These solutions differ slightly in the number and amount of particular electrolytes. A second group provides *replacement* amounts of electrolytes (mainly sodium and chloride) when electrolytes are lost from the body in abnormal amounts. This group includes Normosol-R (Abbott), and Plasma-Lyte 148 (Travenol). These electrolyte preparations are available with dextrose 2.5% to 10%. Ringer's solution is another replacement fluid that is used often. It is manufactured by several different companies; health care agencies use one manufacturer's products for the most part.

Several oral electrolyte solutions (*e.g.,* Lytren, Pedialyte) contain sodium, chloride, potassium, calcium, magnesium, and other electrolytes along with a small amount of dextrose. They are used to supply maintenance amounts of fluids and electrolytes when oral intake is restricted. They are especially useful in children for treatment of diarrhea and may prevent severe fluid and electrolyte depletion. The amount given must be carefully prescribed and calculated to avoid excessive intake. They should not be used in severe circumstances in which IV fluid and electrolyte therapy is indicated. They must be cautiously used with impaired renal function. They should not be mixed with other electrolyte-containing fluids, such as milk or fruit juices.

Routes and Dosage Ranges

Adults: IV 2000–3000 ml/24 h, depending on individual fluid and electrolyte needs
Children: IV, PO, amount individualized according to fluid and electrolyte needs

Nursing Process

Assessment

Assess each client for current or potential mineral–electrolyte or acid–base disorders. This is usually done in an overall assessment of nutritional status. Specific assessment factors related to minerals and electrolytes include the following:

- Deficiency states are probably more common than excess states unless a mineral–electrolyte supplement is being taken. However, deficiencies and excesses may be equally harmful, and both must be assessed.
- Clients with other nutritional deficiencies are likely to have mineral–electrolyte deficiencies as well. Moreover, deficiencies are likely to be multiple, with overlapping signs and symptoms.
- Many drugs influence gains and losses of minerals and electrolytes, including diuretics and laxatives.
- Minerals and electrolytes are lost with gastric suction, polyuria, diarrhea, excessive perspiration, and other conditions.
- Assess laboratory reports when available.
  - Check the complete blood count for decreased red blood cells, hemoglobin, and hematocrit. Reduced values may indicate iron deficiency anemia, and further assessment is needed.
  - Check serum electrolyte reports for increases or decreases. All major minerals can be measured in clinical laboratories. The ones usually measured are sodium, chloride, and potassium; carbon dioxide content, a measure of bicarbonate, is also assessed. Normal values vary to some extent with the laboratory and the method of measurement, but a general range of normal values is sodium, 135 to 145 mEq/L; chloride, 95 to 105 mEq/L; potassium, 3.5 to 5 mEq/L; and carbon dioxide, 22 to 26 mEq/L. Minor differences in these values are insignificant.

Nursing Diagnoses

- Altered Nutrition: Less Than Body Requirements related to mineral–electrolyte deficiency
- Altered Nutrition: More Than Body Requirements related to excessive intake of drug preparations
- Risk for Injury related to mineral–electrolyte deficiency or overdose

- Knowledge Deficit: Importance of adequate mineral–electrolyte intake in normal body functioning
- Knowledge Deficit: Dietary sources of various mineral–electrolyte nutrients

Planning/Goals

The client will:
- Have an adequate dietary intake of minerals and electrolytes
- Avoid mineral–electrolyte supplements unless recommended by a health care provider
- Participate in follow-up procedures and laboratory tests as requested when mineral–electrolyte drugs are prescribed
- Take mineral–electrolyte drugs as prescribed
- Avoid adverse effects of drug preparations

Interventions

Implement measures to prevent mineral–electrolyte disorders:
- Promote a varied diet. A diet adequate in protein and calories generally provides adequate minerals and electrolytes.
- If assessment data reveal potential development of a disorder, start preventive measures as soon as possible. For clients able to eat, foods high in iron may delay onset of iron deficiency anemia, foods high in potassium may prevent hypokalemia with diuretic therapy, and salty foods along with water help to prevent problems associated with excessive perspiration. For people unable to eat, IV fluids and electrolytes are usually given. Generally, oral food intake or tube feeding is preferable to IV therapy.
- Treat underlying disorders that contribute to the mineral–electrolyte deficiency or excess. Measures to relieve anorexia, nausea, vomiting, diarrhea, pain, and other symptoms help to increase intake or decrease output of certain minerals. Measures to increase urine output, such as forcing fluids, help to increase output of some minerals in the urine and therefore prevent excess states from developing.
- Mineral supplements are recommended only for current or potential deficiencies. They provide no beneficial effects in the absence of deficiency, and all are toxic if taken in excessive amounts. When deficiencies are identified, treat with foods when possible. Next, use oral mineral supplements. Use parenteral supplements only for clear-cut indications, because they are potentially the most hazardous.
- For clients who have nasogastric tubes to suction, irrigate the tubes with isotonic sodium chloride solution. The use of tap water is contraindicated because it is hypotonic and would pull electrolytes into the stomach. Electrolytes are then lost in the aspirated and discarded stomach contents. For the same reason, only 2 to 3 teaspoons of ice chips or water are allowed per hour. Clients often request ice chips or water frequently and in larger amounts than desirable; the nurse must explain the reason for the restrictions.
- If tap-water enemas are ordered to be given until clear of feces, give no more than three. Isotonic sodium chloride is preferred to tap water. Still, no more than three enemas should be given consecutively.

Teach clients:
- The best source of minerals and electrolytes is a well-balanced diet with a variety of foods. A well-balanced diet contains all the minerals needed for health in most people. An exception is iron, which is often needed as a dietary supplement in women and children.
- The safest course of action is to take drug preparations only on a health care provider's advice, in the amounts and for the length of time prescribed. All minerals are toxic when taken in excess. Also, there is no benefit to taking more than the body needs.
- To keep all mineral–electrolyte substances out of reach of children to prevent accidental overdose. Acute iron intoxication is a relatively common problem among small children and can be fatal.
- To keep appointments with health care providers for periodic blood tests and other follow-up procedures when mineral–electrolyte supplements are prescribed. This will help prevent ingestion of excessive amounts.

Evaluation

- Interview about and observe the amount and type of food intake in relation to required minerals and electrolytes.
- Interview and observe for signs of mineral–electrolyte deficiency or excess.

Principles of Therapy

Diet Supplements

Some people take mineral preparations as dietary supplements in an effort to promote health and prevent deficiencies. They are rarely needed for this purpose by people who eat a balanced and varied diet; who have no increased need for nutrients, such as growth or pregnancy; and who have no abnormal losses of nutrients, such as those caused by GI diseases. In fact, dietary supplements in a person who eats adequately could exceed nutrient needs by more than 100%. No known benefit to health results from ingesting more mineral nutrients than the body needs, and harm may result because all minerals are toxic at high doses.

Prevention of an Excess State

When a mineral is given to correct a deficiency state, there is a risk of producing an excess state. Because both deficiency and excess states may be harmful, the amount of mineral supplement should be titrated closely to the amount needed by the body. Larger doses are needed to treat deficiency states than are needed to prevent deficiencies from developing. In addition to producing potential toxicity, large doses of one mineral may cause a relative deficiency of another mineral or nutrient.

DRUG SELECTION

Oral drug preparations are preferred, when feasible, for preventing or treating mineral disorders. They are generally safer, less likely to produce toxicity, more convenient to administer, and less expensive than parenteral preparations.

PRINCIPLES OF TREATING SODIUM DISORDERS

Hyponatremia

Treatment of hyponatremia is aimed at restoring normal levels of serum sodium. This can be done with isotonic sodium chloride solution when hyponatremia is caused by sodium depletion and with restriction of water when hyponatremia is caused by fluid volume excess (water intoxication).

Hypernatremia

Treatment of hypernatremia requires administration of sodium-free fluids, either orally or IV, until serum sodium levels return to normal. Milder states usually respond to increased water intake through the GI tract; more severe hypernatremia is likely to require IV administration of 5% dextrose in water.

PRINCIPLES OF TREATING POTASSIUM DISORDERS

Hypokalemia

1. Assess for conditions contributing to hypokalemia, and attempt to eliminate them or reduce their impact. Such conditions are generally inadequate intake, excessive loss, or some combination of the two.
2. Assess the severity of the hypokalemia. This is best done on the basis of serum potassium levels and clinical manifestations. Serum potassium levels alone are inadequate because they may not accurately reflect depletion of body potassium.
3. Potassium supplements are indicated in the following circumstances:
   a. When serum potassium level is below 3 mEq/L on repeated measurements, even if the client is asymptomatic
   b. When serum potassium is 3 to 3.5 mEq/L and clear-cut symptoms or electrocardiogram (ECG) changes indicate hypokalemia. Some clinicians advocate treatment in the absence of symptoms.

   c. In clients receiving digoxin, if necessary to maintain serum potassium levels above 3.5 mEq/L. Such usage is indicated because hypokalemia increases digitalis toxicity.
4. Although opinions differ, potassium supplements are probably not indicated for prevention of hypokalemia except in clients with hypokalemic periodic paralysis, a rare disorder. Thus, use of potassium supplements with diuretic therapy is not indicated unless hypokalemia develops or digoxin is being given.
5. When potassium supplements are necessary, oral administration is preferred. Oral preparations are usually effective and less likely to cause hyperkalemia than IV preparations.
6. Potassium chloride (KCl) is the drug of choice in most instances because it replaces potassium and chloride. Liquids, powders, and effervescent tablets for oral use must be diluted in at least 4 oz of water or juice to improve taste and decrease gastric irritation. Controlled-release tablets or capsules with KCl in a wax matrix or microencapsulated form are preferred by most clients.
7. IV KCl is indicated when a client cannot take an oral preparation or has severe hypokalemia. The serum potassium level should be measured, total body deficit estimated, and adequate urine output established before IV potassium therapy begins.
   a. IV KCl must be well diluted to prevent sudden hyperkalemia, cardiotoxic effects, and phlebitis at the venipuncture site. The usual dilution is KCl 20 to 60 mEq/1000 ml of IV fluid.
   b. Dosage must be individualized. Clients receiving IV fluids only are usually given 40 to 60 mEq of KCl daily. This can be given safely with 20 mEq KCl/l of fluids and a flow rate of 100 to 125 ml/h. In severe deficits, a higher concentration and a higher flow rate may be necessary. In these situations, an infusion pump to control flow rate accurately and continuous cardiac monitoring for detection of hyperkalemia are necessary. Also, serum potassium levels must be checked frequently and dosage adjusted if indicated. No more than 100 to 200 mEq KCl should be given within 24 hours, even if several days are required to replace the estimated deficit.
   c. Do not administer potassium-containing IV solutions into a central venous catheter. There is a risk of hyperkalemia and cardiac arrhythmias or arrest because there is limited time for the solution to be diluted in the blood returning to the heart.
   d. In critical situations, KCl usually should be given in sodium chloride solutions rather than dextrose solutions. Administering dextrose solutions may increase hypokalemia by causing some potassium to leave the serum and enter cells.

Hyperkalemia

1. Eliminate any exogenous sources of potassium, such as potassium supplements, penicillin G potassium, salt substitutes, and blood transfusion with old blood.
2. Treat acidosis if present, because potassium leaves cells and enters the serum with acidosis.
3. Use measures that antagonize the effects of potassium, that cause potassium to leave the serum and reenter cells, and that remove potassium from the body. Appropriate measures are determined mainly by serum potassium levels and ECG changes. Continuous cardiac monitoring is required.

   Severe hyperkalemia (serum potassium above 7 mEq/L and ECG changes indicating hyperkalemia) requires urgent treatment. Immediate IV administration of sodium bicarbonate 45 mEq, over a 5-minute period, causes rapid movement of potassium into cells. This can be repeated in a few minutes if ECG changes persist.

   Calcium gluconate 10%, 5 to 10 ml IV, is also given early in treatment. It acts to decrease the cardiotoxic effects of hyperkalemia. It is contraindicated if the client is receiving digoxin, and it cannot be added to fluids containing sodium bicarbonate because insoluble precipitates are formed.

   The next step is IV infusion of glucose and insulin. This also causes potassium to move into cells, although not as quickly as sodium bicarbonate.
4. When hyperkalemia is less severe or when it has been reduced by the above measures, sodium polystyrene sulfonate, a cation exchange resin, can be given orally or rectally to remove potassium from the body. Each gram of the resin combines with 1 mEq potassium, and both are excreted in feces. The resin is usually mixed with water and sorbitol, a poorly absorbed, osmotically active alcohol that has a laxative effect. The sorbitol offsets the constipating effect of the resin and aids in its expulsion. Oral administration is preferred, and several doses daily may be given until serum potassium is normal. When given as an enema, the solution must be retained from one to several hours, or repeated enemas must be given for therapeutic effect.
5. If the above measures fail to reduce hyperkalemia, peritoneal dialysis or hemodialysis may be used.

PRINCIPLES OF TREATING MAGNESIUM DISORDERS

Hypomagnesemia

1. Prevent, when possible, by giving parenteral fluids with magnesium when the fluids are the only source of nutrients. Multiple electrolyte IV solutions contain magnesium chloride or acetate, and magnesium can be added to solutions for total parenteral nutrition.

2. For mild, asymptomatic hypomagnesemia, oral magnesium preparations may be given. For moderate to severe and symptomatic hypomagnesemia, parenteral (IV or IM) magnesium sulfate may be given daily as long as hypomagnesemia persists or continuing losses occur. Initial dosage may be larger, but the usual maintenance dose is about 8 mEq daily. A 10% solution is available in 10-ml vials that contain 8 mEq of magnesium sulfate for adding to IV solutions. A 50% solution is available in 2-ml vials (8 mEq) for intramuscular (IM) administration.
3. Check serum magnesium levels daily.

Hypermagnesemia

1. Stop any source of exogenous magnesium, such as magnesium sulfate or magnesium-containing antacids, cathartics, or enemas.
2. Have calcium gluconate available for IV administration. It is an antidote for the sedative effects of magnesium excess.
3. Increase urine output by increasing fluid intake, if feasible. This increases removal of magnesium from the body in urine.
4. Clients with chronic renal failure are the most likely to develop hypermagnesemia. They are likely to require peritoneal dialysis or hemodialysis to lower serum magnesium levels.

PRINCIPLES OF TREATING IRON DEFICIENCY AND EXCESS

Iron Deficiency Anemia

1. Anemia is a symptom, not a disease. Therefore, the underlying cause must be identified and eliminated, if possible.
2. Assess the client's intake of and attitude toward foods with high iron content. Encourage increased dietary intake of these foods.
3. Use oral iron preparations when possible. They are generally safe, effective, convenient to administer, and relatively inexpensive. Ferrous preparations (sulfate, gluconate, fumarate) are better absorbed than ferric preparations. Other iron salts do not differ significantly from ferrous sulfate, which is usually the drug of choice for oral iron therapy. Slow-release or enteric-coated products tend to decrease absorption of iron.
4. Dosage is calculated in terms of elemental iron. Iron preparations vary greatly in the amount of elemental iron they contain. Ferrous sulfate, for example, contains 20% iron; thus, each 300-mg tablet furnishes about 60 mg of elemental iron. With the usual regimen of one tablet three times daily, a daily dose of 180 mg of elemental iron is given. For most clients,

probably half that amount (30 mg three times daily) would correct the deficiency. However, tablets are not manufactured in sizes to allow this regimen, and liquid preparations are not popular with clients. Thus, relatively large doses are usually given, but smaller doses may be just as effective, especially if GI symptoms become a problem with higher dosages. Whatever the dose, only about 10% to 15% of the iron is absorbed. Most of the remainder is excreted in feces, which turn dark green or black.

5. Oral iron preparations are better absorbed if taken on an empty stomach. However, because gastric irritation is a common adverse reaction, they are more often given with or immediately after meals.

6. Although normal hemoglobin levels return after about 2 months of oral iron therapy, an additional 6-month period of drug therapy is recommended to replenish the body's iron stores.

7. Reasons for failure to respond to iron therapy include continued blood loss, failure to take the drug as prescribed, or defective iron absorption. These factors must be reevaluated if no therapeutic response is evident within 3 to 4 weeks after drug therapy is begun.

8. Parenteral iron is indicated when oral preparations may further irritate a diseased GI tract, when the client is unable or unwilling to take the oral drugs, or when the anemia must be corrected relatively rapidly.

9. For severe iron deficiency anemia, blood transfusions may be most effective.

Iron Excess

1. Acute iron overdosage requires treatment as soon as possible, even if overdosage is only suspected, and the amount taken is unknown. It is unnecessary to wait until serum iron level is measured.

   If treatment is begun shortly after oral ingestion of iron, induced vomiting or aspiration of stomach contents by nasogastric tube is helpful. This can be followed by lavage with 1% sodium bicarbonate solution to form insoluble iron carbonate compounds. The next step is to instill in the stomach 5 to 8 g of deferoxamine dissolved in 50 ml of distilled water to bind the iron remaining in the GI tract and prevent its absorption. Finally, deferoxamine is given IM or IV to bind with iron in tissues and allow its excretion in the urine. Throughout the treatment period, supportive measures may be needed for GI hemorrhage, acidosis, and shock.

2. For chronic iron overload or hemochromatosis, the first step in treatment is to stop the source of iron, if possible. Phlebotomy is the treatment of choice for most clients because withdrawal of 500 ml of blood removes about 250 mg of iron. Phlebotomy may be

needed as often as weekly and for as long as 2 to 3 years. For clients resistant to or intolerant of phlebotomy, deferoxamine can be given. About 10 to 50 mg of iron is excreted daily in the urine with deferoxamine administration.

PRINCIPLES OF TREATING ACID–BASE DISORDERS

Metabolic Acidosis

1. Assess the presence and severity of acidosis by measuring arterial blood gases. Results reflecting acidosis are decreased pH (less than 7.35) and decreased bicarbonate (less than 22 mEq/L).

2. Assess and treat the underlying condition, such as diabetic ketoacidosis.

3. If this does not relieve acidosis, or if acidosis is severe (arterial blood pH less than 7.2), sodium bicarbonate may be given parenterally to alkalinize the blood. It can be given by direct injection into a vein or as a continuous IV infusion. Ampules and pre-filled syringes are available in 8.4% solution (50 ml contains 50 mEq) or 7.5% solution (50 ml contains 44.6 mEq). IV solutions of 5% and 1.4% sodium bicarbonate are also available in 500-ml bottles.

4. Monitor arterial blood gases and serum potassium levels frequently. Overtreatment of acidosis with sodium bicarbonate will produce alkalosis. Serum potassium levels may change from high to normal levels initially (because acidosis causes potassium to be drawn into the bloodstream) to severely low levels as potassium reenters cells with treatment of acidosis. Thus, potassium replacement is likely to be needed during treatment of acidosis.

5. During severe acidosis, effective ventilation measures are needed along with sodium bicarbonate to remove carbon dioxide from the blood.

6. In lactic acidosis, larger doses of sodium bicarbonate may be required than in other types of acidosis. This is because of continued production of large amounts of lactic acid by body metabolism.

7. Chronic metabolic acidosis may occur with chronic renal failure. Sodium bicarbonate or citrate (which is converted to bicarbonate in the body) can be given orally in a dose sufficient to maintain a normal serum bicarbonate level.

Metabolic Alkalosis

1. Assess the presence and severity of the alkalosis by measuring arterial blood gases. Values indicating alkalosis are increased pH (above 7.45) and increased bicarbonate (above 26 mEq/L).

2. Assess and treat the underlying condition. Often, volume depletion and hypochloremia are present

and can be corrected with isotonic 0.9% sodium chloride solution. If hypokalemia and hypochloremia are present, potassium chloride will likely replace both deficits.

3. In severe alkalosis that does not respond to the above therapy, ammonium chloride can be given, but it must be given cautiously to avoid inducing acidosis.

USE IN CHILDREN

Children need sufficient amounts of minerals and electrolytes to support growth and normal body functioning. In the healthy child, a varied, well-balanced diet is generally preferred over supplements. However, iron deficiency is common in young children and teenage girls, and an iron supplement is often needed.

If supplements are given, dosages should not exceed recommended amounts. All minerals and electrolytes are toxic in overdose and may cause life-threatening adverse effects. All such drugs should be kept out of reach of young children and should never be referred to as "candy."

USE IN OLDER ADULTS

Mineral–electrolyte requirements are the same as for younger adults, but deficiencies of calcium and iron are common in older adults. Numerous factors may contribute to deficiencies, including limited income, anorexia, lack of teeth or ill-fitting dentures, drugs that decrease absorption of dietary nutrients, and disease processes that interfere with the ability to obtain, prepare, or eat adequate amounts of a variety of foods. Diuretic drugs, frequently prescribed for cardiovascular disorders in older adults, may cause potassium deficiency unless serum levels are carefully monitored and preventive measures taken.

Excess states also may occur in older adults. For example, decreased renal function promotes retention of magnesium and potassium. Hyperkalemia also may occur with the use of potassium supplements or salt substitutes. All minerals and electrolytes are toxic in overdose.

Every older adult should be assessed carefully regarding nutritional status and use of drugs that interact with dietary nutrients. Serum levels of minerals and electrolytes should be monitored carefully during illness and measures taken to prevent either deficiency or excess states.

 HOME CARE

The home care nurse has the opportunity to assess household members and the environment for indications of mineral–electrolyte deficiency or excess. Depending on assessment data, teaching may be needed about dietary sources of these nutrients, when mineral supplements are indicated or should be avoided, and safety factors related to iron supplements in homes with small children.

MINERAL-ELECTROLYTE PREPARATIONS

NURSING ACTIONS	RATIONALE/EXPLANATION
1. Administer accurately **a.** Give oral mineral–electrolyte preparations with food or immediately after meals.	To decrease gastric irritation. Iron and possibly some other agents are better absorbed when taken on an empty stomach. However, they are better tolerated when taken with food.
b. Give IV preparations slowly, as a general rule.	The primary danger of rapid IV injection or infusion is a transient excess in serum, which may cause cardiac arrhythmias or other serious problems.
c. Do not mix minerals and electrolytes with any other drug in a syringe.	High risk of physical incompatibility and precipitation of drugs
d. For IV infusion, most minerals and electrolytes are compatible with solutions of dextrose or sodium chloride. Do not mix with other solutions until compatibility is determined.	To avoid physical incompatibility and precipitation of contents

(continued)

NURSING ACTIONS	RATIONALE/EXPLANATION
e. For IV sodium chloride (NaCl) solutions:	
(1) Give fluids at the prescribed flow rate.	Flow rates depend largely on reasons for use. For example, if a client is receiving no oral fluids (NPO) or only small amounts, the flow rate is often 100 to 125 ml/h or 2400 to 3000 ml/24 h. If used as a vehicle for IV antibiotics, the rate is often 50 ml/h or keep open rate (KOR). If the client is dehydrated, 150 to 200 ml/h may be given for a few hours or until a certain amount has been given. (Restrictions in time or amount are necessary to avoid circulatory overload or pulmonary edema.)
(2) Give hypertonic saline solution (3% sodium chloride injection) slowly. Also, give no more than 200 to 400 ml at one time.	To avoid circulatory overload and sclerosing the veins
f. For potassium supplements:	
(1) Mix liquids, powders, and effervescent tablets in at least 4 oz of juice, water, or carbonated beverage.	To dilute, disguise the unpleasant taste, and decrease gastric irritation
(2) Give oral preparations with or after meals.	To decrease gastric irritation
(3) Never give undiluted potassium chloride (KCl) IV.	Transient hyperkalemia may cause life-threatening cardiotoxicity. Severe pain and vein sclerosis also may result.
(4) Dilute IV KCl 20 to 60 mEq in 1000 ml of IV solution, such as dextrose in water. Be sure that KCl is mixed well with the IV solution.	Dilution decreases risks of hyperkalemia and cardiotoxicity. It also prevents or decreases pain at the infusion site.
(5) Generally, give potassium-containing IV solutions at a rate that administers about 10 mEq/h or less.	This is the safest amount and rate of potassium administration. It is also usually effective.
(6) For life-threatening arrhythmias caused by hypokalemia, potassium can be replaced with 20 to 40 mEq/h with appropriate cardiac monitoring.	Risks of hyperkalemia and life-threatening cardiotoxicity are greatly increased with high concentrations or rapid flow rates. Constant electrocardiogram monitoring is the best way to detect hyperkalemia.
g. For magnesium sulfate ($MgSO_4$):	
(1) Read the drug label carefully to be sure you have the correct preparation for the intended use.	$MgSO_4$ is available in concentrations of 10%, 25%, and 50% and in sizes of 2-, 10-, and 20-ml ampules, as well as a 30-ml multidose vial.
(2) For IM administration, small amounts of 50% solution are usually used (1 g $MgSO_4$ = 2 ml of 50% solution).	
(3) For IV use, a 5% or 10% solution is used for direct injection, intermittent infusion, or continuous infusion. Whatever concentration is used, administer no more than 150 mg/min (1.5 ml/min of 10% solution; 3 ml/min of 5% solution).	
h. For sodium bicarbonate ($NaHCO_3$):	
(1) Read the label carefully to be sure you have the correct solution.	$NaHCO_3$ is available in several concentrations and sizes, such as 50-ml ampules or prefilled syringes with 50 mEq drug (8.4% solution) or 44.6 mEq drug (7.5% solution), 500-ml bottles with 297.7 mEq drug (5% solution) or 83 mEq drug (1.4% solution).
(2) Inject directly into the vein or into the tubing of a flowing IV infusion solution in emergencies, such as cardiac arrest.	

NURSING ACTIONS	RATIONALE/EXPLANATION
(3) In nonemergency situations, titrate flow rate of infusions according to arterial blood gases.	To avoid iatrogenic alkalosis
(4) Flush IV lines before and after injecting and do not add any other medications to an IV containing $NaHCO_3$	$NaHCO_3$ is highly alkaline and may cause precipitation of other drugs.
(5) Monitor arterial blood gases for increased pH after each 50 to 100 mEq of $NaHCO_3$.	To avoid overtreatment and metabolic alkalosis
i. For iron preparations:	
(1) Dilute liquid iron preparations, give with a straw, and have the client rinse the mouth afterward	To prevent temporary staining of teeth
(2) To give iron dextran intramuscularly, use a 2- to 3-inch needle and Z-track technique to inject the drug into the upper outer quadrant of the buttock.	To prevent discomfort and staining of subcutaneous tissue and skin
(3) To give iron dextran IV (either directly or diluted in sodium chloride solution and given over several hours), do not use the multidose vial.	The multidose vial contains phenol as a preservative and is not suitable for IV use. Ampules of 2 ml or 5 ml are available without preservative.
j. Refer to the individual drugs or package literature for instructions regarding administration of ammonium chloride, deferoxamine, penicillamine, tromethamine, and multiple electrolyte solutions.	
2. Observe for therapeutic effects **a.** With NaCl, observe for decreased symptoms of hyponatremia and increased serum sodium level.	Therapeutic effects should be evident within a few hours.
b. With KCl or other potassium preparations, observe for decreased signs of hypokalemia and increased serum potassium levels.	
c. With $MgSO_4$, observe for decreased signs of hypomagnesemia, increased serum magnesium levels, or control of convulsions.	
d. With zinc sulfate ($ZnSO_4$), observe for improved wound healing.	
e. With sodium bicarbonate ($NaHCO_3$), observe for decreased manifestations of acidosis and a rise in blood pH and bicarbonate levels.	
f. With iron preparations, observe for:	Therapeutic effects are usually evident within a month unless other problems are also present (*e.g.*, vitamin deficiency, achlorhydria, infection, malabsorption).
(1) Increased vigor and feeling of well-being	
(2) Improved appetite	
(3) Less fatigue	
(4) Increased RBC, hemoglobin, and hematocrit	
(5) With parenteral iron, observe for an average increase in hemoglobin of 1 g/week.	

(continued)

NURSING ACTIONS	RATIONALE/EXPLANATION
3. Observe for adverse effects	
a. Mineral–electrolyte excess states:	These are likely to occur with excessive dosages of supplements. They can usually be prevented by using relatively low doses in nonemergency situations and by frequent monitoring of serum levels of electrolytes and iron.
(1) With NaCl injection, observe for hypernatremia and circulatory overload.	These are most likely to occur with rapid infusion of large amounts or with heart or kidney disease, which decreases water excretion and urine output. They also may occur with hypertonic solutions (*e.g.*, 3% NaCl), but these are infrequently used.
(2) With potassium preparations, observe for hyperkalemia.	This is most likely to occur with rapid IV administration, high dosages or concentrations, or in the presence of renal insufficiency and decreased urine output.
(3) With magnesium preparations, observe for hypermagnesemia.	See potassium preparations, above.
(4) With NaHCO$_3$, observe for metabolic alkalosis.	This is most likely to occur when large amounts of NaHCO$_3$ are given IV.
b. Gastrointestinal (GI) symptoms—anorexia, nausea, vomiting, diarrhea, and abdominal discomfort from gastric irritation	Most oral preparations of minerals and electrolytes are likely to cause gastric irritation. Taking the drugs with food or 8 oz of fluid may decrease symptoms.
c. Cardiovascular symptoms:	
(1) Cardiac arrhythmias	Potentially fatal arrhythmias may occur with hyperkalemia or hypermagnesemia.
(2) Hypotension, tachycardia, other symptoms of shock	May occur with deferoxamine and iron dextran injections
(3) Circulatory overload and possible pulmonary edema	Most likely to occur with large amounts of NaCl or NaHCO$_3$
d. With Kayexalate, observe for hypokalemia, hypocalcemia, hypomagnesemia, and edema.	Although this drug is used to treat hyperkalemia, it removes calcium and magnesium ions as well as potassium ions. Because it acts by trading sodium for potassium, the sodium retention may lead to edema.
4. Observe for drug interactions	
a. Drugs that *increase* effects of minerals and electrolytes and related drugs:	
(1) Acidifying agents (ammonium chloride): effects are increased by sodium chloride, potassium chloride, and ascorbic acid.	Systemic acidification by increased serum chloride; also increased urine acidity
(2) Alkalinizing agents (sodium bicarbonate): effects are increased by antacids, such as magnesium hydroxide, calcium carbonate, and aluminum hydroxide.	Small amounts of antacids may be absorbed to produce additive effects.
(3) Cation exchange resin (Kayexalate): diuretics increase potassium loss; other sources of sodium increase the likelihood of edema.	Additive effects
(4) Iron salts:	
(a) Allopurinol (Zyloprim)	This drug may increase the concentration of iron in the liver. It should not be given concurrently with any iron preparation.
(b) Ascorbic acid (vitamin C)	In large doses of 1 g or more, ascorbic acid increases absorption of iron by acidifying secretions.

NURSING ACTIONS	RATIONALE/EXPLANATION
(5) Potassium salts:	
(a) Spironolactone, triamterene, amiloride	These drugs are potassium-saving diuretics. They should *not* be given with a potassium supplement because of additive risks of producing life-threatening hyperkalemia.
(b) Salt substitutes (*e.g.*, Neo-Curtasol)	These contain potassium rather than sodium and may cause hyperkalemia if given with potassium supplements.
(c) Penicillin G potassium	This potassium salt of penicillin contains 1.7 mEq of potassium per 1 million units. It may produce hyperkalemia if given in combination with potassium supplements.
b. Drugs that *decrease* effects of minerals and electrolytes and related drugs:	
(1) Acidifying agents: effects are decreased by alkalinizing agents.	Alkalinizing agents neutralize the effects of acidifying agents.
(2) Alkalinizing agents: effects are decreased by acidifying drugs.	Acidifying drugs neutralize effects of alkalinizing agents.
(3) Oral iron salts:	
(a) Antacids containing carbonate	The antacids decrease iron absorption by forming an insoluble, nonabsorbable compound of iron carbonate.
(b) Magnesium trisilicate	This antacid decreases absorption of iron.
(c) Pancreatic extracts	These inhibit iron absorption by increasing alkalinity of GI fluids.
(4) Potassium salts:	
(a) Calcium gluconate	Decreases cardiotoxic effects of hyperkalemia and is therefore useful in the treatment of hyperkalemia
(b) Sodium polystyrene sulfonate (Kayexalate)	Used in treatment of hyperkalemia because it removes potassium from the body
5. Teach clients **a.** With iron preparations, teach:	
(1) To take with or after meals, at least initially	To decrease gastric irritation. If no anorexia, nausea, vomiting, or other problems occur, the drug can be tried before meals because it is better absorbed from an empty stomach.
(2) To dilute and take liquid iron preparations through a straw	To avoid staining the teeth
(3) That the drug turns stools dark green or black	
b. Potassium preparations *must* be taken as directed.	The unpleasant taste of oral solutions apparently reduces compliance with physician's orders.
(1) Mix oral solutions or effervescent tablets with at least 4 oz of water or juice.	To improve the taste
(2) Take after meals	To further dilute the drug and decrease gastric irritation
(3) Do *not* stop taking the drug without notifying the physician who prescribed it, especially if also taking digitalis or diuretics.	Serious problems may develop from low levels of potassium in the blood.

REVIEW AND APPLICATION EXERCISES

1. What are the major roles of minerals and electrolytes in normal body functioning?

2. How would you assess a client for hypokalemia?

3. When a client is given potassium supplements for hypokalemia, how do you monitor for therapeutic and adverse drug effects?

4. Identify client populations at risk of developing hyperkalemia.

5. List interventions to decrease risks of developing hyperkalemia.

6. If severe hyperkalemia develops, how is it treated?

7. What are some causes of iron deficiency anemia?

8. In a client with iron deficiency anemia, what information could you provide about good food sources of iron?

9. What are advantages and disadvantages of iron supplements?

SELECTED REFERENCES

Chessman, K.H. & Anderson, J.D. (1997). Pediatric and geriatric nutrition support. In J.T. DiPiro, R.L. Talbert, G.C. Yee, G.R. Matzke, B.G. Wells, & L.M. Posey (Eds.), *Pharmacotherapy: A pathophysiologic approach,* 3rd ed., pp. 2787–2804). Stamford, CT: Appleton & Lange.

Corman, L. C. (1993). The role of nutrition in sickness and in health. *Medical Clinics of North America, 77*(4), 711–724.

Darby, M.K. & Loughead, J.L. (1996). Neonatal nutritional requirements and formula composition: A review. *Journal of Obstetrics, Gynecology, and Neonatal Nursing, 25*(3), 209–217.

Davis, J.R., & Sherer, K. (1994). *Applied nutrition and diet therapy for nurses,* 2nd ed. Philadelphia: W.B. Saunders.

Drug facts and comparisons. (Updated monthly). St. Louis: Facts and Comparisons.

Hillman, R.S. (1996). Hematopoietic agents: Growth factors, minerals, and vitamins. In J.G. Hardman, L.E. Limbird, P.B. Molinoff, & R.W. Ruddon (Eds.), *Goodman & Gilman's The pharmacological basis of therapeutics,* 9th ed., pp. 1311–1340. New York: McGraw-Hill.

Martinez-Maldonado, M. (1997). Approach to the patient with hypokalemia. In W.N. Kelley (Ed.), *Textbook of internal medicine,* 3rd ed., pp. 959–963. Philadelphia: Lippincott-Raven.

Porth, C.M. (1994). *Pathophysiology: Concepts of altered health states,* 3rd ed., pp. 591–627. Philadelphia: J.B. Lippincott.

Schoolwerth, A.C., Feldman, G.M., & Culpepper, R.M. (1997). Approach to the patient with altered magnesium concentration. In W.N. Kelley (Ed.), *Textbook of internal medicine,* 3rd ed., pp. 967–970. Philadelphia: Lippincott-Raven.

Schultz, N.J. & Chitwood, K.K. (1997). Body electrolyte homeostasis. In J.T. DiPiro, R.L. Talbert, G.C. Yee, G.R. Matzke, B.G. Wells, & L.M. Posey (Eds.), *Pharmacotherapy: A pathophysiologic approach,* 3rd ed., pp. 1105–1137. Stamford, CT: Appleton & Lange.

Drugs Used to Treat Infections

33 General Characteristics of Antimicrobial Drugs

Objectives

After studying this chapter, the student will be able to:

1 Identify populations who are at increased risk of developing infections.

2 Discuss common pathogens and methods of infection control.

3 Assess clients for local and systemic signs of infection.

4 Discuss common and potentially serious adverse effects of antimicrobial drugs.

5 Identify clients at increased risk of adverse drug reactions.

6 Discuss ways to increase benefits and decrease hazards of antimicrobial drug therapy.

7 Discuss ways to minimize emergence of drug-resistant microorganisms.

8 State appropriate nursing implications for a client receiving an antimicrobial drug.

9 Discuss important elements of using antimicrobial drugs in children, older adults.

(continued)

Key Terms

Aerobic	**Hypersensitivity**
Anaerobic	**Narrow spectrum**
Anaphylaxis	**Nosocomial**
Bactericidal	**Pathogenic**
Bacteriostatic	**Phlebitis**
Broad spectrum	**Prophylactic**
Chemoprophylaxis	**Pseudomembranous colitis**
Culture and susceptibility studies	**Superinfection**
Drug resistant	

Antimicrobial drugs are used to prevent or treat infections caused by pathogenic (disease-producing) microorganisms. The human body and the environment contain many microorganisms (bacteria, viruses, fungi, and others), most of which live in a state of balance with the human host and do not cause disease. When the balance is upset and infection occurs, characteristics of the infecting microorganism(s) and the adequacy of host defense mechanisms are major factors in the severity of the infection and the person's ability to recover. Conditions that impair defense mechanisms increase the incidence and severity of infections and impede recovery. In addition, use of antimicrobial drugs may lead to serious infections caused by drug-resistant microorganisms. To help prevent infectious diseases and participate effectively in antimicrobial drug therapy, the nurse must be knowledgeable about microorganisms, host responses to microorganisms, and antimicrobial drugs.

Microorganisms and Infections

Organisms are everywhere in the environment, including air, food, water, and soil. They also are present in the human body, especially on the skin and in the upper respiratory tract and colon. In an infection, microorganisms initially attach to host cell receptors (*i.e.*, proteins, carbohydrates, lipids, or combinations of these structures). For example, some bacteria have hair-like structures that attach them to skin and mucous membranes. Most microorganisms preferentially attach themselves to particular body tissues. The microorganisms may then invade tissues, multiply, and produce infection. A major characteristic of microorganisms is their ability to survive in various environments. Bacteria, for example, may form mutant strains, alter their structures and functions, or become embedded in a layer of mucus. These adaptations may protect them from normal body defense mechanisms and antimicrobial drugs. Many bacteria develop drug-resistant strains in the presence of antimicrobial drugs. Classifications, normal microbial flora and common pathogenic microorganisms are described below.

CLASSIFICATIONS

Bacteria are subclassified according to whether they are aerobic (require oxygen) or anaerobic (cannot live in the presence of oxygen), their reaction to Gram's stain (gram-positive or gram-negative), and their shape (cocci [oval], bacilli [rod-shaped], spirilla [spiral]).

Viruses are intracellular parasites that survive only in living tissues. Although they are officially classified according to their structures, they are more commonly described according to origin and the disorders or symptoms they produce. Human pathogens include adenoviruses, herpesviruses, and retroviruses (see Chap. 39).

Fungi are plant-like organisms that live as parasites on living tissue or as saprophytes on decaying organic matter. About 50 species are pathogenic in humans (see Chap. 40).

NORMAL MICROBIAL FLORA

The human body normally has areas that are sterile and areas that are colonized with microorganisms. Sterile areas are body fluids and cavities, the lower respiratory tract (trachea, bronchi, lungs), much of the gastrointestinal (GI) and genitourinary tracts, and the musculoskeletal system. Colonized areas include the skin, upper respiratory tract, and colon.

Normal skin flora includes staphylococci, streptococci, diphtheroids, and transient environmental organisms. The upper respiratory tract contains staphylococci, streptococci, pneumococci, diphtheroids, and *Haemophilus influenzae*. The external genitalia contain skin organisms; the vagina contains lactobacilli, *Candida*, and *Bacteroides*. The colon contains *Escherichia coli*, *Klebsiella*, *Enterobacter*, *Proteus*, *Pseudomonas*, *Bacteroides*, *Clostridia*, lactobacilli, streptococci, and staphylococci. Microorganisms that are part of the normal flora and nonpathogenic in one area of the body may be pathogenic in other parts of the body. For example, *Escherichia coli* often cause urinary tract infections.

Normal flora protects the human host by occupying space and consuming nutrients. This interferes with the ability of potential pathogens to establish residence and proliferate. If the normal flora is suppressed by antimicrobial drug therapy, potential pathogens may thrive. For example, the yeast, *Candida albicans*, is a normal resident of the vagina and intestinal tract. An antibacterial drug may destroy the normal bacterial flora without affecting the fungal organism. Thus, the *Candida* can grow unchecked and become the major organism in these areas. It can then cause infection and severe inflammation in skin and mucous membranes. Thus, much of the normal flora can cause disease under certain conditions, especially in elderly, debilitated, or immunosuppressed individuals. Normal bowel flora also synthesizes vitamin K and vitamin B complex.

INFECTIOUS DISEASES

Colonization involves the presence of microorganisms (normal microbial flora or transient environmental organisms) that do not harm the host. Infection or infectious disease involves the presence of a pathogen plus clinical signs and symptoms indicative of an infection. Accurate assessment and documentation of symptoms can aid in the diagnosis of infectious diseases.

Laboratory Identification of Pathogens

The presence and identification of a probable pathogen can be indicated by laboratory tests such as culture of infected fluids or tissues, serology, or the detection of characteristic antigens or metabolites produced by the pathogen. *Culture* refers to propagation of a microorganism outside the body in artificial growth media. With bacteria, identification is based on microscopic appearance, Gram's stain reaction, shape, texture, and color of the colonies, and other characteristics of the organism. Identification of other microorganisms (*e.g.*, intracellular pathogens such as chlamydiae and viruses) may require different techniques. *Serology* identifies infectious agents indirectly by measuring the antibody level (titer) in the serum of a diseased host. A tentative diagnosis can be made if the antibody level against a specific pathogen rises during the acute phase of the disease and falls during convalescence. *Detection of antigens* uses features of culture and serology but reduces the time required for diagnosis.

Common Human Pathogens

Common human pathogens are viruses, gram-positive enterococci, streptococci and staphylococci, and gram-negative intestinal organisms (*Escherichia coli, Bacteroides, Klebsiella, Proteus, Pseudomonas* species and others; Box 33-1). These microorganisms are usually spread by air, direct contact with an infected person, or contaminated hands, food, water, or objects. Some also may be spread by a carrier (a person who transmits a pathogenic organism but does not have an active infection).

For example, some people "carry" pathogenic strains of staphylococci in their upper respiratory tracts (*e.g.*, anterior nares).

"Opportunistic" microorganisms are usually normal endogenous or environmental flora and nonpathogenic. They become pathogens, however, in hosts whose defense mechanisms are impaired. Opportunistic infections are likely to occur in people with severe burns, cancer, indwelling intravenous (IV) or urinary catheters, and antibiotic or corticosteroid drug therapy. Opportunistic bacterial infections, often caused by drug-resistant microorganisms, are usually serious and may be life threatening. Fungi of the *Candida* genus, especially *Candida albicans*, may cause life-threatening bloodstream or deep tissue infections, such as brain abscesses. Viral infections may cause fatal pneumonia in people with renal or cardiac disorders, and in bone marrow transplant recipients.

Community-Acquired Versus Nosocomial Infections

Infections are often categorized as community-acquired or hospital-acquired (nosocomial). Because the microbial environments differ, the two types of infections often have different etiologies and require different antimicrobial drugs. As a general rule, community-acquired infections are less severe and easier to treat. Nosocomial infections may be more severe and difficult to manage because they often result from drug-resistant microorganisms and occur in people whose resistance to disease is impaired. Drug-resistant strains of staphylococci, *Pseudomonas*, and *Proteus* are common causes of nosocomial urinary tract and surgical wound infections.

ANTIBIOTIC-RESISTANT MICROORGANISMS

The increasing prevalence of bacteria resistant to the effects of antibiotics, in both community-acquired and nosocomial infections, is a major public health concern. Antibiotic resistance commonly occurs in most human pathogens. Infections caused by drug-resistant organisms often require more toxic and more expensive drugs, lead to prolonged illness or hospitalization, and increase mortality rates.

Resistant microorganisms grow and multiply when susceptible organisms (*e.g.*, normal flora) are suppressed by antimicrobial drugs or when normal body defenses are impaired by immunosuppressive disorders or drugs. They may emerge during or after antimicrobial drug therapy. Factors contributing to their development include the following:

1. **Widespread use of antimicrobial drugs, especially broad-spectrum agents.** Antibiotics are among the

BOX 33-1. COMMON BACTERIAL PATHOGENS

Gram-Positive Bacteria

STAPHYLOCOCCI

Staphylococcus aureus organisms are part of the normal microbial flora of the skin and upper respiratory tract and also are common pathogens. Some people carry (are colonized with) the organism in the anterior nares. The organisms are spread mainly by direct contact with people who are infected or who are carriers. The hands of health care workers are considered a major source of indirect spread and nosocomial infections. The organisms also survive on inanimate surfaces for long periods of time.

Staphylococcus aureus organisms cause boils, carbuncles, burn and surgical wound infections, and internal abscesses. Burns or surgical wounds often become infected from clients' own nasal carriage or from health care personnel. The organisms cannot penetrate intact skin or mucous membranes. However, they can penetrate damaged tissues and produce endotoxins that destroy erythrocytes, leukocytes, platelets, fibroblasts, and other human cells. Also, many strains produce enterotoxins that cause food poisoning when ingested. The enterotoxins survive heating at temperatures high enough to kill the organisms. (So reheating foods does not prevent food poisoning.)

High-risk groups for staphylococcal infections include newborns, the elderly, and those who are malnourished, diabetic, or obese. In children, staphylococcal infections of the respiratory tract are most common in those younger than 2 years of age. In adults, staphylococcal pneumonia often occurs in persons with chronic lung disease or as a secondary bacterial infection following influenza. The influenza virus destroys the ciliated epithelium of the respiratory tract and thereby aids bacterial invasion.

Staphylococcus epidermidis organisms are also part of the normal microbial flora of the skin and mucosal surfaces and are increasingly common pathogens. Infections with these organisms are associated with the use of treatment devices such as intravascular catheters, prosthetic heart valves, cardiac pacemakers, orthopedic prostheses, cerebrospinal fluid shunts, and peritoneal catheters. *S epidermidis* infections include endocarditis, bacteremia, and other serious infections and are especially hazardous to neutropenic and immunocompromised persons. Treatment usually requires removal of any infected medical device as well as appropriate antibiotic therapy.

STREPTOCOCCI

S viridans (alpha-hemolytic streptococcus) organisms are part of the normal microbial flora of the throat and nasopharynx in many healthy individuals. Infections are usually spread by inhalation of droplets from the upper respiratory tracts of carriers or people with infections. However, these organisms do not cause disease unless the mucosal barrier is damaged by trauma, previous infection, or surgical manipulation. Such damage allows the organisms to enter the bloodstream and gain access to other parts of the body. For example, the organisms may cause infective endocarditis if they reach damaged heart valves. Streptococcal endocarditis can usually be treated effectively by about 2 weeks of penicillin therapy.

S pneumoniae organisms, often called pneumococci, are common bacterial pathogens. They cause pneumonia, sinusitis, otitis media, and meningitis. Pneumococcal pneumonia usually develops when the mechanisms that normally expel organisms inhaled into the lower airway (*i.e.*, the mucociliary blanket and cough reflex) are impaired by viral infection, smoking, immobility, or other insults. When *S pneumoniae* reach the alveoli, they proliferate, cause acute inflammation, and spread rapidly to involve one or more lobes. Alveoli fill with proteinaceous fluid, neutrophils, and bacteria. When the pneumonia resolves, there is usually no residual damage to the pulmonary parenchyma. Elderly adults have high rates of illness and death from pneumococcal pneumonia, which can often be prevented by pneumococcal vaccine. Pneumococcal vaccine (see Chap. 43) contains 23 strains of the pneumococci that cause most of the serious infections.

Pneumococcal sinusitis and otitis media usually follow a viral illness such as the common cold. The viral infection injures the protective ciliated epithelium and fills the air spaces with nutrient-rich tissue fluid, in which the pneumococci thrive. *S pneumoniae* cause about 35% of cases of bacterial sinusitis. In young children, upper respiratory tract infections may be complicated by acute sinusitis. With otitis media, most children have repeated episodes by 6 years of age and the pneumococcus causes about half of these cases. Recurrent otitis media during early childhood may result in reduced hearing acuity. Otitis media rarely occurs in adults.

Pneumococcal meningitis may develop from sinus or middle ear infections or an injury that allows organisms from the nasopharynx to enter the meninges. *S pneumoniae* are a common cause of bacterial meningitis in adults. Other potential secondary complications include septicemia, endocarditis, pericarditis and empyema.

Susceptible pneumococcal infections may be treated with penicillin G. For people who are allergic to penicillin, a first-generation cephalosporin or erythromycin may be effective for pneumonia, but pneumococcal meningitis should be treated with chloramphenicol.

S pyogenes (beta-hemolytic streptococcus) are often normal flora of the skin and oropharynx. The organisms spread

BOX 33-1. (CONTINUED)

from person to person by direct contact with oral or respiratory secretions. They cause severe pharyngitis ("strep throat"), scarlet fever, rheumatic fever, and infective endocarditis. With streptococcal pharyngitis, persons remain infected with the organism for weeks after symptoms resolve and thus serve as a reservoir for infection.

ENTEROCOCCI

These organisms, formerly Group D streptococci, are now classified as the genus *Enterococcus*, which contains about 12 species. The main pathogens are *E faecalis*, *E faecium*, and *E durans*. The enterococci are normal flora in the human intestine but are also found in soil, food, water, and animals.

Most enterococcal infections occur in hospitalized patients, especially those in critical care units. Risk factors for nosocomial infections include serious underlying disease, prior surgery, renal insufficiency, and the presence of urinary or vascular cathethers. These organisms, especially *E faecalis*, are usually secondary invaders in urinary tract or wound infections. Enterococci may also cause infective endocarditis. This serious infection occurs most often in individuals with underlying heart disease, such as an injured valve. When the organisms reach a heart valve, they multiply and release emboli of foreign particles into the bloodstream. Symptoms of infective endocarditis include fever, heart murmurs, enlarged spleen, and anemia. This infection is diagnosed by isolating enterococci from blood cultures. If not treated promptly and appropriately, infective endocarditis may be fatal. Enterococcal endocarditis is usually treated with a combination of gentamicin and vancomycin.

Gram-negative Bacteria

BACTEROIDES

Bacteroides are anaerobic bacteria normally found in the digestive, respiratory, and genital tracts. They are the most common bacteria in the colon, where they greatly outnumber *E. coli*. *B fragilis* is the major human pathogen in this group. *B fragilis* infections include intra-abdominal and pelvic abscesses (*e.g.*, following surgery or trauma that allows fecal contamination of these tissues), brain abscesses (*e.g.*, from bacteremia or spread from a middle ear or sinus infection), and bacteremia, which may spread the organisms throughout the body.

ESCHERICHIA COLI

E coli inhabit the intestinal tract of humans and animals. They are normally nonpathogenic in the intestinal tract but common pathogens when allowed access to other parts of the body. The organism may be beneficial by synthesizing vitamins and by competitively discouraging growth of possible pathogens.

E coli cause most urinary tract infections. They also cause pneumonia and sepsis in immunocompromised hosts and meningitis and sepsis in newborns. *E coli* pneumonia often occurs in debilitated patients following colonization of the oropharynx with organisms from their endogenous microbial flora. In healthy persons, the normal gram-positive organisms of oral cavities attach to material that coats the surface of oral mucosa and prevents transient *E coli* from establishing residence. Debilitated or severely ill persons produce an enzyme that destroys the material that allows gram-positive flora to adhere to oral mucosa. This allows *E coli* (and other gram-negative enteric bacteria) to compete successfully with the normal gram-positive flora and colonize the oropharynx. Then, droplets of the oral flora are aspirated into the respiratory tract, where impaired protective mechanisms allow survival of the aspirated organisms.

E coli also cause enteric gram-negative sepsis, which is acquired from the normal enteric bacterial flora. When *E coli* and other enteric organisms reach the bloodstream of healthy persons, host defenses eliminate the organisms. When the organisms reach the bloodstream of persons with severe illnesses and conditions such as neutropenia, the host is unable to mount adequate defenses and sepsis occurs. In neonates, *E coli* are the most common gram-negative organisms causing nosocomial septic shock and meningitis.

In addition, *E coli* often cause diarrhea and dysentery. One strain, called 0157:H7, causes hemorrhagic colitis, a disease characterized by severe abdominal cramps, copious bloody diarrhea, and possibly hemolytic-uremia syndrome (hemolytic anemia, thrombocytopenia, and acute renal failure). Hemolytic-uremia syndrome occurs most often in children. The main reservoir of this strain is the intestinal tract of animals, especially cattle, and several epidemics have been associated with ingestion of undercooked ground beef. Other sources include contaminated water and milk and person-to-person spread. Because it cannot survive in nature, the presence of *E coli* in milk or water indicates fecal contamination.

KLEBSIELLA

Klebsiella organisms, which are normal bowel flora, may infect the respiratory tract, urinary tract, bloodstream, burn wounds, and meninges, most often as opportunistic infections in debilitated persons. *K pneumoniae* are a common cause of pneumonia, especially in people with pulmonary disease, bacteremia, and sepsis. Gram-negative pneumo-

(continued)

BOX 33-1. (Continued)

nia and sepsis caused by *Klebsiella* produce the same disease patterns as those caused by *E coli*.

PROTEUS

Proteus organisms are normally found in the intestinal tract and in decaying matter. They most often cause urinary tract and wound infections but may infect any tissue, especially in debilitated persons. Infection usually occurs with antibiotic therapy, which decreases drug-sensitive bacteria and allows drug-resistant bacteria to proliferate. Gram-negative pneumonia and sepsis caused by *Proteus* organisms are essentially the same as those caused by *E coli* and *Klebsiella*.

PSEUDOMONAS

Pseudomonas organisms are found in water, soil, skin, and intestines. They are found in the stools of some healthy individuals and possibly 50% of hospital patients. *P aeruginosa*, the species most often associated with human disease, can cause infections of the respiratory tract, urinary tract, wounds, burns, meninges, eyes, and ears. Because of their resistance to many antibiotics, they can cause severe infections in persons receiving antibiotic therapy for burns, wounds, and cystic fibrosis. *P aeruginosa* colonize the respiratory tract of most individuals with cystic fibrosis and infect about 25% of burn patients. Infection is more likely to occur in hosts who are very young or very old or who have impaired immune systems. Sources of infection include catheterization or other instrumentation of the urinary tract, trauma or procedures involving the brain or spinal cord, and contamination of respiratory ventilators. Gram-negative pneumonia and sepsis caused by *P aeruginosa* are essentially the same as those caused by *E coli* and other gram-negative organisms.

P cepacia infections are increasing, especially in patients with burns, cystic fibrosis, debilitation, or immunosuppression. These infections are especially difficult to treat because the organism is resistant to many of the antibitotics used to treat other gram-negative infections.

SERRATIA

S marcescens organisms are found in infected people, water, soil, milk, and feces. They cause serious nosocomial infections of the urinary tract, respiratory tract, skin, burn wounds, and bloodstream. They also may cause hospital epidemics and produce drug-resistant strains. High-risk patients include newborns, the debilitated, and the immunosuppressed. Pneumonia and sepsis due to *Serratia* organisms produce disease similar to *E coli* and other gram-negative organisms.

SALMONELLA

About 1400 species have been identified; several are pathogenic to humans. The organisms cause gastroenteritis, typhoid fever, septicemia, and a severe, sometimes fatal type of food poisoning. The primary reservoir is the intestinal tract of many animals. Humans become infected through ingestion of contaminated water or food. Water becomes polluted by introduction of feces from any animal excreting salmonellae. Infection by food usually results from ingestion of contaminated meat or by hands transferring organisms from an infected source. In the United States, undercooked poultry and eggs are common sources.

Salmonella enterocolitis is a common cause of food-borne outbreaks of gastroenteritis. Diarrhea usually begins several hours after ingesting contaminated food and may continue for several days, along with nausea, vomiting, headache, and abdominal pain.

SHIGELLA

Shigella species cause gastrointestinal problems ranging from mild diarrhea to severe and sometimes fatal bacillary dysentery. Humans, who seem to be the only natural hosts, become infected after ingestion of contaminated food or water. Effects of shigellosis are attributed to the loss of fluids, electrolytes, and nutrients and to the ulceration that occurs in the colon wall.

---

most frequently prescribed drugs, and their use affects distribution of antibiotic-resistant bacteria in the environment. When an antibiotic is given, it affects not only the bacteria for which it was prescribed, but other bacteria carried by that person as well, including transient organisms, other pathogens, and normal flora. When bacteria of the normal flora are destroyed or suppressed, space and nutrients become available to support the growth of organisms resistant to the effects of that antibiotic. The resistant organisms soon become the predominant strain. Once established, resistant bacteria can cause

superinfection in the original host, spread to other hosts, and even spread their resistance properties for that antibiotic to other species of bacteria. In addition to resistance to the effects of one antibiotic, cross-resistance to similar antibiotics also occurs because most antibiotics are variations of a few basic types.

2. **Interrupted or inadequate antimicrobial treatment of infections.** Consumers often stop taking a prescribed antibiotic when symptoms subside or they feel better. In such circumstances, only the most susceptible bacteria are affected and resistant organisms can become established residents. This often

occurs with tuberculosis, which requires long-term drug therapy for prevention or treatment.

3. **Type of bacteria.** Both gram-positive and gram-negative bacteria are developing more antibiotic-resistant strains. Gram-positive organisms include staphylococci, streptococci, and enterococci. Gram-negative bacteria associated with high rates of antibiotic resistance include *Pseudomonas aeruginosa, Serratia, Enterobacter,* and *Acinetobacter* species. Antibiotic resistance in gram-negative organisms has long been a clinical problem because the organisms are inherently resistant to penetration of antibiotics and acquire resistance by multiple mechanisms. These organisms have outer membranes with openings (porins) that regulate passage of antibiotics. Some gram-negative bacteria (*e.g., Escherichia coli* and most other bowel organisms) have more permeable porins than others (*e.g., Pseudomonas aeruginosa*). *Pseudomonas* organisms have different types of porins, and each type allows the penetration of only a few substances. Thus, *Pseudomonas aeruginosa* organisms are generally resistant to many antibiotics. Those strains resistant to gentamicin may be susceptible to amikacin, ceftazidime, imipenem, ciprofloxacin or aztreonam. Some gram-negative organisms have become increasingly resistant to aminoglycosides, third-generation cephalosporins, and aztreonam, but may be susceptible to imipenem or ciprofloxacin.

4. **Type of infection.** Infections often associated with high rates of resistance include lower respiratory tract infections and those associated with cystic fibrosis or osteomyelitis. These infections are often difficult to treat because they tend to recur, involve multiple, gram-negative, or resistant organisms, and involve anatomic locations that antibiotics do not penetrate well.

5. **Condition of the host.** Patients who are malnourished, severely ill, immunosuppressed, receiving mechanical ventilation, or using other mechanical devices are at high risk for infections, including those caused by antibiotic-resistant organisms.

6. **Location or setting.** Although resistant organisms can develop in essentially any environment, they are especially likely in critical care units and large university or teaching hospitals. In these settings, very ill patients often require extensive antibiotic therapy. The constant presence of antibiotics provides strong pressures for selection and replication of resistant organisms.

Specific resistant organisms and the specific antibiotics to which they develop resistance vary in geographic areas (*e.g.,* from one region to another) and in communities (*e.g.,* from hospital to hospital and from unit to unit within the same institution). These variations stem largely from extensive use of particular antibiotics in particular settings. Nationally, resistant bacterial strains of major concern include penicillin-resistant *Streptococcus pneumoniae,* methicillin-resistant *Staphylococcus aureus* and *Staphylococcus epidermidis,* vancomycin-resistant enterococcus, and multidrug-resistant tuberculosis (MDR-TB). Actually, all of these organisms are resistant to multiple antibiotics. The first three are described in Box 33-2; MDR-TB is discussed in Chapter 38. Viruses and fungi also develop resistance to antimicrobial drugs, as discussed in Chapters 39 and 40.

Mechanisms of Resistance

Bacteria have developed numerous ways to acquire resistance to antimicrobial drugs, including:

- Production of enzymes that destroy or inactivate the drugs. For example, beta-lactamase enzymes change the chemical structure of penicillins and cephalosporins by opening the beta-lactam ring and preventing the antibiotic from binding with its target site (enzymes called penicillin-binding proteins or PBPs) in the bacterial cell wall.
- Genetic mutations that change target enzymes or change the genetic code to produce new enzymes. These changes decrease bacterial susceptibility to an antibiotic, largely by altering binding sites.
- Changing their metabolic pathways to bypass antibiotic activity.
- Changing their cell walls to prevent penetration of the drug (making the drug unable to reach its target sites within the bacterial cell). Drugs usually enter bacterial cells through openings called porins. Some gram-negative bacteria are able to produce porins that restrict antibiotic entry more than usual porins.
- Becoming able to pump drug molecules out of the cell. Multiple nonspecific efflux systems become activated to remove foreign chemicals.
- Transferring genetic material (deoxyribonucleic acid or plasmids) between microorganisms. Bacteria, pathogenic and nonpathogenic, have efficient mechanisms for genetic exchange. This allows them to spread antibiotic resistance from one bacterial strain to another, including different species or types of bacteria. Thus, when a new antibiotic is used, resistance may rapidly appear and be disseminated to multiple bacteria.

Host Defense Mechanisms

Although the numbers and virulence of microorganisms help to determine whether a person colonized or exposed to microorganisms develops an infection,

BOX 33-2. ANTIBIOTIC-RESISTANT STAPHYLOCOCCI, STREPTOCOCCI AND ENTEROCOCCI

Methicillin-resistant Staphylococcus aureus (MRSA)

Penicillin-resistant staphylococci were identified from the early days of penicillin use because the organisms produced beta-lactamase enzymes (penicillinases) that destroyed penicillin. Methicillin was one of five drugs developed to resist the action of beta-lactamase enzymes and thus be effective in treating staphylococcal infections. Eventually, strains of staphylococci became resistant to these drugs as well. The mechanism of resistance in MRSA is alteration of penicillin-binding proteins (PBPs). PBPs, the target sites of penicillins and other beta-lactam antibiotics, are enzymes required for synthesis of cell walls in S aureus organisms. Susceptible S aureus have five PBPs called 1, 2, 3, 3a or 3' and 4. Beta-lactam antibiotics bind to these enzymes and produce defective bacterial cell walls, which kill the organisms. MRSA have an additional PBP called 2a or 2'. Methicillin cannot bind effectively to the PBPs and inhibit bacterial cell wall synthesis except with very high drug concentrations. Consequently, minimum inhibitory concentrations (MICs) of methicillin increased to higher levels that were difficult or impossible to achieve.

The term MRSA is commonly used but misleading because the organisms are widely resistant to penicillins (including all of the antistaphylococcal penicillins, not just methicillin) and cephalosporins. Many strains of MRSA are also resistant to erythromycin, clindamycin, tetracycline, and the aminoglycosides. In addition, the incidence of methicillin-resistant Staphylococcus epidermidis (MRSE) isolates is increasing. MRSE frequently colonize nasal passages of health care workers and are increasing as a cause of nosocomial infections, especially in critical care units.

A major reason for the current concern with infections caused by MRSA and MRSE is that vancomycin is the drug of choice for treatment. Vancomycin has been used extensively to treat infections caused by S epidermidis and enterococci, and vancomycin resistance is increasing in those species. Because resistance genes from the other organisms can be transferred to S aureus, there is concern that vancomycin-resistant MRSA will develop. Overall, infectious disease specialists fear that vancomycin will become ineffective in treating these serious infections. Vancomycin-resistant enterococci (VRE) are discussed below.

Penicillin-resistant Streptococcus pneumoniae (pneumococci)

Penicillin has long been the drug of choice for treating pneumococcal infections (e.g., community-acquired pneumonia, bacteremia, meningitis, and otitis media in children). However, penicillin-resistant strains and multi-antibiotic-resistant strains are being identified with increasing frequency. Risk factors for the development of resistant strains include frequent antibiotic use and prophylactic antibiotics. Once developed, resistant strains spread to other people, especially in children's day care centers and in hospital settings. Children in day care centers are often colonized or infected with antibiotic-resistant S pneumoniae. This is attributed to a high incidence of otitis media, which is often treated with a penicillin or cephalosporin antibiotic. Resistant strains in adults and elderly clients are often associated with previous use of a penicillin or cephalosporin and hospitalization.

S pneumoniae are thought to develop resistance to penicillin by decreasing the ability of their penicillin-binding proteins to bind with penicillin (and other beta-lactam antibiotics). In addition, some penicillin-resistant pneumococci are resistant to third-generation (extended-spectrum) cephalosporins. In pneumococcal infections resistant to penicillins and cephalosporins, vancomycin is the drug of choice. To decrease spread of resistant S pneumoniae, the Centers for Disease Control and Prevention (CDC) have proposed:

- Improved surveillance for drug-resistant pneumococci. This could delineate prevalence by geographic area and assist clinicians in choosing appropriate antimicrobial therapy.
- Rational use of antimicrobial agents to reduce exposures to drug-resistant pneumococci. For example, prophylactic antibiotic therapy for otitis media may increase colonization and infection of young children with resistant organisms.
- Pneumococcal vaccination for persons above 2 years of age with increased risk of pneumococcal infection and for all persons more than 65 years old.

Vancomycin-resistant enterococci (VRE)

Enterococci have intrinsic and acquired resistance to many antibacterial drugs. For example, penicillins and cephalosporins inhibit rather than kill the organisms at achievable concentrations and aminoglycosides (e.g., gentamicin) are ineffective if used alone. Consequently, standard treatment of an enterococcal infection outside of the urinary tract has involved a combination of a penicillin and an aminoglycoside. This combination is often successful because the penicillin damages the bacterial cell wall and allows the aminoglycoside to penetrate the bacterial cell. For penicillin-allergic clients, vancomycin is given with an aminoglycoside.

This treatment is becoming less effective because some strains of enterococci have developed resistance to penicillin, gentamicin and vancomycin. The incidence of multi-antibiotic-resistant and vancomycin-resistant enterococci (VRE) has increased in recent years. Two major types (Van

A and Van B) of vancomycin-resistant enterococci have been described, with different patterns of antimicrobial susceptibility. Van B is susceptible to teicoplanin, a newer agent similar to vancomycin. Van A is resistant to teicoplanin but may be susceptible to minocycline (a tetracycline), ciprofloxacin (a fluoroquinolone), or the investigational agent quinupristin/dalfopristin.

A major contributing factor to VRE is increased use of vancomycin to prevent or treat other infections such as staphylococcal (MRSA and MRSE) infections and antibiotic-associated (pseudomembranous) colitis (caused by toxins released by *Clostridium difficile* organisms). Therefore, to decrease the spread of VRE, the CDC recommend limiting the use of vancomycin. Specific recommendations include avoiding or minimizing use in routine surgical prophylaxis,

empiric therapy for febrile patients with neutropenia (unless the prevalence of MRSA or MSRE is high), systemic or local prophylaxis for intravascular catheter infection or colonization, selective decontamination of the GI tract, eradication of MRSA, primary treatment of antibiotic-associated colitis, and routine prophylaxis for very low birth weight infants or patients on continuous ambulatory peritoneal dialysis. Thorough handwashing and environmental cleaning are also important because VRE can survive for prolonged periods on hands, gloves, stethoscopes, and environmental surfaces. Personnel should remove or change gloves following contact with clients known to be colonized or infected with VRE. Stethoscopes should be used only with an infected patient or cleaned thoroughly between patients if used for both VRE-infected and uninfected patients.

another major factor is the adequacy of the host's ability to defend itself against the would-be invaders.

The major defense mechanisms of the human body are intact skin and mucous membranes, various anti-infective secretions, mechanical movements, phagocytic cells, and the immune and inflammatory processes. The skin prevents penetration of foreign particles, and its secretions and normal bacterial flora inhibit growth of pathogenic microorganisms. Secretions of the GI, respiratory, and genitourinary tracts (*e.g.*, gastric acid, mucus) kill, trap, or inhibit growth of microorganisms. Coughing, swallowing, and peristalsis help to remove foreign particles and pathogens trapped in mucus, as does the movement of cilia. Phagocytic cells in various organs and tissues engulf and digest pathogens and cellular debris. The immune system produces lymphocytes and antibodies (see Chap. 42). The inflammatory process (see Chap. 1) is the body's response to injury by microorganisms, foreign particles, chemical agents, or physical irritation of tissues. Inflammation localizes, destroys, neutralizes, dilutes, or removes the injurious agent so tissue healing can occur.

Many factors impair host defense mechanisms and predispose to infection by disease-producing microorganisms:

1. Breaks in the skin and mucous membranes related to trauma, inflammation, open lesions, or insertion of prosthetic devices, tubes, and catheters for diagnostic or therapeutic purposes
2. Impaired blood supply
3. Neutropenia and other blood disorders
4. Malnutrition
5. Poor personal hygiene

6. Suppression of normal bacterial flora by antimicrobial drugs
7. Suppression of the immune system and the inflammatory response by immunosuppressive drugs, cytotoxic antineoplastic drugs, and adrenal corticosteroids
8. Diabetes mellitus and other chronic diseases
9. Advanced age

Characteristics of Anti-infective Drugs

TERMS AND CONCEPTS

Several terms are used to describe these drugs. *Anti-infective* and *antimicrobial* include antibacterial, antiviral, and antifungal drugs; *antibacterial* and *antibiotic* usually refer only to drugs used in bacterial infections. Most of the drugs in this section are antibacterials. Antiviral and antifungal drugs are discussed in Chapters 39 and 40, respectively.

Additional terms for antibacterial drugs include *broad spectrum,* for those effective against several groups of microorganisms, and *narrow spectrum,* for those effective against a few groups. The action of an antibacterial drug is usually described as *bactericidal* (kills the microorganism) or *bacteriostatic* (inhibits growth of the microorganism). Whether a drug is bactericidal or bacteriostatic often depends on its concentration at the infection site and the susceptibility of the microorganism to the drug. Successful treatment with bacteriostatic antibiotics depends on the ability of the host's immune system to eliminate the inhibited bacteria and an adequate duration of drug therapy. Stopping an antibiotic prematurely can result in rapid resumption of bacterial growth. Bactericidal drugs are preferred in serious infections, especially in persons with impaired immune function.

MECHANISMS OF ACTION

Most antibiotics act on a specific target in the bacterial cell. Almost any structure unique to bacteria, such as proteins or nucleic acids, can be a target for some antibiotic. Specific mechanisms include the following:

1. Inhibition of bacterial cell wall synthesis or activation of enzymes that disrupt bacterial cell walls (*e.g.,* penicillins, cephalosporins, vancomycin)
2. Inhibition of protein synthesis by bacteria or production of abnormal bacterial proteins (*e.g.,* aminoglycosides, clindamycin, erythromycin, tetracyclines). These drugs bind irreversibly to bacterial ribosomes, intracellular structures that synthesize proteins. When antimicrobial drugs are bound to the ribosomes, bacteria cannot synthesize the proteins necessary for cell walls and other structures.
3. Disruption of microbial cell membranes (*e.g.,* antifungals)
4. Inhibition of organism reproduction by interfering with nucleic acid synthesis (*e.g.,* fluoroquinolones, rifampin, anti–acquired immunodeficiency syndrome [AIDS] antivirals)
5. Inhibition of cell metabolism and growth (*e.g.,* sulfonamides, trimethoprim)

INDICATIONS FOR USE

Antimicrobial drugs are used to treat and prevent infections. Because laboratory tests (except Gram's stain) to identify causative organisms usually take 24 hours or longer, empiric therapy against the most likely pathogens is often begun. Once a specific organism is identified, directed therapy is instituted. Prophylactic therapy is generally recommended in only a few circumstances, including the following:

1. Penicillin to prevent group A streptococcal infections and possibly rheumatic fever, rheumatic heart disease, and glomerulonephritis
2. Antibiotics to prevent bacterial endocarditis in clients with cardiac valvular disease who are having dental, surgical or other invasive procedures
3. Isoniazid to prevent tuberculosis (see Chap. 38)
4. Antibiotics during the perioperative period for selected high-risk clients (those whose resistance to infection is lowered due to age, poor nutrition, disease, or drugs) and for selected high-risk surgical procedures (cardiac surgery, GI surgery, certain orthopedic procedures, organ transplants)

5. Antibiotics to prevent sexually transmitted diseases (*e.g.,* gonorrhea, syphilis, chlamydial infections) after exposure has occurred
6. Antibiotics to prevent recurrent urinary tract infections in premenopausal, sexually active women. A single tablet of trimethoprim-sulfamethoxazole, cinoxacin, or cephalexin, taken after sexual intercourse, is often effective.

Nursing Process

Assessment

Assess for current or potential infection:
● General signs and symptoms of infection are the same as those of inflammation, although the terms are not synonymous. Inflammation is the normal response to any injury; infection requires the presence of a microorganism. The two often occur together. Inflammation may weaken tissue, allowing microorganisms to invade and cause infection. Infection (tissue injury by microorganisms) arouses inflammation. Local signs include redness, heat, edema, and pain; systemic signs include fever and leukocytosis. Specific manifestations depend on the site of infection. Common sites are the respiratory tract, surgical or other wounds, and the genitourinary tract.
● Assess each client for the presence of factors that increase risks of infection (see the section entitled Host Defense Mechanisms above).
● Assess culture reports for causative organisms.
● Assess susceptibility reports for appropriate antibacterial drug therapy.
● Assess clients for drug allergies. If present, ask about specific signs and symptoms.
● Assess baseline data about renal and hepatic function and other factors that aid monitoring for therapeutic and adverse drug effects.
● Assess for characteristics that increase risks of adverse drug effects.

Nursing Diagnoses

● Fatigue related to infection
● Self-Care Deficit related to infection
● Activity Intolerance related to fatigue
● Diarrhea related to antimicrobial therapy
● Altered Nutrition: Less Than Body Requirements related to anorexia, nausea, and vomiting associated with antimicrobial therapy
● Risk for Injury related to infection or adverse drug effects
● Risk for Infection related to emergence of drug-resistant microorganisms
● Knowledge Deficit: Methods of preventing infections
● Knowledge Deficit: Appropriate use of antimicrobial drugs

Planning/Goals

The client will:
● Receive antimicrobial drugs accurately when given by health care providers or caregivers
● Take drugs as prescribed and for the length of time prescribed when self-administered as an outpatient

- Experience decreased fever, white blood cell (WBC) count, and other signs and symptoms of infection
- Be monitored regularly for therapeutic and adverse drug effects
- Receive prompt recognition and treatment of potentially serious adverse effects
- Verbalize and practice measures to prevent future infections
- Be safeguarded against nosocomial infections by health care providers

Interventions

- Use measures to prevent and minimize the spread of infection.
  - Wash hands thoroughly and often. This is probably the most effective method of preventing infections.
  - Support natural defense mechanisms by promoting general health measures, such as nutrition, fluid and electrolyte balance, rest, and exercise.
  - Keep the client's skin clean and dry, especially the hands, underarms, groin, and perineum, because these areas harbor large numbers of microorganisms. Also, take care to prevent trauma to the skin and mucous membrane. Damaged tissues are susceptible to infection.
  - Treat all body fluids (*e.g.*, blood, aspirates from abdomen or chest) and body substances (*e.g.*, sputum, feces, urine, wound drainage) as infectious. Major elements of standard precautions to prevent transmission of hepatitis B, human immunodeficiency virus, and other pathogens include wearing gloves when likely to be exposed to any of the above materials and thorough handwashing when the gloves are removed. Rigorous and consistent use of the recommended precautions helps to protect health care providers and clients.
  - Implement isolation procedures appropriately.
  - To prevent spread of respiratory infections, have client wash hands after coughing, sneezing, or contact with infected people; cover mouth and nose with tissues when sneezing or coughing and dispose of tissues by placing them in a paper bag and burning it; expectorate sputum (swallowing may cause reinfection); avoid crowds when possible, especially during influenza season (approximately November through February); recommend annual influenza vaccine to high-risk populations (*e.g.*, people with chronic diseases, such as diabetes, heart, lung, or renal problems; older adults; and health care personnel who are likely to be exposed). Pneumococcal vaccine (see Chap. 43) is recommended as a single dose for the same populations.
  - Assist or instruct clients at risk about pulmonary hygiene measures to prevent accumulation or promote removal of respiratory secretions. These measures include ambulating, turning, coughing and deep-breathing exercises, and incentive spirometry. Retained secretions are good culture media for bacterial growth.
  - Use sterile technique when changing any dressing. If a wound is not infected, sterile technique helps prevent infection; if the wound is already infected, sterile technique avoids introducing new bacteria. For all but the smallest of dressings without drainage, remove the dressing with clean gloves, discard it in a moisture-proof bag, and wash hands before putting on sterile gloves to apply the new dressing.

- To minimize spread of staphylococcal infections, infected personnel with skin lesions should not work until lesions are healed; infected patients should be isolated. Personnel with skin lesions probably spread more staphylococci than clients because personnel are more mobile.
- For clients with infections, monitor temperature for fever increase or decrease, and monitor WBC count for decrease.
- For clients receiving antimicrobial therapy, maintain a total fluid intake of about 3000 ml/24 h, if not contraindicated by the client's condition. An adequate intake and avoidance of fluid volume deficit may help to decrease drug toxicity, especially with aminoglycoside antibiotics. On the other hand, a client receiving IV antibiotics, with 50 to 100 ml of fluid per dose, may be at risk of developing fluid volume overload.

 Teach clients:

- The importance of handwashing, maintaining nutrition and fluid balance, getting adequate rest, and handling secretions correctly. These measures help the body to fight the infection, prevent further infection, and enhance the effectiveness of anti-infective drugs.
- The importance of taking all prescribed doses of an antimicrobial and not stopping when symptoms subside. Reasons include adequate treatment of the current infection and prevention of new infections that may be harder to treat (*e.g.*, infections caused by drug-resistant organisms are usually more serious and often require more expensive and more toxic drugs). If problems occur with taking the drug, report them to the prescribing physician rather than stopping the drug.
- Not to take antimicrobials left over from a previous illness or prescribed for someone else. Even if infection is present and anti-infective treatment appears needed, the likelihood of having the appropriate drug on hand, and in adequate amounts, is extremely small. Thus, taking drugs not prescribed for the particular illness tends to maximize risks and minimize benefits. Also, if the infection is viral, most antimicrobials are ineffective unless a bacterial superinfection develops.
- To report any other drugs being taken to the prescribing physician. Drug interactions may occur, and changes in drug therapy may be indicated.
- To report any drug allergies to all health care providers and wear a medical identification emblem that lists allergens.
- That some antibiotics (*e.g.*, ampicillin, nitrofurantoin, penicillin V, sulfonamides, tetracyclines) decrease the effectiveness of estrogens and oral contraceptives. Women taking these drugs should use another method of contraception. Inadequate blood levels of estrogen may be indicated by breakthrough bleeding and are thought to result from reduced enterohepatic recirculation of estrogens. This, in turn, probably results from drug-induced decreases in intestinal bacterial flora.

Evaluation

- Interview and observe for compliance with instructions for using anti-infective drugs.
- Interview and observe for practices to prevent infection.
- Observe for adverse drug effects.

Principles of Therapy

GOAL OF ANTIMICROBIAL DRUG THERAPY

The goal of treatment for infection is to cure the disease by eradicating the causative microorganism and returning the host to full physiologic functioning. This differs from the goal of most drug therapy, which is to relieve signs and symptoms rather than cure the underlying disorder.

RATIONAL USE OF ANTIMICROBIAL DRUGS

Antimicrobials are among the most frequently used drugs worldwide. Their phenomenal success in saving lives and decreasing severity and duration of infectious diseases has encouraged their extensive use. Some authorities estimate that as much as 50% of antibiotic use is inappropriate and indicates overuse, misuse, or abuse of the drugs. That is, an antibiotic is not indicated at all or the wrong drug, dose, route, or duration is prescribed. Often, potent, broad-spectrum agents are used to treat trivial or self-limiting infections. Inappropriate use of antibiotics increases adverse drug effects, infections with drug-resistant microorganisms, and health care costs. Guidelines to promote more appropriate, rational use of the drugs include:

1. Stop the long-term pattern of use in which a powerful new antimicrobial drug is widely used, then becomes ineffective in some infections because of microbial resistance. Such a pattern began with the penicillins and is evident with currently available antibacterial drugs. Thus, indiscriminant, "routine" use of the most powerful, broadest-spectrum drugs when others may be just as effective leaves no drugs in reserve for serious infections or infections caused by resistant organisms.
2. Give the most narrow-spectrum drug likely to be effective in a given infection. Use of broad-spectrum drugs alters the normal body flora more extensively and increases adverse drug effects and the emergence of drug-resistant microorganisms.
3. Give antibacterial drugs only when a significant bacterial infection is diagnosed or strongly suspected or when there is an established indication for prophylaxis. These drugs should not be used for viral or trivial infections. They are ineffective in viral infections; they expose the client to adverse drug effects and may allow the growth of drug-resistant organisms in trivial infections.
4. Minimize antimicrobial drug therapy for fever unless other clinical manifestations or laboratory data indicate infection.
5. Use the drugs along with other interventions to decrease microbial proliferation, such as universal precautions, medical isolation techniques, frequent and thorough handwashing, and preoperative skin and bowel cleansing.
6. Follow recommendations of the Centers for Disease Control and Prevention (CDC) for prevention and treatment of infections, especially those caused by drug-resistant organisms (*e.g.*, gonorrhea, penicillin-resistant streptococcal infections, methicillin-resistant staphylococcal infections, vancomycin-resistant enterococcal infections, and multidrug-resistant tuberculosis).
7. Consult infectious disease physicians and infection control nurses about local patterns of drug-resistant organisms, treatment of complicated infections, and precautions to prevent spread of infectious diseases.

COLLECTION OF SPECIMENS

Collect specimens for culture and Gram's stain before giving the first dose of an anti-infective. For best results, specimens must be collected accurately and taken directly to the laboratory. If delayed, contaminants may overgrow pathogenic microorganisms.

DRUG SELECTION

Once an infection requiring treatment is diagnosed, numerous factors influence the choice of a specific antimicrobial drug or combination of drugs. Some of these factors are described below.

Initial therapy. Because laboratory tests to identify causative organisms require 48 to 72 hours, the physician usually prescribes for immediate administration a drug that is likely to be effective. This empiric therapy is based on an informed estimate of the most likely pathogen, given the client's signs and symptoms and apparent site of infection. For empiric therapy, a single, broad-spectrum antibiotic or a combination of drugs is often chosen.

Culture and susceptibility studies allow the therapist to "match the drug to the bug." Culture identifies the causative organism; susceptibility tests determine which drugs are likely to be effective against the organism. Culture and susceptibility studies are especially important with suspected gram-negative infections because of the high incidence of drug-resistant microorganisms. However, drug-resistant gram-positive organisms are being identified with increasing frequency.

When a specific organism is identified by a laboratory culture, tests can be performed to measure the organism's susceptibility to particular antibiotics. Laboratory reports indicate whether the organism is sensitive (S) or resistant (R) to the tested drugs. One indication of susceptibility is the minimum inhibitory concentration (MIC). The MIC is the lowest concentration of an antibiotic that prevents visible growth of microorganisms.

Susceptible organisms have low or moderate MICs that can be attained by giving usual doses of an antimicrobial agent. For the drug to be effective, serum and tissue concentrations should generally exceed the MIC of an organism for a period of time. How much and how long drug concentrations need to exceed the MIC depend on the drug class and the bacterial species. With beta-lactam agents (*e.g.,* penicillins, cephalosporins), the drug concentration generally needs to be maintained above the MIC of the infecting organism for the duration of antibiotic therapy. With the aminoglycosides (*e.g.,* gentamicin, others), the drug concentration does not need to be maintained above the MIC. Aminoglycosides have a postantibiotic effect (PAE), defined as a persistent effect of an antimicrobial on bacterial growth after brief exposure of the organisms to a drug. Some studies demonstrate that large doses of aminoglycosides, given once daily, are as effective as more frequent dosing and may cause less nephrotoxicity. *Resistant organisms* have high MICs, perhaps requiring higher concentrations of drug than can be achieved, even if large doses are given. In some cases the minimum bactericidal concentration (MBC) is reported, indicating no growth of the organism in the presence of a particular antibiotic. The MBC is especially desirable for infected hosts with impaired immune functions.

Patients' responses to antimicrobial therapy cannot always be correlated with the MIC of an infecting pathogen. Thus, reports of drug susceptibility testing must be applied in the context of the site of infection, the characteristics of the drug, and the clinical status of the patient, as described below.

Knowledge of antibiotic resistance patterns in the community and agency. Because these patterns change, continuing efforts must be made.

Knowledge of the organisms most likely to infect particular body tissues. For example, urinary tract infections are often caused by *Escherichia coli,* and a drug effective against this organism is indicated.

A drug's ability to penetrate infected tissues. Several antimicrobials are effective in urinary infections because they are excreted in the urine. However, the choice of an effective antimicrobial drug may be limited in infections of the brain, eyes, gallbladder, or prostate gland because many drugs are unable to reach therapeutic concentrations in these tissues.

A drug's toxicity and the risk-to-benefit ratio. Generally, a less toxic drug should be used for mild infections, and the more toxic drugs should be reserved for serious infections.

Drug costs. If an older, less expensive drug meets the criteria for rational drug selection and is likely to be effective in a given infection, it should be used in preference to a more expensive agent. In addition to acquisition costs, personnel costs in relation to preparation and administration should be considered.

ANTIBIOTIC COMBINATION THERAPY

Antimicrobial drugs are often used in combination. One indication for combination therapy is an infection known or thought to be caused by multiple microorganisms (*e.g.,* abdominal and pelvic infections). A second indication is a serious infection in which a combination is synergistic. A commonly used synergistic combination is composed of an aminoglycoside and various other drugs (*e.g.,* a beta-lactam drug, such as an antipseudomonal penicillin for pseudomonal infection; a cephalosporin for gram-negative infection; ampicillin or penicillin G for enterococcal infection; or an antistaphylococcal penicillin for staphylococcal infection). A third indication is the likely emergence of drug-resistant organisms (*e.g.,* tuberculosis is routinely treated with three or more drugs). A fourth indication is fever or other signs of infection in a client whose immune system is suppressed (*e.g.,* a client with cancer and chemotherapy-induced neutropenia, a client with AIDS, or a client with a bone marrow or solid organ transplant). Staphylococci and the gram-negative organisms *Escherichia coli, Klebsiella pneumoniae,* and *Pseudomonas aeruginosa* often cause infections in neutropenic cancer patients. Transplant and AIDS patients may develop a variety of bacterial, viral, or fungal infections.

DOSAGE

Dosage (amount and frequency of administration) should be individualized according to characteristics of the causative organism, the chosen drug and the client's condition. For example, dosage may need to be increased for serious infections or reduced if the client has renal impairment or other disorders that delay drug elimination. The MIC may be used as a guideline for achieving therapeutic blood levels of the antimicrobial agent.

ROUTE OF ADMINISTRATION

Most antimicrobial drugs are given orally or IV for systemic infections. The route of administration depends on the client's condition (*e.g.,* location and severity of the infection, ability to take oral drugs) and the available drug dosage forms. In serious infections, the IV route is usually preferred.

DURATION OF THERAPY

Duration of therapy varies from a single dose to years, depending on the reason for use. For most acute infections, the average duration is about 7 to 10 days or until the recipient has been afebrile and asymptomatic for 48 to 72 hours.

PERIOPERATIVE USE

When used to prevent infections associated with surgery, antimicrobials should be given shortly before the scheduled operation and are often given by the anesthesiologist. This provides effective tissue concentration during the procedure, when contamination occurs. The choice of drug depends on the pathogens most likely to enter the operative area. A first-generation cephalosporin, such as cefazolin (Kefzol), is often used, usually in a single preoperative dose. An antistaphylococcal drug is often given before orthopedic procedures. Repeated doses may be given during surgery for procedures of long duration, procedures involving insertion of prosthetic materials, and contaminated or infected operative sites. Postoperative antimicrobials are indicated with dirty, traumatic wounds or ruptured viscera.

USE IN RENAL INSUFFICIENCY

In renal insufficiency or failure, antimicrobial drug therapy requires extreme caution. Many drugs are excreted primarily by the kidneys; some are nephrotoxic and may further damage the kidneys. In the presence of renal failure, they are likely to accumulate and produce toxic effects. Thus, dosage reductions are necessary for some drugs. Methods of calculating dosage are usually based on rates of creatinine clearance.

The following formula may be used to estimate creatinine clearance:

Males: Weight in kg × (140 minus age), divided by 72 × serum creatinine (mg/100 ml)
Females: 0.85 × above value

Dosage may be reduced by giving smaller individual doses, by increasing the time interval between doses, or both. Anti-infective drugs can be categorized as follows in relation to renal impairment:

1. Drugs that should not be given in the presence of renal disease (*i.e.*, creatinine clearance of less than 30 ml/min) unless the infecting organism is sensitive only to a particular drug. This group includes all tetracyclines except doxycycline (Vibramycin).
2. Drugs that are not used in renal impairment unless the infection is caused by organisms resistant to safer drugs. If used, dosage must be carefully adjusted, renal function must be closely monitored, and the recipient must be closely observed for adverse effects. These drugs include all the aminoglycosides, cephalexin, amphotericin B, ethambutol, flucytosine, and the fluoroquinolones. Serum drug levels are recommended for monitoring aminoglycoside antibiotics.
3. Drugs that require dosage reduction in severe renal failure. These include penicillin G, ampicillin, methicillin, trimethoprim-sulfamethoxazole, and most cephalosporins.
4. Drugs that require little or no dosage adjustment. These include chloramphenicol, clindamycin, dicloxacillin, doxycycline, erythromycin, isoniazid, nafcillin, and rifampin.

An additional factor is important in clients with acute or chronic renal failure who are receiving hemodialysis or peritoneal dialysis: some drugs are removed by dialysis, and an extra dose may be needed during or after dialysis.

USE IN LIVER DISEASE

In severe liver disease, antimicrobial drugs that are excreted by the liver must be reduced in dosage. These include chloramphenicol, clindamycin, and erythromycin. The antitubercular drugs isoniazid and rifampin have longer half-lives in clients with cirrhosis. Overall, dosing in liver disease is not well defined.

USE IN CHILDREN

Antimicrobial drugs are commonly used in hospitals and ambulatory settings for respiratory infections, otitis media, and other infections. General principles of pediatric (see Chap. 4) and antimicrobial drug therapy apply. Other guidelines include the following:

1. **Penicillins and cephalosporins** are considered safe for most age groups. However, they are eliminated more slowly in neonates because of immature renal function and must be used cautiously. Aztreonam (Azactam) and imipenem-cilastatin (Primaxin) have not been established as safe and effective in children under 12 years of age.
2. **Erythromycin,** azithromycin (Zithromax) and clarithromycin (Biaxin) are generally considered safe. The newer macrolide dirithromycin (Dynabac) has not been established as safe and effective in children under 12 years of age.
3. **Aminoglycosides** (*e.g.*, gentamicin and others) may cause nephrotoxicity and ototoxicity in any client population. Neonates are at high risk because of immature renal function.
4. **Tetracyclines** are contraindicated in children under 8 years of age because of drug effects on teeth and bone (see Chap. 36).
5. When **clindamycin** (Cleocin) is given to neonates and infants, liver and kidney function should be monitored.

6. Quinolones such as **ciprofloxacin** (Cipro), **norfloxacin** (Noroxin), and others are not recommended for use in children (younger than 18 years of age) because safety and effectiveness have not been established. In addition, cartilage and function of weight-bearing joints have been impaired in young animals given the drugs.

7. **Isoniazid** (INH) is used to prevent tuberculosis, and isoniazid and rifampin (Rifadin) are used to treat tuberculosis in children as in adults. Ethambutol (Myambutol) is not recommended for children under 13 years of age.

8. **Trimethoprim** (often given in combination with sulfamethoxazole as Bactrim or Septra) has not been proven safe for children under 12 years of age.

USE IN OLDER ADULTS

Antimicrobial drugs are commonly used in all health care settings for infections in older adults as in younger adults. General principles of geriatric (see Chap. 4) and antimicrobial drug therapy apply. Other guidelines include the following:

1. **Penicillins** are generally safe. However, hyperkalemia may occur with large IV doses of penicillin G potassium (1.7 mEq potassium per 1 million units), and hypernatremia may occur with ticarcillin (Ticar), which contains 5.6 mEq sodium per gram. Hyperkalemia and hypernatremia are more likely to occur with impaired renal function, a common condition in older adults.

2. **Cephalosporins** (cefazolin and others) are generally considered safe but may cause or aggravate renal impairment, especially when other nephrotoxic drugs are used concurrently. Dosage of several cephalosporins needs to be reduced in the presence of renal impairment (see Chap. 34).

3. **Macrolides** (erythromycin, azithromycin, clarithromycin and dirithromycin) are generally safe. Dosage of clarithromycin should be reduced with severe renal impairment.

4. **Aminoglycosides** (*e.g.,* gentamicin and others) are contraindicated in the presence of impaired renal function if less toxic drugs are effective against causative microorganisms. Older adults are at high risk of nephrotoxicity and ototoxicity from these drugs. Several specific interventions to decrease adverse drug effects are described in Chapter 35.

5. **Clindamycin** may cause diarrhea and should be used with caution in the presence of GI disease, especially colitis.

6. **Trimethoprim-sulfamethoxazole** (Bactrim, Septra) may cause an increased risk of severe adverse effects in older adults, especially those with impaired liver or kidney function. Severe skin reactions and bone marrow depression are the most frequently reported severe reactions.

7. **Tetracyclines** (except doxycycline) and nitrofurantoin (Macrodantin) are contraindicated in the presence of impaired renal function if less toxic drugs are effective against causative organisms.

HOME CARE

Infections are among the most common illnesses in all age groups, and they are often treated by antibiotic therapy at home, with medications administered by the patient or a family member caregiver. If a home care nurse is involved, responsibilities may include teaching family members how to administer antibiotics (*e.g.,* teaching a parent how to store and measure a liquid antibiotic), care for the person with an infection, and protect other persons in the environment from the infection. General infection control practices include frequent and thorough handwashing, use of gloves when indicated, and appropriate handling and disposal of body substances (*e.g.,* blood, urine, feces, sputum, vomitus, wound drainage).

Increasingly, IV antibiotics are being given in the home. Any patient who needs more than a few days of IV antibiotic therapy may be a candidate for home care. Some infections that require relatively long-term IV antibiotic therapy include endocarditis, osteomyelitis, pyelonephritis, and some surgical wound infections. Numerous people and agencies may be involved in providing this service. First, the patient and family need to be able and willing to manage some aspects of therapy and to provide space for necessary supplies. Second, arrangements must be made for procuring equipment, supplies, and medication. In some areas, nurses employed by equipment companies help families prepare and use IV infusion pumps. Medication is usually obtained from a local pharmacy in a unit-dose package ready for administration.

The role of the home care nurse includes teaching the patient and caregiver to store and administer the medication, monitor the IV site, monitor the infection, manage problems, and report patient responses. Specific responsibilities may vary according to drug administration intermittently or by continuous infusion, whether the patient has a peripheral or central IV line, and other factors. The family should be provided with detailed instructions and emergency telephone numbers of the home care nurse, the pharmacy, and the supply company.

ANTIMICROBIAL DRUGS

NURSING ACTIONS	RATIONALE/EXPLANATION
1. Administer accurately	
a. Schedule at evenly spaced intervals around the clock.	To maintain therapeutic blood levels
b. Give most oral antimicrobials on an empty stomach, about 1 h before or 2 h after meals.	To decrease binding to foods and inactivation by gastric acid.
c. For oral and parenteral solutions from powder forms, follow label instructions for mixing and storing. Check expiration dates.	Several antimicrobial drugs are marketed in powder forms because they are unstable in solution. When mixed, measured amounts of diluent must be added for drug dissolution and the appropriate concentration. Parenteral solutions are usually prepared in the pharmacy. Most solutions require refrigeration to prolong stability. None of the solutions should be used after the expiration date because drug decomposition is likely.
d. Give parenteral antimicrobial solutions alone; do not mix with any other drug in a syringe or IV solution.	To avoid chemical and physical incompatibilities that may cause drug precipitation or inactivation
e. Give IM antimicrobials deeply into large muscle masses (preferably gluteal muscles), and rotate injection sites.	To decrease tissue irritation
f. For IV administration, use dilute solutions, give direct injections slowly and intermittent infusions over 30 to 60 min. After infusions, flush the IV tubing with at least 10 ml of IV solution. For children, check references about individual drugs to avoid excessive concentrations and excessive fluids.	Most antimicrobials that are given IV can be given by intermittent infusion. Although instructions vary with specific drugs, most reconstituted drugs can be further diluted with 50 to 100 ml of IV fluid (D_5W, NS, D_5-¼% or D_5-½% NaCl). Dilution and slow administration minimize vascular irritation and phlebitis. Flushing ensures that the entire dose is given and prevents contact between drugs in the tubing.
2. Observe for therapeutic effects	
a. With local infections, observe for decreased redness, edema, heat, and pain.	Signs and symptoms of inflammation and infection usually subside within about 48 h after antimicrobial therapy is begun. Although systemic manifestations of infection are similar regardless of the cause, local manifestations vary with the type or location of the infection.
b. With systemic infections, observe for decreased fever and white blood cell count, increased appetite, and reports of feeling better.	
c. With wound infections, observe for decreased signs of local inflammation and decreased drainage. Drainage also may change from purulent to serous.	
d. With respiratory infections, observe for decreased dyspnea, coughing, and secretions. Secretions may change from thick and colored to thin and white.	
e. With urinary tract infections, observe for decreased urgency, frequency, and dysuria. If urinalysis is done, check the laboratory report for decreased bacteria and white blood cells.	
f. Absence of signs and symptoms of infection when given prophylactically.	
3. Observe for adverse effects	
a. Hypersensitivity	Reactions are more likely to occur in those with previous hypersensitivity reactions and those with a history of allergy, asthma, or hay fever.

NURSING ACTIONS	RATIONALE/EXPLANATION
(1) Anaphylaxis—hypotension, respiratory distress, urticaria, angioedema, vomiting, diarrhea	Hypersensitivity may occur with most antimicrobial drugs but is more common with penicillins. Anaphylaxis may occur with oral administration but is more likely with parenteral administration and may occur within 5 to 30 min of injection. Hypotension results from vasodilation and circulatory collapse. Respiratory distress results from bronchospasm or laryngeal edema.
(2) Serum sickness—chills, fever, vasculitis, generalized lymphadenopathy, joint edema and inflammation, bronchospasm, urticaria	This is a delayed allergic reaction, occurring 1 wk or more after the drug is started. Signs and symptoms are caused by inflammation.
(3) Acute interstitial nephritis (AIN)—hematuria, oliguria, proteinuria, pyuria	AIN is considered a hypersensitivity reaction that may occur with many antimicrobials, including penicillins, cephalosporins, aminoglycosides, sulfonamides, tetracyclines, and others. It is usually reversible if the causative agent is promptly stopped.
b. Superinfection	Superinfection is a new or secondary infection that occurs during antimicrobial therapy of a primary infection. Superinfections are common and potentially serious because responsible microorganisms are often drug-resistant staphylococci, gram-negative organisms (e.g., *Pseudomonas aeruginosa*) or fungi (e.g., *Candida*).
(1) Recurrence of systemic signs and symptoms (*e.g.,* fever, malaise)	
(2) New localized signs and symptoms—redness, heat, edema, pain, drainage, cough	
(3) Stomatitis or "thrush"—sore mouth, white patches on oral mucosa, black furry tongue	From overgrowth of fungi
(4) Pseudomembranous colitis—severe diarrhea characterized by blood, pus, and mucus in stools	May occur with most antibiotics, but is most often associated with ampicillin, the cephalosporins, and clindamycin. These and other antibiotics suppress normal bacterial flora and allow the overgrowth of *Clostridium difficile*. The organism produces a toxin that kills mucosal cells and produces superficial ulcerations that are visible with sigmoidoscopy. Discontinuing the drug and giving metronidazole or oral vancomycin are curative measures. However, relapses may occur.
(5) Monilial vaginitis—rash in perineal area, itching, vaginal discharge	From overgrowth of yeast organisms
c. Phlebitis at IV sites; pain at IM sites	Many antimicrobial parenteral solutions are irritating to body tissues.
d. Nausea and vomiting	These often occur with oral antimicrobials, probably from irritation of gastric mucosa.
e. Diarrhea	Commonly occurs, caused by irritation of GI mucosa and changes in intestinal bacterial flora, and may range from mild to severe. Pseudomembranous colitis, above, is one type of severe diarrhea.
f. Nephrotoxicity	
(1) See acute interstitial nephritis, above	More likely to occur in clients who are elderly or who have impaired renal function.

(continued)

NURSING ACTIONS	RATIONALE/EXPLANATION
(2) Acute tubular necrosis (ATN)–increased BUN and serum creatinine, decreased creatinine clearance, fluid and electrolyte imbalances	Aminoglycosides are the antimicrobial agents most often associated with ATN.
g. Neurotoxicity–confusion, hallucinations, neuromuscular irritability, convulsive seizures	More likely with large IV doses of penicillins or cephalosporins, especially in clients with impaired renal function.
h. Bleeding–hypoprothrombinemia, platelet dysfunction	Most often associated with penicillins and cephalosporins.
4. Observe for drug interactions	See following chapters. The most significant interactions are those that alter anti-infective effectiveness or increase drug toxicity.
5. Teach clients **a.** Take oral drugs at evenly spaced intervals around the clock.	To maintain effective blood levels
b. Take oral drugs on an empty stomach, 1 h before or 2 h after a meal unless instructed otherwise.	Food decreases absorption of most oral anti-infectives. If the drug causes intolerable nausea or vomiting, a few bites of food (e.g., crackers) may be taken.
c. Take drugs with a full glass of water.	To decrease gastric irritation and increase rates of dissolution and absorption (tablets and capsules)
d. Report nausea, vomiting, diarrhea, skin rash, recurrence of symptoms for which the anti-infective drug was prescribed, or signs of new infection (*e.g.*, fever, cough, sore mouth drainage).	These problems may indicate adverse effects of the drug, lack of therapeutic response to the drug, or a superinfection. Any of these requires evaluation and may indicate changes in drug therapy.

REVIEW AND APPLICATION EXERCISES

1. How does the body defend itself against infection?

2. When assessing a client, what signs and symptoms may indicate an infectious process?

3. Do all infections require antimicrobial drug therapy? Why or why not?

4. With antimicrobial drug therapy, what is meant by the terms bacteriostatic, bactericidal, antimicrobial spectrum of activity, and minimum inhibitory concentration?

5. Why is it important to identify the organism causing an infection?

6. Why are infections of the brain, eye, and prostate gland more difficult to treat than infections of the GI, respiratory, and urinary tracts?

7. What factors promote the development of drug-resistant microorganisms, and how can they be prevented or minimized?

8. What are common adverse effects associated with antimicrobial drug therapy?

9. When teaching a client about a prescribed antibiotic, a common instruction is to take all the medicine and not to stop prematurely. Why is this information important?

10. When a dose of an antibiotic is prescribed to prevent postoperative infection, should it be given before, during, or after surgery? Why?

SELECTED REFERENCES

Antimicrobial prophylaxis in surgery. (1993). *The Medical Letter on Drugs and Therapeutics, 35,* 91–93.

Barg, N. (1994). Antibiotic therapy in 1994: Mechanisms of resistance. *Hospital Formulary, 29*(Suppl. 3), S-13–S-17.

Barriere, S.L. (1993). Selection of antimicrobial regimens. In J.T. DiPiro, R.L. Talbert, P.E. Hayes, G.C. Yee, G.R. Matzke, L.M. Posey (Eds.), *Pharmacotherapy: A pathophysiologic approach,* 2nd ed., pp. 1508–1523. Norwalk, CT: Appleton & Lange.

Briceland, L.L., Cleary, J.D., Fletcher, C.V., Healy, D.P., & Peloquin, C.A. (1995). Recent advances: Antiinfectives. *The Annals of Pharmacotherapy, 29,* 1035–1040.

Burns, J.L. (1995). Mechanisms of bacterial resistance. *Pediatric Clinics of North America, 43*(3), 497–507.

Chambers, H.F. & Sande, M.A. (1996). Antimicrobial agents: General considerations. In J.G. Hardman, L.E. Limbird, P.B. Molinoff, & R.W. Ruddon (Eds.), *Goodman & Gilman's The pharmacological basis of therapeutics,* 9th ed., pp. 1029–1056. New York: McGraw-Hill.

Drug facts and comparisons. (Updated monthly). St. Louis: Facts and Comparisons.

Dudley, M.N. (1993). Use of laboratory tests in infectious diseases. In J.T DiPiro, R.L. Talbert, P.E. Hayes, G.C. Yee, G.R. Matzke, L.M. Posey (Eds.), *Pharmacotherapy: A pathophysiologic approach*, 2nd ed., pp. 1489–1507. Norwalk, CT: Appleton & Lange.

Dunne, W. M. (1994). Mechanisms of infectious disease. In C.M. Porth (Ed.), *Pathophysiology: Concepts of altered health states*, 4th ed., pp. 221–241. Philadelphia: J.B. Lippincott.

Fish, D.N., Piscitelli, S.C., & Danziger, L.H. (1995). Development of resistance during antimicrobial therapy: A review of antibiotic classes and patient characteristics in 173 studies. *Pharmacotherapy, 15*(3), 279–291.

Giamarellou, H. (1995). Empiric therapy for infections in the febrile neutropenic, compromised host. *Medical Clinics of North America, 79*(3), 559–580.

Goldmann, D.A., Weinstein, R.A., Wenzel, R.P., Tablan, O.C., Duma, R.J., Gaynes, R.P., Schlosser, J., & Martone, W.J. (1996). Strategies to prevent and control the emergence and spread of antimicrobial-resistant microorganisms in hospitals. *Journal of the American Medical Association, 275*, 234–240.

Hammerschlag, M.R. (1993). Azithromycin and clarithromycin. *Pediatric Annals, 22*(3), 160–166.

Hoeprich, P.D. (1994). Antibacterial chemotherapy. In P.D. Hoeprich, M.C. Jordan, & A.R. Ronald (Eds.), *Infectious Diseases*, 5th ed., pp. 247–274. Philadelphia: J.B. Lippincott.

Holman, R.G. & Dellinger, E.P. (1996). Fever, infection, and antibiotics. In J.A. Weigelt and F.R. Lewis, Jr. (Eds.), *Surgical Critical Care.* Philadelphia: W.B. Saunders.

Jernigan, D.B., Cetron, M.S., & Breiman, R.F. (1996). Minimizing the impact of drug-resistant *Streptococcus pneumoniae* (DRSP). *Journal of the American Medical Association, 275*, 206–209.

Kunin, C.M. (1993). Resistance to antimicrobial drugs—A worldwide calamity. *Annals of Internal Medicine, 118*, 557–561.

Levy, S.B. (1993). Confronting multidrug resistance. *Journal of the American Medical Association, 269*, 1840–1842.

Lonks, J.R. & Medeiros, A.A. (1995). The growing threat of antibiotic-resistant *Streptococcus pneumoniae. Medical Clinics of North America, 79*(3), 523–535.

Ma, M.Y. & Rho, J.P. (1995). Considerations in antimicrobial prescribing. *Medical Clinics of North America, 79*(3), 537–549.

Mandell, G.L., Bennett, J.E., & Dolin, R. (Eds.) (1995). *Mandell, Douglas, and Bennett's Principles and practice of infectious diseases*, 4th ed. New York: Churchill Livingstone.

Matson, M.A. & Abraham, P.A. (1993). Drug-induced renal disease. In J.T DiPiro, R.L. Talbert, P.E. Hayes, G.C. Yee, G.R. Matzke, L.M.

Posey (Eds.), *Pharmacotherapy: A pathophysiologic approach*, 2nd ed., pp. 701–719. Norwalk, CT: Appleton & Lange.

Merlin, T.L., Gibson, D.W., & Connor, D.H. (1994). Infectious and parasitic diseases. In E. Rubin & J.L. Farber (Eds.), *Pathology*, 2nd ed., pp. 337–452. Philadelphia: J.B. Lippincott.

Moellering, R.C., Jr. (1995). *Enterococcus* species, *Streptococcus bovis*, and *Leuconostoc* species. In G.L. Mandell, J.E. Bennett, & R. Dolin (Eds.), *Mandell, Douglas, and Bennett's Principles and practice of infectious diseases*, 4th ed., pp. 1826–1835. New York: Churchill Livingstone.

Moreira, B.M. & Daum, R.S. (1995). Antimicrobial resistance in staphylococci. *Pediatric Clinics of North America, 42*(3), 619–648.

Morita, M.M. (1993). Methicillin-resistant *Staphylococcus aureus:* Past, present, and future. *Nursing Clinics of North America, 28*(3), 625–637.

Nichols, R.L. (1995). Surgical antibiotic prophylaxis. *Medical Clinics of North America, 79*(3), 509–522.

Peterson, F.Y. & Puhlman, M. (1995). Infectious processes. In L.C. Copstead, *Perspectives on pathophysiology*, pp. 155–171. Philadelphia: W.B. Saunders.

Pinner, R.W., Teutsch, S.M., Simonsen, S., Klug, L.A. Graber, J.M., Clarke, M.J., & Berkelman, R.L. (1996). Trends in infectious diseases mortality in the United States. *Journal of the American Medical Association, 275*, 189–193.

Plouffe, J.F., Breiman, R.F., & Facklam, R.R. (1996). Bacteremia with *Streptococcus pneumoniae:* Implications for therapy and prevention. *Journal of the American Medical Association, 275*, 194–198.

Rupp, M.E. & Archer, G.L. (1994). Coagulase-negative staphylococci: Pathogens associated with medical progress. *Clinical Infectious Diseases, 19*, 231–245.

Schreiber, J.R. & Jacobs, M.R. (1995). Antibiotic-resistant pneumococci. *Pediatric Clinics of North America, 43*(3), 519–537.

Smith, C.E. (1995). Home care environment. In W.J. Phipps, V.L. Cassmeyer, J.K. Sands, & M.K. Lehman (Eds.), *Medical-surgical nursing: Concepts and clinical practice*, 5th ed., pp. 681–705. St. Louis: Mosby-Year Book.

Solomkin, J.S. & Miyagawa, C.I. (1994). Principles of antibiotic therapy. *Surgical Clinics of North America, 74*(3), 497–517.

Thompson, R. (1994). Prevention of nosocomial pneumonia. *Medical Clinics of North America, 78*(5), 1185–1198.

Volk, W.A., Gebhardt, B.M., Hammarskjold, M.L., & Kadner, R.J. (1996). *Essentials of medical microbiology*, 5th ed. Philadelphia, Lippincott-Raven.

Yoshikawa, T.T. & Norman D.C. (1995). Treatment of infections in elderly patients. *Medical Clinics of North America, 79*(3), 651–661.

Beta-Lactam Antibacterials: Penicillins, Cephalosporins, and Others

34

Outline

Objectives

After studying this chapter, the reader will be able to:

1 Describe general characteristics of beta-lactam antibiotics.

2 Discuss penicillins in relation to effectiveness, safety, spectrum of antimicrobial activity, mechanism of action, indications for use, administration, observation of client response, and teaching of clients.

3 Differentiate among extended-spectrum penicillins.

4 Question clients about allergies prior to the initial dose of a penicillin.

(continued)

5 Describe characteristics of beta lactamase inhibitor drugs.

6 State the rationale for combining a penicillin and a beta lactamase inhibitor drug.

7 Discuss similarities and differences between cephalosporins and penicillins.

8 Differentiate among the four generations of cephalosporins in relation to antimicrobial spectrum, indications for use, and adverse effects.

9 Apply principles of using beta lactam antimicrobials in selected client situations.

Key Terms

Anaphylaxis	**Hypersensitivity**
Beta-lactamase enzymes	**Penicillin-binding proteins (PBPs)**

Description

Beta-lactam antibacterials derive their name from the beta-lactam ring that is part of their chemical structure. An intact beta-lactam ring is essential for antibacterial activity. Several gram-positive and gram-negative bacteria produce beta-lactamase enzymes that open the beta-lactam ring and inactivate the drugs. This is a major mechanism by which microorganisms develop resistance to beta-lactam antibiotics. Penicillinase and cephalosporinase are beta-lactamase enzymes that act on penicillins and cephalosporins, respectively.

Despite the common element of a beta-lactam ring, characteristics of beta-lactam antibiotics may differ widely because of variations in side chains and other elements of their chemical structures. More specifically, they may differ in antimicrobial spectrum of activity, routes of administration, susceptibility to beta-lactamase enzymes, and adverse effects. Beta-lactam antibiotics include penicillins, cephalosporins, carbapenems, and monobactams, which are described below. Individual penicillins are listed in Table 34-1, oral cephalosporins are listed in Table 34-2, and parenteral cephalosporins are listed in Table 34-3.

Mechanism of Action

Beta-lactam antibacterial drugs kill bacteria by inhibiting synthesis of the bacterial cell wall. The mechanism of their antibacterial action involves binding of drug molecules to protein molecules (enzymes called penicillin-binding proteins or PBPs) in bacterial cell membranes. This binding produces a defective cell wall that allows intracellular contents to leak out, destroying the microorganism. In sub-bactericidal concentrations, the drugs may inhibit growth, decrease viability, and alter the shape and structure of organisms. The latter characteristic may help to explain the development of mutant strains of microorganisms exposed to the drugs. Beta-lactam antibiotics are most effective when bacterial cells are dividing.

Penicillins

The penicillins are effective, safe, and widely used antimicrobial agents. The group includes natural extracts from the *Penicillium* mold and several semisynthetic derivatives. When penicillin G, the prototype, was introduced, it was effective against streptococci, staphylococci, gonococci, meningococci, *Treponema pallidum*, and other organisms. It had to be given parenterally because it was destroyed by gastric acid, and injections were very painful. With extensive use, strains of drug-resistant staphylococci appeared. Later penicillins were developed to increase gastric acid stability, beta-lactamase stability, and antimicrobial spectrum of activity, especially against gram-negative microorganisms. Semisynthetic derivatives are formed by adding side chains to the penicillin nucleus.

After absorption, penicillins are widely distributed and achieve therapeutic concentrations in most body fluids, including joint, pleural, and pericardial fluids and bile. Therapeutic levels are not usually obtained in intraocular and cerebrospinal fluids (CSF) unless inflammation is present because normal cell membranes act as barriers to drug penetration. Penicillins are rapidly excreted by the kidneys and produce high drug concentrations in the urine (an exception is nafcillin, which is excreted by the liver).

INDICATIONS FOR USE

Clinical indications for use of penicillins include bacterial infections caused by susceptible microorganisms. Generally, they are more effective in infections caused by gram-positive bacteria than those caused by gram-negative bacteria. However, their clinical uses vary according to the subgroup or individual drug and microbial patterns of resistance. The drugs are often useful in respiratory, gastrointestinal (GI), and genitourinary infections. However, the incidence of resistance among streptococci, staphylococci, gonococci, and other microorganisms continues to grow.

TABLE 34-1	PENICILLINS	

	Routes and Dosage Ranges	
Generic / Trade Name	*Adults*	*Children*
Penicillins G and V		
Penicillin G sodium	PO 600,000–3 million U daily	PO 25,000–90,000 U/kg/d in divided doses q6–8h
Penicillin G potassium (Pfizerpen, Pentids, others)	IM 300,000–8 million U daily IV 6–20 million U daily by continuous or intermittent infusion q2–4h. Up to 60 million U daily have been given in certain serious infections.	IM, IV 50,000–250,000 U/kg/d in divided doses q4h
Penicillin G benzathine (Bicillin)	PO 400,000–600,000 U q4–6h IM 1.2–2.4 million U in a single dose Prophylaxis of rheumatic fever, IM 1.2 million U monthly or 600,000 U every 2 wk Treatment of syphilis, IM 2.4 million U (1.2 million U in each buttock) in a single dose	PO 25,000–90,000 U/kg/d in three to six divided doses IM 50,000 U/kg in one dose Prophylaxis of rheumatic fever, IM 1.2 million U monthly or 600,000 U every 1–2 wk
Penicillin G procaine (Wycillin, others)	IM 600,000–1.2 million U daily in 1 or 2 doses Prevention or treatment of uncomplicated gonorrhea, IM 4.8 million U in a single dose, divided into two or more injections and given at different sites. Probenecid 1 g is given 30 min before the penicillin.	IM 25,000–50,000 U/kg/d in divided doses q12h
Penicillin V (V-Cillin K, PenVee K, others)	PO 125–500 mg four to six times daily	Same as adults Infants: PO 15–50 mg/kg/d in three to six divided doses
Penicillinase-Resistant (Antistaphylococcal) Penicillins		
Cloxacillin (Tegopen)	PO 250–500 mg q6h	Weight 20 kg or more: Same as adults Weight under 20 kg: PO 50–100 mg/kg/d in four divided doses q6h
Dicloxacillin (Dynapen)	PO, IM 125–250 mg q6h	Weight 40 kg or more: Same as adults Weight under 40 kg: 12.5–25 mg/kg/d in four divided doses q6h
Methicillin (Staphcillin)	IM 1 g q4–6h IV 1–2 g in 50 ml sodium chloride injection, infused at 10 ml/min q4–6h	IM 100–200 mg/kg/d in four divided doses q6h
Nafcillin (Unipen)	IM 500 mg q4–6h IV 500 mg–2 g in 15–30 ml sodium chloride injection, infused over 5–10 min, q4h; maximal daily dose, 12 g for serious infections	IM, IV 50–100 mg/kg/d in four to six divided doses q4–6h
Oxacillin (Prostaphlin)	PO, IM, IV 500 mg–1 g q4–6h. For direct IV injection, the dose should be well diluted and given over 10–15 min.	Weight over 40 kg: Same as adults Weight 40 kg or less: PO, IM, IV 50–100 mg/kg/d in four divided doses q6h
Ampicillins		
Ampicillin (Omnipen, Penbriten, others)	PO, IM, IV 250–500 mg q6h. In severe infections, doses up to 2 g q4h may be given IV.	Weight over 20 kg: Same as adults Weight 20 kg or less: PO, IM, IV 50–100 mg/kg/d in divided doses q6h
Amoxicillin (Amoxil, Larotid, others)	PO 250–500 mg q8h	Weight over 20 kg: Same as adults Weight 20 kg or less: 20–40 mg/kg/d in divided doses q8h
Bacampicillin (Spectrobid)	PO 400–800 mg q12h	Weight over 25 kg: Same as adults

TABLE 34-1	PENICILLINS	
	Routes and Dosage Ranges	
Generic / Trade Name	**Adults**	**Children**
Extended-Spectrum (Antipseudomonal) Penicillins		
Carbenicillin indanyl sodium (Geocillin)	PO 1–2 tablets (382 mg carbenicillin/tablet) four times daily	PO 30–50 mg/kg/d in divided doses q8h
Ticarcillin (Ticar)	IM, IV 1–3 g q6h. IM injections should not exceed 2 g/injection.	Weight under 40 kg: 100–300 mg/kg/d q6–8h
Mezlocillin (Mezlin)	IM, IV 200–300 mg/kg/d in four to six divided doses. Usual adult dosage, 3 g q4h or 4 g q6h	Age 1 month–12 years: 300 mg/kg/d in six divided doses, q4h
Piperacillin (Pipracil)	IV, IM 200–300 mg/kg/d in divided doses q4–6h. Usual adult dosage, 3–4 g q4–6h; maximal daily dose, 24 g	Age under 12 years: Dosage not established
Penicillin/Beta-Lactamase Inhibitor Combinations		
Ampicillin/sulbactam (Unasyn)	IM, IV 1.5–3 g q6h	Age over 12 years, same as adults Age under 12 years, dosage not established
Amoxicillin/potassium clavulanate (Augmentin)	PO 250–500 mg q8h	Weight under 40 kg: 20–40 mg/kg/d in divided doses q8h
Piperacillin/tazobactam (Zosyn)	IV 3.375 g q6h	Dosage not established
Ticarcillin/clavulanate (Timentin)	IV 3.1 g q4–6h	Weight under 60 kg: 200–300 mg/kg/d in divided doses q4–6h

CONTRAINDICATIONS FOR USE

Contraindications include hypersensitivity or allergic reactions to any penicillin preparation.

SUBGROUPS AND INDIVIDUAL PENICILLINS

Penicillins G and V

Penicillin G, the prototype of the penicillins, is widely used. Because of its effectiveness and minimal toxicity, it is recommended for treatment of infections caused by susceptible microorganisms. Although many strains of staphylococci and gonococci have developed resistance to penicillin G, the drug is still effective in most streptococcal infections. Thus, it is often the drug of choice for the treatment of streptococcal pharyngitis, for prevention of rheumatic fever, a complication of streptococcal pharyngitis, and for prevention of bacterial endocarditis in people with diseased heart valves who undergo dental or some surgical procedures.

Numerous preparations of penicillin G are available for various purposes and routes of administration. They cannot be used interchangeably. Only aqueous preparations can be given intravenously (IV). Preparations containing benzathine or procaine can only be

given intramuscularly (IM). Long-acting repository forms have additives that decrease their solubility in tissue fluids and delay their absorption. When penicillin G is given orally, large doses must be given to offset the portion destroyed by gastric acid.

Penicillin V is derived from penicillin G and has the same antibacterial spectrum. It is not destroyed by gastric acid and is given only by the oral route. It is better absorbed and produces higher blood levels than penicillin G.

Penicillinase-Resistant (Antistaphylococcal) Penicillins

This group includes five drugs (cloxacillin, dicloxacillin, methicillin, nafcillin, and oxacillin) that are effective in some infections caused by staphylococci resistant to penicillin G. The drugs are formulated to resist the penicillinases that inactivate other penicillins. These drugs are recommended for use in known or suspected staphylococcal infections, except for methicillin-resistant *Staphylococcus aureus* (MRSA) infections. Although called "methicillin-resistant," these staphylococcal microorganisms are also resistant to other antistaphylococcal penicillins and antibacterial drugs except vancomycin.

(*text continues on page 462*)

TABLE 34-2	ORAL CEPHALOSPORINS

Generic/Trade Name	Characteristics	Routes and Dosage Ranges	
		Adults	**Children**
First Generation			
Cefadroxil (Duricef, Ultracef)	A derivative of cephalexin with no apparent advantage over the parent drug except that it has a longer half-life and can be given less often	PO 1–2 g twice daily	30 mg/kg/d in two doses q12h
Cephalexin (Keflex)	1. Somewhat less active against penicillinase-producing staphylococci than cephalothin 2. First oral cephalosporin; still used extensively	PO 250–500 mg q6h, increased to 4 g q6h if necessary in severe infections	PO 25–50 mg/kg/d in divided doses q6h
Cephradine (Anspor, Velosef)	Essentially the same as cephalexin, except it also can be given parenterally	PO 250–500 mg q6h, up to 4 g daily in severe infections	PO 25–50 mg/kg/d in divided doses q6h. In severe infections, up to 100 mg/kg/d may be given.
Second Generation			
Cefaclor (Ceclor)	May be more active against *Haemophilus influenzae* and *Escherichia coli* than cephalothin	PO 250–500 mg q8h	PO 20–40 mg/kg/d in three divided doses q8h
Cefuroxime (Ceftin)	1. Can also be given parenterally 2. Available only in tablet form 3. The tablet may be crushed and added to a food (*e. g.,* applesauce), but the crushed tablet leaves a strong, bitter, persistent aftertaste.	PO 250 mg q12h; severe infections, 500 mg q12h; UTI, 125 mg q12h	>12 years, same as adults; <12 years, 125 mg q12h Otitis media, >2 years, 250 mg q12h, <2 years, 125 mg q12h
Cefprozil (Cefzil)	Similar to cefaclor and cefuroxime	PO 250–500 mg q12–24h	PO 15 mg/kg q12h
Loracarbef (Lorabid)	A synthetic drug similar to cefaclor	PO 200–400 mg q12h	PO 15–30 mg/kg/d in divided doses q12h
Third Generation			
Cefixime (Suprax)	First oral third-generation drug	PO 200 mg q12h or 400 mg q24h	PO 4 mg/kg q12h or 8 mg/kg q24h; give adult dose to children 50 kg of weight or 12 years of age or older
Cefpodoxime (Vantin)	Similar to cefixime except has some activity against staphylococci (except methicillin-resistant *Staphylococcus aureus*)	PO 200–400 mg q12h	PO 5 mg/kg q12h Give 10 mg/kg (400 mg or adult dose) to children 13 years or older with skin and soft-tissue infections
Ceftibuten (Cedax)	1. Indicated for bronchitis, otitis media, pharyngitis, or tonsillitis caused by streptococci or *Haemophilus influenzae.* 2. Can be given once daily 3. Available in a capsule for oral use and an oral pediatric suspension that comes in two concentrations (90 mg/5 ml and 180 mg/5 ml). 4. Dosage must be reduced with renal impairment.	PO 400 mg daily for 10 d Renal impairment: creatinine clearance (CrCl) 30–49 ml/min, 200 mg q24h CrCl 5–29 ml/min, 100 mg q24h	Oral suspension with 90 mg/ml *10 kg:* 5 ml daily *20 kg:* 10 ml daily *40 kg:* 20 ml daily *Above 45 kg:* Same as adults Oral suspension with 180 mg/ 5 ml *10 kg:* 2.5 ml daily *20 kg:* 5 ml daily *40 kg:* 10 ml daily *Above 45 kg:* Same as adults

| TABLE 34-3 | PARENTERAL CEPHALOSPORINS | | |

Generic / Trade Name	Characteristics	Routes and Dosage Ranges	
		Adults	**Children**
First Generation			
Cephalothin (Keflin)	1. The first cephalosporin 2. Active against streptococci, staphylococci, *Neisseria*, *Salmonella*, *Shigella*, *Escherichia*, *Klebsiella*, *Listeria*, *Bacillus*, *Haemophilus influenzae*, *Corynebacterium diphtheriae*, *Proteus mirabilis*, and *Bacteroides* (except *Bacteroides fragilis*) 3. Inactive against enterococci, *Enterobacter*, *Pseudomonas*, and *Serratia*	IV, IM 1–2 g q4–6h, depending on severity of infection	IV, IM 75–160 mg/kg/d in divided doses q4–6h
Cefazolin (Kefzol, Ancef)	More active against *Escherichia coli* and *Klebsiella* species than cephalothin	IM, IV 250 mg–1 g q6–8h	IM, IV 50–100 mg/kg/d in three to four divided doses
Cephapirin (Cefadyl)	No significant differences from cephalothin	IV, IM 500 mg–1 g q4–6h, up to 12 g daily, IV, in serious infections	IV, IM 40–80 mg/kg/d in four divided doses (q6h)
Cephradine (Anspor, Velosef)	No significant differences from cephalothin except it also can be given orally	IV, IM 500 mg–1 g two to four times daily, depending on severity of infection	IV, IM 75–125 mg/kg/d in divided doses q6h
Second Generation			
Cefamandole (Mandol)	1. More active against some gram-negative organisms than cephalothin and other first-generation cephalosporins, especially *Haemophilus influenzae*, *Enterobacter* and *Klebsiella* species, indole-positive strains of *Proteus*, and *Escherichia coli* 2. Major clinical usefulness is treatment of gram-negative infections caused by organisms resistant to other cephalosporins	IV, IM 0.5–2 g q4–6h, up to 12 g daily in life-threatening infections	V, IM 50–150 mg/kg/d in four to six divided doses q4–6h
Cefmetazole (Zefazone)	Similar to cefoxitin in antibacterial spectrum and clinical use	IV 2 g q6–12h for 5–14 d Surgical prophylaxis, IV 1 or 2 g 30–90 min before surgery, repeated 8 and 16 h later (total of three doses)	
Cefonocid (Monocid)	1. Antimicrobial spectrum similar to other second-generation cephalosporins 2. Has a long half-life and can therefore be given once daily 3. Not approved for use in children	IV, IM 1 g daily (q24h) Surgical prophylaxis, IV, IM 1 g 1 h before procedure	

(continued)

| TABLE 34-3 | PARENTERAL CEPHALOSPORINS (Continued) | | |

| Generic/Trade Name | Characteristics | Routes and Dosage Ranges | |
		Adults	Children
Ceforanide (Precef)	1. Similar to other second-generation cephalosporins 2. Has a relatively long half-life and can therefore be given twice daily	IV, IM 0.5–1 g q12h Surgical prophylaxis, IV, IM 0.5–1g 1 h before the procedure	20–40 mg/kg/d in divided doses q12h
Cefotetan (Cefotan)	1. Effective against most organisms except *Pseudomonas* 2. Highly resistant to beta-lactamase enzymes 3. Dosage must be reduced with renal failure, according to creatinine clearance.	IV, IM 1–2 g q12h for 5–10 d; maximum dose, 3 g q12h in life-threatening infections Perioperative prophylaxis, IV 1–2 g 30–60 min before surgery	
Cefoxitin (Mefoxin)	1. The first cephamycin (derived from a different fungus than cephalosporins) 2. Compared with cephalothin, cefoxitin is more active against gram-negative bacteria and less active against gram-positive bacteria 3. Compared with cefamandole, cefoxitin is more active against indole-positive *Proteus* and *Serratia* but less active against gram-positive bacteria and gram-negative *Enterobacter* and *Haemophilus influenzae*. 4. A major clinical use may stem from increased activity against *Bacteroides fragilis*, an organism resistant to most other antimicrobial drugs.	IV, IM 1–2 q q4–6h	IV, IM 80–160 mg/kg/d in divided doses q4–6h. Do not exceed 12 g/d.
Second Generation			
Cefuroxime (Ceftin, Kefurox, Zinacef)	1. Similar to other second-generation cephalosporins 2. Penetrates cerebrospinal fluid in presence of inflamed meninges	IV, IM, 750 mg–1.5 g q8h Surgical prophylaxis, IV 1.5 g 30–60 min before initial skin incision, then 750 mg IV or IM q8h if procedure is prolonged	Over 3 mo of age: IV, IM 50–100 mg/kg/d in divided doses q6–8h Bacterial meningitis, IV 200–240 mg/kg/d in divided doses q6–8h, reduced to 100 mg/kg/d on clinical improvement
Third Generation			
Cefoperazone (Cefobid)	1. Active against gram-negative and gram-positive organisms, including gram-negative organisms resistant to earlier cephalosporins	IV, IM 2–4 g/d in divided doses q8–12h	Dosage not established

TABLE 34-3	PARENTERAL CEPHALOSPORINS		
		Routes and Dosage Ranges	
Generic / Trade Name	Characteristics	*Adults*	*Children*
	2. Has increased activity against *Pseudomonas* organisms but cannot be used for single-agent treatment of systemic pseudomonal infections 3. Excreted primarily in bile; half-life prolonged in hepatic failure		
Cefotaxime (Claforan)	1. Antibacterial activity against most gram-positive and gram-negative bacteria, including several strains resistant to other antibiotics. It has activity against some strains of *Pseudomonas aeruginosa* resistant to first- and second-generation cephalosporins. 2. Recommended for serious infections caused by susceptible microorganisms	IV, IM 1g q6–8h; maximum dose, 12 g/24h	Weight >50 kg: same as adults Weight <50 kg and age over 1 mo: IV, IM 50–180 mg/kg/d, in divided doses q4–6h Neonates: up to 1 wk of age, IV 50 mg/kg q12h; 1–4 wk, IV 50 mg/kg q8h
Ceftazidime (Fortaz)	1. Active against gram-positive and gram-negative organisms 2. Especially effective against gram-negative organisms, including *Pseudomonas aeruginosa* and other bacterial strains resistant to aminoglycosides 3. Indicated for serious infections caused by susceptible organisms	IV, IM 1 g q8–12h	1 month to 12 years: IV 30–50 mg/kg q8h, not to exceed 6 g/d Under 1 mo of age: IV 30 mg/kg q12h
Ceftizoxime (Cefizox)	1. Broader gram-negative and anaerobic activity, especially against *Bacteroides fragilis* 2. More active against gram-positive organisms than moxalactam and more active against *Enterobacteriaceae* than cefoperazone 3. Dosage must be reduced with even mild renal insufficiency (creatinine clearance <80 ml/min)	IV, IM 1–2 g q8–12h Gonorrhea, uncomplicated, IM 1 g as a single dose	Over 6 mo of age: IV, IM 50 mg/kg q6–8h, increased to a total daily dose of 200 mg/kg if necessary
Ceftriaxone (Rocephin)	First third-generation cephalosporin approved for once-daily dosing	IV, IM 1–2 g once daily (q24h) Surgical prophylaxis, IV, IM 1 g ½–2 h before the procedure	IV, IM 50–75 mg/kg/d, not to exceed 2 g daily, in divided doses q12h Meningitis, IV, IM 100 mg/kg/d, not to exceed 4 g daily, in divided doses q12h

(continued)

TABLE 34-3 **PARENTERAL CEPHALOSPORINS** (Continued)

Generic/Trade Name	Characteristics	Routes and Dosage Ranges	
		Adults	**Children**
Moxalactam (Moxam)	Antibacterial spectrum is similar to that of cefotaxime, but moxalactam has better activity against anaerobic bacteria and better penetration into cerebrospinal fluid.	IM, IV 1–2 g q8h	Age 1 mo to 12 y: IV, IM 50 mg/kg q6–8h Neonates: up to 1 wk of age, IV 50 mg/kg q12; 1–4 wk, IV 50 mg/kg q8h
Fourth Generation			
Cefepime (Maxipime)	1. Indicated for urinary tract infections caused by *Escherichia coli* or *Klebsiella pneumoniae*; skin and soft tissue infections caused by susceptible streptococci or staphylococci; and pneumonia caused by *Streptococcus pneumoniae* 2. Dosage must be reduced with renal impairment.	IV 0.5–2 g q12h for 10 d IM 0.5–1 g q12h for 7–10 d Renal impairment: creatinine clearance (CrCl) 30–60 ml/min, 0.5–2 g q24h; CrCl 11–29 ml/min, 0.5–1 g q24h; CrCl 10 or below, 250–500 mg q24h	Dosage not established

Ampicillins

Ampicillin is a broad-spectrum, semisynthetic penicillin that is bactericidal for several types of gram-positive and gram-negative bacteria. It has been effective against *Proteus mirabilis, Salmonella, Shigella,* and most strains of *Escherichia coli,* but resistant forms of these organisms are increasing. Ampicillin is not used against gram-positive cocci because penicillin G or V is more effective and less expensive. It is ineffective against penicillinase-producing staphylococci and gonococci. It is excreted mainly by the kidneys; thus, it is useful in urinary tract infections (UTI). Because some is excreted in bile, it is useful in biliary tract infections not caused by biliary obstruction. It is widely used in treatment of bronchitis, sinusitis, and otitis media.

Amoxicillin is similar to ampicillin but is better absorbed and produces therapeutic blood levels more rapidly. It also causes less GI distress. **Bacampicillin** is a "pro-drug" that is converted to ampicillin in the body. It has a long duration of action and can be given twice daily. Dosage should be reduced in the presence of renal insufficiency.

Extended-Spectrum (Antipseudomonal) Penicillins

The drugs in this group (**carbenicillin, ticarcillin, mezlocillin,** and **piperacillin**) have a broad spectrum of antimicrobial activity. They are especially effective against gram-negative organisms such as *Pseudomonas, Proteus,* and *Escherichia coli.* For pseudomonal infections, one of these drugs is usually given concomitantly with an aminoglycoside antibiotic. Carbenicillin is available only as an oral formulation given for UTI or prostatitis caused by susceptible pathogens. The other drugs are usually given by intermittent IV infusion, although most can be given IM. Dosage of these drugs should be reduced in renal failure.

Penicillin/Beta-Lactamase Inhibitor Combinations

Beta-lactamase inhibitors are drugs with a beta-lactam structure but little antibacterial activity. They bind irreversibly and inactivate the beta-lactamase enzymes produced by many bacteria (*e.g., Escherichia coli, Klebsiella, Enterobacter, Bacteroides,* and *Staphylococcus aureus*). When combined with a penicillin, the beta-lactamase inhibitor protects the penicillin from destruction by the enzymes and extends the penicillin's spectrum of antimicrobial activity. Thus, the combination drug may be effective in infections caused by bacteria that are resistant to a beta-lactam antibiotic alone. Potassium clavulanate, sulbactam and tazobactam are the beta-lactamase inhibitors currently available in combinations with penicillins.

Unasyn is a combination of ampicillin and sulbactam available in vials with 1 g of ampicillin and 0.5 g of sulbactam or 2 g of ampicillin and 1 g of sulbactam.

Augmentin contains amoxicillin and potassium clavulanate. It is available in 250-mg and 500-mg tablets, each of which contains 125 mg of potassium clavulanate. Thus, two 250-mg tablets are not equivalent to one 500-mg tablet. **Timentin** is a combination of ticarcillin and clavulanate available in an IV formulation containing 3 g ticarcillin and 100 mg clavulanate. **Zosyn** is a combination of piperacillin and tazobactam in an IV formulation. Three dosage strengths are available with 2 g piperacillin and 0.25 g tazobactam, 3 g piperacillin and 0.375 g tazobactam, or 4 g piperacillin and 0.5 g tazobactam. Dosage of Zosyn should be reduced for clients with creatinine clearance below 40 ml/min and those undergoing hemodialysis.

Cephalosporins

Cephalosporins are a widely used group of antimicrobial drugs that are derived from a fungus. Although technically cefoxitin and cefotetan (cephamycins derived from a different fungus) and loracarbef (a carbacephem) are not cephalosporins, they are categorized with the cephalosporins because of their similarities to the group. Cephalosporins are broad-spectrum antimicrobial agents with a wide range of activity against both gram-positive and gram-negative bacteria. Compared to penicillins, they are generally less active against gram-positive organisms but more active against gram-negative ones.

Once absorbed, cephalosporins are widely distributed into most body fluids and tissues, with maximum concentrations in the liver and kidneys. Many cephalosporins do not reach therapeutic levels in CSF; exceptions are cefuroxime, a second-generation drug, and the third-generation agents. These drugs reach therapeutic levels when meninges are inflamed. Cephalosporins are excreted through the kidneys (except for cefoperazone, which is excreted in bile).

FIRST-GENERATION CEPHALOSPORINS

First-generation cephalosporins have essentially the same spectrum of antimicrobial activity and can be described as a group. They are effective against streptococci, staphylococci (except methicillin-resistant *Staphylococcus aureus*), *Neisseria, Salmonella, Shigella, Escherichia, Klebsiella, Bacillus, Corynebacterium diphtheriae, Proteus mirabilis,* and *Bacteroides* (except *Bacteroides fragilis*). They are not effective against *Enterobacter, Pseudomonas,* and *Serratia.*

SECOND-GENERATION CEPHALOSPORINS

Second-generation cephalosporins are more active against some gram-negative organisms than older drugs. Thus, they may be effective in infections resistant to other antibiotics, including infections caused by *Haemophilus influenzae, Enterobacter, Klebsiella, Escherichia coli,* and some strains of *Proteus.* Because each of these drugs has a somewhat different antimicrobial spectrum, susceptibility tests must be performed for each drug rather than for the entire group, as was feasible with first-generation drugs. Cefoxitin (Mefoxin), for example, is active against *Bacteroides fragilis,* an anaerobic organism resistant to most drugs.

THIRD-GENERATION CEPHALOSPORINS

Third-generation cephalosporins further extend the spectrum of activity against gram-negative organisms. In addition to activity against the usual enteric pathogens (*e.g., Escherichia coli, Proteus, Klebsiella*), they are also active against several strains resistant to other antibiotics and to first- and second-generation cephalosporins. Thus, they may be useful in infections caused by unusual strains of enteric organisms such as *Citrobacter, Serratia, Providencia,* and *Enterobacter.* Another difference is that third-generation cephalosporins penetrate inflamed meninges to reach therapeutic concentrations in CSF. Thus, they may be useful in meningeal infections caused by many common pathogens, including *Haemophilus influenzae, Neisseria meningitidis,* and *Streptococcus pneumoniae.* Although some of the drugs are active against *Pseudomonas* organisms, drug-resistant strains emerge when a cephalosporin is used alone for treatment of pseudomonal infection.

Overall, cephalosporins gain gram-negative activity and lose gram-positive activity as they move from the first to the third generation. The second- and third-generation drugs are more active against gram-negative organisms because they are more resistant to the beta-lactamase enzymes (cephalosporinases) produced by some bacteria to inactivate cephalosporins.

FOURTH-GENERATION CEPHALOSPORINS

Fourth-generation cephalosporins have a greater spectrum of antimicrobial activity and greater stability against breakdown by beta-lactamase enzymes, compared to third-generation drugs. Cefepime is the first fourth-generation cephalosporin to be developed. It is active against both gram-positive and gram-negative organisms. With gram-positive organisms, it is active against streptococci and staphylococci (except for methicillin-resistant staphylococci). With gram-negative organisms, its activity against *Pseudomonas aeruginosa* is similar to that of ceftazidime and its activity against Enterobacteriaceae is greater than that of third-generation cephalosporins. Moreover, cefepime retains activity against strains of *Enterobacteriaceae* and *Pseudomonas aeruginosa* that have developed resistance to third-generation agents.

INDICATIONS FOR USE

Clinical indications include surgical prophylaxis and treatment of infections of the respiratory tract, skin and soft tissues, bones and joints, urinary tract, and bloodstream (septicemia). Cephalosporins are often used as alternative drugs in infections caused by organisms resistant to other drugs. They are most important clinically for gram-negative infections. In most infections with streptococci and staphylococci, penicillins are more effective and less expensive. In infections caused by methicillin-resistant *Staphylococcus aureus*, cephalosporins are not clinically effective even if in vitro testing indicates susceptibility. The fourth-generation drug, cefepime, is indicated for use in severe infections of the lower respiratory and urinary tracts, skin and soft tissue, female reproductive tract, and in febrile neutropenic patients. It should be used as monotherapy for all infections caused by susceptible organisms except *Pseudomonas aeruginosa*; a combination of drugs should be used for serious *Pseudomonas aeruginosa* infections.

CONTRAINDICATIONS FOR USE

A major contraindication to the use of cephalosporins is a previous severe anaphylactic reaction to penicillin. Because cephalosporins are chemically similar to penicillins, there is a risk of cross-sensitivity. However, incidence of cross-sensitivity is thought to be low, especially in clients who have had delayed reactions (*e.g.,* skin rash) to penicillins. Another contraindication is cephalosporin allergy. Immediate allergic reactions with anaphylaxis, bronchospasm, and urticaria occur less often than delayed reactions with skin rash, drug fever, and eosinophilia.

Carbapenems

Carbapenems are broad-spectrum, bactericidal, beta-lactam antimicrobial agents. Like other beta-lactam drugs, they inhibit synthesis of bacterial cell walls by binding with penicillin-binding proteins. The group consists of two drugs.

Imipenem/cilastatin (Primaxin) is given parenterally and distributed in most body fluids. Imipenem is rapidly broken down by an enzyme (dehydropeptidase) in renal tubules and therefore reaches only low concentrations in urine. Cilastatin was synthesized to inhibit the enzyme and increase urine levels of the antibacterial agent. Recommended doses indicate the amount of imipenem; the solution contains an equivalent amount of cilastatin.

The drug is effective in infections caused by a wide range of bacteria, including penicillinase-producing staphylococci, *Escherichia coli*, *Proteus* species, *Enterobacter-Klebsiella-Serratia* species, and *Pseudomonas aeruginosa*. It is effective against *Enterococcus faecalis* (enterococcus) but is not effective against other streptococci. Its main indication for use is treatment of infections caused by organisms resistant to other drugs. Adverse effects are the same as those occurring with other beta-lactam antibiotics. Dosage should be reduced in renal impairment. The solution for IM injection contains lidocaine, a local anesthetic to decrease pain. This solution is contraindicated in persons allergic to this type of local anesthetic or who have severe shock or heart block.

Route and Dosage Ranges

Adults: IV 250–500 mg q6h: IM 500–750 mg q12h
Children below 40 kg weight: IV 60 mg/kg/d in divided doses: Children above 40 kg, use adult dosage

Meropenem (Merrem) is a newer carbapenem. It has a broad spectrum of antibacterial activity and may be used as a single drug for empiric therapy before causative microorganisms are identified. It is reportedly effective against penicillin-susceptible staphylococci and *Streptococcus pneumoniae*, most gram-negative aerobes (*e.g.,* *Escherichia coli*, *Haemophilus influenzae*, *Klebsiella pneumoniae*, *Pseudomonas aeruginosa*), and some anaerobes, including *Bacteroides fragilis*. It is indicated for use in intra-abdominal infections and bacterial meningitis caused by susceptible organisms. Compared to imipenem, meropenem costs more and seems to offer no clinical advantages.

Route and Dosage Ranges

Adults: IV 1 g q8h, as a bolus injection over 3 to 5 minutes or infusion over 15 to 30 minutes. Reduce dosage in patients with impaired renal function (creatinine clearance <50 ml/min).
Children 3 mos and older: IV 20–40 mg/kg q8h. Maximum dose 2 g q8h.

Monobactam

Aztreonam (Azactam) is a monobactam with activity against gram-negative bacteria, including *Enterobacteriaceae* and *Pseudomonas aeruginosa*, and many strains that are resistant to multiple antibiotics. Activity against gram-negative bacteria is similar to that of the aminoglycosides, but the drug does not cause kidney damage or hearing loss. Aztreonam is stable in the presence of beta-lactamase enzymes.

Indications for use include UTI, lower respiratory tract infections, septicemia, and abdominal and gynecologic infections caused by susceptible organisms. Gram-positive and anaerobic bacteria are resistant. Consequently, its ability to preserve normal gram-positive and anaerobic flora may be an advantage over most other antimicrobial agents.

Adverse effects are similar to those for penicillin. Dosage should be reduced in renal impairment.

Routes and Dosage Ranges

Adults: UTI, IM, IV 0.5–1.0 g q8–12h
  Systemic infections, 1–2 g q6–12h
Children: Dosage not established

Nursing Process

General aspects of the nursing process in antimicrobial drug therapy, as described in Chapter 33, apply to the client receiving penicillins, cephalosporins, aztreonam, and imipenem-cilastatin. In this chapter, only those aspects related specifically to these drugs are included.

Assessment

With penicillins, ask clients whether they have ever taken a penicillin and, if so, whether they ever had a skin rash, hives, swelling, or difficulty breathing associated with the drug. With cephalosporins, ask clients if they have ever taken one of the drugs, as far as they know, and whether they ever had a severe reaction to penicillin. Naming a few cephalosporins (*e.g.,* Ceclor, Keflex, Rocephin, Suprax) may help the client identify previous usage.

Nursing Diagnoses

- Risk for Injury: Hypersensitivity reactions with penicillins or cephalosporins
- Risk for Injury: Renal impairment with cephalosporins
- Knowledge Deficit: Correct home-care administration and usage of oral beta-lactams

Planning/Goals

The client will:
- Take oral beta-lactam antibacterials as directed
- Receive parenteral beta-lactam drugs by appropriate techniques to minimize tissue irritation
- Receive prompt and appropriate treatment if hypersensitivy reactions occur

Interventions

- After giving a penicillin parenterally in an outpatient setting, keep the client in the area for at least 30 minutes. Anaphylactic reactions are more likely to occur with parenteral than oral use and within a few minutes after injection.
- In any client care setting, keep emergency equipment and supplies readily available.
- Monitor client response to beta-lactam drugs.
- Monitor dosages of cephalosporins for clients with impaired renal function.

Evaluation

- Observe for improvement in signs of infection.
- Interview and observe for adverse drug effects.

Principles of Therapy: Beta-Lactam Antibacterials

GUIDELINES RELATED TO HYPERSENSITIVITY TO PENICILLINS

1. Before giving the initial dose of any penicillin preparation, ask the client if he or she has ever taken penicillin and, if so, whether an allergic reaction occurred. Penicillin is the most common cause of drug-induced anaphylaxis, a life-threatening hypersensitivity reaction, and a person known to be hypersensitive should generally be given another type of antibiotic.
2. In the rare instance in which penicillin is considered essential, a skin test may be helpful in assessing hypersensitivity. Benzylpenicilloyl polylysine (Pre-Pen) or a dilute solution of the penicillin to be administered (10,000 units/ml) may be applied topically to a skin scratch made with a sterile needle. If the scratch test is negative (no urticaria, erythema, or pruritus), the preparation may be injected intradermally. Allergic reactions, including fatal anaphylactic shock, have occurred with skin tests and following negative skin tests.
3. Because anaphylactic shock may occur with administration of the penicillins, especially by parenteral routes, emergency drugs and equipment must be readily available. Treatment may require parenteral epinephrine, oxygen, and insertion of an endotracheal or tracheostomy tube if laryngeal edema occurs.

DRUG SELECTION

Choice of a beta-lactam antibacterial depends primarily on the organism causing the infection, severity of the infection, and other factors. With penicillins, penicillin G is the drug of choice in many infections; ampicillin is useful in many gram-negative infections; an antipseudomonal penicillin is indicated in most *Pseudomonas* and *Proteus* infections; and an antistaphylococcal penicillin is indicated in staphylococcal infections. Most staphylococcal infections are caused by organisms that produce penicillinase, an enzyme that inactivates most penicillins. Antistaphylococcal penicillins were formulated to resist the enzyme. Nafcillin is the IV agent of choice, and dicloxacillin is the oral agent of choice.

With cephalosporins, *first-generation* drugs are often used for surgical prophylaxis, especially with prosthetic implants, because most postimplant infections are caused by gram-positive organisms such as staphylococci. They may also be used alone for treatment of infections caused by any susceptible organisms in body sites where drug penetration and host defenses are not a problem. Cefazolin (Kefzol) and cephapirin (Cefadyl) are frequently used parenteral agents. Cefazolin reportedly reaches a higher serum concentration, is more protein-bound, and has a slower rate of elimination than other first-generation drugs. These factors prolong serum half-life, so cefazolin can be given in smaller doses or less frequently. Cefazolin is also preferred for IM administration because it is less irritating to body tissues. *Second-generation* cephalosporins are also often used for surgical prophylaxis, especially for gynecologic and colorectal surgery. They are also used for treatment of intra-abdominal infections such as pelvic inflammatory disease, diverticulitis, penetrating wounds of the abdomen, and other infections caused by organisms inhabiting pelvic and colorectal areas. *Third-generation* cephalosporins are recommended for serious infections caused by susceptible organisms that are resistant to first- and second-generation cephalosporins. They are often used in the treatment of infections caused by *Escherichia coli, Proteus, Klebsiella, Serratia,* and other Enterobacteriaceae, especially when the infections occur in body sites not readily reached by other drugs (*e.g.,* CSF, bone) and in clients with immunosuppression. Although these drugs are effective against 50% to 75% of *Pseudomonas* strains, they should not be used alone in treating pseudomonal infections because drug resistance develops. *Fourth-generation* drugs are probably most useful in serious gram-negative infections, especially infections caused by organisms resistant to third-generation drugs. Cefepime is considered interchangeable with ceftazidime in indications for use.

ROUTE OF ADMINISTRATION AND DOSAGE

Choice of route and dosage depends largely on the seriousness of the infection being treated. For serious infections, beta-lactam antibacterials are usually given IV in large doses. With penicillins, most must be given every 4 to 6 hours to maintain therapeutic blood levels, because they are rapidly excreted by the kidneys. The oral route is often used, especially for less serious infections and for long-term prophylaxis of rheumatic fever; the IM route is rarely used in hospitalized clients but may be used in ambulatory settings. With cephalosporins, a few are sufficiently well absorbed for oral administration; these are most often used in mild infections and UTI. Although some cephalosporins can be given IM, the injections cause pain and induration. Cefazolin is preferred for IM administration because it

is less irritating to tissues. Dosages need to be lower with renal failure (except with cefoperazone, which is excreted through the biliary tract).

USE OF PENICILLINS IN SPECIFIC SITUATIONS

Streptococcal Infections

When used for streptococcal infections, penicillins should be given for the full prescribed course to prevent complications such as rheumatic fever, endocarditis, and glomerulonephritis.

Sexually Transmitted Diseases

When penicillins are used for sexually transmitted diseases, it is advisable to refer to the guidelines established by the Centers for Disease Control and Prevention (CDC). Recommendations vary according to patterns of bacterial resistance. For example, penicillin-resistant strains of *Neisseria gonorrhoeae* are being encountered with increasing frequency.

With Probenecid

Probenecid (Benemid) can be given concurrently with penicillins to increase serum drug levels. Probenecid acts by blocking renal excretion of the penicillins. This action may be useful when high serum levels are needed with oral penicillin preparations or when a single large dose is given for prevention or treatment of gonorrhea or syphilis.

With an Aminoglycoside

A penicillin is often given concomitantly with an aminoglycoside antibiotic for serious infections, such as those caused by *Pseudomonas aeruginosa*. In this instance, the drugs should not be mixed in a syringe or an IV solution because that inactivates the aminoglycoside.

POTENTIAL ELECTROLYTE DISTURBANCES

Excessive amounts of potassium or sodium may be ingested during penicillin therapy. Potassium excess may occur with large IV doses of penicillin G potassium, which contains 1.7 mEq of potassium per 1 million units. Hyperkalemia is unlikely with normal renal function but may occur with impaired renal function. Sodium excess may occur when ticarcillin (5.6 mEq sodium/g) is given to clients with renal impairment or congestive heart failure. Hypokalemic metabolic acidosis may occur with ticarcillin in clients whose renal function is impaired. This occurs because potassium loss is enhanced by high sodium intake.

USE OF CEPHALOSPORINS IN SPECIFIC SITUATIONS

Perioperative Use

Many cephalosporins are used in surgical prophylaxis. The particular drug depends largely on the type of organism likely to be encountered in the operative area. First-generation drugs are often used for procedures associated with gram-positive postoperative infections, such as prosthetic implant surgery. Second-generation cephalosporins are often used for abdominal procedures, especially gynecologic and colorectal surgery, in which enteric gram-negative infections may occur postoperatively. Third-generation drugs should not be used for surgical prophylaxis because they are less active against staphylococci than cefazolin, the gram-negative organisms they are most useful against are rarely encountered in elective surgery, widespread usage for prophylaxis promotes emergence of drug-resistant organisms, and they are very expensive.

When used perioperatively, a cephalosporin should be given about 30 to 60 minutes before the first skin incision is made, so the drug has time to reach therapeutic serum and tissue concentrations. A single dose is usually sufficient. In prosthetic implants such as arthroplasty and open-heart surgery, the drug may be continued for 3 to 5 days.

Use in Renal Failure or Impairment

In renal failure (creatinine clearance <20–30 ml/min), dosage of all cephalosporins except cefoperazone should be reduced by 50%. Cefoperazone is excreted primarily through the bile and therefore does not accumulate with renal failure. Dosage of ceftizoxime should be reduced even with moderate renal impairment (creatinine clearance <80 ml/min).

USE IN CHILDREN

Penicillins and cephalosporins are widely used to treat infections in children and are generally safe. They should be used cautiously in neonates because immature kidney function slows their elimination. Dosages should be based on age, weight, severity of the infection being treated, and renal function.

The use of aztreonam and imipenem-cilastatin in children is not well defined. Although no children's dosage has been established for aztreonam, the drug has been given to children with various infections in doses of 30 mg/kg every 6 to 8 hours and in doses of 50 mg/kg every 4 to 6 hours for infections caused by *Pseudomonas aeruginosa*.

USE IN OLDER ADULTS

Beta-lactam antibacterials are relatively safe, although decreased renal function, other disease processes and concurrent drug therapies increase the risks of adverse effects in older adults. With penicillins, hyperkalemia may occur with large IV doses of penicillin G potassium and hypernatremia may occur with ticarcillin (Ticar). Hypernatremia is less likely with other antipseudomonal penicillins such as mezlocillin (Mezlin) and piperacillin (Pipracil). Cephalosporins may aggravate renal impairment, especially when other nephrotoxic drugs are used concurrently. Dosage of most cephalosporins must be reduced in the presence of renal impairment, depending on creatinine clearance. No guidelines have been established for the use of aztreonam or imipenem/cilastatin in older adults.

 ## HOME CARE

Many beta-lactam antibiotics are given in the home setting. With oral agents, the role of the home care nurse is mainly to teach accurate administration and observation for therapeutic and adverse effects. With liquid suspensions for children, shaking to resuspend medication and measuring with a measuring spoon or calibrated device are required for safe dosing. Household spoons should *not* be used because they vary widely in capacity. General guidelines for IV therapy are discussed in Chapter 33; specific guidelines depend on the drug being given.

NURSING ACTIONS

BETA-LACTAM ANTIBACTERIALS

NURSING ACTIONS	*RATIONALE/EXPLANATION*
1. Administer accurately	
a. With penicillins:	
(1) Give most oral penicillins on an empty stomach, about 1 h before or 2 h after a meal. Penicillin V, amoxicillin, amoxicillin/clavulanate, and bacampicillin may be given without regard to meals.	To decrease binding to foods and inactivation by gastric acid. The latter four drugs are not significantly affected by food.
(2) Give oral drugs with a full glass of water, preferably; do not give with orange juice or other acidic fluids.	To promote absorption and decrease inactivation, which may occur in an acidic environment.
(3) Give IM penicillins deeply into a large muscle mass.	To decrease tissue irritation
(4) For IV administration, generally dilute reconstituted penicillins in 50 to 100 mL of 5% dextrose or 0.9% sodium chloride injection and infuse over 30 to 60 min.	To minimize vascular irritation and phlebitis.
(5) Give reconstituted ampicillin IV or IM within 1 h.	The drug is stable in solution for a limited time, after which effectiveness is lost.
b. With cephalosporins:	
(1) Give most oral drugs with food or milk.	To decrease nausea and vomiting. Food delays absorption but does not affect the amount of drug absorbed. An exception is the pediatric suspension of ceftibuten which must be given at least 2 h before or 1 h after a meal.
(2) Give IM drugs deeply into a large muscle mass.	The drugs are irritating to tissues and cause pain, induration, and possibly sterile abscess. The IM route is rarely used.
(3) For IV administration, generally dilute reconstituted drugs in 50 to 100 mL of 5% dextrose or 0.9% sodium chloride injection and infuse over 30 min.	These drugs are irritating to veins and cause thrombophlebitis. This can be minimized by using small IV catheters, large veins, adequate dilution, slow infusion rates, and changing venipuncture sites. Thrombophlebitis is more likely to occur with doses of more than 6 g/d for longer than 3 d.
c. With aztreonam:	
(1) For IM administration, add 3 ml diluent per gram of drug, and inject into a large muscle mass.	
(2) For IV injection, add 6 to 10 ml sterile water, and inject into vein or IV tubing over 3 to 5 min.	
(3) For IV infusion, mix in at least 50 ml of 0.9% NaCl or 5% dextrose injection per gram of drug and give over 20 to 60 min.	
d. With imipenem/cilastatin: IV: Mix reconstituted solution in 100 ml of 0.9% NaCl or 5% dextrose injection. Give 250- to 500-mg doses over 20 to 30 min; give 1-g doses over 40 to 60 min.	
IM: Inject deeply into large muscle mass with 21 gauge, 2 inch needle	
2. Observe for therapeutic effects	See Chapter 33
a. Decreased signs of local and systemic infection	
b. Decreased signs and symptoms of the infection for which the drug is given	

NURSING ACTIONS	RATIONALE/EXPLANATION
c. Absence of signs and symptoms of infection when given prophylactically	
3. Observe for adverse effects:	
a. Hypersensitivity—anaphylaxis, serum sickness, skin rash, urticaria	See Nursing Actions in Chapter 33 for signs and symptoms. Reactions are more likely to occur in those with previous hypersensitivity reactions and those with a history of allergy, asthma, or hay fever. Anaphylaxis is more likely with parenteral administration and may occur within 5 to 30 min of injection.
b. Phlebitis at IV sites and pain at IM sites	Parenteral solutions are irritating to body tissue.
c. Superinfection	See Chapter 33 for signs and symptoms.
d. Nausea and vomiting	May occur with all beta-lactam drugs, especially with high oral doses.
e. Diarrhea, colitis, pseudomembranous colitis	Diarrhea commonly occurs with beta-lactam drugs and may range from mild to severe. The most severe form is pseudomembranous colitis, which is more often associated with ampicillin and the cephalosporins than other beta-lactams.
f. Nephrotoxicity	
(1) Acute interstitial nephritis (AIN)—hematuria, oliguria, proteinuria, pyuria	AIN may occur with any of the beta-lactams, especially with high parenteral doses of penicillins.
(2) Increased BUN and serum creatinine; casts in urine	More likely with cephalosporins, especially in clients who are elderly or have impaired renal function, unless dosage is reduced
g. Neurotoxicity—confusion, hallucinations, neuromuscular irritability, convulsive seizures	More likely with large IV doses of penicillins or cephalosporins, especially in clients with impaired renal function.
h. Bleeding—hypoprothrombinemia, platelet dysfunction	Ticarcillin may cause decreased platelet aggregation. Cefamandole, cefoperazone, cefotetan, and ceftriaxone may cause hypoprothrombinemia (by killing intestinal bacteria that normally produce vitamin K or a chemical structure that prevents activation of prothrombin) or platelet dysfunction. Hypoprothrombinemia can be treated by giving vitamin K. Vitamin K does not restore normal platelet function or normal bacterial flora in the intestines.
4. Observe for drug interactions	
a. Drugs that *increase* effects of penicillins.	
(1) Gentamicin and other aminoglycosides	Synergistic activity against *Pseudomonas* organisms when given concomitantly with extended-spectrum (antipseudomonal) penicillins
	Synergistic activity against enterococci that cause subacute bacterial endocarditis, brain abscess, meningitis, or urinary tract infection
	Synergistic activity against *Staphylococcus aureus* when used with nafcillin or methicillin
(2) Probenecid (Benemid)	Decreases renal excretion of penicillins, thus elevates and prolongs penicillin blood levels

(continued)

NURSING ACTIONS	RATIONALE/EXPLANATION
b. Drugs that *decrease* effects of penicillins	
(1) Acidifying agents (ammonium chloride, ascorbic acid, cranberry juice, methenamine, methionine, orange juice)	Most oral penicillins are destroyed by acids, including gastric acid. Amoxicillin and penicillin V are acid stable.
(2) Erythromycin	Erythromycin inhibits the bactericidal activity of penicillins against most organisms but potentiates activity against resistant strains of *Staphylococcus aureus*.
(3) Tetracyclines	These bacteriostatic antibiotics slow multiplication of bacteria and thereby inhibit the penicillins, which act against rapidly multiplying bacteria.
c. Drugs that *increase* effects of cephalosporins:	
(1) Loop diuretics (furosemide, ethacrynic acid)	Increased renal toxicity
(2) Gentamicin and other aminoglycoside antibiotics	Additive renal toxicity especially in older clients, those with renal impairment, those receiving high dosages, and those receiving probenecid
(3) Probenecid	Increases blood levels by decreasing renal excretion of the cephalosporins. This may be a desirable interaction to increase blood levels and therapeutic effectiveness or allow smaller doses.
d. Drugs that *decrease* effects of cephalosporins Tetracyclines	Tetracyclines are bacteriostatic and slow the rate of bacterial reproduction. Cephalosporins are bactericidal and are most effective against rapidly multiplying bacteria. Thus, tetracyclines should not be given concurrently with cephalosporins.
e. Drugs that *increase* or *decrease* effects of aztreonam and imipenem/cilastatin	Although few interactions have been reported with these drugs, potential interactions are those that occur with other beta-lactam antibiotics.
5. Teach clients: **a.** With penicillins	
(1) Take on an empty stomach (except amoxicillin, amoxicillin/clavulanate, bacampicillin, and penicillin V), with at least 8 oz of water, at regular intervals around the clock.	To increase therapeutic effects and decrease adverse effects
(2) Report skin rash, hives, itching, severe diarrhea, shortness of breath, fever, sore throat, black tongue, or any unusual bleeding.	These symptoms may indicate a need to discontinue the drug.
(3) Discard liquid forms of penicillins after 7 d at room temperature and 14 d when refrigerated.	Liquid forms deteriorate and should not be taken.
b. With oral cephalosporins	
(1) Take with food or milk.	To decrease gastrointestinal upset.
(2) Report the occurrence of diarrhea, especially if it is severe or contains blood, pus, or mucus.	The drug may need to be stopped.

REVIEW AND APPLICATION EXERCISES

1. How do beta-lactam drugs act against bacteria?

2. What adverse effects are associated with beta-lactam drugs and how may they be prevented or minimized?

3. What are beta-lactamase enzymes and what do they do to beta-lactam antibacterial drugs?

4. How are penicillins and other beta-lactam drugs excreted?

5. What are the main differences between penicillin G or V and antistaphylococcal and antipseudomonal penicillins?

6. What is the reason for combining clavulanate, sulbactam, or tazobactam with a penicillin?

7. When giving injections of penicillin in an outpatient setting, it is recommended to keep clients in the area and observe them for at least 30 minutes. Why?

8. When probenecid is given concurrently with a penicillin, what is its purpose?

9. What are the signs and symptoms of anaphylaxis?

10. How do aztreonam (Azactam) and imipenem/cilastatin (Primaxin) differ from penicillins and cephalosporins?

11. For clients with renal insufficiency, which drugs in this chapter require reduced dosages?

12. How do you assess renal function?

13. Which drugs from this chapter may cause pseudomembranous colitis?

14. What are the signs, symptoms, and treatment of pseudomembranous colitis?

SELECTED REFERENCES

Antimicrobial prophylaxis in surgery (1993). *Medical Letter on Drugs and Therapeutics, 35,* 91–93.

Cunha, B.A. & Gill, M.V. (1995). Cefepime. *Medical Clinics of North America, 79*(4), 721–732.

Drug facts and comparisons. (1996). St. Louis: Facts and Comparisons.

Dunne, W.M., Jr. (1994). Mechanisms of infectious disease. In C.M. Porth, *Pathophysiology: Concepts of altered health states,* 4th ed., pp. 221–241. Philadelphia: J.B. Lippincott.

Johnson, D.H. & Cunha, B.A. (1995). Aztreonam. *Medical Clinics of North America, 79*(4), 733–743.

Klein, N.C. & Cunha, B.A. (1995). Third-generation cephalosporins. *Medical Clinics of North America, 79*(4), 705–719.

Kunin, C.M. (1993). Resistance to antimicrobial drugs—A worldwide calamity. *Annals of Internal Medicine, 118,* 557–561.

Mandell, G.L. & Petri, W.A., Jr. (1996). Antimicrobial agents: Penicillins, cephalosporins, and other beta-lactam antibiotics. In J.G. Hardman, L.E. Limbird, P.B. Molinoff, & R.W. Ruddon (Eds.), *Goodman & Gilman's The pharmacological basis of therapeutics,* 9th ed., pp. 1073–1101. New York: McGraw-Hill.

Morita, M.M. (1993). Methicillin-resistant *Staphylococcus aureus:* Past, present and future. *Nursing Clinics of North America, 28*(3), 625–637.

Norrby, S.R. (1995). Carbapenems. *Medical Clinics of North America, 79*(4), 745–759.

Sensakovic, J.W. & Smith, L.G. (1995). Beta-lactamase inhibitor combinations. *Medical Clinics of North America, 79*(4), 695–704.

Stutman, H.R. (1993). Cefprozil. *Pediatric Annals, 22,* 167–174.

Tan, J.S. & File, T.M., Jr. (1995). Antipseudomonal penicillins. *Medical Clinics of North America, 79*(4), 679–693.

35 Aminoglycosides and Fluoroquinolones

Outline

Aminoglycosides
  mechanism of action
  indications for use
  contraindications for use

Fluoroquinolones
  mechanism of action
  indications for use
  contraindications for use

Nursing Process
  assessment
  planning/goals
  interventions
  evaluation

Principles of Therapy: Aminoglycosides and Fluoroquinolones
  choice of drug
  dosage of aminoglycosides
  dosage of fluoroquinolones
  guidelines for reducing toxicity
    of aminoglycosides
  use in children
  use in older adults
  home care

Objectives

After studying this chapter, the student will be able to:

1 Describe characteristics of aminoglycosides in relation to effectiveness, safety, spectrum of antimicrobial activity, indications for use, administration, and observation of client responses.

2 Discuss factors influencing selection and dosage of aminoglycosides.

3 State the rationale for the increasing use of single daily doses rather than multiple daily doses.

4 Discuss the importance of serum drug levels during aminoglycoside therapy.

5 Describe measures to prevent or minimize nephrotoxicity and ototoxicity with aminoglycosides.

6 Describe characteristics, uses, adverse effects, and nursing process implications of fluoro-quinolones.

7 Apply principles of using aminoglycosides and fluoroquinolones in selected client situations.

Key Terms

Audiometry

Nephrotoxicity

Ototoxicity

Peak and trough serum drug levels

Post-antibiotic effect (PAE)

The aminoglycosides are bactericidal drugs that have been widely used to treat serious gram-negative infections for about 30 years. The quinolones were older drugs used only for treatment of urinary tract infections (UTI). Nalidixic acid (Neg-Gram), the prototype, is rarely used (see Chap. 36); cinoxacin (Cinobac) is used for UTI. The fluoroquinolones were synthesized by adding a fluorine molecule to the quinolone structure. This addition increased drug activity against gram-negative microorganisms, broadened the antimicrobial spectrum to include several other microorganisms, and allowed use of the drugs in treating some systemic infections. General characteristics, mechanisms of action, clinical indications for use, contraindications for use, nursing process implications and principles of therapy for these drugs are described below. Individual drugs, with routes of administration and dosage ranges, are listed in Tables 35-1 and 35-2.

Aminoglycosides

The aminoglycoside antibiotics are bactericidal agents with similar pharmacologic, antimicrobial, and toxicologic characteristics. They are used to treat infections caused by gram-negative microorganisms such as *Pseudomonas, Proteus, Escherichia coli,* and *Klebsiella-Enterobacter-Serratia* species.

These drugs are poorly absorbed (5% or less) from the gastrointestinal (GI) tract. Thus, when given orally, they exert local effects in the GI tract. They are well absorbed from intramuscular (IM) injection sites and reach peak effects in 30 to 90 minutes if circulatory status is good. After intravenous (IV) administration, peak effects occur within 30 to 60 minutes. Plasma half-life is 2 to 4 hours with normal renal function.

Following parenteral administration, aminoglycosides are widely distributed in extracellular fluid and reach therapeutic levels in blood, urine, bone, inflamed joints, and pleural and ascitic fluids. They accumulate in high concentrations in the kidney and inner ear. They are poorly distributed to the central nervous system, intraocular fluids, and respiratory tract secretions.

Injected drugs are not metabolized; they are excreted unchanged in the urine, primarily by glomerular filtration. Oral drugs are excreted in feces.

MECHANISM OF ACTION

Aminoglycosides penetrate the cell walls of susceptible bacteria and bind irreversibly to 30S ribosomes, intracellular structures that synthesize proteins. As a result, the bacteria cannot synthesize the proteins necessary for their function and replication.

INDICATIONS FOR USE

The major clinical use of parenteral aminoglycosides is to treat serious, systemic infections caused by susceptible aerobic, gram-negative organisms. Many hospital-acquired infections are caused by gram-negative organisms. These infections have become more common with control of other types of infections, widespread use of antimicrobial drugs, and diseases (*e.g.,* acquired immunodeficiency syndrome [AIDS]) or treatments (*e.g.,* radical surgery and therapy with antineoplastic or immunosuppressive drugs) that lower host resistance. The infections occur in the respiratory and genitourinary tracts, skin, wounds, bowel, and bloodstream. Any infection with gram-negative organisms may be serious and potentially life-threatening. Management is difficult because the organisms are generally less susceptible to antibacterial drugs, and drug-resistant strains develop rapidly. The few drugs that are effective against them are relatively toxic. In pseudomonal infections, an aminoglycoside is often given concurrently with an antipseudomonal penicillin (*e.g.,* ticarcillin) for synergistic therapeutic effects. The penicillin-induced breakdown of the bacterial cell wall makes it easier for the aminoglycoside to reach its site of action inside the bacterial cell. However, the drugs are chemically and physically incompatible. Therefore, they should not be mixed in a syringe or an IV fluid because the aminoglycoside will be deactivated.

A second clinical use is for treatment of tuberculosis. Streptomycin was often used before the development of other effective and less toxic antitubercular drugs such as isoniazid and rifampin. Now, streptomycin is used for treatment of tuberculosis resistant to other antitubercular drugs. Multidrug resistant strains of the tuberculosis organism, including strains resistant to both isoniazid and rifampin, are being identified with increasing frequency. This development is leading some authorities to recommend an aminoglycoside as part of a four- to six-drug regimen.

A third clinical use of aminoglycosides is oral administration to suppress intestinal bacteria. Neomycin and kanamycin may be given before colonoscopy or bowel surgery and to treat hepatic coma. In hepatic coma, intestinal bacteria produce ammonia, which enters the bloodstream and causes encephalopathy. Drug therapy to suppress intestinal bacteria decreases ammonia production. Paromomycin is used mainly in the treatment of intestinal amebiasis.

A few aminoglycosides are administered topically to the eye or to the skin. These are discussed in Chapters 65 and 66, respectively.

CONTRAINDICATIONS FOR USE

Aminoglycosides are contraindicated in infections for which less toxic drugs are effective. The drugs are nephrotoxic and ototoxic and must be used very cau-
(*text continues on page 476*)

TABLE 35-1	AMINOGLYCOSIDES		
		Routes and Dosage Ranges	
Generic/Trade Name	**Characteristics**	**Adults**	**Children**
Amikacin (Amikin)	1. A semisynthetic derivative of kanamycin 2. Has a broader spectrum of antibacterial activity than other aminoglycosides because it resists degradation by most enzymes that inactivate gentamicin and tobramycin 3. Major clinical use is in infections caused by organisms resistant to other aminoglycosides (e.g., *Pseudomonas, Proteus, Escherichia coli, Klebsiella, Enterobacter, Serratia*), whether community or hospital acquired	IM, IV 15 mg/kg q24h, 7.5 mg/kg q12h, or 5 mg/kg q8h	*Older children:* Same as adults *Neonates:* IM, IV 10 mg/kg initially, then 7.5 mg/kg q12h
Gentamicin (Garamycin)	1. A frequently prescribed aminoglycoside 2. Effective against several gram-negative organisms, although some strains have become resistant 3. Acts synergistically with ticarcillin and related penicillins against *Pseudomonas aeruginosa*. The combination also inhibits the emergence of resistant bacteria that may occur when either drug is used alone.	IV, IM 3–5 mg/kg q24h, 1.5–2.5 mg/kg q12h, or 1–1.7 mg/kg q8h	*Children:* IV, IM 6–7.5 mg/kg/d in three divided doses, q8h *Infants and neonates:* IV, IM 7.5 mg/kg/d in three divided doses, q8h *Premature infants and neonates <1 week old:* IV, IM 5 mg/kg/d in two divided doses, q12h
Kanamycin (Kantrex)	1. Occasionally used to decrease bowel organisms prior to surgery, treat hepatic coma, or to treat multidrug-resistant tuberculosis	IV, IM 15 mg/kg/d, in two or three divided doses Suppression of intestinal bacteria PO 1 g every hour for 4 doses, then 1 g q6h for 36 to 72 h Hepatic coma PO 8–12 g daily in divided doses	IV, IM same as adults
Neomycin	1. Given orally or topically only because too toxic for systemic use 2. Although poorly absorbed from GI tract, toxic levels may accumulate in presence of renal failure. 3. Used topically, often in combination with other drugs, to treat infections of the eye, ear, and skin (burns, wounds, ulcers, dermatoses).	Suppression of intestinal bacteria (with erythromycin 1 g) PO 1 g at 19, 18, and 9 h before surgery (3 doses) Hepatic coma PO 4–12 g daily in divided doses	

Drug		Route & Dosage	
Netilmicin (Netromycin)	When used for wound or bladder irrigations, systemic absorption may occur if the area is large or if drug concentration exceeds 0.1%. 1. Similar to gentamicin in antimicrobial spectrum, but is reportedly less active against *Pseudomonas aeruginosa*	IM, IV 4–6.5 mg/kg/d in 2 or 3 divided doses, q8–12h	*Infants and children (6 wk to 12 y):* 5.5 to 8 mg/kg/d in 2 or 3 divided doses, q8–12h *Neonates (under 6 wk):* 4–6.5 mg/kg/d, in 2 divided doses, q12h Intestinal amebiasis; Same as adults
Paromomycin (Humatin)	1. Acts against bacteria and amebae in the intestinal lumen 2. Used to treat hepatic coma and intestinal amebiasis. It is not effective in amebic infections outside the intestine. 3. Usually not absorbed from GI tract and unlikely to cause ototoxicity and nephrotoxicity associated with systemically absorbed aminoglycosides. However, systemic absorption may occur in the presence of inflammatory or ulcerative bowel disease.	Intestinal amebiasis PO 25–35 mg/kg/d, in 3 divided doses, with meals, for 5–10 d. Repeat after 2 wk, if necessary. Hepatic coma PO 4 g/d in divided doses for 5–6 d	
Streptomycin	1. The first aminoglycoside 2. Used in a four- to six-drug regimen for treatment of multidrug-resistant tuberculosis. Also may be used with penicillin to treat streptococcal or enterococcal endocarditis and with tetracycline to treat brucellosis, plague and tularemia. 3. Use declined because of eighth cranial nerve damage and rapid development of drug-resistant microorganisms	IM 15 mg/kg/d (maximum 1 g) or 25–30 mg/kg two or three times weekly (maximum 1.5 g per dose)	IM 20–40 mg/kg/d in 2 divided doses, q12h (maximum dose, 1 g/d)
Tobramycin (Nebcin)	1. Similar to gentamicin in antibacterial spectrum, but may be more active against *Pseudomonas* organisms. 2. May be indicated in serious staphylococcal infections when penicillins or other less toxic drugs are contraindicated or ineffective. 3. Often used with other antibiotics for septicemia and infections of burn wounds, other soft tissues, bone, the urinary tract and the central nervous system.	IV, IM 3–5 mg/kg q24h, 1.5–2.5 mg/kg q12h, or 1–1.7 mg/kg q8h	Same as adults *Neonates (1 wk or less):* IM, IV up to 4 mg/kg/d in 2 divided doses, q12h

TABLE 35-2	FLUOROQUINOLONES	
Generic/Trade Name	**Characteristics**	**Routes and Dosage Ranges**
Cinoxacin (Cinobac)	1. Used only for urinary tract infections (UTI) 2. Effective against most gram-negative bacteria that commonly cause UTI (*Escherichia coli, Klebsiella, Enterobacter, Proteus*)	PO 1 g daily in 2 to 4 divided doses for 7–14 d
Ciprofloxacin (Cipro)	1. Effective in respiratory, urinary tract, GI tract, and skin and soft tissue infections as well as sexually transmitted diseases caused by chlamydiae and gonorrhea organisms 2. Used as one of four to six drugs in treatment of multidrug-resistant tuberculosis	UTI, PO 250 mg q12h Systemic infections, PO 500–750 mg q12h
Enoxacin (Penetrex)	Used only for UTI and uncomplicated gonorrhea	UTI, PO 200–400 mg q12h for 7–14 d Gonorrhea, PO 400 mg as a single dose
Levofloxacin (Levaquin)	A broad-spectrum agent effective for treatment of bronchitis, pneumonia, and sinusitis	PO, IV 250–500 mg once daily. Infuse IV dose slowly, over 60 min
Lomefloxacin (Maxaquin)	1. See ciprofloxacin, above 2. Also approved for prophylactic therapy before transurethral surgical procedures	PO 400 mg once daily Preoperatively, PO 400 mg as a single dose, 2–6 h before surgery
Norfloxacin (Noroxin)	Used only for UTI and uncomplicated gonorrhea	PO 400 mg twice daily
Ofloxacin (Floxin)	See ciprofloxacin, above	PO, IV 200–400 mg q12h for 3–10 d Gonorrhea, PO 400 mg as a single dose

tiously in the presence of renal impairment. Dosages are adjusted according to serum drug levels and creatinine clearance. The drugs must also be used cautiously in clients with myasthenia gravis and other neuromuscular disorders because muscle weakness may be increased.

Fluoroquinolones

Fluoroquinolones are synthetic, bactericidal drugs with activity against gram-negative and gram-positive organisms. Their development was a significant advance in antimicrobial drug therapy because they often allow oral, ambulatory treatment of infections that previously required parenteral therapy and hospitalization. Most fluoroquinolones are given orally. Oral drugs are generally well absorbed, achieve therapeutic concentrations in most body fluids, and are metabolized to some extent in the liver. The kidneys are the main route of elimination, with about 30% to 60% of an oral dose ex-

creted unchanged in the urine. Dosage should be reduced in renal impairment. Ciprofloxacin and ofloxacin may be given orally or IV.

MECHANISM OF ACTION

The drugs act by interfering with deoxyribonucleic acid (DNA) gyrase, an enzyme required for synthesis of bacterial DNA and therefore required for bacterial growth and replication.

INDICATIONS FOR USE

Fluoroquinolones are indicated for a variety of infections caused by aerobic gram-negative and other microorganisms. Thus, they may be used to treat infections of the respiratory, genitourinary, and GI tracts as well as infections of bones, joints, skin, and soft tissues. They are also being used to treat multidrug-resistant tuberculosis (with several other drugs), infections caused by atypical mycobacteria called *Mycobacterium avium* complex (MAC) in AIDS patients, and fever in neutropenic cancer patients. Specific indications for use vary with individual drugs and are listed in Table 35-2.

CONTRAINDICATIONS FOR USE

Fluoroquinolones are contraindicated in children under 18 years of age, in pregnant or lactating women, and in those who have experienced a hypersensitivity reaction.

Nursing Process

General aspects of the nursing process as described in Chapter 33 apply to the client receiving aminoglycosides and fluoroquinolones. In this chapter, only those aspects related specifically to these drugs are included.

Assessment

With aminoglycosides, assess for the presence of factors that predispose to nephrotoxicity or ototoxicity:

- Check laboratory reports of renal function (*e.g.,* serum creatinine, creatinine clearance, blood urea nitrogen [BUN]) for abnormal values.
- Assess for impairment of balance or hearing, including audiometry reports if available.
- Analyze current medications for drugs that interact with aminoglycosides to increase risks of nephrotoxicity or ototoxicity.

  With fluoroquinolones, assess for the presence of factors that increase risks of adverse drug effects (*e.g.,* impaired renal function, inadequate fluid intake, frequent or prolonged exposure to sunlight in usual activities of daily living).
- Assess laboratory tests (*e.g.,* complete blood counts and tests of renal and hepatic function) for abnormal values.

Planning/Goals

The client will:
- Receive aminoglycoside dosages that are individualized by age, weight, renal function, and serum drug levels
- Have serum aminoglycoside levels monitored regularly and accurately
- Have renal function tests performed regularly during aminoglycoside and fluoroquinolone therapy
- Be well hydrated during aminoglycoside and fluoroquinolone therapy
- Be observed regularly for adverse drug effects

Interventions

- With aminoglycosides, weigh clients accurately (dosage is based on weight), monitor laboratory reports of BUN, serum creatinine, serum drug levels, and urinalysis for abnormal values.
- Force fluids to at least 2000 to 3000 ml daily if not contraindicated. Keeping the client well hydrated reduces risks of nephrotoxicity with aminoglycosides and crystalluria with fluoroquinolones.
- Avoid concurrent use of other nephrotoxic drugs when possible.

Evaluation

- Interview and observe for improvement in the infection being treated.
- Interview and observe for adverse drug effects.

Principles of Therapy: Aminoglycosides and Fluoroquinolones

CHOICE OF DRUG

With aminoglycosides, gentamicin is probably the aminoglycoside of choice for systemic infections if resistant microorganisms have not developed in the clinical setting. If gentamicin-resistant organisms have developed, amikacin or tobramycin may be given because they are less susceptible to drug-destroying enzymes. In terms of toxicity, the drugs cause similar effects, except that tobramycin may cause less nephrotoxicity and netilmicin may cause less ototoxicity. With fluoroquinolones, ciprofloxacin is often the drug of first choice.

DOSAGE OF AMINOGLYCOSIDES

Dosage of aminoglycosides must be carefully regulated because therapeutic doses are close to toxic doses. Two major dosing schedules are used, one involving multiple daily doses and one involving a single daily dose. The multiple-dose regimen has been used for many years, and guidelines are well-defined. The single-dose regimen is being used increasingly, and guidelines are still evolving as studies and clinical experience accumulate. These two regimens are described below.

Multiple Daily Dosing

1. An *initial loading dose* is given to achieve therapeutic serum levels rapidly. The amount is based on weight and desired peak serum level. If the client is obese, lean or ideal body weight should be used because aminoglycosides are not significantly distributed in body fat. In clients with normal renal function, the recommended loading dose for gentamicin, tobramycin, and netilmicin is 1.5 to 2 mg/kg of body weight; for amikacin the loading dose is 5 to 7.5 mg/kg.
2. *Maintenance doses* are based on serum drug levels. Peak serum levels should be assessed 30 to 60 minutes after drug administration (5–8 µg/ml for gentamicin and tobramycin, 20–30 µg/ml for amikacin, 4–12 µg/ml for netilmicin). Measurement of both peak and trough levels is needed to establish and maintain therapeutic serum levels without excessive toxicity. For gentamicin and tobramycin, peak levels

above 10 to 12 µg/ml and trough levels above 2 µg/ml for prolonged periods have been associated with nephrotoxicity. For accuracy, blood samples must be drawn at the correct times.

3. *With impaired renal function*, the dosage of aminoglycoside antibiotics must be reduced. Methods of adjusting drug dosage include measuring serum drug levels or lengthening the time interval between doses according to creatinine clearance levels. For specific instructions, consult the manufacturer's literature on gentamicin, tobramycin, amikacin, and netilmicin.

4. *In urinary tract infections*, smaller doses can be used than in systemic infections because the aminoglycosides reach high concentrations in the urine. Also, alkalinizing the urine increases the activity and effectiveness of aminoglycoside therapy.

Single Daily Dosing

There is a growing trend toward once-daily or extended-interval aminoglycoside dosing. Although a violation of the long-held belief that effective antimicrobial drug therapy required near-constant therapeutic serum drug levels, numerous studies indicate that giving aminoglycosides once daily (q24h) is as effective, and probably less toxic, than q8h or q12h dosing.

The concept of once-daily dosing has evolved with increased knowledge about aminoglycosides. Two important characteristics include concentration-dependent bactericidal effects and post-antibiotic effects. The concentration-dependent bactericidal effects mean that the drugs are most effective in killing microorganisms with a large dose and high peak serum concentrations. The post-antibiotic effects mean that aminoglycosides continue killing microorganisms even with low serum concentrations.

These characteristics of aminoglycosides allow administration of high drug doses to achieve high peak serum concentrations and optimal killing of microorganisms. The 24-hour interval until the next dose allows the patient to eliminate the drug to very low serum levels for about 6 hours. During this low-drug period, the post-antibiotic effect is active and there is minimal drug accumulation in body tissues. Reported advantages of this regimen include increased bactericidal effects, less nephrotoxicity, reduced need for serum drug levels, and reduced nursing time for administration. Studies continue to define guidelines and optimal regimens for particular populations

Dosage of Fluoroquinolones

Recommended dosages of fluoroquinolones should not be exceeded in any patients, and dosages should be reduced in the presence of renal impairment.

Guidelines for Reducing Toxicity of Aminoglycosides

In addition to the above recommendations, guidelines to decrease the incidence and severity of adverse effects include the following:

1. Identify clients at high risk of adverse effects (*e.g.*, neonates, older adults, clients with renal impairment, clients with concurrent disease processes or drug therapies that impair blood circulation and renal function).

2. Keep clients well hydrated to decrease drug concentration in serum and body tissues. The drugs reach higher concentrations in the kidneys and inner ears than in other body tissues. This is a major factor in nephrotoxicity and ototoxicity. The goal of an adequate fluid intake is to decrease the incidence and severity of these adverse effects.

3. Avoid concurrent administration of diuretics. Diuretics may increase nephrotoxicity by decreasing fluid volume, thereby increasing drug concentration in serum and tissues. Dehydration is most likely to occur with loop diuretics such as furosemide (Lasix).

4. Give the drug for no longer than 10 days. Clients are most at risk when high doses are given for prolonged periods.

5. Detect adverse effects early and reduce dosage or discontinue the drug. Changes in renal function tests that indicate nephrotoxicity may not occur until the client has received an aminoglycoside for about 5 days. If nephrotoxicity occurs, it is usually reversible if the drug is stopped. Early ototoxicity is detectable only with audiometric tests.

Use in Children

Aminoglycosides must be used cautiously in children as with adults. Dosage must be accurately calculated according to weight and renal function. Serum drug levels must be monitored and dosage adjusted as indicated to avoid toxicity. Neonates may have increased risk of nephrotoxicity and ototoxicity because of their immature renal function. Neomycin is not recommended for use in infants and children. Fluoroquinolones are not recommended for use in children because they have been associated with permanent damage in cartilage and joints.

Use in Older Adults

Aminoglycosides should not be used in the presence of impaired renal function if less toxic drugs are effective against causative organisms. When the drugs are given to older adults, extreme caution is required. Because of impaired renal function, other disease processes, and multiple-drug therapy, older adults are at high risk of developing nephrotoxicity and ototoxicity. Interventions to decrease the incidence and severity of adverse drug effects are listed above. These interventions are important with any client receiving an aminoglycoside, but are especially important with older adults.

Fluoroquinolones are commonly used in older adults for the same indications as in younger adults. In older adults with normal renal function, the drugs should be accompanied by an adequate fluid intake and urine output to prevent drug crystals from forming in the urinary tract. In addition, urinary alkalinizing agents, such as calcium-containing antacids, should be

avoided because drug crystals form more readily in alkaline urine. In those with impaired renal function, a common condition in older adults, the drugs should be used cautiously and in reduced dosages.

HOME CARE

Parenteral aminoglycosides are usually given in a hospital setting. Oral fluoroquinolones are often self-administered at home. The role of the home care nurse is primarily to teach patients or caregivers how to take the drugs effectively and to observe for adverse drug effects.

AMINOGLYCOSIDES AND FLUOROQUINOLONES

NURSING ACTIONS	RATIONALE/EXPLANATION
1. Administer accurately a. With aminoglycosides:	
(1) For IV administration, dilute the drug in 50 to 100 ml of 5% dextrose or 0.9% sodium chloride injection and infuse over 30 to 60 min. The concentration of gentamicin solution should not exceed 1 mg/ml.	To achieve therapeutic blood levels
(2) Give IM aminoglycosides in a large muscle mass, and rotate sites.	To avoid local tissue irritation. This is less likely to occur with aminoglycosides than with most other antibiotics.
b. With fluoroquinolones	
(1) Give norfloxacin and enoxacin 1 h before or 2 h after a meal. Do not give ofloxacin with food. Ciprofloxacin and lomefloxacin may be given without regard to food intake.	To promote therapeutic plasma drug levels. Food in the GI tract interferes with absorption of most oral fluoroquinolones.
(2) Give IV infusions over 60 min.	To decrease vein irritation and phlebitis
(3) When giving ciprofloxacin IV into a primary IV line (e.g., using piggyback or Y connector), stop the primary solution until ciprofloxacin is infused.	To avoid physical or chemical incompatibilities
2. Observe for therapeutic effects **Decreased signs and symptoms of the infection for which the drug is being given**	See Chapter 33
3. Observe for adverse effects a. With aminoglycosides, observe for	Adverse effects are more likely to occur with parenteral administration of large doses for prolonged periods. However, they may occur with oral administration in the presence of renal impairment and with usual therapeutic doses.
(1) Nephrotoxicity—casts, albumin, red or white blood cells in urine, decreased creatinine clearance, increased serum creatinine, increased blood urea nitrogen.	Renal damage is most likely to occur in clients who are elderly, receive high doses or prolonged therapy, have prior renal damage, or receive other nephrotoxic drugs. This is the most serious adverse reaction. Risks of kidney damage can be minimized by using the drugs appropriately, detecting early signs of renal impairment, and keeping clients well hydrated.

(continued)

NURSING ACTIONS	*RATIONALE/EXPLANATION*
(2) Ototoxicity—deafness or decreased hearing, tinnitus, dizziness, ataxia	This results from damage to the eighth cranial nerve. Incidence of ototoxicity is increased in older clients and those with previous auditory damage, high doses or prolonged duration, and concurrent use of other ototoxic drugs.
(3) Neurotoxicity—respiratory paralysis and apnea	This is caused by neuromuscular blockade and is more likely to occur after rapid IV injection, administration to a client with myasthenia gravis, or concomitant administration of general anesthetics or neuromuscular blocking agents (*e.g.*, succinylcholine, tubocurarine). This effect also may occur if an aminoglycoside is administered shortly after surgery, owing to the residual effects of anesthetics or neuromuscular blockers. Neostigmine or calcium may be given to counteract apnea.
(4) Hypersensitivity—skin rash, urticaria	This is an uncommon reaction except with topical neomycin, which may cause sensitization in as many as 10% of recipients.
(5) Nausea, vomiting, diarrhea, peripheral neuritis, paresthesias	Uncommon with parenteral aminoglycosides. Diarrhea often occurs with oral administration.
b. With fluoroquinolones, observe for	The drugs are generally well tolerated and produce relatively few adverse effects.
(1) Allergic reactions (anaphylaxis, urticaria)	Uncommon but some fatalities have been reported.
(2) Nausea, vomiting, diarrhea, pseudomembranous colitis	Nausea is the most common GI symptom.
(3) Headache, dizziness	
(4) Cyrstalluria	Uncommon but may occur with an inadequate fluid intake
(5) Other	Adverse effects involving most body systems have been reported with one or more of the quinolones. Most have a low incidence (<1%) of occurrence.
4. Observe for drug interactions **a.** Drugs that *increase* effects of aminoglycosides:	The listed drugs increase toxicity.
(1) Loop diuretics (furosemide, ethacrynic acid, bumetanide)	Increased nephrotoxicity apparently caused by increased drug concentration in serum and tissues when the client is relatively "dehydrated" by potent diuretics
(2) Methoxyflurane (Penthrane) and nephrotoxic antimicrobial agents (amphotericin B, cephalosporins, colistimethate, polymyxin)	Increased nephrotoxicity
(3) Drugs with neuromuscular blocking activity (methoxyflurane, procainamide, promethazine, quinidine, sodium citrate, succinylcholine, tubocurarine)	Increased neuromuscular blockade with possible paralysis of respiratory muscles and apnea. This is most likely to occur with succinylcholine and tubocurarine.
b. Drugs that *increase* effects of fluoroquinolones: Cimetidine, probenecid	These drugs inhibit elimination of fluoroquinolones and may increase serum drug levels.
c. Drugs that *decrease* effects of fluoroquinolones:	
(1) Antacids, iron preparations, sucralfate, zinc preparations	These drugs interfere with absorption of fluoroquinolones from the GI tract.
(2) Antineoplastic drugs	These drugs may decrease serum levels of fluoroquinolones.

(continued)

NURSING ACTIONS	RATIONALE/EXPLANATION
(3) Bismuth subsalicylate (*e.g.*, Pepto-Bismol) decreases enoxacin absorption if given with or within 1 h after enoxacin.	These drugs should not be taken together or within 1 h of each other.
(4) Nitrofurantoin may decrease the antibacterial effect of norfloxacin in the urinary tract.	

5. Teach clients

  a. With aminoglycosides

(1) Report ringing in the ears, loss of hearing, dizziness, or unsteady gait.	These are symptoms of ototoxicity.
(2) Drink 2000 to 3000 ml of fluid per day if not contraindicated or received by IV infusion.	To reduce damage to the kidneys
(3) Wash hands thoroughly and often, especially after contact with any secretions or urine.	To help prevent spread of infection and emergence of drug-resistant organisms

  b. With fluoroquinolones

(1) Avoid taking antacids containing magnesium or aluminum (*e.g.*, Mylanta or Maalox) or any products containing iron or zinc at the same time, within 4 h before, or within 2 h after a dose of the antibiotic.	These drugs decrease absorption of fluoroquinolones
(2) Drink 2000–3000 ml of fluid per day if not contraindicated.	To prevent drug crystals from developing and damaging the urinary tract
(3) Avoid exposure to sunlight during and for several days after taking a fluoroquinolone. Stop taking the drug and notify the prescribing physician if skin burning, redness, swelling, rash, or itching occurs.	To avoid reactions to sunlight. Sunscreen lotions do not prevent photosensitivity reactions.

 REVIEW AND APPLICATION EXERCISES

1. How do aminoglycosides exert bactericidal effects?

2. Why must aminoglycosides be given parenterally for systemic infections?

3. How are aminoglycosides excreted?

4. What are risk factors for aminoglycoside-induced nephrotoxicity and ototoxicity?

5. How would you assess a client for nephrotoxicity or ototoxicity?

6. What is the reason for giving an aminoglycoside and an antipseudomonal penicillin in the treatment of serious infections caused by *Pseudomonas aeruginosa*?

7. Why should an aminoglycoside and an antipseudomonal penicllin *not* be combined in a syringe or IV fluid for administration?

8. Which laboratory tests need to be monitored regularly for a client receiving a systemic aminoglycoside?

9. When neomycin is given orally, what is the desired effect?

10. What is the rationale for giving an oral aminoglycoside to treat hepatic coma?

11. How do fluoroquinolones exert their antibacterial effects?

12. What are the main clinical uses of fluoroquinolones?

13. What are adverse effects of fluoroquinolones and how may they be prevented or minimized?

14. Why is it important to maintain an adequate fluid intake and urine output with the fluoroquinolones?

15. Why are fluoroquinolones not given to children?

SELECTED REFERENCES

Chambers, H.F. & Sande, M.A. (1996). Antimicrobial agents: The aminoglycosides. In J.G. Hardman, L.E. Limbird, P.B. Molinoff, & R.W. Ruddon (Eds.), *Goodman & Gilman's The pharmacological basis of therapeutics*, 9th ed., pp. 1103–1121. New York: McGraw-Hill.

Craig, W.A. (1997). Antimicrobial therapeutic agents. In W.N. Kelley (Ed.), *Textbook of internal medicine*, 3rd ed., pp. 1843–1852). Philadelphia: Lippincott-Raven.

Drug facts and comparisons. (Updated monthly). St. Louis: Facts and Comparisons.

Lortholary, O., Tod, M., Cohen, Y., & Petitjean, O. (1995). Aminoglycosides. *Medical Clinics of North America, 79*(4), 761–787.

Mandell, G.L. & Petri, W.A., Jr. (1996). Antimicrobial agents: Sulfonamides, trimethoprim-sulfamethoxazole, quinolones, and agents for urinary tract infections. In J.G. Hardman, L.E. Limbird, P.B. Molinoff, & R.W. Ruddon (Eds.), *Goodman & Gilman's The pharmacological basis of therapeutics*, 9th ed., pp. 1057–1072). New York: McGraw-Hill.

Preston, S.L. & Briceland, L.L. (1995). Single daily dosing of aminoglycosides. *Pharmacotherapy, 15*(3), 297–316.

Suh, B., & Lorber, B. (1995). Quinolones. *Medical Clinics of North America, 79*(4), 869–894.

Tetracyclines, Sulfonamides and Urinary Agents

Outline

Objectives

After studying this chapter, the student will be able to:

1 Discuss major characteristics and clinical uses of tetracyclines.

2 Recognize doxycycline as the only tetracycline safe for use in clients with renal failure.

3 Discuss characteristics, clinical uses, adverse effects, and nursing implications of selected sulfonamides.

4 Describe non-pharmacologic interventions to prevent and treat urinary tract infections.

5 Recognize sulfamethoxazole/trimethoprim as a combination drug that is commonly used for urinary tract and systemic infections.

6 Describe the use of urinary antiseptics in the treatment of urinary tract infections.

7 Teach clients strategies for preventing, recognizing, and treating urinary tract infections.

Key Terms

Antianabolic effect	**Crystalluria**
Antimetabolite	**Mineralization**
Azotemia	

Tetracyclines and sulfonamides are older, broad-spectrum, bacteriostatic drugs that are infrequently used for systemic infections because of microbial resistance and the development of more effective or less toxic drugs. Despite these limitations, however, the drugs are useful in selected infections. Urinary antiseptics are used only in urinary tract infections (UTI). Each group is discussed below in terms of mechanism of action, indications for use, and contraindications for use; individual drugs, including characteristics, routes of administration, and dosage ranges, are listed in Tables 36-1, 36-2, and 36-3.

Tetracyclines

The tetracyclines are similar in chemical structure, pharmacologic properties, and antimicrobial activity. They are effective against a wide range of gram-positive and gram-negative organisms as well as rickettsiae, mycoplasmas, some protozoa, spirochetes, and others. They are widely distributed into most body tissues and fluids. The older tetracyclines are excreted mainly in urine, the newer ones (doxycycline and minocycline) mainly in feces.

TABLE 36-1	**TETRACYCLINES**		

| | | **Routes and Dosage Ranges** | |
Generic/Trade Name	**Characteristics**	**Adults**	**Children**
Tetracycline hydrochloride (Achromycin, others)	1. Prototype drug 2. Marketed under generic and numerous trade names	PO 250–500 mg q6h	PO 22–44 mg/kg/d in four divided doses
Demeclocycline (Declomycin)	1. Has a longer half-life than tetracycline, and smaller doses produce therapeutic serum levels 2. The tetracycline most likely to cause photosensitivity 3. May be used to promote diuresis when fluid retention is caused by inappropriate secretion of antidiuretic hormone	PO 150 mg q6h or 300 mg q12h Gonorrhea in penicillin-sensitive clients, PO 600 mg initially, followed by 300 mg q12h for 4 d	Age over 8 y: PO 3–6 mg/kg/d in two to four divided doses
Doxycycline (Vibramycin)	1. Well absorbed from the gastrointestinal tract. Oral administration yields serum drug levels equivalent to those obtained by parenteral administration. 2. Highly lipid-soluble; therefore, reaches therapeutic levels in cerebrospinal fluid (CSF), the eye, and the prostate gland 3. Can be given in smaller doses and less frequently than other tetracyclines because of long serum half-life (about 18 h) 4. Excreted by kidneys to a lesser extent than other tetracyclines and is the only tetracycline considered safe for clients with impaired renal function	PO 100 mg q12h for two doses, then once daily or in divided doses; severe infections, 100 mg q12h IV 200 mg the first day, then 100–200 mg daily in one or two doses	PO, IV same as adults for children weighing at least 45 kg Those weighing less than 45 kg: PO 4.4 mg/kg (2 mg/lb) q12h for two doses, then 1 mg/kg/d in a single dose; severe infections, 2 mg/kg q12h IV 4.4 mg/kg/d in one or two doses, then 1–2 mg/kg/d, depending on severity of infection
Minocycline (Minocin)	1. Well absorbed after oral administration 2. Like doxycycline, readily penetrates CSF, the eye, and the prostate 3. Metabolized more than other tetracyclines, and smaller amounts are excreted in urine and feces	PO, IV 200 mg initially, then 100 mg q12h	Over 12 y old: PO, IV same as adults Under 12 y old: PO, IV 4 mg/kg initially, then 2 mg/kg q12h

TABLE 36-2 SULFONAMIDE PREPARATIONS

Generic/ Trade Name	Characteristics	Clinical Indications	Routes and Dosage Ranges	
			Adults	*Children*
Single Agents				
Sulfacytine (Renoquid)	A short-acting agent that is rapidly absorbed and rapidly excreted	Urinary tract infections	PO 500 mg initially, then 250 mg four times daily	
Sulfadiazine (Microsulfon)	1. A short-acting, rapidly absorbed, rapidly excreted agent for systemic infections 2. Low solubility 3. Therapeutic blood levels are 10–15 mg/100 ml.	1. Urinary tract infections 2. Prophylaxis of rheumatic fever in clients allergic to penicillin 3. Nocardiosis 4. Meningococcal meningitis	PO 2–4 g initially, then 2–4 g daily in three to six divided doses	Over 2 mo of age: PO 75 mg/kg initially, then 150 mg/kg/d in four to six divided doses: maximal daily dose, 6 g Prophylaxis of rheumatic fever, PO 500 mg once daily for children weighing less than 30 kg, 1 g daily for children weighing over 30 kg
Sulfamethizole (Thiosulfil)	A highly soluble, rapidly absorbed, and rapidly excreted agent that is similar to sulfisoxazole in actions and uses	Urinary tract infections	PO 500 mg–1 g three or four times daily	Over 2 mo of age: PO 30–45 mg/kg/d in four divided doses
Sulfamethoxazole (Gantanol)	1. Similar to sulfisoxazole in therapeutic effects but absorbed and excreted more slowly. More likely to produce excessive blood levels and crystalluria than sulfisoxazole. 2. An ingredient in mixtures with trimethoprim (see Combination Agent, below)	1. Systemic infections 2. Urinary tract infections	PO 2 g initially, then 1–2 g two or three times daily	Over 2 mo of age: PO 50–60 mg/kg initially, then 30 mg/kg q12h; maximal daily dose, 75 mg/kg
Sulfasalazine (Azulfidine)	1. Poorly absorbed, acts within the bowel lumen 2. Does not alter normal bacterial flora in the intestine. Effectiveness in ulcerative colitis may be due to antibacterial (sulfapyridine) and anti-inflammatory (aminosalicylic acid) metabolites.	1. Ulcerative colitis 2. Regional enteritis (Crohn's disease)	PO 3–4 g daily in divided doses initially; 2 g daily in four doses for maintenance; maximal daily dose, 8 g	PO 40–60 mg/kg/d in three to six divided doses initially, followed by 30 mg/kg/d in four divided doses
Sulfisoxazole (Gantrisin)	1. A rapidly absorbed, rapidly excreted sulfonamide that is widely used 2. Highly soluble and less likely to cause crystalluria than most other sulfonamides 3. Available in tablets, parenteral solution, oral suspension and syrup, vaginal cream, and ophthalmic solution and ointment	1. Urinary tract infections 2. Systemic infections 3. Vaginitis 4. Ocular infections 5. Nocardiosis	PO, IV, SC 2–4 g initially, then 4–8 g daily in three to six divided doses Intravaginally, 2.5–5 g of vaginal cream (10%) twice daily	Over 2 mo of age: PO 75 mg/kg of body weight initially, then 150 mg/kg/d in four to six divided doses; maximal daily dose, 6 g

(continued)

TABLE 36-2	SULFONAMIDE PREPARATIONS (Continued)

Generic/ Trade Name	Characteristics	Clinical Indications	Routes and Dosage Ranges	
			Adults	**Children**

Combination Agent

Generic/ Trade Name	Characteristics	Clinical Indications	Adults	Children
Sulfamethoxazoletrimethoprim (Bactrim, Septra, others)	1. Synergistic effectiveness against many gram-positive and gram-negative organisms, including streptococci (*Streptococcus pneumoniae, Streptococcus viridans, Enterococcus faecalis*); staphylococci (*Staphylococcus epidermidis, Staphylococcus aureus*): *Escherichia coli; Proteus; Enterobacter; Salmonella; Shigella; Serratia; Klebsiella, Nocardia*: and others. Most strains of *Pseudomonas* are resistant. 2. The two drugs have additive antibacterial effects because they interfere with different steps in bacterial synthesis and activation of folic acid, an essential nutrient. 3. The combination is less likely to produce resistant bacteria than either agent alone. 4. Oral preparations contain different amounts of the two drugs, as follows: a. "Regular" tablets contain trimethoprim 80 mg and sulfamethoxazole 400 mg. b. Double-strength tablets (*e.g.*, Bactrim D.S., Septra D.S.) contain trimethoprim 160 mg and sulfamethoxazole 800 mg. c. The oral suspension contains trimethoprim 40 mg and sulfamethoxazole 200 mg in each 5 ml. 5. The intravenous preparation contains trimethoprim 80 mg and sulfamethoxazole 400 mg in 5 ml. 6. Dosage must be reduced in renal insufficiency. 7. The preparation is contraindicated if creatinine clearance is less than 15 ml/min.	1. Acute and chronic urinary tract infections 2. Acute exacerbations of chronic bronchitis 3. Acute otitis media (in children) and acute maxillary sinusitis (in adults) caused by susceptible strains of *Haemophilus influenzae* and *Streptococcus pneumoniae* 4. Shigellosis 5. Typhoid fever 6. Salmonella infections 7. Infection by *Pneumocystis carinii* (prevention and treatment) 8. Acute gonococcal urethritis 9. Intravenous preparation indicated for *Pneumocystis carinii* pneumonia, severe urinary tract infections, and shigellosis	Urinary tract infections, trimethoprim 160 mg and sulfamethoxazole 800 mg PO q12h for 10–14 d Shigellosis, same dose as above for 5 d Severe urinary tract infections, PO 8–10 mg (trimethoprim component) per kg/d in two to four divided doses, up to 14 d *Pneumocystis carinii* pneumonia, IV 15–20 mg (trimethoprim component) per kg/d in three or four divided doses, q6–8h up to 14 d	Urinary tract infections, otitis media, and shigellosis, PO 8 mg/kg trimethoprim and 40 mg/kg sulfamethoxazole in two divided doses q12h for 10 d Severe urinary tract infections, IV 8–10 mg (trimethoprim component)/kg in two to four divided doses q6–8h or q12h up to 14 d *Pneumocystis carinii* pneumonia, IV 15–20 mg (trimethoprim component) per kg/d in three or four divided doses, q6–8h up to 14 d

TABLE 36-2 SULFONAMIDE PREPARATIONS

Generic/ Trade Name	Characteristics	Clinical Indications	Routes and Dosage Ranges Adults	Children
Topical Sulfonamides				
Mafenide (Sulfamylon)	1. Effective against most gram-negative and gram-positive organisms, especially *Pseudomonas* 2. Application causes pain and burning. 3. Mafenide is absorbed systemically and may produce metabolic acidosis.	Prevention of bacterial colonization and infection of severe burn wounds	Topical application to burned area, once or twice daily, in a thin layer	Same as adults
Silver sulfadiazine (Silvadene)	1. Effective against most *Pseudomonas* species, the most common pathogen in severe burn sepsis, *Escherichia coli, Klebsiella, Proteus,* staphylococci, and streptococci 2. Application is painless. 3. Does not cause electrolyte or acid-base imbalances 4. Significant amounts may be absorbed systemically with large burned areas and prolonged use.	Same as mafenide. Usually the preferred drug.	Same as mafenide	Same as mafenide

MECHANISM OF ACTION

Tetracyclines penetrate microbial cells by passive diffusion and an active transport system. Intracellularly, they bind to 30S ribosomes, like the aminoglycosides, and inhibit microbial protein synthesis.

INDICATIONS FOR USE

Despite a broad spectrum of antimicrobial activity, a tetracycline is the first drug of choice in only a few infections (*e.g.*, cholera, granuloma inguinale, chancroid, Rocky Mountain spotted fever, psittacosis, typhus, trachoma). Other drugs (*e.g.*, penicillin) are usually preferred in gram-positive infections, and most gram-negative organisms are resistant to tetracyclines. However, a tetracycline may be used if bacterial susceptibility is confirmed. Specific clinical indications for tetracyclines include:

1. Treatment of uncomplicated urethral, endocervical, or rectal infections caused by *Chlamydia* organisms.
2. Adjunctive treatment, with other antimicrobials, in the treatment of pelvic inflammatory disease and sexually transmitted diseases.

3. Long-term treatment of acne. They interfere with the production of free fatty acids and decrease *Corynebacterium* in sebum. These actions decrease the inflammatory, pustular lesions associated with severe acne.
4. As a substitute for penicillin in penicillin-allergic clients. They may be effective in treating gonorrhea and syphilis when penicillin cannot be given. They should not be substituted for penicillin in treating streptococcal pharyngitis because microbial resistance is common, and tetracyclines do not prevent rheumatic fever. In addition, they should not be substituted for penicillin in any serious staphylococcal infection because microbial resistance commonly occurs.
5. Doxycycline may be used to prevent traveler's diarrhea due to enterotoxic strains of *Escherichia coli.*
6. Demeclocycline may be used to inhibit antidiuretic hormone in the management of chronic inappropriate antidiuretic hormone secretion.

CONTRAINDICATIONS FOR USE

The major contraindication is renal failure. High concentrations of tetracyclines inhibit protein synthesis in human cells. This antianabolic effect increases tissue breakdown (catabolism) and the amount of waste

TABLE 36-3	MISCELLANEOUS DRUGS FOR URINARY TRACT INFECTIONS

| Generic/Trade Name | Characteristics | Routes and Dosage Ranges | |
		Adults	Children
Methenamine mandelate (Mandelamine)	1. Antibacterial activity only at a urine pH below 5.5. In acidic urine, the drug forms formaldehyde, which is the antibacterial component. Acidification of urine (*e.g.,* with ascorbic acid) is usually needed. 2. Formaldehyde is active against several gram-positive and gram-negative organisms, including *Escherichia coli*. It is most useful for long-term suppression of bacteria in chronic, recurrent infections. 3. It is not indicated in acute infections because other drugs are more effective. It should also not be used to prevent UTI in clients with indwelling urinary catheters. Several hours are required for methenamine to be hydrolyzed into formaldehyde and become bacteriostatic. Because catheters continuously empty the bladder, the drug hydrolyzes in the urine drainage bag rather than the bladder. 4. Contraindicated in renal failure	PO 1 g four times daily	Age 6–12 y: PO 500 mg four times daily Age under 6 y: PO 50 mg/kg/d, in three divided doses
Methenamine hippurate (Hiprex)	See methenamine mandelate, above	PO 1 g twice daily	PO 500 mg–1 g twice daily
Nalidixic acid (NegGram)	1. Prototype of quinolones 2. Active against most gram-negative organisms that cause UTI, but rarely used because organisms develop resistance rapidly and other effective drugs are available.	PO 4 g daily in four divided doses for 1–2 wk, then 2 g/d if long-term treatment is required	PO 55 mg/kg/d in four divided doses, reduced to 33 mg/kg/d for long-term use in children under 12 y of age. Contraindicated in infants under 3 months of age
Nitrofurantoin (Furadantin, Macrodantin)	1. Anti-bacterial activity against *Escherichia coli* and most other organisms that cause UTI. 2. Used for short-term treatment of UTI or long-term suppression of bacteria in chronic, recurrent UTI. 3. Bacterial resistance develops slowly and to a limited degree. 4. Contraindicated in severe renal disease	PO 50–100 mg four times daily Prophylaxis of recurrent UTI in women, PO 50–100 mg at bedtime	Age over 3 months: PO 5–7 mg/kg/d, in four divided doses
Phenazopyridine (Pyridium)	1. An azo dye that acts as a urinary tract analgesic and relieves symptoms of dysuria, burning, and frequency and urgency of urination, which occur with UTI. 2. It has no anti-infective action.	PO 200 mg three times daily after meals	6–12 y of age: PO 12 mg/kg/d, in three divided doses

TABLE 36-3	MISCELLANEOUS DRUGS FOR URINARY TRACT INFECTIONS		
		Routes and Dosage Ranges	
Generic/Trade Name	**Characteristics**	*Adults*	*Children*
	3. It turns urine orange-red, which may be mistaken for blood. 4. It is contraindicated in renal insufficiency and severe hepatitis. 5. Available alone or in fixed-dose combinations with sulfamethoxazole and sulfisoxazole. When indicated, phenazopyridine is better given alone. It can usually be discontinued after 2 to 3 d, whereas the sulfonamide component is given longer.		
Trimethoprim (Proloprim, Trimpex)	1. A folate antagonist drug with antibacterial effects. 2. Available as a single agent for treatment of UTI caused by susceptible strains of *Escherichia coli*, and other gram-negative organisms 3. Most often used in a fixed-dose combination with sulfamethoxazole (Bactrim, Septra) 4. Contraindicated in clients with hypersensitivity to trimethoprim or megaloblastic anemia due to folate deficiency. 5. Rash and pruritus are the most common adverse effects. Nausea, vomiting, glossitis, thrombocytopenia, leukopenia, and methemoglobinemia occasionally occur.	PO 100 mg q12h for 10 d	

products to be excreted by the kidneys. The increased workload can be handled by normally functioning kidneys, but waste products are retained when renal function is impaired. This leads to azotemia, increased blood urea nitrogen (BUN), hyperphosphatemia, hyperkalemia, and acidosis. If a tetracycline is necessary because of an organism's sensitivity or the host's inability to take other antimicrobial drugs, doxycycline or minocycline should be given.

Tetracyclines are also contraindicated in pregnant women and in children up to 8 years of age. During pregnancy, tetracyclines may cause fatal hepatic necrosis in the mother. In the fetus and young child, tetracyclines are deposited in bones and teeth along with calcium. If given during active mineralization of these tissues, tetracyclines can cause permanent brown coloring (mottling) of tooth enamel and can depress bone growth. Tetracyclines should not be used in children unless other drugs are ineffective or contraindicated.

Sulfonamides

Sulfonamides were the first synthetic antibacterial agents to be developed. They are bacteriostatic against a wide range of bacteria, including pneumococci, *Neisseria*, *Escherichia coli*, *Klebsiella*, *Proteus*, *Enterobacter*, and *Haemophilus influenzae*.

Individual drugs vary in extent of systemic absorption and clinical indications. Some are well absorbed and can be used in systemic infections; others are poorly absorbed and exert more local effects. In systemic infections, sulfonamides have largely been replaced by newer, more effective antibacterial agents.

MECHANISM OF ACTION

Sulfonamides act as antimetabolites of para-aminobenzoic acid (PABA), which microorganisms require to produce folic acid; folic acid, in turn, is required for the production of bacterial intracellular proteins. Sulfonamides enter into the reaction instead of PABA, compete for the enzyme involved, and cause formation of nonfunctional derivatives of folic acid. Thus, sulfonamides halt multiplication of new bacteria but do not kill mature, fully formed bacteria. With the exception of the topical sulfonamides used in burn therapy, the presence of pus, serum, or necrotic tissue interferes with sulfonamide action because these materials contain PABA. Some bacteria can change their metabolic pathways to use precursors or other forms of folic acid and thereby develop resistance to the antibacterial action of sulfonamides. Once resistance to one sulfonamide develops, cross-resistance to others is common.

INDICATIONS FOR USE

A major clinical use of sulfonamides is in UTI caused by *Escherichia coli*, *Proteus* or *Klebsiella* organisms. These drugs are most useful in the treatment of acute and chronic cystitis. They are also used in asymptomatic bacteriuria. In acute pyelonephritis, other agents are usually preferred. Additional uses include ulcerative colitis and uncommon infections such as chancroid, lymphogranuloma venereum, nocardiosis, toxoplasmosis, and trachoma. Topical sulfonamides are used in prevention of burn wound infections and in treatment of ocular, vaginal, and other soft-tissue infections. For specific clinical indications of individual drugs, see Table 36-2.

Urinary antiseptics are used only for UTI.

CONTRAINDICATIONS FOR USE

Sulfonamides are contraindicated in people who have had hypersensitivity reactions to them or to chemically related drugs such as thiazide diuretics or antidiabetic sulfonylureas. They are also contraindicated in renal failure, late pregnancy, lactation, and children under 2 months of age (except for treatment of congenital toxoplasmosis). Sulfasalazine (Azulfidine) is contraindicated in people who are allergic to salicylates, children under 2 years old, and people with intestinal or urinary tract obstruction. The drugs must be used cautiously in the presence of liver or kidney impairment or blood dyscrasias.

Urinary Drugs

Urinary antiseptics are antibacterial drugs used only to prevent or treat UTI. They are not used in systemic infections because they do not attain therapeutic plasma levels. They are potentially bactericidal for sensitive organisms in the urinary tract because they are concentrated in renal tubules and reach high levels in urine.

An additional drug, phenazopyridine, is given to relieve pain and other symptoms associated with UTI. It has no antibacterial activity.

Nursing Process

General aspects of the nursing process in antimicrobial drug therapy, as described in Chapter 33, apply to the client receiving tetracylines, sulfonamides, and urinary antiseptics. In this chapter, only those aspects related specifically to these drugs are included.

Assessment

With tetracyclines, assess for conditions in which the drugs must be used cautiously or are contraindicated, such as impaired renal or hepatic function.

With sulfonamides assess for signs and symptoms of disorders for which the drugs are used:

- For *UTI*, assess urinalysis reports for white blood cells and bacteria, urine culture reports for type of bacteria, and symptoms of dysuria, frequency and urgency of urination.
- For *burns*, assess the size of the wound, amount and type of drainage, presence of edema, and amount of eschar.
- Ask clients specifically if they have ever taken a sulfonamide and, if so, whether they had an allergic reaction.
- With urinary antiseptics, assess for signs and symptoms of UTI.

Nursing Diagnoses

- Risk for Injury: Hypersensitivity reaction, kidney, liver, or blood disorders with sulfonamides
- Knowledge Deficit: Correct administration and usage of tetracyclines, sulfonamides, and urinary antiseptics

Planning/Goals

The client will:
- Receive or self-administer the drugs as directed
- Receive prompt and appropriate treatment if adverse effects occur

Interventions

- During tetracycline therapy for systemic infections, monitor laboratory tests of renal function for abnormal values.
- During sulfonamide therapy, encourage sufficient fluids to produce a urine output of at least 1200 to 1500 ml daily. A high fluid intake decreases the risk of crystalluria (precipitation of crystals in the urine).
- Avoid urinary catheterization when possible. If catheterization is necessary, use sterile technique. The urinary tract is normally sterile except for the lower third of the urethra. Introduction of any bacteria into the bladder may cause infection.
  - A single catheterization may cause infection. With indwelling catheters, bacteria colonize the bladder and produce infection within 2 to 3 weeks, even with meticulous care.
  - When indwelling catheters must be used, measures to decrease the incidence and severity of UTI include the following: using a closed drainage system; keeping the per-

ineal area clean; forcing fluids, if not contraindicated, to maintain a dilute urine; and removing the catheter as soon as possible, because infection occurs if the catheter is in place more than a few days. Do not disconnect the system and irrigate the catheter unless obstruction is suspected. *Never* raise the urinary drainage bag above bladder level.

- Force fluids in anyone with a UTI unless contraindicated. Bacteria do not multiply as rapidly in dilute urine. In addition, emptying the bladder frequently allows it to refill with uninfected urine. This decreases the bacterial population of the bladder.
- Teach women to cleanse themselves from the urethral area toward the rectum after voiding or defecating to avoid contamination of the urethral area with bacteria from the vagina and rectum. Also, voiding after sexual intercourse probably helps cleanse the lower urethra and prevent UTI.

Evaluation

- Observe for improvement in signs of the infection for which drug therapy was given.
- Interview and observe for adverse drug effects.

Principles of Therapy: Tetracyclines

1. Culture and sensitivity studies are needed before tetracycline therapy is started because many strains of organisms are either resistant or vary greatly in drug susceptibility. Cross-sensitivity and cross-resistance are common among tetracyclines .
2. The oral route of administration is usually effective and preferred. Intravenous therapy is used when oral administration is contraindicated or for initial treatment of severe infections.
3. Tetracyclines decompose with age, exposure to light, and extreme heat and humidity. Because the breakdown products may be toxic, it is very important to store these drugs correctly. Also, the manufacturer's expiration dates on containers should be noted and outdated drugs should be discarded.

USE IN CHILDREN

Tetracyclines should not be used in children under 8 years of age because of their effects on teeth and bones. In teeth, the drugs interfere with enamel development and may cause a permanent yellow, gray, or brown discoloration. In bone, the drugs form a stable compound in bone-forming tissue and may interfere with bone growth.

USE IN OLDER ADULTS

Doxycycline or minocycline should be given because impaired renal function is common in this population. Other tetracyclines are contraindicated with impaired renal function.

Principles of Therapy: Sulfonamides and Urinary Antiseptics

1. With systemically absorbed sulfonamides, an initial loading dose may be given to produce therapeutic blood levels (12 to 15 mg/100 ml) more rapidly. The amount is usually twice the maintenance dose.
2. Urine pH is important in drug therapy with sulfonamides and urinary antiseptics.
   a. With sulfonamide therapy, alkaline urine increases drug solubility and helps prevent crystalluria. It also increases the rate of sulfonamide excretion and the concentration of sulfonamide in the urine. The urine can be alkalinized by giving sodium bicarbonate. Alkalinization is not needed with sulfisoxazole (because the drug is highly soluble) or sulfonamides used to treat intestinal infections or burn wounds (because there is little systemic absorption).
   b. With mandelamine therapy, urine pH must be acidic (below 5.5) for the drug to be effective. At a higher pH, mandelamine does not hydrolyze to formaldehyde, the antibacterial component. Urine can be acidified by concomitant administration of ascorbic acid.
3. Urine cultures and sensitivity tests are indicated in suspected UTI because of the great variability in possible pathogens and their susceptibility to antibacterial drugs, even within the same species or organism. Best results are obtained by using drug therapy indicated by the microorganisms isolated from each client.

USE IN CHILDREN

Systemic sulfonamides are contraindicated during late pregnancy and lactation and in children under 2 months old. If a fetus or young infant receives a sulfonamide by placental transfer, in breast milk, or by direct administration, the drug displaces bilirubin from binding sites on albumin. As a result, bilirubin may accumulate in the bloodstream (hyperbilirubinemia) and central nervous system (kernicterus) and cause life-threatening toxicity.

Sulfonamides are often used to treat UTI and acute otitis media in children older than 2 months. Few data are available regarding the effects of long-term or recurrent use of sulfamethoxazole (Gantanol) in children under 6 years of age with chronic renal disease. Sulfamethoxazole is often given in combination with trimethoprim (Bactrim, Septra), although trimethoprim has not been established as safe and effective in children under 12 years of age. Sulfacytine (Renoquid) is not recommended for use in children under 14 years of age.

USE IN OLDER ADULTS

Renal function is often impaired in older adults, and a major concern is that sulfonamides may cause further damage. As with younger adults, a fluid intake of about 2 liters daily is needed to reduce formation of crystals and stones in the urinary tract.

With the combination of sulfamethoxazole and trimethoprim (Bactrim, Septra), older adults are at increased risk of severe adverse effects. Severe skin reactions and bone marrow depression are most often reported. Folic acid deficiency may also occur because both of the drugs interfere with folic acid metabolism.

NURSING ACTIONS

TETRACYCLINES, SULFONAMIDES, AND URINARY AGENTS

NURSING ACTIONS	RATIONALE/EXPLANATION
1. Administer accurately **a.** With tetracyclines	
(1) Give oral drugs with food that does not contain dairy products; do not give with or within 2 h of dairy products, antacids, or iron supplements.	To decrease nausea and other GI symptoms. Tetracyclines combine with metallic ions (*e.g.*, aluminum, calcium, iron, magnesium) and are not absorbed.
(2) For IV administration, dilute with an appropriate type and amount of IV solution, and infuse over 1–4 h.	Rapid administration should be avoided. IV doses are usually mixed in hospital pharmacies.
b. With sulfonamides	
(1) Give oral drugs before or after meals, with a full glass of water.	Absorption is better when taken on an empty stomach; however, taking with food decreases GI upset.
(2) Infuse IV trimethoprim-sulfamethoxazole (diluted in 125 ml of 5% dextrose in water) over 60–90 min. Do not mix with other drugs or solutions and flush IV lines to remove any residual drug.	Manufacturer's recommendations
(3) For topical sulfonamides to burn wounds, apply a thin layer with a sterile gloved hand after the surface has been cleansed of previously applied medication.	Burn wounds may be cleansed by whirlpool, shower, or spot cleansing with sterile saline, gauze pads, and gloves.
c. Give nitrofurantoin with or after meals.	Food decreases nausea, vomiting, and diarrhea.
2. Observe for therapeutic effects	Therapeutic effects depend on the reason for use.
a. With tetracyclines, observe for decreased signs and symptoms of the infection for which the drug is being given.	
b. With sulfonamides, observe for decreased symptoms of UTI, decreased diarrhea when given for ulcerative colitis or bacillary dysentery, lack of fever and wound drainage and evidence of healing in burn wounds.	Topical sulfonamides for burns are used to prevent rather than treat infection.
c. With urinary antiseptics, observe for decreased symptoms of UTI.	
3. Observe for adverse effects **a.** Nausea, vomiting, diarrhea	Commonly occur with tetracyclines, sulfonamides, and urinary antiseptics, probably from local irritation of GI mucosa. After several days of an oral tetracycline, diarrhea may be caused by superinfection.
b. Hematologic disorders—anemia, neutropenia, thrombocytopenia	

NURSING ACTIONS	RATIONALE/EXPLANATION
c. Hypersensitivity—anaphylaxis, skin rash, urticaria, serum sickness	
d. Photosensitivity—sunburn reaction	This can be prevented or minimized by avoiding exposure to sunlight or other sources of ultraviolet light, wearing protective clothing, and using sunscreen lotions.
e. Thrombophlebitis at IV infusion sites	These drugs are irritating to tissues. Irritation can be decreased by diluting the drugs and infusing them at the recommended rates.
f. Nephrotoxicity—increased BUN and serum creatinine, hematuria, proteinuria, crystalluria	Nephrotoxicity is more likely to occur in people who already have impaired renal function. Keeping patients well hydrated may help prevent renal damage.
g. Hepatotoxicity—elevated aspartate aminotransferase and other enzymes	Hepatitis, cholestasis, and other serious liver disorders rarely occur with these drugs.
h. Superinfection—sore mouth, white patches on oral mucosa, black furry tongue, diarrhea, skin rash, itching in the perineal area, pseudomembranous colitis	Superinfection may occur with tetracyclines because of their broad spectrum of antimicrobial activity. Signs and symptoms usually indicate monilial infection. Meticulous oral and perineal hygiene helps prevent these problems. The drug should be stopped if severe diarrhea occurs, with blood, mucus, or pus in stools.
4. Teach clients **a.** Take medications as prescribed, for the length of time prescribed. Avoid taking tetracyclines within about 2 h of ingesting dairy products, antacids, or iron supplements.	Tetracyclines, sulfonamides, and urinary antiseptics are bacteriostatic agents in most infections and must be taken correctly to achieve therapeutic effects.
b. Drink 2 to 3 quarts of fluid daily, if not contraindicated.	Maintaining a good fluid intake helps the drugs to be more effective, especially in UTI, and to decrease the likelihood of damaging the kidneys.
c. Avoid intense or prolonged exposure to sunlight or artificial ultraviolet light. If exposure is unavoidable, wear protective clothing and a sunscreen lotion.	To avoid sunburn from a photosensitivity reaction
d. With tetracyclines, report severe nausea, vomiting, diarrhea, skin rash, or perineal itching to the prescribing physician.	These symptoms may indicate a need for changing or stopping the tetracycline.
e. With sulfonamides, report skin rash, fever, sore throat, abnormal bleeding (blood in urine, nose bleed, bruises).	These symptoms may indicate adverse drug effects and the need to stop or reduce dosage of the drug.
f. With phenazopyridine, inform the client that the drug turns urine orange-red.	To prevent the client from mistaking the discolored urine for blood from the urinary tract.

REVIEW AND APPLICATION EXERCISES

1. What foods and drugs interfere with absorption of oral tetracyclines? How can interference be prevented or minimized?

2. What are potentially serious adverse effects of tetracyclines?

3. What is the rationale for long-term, low-dose administration of a tetracycline for acne?

4. Which tetracyclines may be given with renal insufficiency?

5. Why are sulfonamides often effective in UTI?

6. What are major adverse effects of sulfonamides and how may they be prevented or minimized?

7. What is the rationale for combining sulfamethoxazole and trimethoprim?

8. What are important characteristics of urinary antiseptics?

SELECTED REFERENCES

Drug facts and comparisons (1996). St. Louis: Facts and Comparisons.

Kapusnik-Uner, J.E., Sande, M.A., & Chambers, H.F. (1996). Antimicrobial agents: Tetracyclines, chloramphenicol, erythromycin, and miscellaneous antibacterial agents. In J.G. Hardman, L.E. Limbird, P.B. Molinoff, & R.W. Ruddon (Eds.), *Goodman & Gilman's The pharmacological basis of therapeutics*, 9th ed., pp. 1123–1153. New York: McGraw-Hill.

Klein, N.C. & Cunha, B.A. (1995). Antimicrobial therapy II: Tetracyclines. *Medical Clinics of North America, 79*(4), 789–801.

Mandell, G.L., Douglas, R.G. Jr., & Bennett, J.E. (Eds.) (1995). *Principles and practice of infectious diseases*, 4th ed. New York: Churchill Livingstone.

Mandell, G.L. & Petri, W.A. Jr., (1996). Antimicrobial agents: Sulfonamides, trimethoprim-sulfamethoxazole, quinolones, and agents for urinary tract infections. In J.G. Hardman, L.E. Limbird, P.B. Molinoff, & R.W. Ruddon (Eds.), *Goodman & Gilman's The pharmacological basis of therapeutics*, 9th ed., pp. 1057–1072. New York: McGraw-Hill.

Macrolides and Miscellaneous Antibacterials

Outline

Macrolides
    mechanism of action
    indications for use
    contraindications for use

Miscellaneous Antibacterial Drugs
    chloramphenicol
    clindamycin
    metronidazole
    spectinomycin
    vancomycin and teicoplanin

Nursing Process
    assessment
    nursing diagnoses
    planning/goals
    interventions

Principles of Therapy: Macrolides and Miscellaneous Antibacterials
    culture and susceptibility studies
    effects of erythromycin on other drugs
    preventing toxicity with chloramphenicol
    preventing toxicity with clindamycin
    preventing toxicity with parenteral vancomycin
    use in renal failure
    use in liver disease
    use in children
    use in older adults
    home care

Objectives

After studying this chapter, the student will be able to:

1 Discuss characteristics and specific uses of erythromycin and other macrolides.

2 Compare and contrast macrolides with other commonly used antibacterial drugs.

3 Describe the interference of erythromycin with the metabolism of other drugs.

4 Apply principles of using macrolides in selected client situations.

5 Discuss characteristics, indications for use, and precautions for using chloramphenicol, clindamycin, metronidazole, teicoplanin, and vancomycin.

6 Discuss the roles of metronidazole and oral vancomycin in the treatment of pseudomembranous colitis.

Key Terms

Cytochrome P450 enzymes

Hepatotoxicity

Pseudomembranous colitis

The drugs described in this chapter are heterogeneous in their antimicrobial spectrum, characteristics, and clinical uses. Some are used often; some are used only in specific circumstances. The macrolides and other drugs are described below.

Macrolides

The macrolide antibiotics include erythromycin, azithromycin (Zithromax), clarithromycin (Biaxin), and dirithromycin (Dynabac). Erythromycin, the prototype, is available in several preparations. Oral forms, except the estolate salt, are coated or buffered to prevent destruction by gastric acid. The estolate salt is stable in gastric acid. Topical and ophthalmic preparations are discussed in Chapters 65 and 66. Individual erythromycin formulations and other macrolides are listed in Table 37-1.

Erythromycin is now used less often because of microbial resistance and the development of newer macrolides. Although the drugs differ somewhat in chemical structure, they have the same mechanism of action and similar antimicrobial activity. They may be bacteriostatic or bactericidal, depending largely on drug concentration in infected tissues. They are effective against gram-positive cocci, including group A streptococci, pneumococci, and most staphylococci. They are also effective against species of *Corynebacterium*, *Treponema*, *Neisseria*, and *Mycoplasma* and against some anaerobic organisms such as *Bacteroides* and *Clostridia*. Compared to erythromycin, azithromycin is less active and clarithromycin is more active against most streptococci and staphylycocci. However, streptococci and staphylococci that are resistant to erythromycin are also resistant to azithromycin and clarithromycin.

In addition to the above antimicrobial activity, azithromycin and clarithromycin also are active against the atypical mycobacteria that cause *Mycobacterium avium* complex (MAC) disease. MAC is an opportunistic infection that occurs mainly in people with advanced human immunodeficiency virus (HIV) infection. The newer drugs require less frequent administration and cause less nausea, vomiting, and diarrhea than erythromycin. Clinical experience with dirithromycin is limited.

The macrolides are widely distributed in body tissues and fluids, including pleural fluid and sputum, ascitic fluid, and middle-ear exudates. The drugs may enter cerebrospinal fluid (CSF) when meninges are inflamed. Erythromycin is metabolized primarily in the liver and excreted in bile, with some reabsorption from the gastrointestinal (GI) tract. About 20% is excreted in urine. Azithromycin and dirithromycin are mainly excreted in bile, and clarithromycin is metabolized to an active metabolite in the liver and excreted in urine.

MECHANISM OF ACTION

The macrolides enter microbial cells and attach to 50S ribosomes, thereby inhibiting microbial protein synthesis.

INDICATIONS FOR USE

Erythromycin is considered safer than many other antibiotics and is used as a penicillin substitute in clients who are allergic to penicillin. Other clinical indications include the following when caused by susceptible organisms:

1. Respiratory tract infections caused by *Streptococcus pyogenes*, *Streptococcus pneumoniae*, and *Mycoplasma pneumoniae*
2. Legionnaire's disease. Erythromycin is the drug of choice for this pneumonia-like disease caused by the gram-negative bacillus *Legionella pneumophila*.
3. Skin and skin structure infections caused by *Streptococcus pyogenes* or *Staphylococcus aureus*
4. Prevention of pertussis (whooping cough) in household contacts
5. Elimination of the diphtheria carrier state as an adjunct to diphtheria antitoxin
6. Substitute for penicillin in prophylaxis of rheumatic fever, gonorrhea, and syphilis and in treatment of pneumococcal pneumonia, streptococcal pharyngitis, and syphilis for people who are allergic to penicillin
7. Infections cause by *Chlamydia trachomatis* (*e.g.*, prevention and treatment of conjunctivitis in newborns [ophthalmic ointment], genitourinary infections)
8. Treatment of intestinal amebiasis caused by *Entamoeba histolytica* (oral erythromycin only)

Azithromycin and clarithromycin are indicated for treatment of respiratory tract infections caused by susceptible organisms (*e.g.*, *Streptococcus pyogenes* or *pneumoniae*) and skin/soft tissue infections caused by susceptible *Staphylococcus aureus* or *Streptococcus pyogenes*. In addition, azithromycin is approved for treatment of urethritis and cervicitis caused by *Chlamydia trachomatis* organisms, and clarithromycin is approved for prevention and treatment of *Mycobacterium avium* complex (MAC) disease. For prevention, clarithromycin may be used alone; for treatment, it is combined with one or two other drugs (*e.g.*, ethambutol and/or rifabutin) to prevent the emergence of drug-resistant organisms.

TABLE 37-1 **MACROLIDES**

Generic/Trade Name	Usual Routes and Dosage Ranges	
	Adults	*Children*
Azithromycin (Zithromax)	Respiratory and skin infections, PO 500 mg as a single dose on the first day, then 250 mg once daily for 4 d. Nongonococcal urethritis and cervicitis caused by *Chlamydia trachomatis*, give 1 g as a single dose.	6 months and older: Acute otitis media PO, 10 mg/kg as a single dose (not to exceed 500 mg) on the first day, then 5 mg/kg (not to exceed 250 mg) once daily for 4 d 2 y and older: Pharyngitis/tonsillitis, PO 12 mg/kg (not to exceed 500 mg) once daily for 5 d
Clarithromycin (Biaxin)	PO 250–500 mg q12h for 7 to 14 d. Prevention or treatment of *Mycobacterium avium* complex (MAC), PO 500 mg q12h	PO 7.5 mg/kg q12h, not to exceed 500 mg q12h Prevention or treatment of MAC. Same as above
Dirithromycin (Dynabac)	Bronchitis caused by *Streptococcus pneumoniae* or *Moraxella catarrhalis* and skin infections caused by methicillin-susceptible *Staphylococcus aureus*, PO 500 mg once daily for 7 d Pharyngitis/tonsillitis caused by *Streptococcus pyogenes*, PO 500 mg once daily for 10 d Community-acquired pneumonia caused by *Legionella pneumophila*, *Mycoplasma pneumoniae* or *Streptococcus pneumoniae* PO 500 mg once daily for 14 d	Dosage not established
Erythromycin base (E-mycin)	PO 250–500 mg q6h; severe infections, up to 4 g or more daily in divided doses	PO 30–50 mg/kg/d in divided doses q6–12h, severe infections, 100 mg/kg/d in divided doses
Erythromycin estolate (Ilosone)	PO 250 mg q6h; maximal daily dose, 4 g	Weight over 25 kg, PO same as adults Weight 10–25 kg, PO 30–50 mg/kg/d in divided doses Weight under 10 kg, PO 10 mg/kg/d in divided doses q6–12h Dosages may be doubled in severe infections.
Erythromycin ethylsuccinate (E.E.S.)	PO 400 mg four times daily; severe infections, up to 4 g or more daily in divided doses	PO 30–50 mg/kg/d in four divided doses q6h. Severe infections, 60–100 mg/kg/d in divided doses
Erythromycin lactobionate	IV 15–20 mg/kg/d in divided doses; severe infections, up to 4 g daily	IV same as adults
Erthromycin stearate (Erythrocin stearate)	PO 250 mg q6h or 500 mg q12h; severe infections, up to 4 g daily	PO 30–50 mg/kg/d in four divided doses q6h; severe infections, 60–100 mg/kg/d

Clarithromycin is also used to treat *Helicobacter pylori* infections associated with peptic ulcer disease. Azithromycin is also being used for the prevention and treatment of MAC disease, although it is not yet FDA-approved for this indication.

CONTRAINDICATIONS FOR USE

The drugs are contraindicated in persons who have hypersensitivity reactions to macrolides. They are also contraindicated or must be used with caution in clients with pre-existing liver disease.

Miscellaneous Antibacterial Drugs

CHLORAMPHENICOL

Chloramphenicol is a broad-spectrum, bacteriostatic antibiotic that is active against most gram-positive bacteria, most gram-negative bacteria, rickettsiae, chlamydiae, and treponemes. Chloramphenicol acts by interfering with microbial protein synthesis. It is well absorbed and diffuses well into body tissues and fluids, including CSF, but low drug levels are obtained in urine. It is metabolized in the liver and excreted in the urine.

Chloramphenicol is rarely used in infections caused by gram-positive organismms because of the effectiveness and low toxicity of penicillins, cephalosporins, and macrolides. It is the drug of choice only in typhoid fever. Otherwise, it is indicated for use in serious infections for which no adequate substitute drug is available. Specific infections include meningococcal, pneumococcal, or *Haemophilus* meningitis in penicillin-allergic clients; anaerobic brain abscess; *Bacteroides fragilis* infections; rickettsial infections and brucellosis when tetracyclines are contraindicated; and *Klebsiella* and *Haemophilus* infections that are resistant to other drugs.

Routes and Dosage Ranges

Adults: PO, IV 50–100 mg/kg/d, in four divided doses, q6h

Children and full-term infants >2 weeks old: PO 50 mg/kg/d, in three or four divided doses, q6–8h

CLINDAMYCIN

Clindamycin is similar to erythromycin and other macrolides in its mechanism of action and antimicrobial spectrum. It is bacteriostatic in usual doses. It is effective against gram-positive cocci, including group A streptococci, pneumococci, and most staphylococci. It is also effective against species of *Corynebacterium*, *Treponema*, *Neisseria*, and *Mycoplasma* and against some anaerobic organisms such as *Bacteroides* and *Clostridia*. Clindamycin enters microbial cells and attaches to 50S ribosomes, thereby inhibiting microbial protein synthesis.

Clindamycin is the drug of choice in infections caused by *Bacteroides fragilis*. Because these bacteria are usually mixed with gram-negative organisms from the gynecologic or GI tracts, clindamycin is usually given with another drug, such as gentamicin, to treat mixed infections. The drug may be useful as a penicillin substitute in clients who are allergic to penicillin and who have streptococcal, staphylococcal, or pneumococcal infections in which the causative organism is sensitive to clindamycin. A topical solution is used in the treatment of acne, and a vaginal cream is available. Despite its effectiveness in infections caused by gram-positive microorganisms, clindamycin should be used only in infections in which it is clearly more effective than other drugs (*e.g.*, anaerobic infections) because of the diarrhea and pseudomembranous colitis associated with its use. Clindamycin does not reach therapeutic concentrations in the central nervous system (CNS) and should not be used for treating meningitis.

Clindamycin is well absorbed with oral administration and reaches peak plasma levels within 1 hour after a dose. It is widely distributed in body tissues and fluids, except CSF, and crosses the placenta. It is highly bound (90% or more) to plasma proteins. It is metabolized in the liver, and the metabolites are excreted in bile and urine. Dosage may need to be reduced in patients with severe hepatic failure, to prevent accumulation and toxic effects.

Clindamycin Hydrochloride
Route and Dosage Ranges

Adults: PO 150–300 mg q6h; up to 450 mg q6h for severe infections

Children: PO 8–16 mg/kg/d in three or four divided doses, q6–8h; up to 20 mg/kg/d in severe infections

Clindamycin Phosphate
Routes and Dosage Ranges

Adults: IM 600 mg–2.7 g/d in two to four divided doses, q6–12h

IV 600 mg–2.7 g/d in two to four divided doses; up to 4.8 g/d in life-threatening infections

Children: IM, IV 15–40 mg/kg/d in three or four divided doses, q6–8h; up to 40 mg/kg/d in severe infections

Clindamycin palmitate hydrochloride (Cleocin Pediatric—75 mg/ml)
Route and Dosage Ranges

Children: PO 8–12 mg/kg/d in three or four divided doses; up to 25 mg/kg/d in very severe infections. For children weighing 10 kg or less, the minimum dose is 37.5 mg, three times per day

METRONIDAZOLE

Metronidazole (Flagyl) is effective against anaerobic bacteria, including gram-negative bacilli such as *Bacteroides*, gram-positive bacilli such as *Clostridia*, and gram-positive cocci such as *Peptococcus* and *Peptostreptococcus*. It is also effective against protozoa that cause amebiasis, giardiasis, and trichomoniasis (see Chap. 41)

Clinical indications for use of metronidazole include prevention or treatment of anaerobic bacterial infections (*e.g.*, in colorectal surgery and intra-abdominal infections), treatment of *Helicobacter pylori* infections associated with peptic ulcer disease, and treatment of *Clostridium difficile* infections associated with pseudomembranous colitis. It is generally contraindicated during the first trimester of pregnancy and must be used with caution in clients with CNS or blood disorders.

Metronidazole is carcinogenic in rodents, if given in high doses for prolonged periods, and mutagenic activity is associated with the drug and metabolites found in the urine of clients who have received therapeutic doses. However, there is no evidence that people treated with therapeutic doses have an increased risk of developing cancer. Metronidazole is widely distributed in body fluids and tissues, metabolized in the liver, and excreted mostly (60% to 80%) in urine, with a small amount excreted in feces.

Routes and Dosage Ranges

Adults: Anaerobic bacterial infection, IV 15 mg/kg (about 1 g for a 70-kg adult) as a loading dose, infused over 1 hour, followed by 7.5 mg/kg (about 500 mg for a 70-kg adult) q6h as a maintenance dose, infused over 1 hour; duration usually 7–10 days; maximum dose 4 g/24 h.

Surgical prophylaxis, colorectal surgery, IV 15 mg/kg, infused over 30–60 minutes, infusion to be completed about 1 hour before surgery, followed by 7.5 mg/kg, infused over 30–60 minutes, at 6 hours and 12 hours after the initial dose

Helicobacter pylori infection and Clostridium difficile colitis, PO 1–2 g daily for 7–10 days

SPECTINOMYCIN

Spectinomycin is used for treatment of gonococcal exposure or infection in people who are allergic to or unable to take preferred drugs (the cephalosporins ceftriaxone or cefixime, or the quinolones ciprofloxacin or ofloxacin). It may be used during pregnancy when patients cannot tolerate cephalosporins and when quinolones are contraindicated. Spectinomycin has no activity against infections caused by *Chlamydia* organisms, which often accompany gonorrhea.

Route and Dosage Range

Adults: IM 2 g in a single dose

VANCOMYCIN AND TEICOPLANIN

Vancomycin and **teicoplanin** (Targocid) are active only against gram-positive microorganisms. They act by inhibiting cell-wall synthesis. Vancomycin is indicated only for the treatment of severe infections. Parenteral vancomycin has been used extensively in the treatment of infections caused by methicillin-resistant *Staphylococcus aureus* (MRSA) and *Staphylococcus epidermidis* (MRSE) and endocarditis caused by *Streptococcus viridans* (in patients allergic to or with infections resistant to penicillins and cephalosporins) or *Enterococcus faecalis* (with an aminoglycoside). The drug has also been widely used for prophylaxis of gram-positive infections in patients requiring long-term use of intravascular catheters and other invasive treatment or monitoring devices. Oral drug has been used extensively to treat pseudomembranous colitis caused by *Clostridium difficile* organisms and staphylococcal enterocolitis. Vancomycin is being used to treat infections caused by penicillin-resistant *Streptococcus pneumoniae.*

Partly because of this widespread use, vancomycin-resistant enterococci (VRE) are being encountered more often, especially in critical care units, and treatment options for infections caused by these organisms are very limited. To decrease the spread of VRE, the Centers for Disease Control and Prevention (CDC) recommend limiting the use of vancomycin. Specific recommendations include avoiding or minimizing use in empiric treatment of febrile patients with neutropenia (unless the prevalence of MRSA or MRSE is high), initial treatment for *Clostridium difficile* colitis (metronidazole is preferred), and prophylaxis for surgery, low birthweight infants, intravascular catheter colonization or infection, and peritoneal dialysis.

For systemic infections, vancomycin is given intravenously (IV) and reaches therapeutic plasma levels within 1 hour after infusion. It is very important to give IV infusions slowly, over 1 to 2 hours, to avoid an adverse reaction characterized by hypotension and possibly flushing and skin rash. This reaction, sometimes called "red man syndrome" is attributed to histamine release. Vancomycin is excreted through the kidneys; dosage should be reduced in the presence of renal impairment. For bacterial colitis, vancomycin is given orally because it is not absorbed from the GI tract and acts within the bowel lumen. Large amounts of vancomycin are excreted in the feces after oral administration.

Teicoplanin is a newer drug that is similar to vancomycin in antimicrobial spectrum, mechanism of action, and indications for use. It is reportedly as effective as vancomycin in the treatment of streptococcal and staphylococcal infections, and it may be effective in some enterococcal infections that are resistant to vancomycin. It is excreted almost entirely by the kidneys, and dosage should be reduced with renal impairment. Teicoplanin differs from vancomycin in that it can be given intramuscularly (IM) as well as IV for systemic infections, it does not cause "red man syndrome," and it can be given once daily for most infections because it has a long serum half-life.

Routes and Dosage Ranges

Vancomycin
Adults: PO 500 mg q6h or 1 g q12h; maximum dose, 4 g/d
IV 2 g/d in two to four divided doses, q6–12h
Children: PO, IV 40 mg/kg/d in divided doses
Teicoplanin
Adults: 6 mg/kg/d, up to 30 mg/kg/d for serious staphylococcal infections

Nursing Process

Assessment

- Assess for infections that macrolides and the designated miscellaneous drugs are used to prevent or treat.
- Assess each client for signs and symptoms of the specific current infection.
- Assess culture and susceptibility reports when available.
- Assess each client for risk factors that increase risks of infection (*e.g.,* immunosuppression) or risks of adverse drug reactions (*e.g.,* impaired renal function).

Nursing Diagnoses

- Knowledge Deficit related to type of infection
- Knowledge Deficit related to appropriate use of prescribed antimicrobial drugs
- Risk for Injury related to adverse drug effects
- Risk for Injury related to infection with antibiotic-resistant microorganisms

Planning/Goals

The client will:

- Take or receive macrolides and miscellaneous antimicrobials accurately, for the prescribed length of time
- Experience absent or decreased signs and symptoms of the infection being treated
- Be monitored regularly for theraputic and adverse drug effects
- Verbalize and practice measures to prevent recurrent infection

Interventions

- Use measures to prevent and minimize the spread of infection (see Chap. 33).
- Monitor for fever and other signs and symptoms of infection.
- Monitor laboratory reports for indications of the client's response to drug therapy (*e.g.,* white blood cells (WBC), tests of renal function).
- Encourage fluid intake to decrease fever and maintain good urinary tract function.
- Provide foods and fluids with adequate nutrients to maintain or improve nutritional status, especially if febrile and hypermetabolic.

Teach clients:

- Ways to prevent or minimize infections with streptococci, staphylococci, and other gram-positive organisms
- To report symptoms that recur or develop during antibiotic therapy to a health care provider

- That the fastest and most complete relief of infections occurs with accurate usage of antibiotics, and that inaccurate use may cause other, potentially more severe infections.

Principles of Therapy: Macrolides and Miscellaneous Antibacterials

CULTURE AND SUSCEPTIBILITY STUDIES

Specimens for culture and sensitivity studies should be obtained before the first dose of macrolides and clindamycin because these drugs have a narrow spectrum of antibacterial activity. They are mainly effective against gram-positive organisms, and a number of organisms are resistant. Drug therapy is often started before results are available, especially with serious infections.

EFFECTS OF ERYTHROMYCIN ON OTHER DRUGS

Erythromycin interferes with the elimination of several drugs, especially those metabolized by the cytochrome P450 enzymes in the liver. As a result, the affected drugs are eliminated more slowly, their serum levels are increased, and they are more likely to cause adverse effects and toxicity unless dosage is reduced. Interacting drugs include alfentanil (Alfenta), astemizole (Hismanal), bromocriptine (Parlodel), carbamazepine (Tegretol), cyclosporine (Sandimmune), digoxin (Lanoxin), disopyramide (Norpace), methylprednisolone (Medrol), terfenadine (Seldane), theophylline (Theo-Dur), triazolam (Halcion), and warfarin (Coumadin). These drugs represent a variety of drug classes. When erythromycin has been given concurrently with the nonsedating antihistamines, astemizole or terfenadine, serious ventricular arrhythmias and fatalities have been reported. These interactions are less likely to occur with azithromycin, clarithromycin, and dirithromycin.

PREVENTING TOXICITY WITH CHLORAMPHENICOL

Clients taking chloramphenicol need a complete blood count, platelet count, reticulocyte count, and serum iron every 3 days. These tests are necessary because chloramphenicol may lead to serious bone marrow depression, including aplastic anemia. In addition, periodic measurements of serum drug levels are recommended. Therapeutic levels are 10 to 20 µg/ml.

PREVENTING TOXICITY WITH CLINDAMYCIN

If a client receiving clindamycin develops diarrhea, stools should be checked for WBC, blood, and mucus, and a proctoscopy should be done to determine whether the client has pseudomembranous colitis, a potentially fatal adverse reaction. If lesions are seen on proctoscopy, the drug should be stopped immediately. Although pseudomembranous colitis may occur with any antibiotic, it has often been associated with clindamycin therapy.

PREVENTING TOXICITY WITH PARENTERAL VANCOMYCIN

Dosage should be reduced in clients with renal impairment, and renal function should be monitored during IV vancomycin therapy. Serum vancomycin levels should also be monitored; therapeutic levels are 10 to 25 µg/ml.

USE IN RENAL FAILURE

Dosage of erythromycin and clindamycin does not need reduction in renal failure because the drugs are excreted primarily by the liver. With clarithromycin, dosage should be reduced; no data are available about azithromycin dosage in renal failure. Dosage of vancomycin should be reduced.

USE IN LIVER DISEASE

Macrolides, clindamycin, and chloramphenicol should be used cautiously, if at all, in the presence of liver disease. Because these drugs are eliminated through the liver, they may accumulate and cause toxic effects. When feasible, other drugs should be substituted. If no effective substitutes are available, dosage should be reduced. The dosage of metronidazole should be reduced with alcoholic cirrhosis or severe obstructive liver disease.

USE IN CHILDREN

Erythromycin is generally considered safe for treatment of infections caused by susceptible organisms. The newer macrolides, azithromycin, clarithromycin,

and dirithromycin, are approved for use in children under 12 years of age. Dosage of chloramphenicol must be reduced in premature infants and in full-term infants less than 2 weeks old, because impaired metabolism may lead to accumulation and adverse effects. Clindamycin should be given to neonates and infants only if clearly indicated, and then liver and kidney function must be monitored. Diarrhea and pseudo-membranous colitis may occur with topical clindamycin for treatment of acne. The safety and efficacy of metronidazole have been established in children only for the treatment of amebiasis. Vancomycin is often used in children, including preterm and full-term neonates, for the same indications as in adults. Monitoring serum drug levels is recommended with IV vancomycin.

USE IN OLDER ADULTS

Erythromycin is generally considered safe. Because it is metabolized in the liver and excreted in bile, it may be useful in clients with impaired renal function. Little information is available about the use of azithromycin and clarithromycin in older adults. A small group given high doses of clarithromycin (1000 mg q12h) for chronic mycobacterial (*Mycobacterium avium* complex and/or *Mycobacterium abscessus*) lung disease experienced a high incidence of adverse effects, including elevated liver enzymes. The group tolerated smaller doses of 500 mg q12h.

The miscellaneous drugs are used in older adults for the same indications as in younger adults. Dosage may need to be reduced when renal function is impaired, a common condition in older adults.

 HOME CARE

Most of the macrolides and miscellaneous drugs may be taken in the home setting, including IV vancomycin. The role of the home care nurse is generally the same as with other antibiotic therapy. That is, the nurse may need to teach clients or caregivers about drug administration and expected effects. For clients taking oral metronidazole or vancomycin for pseudo-membranous colitis, stool specimens may need to be collected and tested in the laboratory for *Clostridium difficile* organisms or toxins.

NURSING ACTIONS

MACROLIDES AND MISCELLANEOUS ANTIBACTERIALS

NURSING ACTIONS	*RATIONALE/EXPLANATION*
1. Administer accurately.	
a. Give oral erythromycin and azithromycin capsules on an empty stomach 1 h before or 2 h after a meal. Give clarithromycin without regard to food intake.	To aid absorption and maintenance of therapeutic serum drug levels. Food in the GI tract decreases absorption of erythromycin and azithromycin but does not interfere with absorption of clarithromycin.
b. For IV erythromycin, consult the manufacturer's instructions for dissolving, diluting, and administering the drug. Infuse continuously or intermittently (*e.g.*, q6h over 30–60 min).	The IV formulation has limited stability in solution, and instructions must be followed carefully to achieve therapeutic effects. Also, instructions differ for intermittent and continuous infusions. IV erythromycin is the treatment of choice for Legionnaire's disease. Otherwise, it is rarely used.
c. With chloramphenicol:	
(1) Give oral drug 1 h before or 2 h after meals, q6h around the clock. If GI upset occurs, give with food.	To increase absorption and maintain therapeutic blood levels
(2) Mix IV chloramphenicol in 50–100 ml of 5% dextrose in water and infuse over 15–30 min.	
d. With clindamycin:	
(1) Give capsules with a full glass of water.	To avoid esophageal irritation
(2) Do not refrigerate reconstituted oral solution.	Refrigeration is not required for drug stability and may thicken the solution, making it difficult to measure and pour accurately.
(3) Give IM injections deeply, and rotate sites. Do not give more than 600 mg in a single injection.	To decrease pain, induration, and abscess formation
(4) For IV administration, dilute 300 mg in 50 ml of IV fluid and give over 10 min, or dilute 600 mg in 100 ml and give over 20 min. *Do not* give clindamycin undiluted or by direct injection.	Dilution decreases risks of phlebitis. Cardiac arrest has been reported with bolus injections of clindamycin.
e. With IV metronidazole, check the manufacturer's instructions.	The drug requires specific techniques for preparation and administration.
f. With vancomycin, dilute 500-mg doses in 100 ml and 1-g doses in 200 ml of 0.9% NaCl or 5% dextrose injection and infuse over at least 60 min.	To decrease hypotension and flushing (*i.e.,* "red man syndrome") that may occur with more rapid IV administration. This reaction is attributed to histamine release and may be prevented by prior administration of diphenhydramine, an antihistamine. Dilution also decreases pain and phlebitis at the injection site.
2. Observe for therapeutic effects	
a. Decreased local and systemic signs of infection	See Chapter 33.
b. Decreased signs and symptoms of the specific infection for which the drug is being given	
3. Observe for adverse effects	
a. With macrolides:	
(1) Nausea, vomiting, diarrhea	These are the most frequent adverse reactions, reportedly less common with azithromycin and clarithromycin than with erythromycin.
(2) With IV erythromycin, phlebitis at the IV infusion site	The drug is very irritating to body tissues. Phlebitis can be minimized by diluting the drug well, infusing it slowly, and not using the same vein more than 48–72 h, if possible.

NURSING ACTIONS	RATIONALE/EXPLANATION
(3) Hepatotoxicity—nausea, vomiting, abdominal cramps, fever, leukocytosis, abnormal liver function, and possibly jaundice	More likely to occur with the estolate formulation of erythromycin, but has been reported with other preparations as well
(4) Allergic reactions (anaphylaxis, skin rash, urticaria)	Potentially serious but infrequent
b. With chloramphenicol:	
(1) Anemia, leukopenia, thrombocytopenia	Blood dyscrasias are the most serious adverse reaction to chloramphenicol. They are caused by bone marrow depression.
(2) Clinical signs of infection or bleeding	
c. With clindamycin:	
(1) Nausea, vomiting, diarrhea	These are the most frequent adverse effects and may be severe enough to require stopping the drug.
(2) Pseudomembranous colitis (also called antibiotic-associated colitis)—severe diarrhea, fever, stools containing neutrophils and shreds of mucous membrane	May occur with most antibiotics but is more common with oral clindamycin. It is caused by *Clostridium difficile*. The organism produces a toxin that kills mucosal cells and produces superficial ulcerations that are visible with sigmoidoscopy. Discontinuing the drug and giving oral metronidazole are curative measures.
d. With metronidazole:	
(1) CNS effects—convulsive seizures, peripheral paresthesias, ataxia, confusion, dizziness, headache	Convulsions and peripheral neuropathy may be serious effects; GI effects are most common.
(2) GI effects—nausea, vomiting, diarrhea	
(3) Dermatologic effects—skin rash, pruritus, thrombophlebitis at infusion site	
e. With vancomycin:	
(1) Nephrotoxicity—oliguria, increased blood urea nitrogen and serum creatinine	Uncommon. Most likely to occur with large doses, concomitant administration of an aminoglycoside antibiotic, or pre-existing renal impairment. Usually resolves when vancomycin is discontinued.
(2) Ototoxicity—hearing loss, tinnitus	Most likely to occur in people with renal impairment or a pre-existing hearing loss
(3) "Red man syndrome"—hypotension, skin flushing	Occurs with rapid infusion of IV vancomycin. Can be prevented by adequate dilution and infusing over 1–2 h or premedicating with diphenhydramine (an antihistamine). This reaction does not occur with teicoplanin.

4. Observe for drug interactions
  a. Drugs that *decrease* effects of azithromycin

(1) Antacids	Antacids decrease peak serum levels

  b. Drug that *increases* effects of clarithromycin

  (1) Fluconazole

  c. Drugs that *increase* effects of dirithromycin

(1) Antacids, histamine$_2$ (H$_2$) receptor antagonists	These agents raise gastric pH and slightly increase absorption of dirithromycin.

  d. Drugs that *increase* effects of erythromycin

(1) Chloramphenicol	The combination is effective against some strains of resistant *Staphylococcus aureus*.

(continued)

NURSING ACTIONS	RATIONALE/EXPLANATION
(2) Streptomycin	The combination is effective against the enterococcus in bacteremia, brain abscess, endocarditis, meningitis, and UTI.
e. Drugs that *decrease* effects of chloramphenicol:	
(1) Barbiturates, rifampin	Reduce serum levels, probably by accelerating liver metabolism of chloramphenicol
f. Drugs that *decrease* effects of clindamycin:	
(1) Erythromycin	
(2) Kaolin-pectin	Delays absorption
g. Drug that *increases* effects of metronidazole:	
(1) Cimetidine	Inhibits hepatic metabolism
h. Drugs that *decrease* effects of metronidazole:	
(1) Phenobarbital, phenytoin, prednisone, rifampin	These drugs induce hepatic enzymes and decrease effects of metronidazole by accelerating its rate of hepatic metabolism.
5. Teach clients:	
a. Take azithromycin capsules and oral solution on an empty stomach, 1 h before or 2 h after a meal; take tablets without regard to meals. Do not take with an antacid.	To promote absorption and therapeutic effects
b. Take clarithromycin without regard to meals. With the oral suspension, do not refrigerate, and shake well before measuring the dose.	Refrigeration is not required for the oral suspension, and it thickens the drug so accurate measurement is difficult.
c. Take dirithromycin with food or within 1 h of having eaten. Do not cut, chew, or crush the tablets.	
d. Take erythromycin according to instructions, with 6 to 8 oz of water, preferably at evenly spaced intervals around the clock.	Some preparations should be taken on an empty stomach whereas others may be taken without regard to meals.
e. Take chloramphenicol on an empty stomach, 1 h before or 2 h after a meal, at evenly spaced intervals around the clock.	May be taken with food if GI upset occurs
f. Take clindamycin with a full glass of water, without regard to meals. Notify prescriber if diarrhea occurs; do not treat with over-the-counter drugs.	The drug may need to be stopped if severe diarrhea occurs.
g. Take metronidazole with food; do not drink alcoholic beverages while taking metronidazole.	Taking with food decreases GI upset; drinking alcohol may cause abdominal discomfort, vomiting, flushing, or headache.
h. Take all prescribed doses of oral vancomycin	Most often prescribed for antibiotic-induced diarrhea and colitis. Relapses may occur, especially if vancomycin is stopped prematurely

 REVIEW AND APPLICATION EXERCISES

1. Why is erythromycin called a penicillin substitute?

2. What are adverse effects with erythromycin and how may they be prevented or minimized?

3. Why is erythromycin seldom given parenterally?

4. How are the macrolides excreted? What difference does this make in client care?

5. How do the newer macrolides differ from erythromycin?

6. Why is the use of chloramphenicol limited?

7. How would you recognize pseudomembranous colitis in a client? What would you do if you thought a client might have it? Why?

8. Why is metronidazole preferred over vancomycin for initial treatment of pseudomembranous colitis?

9. Which antibacterial drug is considered the drug of choice for MRSA and MRSE?

10. What is "red man syndrome" and how can it be prevented or minimized?

SELECTED REFERENCES

Belliveau, R.P., Rothman, A.L., & Maday, C.E. (1996). Limiting vancomycin use to combat vancomycin-resistant *Enterococcus faecium*. *American Journal of Health-System Pharmacy, 53,* 1570–1575.

Drug facts and comparisons. (Updated monthly). St. Louis: Facts and Comparisons.

Hammerschlag, M.R. (1993). Azithromycin and clarithromycin. *Pediatric Annals, 22,* 161–166.

Horsburgh, C.R., Jr. (1996). Advances in the prevention and treatment of *Mycobacterium avium* disease (editorial). *New England Journal of Medicine, 335*(6), 428–429.

Kapusnik-Uner, J.E., Sande, M.A., & Chambers, H.F. (1996). Antimicrobial agents: Tetracyclines, chloramphenicol, erythromycin, and miscellaneous antibacterial agents. In J.G. Hardman, L.E. Limbird, P.B. Molinoff, & R.W. Ruddon (Eds.), *Goodman & Gilman's The pharmacological basis of therapeutics,* 9th ed., pp. 1123–1153). New York: McGraw-Hill.

Pierce, M., Crampton, S., Henry, D., et al (1996). A randomized trial of clarithromycin as prophylaxis against disseminated *Mycobacterium avium* complex infection in patients with advanced acquired immunodeficiency syndrome. *New England Journal of Medicine, 335*(6), 384–391.

Wallace, R.J., Jr., Brown, B.A., & Griffith, D.E. (1993). Drug intolerance to high-dose clarithromycin among elderly patients. *Diagnostic Microbiology and Infectious Disease, 16,* 215–221.

38

Drugs for Tuberculosis and Mycobacterium Avium Complex (MAC) Disease

Outline

Tuberculosis

Prevention and Treatment of Tuberculosis

Characteristics of Antitubercular Drugs
    mechanism of action
    indications for use
    contraindications for use

Individual Antitubercular Drugs
    primary drugs
      INH
      rifampin
      ethambutol
      pyrazinamide
      streptomycin
    secondary drugs
      para-aminosalicylic acid
      capreomycin
      cycloserine
      ethionamide
    other drugs used in MDR-TB
    combination antitubercular drugs

***Mycobacterium avium* Complex (MAC) Disease**
    rifabutin

Nursing Process
    assessment
    nursing diagnoses
    planning/goals
    interventions
    evaluation

Principles of Therapy
    drug-susceptible tuberculosis
    multi-drug resistant tuberculosis

    increasing compliance with antituberculosis
      drug therapy
    use in HIV infection
    use in renal disease
    use in liver disease
    use in children
    use in older adults
    home care

Objectives

After studying this chapter, the student will be able to:

1 Describe unique characteristics of tuberculosis infection.

2 Discuss the increased incidence of tuberculosis, especially multi-drug resistant tuberculosis (MDR-TB).

3 Identify populations at high risk of developing tuberculosis

4 List characteristics, uses, effects, and nursing implications of using isoniazid (INH), rifampin, and pyrazinamide.

5 Describe the rationale for multiple drug therapy in treatment of tuberculosis.

6 Discuss common problems associated with drug therapy of drug-susceptible and MDR-TB.

7 Discuss the use of aminoglycosides and fluoro-quinolones in the treatment of MDR-TB.

8 Describe *Mycobacterium avium* complex (MAC) disease and the drugs used to prevent or treat it.

Key Terms

Dormant	**Jaundice**
Hepatitis	**Peripheral neuritis**

Tuberculosis

Tuberculosis is an infectious disease that usually affects the lungs but may involve the kidneys, meninges, bone, adrenal glands, and gastrointestinal (GI) tract. It is caused by *Mycobacterium tuberculosis,* the tubercle bacillus. These organisms have unique characteristics that influence the disease process and drug therapy. They multiply slowly; they may lie dormant within the body for many years, encapsulated in calcified tubercles; they resist phagocytosis and survive within phagocytic cells; they rapidly develop resistance to single-drug therapies; and they develop resistance to multiple drugs when treatment is inadequate or incomplete.

In any population of *Mycobacterium tuberculosis* microorganisms, including those that have not been exposed to an antitubercular drug, there are some randomly produced mutant organisms that are inherently drug resistant. In persons with infection who receive antitubercular drugs, drug-resistant mutants continue to occur and reproduce in the presence of the drugs. These strains may become predominant as the drugs eliminate susceptible strains and provide more space and nutrients for resistant strains. Most drug-resistant strains develop when previously infected clients do not take the drugs and doses prescribed for the length of time prescribed. However, drug-resistant strains can be spread from one person to another and cause new infections, especially in individuals whose immune systems are suppressed by disease (*e.g.,* advanced human immunodeficiency virus [HIV] infection) or drugs (*e.g.,* antineoplastic drugs and those used to prevent rejection of organ transplants). Tuberculosis has increased during recent years. This increase is largely attributed to a high incidence in people with acquired immunodeficiency syndrome (AIDS) and in immigrants from Southeast Asia, where the disease is endemic. In addition to the increase in number of cases, a major concern is the increase in multidrug-resistant tuberculosis (MDR-TB). MDR-TB indicates organisms that are resistant to two or more antitubercular drugs and often include both INH and rifampin, the most effective drugs available. As with single-drug resistance, MDR-TB develops in infected people who receive inadequate drug therapy and it can be transmitted to previously uninfected contacts. Several outbreaks have occurred in prisons and hospitals, mostly in large urban areas.

Prevention and Treatment of Tuberculosis

Drug therapy is the only effective method for prevention and treatment of tuberculosis. If effective preventive therapy is implemented, active tuberculosis does not occur. If effective drug therapy is implemented for active disease, most patients show clinical improvement within about 2 weeks, with decreased fever and cough, weight gain and feeling better, and improved chest x-rays. With optimal treatment, most clients will have negative sputum cultures within 3 to 6 months. If the client is symptomatic or the culture is positive after 3 months, noncompliance or drug resistance must be considered. Cultures that are positive after 6 months often include drug-resistant organisms, and an alternative drug therapy regimen is probably needed.

For many years, isoniazid (INH) was the only drug prescribed for chemoprophylaxis of tuberculosis (usually for 6 to 12 months), and it is still the drug of choice when INH-susceptible organisms predominate in the client's community. With the increasing prevalence of INH-resistant and multidrug-resistant tuberculosis, optimal drug therapy for chemoprophylaxis has not been established, and various regimens are being tried. For persons with positive tuberculin reactions who have been exposed to someone with INH-resistant tuberculosis, rifampin may be given alone or in combination with ethambutol or pyrazinamide for 12 months. For persons with exposure to someone with documented MDR-TB, a combination of pyrazinamide (25–30 mg/kg/d) and ofloxacin (400 mg twice daily) may be given.

For several years, also, initial treatment of new cases of active tuberculosis involved a three-drug regimen (INH, rifampin, and pyrazinamide daily for 2 months, followed by continued INH and rifampin for 4 additional months, daily or twice weekly). Organism susceptibility to INH and rifampin was assumed and usually validated by effectiveness of treatment. This regimen may still be used in communities with rare isolates of drug-resistant organisms. In the twice-weekly schedule, health care providers either administer the drugs or observe the client taking them. This schedule was developed for clients unable or unwilling to self-administer the drugs independently.

With the increasing prevalence of MDR-TB, guidelines for treatment have changed and continue to evolve in the attempt to promote client adherence to treatment and to manage MDR-TB, two of the major problems in drug therapy of tuberculosis. Some of the current treatment regimens are described below:

- The Centers for Disease Control and Prevention (CDC) recommend performing culture and susceptibility tests with all cases; prescribing four antitubercular drugs (INH, rifampin, pyrazinamide, and either ethambutol or streptomycin) until susceptibility reports become available (usually several weeks); directly observing therapy to ensure that the client actually takes the drugs; and continuing treatment at least 6 months or 3 months following negative cultures. This four-drug regimen is indicated for clients in areas where drug-resistant organisms have been isolated, and for clients who require intensive treatment (*e.g.,* those with advanced HIV infection). (A five- or six-drug regimen, including two or three drugs not taken before, is recommended for clients who have received several courses of drug therapy and are therefore at high risk of having MDR-TB.)

- This four-drug regimen is evaluated when culture and susceptibility reports become available. If the causative strain of *Mycobacterium tuberculosis* is susceptible to INH, rifampin, and pyrazinamide, the regimen is continued as with the three-drug regimen described above and the fourth drug (ethambutol or streptomycin) is discontinued.
- If the causative organism is resistant to INH, rifampin and ethambutol are given for 12 months. Opinions differ about adding INH, with some clinicians believing INH should be a component of all treatment regimens.
- If the causative organism is resistant to rifampin, INH and ethambutol are given for 18 months, with pyrazinamide also being given during the first 2 months.
- When culture reports identify MDR-TB, a five- or six-drug regimen, individualized according to susceptibility reports and containing at least three drugs to which the organism is susceptible, should be instituted. Such regimens include second-line antitubercular drugs and other drugs with activity against *Mycobacterium tuberculosis* organisms, such as amikacin, ciprofloxacin, or ofloxacin. Some clinicians include at least one injectable agent. The drugs should be given for 1 to 2 years after cultures become negative, preferably with direct observation. Intermittent administration is not recommended for MDR-TB.
- For patients who are unable to tolerate pyrazinamide, INH and rifampin may be given for 9 months.
- During pregnancy, a three-drug regimen of INH, rifampin, and ethambutol is generally considered safe.

Characteristics of Antitubercular Drugs

Antitubercular drugs are divided into primary and secondary agents. Primary drugs (INH, rifampin, pyrazinamide, ethambutol, streptomycin) are used in the initial treatment of tuberculosis. Secondary drugs, used when organisms develop resistance to primary drugs, are less effective, more toxic, or both. Amikacin, ciprofloxacin, and ofloxacin (see Chap. 35) are not usually considered antitubercular drugs, but they are used in prevention and treatment of MDR-TB.

MECHANISMS OF ACTION

INH inhibits formation of cell walls in mycobacteria. The drug is actively transported into the bacterium, where it kills actively growing organisms and inhibits the growth of dormant organisms in macrophages and tuberculous lesions. Its exact mechanism of action is unknown, but it is thought to combine with an enzyme needed by INH-susceptible tuberculosis organisms. Rifampin inhibits synthesis of RNA in mycobacterial cells, thereby causing defective, nonfunctional proteins to be produced. It also penetrates intact cells and kills intracellular bacteria. This unique ability contributes to its effectiveness in treating tuberculosis because mycobacteria are harbored within host cells. Thus, it acts synergistically with INH. Pyrazinamide is bactericidal against actively growing mycobacteria within macrophages, but its exact mechanism of action is unknown. Ethambutol probably inhibits bacterial synthesis of ribonucleic acid (RNA). Streptomycin acts only against extracellular organisms; it does not penetrate macrophages and tuberculous lesions.

INDICATIONS FOR USE

INH is used to prevent and treat tuberculosis. Because the drug may cause hepatotoxicity, there is some controversy about who should receive prophylaxis. Generally, though, candidates include the following groups who are at high risk for developing active disease:

1. Household and other close contacts of clients with recently diagnosed tuberculosis. These people should receive INH for 3 months. Then, if a skin test and chest x-ray are negative, the drug may be stopped. If the tests are positive, INH should be continued for 9 additional months.
2. People who are considered newly infected (recent converters from negative to positive skin tests)
3. People with positive skin tests and additional risk factors (lung lesions on chest x-ray; diseases such as diabetes mellitus, silicosis, AIDS, leukemia, or lymphoma; alcoholism; postgastrectomy status; on chronic hemodialysis; on corticosteroid or other immunosuppressive drugs; immigrants from Southeast Asia)
4. Children and adults under 35 years of age with positive skin tests

In chemotherapy of active tuberculosis, INH is included in most drug regimens. It is always used in conjunction with one or two other primary antitubercular drugs to inhibit emergence of drug-resistant organisms. Historically, rifampin, pyrazinamide, and ethambutol were used only for treatment of active disease. Now, they are being used for chemoprophylaxis with drug-resistant tuberculosis. Streptomycin is used in the treatment of active tuberculosis.

Rifampin also is a drug of choice for prophylaxis of meningitis in close contacts of clients with meningitis. It is being investigated for use in other infections as well, including those caused by some staphylococci, atypical mycobacteria, viruses, and fungi.

CONTRAINDICATIONS FOR USE

Chemoprophylaxis with INH is contraindicated in clients with hepatic disease, in those who have had reactions to the drug, and in pregnant women. Rifampin is contraindicated in people who have had hypersensitivity reactions and must be used with caution in the presence of liver disease. Pyrazinamide should be used in the presence of liver disease only if necessary.

Individual Antitubercular Drugs

PRIMARY DRUGS

INH is the most important antitubercular drug. It penetrates body cells and is effective against bacilli growing within cells. Although it can be used alone for chemoprophylaxis of tuberculosis, it must be used with one or two other antitubercular drugs for treatment of active disease. Drug-resistant mutant organisms develop readily in the presence of INH when the drug is used alone.

INH is well absorbed from the GI tract and widely distributed in body tissues and fluids, including cerebrospinal fluid (CSF). It is acetylated in the liver to acetylisoniazid, which is more efficiently excreted by the kidneys. Metabolism of INH is genetically determined; some people are "slow acetylators" and others are "rapid acetylators." A person's rate of acetylation may be significant in determining response to INH. Slow acetylators have less N-acetyltransferase, the acetylating enzyme, in their livers. In these clients, INH is more likely to accumulate to toxic concentrations, and the development of peripheral neuropathy is more likely. However, there is no significant difference in the clinical effectiveness of INH. Rapid acetylators may require unusually high doses of INH. They also may be more susceptible to serious liver injury related to the formation of hepatotoxic metabolites.

Potentially serious adverse effects include hepatotoxicity and peripheral neuropathy. Hepatotoxicity may be manifested by symptoms of hepatitis (*e.g.*, anorexia, nausea, fatigue, malaise, and jaundice) or elevated liver enzymes. The drug should be stopped if hepatitis develops or liver enzymes are more than five times the normal values. Hepatitis is more likely to occur during the first 8 weeks of INH therapy. Patients receiving INH should be monitored monthly for signs and symptoms of hepatitis. Some clinicians also monitor liver enzymes monthly. Because of the risk of hepatotoxicity, INH should not be used for prophylaxis and should be used very cautiously for treatment of patients with pre-existing liver disease. Peripheral neuropathy may be manifested by numbness and tingling in the hands and feet. It is most likely to occur in patients who are malnourished or elderly, or who have alcoholism, diabetes mellitus, or uremia. Pyridoxine 15 to 50 mg daily should be given with INH to minimize peripheral neuropathy in susceptible groups.

Routes and Dosage Ranges

Adults: Treatment of active disease, PO, IM 4–5 mg/kg/d in a single dose (maximum dose, 300 mg/d), for at least 6 months or daily for 2 months, then 15 mg/kg twice weekly for 4 months

Chemoprophylaxis, PO, IM 300 mg/d in a single dose for 3–12 months

Disseminated tuberculosis or pulmonary disease resulting from atypical mycobacteria, PO, IM 10–20 mg/kg/d, perhaps for years

Children: Treatment of active disease, PO, IM 10–20 mg/kg/d; maximum dose, 300 mg/d for at least 6 months

Chemoprophylaxis, 10 mg/kg/d in a single dose (maximum dose, 300 mg/d), for 3–12 months

Rifampin is a semisynthetic antibacterial drug that inhibits growth of many gram-positive and gram-negative bacteria, including *Escherichia coli, Pseudomonas, Proteus, Klebsiella, Staphylococcus aureus,* and meningococci, as well as mycobacteria causing tuberculosis. It is bactericidal for both intracellular and extracellular tuberculosis organisms.

Rifampin is well absorbed following oral administration and diffuses well into body tissues and fluids, with highest concentrations in the liver, lungs, gallbladder, and kidneys. It is metabolized in the liver and excreted primarily in bile; a small amount is excreted in urine. The drug causes a harmless red-orange discoloration of body secretions, including urine, tears, saliva, sputum, perspiration, and feces.

Rifampin induces hepatic microsomal enzymes and accelerates the metabolism of numerous other drugs, thereby decreasing their half-lives and therapeutic effects. Affected drugs include acetaminophen, benzodiazepines, oral contraceptives, corticosteroids, cyclosporine, estrogens, fluconazole, ketoconazole, mexilitene, methadone, metoprolol, phenytoin, propranolol, quinidine, oral sul-fonylureas, theophylline, verapamil, and warfarin. With warfarin, decreased anticoagulant effect occurs about 5 to 8 days after rifampin is started and lasts for 5 to 7 days after rifampin is stopped. With methadone, concurrent administration with rifampin may precipitate signs and symptoms of opiate withdrawal.

Rifampin is always used with other drugs to mini-mize the occurrence of drug-resistant organisms. Ri-fampin and INH in combination eliminate tuberculosis bacilli from sputum and produce clinical improvement faster than any other drug regimen, unless organisms resistant to one or both drugs are causing the disease. Rifampin may also be given with trimethoprim-sulfamethoxazole (Bactrim) to treat methicillin-resistant staphylococcal infections and with cefotaxime or ceftri-axone to treat central nervous system infections caused by strains of *Streptococcus pneumoniae* that are resistant to penicillins and cephalosporins.

Route and Dosage Range

Adults: Treatment of tuberculosis, PO 600 mg or 10–20 mg/kg/d in a single dose for at least 6 months or daily for 2 months, then 10 mg/kg twice weekly for 4 months
Children: Treatment of tuberculosis, PO 10–20 mg/kg once daily; maximum dose, 600 mg/d for at least 6 months

Ethambutol is a tuberculostatic drug that inhibits synthesis of ribonucleic acid and thus interferes with mycobacterial protein metabolism. It is well absorbed from the GI tract, even when given with food. The ex-tent of tissue distribution is unclear except that diffu-sion into CSF is limited. It is excreted primarily by the kidneys, either unchanged or as metabolites. Myco-bacterial resistance to ethambutol develops slowly. Ethambutol may be a component in a four-drug regi-men for initial treatment of tuberculosis that may be caused by multidrug-resistant organisms.

Dosage is determined by body weight because no practical method of measuring serum drug levels is available. Also, dosage is changed during treatment if significant changes in body weight occur. Dosage must be reduced with impaired renal function. To obtain therapeutic serum levels, the total daily dose is given at one time. Ethambutol is not recommended for young children (*e.g.*, under 5 years of age) whose visual acuity cannot be monitored but may be considered for chil-dren of any age when organisms are susceptible to ethambutol and resistant to other drugs.

A major adverse effect is optic neuritis, which de-creases visual acuity and ability to differentiate red from green. Tests of visual acuity and red-green discrimina-tion are recommended before starting ethambutol and periodically during therapy. If optic neuritis develops,

the drug should be promptly stopped. Recovery usually occurs when ethambutol is discontinued.

Route and Dosage Range

Adults and children >13 years: Initial treatment, PO 15 mg/kg/d in a single dose
Retreatment, 25 mg/kg/d for 2 months, then 15 mg/kg/d
Children 6–12 years: PO 10–15 mg/kg/d

Pyrazinamide is recommended for the first 2 months of tuberculosis treatment, along with INH and rifampin. It is well absorbed with oral administration and widely distributed through the body. It is excreted mainly through the kidneys.

A major adverse effect is hepatotoxicity, and the drug should not be given to a client with pre-existing liver impairment unless it is considered absolutely essential. For clients without liver impairment, liver function studies should be done before starting pyra-zinamide and periodically during treatment. Increased plasma levels of alanine and aspartate aminotrans-ferases (ALT, AST) are usually the first clinical signs of liver damage. If significant liver damage is indicated, pyrazinamide should be stopped.

Pyrazinamide inhibits urate excretion. This charac-teristic causes hyperuricemia in most patients and may cause acute attacks of gout.

Route and Dosage Range

Adults: PO 15–30 mg/kg/d, in a single dose, to a maximum dose of 3 g/d or 50–70 mg/kg twice weekly to a maximum dose of 4 g, for the initial 2 months of antitubercular drug therapy
Children: Same as for adults, to a maximum dose of 2 g/d

Streptomycin, an aminoglycoside (see Chap. 35), is mainly used in a regimen of four to six drugs in the treatment of tuberculosis suspected or known to be resistant to INH, rifampin, or both. It may be discon-tinued when cultures become negative or after a few months of therapy.

Route and Dosage Range

Adults: IM 15 mg/kg/d, in divided doses, q12h, not to exceed 2 g/d for 2 months, then 1 g twice weekly
Children: IM 20–40 mg/kg/d, in divided doses, q12h, not to exceed 2 g/d

SECONDARY DRUGS

Para-aminosalicylic acid (PAS), **capreomycin** (Capa-stat), **cycloserine** (Seromycin), and **ethionamide** (Tre-cator SC) are diverse drugs that share tuberculostatic properties. These drugs are generally less effective or more toxic than primary drugs. They are indicated for use only when other agents are contraindicated or in disease caused by drug-resistant organisms. They must be given concurrently with other tuberculostatic drugs to inhibit emergence of resistant mycobacteria.

Para-aminosalicylic Acid, Sodium Aminosalicylate
Route and Dosage Range

Adults: PO 10–12 g/d in two or three divided doses
Children: PO 150–300 mg/kg/d in three or four divided doses

Capreomycin
Route and Dosage Range

Adults: IM (deep) 15–30 mg/kg or up to 1 g daily for 2–4 wk, then 1 g two or three times weekly for 6–12 months or longer
Children: No dosage established

Cycloserine
Route and Dosage Range

Adults: PO 250–500 mg twice daily
Children: No dosage established

Ethionamide
Route and Dosage Range

Adults: PO 250 mg twice daily, increased by 125 mg/d every 5 days until a dose of 15–20 mg/kg/d is reached. Maximal daily dose, 1 g
Children: PO 15–20 mg/kg/d, in two divided doses; maximum dose, 1 g/d

OTHER DRUGS USED IN MDR-TB

Amikacin and kanamycin are aminoglycoside antibiotics with activity against mycobacteria. Although they are not usually considered antitubercular drugs, one may be a component of a four- to six-drug regimen to treat suspected or known multidrug-resistant tuberculosis. Similarly, the fluoroquinolones ciprofloxacin and ofloxacin have antimycobacterial activity and may be used to prevent or treat multidrug-resistant tuberculosis.

COMBINATION ANTITUBERCULAR DRUGS

Rifamate and **Rifater** are combination products developed to increase convenience to clients and promote adherence to the prescribed drug therapy regimen (for drug-susceptible tuberculosis). Each Rifamate tablet contains INH 150 mg and rifampin 300 mg, and two tablets daily provide the recommended doses for a 6-month, short-course treatment regimen. Rifater contains INH 50 mg, rifampin 120 mg, and pyrazinamide 300 mg and is approved for the first 2 months of a 6-month, short-course treatment regimen. Dosage depends on weight, with 4 tablets daily for patients weighing 44 kg or less, 5 tablets daily for those weighing 45 to 54 kg, and 6 tablets daily for those weighing 55 kg or more.

Mycobacterium avium Complex (MAC) Disease

Mycobacterium avium and *Mycobacterium intracellulare* are different types of mycobacteria that resemble each other so closely they are usually grouped together as *Mycobacterium avium* complex (MAC). These atypical mycobacteria are found in water and soil throughout the United States. The organisms are thought to be transmitted by inhalation of droplets of contaminated water; there is no evidence of spread to humans from animals or other humans.

Mycobacterium avium complex rarely causes significant disease in immunocompetent persons but causes an opportunistic pulmonary infection in about 50% of patients with advanced HIV infection. Symptoms include a productive cough, weight loss, hemoptysis, and fever. As the disease becomes disseminated through the body, chronic lung disease develops and the organism is found in the blood, bone marrow, liver, lymph nodes, and other body tissues.

MAC disease was formerly treated with a combination of antitubercular drugs. However, these drugs are not very effective because of high rates of drug resistance and relapse. Newer drugs used in prevention and treatment of MAC disease are the macrolides, azithromycin and clarithromycin (see Chap. 37) and rifabutin. Prophylactic drug therapy is recommended to be lifelong, and azithromycin or clarithromycin should be included in any treatment regimen.

RIFABUTIN

Rifabutin (Mycobutin) is an antimycobacterial drug that is chemically related to rifampin, an antituberculosis drug. Rifabutin is approved for prevention of *Mycobacterium avium* complex (MAC) disease in patients with advanced HIV infection. Although opinions differ, rifabutin may be started when CD4+ cell counts are below 100 cells/mm³. Rifabutin has no advantage over rifampin in treatment of tuberculosis but may be given concurrently with isoniazid (INH) to patients who need prophylaxis against both *Mycobacterium tuberculosis* and *Mycobacterium avium.*

Rifabutin is absorbed from the GI tract, metabolized in the liver, and eliminated in urine and bile. The drug and its metabolites may cause a brownish-orange discoloration of urine, feces, saliva, sputum, perspiration, tears, and skin. Soft contact lenses may be permanently discolored. Like rifampin, rifabutin induces drug-metabolizing enzymes in the liver and accelerates metabolism of several drugs, including ketoconazole, phenytoin, prednisone, propranolol, quinidine, warfarin, and zidovudine. The drug is generally well tolerated. Adverse effects include skin rash, nausea, vomiting, diarrhea, neutropenia, and uveitis (an eye disorder characterized by inflammation, pain, and impaired vision). Safety and effectiveness in children have not been established.

Route and Dosage Range

Adults: PO 300 mg once daily

Nursing Process

Assessment

Assess for current or potential tuberculosis:

- For current disease, clinical manifestations include fatigue, weight loss, anorexia, malaise, fever, and a productive cough. In early phases, however, there may be no symptoms. If available, check diagnostic test reports for indications of tuberculosis (chest x-ray, tuberculin skin test, and sputum smear and culture).
- For potential tuberculosis, identify high-risk clients: those who are close contacts of someone with active tuberculosis; those who are elderly or undernourished; those who have diabetes mellitus, silicosis, Hodgkin's disease, leukemia, or AIDS; those who are alcoholics; and those who are receiving immunosuppressive drugs. Most new cases of tuberculosis develop in people previously infected, including immigrants from Southeast Asia and other parts of the world where the disease is endemic. However, the number of new cases with primary infection by multidrug-resistant organisms and rapid progression to active disease is increasing.
- Assess for signs and symptoms of *Mycobacterium avium* complex disease, especially in clients with advanced HIV infection who have a CD4+ cell count of 100/mm³ or less.

Nursing Diagnoses

- Anxiety or Fear related to chronic illness and long-term drug therapy
- Knowledge Deficit: Disease process and need for treatment
- Noncompliance related to adverse drug effects and need for long-term treatment
- Knowledge Deficit: Consequences of noncompliance with the drug therapy regimen
- Risk for Injury: Adverse drug effects

Planning/Goals

The client will:

- Take drugs as prescribed
- Keep appointments for follow-up care

- Report adverse drug effects
- Act to prevent spread of tuberculosis

Interventions

Use measures to prevent the spread of tuberculosis:

- Isolate suspected or newly diagnosed hospitalized clients in a private room for 2 or 3 weeks, until drug therapy has rendered them noninfectious.
- Wear masks with close contact, and wash hands thoroughly afterward.
- Have clients wear masks when out of the room for diagnostic tests.
- Assist clients to take antitubercular drugs as prescribed, for the length of time prescribed.

 Teach clients:

- About the disease process and the necessity for long-term treatment and follow-up. This is extremely important for the client and the community, because lack of knowledge and failure to comply with the therapeutic regimen lead to disease progression and spread. The American Lung Association publishes many helpful pamphlets, written for the general public, that can be obtained from a local chapter and given to clients and their families. Do not use these as a substitute for personal contact, however.
- Measures to prevent spread of tuberculosis:
  - Cover mouth and nose when coughing or sneezing. This prevents the expulsion of droplet nuclei containing the tubercle bacillus into the surrounding air, where they can be inhaled by and infect others.
  - Cough and expectorate sputum into at least two layers of tissue. Place the used tissues in a waterproof bag, and dispose of the bag, preferably by burning.
  - Wash hands after coughing or sneezing.
- The importance of nutrition and rest in promoting healing
- The risk factors and consequences of developing multi-drug-resistant tuberculosis (*i.e.,* longer treatment with drugs that cause more adverse effects, spread of the disease to others)
- The need for follow-up sputum cultures, blood tests, and so forth

Evaluation

- Observe for improvement in signs and symptoms of tuberculosis and MAC disease.
- Interview and observe for adverse drug effects; check laboratory reports of hepatic and renal function, when available.
- Question regarding compliance with instructions for taking antitubercular drugs and anti-MAC drugs.

Principles of Therapy

DRUG-SUSCEPTIBLE TUBERCULOSIS

1. Sputum culture and susceptibility reports require 6 to 8 weeks because the tubercle bacillus multiplies slowly. Consequently, initial drug therapy is based

on other factors, such as the extent of disease, whether the client has previously received antitubercular drugs, and whether multidrug-resistant strains are being isolated in the particular community.

2. Multiple drugs are required to inhibit emergence of drug-resistant organisms.

3. Duration of drug therapy varies with the purpose, extent of disease, and clinical response. INH for positive tuberculin reactors is given for 6 to 12 months. Treatment of active disease with multiple drugs ranges from 6 months to 1 year or more, depending on clinical response and culture reports.

MULTIDRUG-RESISTANT TUBERCULOSIS

1. Multidrug-resistant strains may occur anywhere. However, in the United States, they have been most evident in populations with AIDS, in closed environments (*e.g.,* hospitals, prisons), and in large urban areas.

2. Drug therapy regimens for persons exposed to someone with MDR-TB or suspected of having MDR-TB should be designed in consultation with infectious disease specialists.

3. Prevention or treatment of MDR-TB requires concurrent administration of more drugs, for a longer period of time, than drug-susceptible tuberculosis, and may require 2 years or longer.

4. All drug therapy for suspected or known MDR-TB should involve daily administration and directly observed therapy (DOT). Intermittent schedules of drug administration are not recommended.

5. The fluoroquinolones are not recommended for use in children.

INCREASING COMPLIANCE WITH ANTITUBERCULOSIS DRUG THERAPY

1. Close supervision by a health care provider is needed during chemoprophylaxis and treatment regimens to monitor the client's response and compliance. In addition, continued contact is needed during the year after completion of drug therapy, because most relapses occur during that time.

2. Intermittent dosing (*e.g.,* twice weekly rather than daily) and directly observed therapy (*i.e.,* a health care provider watching a person take a drug dose) are two strategies designed to increase compliance with drug therapy and decrease drug-resistant tuberculosis. All intermittent regimens should be administered under direct observation. In addition, alcoholics, drug abusers, homeless persons, and others at high risk for noncompliance should be treated under directly observed therapy.

3. Combinations of drugs may reduce the number of pills to be taken per dose and promote compliance.

However, they are more expensive than purchasing each drug separately.

USE IN HIV INFECTION

Tuberculosis is a common opportunistic infection in people with advanced HIV infection and may develop from an initial infection or reactivation of an old infection. Because of the damaged immune system, treatment is difficult and long term (2 to 3 years). Patients with AIDS do not absorb most antitubercular drugs very well, and this may lead to treatment failures and drug-resistant organisms. These patients are also at high risk of developing primary infection with multidrug-resistant organisms.

USE IN RENAL DISEASE

Dosage of amikacin, capreomycin, cycloserine, ethambutol, fluoroquinolones, and streptomycin should be reduced in patients with impaired renal function. Cycloserine is contraindicated in severe renal impairment.

USE IN LIVER DISEASE

Most antitubercular drugs are metabolized in the liver and several (*e.g.,* INH, rifampin, and pyrazinamide) are hepatotoxic. To detect hepatotoxicity as early as possible, plasma alanine aminotransferase (ALT) and aspartate aminotransferase (AST) should be measured before starting and periodically during drug therapy. If hepatitis develops, these enzymes usually increase before other signs and symptoms develop.

With INH, mild increases in AST and ALT occur in about 10% to 20% of patients but are not considered significant and usually resolve without stopping the drug. Occasionally, hepatitis and progressive liver damage occur, usually in middle-age and older adults. Patients should be assessed monthly for symptoms of hepatitis (anorexia, nausea, fatigue, malaise, and jaundice). If symptoms occur or if AST and ALT increase significantly, INH should be discontinued. INH should be given very cautiously to people with pre-existing hepatic disease.

With rifampin, liver damage is most likely to occur with pre-existing liver disease or concurrent use of other hepatotoxic drugs. AST and ALT should be measured before starting rifampin and every 2 to 4 weeks during rifampin therapy. The drug should be stopped if signs of liver damage occur.

With pyrazinamide, the earliest signs of liver injury are increased ALT and AST values. If significant elevations occur or if other evidence of liver damage becomes apparent, the drug must be stopped. For a patient with pre-existing liver dysfunction, pyrazinamide should not be given unless considered absolutely necessary.

USE IN CHILDREN

Tuberculosis occurs in children of all ages. Infants and preschool-age children are especially in need of early recognition and treatment because they can rapidly progress from primary infection to active pulmonary disease and perhaps to extrapulmonary involvement. Tuberculosis is usually discovered during examination of a sick child or investigation of the contacts of someone with newly diagnosed active tuberculosis. Children in close contact with a case of tuberculosis should receive skin testing, a physical examination, and a chest x-ray.

When children require antitubercular drugs for prevention or treatment, treatment is mainly empirical. For example, some drugs are not established as safe or effective or are not recommended for use in children. For drugs that are used, dosage ranges are not well defined because few data are available about the pharmacokinetics of antitubercular drugs in children. In addition, most of the drugs are not available in pediatric dosage forms and are given as crushed portions of adult dosage forms. INH is available as a solution, but it contains sorbitol and may cause diarrhea.

As with adults, drug therapy regimens vary with particular circumstances and continue to evolve. Health care providers need to follow current recommendations of the CDC and pediatric infectious disease specialists. Children with exposure to tuberculosis but negative skin tests should be given INH for 3 months. If exposure stops and the skin test and examination remain negative, the INH can be stopped. For older children and adolescents with negative skin tests and no symptoms, chemoprophylaxis may be omitted or delayed until skin tests become positive or other signs and symptoms develop.

Children who are infected but without disease (*i.e.,* have positive skin tests) should receive preventive therapy. If the infection to which the child was exposed was drug susceptible, INH should be given daily for about 9 months (12 months or longer for children with HIV infection or immunosuppression). If the causative strain in the index case was INH resistant, rifampin may be given empirically. Children with suspected disease should receive multidrug treatment until infection can be ruled out.

If the drug-susceptibility patterns of the *Mycobacterium tuberculosis* strain causing the index case are known, the child is treated with those drugs; if this information is not available, the pattern of drug resistance in the community where the child likely became infected should be the guide for selecting the drug therapy regimen. As in adults, drug-susceptible tuberculosis is treated with INH, rifampin and pyrazinamide for 2 months. Then, pyrazinamide is stopped and the INH and rifampin are continued for 4 more months. If drug-resistant organisms have been identified in the com-

munity, the CDC recommends a fourth drug, ethambutol or streptomycin, until the patient's culture and susceptiblilty data become available. If pyrazinamide is not given, INH and rifampin are recommended for 9 months. When INH or rifampin cannot be used, therapy should continue for 12 to 24 months.

Drug-resistant tuberculosis in children is usually acquired from an adult family member or other close contact with active, drug-resistant disease. For children exposed to MDR-TB, there is no proven preventive therapy. Several regimens are used empirically, including ethambutol and pyrazinamide or ethionamide and cycloserine. When INH and rifampin cannot be given because of MDR-TB, drug therapy should continue for 24 months after sputum smears or cultures become negative. Ciprofloxacin and ofloxacin are used for prevention and treatment of MDR-TB in adults, but are not recommended for use in children because of possible cartilage damage, especially in weight-bearing joints. If they are used, children must be monitored often for joint pain or swelling. Patients with MDR-TB may require months of treatment before sputum smears become negative, and they are infectious during this period. To guide dosage and minimize adverse drug effects, serum drug levels should be measured periodically, especially in patients with GI, renal or hepatic disease or with advanced HIV infection.

USE IN OLDER ADULTS

Potentially fatal hepatitis may occur with INH, especially in people who drink alcoholic beverages daily. Liver function tests should be monitored regularly, and the drug should be discontinued if signs and symptoms of hepatotoxicity occur. Pyrazinamide and rifampin also may cause hepatotoxicity. Because these are the drugs of first choice for the first 2 months of tuberculosis therapy, clients must be observed closely for signs of liver dysfunction. In older adults with suspected or known MDR-TB, the drug therapy regimen is determined by personal or local patterns of drug-resistant strains of *Mycobacterium tuberculosis*.

HOME CARE

The home care nurse has major roles to play in the health care of clients, families, and communities. With individual clients receiving preventive or therapeutic antitubercular drugs, the home care nurse needs to assist in taking the drugs as directed. Specific interventions vary widely and may include administering the drug(s) (directly observed therapy or DOT); teaching about the importance of taking the drugs and the possible consequences of not taking them (*i.e.,* more severe disease, longer treatment regimens with more toxic drugs, spreading the disease to others); monitoring for adverse drug effects and assisting the client to manage them or reporting them to the health care provider who is prescribing the drugs; assisting in obtaining the drugs; and keeping follow-up appointments for blood tests, chest x-rays; and others. Family members may also need teaching related to preventing spread of the disease and assisting the client to obtain adequate treatment. In relation to community needs, the nurse needs to be active in identifying cases, investigating contacts of newly diagnosed cases, and promoting efforts to manage tuberculosis effectively.

NURSING ACTIONS   ANTITUBERCULAR DRUGS

NURSING ACTIONS	RATIONALE/EXPLANATION
1. Administer accurately **a.** Give INH, ethambutol, and rifampin in a single dose once daily.	A single dose with the resulting higher blood levels is more effective. Also, fewer doses may increase client compliance with drug therapy.
b. Give PAS and ethionamide with food.	To minimize nausea, vomiting, and diarrhea.
c. Give rifampin 1 h before or 2 h after a meal.	Food delays absorption.
d. Give capreomycin and parenteral INH by deep intramuscular injection into a large muscle mass, and rotate injection sites.	To decrease local pain and tissue irritation.
2. Observe for therapeutic effects	Therapeutic effects are usually apparent within the first 2 or 3 weeks of drug therapy.
a. Clinical improvement	
(1) Decreased cough, sputum, fever, night sweats, and fatigue	
(2) Increased appetite, weight, and feeling of well-being.	
b. Negative sputum smear and culture	
c. Improvement in chest x-ray studies	
3. Observe for adverse effects **a.** Nausea, vomiting, diarrhea	These symptoms are likely to occur with any of the oral antitubercular drugs and are usually most severe with PAS.
b. Neurotoxicity:	
(1) Eighth cranial nerve damage—vertigo, tinnitus, hearing loss	A major adverse reaction to aminoglycoside antibiotics
(2) Optic nerve damage—decreased vision and color discrimination	The major adverse reaction to ethambutol
(3) Peripheral neuritis—tingling, numbness, paresthesias	Often occurs with INH but can be prevented by administering pyridoxine (vitamin B_6). Also may occur with ethambutol.
(4) CNS changes—confusion, convulsions, depression	More often associated with INH but similar changes may occur with ethambutol.
c. Hepatotoxicity—increased serum aspartate aminotransferase (AST), alanine aminotransferase (ALT), and serum bilirubin; jaundice; and other symptoms of hepatitis	May occur with INH, rifampin, and pyrazinamide, especially if the client already has liver damage.

NURSING ACTIONS	RATIONALE/EXPLANATION
d. Nephrotoxicity—increased blood urea nitrogen and serum creatinine, cells in urine, oliguria	A major adverse reaction to aminoglycosides
e. Hypersensitivity—fever, tachycardia, anorexia, and malaise are early symptoms. If the drug is not discontinued, exfoliative dermatitis, hepatitis, renal abnormalities, and blood dyscrasias may occur.	Hypersensitivity reactions are more likely to occur between the third and eighth weeks of drug therapy. Early detection and drug discontinuation are necessary to prevent progressive worsening of the client's condition. Severe reactions can be fatal.

4.　Observe for drug interactions

NURSING ACTIONS	RATIONALE/EXPLANATION
a. Drugs that *increase* effects of antitubercular drugs: Other antitubercular drugs	Potentiate antitubercular effects. These drugs are always used in combination of two or more for treatment of tuberculosis. For chemoprophylaxis, INH is used alone.
b. Drugs that *alter* the effects of INH:	
(1) Alcohol and oral antacids decrease effects.	Alcohol induces hepatic enzymes, which accelerate the rate of isoniazid metabolism and may increase the likelihood of toxicity. Oral antacids may decrease absorption of oral INH.
(2) Disulfiram	May cause behavioral changes and impairments in coordination
(3) Pyridoxine (vitamin B$_6$)	Pyridoxine decreases peripheral neuritis, a common adverse effect of INH, and is usually combined with INH for this purpose.
(4) Sympathomimetics	May result in increased blood pressure owing to the MAO inhibitory activity of INH
c. Drugs that *alter* effects of rifampin: Halothane and INH *increase* effects.	Additive risk of hepatotoxicity
d. Drugs that *alter* effects of aminoglycosides.	See Chapter 35

5. Teach clients

NURSING ACTIONS	RATIONALE/EXPLANATION
a. Report adverse reactions to drug therapy:	
(1) Severe gastrointestinal problems	
(2) Yellowing of sclera, dark urine, clay-colored stools	Characteristics of jaundice and possible liver damage
(3) Any changes in vision or hearing	May indicate need to change dosage or discontinue drugs
(4) Numbness or tingling of hands or feet	May indicate peripheral neuritis, which can usually be controlled by taking pyridoxine (vitamin B$_6$).
(5) Any other changes in usual patterns such as drowsiness, dizziness, decreased urine output, skin rash, or fever	These may indicate adverse reactions to drugs that must be evaluated by the physician because they may be caused by other conditions as well.
b. If taking PAS, discard any tablets that turn brownish or purplish.	PAS deteriorates rapidly in contact with water, heat, and sunlight. Deterioration is manifested by discoloration of the tablets.
c. If taking rifampin, urine, tears, saliva, and other body secretions become red. Discoloration of secretions is harmless, except that contact lenses may be permanently stained.	

REVIEW AND APPLICATION EXERCISES

1. How do tuberculosis infections differ from most other bacterial infections?

2. Why are AIDS patients at high risk of developing tuberculosis?

3. What are the main risk factors for developing drug-resistant tuberculosis?

4. Who should receive INH to prevent tuberculosis? Who should not be given INH? Why?

5. When INH is given alone for prophylaxis, how long should it be taken?

6. If you worked in a health department with clients on INH prophylaxis, what are some interventions to promote client adherence to the drug regimen?

7. Why is active, symptomatic tuberculosis always treated with multiple drugs?

8. In a client with tuberculosis newly started on drug therapy, how could you explain the emergence of drug-resistant organisms and the importance of preventing this problem?

9. What are advantages and disadvantages of short-course (6 to 9 months) treatment programs?

10. For which clients would intermittent, direct administration of antitubercular drugs be preferred?

11. What adverse effects are associated with INH, rifampin, pyrazinamide, and ethambutol, and how may they be prevented or minimized?

12. In a client with multidrug-resistant tuberculosis, what are nursing implications?

SELECTED REFERENCES

Boutotte, J. (1993). TB. The second time around . . . and how you can help control it. *Nursing 93, 23,* 42–49.

Centers for Disease Control and Prevention. (1993). Initial therapy for tuberculosis in the era of multidrug resistance. Recommendations of the Advisory Council for the Elimination of Tuberculosis. *Morbidity and Mortality Weekly Report, 42*(No. RR-7), 1–7.

Ebert, S.C. (1997). Tuberculosis. In J.T. DiPiro, R.L. Talbert, G.C. Yee, G.R. Matzke, B.G. Wells, & L.M. Posey (Eds.), *Pharmacotherapy: A pathophysiologic approach,* 3rd ed., pp. 2101–2124). Stamford, CT: Appleton & Lange.

Horsburgh, C.R. (1996). Advances in the prevention and treatment of *Mycobacterium avium* complex disease (Editorial). *The New England Journal of Medicine, 335*(6), 428–429.

Humma, L.M. (1996). Prevention and treatment of drug-resistant tuberculosis. *American Journal of Health-System Pharmacy, 53,* 2291–2298.

Iseman, M.D. (1993). Treatment of multidrug-resistant tuberculosis. *The New England Journal of Medicine, 329*(11), 784–791.

Mandell, G.L. & Petri, W.A., Jr. (1996). Drugs used in the chemotherapy of tuberculosis, *Mycobacterium avium* complex disease, and leprosy. In J.G. Hardman, L.E. Limbird, P.B. Molinoff, & R.W. Ruddon (Eds.), *Goodman and Gilman's The pharmacological basis of therapeutics,* 9th ed., pp. 1155–1174. New York: McGraw-Hill.

Peloquin, C.A. & Berning, S.E. (1995). Tuberculosis and multidrug resistant tuberculosis in children. *Pediatric Nursing, 21*(6), 566–572.

Porth, C.M. (1994). *Pathophysiology: Concepts of altered health states,* 4th ed., pp. 523–569. Philadelphia: J.B. Lippincott.

Toossi, Z. & Ellner, J.J. (1997). Tuberculosis. In W.N. Kelley (Ed.), *Textbook of internal medicine,* 3rd ed., pp. 1687–1696. Philadelphia: Lippincott-Raven.

Antiviral Drugs

Outline

Objectives

After studying this chapter, the student will be able to:

1 Describe characteristics of viruses and common viral infections.

2 Discuss difficulties in developing and using antiviral drugs.

3 Identify clients at risk of developing systemic viral infections.

4 Differentiate types of antiviral drugs used for herpes infections, human immunodeficiency virus (HIV) infections, influenza A, and respiratory syncytial virus (RSV) infections.

5 Describe commonly used antiviral drugs in terms of indications for use, adverse effects, and nursing process implications.

6 Discuss the rationale for using combinations of drugs in treating HIV infection.

7 Teach clients techniques to prevent viral infections.

Key Terms

Acquired immunodeficiency syndrome (AIDS)

Cytomegalovirus (CMV) retinitis

Genital herpes

Human immunodeficiency virus (HIV)

Immunocompromised

Virucidal

Virustatic

General Characteristics of Viruses and Viral Infections

Viruses produce many diseases, including acquired immunodeficiency syndrome (AIDS), hepatitis, encephalitis, pneumonia, rhinitis, skin and mucous membrane diseases, and other disorders that affect almost every body system. Many potentially pathogenic viral strains exist. For example, more than 150 distinct viruses infect the human respiratory tract, including about 100 types of rhinovirus that cause the common cold. Viruses are spread by secretions from infected people, ingestion of contaminated food or water, breaks in skin or mucous membrane, blood transfusions, sexual contact, pregnancy, breast-feeding, and organ transplantation. Viral infections vary from mild, localized disease with few symptoms to severe systemic illness and death. Severe infections are more common when host defense mechanisms are impaired by disease or drugs. Additional general characteristics of viruses and viral infections are listed below; specific characteristics of selected viral infections are described in Box 39-1:

1. Viruses are intracellular parasites that can live and reproduce only while inside other living cells. They gain entry to human host cells by binding to specific receptors on cell membranes. All human cells do not have receptors for all viruses; cells that lack receptors for a particular virus are resistant to infection by that virus. Thus, the locations and numbers of the receptors determine which host cells can be infected by a particular virus. For example, the mucous membranes lining the tracheobronchial tree have receptors for the influenza A virus and certain white blood cells (helper T lymphocytes and monocyte/macrophages) have CD4 molecules, which are the receptors for the human immunodeficiency virus (HIV).
2. Once inside host cells, viruses use cellular metabolic activities for their own survival and replication. Viral replication involves dissolution of the protein coating and subsequent exposure of the genetic material (deoxyribonucleic acid [DNA] or ribonucleic acid [RNA]). With DNA viruses, the viral DNA enters the host cell's nucleus, where it becomes incorporated into the host cell's chromosomal DNA. Then, host cell genes are coded to produce new viruses. In addition, the viral DNA incorporated with host DNA is transmitted to the host's daughter cells during host cell mitosis and becomes part of the inherited genetic information of the host cell and its progeny. With RNA viruses (e.g., HIV), the viral RNA must be converted to DNA by an enzyme called reverse transcriptase before replication can occur.

   Once new viruses are formed, they may be released from the infected cell by budding out and breaking off from the cell membrane (leaving the host cell intact) or by causing lysis of the cell. When the cell is destroyed, the viruses are released into the blood and surrounding tissues, from which they can transmit the viral infection to other host cells.
3. Viruses induce antibodies and immunity. Antibodies are proteins that defend against microbial or viral invasion. They are very specific (i.e., an antibody will protect only against a specific virus or other antigen). For instance, a person who has had measles develops antibody protection (immunity) against future infection by the measles virus but does not develop immunity against other viral infections, such as chickenpox or hepatitis.

   The protein coat of the virus allows the immune system of the host to recognize the virus as a "foreign invader" and to produce antibodies against it. This system works efficiently for most viruses but does not work for the influenza A virus. Apparently, the influenza A virus can alter its protein covering so much and so often that the immune system does not recognize it as foreign to the body. Thus, last year's antibody cannot recognize and neutralize this year's virus.

   Antibodies against infecting viruses can prevent their reaching the bloodstream or, if they have reached the bloodstream, prevent their invasion of host cells. Once the virus has penetrated the cell, it is protected from antibody action, and the host depends on cell-mediated immunity (lymphocytes and macrophages) to eradicate the virus along with the cell harboring it.
4. Viral infection may occur without signs and symptoms of illness. If illness does occur, the clinical course is usually short and self-limited. Recovery occurs as the virus is eliminated from the body. Some viruses (e.g., herpesviruses) can survive in host cells for many years and cause a chronic, latent infection that periodically becomes reactivated. Also, autoimmune diseases may be caused by viral alteration of host cells so lymphocytes are fooled into thinking the host's own tissues are foreign.
5. Symptoms usually associated with acute viral infections include fever, headache, cough, malaise, muscle pain, nausea and vomiting, diarrhea, insomnia, and photophobia. White blood cell count is usually normal. Other signs and symptoms vary with the type of virus and the body organs involved.

Antiviral Drugs

Until the AIDS epidemic in the 1980s, there were only a few clinically useful antiviral drugs. Since then, numerous new agents have been developed to treat HIV infection and opportunistic viral infections that occur in hosts whose immune systems are suppressed by AIDS or immunosuppressant drugs given to organ transplant

BOX 39-1. SELECTED VIRAL INFECTIONS

Herpesvirus Infections

CYTOMEGALOVIRUS DISEASE AND RETINITIS

Cytomegalovirus (CMV) infection is extremely common, and most persons become infected by adulthood. Infection is usually asymptomatic in healthy, immunocompetent adults. Like other herpesviruses, CMV can cause a primary infection, then remain latent in body tissues, probably for life. This means the virus can be shed in secretions of an asymptomatic host and spread to others by contact with infected saliva, blood, urine, semen, breast milk, and cervical secretions. It also means the virus is ready to cause an opportunistic infection when the host becomes immunosuppressed. During pregnancy, CMV is transmitted to the fetus across the placenta and may cause infection in the brain, inner ears, eyes, liver, and bone marrow. Learning disabilities and mental retardation may result from congenital CMV infection. Children spread the virus to each other in saliva or urine; adolescents and adults transmit the virus mainly through sexual contact.

Major populations at risk for developing CMV infection are cancer patients who receive immunosuppressant drugs; organ transplant recipients, who must receive immunosuppressant drugs to prevent their body's rejection of the transplanted organ; and those with advanced HIV infection. Systemic CMV infection occurs mainly from reactivation of endogenous virus, although it may occur from an exogenous source, and it may cause cellular necrosis and inflammation in various body tissues. Common disorders are pneumonitis, hepatitis, encephalitis, adrenal insufficiency, and gastrointestinal inflammation and ulcers.

In the eye, CMV infection produces retinitis, usually characterized by blurred vision and decreased visual acuity. Visual impairment is progressive and irreversible, if untreated, and causes blindness in one or both eyes. CMV retinitis may also indicate systemic CMV disease, or it may be asymptomatic or discovered at autopsy.

GENITAL HERPES INFECTION

Genital herpes infection is caused by the herpes simplex virus type 2 (HSV-2) and produces recurrent, painful, blister-like eruptions of the skin and mucous membranes. The virus is usually transmitted from person to person by direct contact with open lesions or secretions, including genital secretions. Primary infection occurs at a site of viral entry, where the virus infects epithelial cells, produces progeny viruses, and destroys the infected cells. Recovery from the primary infection leaves latent infection in sensory nerve cells. In response to various stimulii, such as intense sunlight, emotional stress, febrile illness, or menstruation, the latent infection is reactivated periodically, with viral reproduction and shedding.

In the fetus, the HSV-2 virus may be transmitted from an infected birth canal, and neonatal herpes is a serious complication of maternal genital herpes. Neonatal herpes usually becomes evident within the first week of life and may be manifested by the typical clusters of blister-like lesions on skin or mucous membranes. Irritability, lethargy, jaundice, bleeding problems, respiratory distress, seizures, or coma may also occur. The lesions heal in 1 to 2 weeks, but neonatal herpes still carries a high mortality rate. In immunosuppressed persons, HSV-2 infection may result in severe, systemic disease.

HERPES ZOSTER

Herpes zoster is caused by the varicella-zoster virus, which is highly contagious and present worldwide. Most children in the United States are infected by early school age. The virus produces chickenpox on first exposure and is spread from person to person by the respiratory route or by contact with secretions from the skin lesions. Recovery from the primary infection leaves latent infection in nerve cells. Reactivation of the latent infection causes herpes zoster (commonly called shingles), a localized cluster of painful, blister-like skin eruptions. The skin lesions have the same appearance as those of chickenpox and genital herpes. Over several days, the vesicles become pustules, then rupture and heal. Because the virus remains in sensory nerve cells, pain can persist for months after the skin lesions heal. Most cases of herpes zoster infection occur among the elderly and the immunocompromised.

HUMAN IMMUNODEFICIENCY VIRUS (HIV) INFECTION

HIV infection is caused by a retrovirus that attacks the immune system. Two types of HIV virus have been identified. Most infections are caused by HIV-1; HIV-2 infections occur mainly in Africa. HIV-1 binds to a receptor protein (CD4 molecule) on the surface of susceptible cells, primarily T-lymphocytes (also called helper T cells and CD4 cells) and monocyte/macrophages. The infection and destruction of CD4 cells lead to the severe impairment of the immune system.

Progression of HIV-1 infection to acquired immunodeficiency syndrome (AIDS) occurs during phases of disease development. One phase is characterized by the primary infection, during which influenza-like symptoms (*e.g.*, fever, chills, muscle aches) may last several weeks. During this time, the virus is rapidly growing and spreading to lymphoid and other body tissues. The next phase is characterized by a dramatic decline in the rate of viral replication, attributed to a partially effective immune system response, and no visible manifestations of HIV infection. However, there is continued replication of HIV in body tissues, destruction of lymphoid tissues, and the presence of HIV antibodies in the blood

BOX 39-1. (CONTINUED)

(called seroconversion). During this period, which may last 5 to 10 years, the person is seropositive (HIV+) and infectious but asymptomatic. Eventually, the immune system is substantially damaged and the rate of viral reproduction accelerates. When the viral load and immunodeficiency reach significant levels, the illness is called advanced HIV infection or AIDS. This phase is characterized by decreased CD4+ cell counts, loss of immune responses, and clinical disease most often manifested by opportunistic infections such as *Pneumocystis carinii* pneumonia (PCP).

HIV can spread to a new host during any phase of infection and is spread by sexual intercourse, injection of IV drugs with contaminated needles, mucous membrane contact with blood or body fluids containing HIV, and perinatally, from mother to fetus. Although the virus has been found in most body fluids, blood, semen, or vaginal secretions have been associated with most infections. Health care workers have been infected by needle stick injuries. The virus is not spread through casual contact.

RESPIRATORY SYNCYTIAL VIRUS (RSV) INFECTION

The respiratory syncytial virus is present worldwide, is highly contagious, and infects most children by school age. Epidemics of RSV infection may occur in nurseries, day care centers, and pediatric hospital units during winter months. This virus infects and destroys respiratory epithe-

lium in the bronchi, bronchioles, and alveoli. It is spread by respiratory droplets and secretions, direct contact with an infected person, and contact with fomites, including the hands of caregivers.

RSV is the most common cause of bronchiolitis and pneumonia in infants and causes the most severe illness in those under 6 months old. These infants usually have wheezing, cough, and respiratory distress, and may have fever. The infection is usually self-limited and resolves in 1 to 2 weeks. Antiviral therapy with ribavirin is used in some cases. The mortality rate from RSV infection is low in children who are generally healthy but increases substantially in those with congenital heart disease or immunosuppression. Recurrent infection occurs but is usually less severe than the primary infection. In older children, RSV infection produces much milder disease but may be associated with acute exacerbations of asthma.

In adults, RSV infection causes colds and bronchitis, with symptoms of fever, cough, and nasal congestion. Infection occurs most often in those with household or other close contact with children, including pediatric health care workers. In elderly adults, RSV infection may cause pneumonia and require hospitalization. In immunocompromised patients, RSV infection may cause severe and potentially fatal pneumonia.

---

recipients. Because of the seriousness of HIV infection, the Food & Drug Administration (FDA) accelerated its review and approval process for anti-AIDS drugs.

Despite the increased numbers of antiviral drugs, drug therapy for viral infections is still limited and primarily geared toward relieving symptoms or slowing progress of the disease. Development of effective antiviral drugs is extremely difficult owing to the relationship between viruses and their host cells. Viruses depend on the enzymatic, genetic, and nutritional systems of the host cells for all their own vital functions. Consequently, relatively few drugs suppress multiplication or transmission of viruses without being excessively toxic to host tissues. The drugs inhibit viral reproduction but do not eliminate viruses from tissues. Available antiviral drugs are expensive, relatively toxic, and effective in a limited number of specific infections. They are of potential use in treating an established infection if given promptly and in chemoprophylaxis if given before or soon after exposure. Protection conferred by chemoprophylaxis is immediate but lasts only while the drug is being taken. Subgroups of antiviral drugs are described below; specific drugs, with their indications for use and dosage ranges, are listed in Table 39-1.

DRUGS FOR HERPESVIRUS INFECTIONS

Acyclovir, famciclovir, and valacyclovir penetrate virus-infected cells, become activated by an enzyme, and inhibit viral DNA reproduction. They are used in the treatment of herpes simplex and herpes zoster infections. Acyclovir is used to treat genital herpes, in which it decreases viral shedding and the duration of skin lesions and pain. It does not eliminate inactive virus in the body and thus does not prevent transmission or recurrence of the disease unless oral drug therapy is continued. Acyclovir is also used for treatment of herpes labialis ("cold sores" or "fever blisters") or other herpes simplex infections in immunocompromised clients. Prolonged or repeated courses of acyclovir therapy may result in the emergence of acyclovir-resistant viral strains. This is most likely to occur in immunocompromised clients. Acyclovir can be given orally, intravenously (IV), or applied topically to lesions. IV use is recommended only for severe genital herpes in nonimmunocompromised clients and any herpes infections in immunocompromised clients.

(text continues on page 524)

TABLE 39-1	DRUGS FOR PREVENTION OR TREATMENT OF VIRAL INFECTIONS

| Generic/ Trade Name | Indications for Use | Routes and Dosage Ranges | |
		Adults	Children
Herpes Virus Infections			
Acyclovir (Zovirax)	Oral mucocutaneous lesions (*e.g.*, cold sores, fever blisters) Genital herpes Herpes simplex encephalitis Varicella (chickenpox) in immunocompromised hosts Herpes zoster (shingles) in normal and immunocompromised hosts	Genital herpes, PO 200 mg q4h, five times daily for 10 d for initial infection; 400 mg two times daily to prevent recurrence of chronic infection; 200 mg q4h five times daily for 5 d to treat recurrence Herpes zoster, PO 800 mg q4h five times daily for 7–10 d Chickenpox, PO 20 mg/kg (maximum dose 800 mg) four times daily for 5 d Mucosal and cutaneous herpes simplex virus (HSV) infections in immunocompromised hosts (ICH), IV 5 mg/kg infused at constant rate over 1 h, q8h for 7 d Varicella-zoster infections in ICH, IV 10 mg/kg, infused as above, q8h for 7 d HSV encephalitis, IV 10 mg/kg infused as above, q8h for 10 d Topically to lesions q3h, six times daily for 7 d	Children under 12 y: IV 250 mg/m^2 q8h for 7 d
Famciclovir (Famvir)	Acute herpes zoster Genital herpes, recurrent episodes	*Herpes zoster*, PO 500 mg q8h for 7 d *Genital herpes*, PO 125 mg twice daily for 5 d	Dosage not established
Foscarnet (Foscavir)	Treatment of CMV retinitis in persons with AIDS Treatment of acyclovir-resistant mucocutaneous HSV infections in immunocompromised patients	CMV retinitis, IV 60 mg/kg q8h for 2–3 wk, depending on clinical response, then 90–120 mg/kg/d for maintenance HSV infections, IV 40 mg/kg q8–12h for 2–3 wk or until lesions are healed Reduce dosage with impaired renal function	
Ganciclovir (Cytovene)	CMV retinitis in immunocompromised patients Prevention of CMV disease in persons with organ transplants or advanced HIV infection	CMV retinitis, IV 5 mg/kg q12h for 14 to 21 d, then 5 mg/kg once daily for 7 d/wk or 6 mg/kg once daily for 5 d/wk or PO 1000 mg three times daily for maintenance Prevention in transplant patients, IV 5 mg/kg once daily 7 d/wk or 6 mg/kg once daily 5 d/wk Prevention in patients with HIV infection, PO 1000 mg three times daily	
Idoxuridine (Herplex)	Keratoconjunctivitis caused by herpes viruses	Topically to eye, 0.1% solution, 1 drop q1h daytime and q2h during the night until improvement, then 1 drop q2h daytime and q4h during the night; 0.5% ointment, apply q4h during the day and at bedtime. Continue for 5 d after healing is complete.	
Trifluridine (Viroptic)	Keratoconjunctivitis caused by herpes viruses	Topically to eye, 1% ophthalmic solution, 1 drop q2h while awake (maximum 9 drops/d) until re-epithelialization of corneal ulcer occurs; then 1 drop q4h (maximum 5 drops/d) for 7 d	
Valacyclovir (Valtrex)	Herpes zoster and recurrent genital herpes in immunocompetent patients	Herpes zoster, PO 1 g q8h for 7 d Recurrent genital herpes, PO 500 mg q12h daily for 5 d Reduce dosage with renal impairment (creatinine clearance below 50 ml/min)	

TABLE 39-1 DRUGS FOR PREVENTION OR TREATMENT OF VIRAL INFECTIONS

Generic/ Trade Name	Indications for Use	Routes and Dosage Ranges	
		Adults	*Children*
Vidarabine (Vira-A)	Keratoconjunctivitis caused by herpes viruses	IV 15 mg/kg/d dissolved in 2500 ml of fluid and given over 12–24 h daily for 10 d Topically to eye, 3% ophthalmic ointment, applied q3h until re-epithelialization, then twice daily for 7 d	
Human Immunodeficiency Virus (HIV) Infection			
Didanosine (**ddI**) (Videx)	Advanced HIV infection in people who cannot tolerate zidovudine or whose condition worsens while receiving zidovudine	35–49 kg: PO 125 mg q12h 50–74 kg: PO 200 mg q12h 75 kg or more: PO 300 mg q12h	<0.4 m² body surface area (BSA): PO 25 mg q12h 0.5–0.7 m² BSA: PO 50 mg q12h 0.8–1 m² BSA: PO 75 mg q12h 1.1–1.4 m² BSA: PO 100 mg q12h
Indinavir (Crixivan)	HIV infection in adults, alone or with other antiretroviral agents	PO 800 mg q8h	Dosage not established
Lamivudine (Epivir)	HIV infection, in combination with zidovudine	PO 150 mg twice daily Weight below 50 kg (110 lb): PO 2 mg/kg twice daily Reduce dosage with renal impairment (creatinine clearance below 50 ml/min).	3 mo to 12 y: PO 4 mg/kg twice daily 12 to 16 y: PO same as adults
Nevirapine (Viramune)	HIV infection in combination withzidovudine and related drugs	PO 200 mg once daily for 2 wk, then 200 mg twice daily	Dosage not established
Ritonavir (Norvir)	HIV infection, alone or with reverse transcriptase inhibitors	PO 600 mg twice daily	Dosage not established
Saquinavir (Invirase)	Advanced HIV infection, combined with reverse transcriptase inhibitors	PO 600 mg q8h (with zalcitabine 0.75 mg or zidovudine 200 mg)	Dosage not established
Stavudine (Zerit)	HIV infection in adults who do not improve with or do not tolerate other anti-HIV medications	Patients weighing 60 kg or more, PO 40 mg q12h Patients weighing <60 kg, PO 30 mg q12h. Reduced dosage with renal impairment (creatinine clearance <50 ml/min)	Dosage not established
Zalcitabine (Hivid)	Advanced HIV infection in people whose condition worsens while receiving zidovudine Given concurrently with zidovudine	PO 0.75 mg q8h (2.25 mg/d) with zidovudine 200 mg q8h (600 mg/d)	Children weighing 30 kg or more: PO same as adults Children weighing <30 kg: PO reduce doses proportionately
Zidovudine (Retrovir)	Prevention of maternal–fetal transmission of HIV Treatment of HIV infection in children and adults	Symptomatic HIV infection, PO 100 mg q4h (total daily dose, 600 mg), IV 1–2 mg/kg q4h around the clock Asymptomatic HIV infection, PO q4h while awake (total daily dose, 500 mg) Maternal dose after 14 weeks of pregnancy, PO 100 mg five times daily until labor begins. During labor and delivery, IV 2 mg/kg over 1 h, then IV 1 mg/kg/h until umbilical cord clamped	Children 3 mo to 12 y: 180 mg/m² q6h (not to exceed 200 mg q6h) Neonate born of HIV-infected mother who took zidovudine during pregnancy, labor and delivery PO 2 mg/kg q6h starting within 12 h of birth and

(continued)

| TABLE 39-1 | DRUGS FOR PREVENTION OR TREATMENT OF VIRAL INFECTIONS (Continued) |

Generic/Trade Name	Indications for Use	Routes and Dosage Ranges	
		Adults	*Children*
			continuing until 6 wk old. If unable to take oral drug, give 1.5 mg/kg IV q6h, infused over 30 min

Influenza Virus Infection

Generic/Trade Name	Indications for Use	*Adults*	*Children*
Amantadine (Symmetrel)	Prevention or treatment of influenza A infection	PO 200 mg once daily or 100 mg twice daily Reduce dosage with renal impairment (creatinine clearance <50 ml/min)	9 to 12 y: PO 100 mg twice daily 1 to 9 y: PO 4.4 to 8.8 mg/kg/d given in one single dose or two divided doses, not to exceed 150 mg/d
Rimantadine (Flumadine)	Prevention or treatment of influenza A infection in adults Prophylaxis of influenza A in children	PO 100 mg twice daily	Under 10 y of age: 5 mg/kg once daily, not exceeding 150 mg Over 10 y of age: Same as adults

Respiratory Syncytial Virus (RSV) Infection

Generic/Trade Name	Indications for Use	*Adults*	*Children*
Ribavirin (Virazole)	Treatment of hospitalized infants and young children with severe lower respiratory tract infections		Inhalation; diluted to a concentration of 20 mg/ml for 12 to 18 h/d for 3 to 7 d

Acyclovir is excreted mainly in urine, and dosage should be decreased in clients who are elderly or have renal impairment.

Famciclovir and valacyclovir are newer oral drugs approved to treat herpes zoster and recurrent genital herpes. Famciclovir is metabolized to penciclovir, its active form, and excreted mainly in the urine. Valacyclovir is metabolized to acyclovir by enzymes in the liver or intestine or both, and excreted in the urine. As with acyclovir, dosage of these drugs must be reduced in the presence of renal insufficiency. Safety and effectiveness of these drugs during pregnancy and lactation have not been established.

Ganciclovir and **foscarnet** also inhibit viral reproduction after activation by a viral enzyme found in virus-infected cells. Ganciclovir is approved for prevention of disseminated cytomegalovirus (CMV) disease in people who are at risk, mainly those with organ transplants or advanced HIV infection. It is also approved for treatment of CMV retinitis in immunocompromised clients, including those with AIDS. Ganciclovir may improve but does not cure CMV retinitis. Ganciclovir causes hematologic toxicity (*e.g.*, granulocytopenia and thrombocytopenia) in about 20% to

40% of recipients. These effects may occur at any time during therapy but often occur during the first 2 weeks. If severe bone marrow depression occurs, ganciclovir should be discontinued. Recovery usually occurs within a week of stopping the drug. Foscarnet is approved for treatment of CMV retinitis in persons with AIDS and acyclovir-resistant mucocutaneous herpes simplex viral infections in persons with impaired immune functions. Foscarnet causes renal impairment in most recipients, and dosage of both ganciclovir and foscarnet must be reduced with renal impairment.

Idoxuridine, trifluridine, and **vidarabine** are applied topically to treat infections of the eye, such as keratoconjunctivitis and corneal ulcers caused by the herpes simplex virus (herpetic keratitis). Trifluridine may promote more rapid healing of corneal ulcers but should not be used longer than 21 days because of possible ocular toxicity. Vidarabine is as effective as idoxuridine for keratoconjunctivitis and causes less tissue irritation. Vidarabine also is given IV to treat herpes zoster infections in clients whose immune systems are impaired and encephalitis caused by herpes simplex viruses. IV dosage must be reduced with impaired renal function.

DRUGS FOR HIV INFECTION AND AIDS

Nucleoside Reverse Transcriptase Inhibitors

Didanosine, lamivudine, stavudine, zalcitabine, and **zidovudine** are used to treat HIV infection and AIDS. They are usually called nucleoside analogs or nucleoside reverse transcriptase inhibitors. Chemically, the drugs are similar in structure to one of the component parts of DNA (adenosine, cytosine, guanosine, or thymidine) and thus are able to enter human cells and viruses within human cells. Zidovudine, for example, is able to substitute for thymidine. Within the infected cell, these drugs inhibit reverse transcriptase, an enzyme required by retroviruses to convert RNA to DNA and allow replication. These drugs are most active in preventing acute infection of cells and less active in chronically infected cells, which means they slow progression of HIV infection to AIDS, but do not cure HIV infection. In addition, they do not prevent transmission of the virus through sexual contact or blood contamination.

Zidovudine (also called AZT or azidothymidine) was the first anti-HIV drug to be developed and has been the most extensively used. It is usually the first drug of choice for HIV infection, and it also is used to prevent transmission of HIV to the fetus during pregnancy. Zidovudine is rapidly absorbed with oral administration, and peak serum levels occur within approximately 1.5 hours. It penetrates cerebrospinal fluid and crosses the placenta. It is metabolized in the liver to an inactive metabolite, which is excreted in urine. Zidovudine often causes severe anemia and granulocytopenia. These hematologic effects are dose-related and usually occur within a few weeks of starting drug therapy. Management may include reducing drug dosage, discontinuing the drug, giving blood transfusions, or giving colony stimulating factors (*e.g.,* filgrastim or sargramostim) to hasten bone marrow recovery. Zidovudine may also cause peripheral neuropathy and pancreatitis. In current treatment regimens, zidovudine is usually given in combination with another reverse transcriptase inhibitor and a protease inhibitor.

Didanosine (also called ddI), considered a second-line drug, replaces an adenosine-based nucleoside. It is approved for treatment of adults and children (older than 6 months) with advanced HIV infection who do not respond to or cannot tolerate zidovudine. Lamivudine is a newer drug approved for combination therapy with zidovudine in advanced HIV infection in adults whose condition continues to deteriorate while receiving zidovudine. It is rapidly absorbed with oral administration and mainly eliminated unchanged in urine. Dosage should be reduced with renal insufficiency. Stavudine may be useful in treating strains of HIV that have developed resistance to zidovudine. In addition, about 40% of stavudine is eliminated through the kidneys, and dosage should be reduced with renal impairment. Zalcitabine (also called dideoxycytidine or ddC) is approved for combination therapy with zidovudine in advanced HIV infection in adults whose condition continues to deteriorate while receiving zidovudine. Didanosine, stavudine, and zalcitabine may cause peripheral neuropathy, and stavudine should not be given to patients who are receiving didanosine or zalcitabine because of increased risk of severe peripheral neuropathy.

Non-nucleoside Reverse Transcriptase Inhibitor

Nevirapine directly inhibits the activity of reverse transcriptase, an enzyme required by retroviruses to convert RNA to DNA and allow replication. It is indicated for treatment of patients with advanced HIV infection whose clinical status is worsening. It is used in combination with the nucleoside reverse transcriptase inhibitors described above. The two types of drugs act by different mechanisms to inhibit replication of HIV and therefore have synergistic antiviral effects. Nevirapine is not recommended for combination therapy with protease inhibitors because studies have not been done.

Nevirapine was generally well tolerated in clinical trials. The most common adverse effects were fever, headache, nausea, and skin rash. The drug did not cause the severe adverse effects associated with other anti-AIDS drugs (*e.g.,* blood dyscrasias, peripheral neuropathy, pancreatitis).

Protease Inhibitors

Indinavir, ritonavir, and **saquinavir** are protease inhibitors, drugs that attack the HIV at a different phase of its life cycle than the reverse transcriptase inhibitors described above. Protease is an enzyme in HIV-infected cells that is required to process protein precursors into mature viral particles capable of infecting other cells. The drugs inhibit the enzyme by binding to the protease-active site. This inhibition causes the production of immature, non-infectious viral particles. These drugs are active in both acutely and chronically infected cells because they block viral maturation.

Indinavir is rapidly absorbed and about 60% bound to plasma proteins. Saquinavir has low bioavailability, partly from incomplete absorption and partly from extensive first-pass metabolism in the liver. It is highly bound to plasma proteins. All three drugs are metabolized in the liver and excreted mainly in feces. These drugs are generally well tolerated but may cause gastrointestinal (GI) upset. In addition, indinavir may cause kidney stones composed of precipitated indinavir. Nephrolithiasis is more likely to occur if the patient is not well hydrated.

The protease inhibitors are metabolized in the liver by the cytochrome P450 enzyme system and should be used cautiously in patients with impaired liver function. They should be used only if necessary in pregnant women because no studies have been done. It is unknown whether the drugs are excreted in breast milk. However, the Centers for Disease Control and Prevention (CDC) advises women with HIV infection to avoid breast-feeding because HIV may be transmitted to an uninfected infant. Safety and efficacy of protease inhibitors in children have not been established.

The long-term effects of these drugs are unknown because they were approved within a few months under the FDA's accelerated process for anti-AIDS drugs. Two major concerns are viral resistance and drug interactions. Viral resistance develops fairly rapidly, with about half of recipients developing resistant strains within a year of drug therapy. It is unknown whether a viral strain resistant to one protease inhibitor will be resistant to others, although cross-resistance among protease inhibitors has been described. In relation to drug interactions, several have been identified between these drugs and others metabolized by the cytochrome P450 enzymes in the liver. The protease inhibitors interfere with metabolism, increase plasma concentrations, and increase risks of toxicity if taken with numerous other drugs. Not all interactions have been reported with all of the protease inhibitors. The most interactions have been observed with ritonavir, which is expected to increase plasma concentrations of amiodarone, astemizole, bepridil, bupropion, cisapride, clozapine, flecainide, meperidine, piroxicam, propafenone, propoxyphene, quinidine, rifabutin, and terfenadine. None of these drugs should be given concomitantly with ritonavir because high plasma concentrations may cause cardiac arrhythmias, hematologic abnormalities, seizures, and other potentially serious adverse effects. In addition, ritonavir may increase sedation and respiratory depression with the benzodiazepine antianxiety and sedative/hypnotic drugs (*e.g.,* alprazolam, clorazepate, diazepam, estazolam, flurazepam, midazolam, triazolam) and zolpidem, and should not be given concomitantly with these drugs. Indinavir increases plasma concentrations of several of the same drugs listed above (*e.g.,* astemizole, cisapride, midazolam, terfenadine, triazolam) and should not be given concomitantly with them because of potentially serious adverse effects such as cardiac arrhythmias or prolonged sedation. Saquinavir may produce fewer interactions because it inhibits the cytochrome P450 enzyme system to a lesser extent than indinavir and ritonavir. However, saquinavir should not be given concomitantly with the nonsedating antihistamines, astemizole and terfenadine, because of possible cardiac arrhythmias. In addi-

tion, if the drug is given concomitantly with clindamycin, quinidine, triazolam, or a calcium channel blocker, patients should be monitored closely for increased plasma levels and adverse drug effects.

DRUGS FOR INFLUENZA A

Amantadine and **rimantadine** inhibit replication of the influenza A virus and are used to prevent or treat influenza A infections. Postexposure prophylaxis with either drug protects contacts of persons with influenza A infections. Seasonal prophylaxis may be used in high-risk patients if the influenza vaccine cannot be given or may be ineffective. In epidemics of influenza A infections, one of the drugs is recommended for clients at high risk who have not been vaccinated. The high-risk population includes older adults, those who have chronic lung disease, and those who have immunodeficiency disorders. During an epidemic, amantadine or rimantadine may be given about 2 weeks if the client is vaccinated at the beginning of drug therapy or about 4 to 8 weeks if the client is not vaccinated. Protection is lost within a few days after drug therapy is stopped. For treatment of influenza A infection, either drug may shorten the illness if started as early as possible after onset and continued for 5 days. The drugs may also decrease viral shedding and spread of the disease.

Amantadine and rimantadine are well absorbed after oral administration. Amantadine is excreted in the urine unchanged. It accumulates in the body of elderly adults and others with impaired renal function, thus dosage should be reduced in these groups. Rimantadine is extensively metabolized, with small amounts excreted in the urine. The most common adverse effects of the drugs are GI (anorexia, nausea) and central nervous system (CNS; nervousness, lightheadedness, difficulty concentrating) symptoms. CNS effects are more likely to occur with amantadine than rimantadine, and high plasma levels of amantadine have been associated with delirium, hallucinations, seizures, coma, and cardiac arrhythmias. Amantadine has also been associated with exacerbations of pre-existing seizure disorders and psychiatric symptoms. Amantadine is teratogenic in animals, and neither drug has been established as safe for pregnant women.

Amantadine is also used in the treatment of Parkinson's disease and extrapyramidal symptoms associated with the use of some antipsychotic drugs (see Chap. 12).

DRUG FOR RESPIRATORY SYNCYTIAL VIRUS (RSV) RESPIRATORY TRACT INFECTIONS

Ribavirin is used for the treatment of severe infections of the lower respiratory tract (*e.g.,* bronchiolitis or pneumonia) caused by the RSV. It is used mainly in hospitalized infants and young children and given by inhalation with the Viratek Small Particle Aerosol Generator. The drug is not recommended for clients on ventilators because it precipitates and blocks tubes, including endotracheal tubes. Deterioration of pulmonary function is a common adverse effect. The drug is absorbed systemically following administration by aerosol. Most infants and children with RSV infections have mild, self-limited disease that does not involve the lower respiratory tract and does not require hospitalization or ribavirin therapy.

Nursing Process

Assessment

- Assessment varies with the type of viral infection and may include signs and symptoms of influenza or other viral infections of the respiratory tract, genital herpes, viral infections of the eye, or other conditions.
- Assess renal function and adequacy of fluid intake.
- With HIV infection, assess baseline data to assist in monitoring and evaluating response to drug therapy. Baseline data may include vital signs, weight and nutritional status, signs and symptoms of the disease, signs and symptoms of opportunistic infections associated with the disease and immunosuppression, and available reports of laboratory tests (*e.g.*, complete blood count, CD4+ lymphocyte counts, plasma levels of viral RNA, blood urea nitrogen and serum creatinine).

Nursing Diagnoses

- Self-Care Deficit related to systemic infection
- Anxiety related to a medical diagnosis of HIV infection, genital herpes, or CMV retinitis
- Altered Sexuality Patterns related to sexually transmitted viral infections (HIV infection, genital herpes)
- Body Image Disturbance related to sexually transmitted infection
- Social Isolation related to a medical diagnosis of HIV infection or genital herpes
- Knowledge Deficit: Disease process and methods of spread
- Knowledge Deficit: Availability of vaccines and other prophylactic interventions
- Risk for Injury: Recurrent infection
- Risk for Injury: Adverse drug effects
- Risk for Injury: Infections and other problems associated with compromised immune systems in HIV infection

Planning/Goals
The client will:
- Receive or take antiviral drugs as prescribed
- Be safeguarded against new or recurrent infection
- Act to prevent spread of viral infection to others and recurrence in self
- Avoid preventable adverse drug effects
- Receive emotional support and counseling to assist in coping with HIV infection or genital herpes

Interventions

- Follow recommended policies and procedures for preventing spread of viral infections.
- For clients receiving systemic antiviral drugs, monitor serum creatinine and other tests of renal function, complete blood count, and fluid balance.
- Spend time with the client when indicated to reduce anxiety and support usual coping mechanisms.
- For clients with HIV infection, monitor for changes in baseline data during each contact.

 Teach clients:

- Ways to control spread and recurrence of viral infection
- To maintain immunizations against viral infections as indicated
- To avoid sexual intercourse when genital herpes lesions are present because drug therapy does not eliminate the causative virus or prevent its transmission to other people
- That drug therapy for HIV does not prevent the causative virus from being transmitted to other people or the opportunistic infections and other disorders associated with the disease
- That HIV infection is a chronic, progressive illness that requires close collaboration between clients and health care providers for optimal results
- Ways to prevent or manage signs and symptoms of HIV infection, opportunistic infections, and adverse drug effects
- About available community resources

Evaluation

- Observe for improvement in signs and symptoms of the viral infection for which a drug is given.
- Interview outpatients regarding their compliance with instructions for taking antiviral drugs.
- Interview and observe for use of infection-control measures.
- Interview and observe for adverse drug effects.
- Observe the extent and severity of any symptoms in clients with HIV infection.

Principles of Therapy

PREVENTION OF VIRAL INFECTIONS

General preventive measures include vaccination, handwashing, teaching infected clients to cover their mouth and nose when coughing or sneezing, treatment of symptoms, and recognition and treatment of complications.

VIRAL VACCINES

Viral vaccines are used for active immunization of clients before exposure or to control epidemics of viral disease in a community. Vaccines for prevention of poliomyelitis, measles, rubella, mumps, smallpox, and yellow fever and for protection against influenza and rabies are available (see Chap. 43). Live attenuated viral vaccines are generally safe and nontoxic. However, they probably should not be used in clients who are pregnant, immunodeficient, or receiving corticosteroids, antineoplastic or immunosuppressive drugs, or irradiation. Influenza vaccines prevent infection in most clients. If infection does occur, less virus is shed in respiratory secretions. Thus, vaccination reduces transmission of influenza by decreasing the number of susceptible people and by decreasing transmission by immunized people who still become infected. The multiplicity of rhinoviruses (common cold), enteroviruses, and respiratory viruses precludes imminent development of practical vaccines for these common diseases.

USE OF ANTIMICROBIAL DRUGS IN VIRAL INFECTIONS

Antiviral drugs are available to prevent or treat a few specific viral infections. They should not be used unless the etiologic diagnosis is certain. Antibacterial drugs should not be used in viral infections in the hope of preventing complications. They do have a role, however, in treating bacterial complications of viral infections. For example, bacterial pneumonia may develop as a complication of influenza.

USE OF ANTIVIRAL DRUGS IN HIV INFECTION

1. Treatment of HIV infection is very dynamic, and recommendations change often as new drugs and research reports become available. Thus, one important principle for health care providers who work with clients with HIV infection is to consult current sources of information frequently.
2. Drug therapy should be started very early in the course of the infection. As a general rule, the initial infection is manifested by an illness similar to influenza, with fever, chills, and muscle aches that may last for several weeks. This period is usually followed by a quiescent phase, which may last up to 10 years, during which there may be no clinical manifestations. This quiescent phase was formerly thought to indicate viral latency and inactivity. However, research has shown that the initial infection is characterized by explosive viral growth and spread to various body tissues, especially the lymphoid system, and including the brain. The period following the initial infection is characterized by a partially effective immune system response, which decreases viral replication. However, some viral replication and destruction of lymphoid tissue continue during this period. Early treatment that reduces the viral load or burden of the body may delay progression of the disease and development of clinical signs and symptoms.
3. A combination of two or three drugs should be used to treat HIV infection. Numerous combinations are being investigated, and optimal therapy is still evolving. However, research indicates that a combination of drugs is more effective than any currently available single drug. Some clinicians prescribe two reverse transcriptase inhibitors; some add a protease inhibitor as a third drug.
4. Monitor appropriate laboratory tests to evaluate response to therapy. The preferred test (called HIV RNA levels or copies) measures the number of HIV in the blood. The extent of viremia or viral load usually decreases within a month of starting or changing anti-HIV drug therapy. Note that this test measures the virus in the blood; it does not measure viral levels in tissues, where viral reproduction may be continuing. CD4+ cell counts may also be used and would be expected to increase with effective drug therapy. Complete blood counts, tests of renal and hepatic function, and other tests are also needed.
5. Prevent opportunistic infections when possible. Therapies are available to prevent or manage several opportunistic infections that commonly occur with HIV infection (*e.g.*, CMV retinitis, herpes infections).
6. Manage signs and symptoms of HIV infection, disease complications, and adverse effects of drug therapy to promote quality of life .

USE IN CHILDREN

Most systemic antiviral drugs have not been established as safe and effective for use in children. Amantadine is given to prevent or treat influenza A in children 1 year old or older, and rimantadine is given only for prevention in children. The optimal dose and duration of amantadine or rimantadine therapy have not been established.

There are few guidelines for the use of anti-HIV drugs in children. Most HIV infections in children result from perinatal transmission. Thus, pregnant women with possible exposure to HIV should be tested and, if HIV positive, should receive zidovudine to prevent perinatal transmission. Following delivery, zidovudine is given to the infant for the first 6 weeks of life. If perinatal infection occurs, the infant usually develops symptoms (*e.g.*, an opportunistic infection or failure to thrive) within the first 3 to 8 months of life and the disease continues to progress rapidly. Zidovudine is approved for treatment of HIV infection in children and is usually the drug of choice. As in adults, anemia and neutropenia are common adverse effects of zidovudine.

For children who do not respond to zidovudine, didanosine may be given. Zalcitabine is approved for combination therapy with zidovudine in adolescents but not children. Newer drugs are being studied for use in children.

USE IN OLDER ADULTS

Most of the systemic antiviral drugs are excreted by the kidneys. Because renal impairment is common in older adults, there probably are greater risks of toxicity. These risks may be minimized by reducing drug dosage when indicated by decreased creatinine clearance, close monitoring of renal function, and maintaining adequate fluid intake. When amantadine is given to prevent or treat influenza A, dosage should be reduced with renal impairment, and older adults must be monitored closely for CNS effects (*e.g.*, hallucinations, depression, confusion) and cardiovascular effects (*e.g.*, congestive heart failure, orthostatic hypotension). Rimantadine reportedly causes fewer CNS effects.

HOME CARE

Most antiviral drugs are self-administered by clients or given by caregivers in the home setting. Precautions to prevent viral infections from occurring or spreading are especially important because of the close contacts among members of a household. The home care nurse may need to teach infection control precautions to household members. In addition, the home care nurse needs to assess the immunization status of all household members. If immunizations are indicated, the nurse may need to teach, encourage, provide, or somehow facilitate their accomplishment.

Home care of clients with HIV infection may include a variety of activities such as assisting with drug therapy for HIV infection or opportunistic infections, coordinating medical and social services, managing symptoms of the disease or adverse drug effects, preventing or minimizing opportunistic infections, teaching clients and others that HIV infection is a chronic illness that progresses differently among individuals, and making referrals for hospitalization or hospice care when indicated.

NURSING ACTIONS	RATIONALE/EXPLANATION
1. Administer accurately **a.** Give most oral antiviral drugs without regard to meals; give ganciclovir, ritonavir and saquinavir with food; give indinavir on an empty stomach if possible	Manufacturers' recommendations to promote absorption and bioavailability
b. Give IV acyclovir, ganciclovir and foscarnet over 1 h	To decrease tissue irritation and increased toxicity from high plasma levels
c. With topical acyclovir, wear a glove to apply	To prevent spread of infection, because lesions contain herpesvirus
d. With ribavarin, follow the manufacturer's instructions	Specific techniques are required for accurate usage
2. Observe for therapeutic effects **a.** With acyclovir for genital herpes, observe for fewer recurrences when given for prophylaxis; observe for healing of lesions and decreased pain and itching when given for treatment.	
b. With amantadine, observe for absence of symptoms when given for prophylaxis of influenza A and decreased fever, cough, muscle aches, and malaise when given for treatment.	
c. With ganciclovir or foscarnet for CMV retinitis, observe for improved vision.	

(continued)

NURSING ACTIONS	*RATIONALE/EXPLANATION*
d. With idoxuridine and other ophthalmic drugs, observe for decreased signs of eye infection.	
e. With anti-HIV drugs, observe for improved clinical status (fewer signs and symptoms) and improved laboratory markers (*e.g.*, decreased viral load, increased CD4+ cell count)	
3. Observe for adverse effects	
a. General effects—anorexia, nausea, vomiting, diarrhea, fever, headache	These effects occur with most systemic antiviral drugs and may range from mild to severe.
b. With IV acyclovir—phlebitis at injection site, skin rash, urticaria, increased BUN or serum creatinine, encephalopathy manifested by confusion, coma, lethargy, seizures, tremors	Encephalopathy is rare but potentially serious; other effects commonly occur.
c. With topical acyclovir—burning or stinging and pruritus	These effects are usually transient.
d. With amantadine and rimantadine—CNS effects with anxiety, ataxia, dizziness, hyperexcitability, insomnia, mental confusion, hallucinations, slurred speech	CNS symptoms are reportedly more likely with amantadine than with rimantadine and may be similar to those caused by atropine and CNS stimulants. Adverse reactions are more likely to occur in older adults and those with renal impairment.
e. With didanosine and zalcitabine—peripheral neuropathy (numbness, burning, pain in hands and feet), pancreatitis (abdominal pain, severe nausea and vomiting, elevated serum amylase)	Peripheral neuropathy may be more likely with zalcitabine, and the drug should be stopped promptly if symptoms appear, to avoid irreversible neuropathy. Pancreatitis may be more likely with didanosine, especially in those with previous episodes, alcohol consumption, elevated serum triglycerides, or advanced HIV infection. Didanosine should be stopped promptly if symptoms of pancreatitis occur.
f. With ganciclovir and foscarnet—bone marrow depression (anemia, leukopenia, neutropenia, thrombocytopenia), renal impairment (increased serum creatinine and decreased creatinine clearance), neuropathy	Renal impairment may be more likely to occur with foscarnet.
g. With indinavir, ritonavir, and saquinavir—circumoral and peripheral paresthesias, debilitation, fatigue	The most frequent adverse effects are the general ones listed above. Most are relatively mild. However, other adverse reactions may emerge with more extensive clinical usage.
h. With lamivudine and stavudine—peripheral neuropathy, flu-like syndrome (fever, malaise, muscle and joint aches or pain), dizziness, insomnia, depression	
i. With ribavirin—increased respiratory distress	Pulmonary function may deteriorate.
j. With zidovudine—bone marrow depression (anemia, leukopenia, granulocytopenia, thrombocytopenia); anemia and neutropenia in newborn infants	Anemia may occur within 2–4 wk of starting the drug; granulocytopenia is more likely after 6–8 wk. A complete blood count should be done every 2 wk. Dosage should be reduced with moderate bone marrow depression (BMD), and the drug should be stopped with severe BMD (hemoglobin below 7.5 g/dl; granulocyte count below 750 mm^3), until the bone marrow recovers. Colony-stimulating factors (filgrastim or sargramostim) may be given to aid recovery of bone marrow function. Blood transfusions may be given for anemia.
	The hematologic effects on newborn infants may occur when the mothers received zidovudine during pregnancy.
k. With ophthalmic antiviral drugs—pain, itching, edema, or inflammation of the eyelids	These symptoms are more likely to occur with idoxuridine than with vidarabine. They result from tissue irritation or hypersensitivity reactions.

NURSING ACTIONS	*RATIONALE/EXPLANATION*
4. Observe for drug interactions	Antiviral drugs are often given concomitantly with each other and with many other drugs, especially those used to treat opportunistic infections and other illnesses associated with HIV infection and organ transplantation. In general, combinations of drugs that cause similar, potentially serious adverse effects (*e.g.*, bone marrow depression, peripheral neuropathy) should be avoided, when possible.
a. Drugs that *increase* effects of acyclovir	
(1) Probenecid	May increase blood levels of acyclovir by slowing its renal excretion
(2) Zidovudine	Severe drowsiness and lethargy may occur.
b. Drugs that *increase* effects of amantadine and rimantadine	
(1) Anticholinergics—atropine, first-generation antihistamines, antipsychotics, tricyclic antidepressants	These drugs add to the anticholinergic effects (*e.g.*, blurred vision, mouth dryness, urine retention, constipation, tachycardia) of the antiviral agents.
(2) CNS stimulants	These drugs add to the CNS-stimulating effects (*e.g.*, confusion, insomnia, nervousness, hyperexcitability) of the antiviral agents.
c. Drugs that *increase* effects of foscarnet	
Aminoglycoside antibiotics, amphotericin B, didanosine, IV pentamidine	These drugs are nephrotoxic and may increase risks of nephrotoxicity with foscarnet by impairing its elimination. Foscarnet should not be combined with nephrotoxic agents unless expected benefits outweigh potential risks.
d. Drugs that *increase* effects of ganciclovir	
(1) Imipenem/cilastatin	Increased risk of seizures; avoid the combination if possible.
(2) Nephrotoxic drugs (*e.g.*, amphotericin B, cyclosporine)	Increased serum creatinine and potential nephrotoxicity
(3) Probenecid	May increase blood levels of ganciclovir by decreasing its renal excretion
e. Drugs that *increase* effects of indinavir	
Clarithromycin, ketoconazole, quinidine, zidovudine	Increase blood levels of indinavir, probably by decreasing its metabolism and elimination
f. Drugs that *decrease* effects of indinavir	
(1) Didanosine	Didanosine increases gastric pH and decreases absorption of indinavir. If the two drugs are given concurrently, give at least 1 h apart, on an empty stomach.
(2) Fluconazole	Decreases blood levels of indinavir
(3) Rifampin, rifabutin	These drugs speed up metabolism of indinavir by inducing hepatic drug-metabolizing enzymes
g. Drug that *increases* the effects of lamivudine	
Trimethoprim/sulfamethoxazole	Decreases elimination of lamivudine
h. Drugs that *increase* the effects of ritonavir	
Clarithromycin, fluconazole, fluoxetine	Increase blood levels, probably by slowing metabolism of ritonavir

(continued)

NURSING ACTIONS	RATIONALE/EXPLANATION
i. Drug that *decreases* the effects of ritonavir	
Rifampin	Accelerates metabolism of ritonavir by inducing drug-metabolizing enzymes in the liver
j. Drug that *increases* the effects of saquinavir	
Ketoconazole	Increases blood levels of saquinavir
k. Drugs that *decrease* the effects of saquinavir	
Rifampin, rifabutin	Accelerate metabolism of ritonavir by inducing drug-metabolizing enzymes in the liver
l. Drugs that *increase* the effects of zalcitabine	
(1) Chloramphenicol, cisplatin, didanosine, ethionamide, isoniazid, metronidazole, nitrofurantoin, phenytoin, ribavirin, vincristine	Zalcitabine and these drugs are associated with peripheral nephropathy; concomitant use increases risks of this adverse effect. Didanosine and zalcitabine should not be used concomitantly.
(2) Cimetidine, probenecid	Increase blood levels of zalcitabine by decreasing its elimination
(3) Pentamidine (IV)	Increased risk of pancreatitis. If IV pentamidine is used to treat *Pneumocystis carinii* pneumonia, zalcitabine should be interrupted.
m. Drugs that *decrease* effects of zalcitabine	
Antacids, metoclopramide	Decrease absorption. Do not give antacids at the same time as zalcitabine.
n. Drugs that *increase* effects of zidovudine	
(1) Doxorubicin, vincristine, vinblastine	Increased bone marrow depression, including neutropenia
(2) Amphotericin B, flucytosine	Increased nephrotoxicity
(3) Ganciclovir and pentamidine	Increased neutropenia
(4) Probenecid, trimethoprim	May increase blood levels of zidovudine, probably by decreasing renal excretion
o. Drugs that *decrease* effects of zidovudine	
Rifampin, rifabutin	Accelerate metabolism of zidovudine
5. Teach clients:	
a. With acyclovir, famciclovir, and valacyclovir for genital herpes:	The drugs do not cure or prevent transmission of herpesvirus infections.
(1) Avoid sexual intercourse when visible lesions are present.	
(2) Always wash hands after touching any lesion.	
(3) Start oral drugs for recurrent lesions as soon as signs and symptoms begin.	
(4) Use gloves to apply acyclovir ointment to lesions.	
b. With foscarnet or ganciclovir for CMV retinitis	
(1) Have eye examinations about every 6 wk	These drugs do not cure or prevent progression of CMV retinitis.

NURSING ACTIONS	RATIONALE/EXPLANATION
c. With didanosine, lamivudine, stavudine, zalcitabine, zidovudine for HIV infection:	These drugs do not cure HIV infection or prevent illnesses associated with AIDS.
(1) Take medications exactly as prescribed.	To increase therapeutic effects and minimize adverse effects
(2) Use appropriate precautions to prevent spread of HIV infection.	These drugs do not prevent transmission of HIV infection by sexual intercourse or blood contamination.
(3) Have regular blood tests of viral load, CD4+ cell count, CBC, and others as indicated.	These tests are required to assess therapeutic and adverse effects of the drugs.
(4) Report signs and symptoms of bone marrow depression, peripheral neuropathy, pancreatitis, hepatotoxicity, and other adverse drug effects to a health care provider.	
d. With indinavir, ritonavir, or saquinavir:	These drugs do not cure HIV infection, prevent illnesses associated with AIDS, or prevent transmission of HIV infection by sexual intercourse or blood contamination.
(1) How to take in relation to food.	
(2) Take every day; do not change the dose or stop taking without consulting a health care provider. If a dose is missed, do not double the next dose.	To increase therapeutic effects and minimize adverse effects
(3) Report any other medications being taken.	These drugs, especially ritonavir, interact to increase or decrease the effects of several other drugs.

REVIEW AND APPLICATION EXERCISES

1. Why is it difficult to develop clinically useful antiviral drugs?

2. What is the major effect of antiviral drugs on susceptible viruses?

3. Which viral infections may be prevented by administration of an antiviral drug?

4. What are the major adverse effects associated with commonly used antiviral drugs? How would you assess for each of the adverse effects?

5. Why is it important to monitor renal function in any client receiving a systemic antiviral drug?

6. What is the advantage of combination drug therapy for HIV infection?

7. List nursing interventions to prevent or minimize adverse effects of anti-HIV drugs.

SELECTED REFERENCES

Carpenter, C.C., Fischl, M.A., Hammer, S.M. et al.(1996). Antiretroviral therapy for HIV infection in 1996: Recommendations of an international panel. *Journal of the American Medical Association, 276*(2), 146–154.

Collier, A.C. (1996). Efficacy of combination antiretroviral therapy. In J. Mills, P.A. Volberding & L. Corey (Eds.), *Antiviral chemotherapy*, pp. 355–372. New York: Plenum Press.

Crumpacker, C.S. (1996). Ganciclovir. *The New England Journal of Medicine, 335*(10), 721–729.

Deitz, S.E. (1994). Acquired immunodeficiency syndrome (AIDS). In C.M. Porth, *Pathophysiology: Concepts of altered health states*, 4th ed., pp. 283–296. Philadelphia: J.B. Lippincott.

Drug facts and comparisons. (Updated monthly). St. Louis: Facts and Comparisons.

Goldschmidt, R.H. & Moy, A. (1996). Antiretroviral drug treatment for HIV/AIDS. *American Family Physician, 54*(2), 574–580.

Hayden, F.G. (1996). Antiviral agents. In J.G. Hardman, L.E. Limbird, P.B. Molinoff & R.W. Ruddon (Eds.), *Goodman & Gilman's The pharmacological basis of therapeutics*, 9th ed., pp. 1191–1223. New York: McGraw-Hill.

Hoernle, E.H. & Reid, T.E. (1995). Human immunodeficiency virus infection in children. *American Journal of Health-System Pharmacy, 52*, 961–979.

Tartaglione, T.A., Fletcher, C.V. & Collier, A.C. (1993). Principles and management of the acquired immunodeficiency syndrome. In J.T. Dipiro, R.L. Talbert, P.E. Hayes, G.C. Yee, G.R. Matzke & L.M. Posey (Eds.). *Pharmacotherapy: A pathophysiologic approach*, 2nd ed., pp. 1837–1867. Norwalk, CT: Appleton & Lange.

Volk, W.A., Gebhardt, B.M., Hammarskjold, M.L. & Kadner, R.J. (1996). *Essentials of medical microbiology*, 5th ed. Philadelphia: Lippincott-Raven.

Antifungal Drugs

Outline

Fungi and Fungal Infections

Antifungal Drugs
mechanism of action

Nursing Process
assessment
nursing diagnoses
planning/goals
interventions
evaluation

Principles of Therapy
diagnostic and therapeutic factors
decreasing adverse effects of amphotericin B
use in children
use in older adults
home care

Objectives

After studying this chapter, the student will be able to:

1 Describe distinctive characteristics of fungi and fungal infections.

2 Discuss antibacterial drug therapy and immunosuppression as risk factors for developing fungal infections.

3 Describe commonly used antifungal drugs in terms of indications for use, adverse effects, and nursing process implications.

4 Differentiate between adverse effects associated with systemic and topical antifungal drugs.

5 List interventions to decrease adverse effects of IV amphotericin B.

Key Terms

Candidiasis	**Mycoses**
Dermatophytes	

Fungi and Fungal Infections

Fungi are plant-like, parasitic microorganisms that are widely dispersed in the environment. Humans are often unavoidably exposed to fungi; conditions in which exposure is followed by infection are not fully known. Mechanisms of infection include inhalation of air-borne spores, oral ingestion, and implantation of the fungus under the skin as a result of injury. Fungal infections (mycoses) range from mild, superficial infections to life-threatening systemic infections. Serious systemic fungal infections have become more common, largely because of acquired immunodeficiency syndrome (AIDS), the use of immunosuppressant drugs to treat cancer and organ transplant recipients, the use of indwelling intravenous (IV) catheters for prolonged drug therapy or parenteral nutrition, more frequent implantation of prosthetic devices, and widespread use of broad-spectrum antibacterial drugs. Additional characteristics of fungi and fungal infections include the following:

1. Fungi that cause superficial infections of the skin, hair, and nails are called *dermatophytes*. These fungi are often present on the body without causing infection. They obtain nourishment from keratin, a protein in skin, hair, and nails. Dermatophytic infections include tinea pedis (athlete's foot) and tinea capitis (ringworm of the scalp; see Chap. 66).
2. *Candida albicans* is usually part of the indigenous microbial flora of the skin, mouth, intestine, and vagina. It causes infection in certain circumstances. Vaginal candidiasis is common in women who are pregnant, have diabetes mellitus, or take oral contraceptives. Oral candidiasis (thrush) is common in newborns. Oral, intestinal, vaginal, and systemic candidiasis can occur with antibiotic, antineoplastic, corticosteroid, and immunosuppressant drug therapy. Systemic candidiasis also occurs in clients receiving parenteral nutrition and in those with burn wounds, organ transplants, and immune disorders, such as AIDS. *Candida* may cause endocarditis after insertion of a prosthetic heart valve.
3. Fungi that cause other serious infections are not part of the indigenous microbial flora. These fungi grow independently in soil and decaying organic matter. Fungal infections, such as histoplasmosis, coccidioidomycosis, and blastomycosis, usually occur as pulmonary disease but may be systemic. Severity of disease increases with intensity of exposure.
   a. Histoplasmosis is endemic in many parts of the world. Most infections are asymptomatic or produce minimal symptoms for which treatment is not sought. Clinically evident symptoms are usually those of an acute, influenza-like respiratory infection. The disease occasionally occurs as a rapidly fatal infection involving the liver, spleen, and other organs. Healed lung lesions may calcify and be confused with the lesions of tuberculosis. The fungus causing histoplasmosis is found in soil and organic debris, especially around chicken houses, bird roosts, and caves inhabited by bats.
   b. Coccidioidomycosis usually occurs as an acute, self-limiting respiratory infection but may occur as a chronic, diffuse disease involving almost any body part.
   c. Blastomycosis most often causes respiratory infection that resembles pneumonia or tuberculosis. Other organs may be involved, however, especially the skin. Skin pustules, ulcerations, and abscesses may occur.

Antifungal Drugs

Drugs for superficial fungal infections of skin and mucous membranes are usually applied topically. Numerous preparations are available, many without a prescription. Drugs for systemic infections are given IV or orally. Amphotericin B is considered the drug of choice for most serious fungal infections. It must be given IV and produces numerous adverse effects in most recipients. The azole antifungal agents (*e.g.*, fluconazole, itraconazole, ketoconazole) are also widely used and may be better tolerated by most patients. Fluconazole can be given orally or IV; the others are given orally. Fluconazole and itraconazole increase serum levels, prolong half-lives, or decrease the clearance of numerous drugs. These drug interactions increase the risks of adverse effects with nonsedating antihistamines (*e.g.*, terfenadine, astemizole), cyclosporine, phenytoin, sulfonylureas, theophylline, warfarin and zidovudine. Indications for use and dosages of individual antifungal drugs are listed in Table 40-1.

MECHANISM OF ACTION

Most antifungal drugs bind with essential components in fungal cell membranes. This binding increases permeability of the cell membrane and allows intracellular contents to leak out.

Nursing Process

Assessment

Assess for fungal infections. Specific signs and symptoms vary with location and type of infection.
● Superficial lesions of skin, hair, and nails are usually characterized by pain, burning, and itching. Some lesions are moist;

TABLE 40-1 **SELECTED ANTIFUNGAL DRUGS**

Generic/ Trade Name	Clinical Indications	Routes and Dosage Ranges Adults	Children
Amphotericin B (Fungizone, Abelcet)	Systemic mycoses (*e.g.*, candidiasis, histoplasmosis, blastomycosis, others) Cutaneous candidiaisis	IV, individualized according to disease severity and client tolerance. Optimal dose unknown; average dose 0.25–0.5 mg/kg/d Topically to skin lesions, two to four times daily for 1–4 wk (Abelcet) IV, 5 mg/kg/d	Same as for adults Same as for adults
Butoconazole (Femstat)	Vaginal candidiasis	Intravaginally, once daily for 3 d	
Ciclopirox (Loprox)	Tinea infections, cutaneous candidiasis	Topically to skin lesions, twice daily for 2–4 wk	
Clotrimazole (Lotrimin, Mycelex, Gyne-Lotrimin)	Cutaneous dermatophytosis; oral, cutaneous, and vaginal candidiasis	Orally, 1 troche dissolved in mouth five times daily Topically to skin twice daily Intravaginally, once daily	Same as for adults Dosage not established
Econazole (Spectazole)	Tinea infections, cutaneous candidiasis	Topically to skin lesions, once or twice daily for 2-4 wk	
Fluconazole (Diflucan)	Oropharyngeal, esophageal, and systemic candidiasis; cryptococcal meningitis	Oral or esophageal infection, PO, IV 200 mg on first day, then 100 mg daily for 2–3 wk Systemic infection, PO, IV 400 mg on first day, then 200 mg daily for at least 4 wk and 2 wk after symptoms subside Cryptococcal meningitis, PO, IV 400 mg on first day, then 200 mg daily for 10–12 wk after cultures of cerebrospinal fluid become negative	
Flucytosine (Ancobon)	Systemic mycoses due to *Candida* species or *Cryptococcus neoformans*	PO 50–150 mg/kg/d in divided doses q6h. Dosage must be decreased with impaired liver function	Same as for adults
Griseofulvin (Fulvicin)	Dermatophytosis (skin, hair, nails)	Microsize, PO 500 mg–1 g daily in divided doses q6h Ultramicrosize, PO 250–500 mg daily	Microsize, PO 10 mg/kg in divided doses q6h Ultramicrosize, PO 5–7 mg/kg/d
Haloprogin (Halotex)	Dermatophytosis, mainly tinea pedis (athlete's foot), cutaneous candidiasis	Topically to skin, 1% cream or solution twice daily for 2–4 wk	Dosage not established
Itraconazole (Sporanox)	Systemic fungal infections, including aspergillosis, in neurotropenic and immunocompromised hosts	PO 200 mg once or twice daily	
Ketoconazole (Nizoral)	Candidiasis, histoplasmosis, coccidioidomycosis, paracoccidioidomycosis	PO 200 mg once daily, increased to 400 mg once daily if necessary in severe infections	Weight above 40 kg: PO 200 mg once daily Weight 20–40 kg: PO 100 mg (1/2 tablet) once daily Weight under 20 kg: PO 50 mg (1/4 tablet) once daily
Miconazole (Monistat)	Systemic mycoses Dermatophytosis, cutaneous and vulvovaginal candidiasis	IV 600 mg–1 g q8h Topically to skin, once or twice daily for 4 wk Intravaginally, once daily for 1–2 wk	IV 20–40 mg/kg/d in divided infusions

TABLE 40-1   SELECTED ANTIFUNGAL DRUGS (Continued)

Generic/ Trade Name	Clinical Indications	Routes and Dosage Ranges	
		Adults	*Children*
Naftifine (Naftin)	Tinea infections (athlete's foot, jock itch, ringworm)	Topically to skin, once daily (cream) or twice daily (gel)	Safety and efficacy not established
Natamycin (Natacyn)	Fungal infections of the eye	Topically to eye, 1 drop q1–2h for 3–4 d, then 1 drop six to eight times daily for 14–24 d	
Nystatin (Mycostatin)	Candidiasis of skin, mucous membrane, and intestinal tract	Oral or intestinal infection, PO 400,000–600,000 U four times daily Topically to skin lesions, two or three times daily, continued for 1 wk after cure Intravaginally, 1 vaginal tablet once daily for 14 d	Oral infection, PO 100,000 U three or four times daily
Oxiconazole (Oxistat)	Tinea infections	Topically to skin lesions, once daily in evening, for 2–4 wk	
Sulconazole (Exelderm)	Tinea infections	Topically to skin lesions once or twice daily for 3 to 4 wk	Safety and efficacy not established
Terconazole (Terazol)	Vaginal candidiasis	Intravaginally, 1 applicator once daily at bedtime for 7 doses	
Terbinafine (Lamisil)	Tinea infections Onychomycosis of fingernails or toenails	*Tinea infections*, topically to skin, once or twice daily for at least 1 wk and no longer than 4 wk *Fingernail infections*, PO 250 mg daily for 6 wk *Toenail infections*, PO 250 mg daily for 12 wk	Same as for adults Dosage not established
Tioconazole (Vagistat)	Vaginal candidiasis	Intravaginally, 1 applicator at bedtime	
Tolnaftate (Tinactin)	Cutaneous mycoses (dermatophytosis)	Topically to skin lesions, twice daily for 2–6 wk	Same as for adults
Triacetin (Fungoid)	Dermatophytosis (*e.g.,* athlete's foot), cutaneous candidiasis	Topically to skin lesions, twice daily until 1 wk after symptoms are relieved	Same as for adults
Zinc undecylenate (Desenex)	Dermatophytosis	Topically to skin twice daily for 2–4 wk	Same as for adults

others are dry and scaling. They also may appear inflamed or discolored.

- Candidiasis occurs in warm, moist areas of the body. Skin lesions are likely to occur in perineal and intertriginous areas. They are usually moist, inflamed, pruritic areas with vesicles and pustules. Oral lesions are white patches that adhere to the buccal mucosa. Vaginal infection causes a cheesy vaginal discharge, burning, and itching. Intestinal infection causes diarrhea.
- Histoplasmosis, coccidioidomycosis, and blastomycosis often simulate influenza, pneumonia, or tuberculosis, with cough, fever, malaise, and other pulmonary manifestations.
- Systemic mycoses are confirmed by recovery of organisms from specimens of body tissues or fluids.

Nursing Diagnoses

- Self-Care Deficit related to systemic infection
- Knowledge Deficit: Prevention and treatment of fungal infection

- Knowledge Deficit: Accurate drug usage
- Noncompliance related to the need for long-term therapy
- Risk for Injury: Adverse drug effects with systemic antifungal drugs

Planning/Goals

The client will:
- Receive systemic antifungal drugs as prescribed
- Apply topical drugs accurately
- Act to prevent recurrence of fungal infection
- Avoid preventable adverse effects from systemic drugs

Interventions

Use measures to prevent spread of fungal infections. Superficial infections (*e.g.,* ringworm or tinea) are highly contagious and can be spread by sharing towels and hairbrushes. Systemic mycoses are not contagious.

With neutropenic and other immunocompromised clients, try to decrease exposure to environmental fungi. For example, do not allow soil-containing plants and request regular cleaning and inspection of air conditioning systems. Aspergillosis has occurred following inhalation of air-borne spores from air conditioning units.

Teach clients:

- With skin lesions, wash hands often; do not share towels, hairbrushes, or other personal items.
- With histoplasmosis and other potentially serious fungal infections, avoid or minimize future exposure to chicken, pigeon, and bat excreta.

Evaluation

- Observe for relief of symptoms for which an antifungal drug was prescribed.
- Interview outpatients regarding their compliance with instructions for using antifungal drugs.
- Interview and observe for adverse drug effects with systemic antifungal agents.

Principles of Therapy

DIAGNOSTIC AND THERAPEUTIC FACTORS

1. An etiologic diagnosis should be made before an antifungal drug is used. Local infections can be caused by bacteria, fungi, or both. Most antifungal drugs are ineffective in bacterial infections. Antifungal drugs effective in candidiasis are not usually effective in dermatophytic infections and vice versa.
2. Candidal infections of blood or urine often respond to the removal of predisposing factors, such as antibiotics, corticosteroids or other immunosuppressive drugs, and indwelling IV or bladder catheters. Candidal endocarditis, which may occur after prosthetic heart valve replacement, is best treated by surgical removal of the infected prosthesis and administration of amphotericin B.
3. Most antifungal drug therapy is long term (several weeks to months).

DECREASING ADVERSE EFFECTS OF AMPHOTERICIN B

Several recommendations for reducing toxicity of IV amphotericin B have evolved, but most of them have not been tested in controlled studies. Recommendations to decrease fever and chills include premedication with acetaminophen, aspirin or ibuprofen, diphenhydramine, IV corticosteroid, and meperidine. Recommendations to decrease nephrotoxicity include

IV administration of a liter of sodium chloride 0.9% solution and monitoring serum creatinine and blood urea nitrogen (BUN) at least weekly. The drug should be stopped or dosage should be reduced until renal function recovers if the BUN exceeds 40 mg/dl or the serum creatinine exceeds 3 mg/dl. Recommendations to decrease phlebitis at injection sites include administering on alternate days, adding 500 to 2000 units of heparin to the infusion, rotating infusion sites, and administering through a large central vein. Supplemental potassium may be used to treat hypokalemia, and recombinant erythropoietin may be used to treat anemia, if the client has a low plasma level of erythropoietin.

USE IN CHILDREN

Antifungal drugs are used in children for the same indications as for adults. Few studies with oral and parenteral drugs have been done in children. Dosages are often listed for children older than 1 or 2 years.

No pediatric guidelines have been established for IV amphotericin B (Fungizone), a highly toxic drug often used for serious systemic infections. As with adults, children receiving this drug must be monitored closely to reduce the incidence and severity of nephrotoxicity, hypokalemia, and other adverse effects.

Guidelines for topical agents are the same as those for adults.

USE IN OLDER ADULTS

No geriatric guidelines have been established for antifungal drugs. The main concern is with oral or parenteral drugs, because topical agents produce few adverse effects.

Virtually all adults receiving IV amphotericin B experience kidney damage and other adverse effects. With the impaired renal and cardiovascular functions that usually accompany aging, older adults are especially vulnerable to serious adverse effects. They must be monitored closely to reduce the incidence and severity of nephrotoxicity, hypokalemia, and other adverse drug reactions.

 HOME CARE

Antifungal drugs may be taken at home by a variety of routes. For topical and oral routes, the role of the home care nurse may be teaching correct usage and encouraging clients to persist with the long-term treatment usually required. With IV antifungal drugs for serious infections, the home care nurse may need to assist in administration and monitoring for adverse reactions.

ANTIFUNGAL DRUGS

NURSING ACTIONS	RATIONALE/EXPLANATION

1. Administer accurately

a. Give conventional IV amphotericin B in 5% dextrose in water, over 4–6 h; give the liposomal preparation (Abelcet) over 2 h.

These drug infusions should be prepared in a pharmacy, according to manufacturers' instructions.

b. With IV fluconazole, follow instructions for preparation carefully; give as a continuous infusion at a maximum rate of 200 mg/h.

c. For IV miconazole, dilute in at least 200 ml of 0.9% saline or 5% dextrose and infuse over 60 min or longer.

To prevent cardiorespiratory toxicity during infusion

d. For ketoconazole, do not give antacids, anticholinergics, or cimetidine within 2 h of administration of ketoconazole. For clients with achlorhydria, dissolve ketoconazole tablets in 4 ml aqueous solution of 0.2 N hydrochloric acid, and have them drink the mixture through a straw and then drink 8 oz of tap water.

The drug is dissolved and absorbed only in an acid environment.

e. For nystatin, the suspension should be swished in the mouth for a few minutes before swallowing.

To increase contact with oral lesions

2. Observe for therapeutic effects

a. Decreased fever and malaise with systemic mycoses

b. Healing of lesions on skin and mucous membranes

c. Diminished diarrhea with intestinal candidiasis

d. Decreased vaginal discharge and discomfort with vaginal candidiasis

3. Observe for adverse effects

a. With amphotericin B, observe for fever, chills, anorexia, nausea, vomiting, renal damage (elevated blood urea nitrogen and serum creatinine), hypokalemia, hypomagnesemia, headache, stupor, coma, convulsions, anemia from bone marrow depression, phlebitis at venipuncture sites, anaphylaxis.

Amphotericin B is a highly toxic drug, and most recipients develop some adverse reactions, including some degree of renal damage. Antipyretic and antiemetic drugs may be given to help minimize adverse reactions and promote patient comfort. Adequate hydration may decrease renal damage.

b. With flucytosine, observe for nausea, vomiting, and diarrhea.

These are common effects. Hepatic, renal, and hematologic functions also may be affected. Drug resistance often develops when flucytosine is used alone.

c. With IV miconazole, observe for nausea, phlebitis, anemia, thrombocytopenia, and pruritus.

d. With ketoconazole, observe for nausea, vomiting, pruritus, and abdominal pain.

Adverse effects are mild and transient.

e. With griseofulvin, observe for gastrointestinal symptoms, hypersensitivity (urticaria, photosensitivity, skin rashes, angioedema), headache, mental confusion, fatigue, dizziness, peripheral neuritis, and blood dyscrasias (leukopenia, neutropenia, granulocytopenia).

Incidence of serious reactions is very low.

f. With oral terbinafine, observe for diarrhea, dyspepsia, headache, skin rash or itching, liver enzyme abnormalities.

(continued)

NURSING ACTIONS	RATIONALE/EXPLANATION
g. With topical drugs, observe for skin rash and irritation.	Adverse reactions are usually minimal with topical drugs, although hypersensitivity may occur.
4. Observe for drug interactions:	
a. Drugs that increase effects of amphotericin B:	
(1) Antineoplastic drugs	May increase risks of nephrotoxicity, hypotension, and bronchospasm
(2) Corticosteroids	May potentiate hypokalemia and precipitate cardiac dysfunction.
(3) Zidovudine	Increases renal and hematologic adverse effects of the liposomal formulation of amphotericin B. Renal and hematologic functions should be monitored closely.
b. Drug that *increases* effects of fluconazole: Hydrochlorothiazide	Increased serum level of fluconazole, attributed to decreased renal excretion
c. Drugs that *decrease* effects of fluconazole Cimetidine, rifampin	Decrease serum levels
d. Drugs that *decrease* effects of griseofulvin: Barbiturates and other drugs that induce liver enzymes	Enzyme inducers inhibit effects of griseofulvin by increasing its rate of metabolism.
e. Drugs that *decrease* effects of itraconazole Histamine H$_2$ antagonists, phenytoin, rifampin	Decrease serum levels
f. Drugs that *decrease* effects of ketoconazole:	
(1) Antacids, histamine H$_2$ antagonists	These drugs increase gastric pH; this may inhibit absorption of ketoconazole.
(2) Isoniazid, rifampin	Decrease serum levels
g. Drug that *decreases* effects of terbinafine Rifampin	Causes rapid clearance of terbinafine
5. Teach clients	
a. Take drugs as prescribed.	To avoid recurrence of the infection. Drugs often must be taken several weeks after symptoms subside.
b. Report severe adverse effects.	Drug administration may need to be altered or discontinued.
c. With topical skin preparations, wash and dry the area before each application of medication.	
d. With vaginal antifungal preparations	
(1) Read instructions carefully, with prescribed and over-the-counter drugs.	
(2) Insert high into the vagina (except during pregnancy).	
(3) Continue use through menstruation.	
(4) Wear a minipad to avoid staining clothing; do not use a tampon.	
(5) Wash applicator with mild soap and rinse thoroughly after each use.	
(6) Avoid sexual intercourse while using the drug.	

REVIEW AND APPLICATION EXERCISES

1. What environmental factors predispose clients to develop fungal infections?

2. What signs and symptoms occur with candidiasis, and how would you assess for these?

3. What are the clinical indications for use of IV amphotericin B?

4. What are nursing interventions to decrease adverse effects of IV amphotericin B?

5. What are the clinical indications for use of oral antifungal drugs?

SELECTED REFERENCES

Armstrong, D. (1993). Treatment of opportunistic fungal infections. *Clinical Infectious Diseases, 16,* 1–9.

Bennett, J.E. (1996). Antifungal agents. In J.G. Hardman, L.E. Limbird, P.B. Molinoff & R.W. Ruddon (Eds.), *Goodman & Gilman's The pharmacological basis of therapeutics,* 9th ed., pp. 1175–1190. New York: McGraw-Hill.

Carver, P.L. (1997). Invasive fungal infections. In J.T. DiPiro, R.L. Talbert, G.C. Yee, G.R. Matzke, B.G. Wells & L.M. Posey (Eds.), *Pharmacotherapy: A pathophysiologic approach,* 3rd ed., pp. 2251–2279. Stamford, CT: Appleton & Lange.

Drug facts and comparisons. (Updated monthly.) St. Louis: Facts and Comparisons.

Rex, J.H. (1997). Approach to the treatment of systemic fungal infections. In W.N. Kelley (Ed.), *Textbook of internal medicine,* 3rd ed., pp. 1853–1854. Philadelphia: Lippincott-Raven.

Volk, W.A., Gebhardt, B.M., Hammarskjold, M.L. & Kadner, R.J. (1996). *Essentials of medical microbiology,* 5th ed. Philadelphia: Lippincott-Raven.

41 Antiparasitics

Outline

Objectives

After studying this chapter, the student will be able to:

1 Describe environmental and other major factors in prevention and recognition of selected parasitic diseases.

2 Discuss assessment and treatment of pinworm infestations and pediculosis in school-age children.

3 Discuss the drugs used to treat *Pneumocystis carinii* pneumonia (PCP) in clients with acquired immunodeficiency syndrome (AIDS).

4 Teach preventive interventions to clients planning travel to a malarious area.

Key Terms

Amebicide	**Pediculocide**
Anthelmintic	**Plasmodia**
Giardiasis	**Pneumocystosis**
Larvae	

A parasite is a living organism that survives at the expense of another organism, called the host. Parasitic infestations are common human ailments worldwide. The effects of parasitic diseases on human hosts vary from minor and annoying to major and life-threatening. Parasitic diseases in this chapter are those caused by protozoa, helminths (worms), the itch mite, and pediculi (lice). Protozoa and helminths can infect the digestive tract and other body tissues; the itch mite and pediculi affect the skin.

Protozoal Infections

AMEBIASIS

Amebiasis is a common disease in Africa, Asia, and Latin America, but it can occur in any geographic region. In the United States it is most likely to occur in residents of institutions for the mentally retarded, homosexual and bisexual men, and residents or travelers in countries with poor sanitation.

Amebiasis is caused by the pathogenic protozoan *Entamoeba histolytica,* which exists in two forms. The cystic form is inactive and resistant to drugs, heat, cold, and drying and can live outside the body for long periods. Amebiasis is transmitted by the fecal–oral route, such as ingesting food or water contaminated with human feces containing amebic cysts. Once ingested, some cysts break open in the ileum to release amebae, which produce trophozoites. Other cysts remain intact to be expelled in feces and continue the chain of infection. Trophozoites are active amebae that feed, multiply, move about, and produce clinical manifestations of amebiasis. Trophozoites produce an enzyme that allows them to invade body tissues. They may form erosions and ulcerations in the intestinal wall and cause diarrhea (this form of the disease is called *intestinal amebiasis* or *amebic dysentery*), or they may penetrate blood vessels and be carried to other organs, where they form abscesses. These abscesses are usually found in the liver (hepatic amebiasis), but they also may occur in the lungs or brain.

Drugs used to treat amebiasis (amebicides) are classified according to their site of action. Some drugs (*e.g.,* iodoquinol, paromomycin) are called *intestinal amebicides* because they act within the lumen of the bowel. Other drugs (*e.g.,* chloroquine, emetine) are called *tissue* or *extraintestinal amebicides* because they act in the bowel wall, liver, and other tissues. Metronidazole (Flagyl) is effective in intestinal and extraintestinal amebiasis. No available amebicides are recommended for prophylaxis of amebiasis.

GIARDIASIS

Giardiasis is caused by *Giardia lamblia,* a common intestinal parasite. It is spread by food or water contaminated with human feces containing encysted forms of the organism or by contact with infected people or animals. Person-to-person spread often occurs among children in day care centers, institutionalized persons, and male homosexuals. The organism is also found in people who camp or hike in wilderness areas or who drink untreated well water in areas where sanitation is poor. Giardiasis may affect children more than adults, and it has caused community outbreaks of diarrhea.

Giardial infections occur 1 to 2 weeks after ingestion of the cysts and may be asymptomatic or produce diarrhea, abdominal cramping, and distention. If untreated, giardiasis may resolve spontaneously or progress to a chronic disease with anorexia, nausea, malaise, weight loss, and continued diarrhea with large, foul-smelling, light-colored, fatty stools. Deficiencies of vitamin B_{12} and fat-soluble vitamins may occur. Adults and children older than 8 years with symptomatic giardiasis should be treated with oral metronidazole.

MALARIA

Malaria is a common cause of morbidity and mortality in many parts of the world, especially in tropical regions. In the United States, malaria is rare and affects travelers or immigrants from malarious areas.

Malaria is caused by four species of protozoa of the genus *Plasmodium.* The human being is the only natural reservoir of these parasites. All types of malaria are transmitted only by *Anopheles* mosquitoes. *Plasmodium vivax, Plasmodium malariae,* and *Plasmodium ovale* cause recurrent malaria by forming reservoirs in the human host. In these types of malaria, signs and symptoms may occur months or years after the initial attack. *Plasmodium falciparum* causes the most life-threatening type of malaria but does not form a reservoir. This type of malaria may be cured and prevented from recurring.

Plasmodia have a life cycle in which one stage of development occurs within the human body. When a mosquito bites a person with malaria, it ingests blood that contains gametocytes (male and female forms of the protozoan parasite). From these forms, sporozoites are produced and transported to the mosquito's salivary glands. When the mosquito bites the next person, the sporozoites are injected into that person's bloodstream. From the bloodstream, the organisms lodge in the liver and other tissues, where they reproduce asexually and form merozoites. The liver cells containing the parasite eventually rupture and release the merozoites into the bloodstream, where they invade red blood cells. After a period of growth and asexual reproduction, merozoites rupture red blood cells, invade other erythrocytes, form gametocytes, and continue the cycle. After several cycles, clinical manifestations of malaria occur because of the large numbers of parasites. The characteristic cycles of chills and fever correspond to the release of merozoites from erythrocytes.

Antimalarial drugs act at different stages in the life cycle of plasmodial parasites. Some drugs (*e.g.,* chloroquine) are effective against erythrocytic forms and are therefore useful in preventing or treating acute attacks of malaria. These drugs do not prevent infection with the parasite, but they do prevent clinical manifestations. Other drugs (*e.g.,* primaquine) act against exoerythrocytic or tissue forms of the parasite to prevent initial infection and recurrent attacks or to cure some types of malaria. Combination drug therapy, administered concomitantly or consecutively, is common with antimalarial drugs.

PNEUMOCYSTOSIS

Pneumocystosis is caused by *Pneumocystis carinii,* a parasitic organism formerly considered a protozoan but now considered a fungus. Sources and routes of spread have not been clearly delineated. It is apparently widespread in the environment, and most people are exposed at an early age. Infections are mild or asymptomatic in immunocompetent persons. However, the organism can form cysts in the lungs, persist for long periods, and become activated in immunocompromised hosts. Activation produces *Pneumocystis carinii pneumonia* (PCP), an acute, life-threatening respiratory infection characterized by cough, fever, dyspnea, and finding the organism in sputum. Groups at risk include those with acquired immunodeficiency syndrome (AIDS), those receiving corticosteroids, antineoplastics, and other immunosuppressive drugs, and probably caregivers of infected people. PCP is often the cause of death in people with AIDS. PCP is discussed in this chapter because antiprotozoan rather than antifungal drugs are used to treat the condition.

TOXOPLASMOSIS

Toxoplasmosis is caused by *Toxoplasma gondii,* a parasite spread by ingesting undercooked meat or other food containing encysted forms of the organism, by contact with feces from infected cats, and by congenital spread from mothers with acute infection. Once infected, the organism may persist in tissue cysts for the life of the host. However, symptoms rarely occur unless the immune system is impaired or becomes impaired at a later time. Although symptomatic infection may occur in anyone with immunosuppression (*e.g.,* persons with cancer or organ transplants), it is especially common and serious in people with AIDS, in whom it often causes encephalitis and death.

TRICHOMONIASIS

The most common form of trichomoniasis is a vaginal infection caused by *Trichomonas vaginalis.* The disease is usually spread by sexual intercourse. Antitrichomonal drugs may be administered systemically (*i.e.,* metronidazole) or applied locally as douche solutions or vaginal creams.

Helminthiasis

Helminthiasis, an infestation with parasitic worms, is a major disease in many parts of the world. Helminths are most often found in the gastrointestinal (GI) tract. However, several types of parasitic worms penetrate body tissues or produce larvae, which migrate to the blood, lymph channels, lungs, liver, and other body tissues. Specific types of helminthiasis include the following:

1. **Hookworm infections** are caused by *Necator americanus,* a species found in the United States, and *Ancylostoma duodenale,* a species found in Europe, the Middle East, and North Africa. Hookworm is spread by ova-containing feces from infected people. Ova develop into larvae when deposited on the soil. Larvae burrow through the skin (*e.g.,* if the person walks on the soil with bare feet), enter blood vessels, and migrate through the lungs to the pharynx, where they are swallowed. Larvae develop into adult hookworms in the small intestine and attach themselves to the intestinal mucosa.
2. **Pinworm infections** (enterobiasis), caused by *Enterobius vermicularis,* are the most common parasitic worm infections in the United States. Pinworm infections are highly communicable; they often involve school children and household contacts. Infection occurs from contact with ova in food or water or on bed linens. The female pinworm migrates from the bowel to the perianal area to deposit eggs, especially at night. Touching or scratching the perianal area deposits ova on hands and any objects touched by the contaminated hands.
3. **Roundworm infections** (ascariasis), caused by *Ascaris lumbricoides,* are the most common parasitic worm infections in the world. They occur most often in tropical regions but may occur wherever sanitation is poor. The infection is transmitted by ingesting food or water contaminated with feces from infected people. Ova are swallowed and hatch into larvae in the intestine. Like the hookworm larvae, roundworm larvae penetrate blood vessels and migrate through the lungs before returning to the intestines, where they develop into adult worms.
4. **Tapeworms** attach themselves to the intestinal wall and may grow as long as several yards. Segments called proglottids, which contain tapeworm eggs, are expelled in feces. Tapeworms are transmitted by ingestion of contaminated, raw, or improperly cooked beef, pork, or fish. Beef and fish tapeworm infections are not usually considered serious illnesses. Pork

tapeworm, which is uncommon in the United States, is more serious because it produces larvae that enter the bloodstream and migrate to other body tissues (*i.e.*, muscles, liver, lungs, and brain).

5. **Threadworm infections** (strongyloidiasis), caused by *Strongyloides stercoralis*, are potentially serious infections. This parasitic worm burrows into the mucosa of the small intestine, where the female lays eggs. The eggs hatch into larvae that can penetrate all body tissues.
6. **Trichinosis,** a parasitic worm infection caused by *Trichinella spiralis,* occurs worldwide. It is caused by inadequately cooked meat, especially pork. Encysted larvae are ingested in infected pork. In the intestine, the larvae excyst, mature, and produce eggs that hatch into new larvae. The larvae enter blood and lymphatic vessels and are transported throughout the body. They penetrate various body tissues (*e.g.*, muscles and brain) and evoke inflammatory reactions. Eventually, the larvae are re-encysted or walled off in the tissues and may remain for 10 years or longer.
7. **Whipworm infections** (trichuriasis) are caused by *Trichuris trichiura.* Whipworms attach themselves to the wall of the colon.

Drugs used for treatment of helminthiasis are called *anthelmintics.* Most anthelmintics act locally to kill or cause expulsion of parasitic worms from the intestines; some anthelmintics act systemically against parasites that have penetrated various body tissues. The goal of anthelmintic therapy may be to eradicate the parasite completely or to decrease the magnitude of infestation ("worm burden").

Scabies and Pediculosis

Scabies and pediculosis are parasitic infestations of the skin. Scabies is caused by the itch mite (*Sarcoptes scabiei*), which burrows into the skin and lays eggs that hatch in 4 to 8 days. The burrows may produce visible skin lesions, most often between the fingers and on the wrists, but other parts of the body may be affected as well.

Pediculosis is caused by three types of lice, which are blood-sucking insects. Pediculosis capitis (head lice) is the most common type of pediculosis in the United States. It is diagnosed by finding louse eggs (nits) attached to hair shafts close to the scalp. Pediculosis corporis (body lice) is diagnosed by finding lice in clothing, especially in seams. Body lice can transmit typhus and other diseases. Pediculosis pubis (pubic or crab lice) is diagnosed by finding lice in the pubic and genital areas. Occasionally, these lice infest the axillae, mustache, or eyelashes. Pediculosis is usually associated with poor personal hygiene and spread by social and sexual contact.

Although scabies and pediculosis are caused by different parasites, the conditions have several characteristics in common:

1. Scabies and pediculosis are more likely to occur in areas of poverty, overcrowding, and poor sanitation. However, they may occur in any geographic area and socioeconomic group.
2. Scabies and pediculosis are highly communicable. The diseases are transmitted by direct contact with an infected person or the person's personal effects (*e.g.*, clothing, combs and hairbrushes, bed linens).
3. Pruritus is usually the major symptom of scabies and pediculosis. It results from an allergic reaction to parasite secretions and excrement. In addition to the intense discomfort associated with pruritus, scratching is likely to cause skin excoriation with secondary bacterial infection and formation of vesicles, pustules, and crusts.
4. Some of the same medications, applied topically, are used in both scabies and pediculosis.

Individual Antiparasitic Drugs

AMEBICIDES

Chloroquine (Aralen) is a drug used primarily for its antimalarial effects. When used as an amebicide, the drug is effective in extraintestinal amebiasis (*i.e.*, hepatic amebiasis) but generally ineffective in intestinal amebiasis. The phosphate salt is given orally. When the oral route is contraindicated, severe nausea and vomiting occur, or the infection is severe, the hydrochloride salt can be given intramuscularly. Treatment is usually combined with an intestinal amebicide.

Chloroquine Phosphate
Route and Dosage Ranges

Adults: PO 1 g/d for 2 days, then 500 mg/d for 2 to 3 weeks
Children: PO 20 mg/kg/d, in two divided doses, for 2 days, then 10 mg/kg/d for 2 to 3 weeks

Chloroquine Hydrochloride
Route and Dosage Ranges

Adults: IM 200 to 250 mg/d for 10 to 12 days
Children: IM 15 mg/kg/d for 2 days, then 7.5 mg/kg/d for 2 to 3 weeks

Iodoquinol or diiodohydroxyquin (Yodoxin) is an iodine compound that acts against active amebae (trophozoites) in the intestinal lumen. Iodoquinol may be used alone in asymptomatic intestinal amebiasis to decrease the number of amebic cysts passed in the feces. When given for symptomatic intestinal amebiasis (*e.g.,* amebic dysentery), iodoquinol is usually given with other amebicides in concurrent or alternating courses. Iodoquinol is ineffective in amebic hepatitis and abscess formation. Its use is contraindicated with iodine allergy and liver disease.

Route and Dosage Ranges

Adults: Asymptomatic carriers, PO 650 mg/d
   Symptomatic intestinal amebiasis, PO 650 mg three times per day after meals for 20 days. If necessary, the 20-day course of therapy may be repeated after a drug-free interval of 2 to 3 weeks.
Children: PO 40 mg/kg/d in three divided doses for 20 days (maximum dose, 2 g/d); repeat after 2 to 3 weeks if necessary

Metronidazole (Flagyl) is effective against protozoa that cause amebiasis, giardiasis, and trichomoniasis and against anaerobic bacilli, such as *Bacteroides* and *Clostridia* (see Chap. 37). In amebiasis, metronidazole is amebicidal at intestinal and extraintestinal sites of infection. It is probably the drug of choice for all forms of amebiasis except asymptomatic intestinal amebiasis (in which amebic cysts are expelled in the feces). In trichomoniasis, metronidazole is the only systemic trichomonacide available, and it is more effective than any locally active agent. Because trichomoniasis is transmitted by sexual intercourse, partners should be treated simultaneously to prevent reinfection.

Metronidazole is generally contraindicated during the first trimester of pregnancy and must be used with caution in clients with central nervous system (CNS) or blood disorders.

Route and Dosage Ranges

Adults: Amebiasis, PO 500 to 750 mg three times per day for 5 to 10 days
   Giardiasis, PO 250 mg three times daily for 7 days
   Trichomoniasis, PO 250 mg three times per day for 7 days, 1 g twice daily for 1 day, or 2 g in a single dose. If necessary, the course of treatment may be repeated after 4 to 6 weeks.
   Gardnerella vaginalis vaginitis, PO 500 mg twice daily for 7 days
Children: Amebiasis, PO 35 to 50 mg/kg/d in three divided doses, for 10 days
   Giardiasis, PO 15 mg/kg/d in three divided doses, for 7 days

Tetracycline and **doxycycline** are antibacterial drugs (see Chap. 36) that act against amebae in the in-

testinal lumen by altering the bacterial flora required for amebic viability. One of these drugs may be used with other amebicides in the treatment of all forms of amebiasis except asymptomatic intestinal amebiasis.

Route and Dosage Ranges

Adults: PO 250 to 500 mg q6h, up to 14 days
Children: PO 25 to 50 mg/kg/d in four divided doses for 7 to 10 days

ANTIMALARIAL AGENTS

Chloroquine is one of the most widely used antimalarial agents. Chloroquine acts against erythrocytic forms of plasmodial parasites to prevent or treat malarial attacks. When used for prophylaxis, chloroquine is given before, during, and after travel or residence in endemic areas. When used for treatment of malaria caused by *Plasmodium vivax, Plasmodium malariae,* or *Plasmodium ovale,* chloroquine relieves symptoms of the acute attack. However, chloroquine does not prevent recurrence of malarial attacks because the drug does not act against the tissue (exoerythrocytic) forms of the parasite. When used for treatment of malaria caused by *Plasmodium falciparum,* chloroquine relieves symptoms of the acute attack and eliminates the parasite from the body because *Plasmodium falciparum* does not have tissue reservoirs. However, chloroquine-resistant strains of *Plasmodium falciparum* have developed in some geographic areas.

Chloroquine also is used in protozoal infections other than malaria, including extraintestinal amebiasis and giardiasis. Chloroquine should be used with caution in clients with hepatic disease or severe neurologic, GI, or blood disorders.

Hydroxychloroquine sulfate (Plaquenil) is a derivative of chloroquine with essentially the same actions, uses, and adverse effects as chloroquine. It is also used to treat rheumatoid arthritis and lupus erythematosus.

Chloroquine Phosphate
Route and Dosage Ranges

Adults: Prophylaxis of malaria, PO 5 mg/kg (base) weekly (maximum of 300 mg of chloroquine base weekly), starting 2 weeks before entering a malarious area and continuing for 8 weeks after return
   Treatment of an acute attack of malaria, PO 1 g (600 mg of base) initially, then 500 mg (300 mg of base) after 6 to 8 hours, then 500 mg daily for 2 days (total of 2.5 g in four doses)
Children: Treatment of an acute attack of malaria, PO 10 mg/kg of chloroquine base initially, then 5 mg/kg after 6 hours, then 5 mg/kg/d for 2 days (total of four doses)

Chloroquine Hydrochloride
Route and Dosage Ranges

Adults: Treatment of malarial attacks, IM 250 mg (equivalent to 200 mg of chloroquine base) initially, repeated q6h if necessary, to a maximal dose of 800 mg of chloroquine base in 24 hours
Children: Treatment of malarial attacks, IM 5 mg/kg chloroquine base initially, repeated after 6 hours if necessary; maximal dose, 10 mg/kg/24 h

Hydroxychloroquine Sulfate
Route and Dosage Ranges

Adults: Prophylaxis, PO 5 mg/kg, not to exceed 310 mg (of hydroxychloroquine base), once weekly for 2 weeks before entry to and 8 weeks after return from malarious areas
  Treatment of acute malarial attacks, PO 620 mg initially, then 310 mg 6 hours later, and 310 mg/d for 2 days (total of four doses)
Children: Prophylaxis, PO 5 mg/kg (of hydroxychloroquine base) once weekly for 2 weeks before entry to and 8 weeks after return from malarious areas
  Treatment of acute malarial attacks, PO 10 mg/kg initially, then 5 mg/kg 6 hours later, and 5 mg/kg/d for two doses (total of four doses)

Chloroquine with **primaquine** is a mixture available in tablets containing chloroquine phosphate 500 mg (equivalent to 300 mg of chloroquine base) and primaquine phosphate 79 mg (equivalent to 45 mg of primaquine base). This combination is effective for prophylaxis of malaria and may be more acceptable to clients. It also may be more convenient for use in children, because no pediatric formulation of primaquine is available.

Route and Dosage Ranges

Adults: Prophylaxis of malaria, PO 1 tablet weekly on the same day each week for 2 weeks before entering and 8 weeks after leaving malarious areas
Children: PO same as adults for children weighing over 45 kg; ½ tablet for children weighing 25 to 45 kg. For younger children, a suspension is prepared, using the tablets and chocolate syrup or fruit juice. The usual concentration is 40 mg of chloroquine base and 6 mg of primaquine base in 5 ml of suspension. Dosages are then 2.5 ml for children weighing 5 to 7 kg, 5 ml for 8 to 11 kg, 7.5 ml for 12 to 15 kg, 10 ml for 16 to 20 kg, and 12.5 ml for 21 to 24 kg. These dosages are administered weekly, on the same day of the week, for 2 weeks before entering and 8 weeks after leaving malarious areas.

Halofantrine (Halfan) is indicated for treatment of malaria caused by *Plasmodium falciparum* or *Plasmodium vivax*, including chloroquine or multidrug-resistant strains.

Route and Dosage Ranges

Adults: PO 500 mg q6h for three doses, repeat in 1 week for clients without previous exposure to malaria (*e.g.*, travelers)
Children <40 kg: PO 8 mg/kg according to the schedule for adults

Mefloquine (Lariam) is used to prevent *Plasmodium falciparum* malaria, including chloroquine-resistant strains, and to treat acute malaria caused by *Plasmodium falciparum* or *Plasmodium vivax*.

Route and Dosage Ranges

Adults: Prophylaxis, PO 250 mg 1 week before travel, then 250 mg weekly during travel and for 4 weeks after leaving a malarious area
  Treatment, 1250 mg (5 tablets) as a single dose
Children: Prophylaxis, PO ¼ tablet for 15 to 19 kg weight; ½ tablet for 20 to 30 kg; ¾ tablet for 31 to 45 kg; and 1 tablet for more than 45 kg, according to the schedule for adults

Primaquine is an antimalarial agent used to prevent the initial occurrence of malaria; to prevent recurrent attacks of malaria caused by *Plasmodium vivax, Plasmodium malariae*, and *Plasmodium ovale*; and to achieve "radical cure" of these three types of malaria. (Radical cure involves eradicating the exoerythrocytic forms of the plasmodium and preventing the survival of the blood forms.) The clinical usefulness of primaquine stems primarily from its ability to destroy tissue (exoerythrocytic) forms of the malarial parasite. Primaquine is especially effective in vivax malaria. Thus far, plasmodial strains causing the three relapsing types of malaria have not developed resistance to primaquine. When used to prevent initial occurrence of malaria (causal prophylaxis), primaquine is given concurrently with a suppressive agent (*e.g.*, chloroquine or hydroxychloroquine) after the client has returned from a malarious area. Primaquine is not effective for treatment of acute attacks of malaria.

Route and Dosage Ranges

Adults: Prophylaxis, PO 26.3 mg (equivalent to 15 mg of primaquine base) daily for 14 days, beginning immediately after leaving a malarious area, or 79 mg (45 mg of base) once a week for 8 weeks. To prevent relapse (*i.e.*, acute malarial attacks), the same dose is given with chloroquine or a related drug daily for 14 days.

Children: Prophylaxis of the disease and relapse, PO 0.3 mg of base/kg/d for 14 days, according to the schedule outlined above, or 0.9 mg of base/kg/ wk for 8 weeks

Pyrimethamine (Daraprim) is a folic acid antagonist used to prevent malaria caused by susceptible strains of plasmodia. Pyrimethamine is sometimes used with a sulfonamide and quinine to treat chloroquine-resistant strains of *Plasmodium falciparum*. Folic acid antagonists and sulfonamides act synergistically against plasmodia because they block different steps in the synthesis of folic acid, a nutrient required by the parasites.

Route and Dosage Ranges

Adults: Prophylaxis, PO 25 mg once weekly, starting 2 weeks before entering and continuing for 8 weeks after returning from malarious areas
Children: Prophylaxis, PO 25 mg once weekly, as above, for children over 10 years; 6.25 to 12.5 mg once weekly for children under 10 years

Quinine (Quinamm) is derived from the bark of the cinchona tree. Quinine was the primary antimalarial drug for many years but has been largely replaced by synthetic agents that cause fewer adverse reactions. However, it may still be used in the treatment of chloroquine-resistant falciparum malaria, usually in conjunction with pyrimethamine and a sulfonamide. Quinine also relaxes skeletal muscles and is used for prevention and treatment of nocturnal leg cramps.

Route and Dosage Ranges

Adults: Treatment of malaria, PO 650 mg q8h for 10 to 14 days
Leg cramps, PO 200 to 300 mg at bedtime
Children: Treatment of malaria, PO 25 mg/kg/d in divided doses q8h for 10 to 14 days

ANTITRICHOMONAL AGENT

For information about **Metronidazole** (Flagyl), see amebicides above.

ANTI–*PNEUMOCYSTIS CARINII* AGENTS

Trimethoprim-sulfamethoxazole or **TMP-SMX** (Bactrim, others; see Chap. 36) is the drug of choice for prevention and treatment of PCP. Prophylaxis is indicated for adults and adolescents with human immunodeficiency virus (HIV) infection and a low CD4+ T-helper cell count (below 200); children with HIV; newborns whose mothers have HIV; organ transplant recipients; patients with leukemia or lymphoma who are receiving cytotoxic chemotherapy; and for patients receiving

high doses of corticosteroids (equivalent to 20 mg or more daily of prednisone), including the tapering period, and for 1 month after the corticosteroid is stopped.

Adverse effects include nausea, fever, skin rash, and others, with some attributed to hypersensitivity reactions to the sulfamethoxazole. These effects seem to be more severe in patients with HIV infection.

Routes and Dosage Ranges

Adults: Prophylaxis, PO 1 double strength tablet (160 mg trimethoprim and 800 mg sulfamethoxazole) q24h
   Treatment, IV 15 to 20 mg/kg/d (based on trimethoprim) q6–8 h, for up to 14 days; PO 15 to 20 mg/ kg TMP/100 mg/kg SMX per day, in divided doses, q6h, for 14 to 21 days
Children: Prophylaxis, PO 150 mg/m² TMP/750 mg/ m² SMX per day, in equally divided doses q12h, on 3 consecutive days per week. Maximum daily dose, 320 mg TMP/1600 mg SMX.
   Treatment, IV 15 to 20 mg/kg/d (based on trimethoprim) q6–8 h, for up to 14 days; PO 15 to 20 mg/ kg TMP/100 mg/kg SMX per day, in divided doses, q6h, for 14 to 21 days

Atovaquone (Mepron) is used for treatment of PCP in people who are unable to take trimethoprim-sulfamethoxazole. Adverse effects include nausea, vomiting, diarrhea, fever, insomnia, and elevated hepatic enzymes.

Route and Dosage Range

Adults: PO 750 mg three times daily with food

Trimetrexate (Neutrexin) is a folate antagonist (which must be used with leucovorin rescue) approved only for treatment of moderate to severe PCP in immunocompromised patients, including those with advanced HIV infection, who are unable to take trimethoprim-sulfamethoxazole. Hematologic toxicity is the main dose-limiting adverse effect. Leucovorin must be given daily during trimetrexate therapy and for 72 hours after the last trimetrexate dose. Dosage of trimetrexate must be reduced and dosage of leucovorin must be increased with significant neutropenia or thrombocytopenia.

Routes and Dosage Ranges

Trimetrexate
Adults: IV infusion 45 mg/m² daily, over 60 to 90 minutes, for 21 days
Leucovorin
Adults: PO, IV 20 mg/m² q6h for 24 days. Give IV doses over 5 to 10 minutes.

Pentamidine isethionate (Pentam 300, NebuPent) is used to prevent or treat PCP. Pentamidine interferes with production of ribonucleic acid (RNA) and deoxyribonucleic acid (DNA) by the organism. The drug is given parenterally for treatment of PCP and by inhalation for prophylaxis. It is excreted by the kidneys and accumulates in the presence of renal failure, so dosage should be reduced with renal failure. With parenteral pentamidine, appropriate tests should be performed before, during, and after treatment (*e.g.,* complete blood count, platelet count, serum creatinine, blood urea nitrogen, blood glucose, serum calcium, and electrocardiogram).

Routes and Dosage Ranges

Adults: IM, IV 4 mg/kg once daily for 14 days
  Inhalation, 300 mg every 4 weeks
Children: IM, IV same as adults
  Inhalation, dosage not established

ANTHELMINTICS

Mebendazole (Vermox) is a broad-spectrum anthelmintic used in the treatment of parasitic infections by hookworms, pinworms, roundworms, and whipworms. It is also useful but less effective in tapeworm infection. Mebendazole kills helminths by preventing uptake of the glucose necessary for parasitic metabolism. The helminths become immobilized and die slowly, so they may be expelled from the GI tract up to 3 days after drug therapy is completed. Mebendazole acts locally within the GI tract, and less than 10% of the drug is absorbed systemically.

Mebendazole is usually the drug of choice for single or mixed infections caused by the above parasitic worms. The drug is contraindicated during pregnancy because of teratogenic effects in rats; it is relatively contraindicated in children under 2 years of age because it has not been extensively investigated for use in this age group.

Route and Dosage Range

Adults and children: Most infections, PO 100 mg morning and evening for 3 consecutive days. For pinworms, a single 100-mg dose may be sufficient. A second course of therapy may be administered in 3 weeks, if necessary.

Pyrantel (Antiminth) is effective in infestations of roundworms, pinworms, and hookworms. The drug acts locally to paralyze worms in the intestinal tract. Pyrantel is poorly absorbed from the GI tract, and most of an administered dose may be recovered in feces. Pyrantel is contraindicated in pregnancy and is not recommended for children under 1 year of age.

Route and Dosage Range

Adults and children: Roundworms and pinworms, PO 11 mg/kg (maximal dose, 1 g) as a single dose; for hookworms, the same dose is given daily for 3 consecutive days. The course of therapy may be repeated in 1 month, if necessary.

Thiabendazole (Mintezol) is an anthelmintic agent that is most effective against threadworms and pinworms. It is useful but less effective against hookworms, roundworms, and whipworms. Because of the broad spectrum of anthelmintic activity, thiabendazole may be especially useful in mixed parasitic infestations. In trichinosis, thiabendazole decreases symptoms and eosinophilia but does not eliminate larvae from muscle tissues. The mechanism of anthelmintic action is uncertain but probably involves interference with parasitic metabolism. The drug is relatively toxic compared to other anthelmintic agents.

Thiabendazole is a first drug of choice for threadworm infestations. For other types of helminthiasis, it is usually considered an alternative drug. Thiabendazole is rapidly absorbed after oral administration. Most of the drug is excreted in urine within 24 hours. Thiabendazole should be used with caution in clients with liver or kidney disease.

Route and Dosage Range

Adults and children: PO 22 mg/kg (maximal single dose, 3 g) twice daily after meals; 1 day for pinworms, repeated after 1 to 2 weeks; 2 days for other infections, except trichinosis, which requires about 5 days

SCABICIDES AND PEDICULICIDES

Permethrin is the drug of choice for both pediculosis and scabies. A single application eliminates parasites and ova and is usually curative. For pediculosis, permethrin is used in a 1% liquid (Nix), a nonprescription drug. For scabies, it is used in a 5% cream (Elimite), which requires a prescription. Permethrin is safer than other scabicides and pediculicides, especially for infants and children.

Permethrin is derived from a chrysanthemum plant, and persons with a history of allergy to ragweed or chrysanthemum flowers should use it cautiously. The most frequent adverse effect is pruritus; burning, stinging, and tingling may also occur.

To avoid reinfection, close contacts should be treated simultaneously. With pediculosis, clothing and bedding should be sterilized by boiling or steaming and seams of clothes should be examined to verify that all lice are eliminated.

Route and Dosage Range

Adults and children:

> Scabies, massage Elmite into the skin over the entire body except the face, leave on for 8 to 14 hours, wash off.
>
> Pediculosis, apply Nix after shampooing, rinsing, and towel drying hair. Saturate the hair and scalp, leave on for 10 minutes, rinse off with water.

Gamma benzene hexachloride (Kwell, Lindane) is a second-line drug for scabies and pediculosis. It may be used for people who have hypersensitivity reactions to permethrin. It is applied topically, and substantial amounts are absorbed through intact skin. CNS toxicity has been reported with excessive use, especially in infants and children. The drug is available in a 1% concentration in a cream, lotion, and shampoo.

Route and Dosage Range

Adults and children:

> *Scabies,* apply topically to entire skin except the face, neck, and scalp, leave in place for 24 hours, then remove by shower
>
> *Pediculosis,* use the cream or lotion (rub into the affected area, leave in place for 12 hours, then wash thoroughly) or shampoo (rub into the affected area for 4 minutes and rinse thoroughly)

Malathion (Ovide) is a pediculicide used in the treatment of head lice. It is sprinkled on the hair and rubbed in until the hair is thoroughly moistened. Allow the hair to dry naturally; keep uncovered and do not apply heat or a hair dryer. After 8 to 12 hours, the hair should be shampooed, rinsed, and combed with a fine-toothed comb to remove dead lice and eggs. If necessary, treatment can be repeated in 7 to 9 days.

Pyrethrin preparations (*e.g.,* Barc, RID) are available over-the-counter as gels, shampoos, and liquid suspensions for treatment of pediculosis.

Crotamiton (Eurax) is used as a 10% cream or lotion for scabies.

Nursing Process

Assessment

Assess for conditions in which antiparasitic drugs are used.

- Assess for exposure to parasites. Although exposure is influenced by many variables (*e.g.,* geographic location, personal hygiene, environmental sanitation), some useful questions may include the following:
  - Does the person live in an institution, an area of poor sanitation, an underdeveloped country, a tropical region, or an area of overcrowded housing? These conditions predispose to parasitic infestations with lice, the itch mite, protozoa, and worms.
  - Are parasitic diseases present in the person's environment? For example, head lice, scabies, and pinworm infestations often affect school children and their families.
  - Has the person recently traveled (within the previous 1 to 3 weeks) in malarious regions? If so, were prophylactic measures used appropriately?
  - With vaginal trichomoniasis, assess in relation to sexual activity. The disease is spread by sexual intercourse, and sexual partners need simultaneous treatment to prevent reinfection.
  - With pubic (crab) lice, assess sexual activity. Lice may be transmitted by sexual and other close contact and by contact with infested bed linens.
- Assess for signs and symptoms. These vary greatly, depending on the extent of parasitic infestation.
  - **Amebiasis.** The person may be asymptomatic, have nausea, vomiting, diarrhea, abdominal cramping, and weakness or experience symptoms from ulcerations of the colon or abscesses of the liver (amebic hepatitis) if the disease is severe, prolonged, and untreated. Amebiasis is diagnosed by identifying cysts or trophozoites of *Entamoeba histolytica* in stool specimens.
  - **Malaria.** Initial symptoms may resemble those produced by influenza (*e.g.,* headache, myalgia). Characteristic paroxysms of chills, fever, and copious perspiration may not be present in early malaria. During acute malarial attacks, the cycles occur every 36 to 72 hours. Additional symptoms include nausea and vomiting, splenomegaly, hepatomegaly, anemia, leukopenia, thrombocytopenia, and hyperbilirubinemia. Malaria is diagnosed by identifying the plasmodial parasite in peripheral blood smears (by microscopic examination).
  - **Trichomoniasis.** Females usually have vaginal burning, itching, and yellowish discharge; males may be asymptomatic or have symptoms of urethritis. The condition is diagnosed by finding *Trichomonas vaginalis* organisms in a wet smear of vaginal exudate, semen, prostatic fluid, or urinary sediment (by microscopic examination). Cultures may be necessary.
  - **Helminthiasis.** Light infestations may be asymptomatic. Heavy infestations produce symptoms according to the particular parasitic worm. Hookworm, roundworm, and threadworm larvae migrate through the lungs and may cause symptoms of pulmonary congestion. The hookworm may cause anemia by sucking blood from the intestinal mucosa; the fish tapeworm may cause megaloblastic or pernicious anemia by absorbing folic acid and vitamin B_{12}. Large masses of roundworms or tapeworms have caused intestinal obstruction. The major symptom usually associated with pinworms is intense itching in the perianal area (pruritus ani). Helminthiasis is diagnosed by microscopic identification of parasites or ova in stool specimens. Pinworm infestation is diagnosed by identifying ova on anal swabs, obtained by touching the sticky side of cellophane tape to the anal area. (Early morning swabs are best because the female pinworm deposits eggs during sleeping hours.)
  - **Scabies and pediculosis.** Pruritus is usually the primary symptom. Secondary symptoms result from scratching and often include skin excoriation and infection (*i.e.,* vesicles, pustules, and crusts). Pediculosis is diagnosed by visual identification of lice or ova (nits) on the client's body or clothing.

Nursing Diagnoses

- Knowledge Deficit: Management of disease process and prevention of recurrence
- Knowledge Deficit: Accurate drug administration
- Altered Nutrition: Less Than Body Requirements related to parasitic disease or drug therapy
- Self-Esteem Disturbance related to a medical diagnosis of parasitic infestation
- Noncompliance related to need for hygienic and other measures to prevent and treat parasitic infestations

Planning/Goals

The client will:

- Experience relief of symptoms for which antiparasitic drugs were taken
- Self-administer drugs accurately
- Avoid preventable adverse effects
- Act to prevent recurrent infestation
- Keep appointments for follow-up care

Interventions

Use measures to avoid exposure to or prevent transmission of parasitic diseases.

- Environmental health measures include the following:
  - Sanitary sewers to prevent deposition of feces on surface soil and the resultant exposure to helminths
  - Monitoring of community water supplies, food-handling establishments, and food-handling personnel
  - Follow-up examination and possibly treatment of household and other close contacts of people with helminthiasis, amebiasis, trichomoniasis, scabies, and pediculosis
  - Mosquito control in malarious areas and prophylactic drug therapy for travelers to malarious areas. In addition, teach travelers to decrease exposure to mosquito bites (*e.g.,* wear long-sleeved, dark clothing; use an effective insect repellent such as DEET; and sleep in well-screened rooms or under mosquito netting). These measures are especially needed at dusk and dawn, the maximal feeding times for mosquitoes.
- Personal and other health measures include the following:
  - Maintain personal hygiene (*i.e.,* regular bathing and shampooing, handwashing before eating or handling food and after defecation or urination).
  - Avoid raw fish and undercooked meat. This is especially important for anyone with immunosuppression.
  - Avoid contaminating streams or other water sources with feces.
  - Control flies and avoid foods exposed to flies.
  - With scabies and pediculosis infestations, drug therapy must be accompanied by adjunctive measures to avoid reinfection or transmission to others. For example, close contacts should be examined carefully and treated if indicated. Clothes, bed linens, and towels should be washed and dried on hot cycles. Clothes that cannot be washed should be dry cleaned. With head lice, combs and brushes should be cleaned and disinfected; carpets and upholstered furniture should be vacuumed.
  - With pinworms, clothing, bed linens, and towels should be washed daily on hot cycles. Toilet seats should be disinfected daily.
  - Ensure follow-up measures, such as stool specimens, vaginal examinations, anal swabs, smears, and cultures.

- With vaginal infections, avoid sexual intercourse, or have the male partner use a condom.

Evaluation

- Interview and observe for relief of symptoms.
- Interview outpatients regarding compliance with instructions for taking antiparasitic drugs and measures to prevent recurrence of infestation.
- Interview and observe for adverse drug effects.
- Interview and observe regarding food intake or changes in weight.

Principles of Therapy

1. Antiparasitic drugs should be used along with personal and public health control measures to prevent spread of parasitic infestations. Specific measures vary according to the type of organism, the environment, and the host.
2. Many of the drugs described in this chapter are quite toxic; they should be used only when clearly indicated (*i.e.,* laboratory documentation of parasitic infestation or infection).

USE IN CHILDREN

Children often receive an antiparasitic drug for head lice or worm infestations. These should be used exactly as directed and with appropriate precautions to prevent reinfection. Malaria is usually more severe in children than in adults, and children should be protected from exposure when possible. When chemoprophylaxis or treatment for malaria is indicated, the same drugs are used for children as for adults, with appropriate dosage adjustments. An exception is that tetracyclines should not be given to children under 8 years old. Giardiasis seems to be more common in children than adults.

USE IN OLDER ADULTS

Older adults are more likely to experience adverse effects of antiparasitic drugs because they often have impaired renal and hepatic function.

 HOME CARE

Most antiparasitic drugs are given primarily in the home setting. The home care nurse may need to examine close contacts of the infected person and assess their need for treatment, assist parents and patients to use the drugs appropriately, and teach personal and environmental hygiene measures to prevent reinfection. When children have parasitic infestations, the home care nurse may need to collaborate with day care centers and schools to prevent or control outbreaks.

ANTIPARASITICS

NURSING ACTIONS	RATIONALE/EXPLANATION
1. Administer accurately	
a. Give atovaquone, chloroquine and related drugs, iodoquinol, and oral metronidazole with or after meals.	Food improves absorption of atovaquone and decreases GI irritation of the other drugs.
b. With pentamidine:	
(1) For IM administration, dissolve the drug in 3 ml of sterile water for injection and inject deeply in a large muscle mass.	IM administration is painful and may cause sterile abscesses.
(2) For IV administration, dissolve the calculated dose in 3–5 ml of sterile water or 5% dextrose in water. Dilute further with 50–250 ml of 5% dextrose solution and infuse over 60 min.	
(3) For aerosol use, dissolve the contents of 1 vial in 6 ml of sterile water, place the solution in the nebulizer chamber of a Respirgard II device, and deliver by way of oxygen or compressed air flow until the nebulizer chamber is empty (about 30–45 min).	
c. Give anthelmintics without regard to mealtimes or food ingestion. Mebendazole tablets may be chewed, swallowed, or crushed and mixed with food.	Food in the GI tract does not decrease effectiveness of most anthelmintics.
d. For pediculicides and scabicides, follow the label or manufacturer's instructions.	Instructions vary among preparations.
2. Observe for therapeutic effects	
a. With chloroquine for acute malaria, observe for relief of symptoms and negative blood smears.	Fever and chills usually subside within 24–48 h, and blood smears are negative for plasmodia within 48–72 h.
b. With amebicides, observe for relief of symptoms and negative stool examinations.	Relief of symptoms does not indicate cure of amebiasis; laboratory evidence is required. Stool specimens should be examined for amebic cysts and trophozoites periodically for about 6 mo.
c. With anti-*Pneumocystis carinii* agents for prophylaxis, observe for absence of symptoms; when used for treatment, observe for decreased fever, cough, and respiratory distress.	
d. With anthelmintics, observe for relief of symptoms, absence of the parasite in blood or stool for three consecutive examinations, or a reduction in the number of parasitic ova in the feces.	The goal of anthelmintic drug therapy may be complete eradication of the parasite or reduction of the "worm burden."
e. With pediculicides, inspect affected areas for lice or nits.	For most clients, one treatment is effective. For others, a second treatment may be necessary.
3. Observe for adverse effects	
a. With amebicides, observe for anorexia, nausea, vomiting, epigastric burning, diarrhea.	GI effects may occur with all amebicides.
(1) With iodoquinol, observe for agitation, amnesia, peripheral neuropathy, and optic neuropathy.	These effects are most likely to occur with large doses or long-term drug administration.
b. With antimalarial agents, observe for nausea, vomiting, diarrhea, pruritus, skin rash, headache, central nervous system (CNS) stimulation.	These effects may occur with most antimalarial agents. However, adverse effects are usually mild because small doses are used for prophylaxis, and the larger doses required for

NURSING ACTIONS	RATIONALE/EXPLANATION
	treatment of acute malarial attacks are given only for short periods. When chloroquine and related drugs are used for long-term treatment of rheumatoid arthritis or lupus erythematosus, adverse effects increase (*e.g.*, blood dyscrasias, retinal damage).
(1) With pyrimethamine, observe for anemia, thrombocytopenia, and leukopenia.	This drug interferes with folic acid metabolism.
(2) With quinine, observe for signs of cinchonism (headache, tinnitus, decreased auditory acuity, blurred vision).	These effects occur with usual therapeutic doses of quinine. They do not usually necessitate discontinuance of quinine therapy.
c. With metronidazole, observe for convulsions, peripheral paresthesias, nausea, diarrhea, unpleasant taste, vertigo, headache, and vaginal and urethral burning sensation.	CNS effects are most serious: GI effects are most common.
d. With parenteral pentamidine, observe for leukopenia, thrombocytopenia, hypoglycemia, hypocalcemia, hypotension, acute renal failure, ventricular tachycardia, and Stevens-Johnson syndrome.	Severe hypotension may occur after a single parenteral dose. Deaths from hypotension, hypoglycemia, and cardiac arrhythmias have been reported.
e. With aerosol pentamidine, observe for fatigue, shortness of breath, bronchospasm, cough, dizziness, rash, anorexia, nausea, vomiting, chest pain.	These are the most common adverse effects.
f. With atovaquone, observe for nausea, vomiting, diarrhea, fever, headache, skin rash.	
g. With trimetrexate, observe for anemia, neutropenia, thrombocytopenia, increased bilirubin and liver enzymes (AST, ALT, alkaline phosphatase), fever, skin rash, pruritus, nausea, vomiting, hyponatremia, hypocalcemia.	
h. With tropical antitrichomonal agents, observe for hypersensitivity reactions (*e.g.*, rash, inflammation), burning, and pruritus.	Hypersensitivity reactions are the major adverse effects. Other effects are minor and rarely require that drug therapy be discontinued.
i. With permethrin, observe for pruritus, burning, or tingling; with Lindane, observe for CNS stimulation (nervousness, tremors, insomnia, convulsions).	Antihistamines or topical corticosteroids may be used to decrease itching. CNS toxicity is more likely to occur with excessive use of Lindane (*i.e.*, increased amounts, leaving in place longer than prescribed, or applying more frequently than prescribed).
4. **Observe for drug interactions**	Few clinically significant drug interactions occur because many antiparasitic agents are administered for local effects in the GI tract or on the skin. Most of the drugs also are given for short periods.
a. Drugs that alter effects of chloroquine:	
(1) Acidifying agents (*e.g.*, ascorbic acid).	Inhibit chloroquine by increasing the rate of urinary excretion
(2) Alkalinizing agents (*e.g.*, sodium bicarbonate)	Potentiate chloroquine by decreasing the rate of urinary excretion
(3) MAO inhibitors	Increase risk of toxicity and retinal damage by inhibiting hepatic enzymes.
b. Drugs that alter effects of metronidazole:	
(1) Phenobarbital, phenytoin	These drugs induce hepatic enzymes and decrease effects of metronidazole by accelerating its rate of hepatic metabolism.

(continued)

NURSING ACTIONS	RATIONALE/EXPLANATION
(2) Cimetidine	May increase effects by inhibiting hepatic metabolism of metronidazole.
c. Drugs that decrease effects of atovaquone and trimetrexate: Rifampin and other drugs that induce P450 drug-metabolizing enzymes in the liver	Although few interactions have been reported, any enzyme-inducing drug can potentially decrease effects of atovaquone and trimetrexate by accelerating their metabolism in the liver.
5. Teach clients	
a. Use antiparasitic drugs as prescribed	To achieve therapeutic effects without adverse effects
b. Measures to prevent parasitic infection or reinfection	

REVIEW AND APPLICATION EXERCISES

1. What groups are at risk of developing parasitic infections (*e.g.,* amebiasis, malaria, pediculosis, helminthiasis)?

2. What interventions are needed to prevent parasitic infections?

3. How would you assess for a parasitic infection in a client who has been in an environment associated with a particular infestation?

4. How can you assess a client's personal hygiene practices and environmental sanitation facilities?

5. How would you instruct a mother about treatment and prevention of reinfection with head lice or pinworms?

6. What are adverse effects of commonly used antiparasitic drugs, and how may they be prevented or minimized?

SELECTED REFERENCES

Anandan, J.V. (1997). Parasitic diseases. In J.T. DiPiro, R.L. Talbert, G.C Yee, G.R. Matzke, B.G. Wells & L.M. Posey (Eds.), *Pharmacotherapy: A pathophysiologic approach,* 3rd ed., pp. 2161–2170. Stamford, CT: Appleton & Lange.

Drug facts and comparisons. Updated monthly. St. Louis: Facts and Comparisons.

Grubman, S. & Simonds, R.J. (1996). Preventing *Pneumocystis carinii* pneumonia in human immunodeficiency virus-infected children: New guidelines for prophylaxis. *Pediatric Infectious Disease Journal, 15,* 165–168.

Kelley, W.N. (1997). *Textbook of internal medicine,* 3rd ed. Philadelphia: Lippincott-Raven.

Peterson, C.M. & Eichenfield, L.F. (1996). Scabies. *Pediatric Annals, 25*(2), 97–100.

Smeltzer, S.C. & Bare, B.G. (1996). *Brunner and Suddarth's Textbook of medical-surgical nursing,* 8th ed. Philadelphia: Lippincott-Raven.

Tracy, J.W. & Webster, L.T., Jr. (1996). Chemotherapy of parasitic infections. In J.G. Hardman, L.E. Limbird, P.B. Molinoff & R.W. Ruddon (Eds.), *Goodman and Gilman's The pharmacological basis of therapeutics,* 9th ed., pp. 955–1026. New York: McGraw-Hill.

Drugs Affecting the Immune System

42 Physiology of the Immune System

Objectives

After studying this chapter, the student will be able to:

1 Review body defense mechanisms.

2 Differentiate between cellular and humoral types of immunity.

3 Describe the antigen–antibody reaction.

4 Discuss similarities and differences between inflammation and the immune response.

5 Discuss roles of various white blood cells in the immune response.

6 Describe the functions of cytokines.

Key Terms

Acquired immunity

Antibody

Antigen

Complement

Cytokine

Immunoglobulin (IG)

Innate or natural immunity

Macrophage

Phagocytosis

Overview of Body Defense Mechanisms

The immune system is one of several mechanisms that protect the body from potentially harmful substances, including pathogenic microorganisms. The body's primary external defense mechanism is intact skin, which prevents entry of foreign substances and produces secretions that inhibit microbial growth. The mucous membranes lining the gastrointestinal (GI) and respiratory tracts are internal defense mechanisms that act as physical barriers and produce mucus that traps foreign substances so they may be expelled from the body. Mucous membranes also produce other secretions (*e.g.*, gastric acid) that kill ingested microorganisms. Additional internal mechanisms include the normal microbial population, which is usually nonpathogenic and controls potential pathogens, and secretions (*e.g.*, perspiration, tears, and saliva) that contain lysozyme, an enzyme that destroys the cell walls of gram-positive bacteria.

If a foreign substance gets through the above defenses and penetrates body tissues, an inflammatory response begins immediately. Inflammation is a generalized reaction to cellular injury from any cause. It involves phagocytic leukocytes and chemical substances that destroy the foreign invader.

The final defense mechanism is the immune response, a specific reaction that stimulates production of antibodies and activated lymphocytes, which then destroy foreign invaders. Immune responses occur more slowly than inflammatory responses. Inflammatory and immune responses interact in complex ways and share a number of processes, including phagocytosis. As a result, understanding inflammation promotes understanding of immunity and vice versa. Cellular physiology and inflammation as a response to cellular injury are discussed in Chapter 1.

Immunity

Immunity indicates protection from a disease, and the major function of the immune system is to detect and eliminate foreign substances that may cause tissue injury or disease. To perform this function, the immune system must be able to differentiate body tissues (self) from foreign substances (nonself). Self tissues are recognized by distinctive protein molecules on the surface membranes of essentially all body cells. These molecules or markers (also called autoantigens) are encoded by a group of genes called the major histocompatibility complex (MHC). MHC markers are essential to immune system function because they regulate the antigens to which a person responds and

allow immune cells (*e.g.*, lymphocytes and macrophages) to recognize and communicate with each other. Nonself or foreign substances are also recognized by distinctive molecules, called epitopes, on their surfaces. Epitopes vary widely in type, number, and ability to elicit an immune response.

A normally functioning immune system does not attack body tissues labeled as self but attacks nonself substances. In most instances, a normally functioning immune system is highly desirable. With organ or tissue transplants, however, the system responds appropriately but undesirably when it attacks the nonself grafts. An abnormally functioning immune system causes numerous diseases. When the system is hypoactive, immunodeficiency disorders develop in which the person is highly susceptible to infectious and neoplastic diseases. When the system is hyperactive, it perceives ordinarily harmless environmental substances (*e.g.*, foods, plant pollens) as harmful and induces allergic reactions. When the system is inappropriately activated (it loses its ability to distinguish between self and nonself, so an immune response is aroused against the host's own body tissues), the result is autoimmune disorders, such as systemic lupus erythematosus and rheumatoid arthritis. Many other disorders, including diabetes mellitus and myasthenia gravis, are thought to involve autoimmune mechanisms. To aid understanding of the immune response and drugs used to alter immune response, more specific characteristics, processes, and functions of the immune system are described.

TYPES OF IMMUNITY

Innate immunity, which includes the general protective mechanisms described above, is not produced by the immune system. It is often described as species dependent. Thus, humans have an inborn resistance to many infectious diseases that affect other species because human tissues do not provide a suitable environment for growth of the causative microorganisms.

Acquired immunity develops during gestation or after birth and may be active or passive. *Active immunity* is produced by the person's own immune system in response to a disease caused by a specific antigen or administration of an antigen (*e.g.*, a vaccine) from a source outside the body, usually by injection. The immune response stimulated by the antigen produces activated lymphocytes and antibodies against the antigen. When an antigen is present for the first time, production of antibodies requires several days. As a result, the serum concentration of antibodies does not reach protective levels for about 7 to 10 days, and the host develops the disease. When the antigen is eliminated, the antibody concentration gradually decreases over several weeks.

The duration of active immunity may be relatively brief (*e.g.,* to influenza viruses), or it may last for years or a lifetime. Long-term active immunity has a unique characteristic called *memory.* When the host is re-exposed to the antigen, lymphocytes are activated and antibodies are produced rapidly, and the host does not develop the disease. This characteristic allows "booster" doses of antigen to increase antibody levels and maintain active immunity against some diseases.

Passive immunity occurs when antibodies are formed by the immune system of another person or animal and transferred to the host. For example, an infant is normally protected for several months by maternal antibodies received through the placenta during gestation. Also, antibodies previously formed by a donor can be transferred to the host by an injection of immune serum. These antibodies act against antigens immediately. Passive immunity is short term, lasting only a few weeks or months.

Types of acquired immunity have traditionally been separated into cellular immunity (mainly involving activated T lymphocytes in body tissues) and humoral immunity (mainly involving B lymphocytes and antibodies in the blood). However, it is now known that the two types are closely connected, that virtually all antigens elicit both cellular and humoral responses, and that most humoral (B cell) responses require cellular (T cell) stimulation.

Although most humoral immune responses occur when antibodies or B cells encounter antigens in blood, some occur when antibodies or B cells encounter antigens in other body fluids (*e.g.,* tears, sweat, saliva, mucus, and breast milk). The antibodies in body fluids other than blood are produced by a part of humoral immunity sometimes called the secretory or mucosal immune system. The B cells of the mucosal system migrate through lymphoid tissues of tear ducts, salivary glands, breasts, bronchi, intestines, and genitourinary structures. The antibodies (mostly immunoglobulin A [IgA], some IgM and IgG) secreted at these sites act locally rather than systemically. This local protection combats foreign substances, especially pathogenic microorganisms, that are inhaled, swallowed, or otherwise come in contact with external body surfaces. When the foreign substances bind to local antibodies, they are unable to attach to and invade mucosal tissue.

ANTIGENS

Antigens are the foreign (nonself) substances, usually microorganisms, other proteins, or polysaccharides, that initiate immune responses. Antigens have specific sites that interact with immune cells to induce the immune response. The number of antigenic sites on a molecule depends largely on its molecular weight. Large protein and polysaccharide molecules are com-plete antigens because of their complex chemical structures and multiple antigenic sites. Smaller molecules (*e.g.,* animal danders, plant pollens, and most drugs) are incomplete antigens (called haptens) and cannot act as antigens by themselves. However, they have antigenic sites and can combine with carrier substances to become antigenic. Antigens also may be called immunogens, which is a more accurate term because an antigen may be too weak to arouse an immune response. In discussions of allergic conditions, antigens are often called allergens.

Immune Responses to Antigens

The immune response involves antigens that induce the formation of antibodies or sensitized T lymphocytes. The initial response occurs when an antigen is first introduced into the body. B lymphocytes recognize the antigen as foreign and develop antibodies against it. Antibodies are proteins called immunoglobulins that interact with specific antigens. Antigen–antibody interactions may result in formation of antigen–antibody complexes, agglutination or clumping of cells, neutralization of bacterial toxins, destruction of pathogens or cells, attachment of antigen to immune cells, activation of complement (a group of plasma proteins essential to normal inflammatory and immunologic responses), and coating of the antigen so that it is more readily phagocytized (opsonization). With a later exposure to the antigen, antibody is rapidly produced.

The exact number of exposures required to produce enough antibodies to bind a significant amount of antigen is unknown. Thus, an allergic reaction may occur with the second exposure or after several exposures, when sufficient antibodies have been produced. Antigen–T lymphocyte interactions stimulate production and function of other T lymphocytes and help to regulate immunoglobulin production by B lymphocytes. T cells are involved in delayed hypersensitivity reactions, rejection of tissue or organ transplants, and response to neoplasms and some infections.

Immune Cells

Immune cells (Fig. 42-1) are white blood cells (WBCs) found throughout the body in lymphoid tissues (bone marrow, spleen, thymus, tonsils and adenoids, Peyer's patches in the small intestine, lymph nodes, and blood and lymphatic vessels that transport the cells). When exposure to an antigen occurs and an immune response is aroused, WBCs are attracted to the antigen in a process called chemotaxis. Once WBCs reach the area, they phagocytize the antigen. Specific WBCs are granulocytes (neutrophils, eosinophils, basophils), monocytes, and lymphocytes. Although all WBCs play a role,

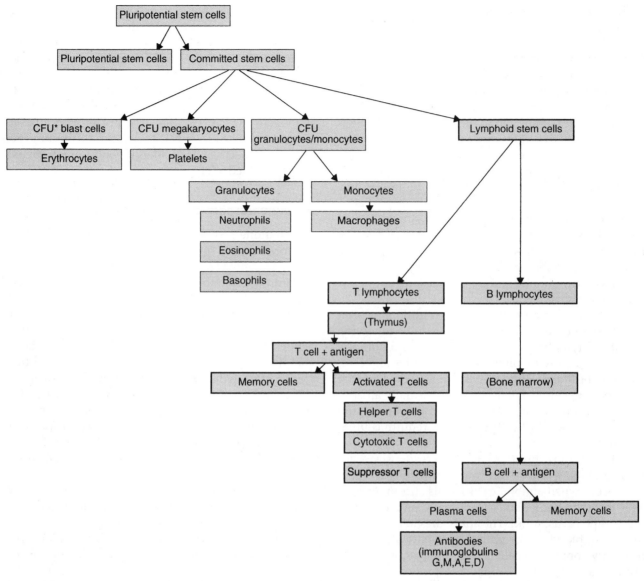

Figure 42-1
Hematopoiesis and formation of immune cells.

neutrophils, monocytes, and lymphocytes are especially important in phagocytic and immune processes.

Neutrophils arrive first and start phagocytosis; *monocytes* arrive several hours later. In comparison to neutrophils, monocytes are larger, can ingest larger amounts of antigen, and have a much longer life span. In addition to their activity in the bloodstream, monocytes can enter tissue spaces (then called tissue macrophages). Tissue macrophages are widely distributed throughout the body and form the mononuclear phagocyte system (formerly called the reticuloendothelial system). Both mobile monocytes and fixed monocyte–macrophages can initiate the immune response by activating lymphocytes. They perform this function as part of phagocytosis in which they engulf a circulating antigen, break it into fragments, and return antigenic fragments to the cell surface. The antigenic fragments are recognized as foreign material by circulating T and B lymphocytes, and an immune response is initiated. Because the monocytes prepare the antigen to interact with T and B lymphocytes, they are called antigen-processing and antigen-presenting cells.

Lymphocytes are the main immunocytes, and those in tissues are in dynamic equilibrium with those in circulating blood. These cells continuously travel through blood and lymph vessels from one lymphoid organ to another. The three types of lymphocytes are natural killer cells, T cells, and B cells.

Natural killer cells, so called because they do not need to interact with a specific antigen to become activated, destroy infectious microorganisms and malignant cells by releasing powerful chemicals. T lymphocytes are especially able to combat intracellular infections (*e.g.,* virally infected cells), whereas B lymphocytes secrete antibodies that can neutralize pathogens before their entry into host cells. Both T and B cells must be activated by antigens before they can fulfill their immune functions, and both have proteins on their cell membrane surfaces that act as receptors for antigens.

Each T or B lymphocyte reacts only with a specific type of antigen and is capable of forming only one type of antibody or one type of T cell. When a specific antigen attaches to cell membrane receptors to form an antigen–antibody complex, the complex activates the lymphocyte to form tremendous numbers of duplicate lymphocytes (clones) that are exactly like the parent cell. Clones of a B lymphocyte eventually secrete antibodies that circulate throughout the body. Clones of a T lymphocyte are sensitized T cells that are released into lymphatic ducts, carried to the blood, circulated through all tissue fluids, then returned to lymphatic ducts and recirculated. Additional participants in the activation process are phagocytic macrophages and helper T cells, which secrete substances called cytokines that regulate the growth, reproduction, and function of lymphocytes.

T LYMPHOCYTES

T lymphocytes are the primary regulators of immune responses because they direct the activities of B cells and macrophages. They originate in pluripotential stem cells in the bone marrow and differentiate into immune cells in the thymus gland. The thymus produces a substance called thymosin, which is necessary for T cell maturation. When T cells bind with an antigen, specific genes are activated to produce substances that direct T cell proliferation and differentiation. One such substance is interleukin-2 (IL-2), which stimulates T cell deoxyribonucleic acid (DNA) replication and mitosis. Cell division is necessary for production of large numbers of antigen-reactive cells and for cellular changes associated with the different subgroups of T cells. Specific types and functions of T cells include the following:

- *Helper T cells* (also called T4 or CD4 cells), the largest subgroup, regulate virtually all immune functions by producing protein substances called lymphokines (cytokines produced by lymphocytes). Lymphokines stimulate the growth of bone marrow and other cells of the immune system (*e.g.,* cytotoxic and suppressor T cells and B cells). They also activate macrophages and facilitate phagocytosis. Important lymphokines include IL-2, -3, -4, -5, -6, granulocyte-macrophage colony-stimulating factor (CSF), and interferon-gamma. The devastating effects of acquired immunodeficiency syndrome (AIDS) result primarily from the ability of the human immunodeficiency virus (HIV) to destroy helper T cells.
- *Cytotoxic T cells* (also called killer T cells) are recruited and activated by helper T cells. More specifically, helper T cells secrete IL-2, which is necessary for activation and proliferation (clonal expansion) of cytotoxic T cells. Once activated by antigen and IL-2, cytotoxic T cells bind to antigens on surfaces of target cells and release substances that form large holes in the target cell membrane. The damaged cell membrane allows water, electrolytes, and other molecules to enter the cell, resulting in cellular edema and death. Once these cytotoxic cells have damaged the target cells, they can detach themselves and attack other target cells.

  Cytotoxic T cells are especially lethal to virally infected cells because virus particles become entrapped in the membranes of the cells and act as strong antigens that attract the T cells. These cells persist in tissues for months, even after destruction of all the invaders that elicited the original cytotoxic activity. Thus, T cells are especially important in killing body cells that have been invaded by foreign microorganisms or cells that have become malignant. Cytotoxic T cells also play a role in the destruction of transplanted organs and delayed hypersensitivity reactions.
- *Suppressor T cells* (also called T8 or CD8 cells) stop the immune response when an antigen has been destroyed by decreasing the activities of B cells and other T cells. This function is important in preventing further tissue damage. In autoimmune disorders, suppressor T cell function is impaired, and extensive tissue damage may result.

B LYMPHOCYTES

B lymphocytes originate in stem cells in the bone marrow, differentiate into cells capable of forming antibodies (also in the bone marrow), and migrate to the spleen, lymph nodes, or other lymphoid tissue. In lymphoid tissue, the cells may be dormant until exposed to an antigen. In response to an antigen and IL-2 from helper T cells, B cells multiply rapidly, enlarge, and differentiate into plasma cells, which then produce antibodies (immunoglobulins) to oppose the antigen. Immunoglobulins are secreted into lymph and transported to the bloodstream for circulation throughout the body. There are five main classes of immunoglobulins:

- *IgG* is the most abundant immunoglobulin, constituting about 80% of the antibodies in human serum. Molecules of IgG combine with molecules of antigen, and the antigen–antibody complex activates complement. Activated complement causes an inflammatory reaction, promotes phagocytosis, and inactivates or destroys the antigen. IgG also crosses the placenta to provide maternally acquired antibodies (passive immunity) to the infant.

- *IgA* is located primarily in secretions of the respiratory and GI tracts, where it acts against antigens entering those areas.
- *IgM* constitutes about 10% of serum antibodies and reacts with antigens in the bloodstream because its large molecular size prevents transport through capillary walls. It activates complement to destroy microorganisms.
- *IgE* is located mainly in tissues and is thought to be responsible for allergic reactions, including anaphylaxis. IgE sensitizes mast cells, which then release histamine and other chemical mediators that cause bronchoconstriction, edema, urticaria, and other manifestations of allergic reactions. IgE does not activate complement. The production of IgE is stimulated by T lymphocytes and lymphokines (mainly IL-4, -5, and -6) and inhibited by the interferons. Small amounts of IgE are present in the serum of nonallergic people; larger amounts are produced by people with allergies.
- *IgD* is present in serum in trace amounts and probably functions in recognition of antigens.

CYTOKINES

Cytokines are protein growth factors secreted by WBCs that act on the secreting cells or other leukocytes to stimulate leukocyte replication and function. Generally, cytokines act as messengers between cells through receptors on cell surfaces and interact synergistically with other growth factors. More specifically, cytokines regulate tissue inflammation and repair and immune responses.

In the immune system, cytokines regulate growth, mobility and differentiation of leukocytes. Although the process is not completely clear, it appears that cytokines formed by activated macrophages enter the bone marrow where they induce the synthesis and release of other cytokines that activate resting stem cells to produce more granulocytes and monocyte–macrophages. Newly formed granulocytes and monocytes leave the bone marrow and enter the circulating blood in about 3 days. Cytokines produced by lymphocytes are called lymphokines, and those produced by monocyte–macrophages are called monokines.

Lymphokines enhance macrophage activity by two main mechanisms. First, they cause macrophages to accumulate in damaged tissues by delaying or stopping macrophage migration from the area. Second, they increase the capacity and effectiveness of phagocytosis.

Some lymphokines, especially IL-2, directly stimulate helper T cells and enhance their antiantigenic activity. They also enhance the antiantigenic activity of the entire immune system. Several types of cytokines have been identified, including CSF, interferons, interleukins, and tumor necrosis factor. Cytokines are described further below and in Table 42-1.

Colony-Stimulating Factors

Colony-stimulating factors (CSF) stimulate the growth and function of hematopoietic cells. All blood cells originate in bone marrow in stem cells that are capable of becoming different types of blood cells. As these pluripotential stem cells reproduce during the life of the host, some reproduced cells are exactly like the original multipotential cells and are retained in bone marrow to maintain a continuing supply. However, most reproduced stem cells differentiate to form other types of cells. The early offspring are committed to become a particular type of cell, and a committed stem cell that will produce a cell type is called a colony-forming unit (CFU), such as CFU-erythrocyte or CFU-granulocyte. CSF control the growth, differentiation and reproduction of the CFU.

Four major CSF have been identified. One (multi-CSF or IL-3) promotes the growth of virtually all types of stem cells; the other three induce the growth of specific types of committed stem cells, such as granulocytes and macrophages. Although most cytokines were initially defined by their action on one lineage, they actually act on different lineages. For example, G-CSF was initially labeled as a granulocyte-colony stimulator, but it also affects erythrocyte, megakaryocyte (platelet precursor), macrophage, and pre–B cell lineages. These growth factors also may stimulate cell division in neoplastic counterparts of their target cells, including the cancerous cells of acute myelocytic leukemia, lymphomas, and multiple myeloma.

Interferons

Interferons "interfere" with the ability of viruses in infected cells to replicate and spread to uninfected cells. They also inhibit reproduction and growth of other cells, including tumor cells, and activate natural killer cells. These antiproliferative and immunomodulatory activities play important roles in normal host defense mechanisms.

Interleukins

Interleukins stimulate growth and differentiation of early lymphoid and multilineage stem cells into lymphocytes, for the most part. IL-3, also known as multi-CSF, stimulates pluripotential stem cells to produce

TABLE 42-1 CYTOKINES

Type	Name	Main Source	Main Functions
Colony-stimulating factors (CSF)	G-CSF	Leukocytes	Stimulates growth of bone marrow Generates neutrophils
	M-CSF		Generates macrophages Stimulates growth of macrophages
	GM-CSF		Stimulates growth of monocyte–macrophages
Interferons (IFN)	IFN-alpha	Leukocytes	Antiviral, antiproliferative, and immunomodulating effects Stimulates macrophages and natural killer (NK) cells
	IFN-beta	Fibroblasts	Antiviral and immunoregulatory effects
	IFN-gamma	Circulating T cells and NK cells	Induces cell membrane antigens (*e.g.*, major histocompatibility complex) Influences functions of basophils and mast cells by increasing their ability to release histamine and decreasing their capacity for growth
Interleukins (IL)	IL-1	Monocytes	Interacts with tumor necrosis factor to induce other growth factors Stimulates growth of blood cells, especially B and T lymphocytes Enhances interactions between monocytes and lymphocytes Causes inflammation Causes fever
	IL-2	T lymphocytes	Promotes growth of T cells Activates T and B cells and NK cells Augments production of other lymphokines, such as interferon-gamma Influences the expression of histocompatibility antigens May inhibit granulocyte–macrophage colony formation and erythropoiesis.
	IL-3 (Multi-CSF)	T lymphocytes	Stimulates bone marrow; growth factor for all blood cells Stimulates growth of macrophages, eosinophils, and mast cells
	IL-4	Helper T cells	Stimulates growth of T and B cells and mast cells Promotes immunoglobulin synthesis and reactions Interacts with other cytokines to stimulate granulocytes, macrophages, mast cells, and other cells
	IL-5	Helper T cells	Stimulates B cell growth, differentiation, and antibody secretion Stimulates eosinophils; promote eosinophilia Stimulates T cell replacement
	IL-6	Fibroblasts and others	Interacts with other growth factors to stimulate growth and differentiation of B and T cells and production of antibodies Augments inflammatory and immune responses Augments colony formation induced by other growth factors Stimulates granulocyte–macrophage and megakaryocyte colony formation
	IL-7 (lymphopoietin-1)	Stromal cells	Generates pre–B and pre–T cells Stimulates lymphocyte growth Activates B and T cells

(continued)

TABLE 42-1 CYTOKINES (Continued)

Type	Name	Main Source	Main Functions
	IL-8	Macrophages and others	Regulates growth and movement of neutrophils and lymphocytes Induces immediate inflammatory responses
	IL-9		Stimulates production of red blood cells and platelets
	IL-10		?
	IL-11		Stimulates growth of megakaryocytes, B cells and blast cells
Tumor necrosis factor (TNF)	TNF-alpha	Monocytes	Inflammatory, immunoenhancing, and tumoricidal Causes vascular thromboses and tumor necrosis
	TNF-beta (lymphotoxin)	T lymphocytes	?
T lymphocyte growth factor (TGF)	TGF-beta	Platelets, bone, other tissue	Fibroplasia and immunosuppression Wound healing and bone remodeling

all types of blood cells. Most interleukins stimulate B lymphocyte activity, but IL-4, -5, and -6 are especially important in B cell activities.

Tumor Necrosis Factor

Tumor necrosis factor is produced by activated macrophages and other cells and acts on many immune and nonimmune target cells. It participates in the inflammatory response and causes hemorrhagic necrosis in several types of tumor cells. It is structurally the same as cachectin, a substance associated with debilitation and weight loss in patients with cancer.

Patient-Related Factors That Influence Immune Function

AGE

Immune Function During Fetal and Neonatal Periods

During the first few months of gestation, the fetal immune system is deficient in antibody production and phagocytic activity. During the last trimester, the fetal immune system may be able to respond to infectious antigens, such as cytomegalovirus, rubella virus, and toxoplasmosis. However, most fetal protection against infectious microorganisms is by maternal antibodies that reach the fetal circulation through the placenta. In the placenta, maternal blood and fetal blood are separated only by a layer of specialized cells called trophoblasts. Because antibodies are too large to diffuse across the trophoblastic layer, they are actively trans-

ported from the maternal to the fetal circulation by the trophoblastic cells.

At birth, the neonatal immune system is still immature, but IgG levels (from maternal blood) are near adult levels in umbilical cord blood. However, the source of maternal antibodies is severed at birth. Antibody titers in infants decrease over approximately 6 months as maternal antibodies are catabolized. Although the infant does start producing IgG, the rate of production is lower than the rate of breakdown of maternal antibodies. Cell-mediated immunity is probably completely functional at birth.

Immune Function in Older Adults

Both humoral and cell-mediated immune functions decline with aging, and this decline is probably a major factor in the older adult's increased susceptibility to infections and tumors. The regulation of immunologic functions also declines with age, which may account for the greater frequency of autoimmune diseases in this age group. Lymphocytes are less able to proliferate in response to antigenic stimulation and a relative state of immunodeficiency prevails. With T lymphocytes, function is impaired, and the numbers are possibly decreased in peripheral blood. The functional impairment includes decreased activity of helper T cells and increased activity of suppressor T cells. With B lymphocytes, the numbers probably do not decrease, but the cells are less able to form antibodies in response to antigens. Abnormal antibody production results from impaired function of B cells and helper T cells. In addition, older adults have increased blood levels of antibodies against their own tissues (autoantibodies).

Impaired immune mechanisms have several implications for clinicians who care for elderly patients, including the following:

- Older adults are more susceptible to develop infections and less able to recover from them. Therefore, older adults need protective measures, such as rigorous personal hygiene; good nutrition; adequate exercise, rest, and sleep; minimal exposure to potential pathogens, when possible; and appropriate immunizations (*e.g.,* influenza, pneumonia, tetanus). When older adults develop an infection, signs and symptoms (*e.g.,* fever and drainage) may be absent or less pronounced than in younger adults.
- Older adults have impaired immune responses to antigens. Thus, higher doses of immunizing antigens may be needed in older adults to achieve protective antibody titers than in younger adults.
- Older adults often exhibit a less intense positive reaction in skin tests for tuberculosis (indicating a decreased delayed hypersensitivity response).

NUTRITIONAL STATUS

Nutritional status can have profound effects on immune function. Adequate nutrient intake contributes to immunocompetence (ability of the immune system to function effectively). Malnutrition contributes to immunodeficiency. A severe lack of calories or protein decreases numbers and functions of T cells, complement activity, neutrophil chemotaxis, and phagocytosis. An inadequate zinc intake can depress the functions of T and B cells. Zinc is a cofactor for many enzymes, some of which are found in lymphocytes and are required for lymphocyte function. Zinc deficiency also may result from inadequate absorption in the GI tract or excessive losses in urine, feces, or through the skin with such disorders as chronic renal disease, chronic diarrhea, burns, or severe psoriasis. Vitamin deficiencies may also depress T- and B-cell function because several (*e.g.,* A, E, folic acid, pantothenic acid, and pyridoxine) also are enzyme cofactors in lymphocytes.

STRESS

There is evidence that stress depresses immune function and therefore increases risks of developing infection and cancer. The connection between the stress response and the immune response is thought to involve neuroendocrine mechanisms. The stress response is characterized by increased activity of catecholamine neurotransmitters in the central and autonomic nervous systems (*e.g.,* norepinephrine, epinephrine) and increased secretion of cortisol from the adrenal cortex.

Cortisol and other corticosteroids are well known to suppress immune function and are used therapeutically for that purpose. The immune response is affected by these neuroendocrine influences on lymphoid organs and lymphocyte functions because lymphocytes have receptors for many neurotransmitters and hormones.

Immune Disorders

Dysfunction of the immune system is related to many different disease processes, including allergic, autoimmune, immunodeficiency, and neoplastic disorders. Each of these is described below to assist in understanding the use of drugs to alter immune functions:

- In *allergic disorders,* the body erroneously perceives normally harmless substances (*e.g.,* foods, pollens) as antigens and mounts an immune response. More specifically, IgE binds to antigen on the surface of mast cells and causes the release of chemical mediators (*e.g.,* histamine) that produce the allergic manifestations. This reaction may cause tissue damage ranging from mild skin rashes to life-threatening anaphylaxis.
- In *autoimmune disorders,* the body erroneously perceives the person's own body tissues as antigens and elicits an immune response, often inflammatory in nature. Rheumatoid arthritis and systemic lupus erythematosus have long been considered autoimmune disorders. More recently, insulin-dependent diabetes mellitus, myasthenia gravis, and several other disorders have been added to the list. Autoimmune processes may damage virtually every body tissue.
- In *immunodeficiency disorders,* the body is especially susceptible to infections and neoplastic diseases. A major immunodeficiency disorder is caused by infection with HIV, which decreases the numbers and almost all functions of T lymphocytes and several functions of B lymphocytes and monocytes. Immunodeficiency also is induced by severe malnutrition, cancer, and immunosuppressant drugs.
- In *neoplastic disease,* immune cells apparently lose their ability to destroy mutant cells or early malignant cells. This effect could result from immunodeficiency states or from cancer cells that are overwhelming in number or highly malignant. Mutant cells constantly occur during cell division, but few survive or lead to cancer. Most mutant cells simply die; some survive but retain the normal controls that prevent excessive growth; and some are destroyed by immune processes activated by abnormal proteins found in most mutant cells.

Immunotherapy

Immunotherapy involves alteration of the immune response for therapeutic purposes. Immunotherapy is mainly used to prevent or treat rejection of transplanted tissues or organs and to treat immunodeficiency disorders and some cancers. Methods include administering exogenous antigens (*e.g.,* immunizations and desensitization procedures), strengthening antigens (*e.g.,* an antigen that is too weak to elicit an immune response), or suppressing the normal response to an antigen. In desensitization procedures, weak extracts of antigenic substances (*e.g.,* foods, plant pollens, penicillin) are prepared as drugs and administered in small, increasing amounts so the patient develops a tolerance for the substances and avoids serious allergic reactions.

Drugs can be given to stimulate immune responses (immunizing agents [see Chap. 43] and other immunostimulants [see Chap. 44]) or to suppress the normal response (immunosuppressants [see Chap. 45]).

REVIEW AND APPLICATION EXERCISES

1. What is the difference between innate and acquired immunity?

2. What are methods of producing active acquired immunity?

3. Which WBCs are phagocytes?

4. Describe phagocytosis.

5. Where are T lymphocytes formed, and what are their functions?

6. Where are B lymphocytes formed, and what are their functions?

7. What are antigens, and how do they elicit an immune response?

8. What are cytokines, and how do they function in the immune response?

9. What is complement, and how does it function in the immune response?

SELECTED REFERENCES

Boon, T. (1993). Teaching the immune system to fight cancer. *Scientific American, 266*(3), 82–89.

Guyton, A.C. & Hall, J.E. (1996). *Textbook of medical physiology,* 9th ed. Philadelphia: W.B. Saunders.

Hall, P.D. & Tami, J.A. (1997). Function and evaluation of the immune system. In J.T. DiPiro, R.L. Talbert, G.C. Yee, G.R. Matzke, B.G. Wells, & L.M. Posey (Eds.), *Pharmacotherapy: A pathophysiologic approach,* 3rd ed., pp. 1647–1660. Stamford, CT: Appleton & Lange.

Porth, C.M. (1994). *Pathophysiology: Concepts of altered health states,* 4th ed. Philadelphia: J.B. Lippincott.

Rich, R.R., Fleisher, T.A., Schwartz, B.D., Shearer, W.T. & Strober, W. (Eds.). (1996). *Clinical immunology: Principles and practice.* St. Louis: C.V. Mosby.

Sahai, J. & Louie, S.G. (1993). Overview of the immune and hematopoietic systems. *American Journal of Hospital Pharmacy, 50*(Suppl. 3), S4–S9.

Winchester, R. (1996). Principles of the immune response. In W.N. Kelley (Ed.), *Textbook of internal medicine,* 3rd ed., pp. 18–24. Philadelphia: Lippincott-Raven.

Immunizing Agents

Outline

Immunization

Agents for Active Immunity
indications for use
contraindications for use

Agents for Passive Immunity

Individual Immunizing Agents

Nursing Process
assessment
nursing diagnoses
planning/goals
interventions
evaluation

Principles of Therapy
sources of information
selection of preparation
storage of vaccines
use in children
use in healthy adolescents, young adults,
   and middle-age adults
use in older adults
use in immunosuppression

Objectives

After studying this chapter, the student will be able to:

1 Discuss common characteristics of immunizations.

2 Discuss the importance of immunizations in promoting health and preventing disease.

3 Identify immunizations recommended for adults.

4 Identify immunizations recommended for children.

5 Discuss ways to promote immunization of children.

6 Teach parents about recommended immunizations and record keeping.

Key Terms

Active immunity **Toxoid**

Immunization **Vaccine**

Passive immunity

Immune responses and types of immunity are described in Chapter 42. Many antigens that activate the immune response are microorganisms that cause infectious diseases. Early scientists observed that people who developed certain diseases were thereafter protected despite repeated exposure to the disease. As knowledge evolved, it was discovered that protection stemmed from body substances called antibodies and that antibodies could also be induced by deliberate, controlled exposure to the antigen. Subsequently, immunization techniques were developed.

Immunization

Immunization or vaccination involves administration of an antigen to induce antibody formation (for active immunity) or serum from immune people or animals (for passive immunity). Preparations used for immunization are biologic products prepared by pharmaceutical companies and regulated by the Food & Drug Administration (FDA).

Agents for Active Immunity

The biologic products used for active immunity are vaccines and toxoids. *Vaccines* are suspensions of microorganisms that have been killed or attenuated (weakened or reduced in virulence) so that they can induce antibody formation while preventing or causing very mild forms of the disease. *Toxoids* are bacterial toxins that have been modified to destroy toxicity while retaining antigenic properties (*i.e.,* ability to induce antibody formation). For maximum effectiveness, vaccines and toxoids must be given before exposure to the pathogenic microorganism.

INDICATIONS FOR USE

Clinical indications for use of vaccines and toxoids include the following:

1. Routine immunization of all children against diphtheria, hepatitis B, tetanus, pertussis (whooping cough), rubeola ("red" measles), rubella (German measles), mumps, and poliomyelitis
2. Immunization of adults against tetanus
3. Immunization of prepubertal girls or women of childbearing age against rubella. Rubella during the first trimester of pregnancy is associated with a high incidence of birth defects in the newborn.
4. Immunization of people at high risk of serious morbidity or mortality from a particular disease. For

example, hepatitis B, influenza, and pneumococcal vaccines are recommended for selected groups of people (Table 43-1).
5. Immunization of adults and children at high risk of exposure to a particular disease. For example, several diseases (*e.g.,* yellow fever, cholera) rarely occur in most parts of the world. Thus, immunization is recommended only for people who live in or travel to geographic areas where the disease can be contracted.

CONTRAINDICATIONS FOR USE

Vaccines and toxoids are generally contraindicated during febrile illnesses; immunosuppressive drug therapy (see Chap. 45); immunodeficiency states; leukemia, lymphoma, or generalized malignancy; and pregnancy.

Agents for Passive Immunity

The biologic products used for passive immunity are immune serums and antitoxins. These substances may be obtained from human or animal sources, and they may consist of whole serum or the immunoglobulin portion of serum in which the specific antibodies are concentrated. When possible, human serum is preferred to animal serum because risks of severe allergic reactions are reduced. Also, immunoglobulin fractions are preferred over whole serum because they are more likely to be effective. Human immunoglobulins are available for measles, hepatitis, rabies, respiratory syncytial virus (RSV), rubella, tetanus, and varicella-zoster infections.

To obtain antitoxins or animal immune serums, an animal such as a horse is injected with a purified toxin or toxoid. After antibodies have had time to develop, blood is withdrawn from the animal and prepared for clinical use. Antitoxins are available for rabies, botulism, diphtheria, gas gangrene, and tetanus. A major disadvantage of antitoxins is that a relatively high number of people are allergic to horse serum.

Immune serums and antitoxins are used to provide temporary immunity in people exposed to or experiencing a particular disease. The goal of therapy is to prevent or modify the disease process (*i.e.,* decrease incidence and severity of symptoms). Antitoxins are contraindicated in clients allergic to horse serum.

Individual Immunizing Agents

Vaccines and toxoids are listed in Table 43-1; immune serums and antitoxins are listed in Table 43-2.

(*text continues on page 576*)

TABLE 43-1 VACCINES AND TOXOIDS FOR ACTIVE IMMUNITY

Generic/Trade Name	Characteristics	Clinical Indications	Adults	Children
Cholera vaccine	Sterile suspension of killed cholera organisms. Protects about 50% of recipients for 3–6 mo. Does not prevent transmission of cholera. Protection begins about 1 wk after the initial dose.	Travel to endemic areas (Asia, Africa, Middle East). Living in endemic areas	IM, SC 0.5 ml initially, 0.5 ml 4 wk later, then 0.5 ml every 6 mo if indicated	Over age 10 y, same as adults. Age 5–10 y, IM, SC 0.3 ml initially, 0.3 ml 4 wk later, then 0.3 ml every 6 mo if indicated. Age 6 mo–4 y, IM, SC 0.2 ml initially, 0.2 ml 4 wk later, then 0.2 ml every 6 mo if indicated
Haemophilus b conjugate vaccine (HibTITER, PedvaxHIB, ProHibit)	Formed by conjugating a derivative of the organism with a protein	To prevent infection with Hib, a common cause of serious bacterial infections, including meningitis, in children under 5 years of age		HibTITER age 2–5 mo, IM 0.5 ml q2 mo for 3 doses; age 15 mo, 0.5 ml as a single booster dose. Age 7–11 mo, IM 0.5 ml q2 mo for two doses; age 15 mo, 0.5 ml as a single booster dose. Age 12–14 mo, IM 0.5 ml as single dose; age 15 mo, 0.5 ml as a single booster dose, at least 2 mo after the first dose. Age 15–59 mo, IM 0.5 ml as a single dose (no additional booster dose). Pedvax HIB age 2–6 mo, IM 0.5 ml q2 mo for two doses; age 12 mo, 0.5 ml as a booster dose. Age 7–11 mo, IM 0.5 ml q2 mo for two doses; age 15 mo, 0.5 ml as booster dose. Age 12–14 mo, IM 0.5 ml as single dose; age 15 mo, 0.5 ml as a single booster dose, at least 2 mo after the first dose

(continued)

TABLE 43-1	VACCINES AND TOXOIDS FOR ACTIVE IMMUNITY (Continued)			
			Routes and Dosage Ranges	
Generic/Trade Name	**Characteristics**	**Clinical Indications**	*Adults*	*Children*
				Age 15–59 mo, IM 0.5 ml as a single dose (no additional booster dose) ProHiBit Age 15–59 mo, IM 0.5 ml as a single dose (no additional booster dose)
Hepatitis A vaccine (Havrix)	Inactivated whole virus More than 90% effective Duration of protection unknown Contraindicated during febrile illness, immunosuppression The adult formulation contains 1440 units in 1 ml; the pediatric formulation contains 360 units in 0.5 ml	Workers in day care centers, laboratories, food-handling establishments; homosexual males; IV drug users; military personnel; travelers to areas where hepatitis A is endemic; community residents during an outbreak	IM one dose of 1440 units Booster dose 6–12 mo after initial dose	2–18 y, IM, two doses of 360 units each, given 1 mo apart Booster dose 6–12 mo after initial dose
Hepatitis B vaccine (recombinant) (Recombivax HB, Engerix-B)	Prepared by recombinant DNA techniques of inserting the gene coding for production of hepatitis B surface antigen (HBsAG) into yeast cells Contains no blood or blood products About 96% effective in children and young adults; about 88% effective in adults >40 y Duration of protection unknown; can measure serum antibody levels periodically (protective levels about 10 million U/ml)	Pre-exposure immunization of high-risk groups, such as health care providers (nurses, physicians, dentists, laboratory workers); clients with cancer, organ transplants, hemodialysis, immunosuppressant drug therapy, or multiple infusions of blood or blood products; male homosexuals; intravenous drug abusers; residents and staff of institutions for mentally handicapped people	Engerix, IM 20 μg (1 ml) × three doses, initially and at 1 mo and 6 mo after the first dose Booster, IM 20 μg × one dose Dialysis patients, IM 40 μg (2 ml) × four doses, initially and at 1, 2, and 6 mo after the first dose Recombivax, IM 10 μg (1 ml) × three doses, initially and at 1 mo and 6 mo after the first dose Booster 10 μg × one dose Dialysis formulation, IM 40 μg (1 ml) × three doses, initially and at 1 mo and 6 mo after the first dose Booster 40 μg × one dose if antibody level <10 million U/ml 1–2 mo after third dose of above schedule	Engerix, neonates to 10 y, IM 10 μg (0.5 ml) × three doses, initially and at 1 mo and 6 mo after first dose Booster, IM 10 μg × one dose Children >10 years, IM 20 μg (1 ml) × three doses, same schedule as above Booster, IM 20 μg × one dose Recombivax, birth to 10 years, IM 2.5 μg (0.25 ml) × three doses, initially and at 1 mo and 6 mo after the first dose 11–19 y, IM 5 μg (0.5 ml) × three doses, same schedule as above

TABLE 43-1   **VACCINES AND TOXOIDS FOR ACTIVE IMMUNITY (Continued)**

Generic/Trade Name	Characteristics	Clinical Indications	Routes and Dosage Ranges	
			Adults	*Children*
Influenza vaccine (Fluogen)	Inactivated strains of A and B influenza viruses, reformulated annually to include current strains Protects 60%–75% of recipients for a few months. Maximal antibody production occurs the second week after vaccination; the titer remains constant for about 1 mo, then gradually declines Grown in chick embryos; therefore, contraindicated in clients who are highly allergic to eggs	Recommended annually for health care providers; older adults; and people chronically ill with pulmonary, cardiovascular, or renal disorders, diabetes mellitus, or adrenocortical insufficiency	IM 0.5 ml as single dose	<3 years, IM 0.25 ml as single dose >3 years, IM 0.5 ml as single dose Note: Children <9 years not previously immunized need two doses, at least 1 mo apart
Measles vaccine (Attenuvax)	Sterile preparation of live, attenuated measles (rubeola) virus Protects approximately 95% of recipients for several years or lifetime Usually given with mumps and rubella vaccines. A combination product containing all three antigens is available and preferred. Measles vaccine should not be given for 3 mo after administration of immune serum globulin, plasma, or whole blood	Routine immunization of children 1 y of age or older Immunization of adults not previously immunized	SC 0.5 ml in a single dose	SC, same as adults
Measles and rubella vaccine (M-R-Vax II)	Mixture of live attenuated rubeola virus (Attenuvax) and rubella (German measles) virus	Immunization of 15-mo-old children against rubeola and rubella		SC, total volume of reconstituted vial
Measles, mumps, and rubella vaccine (M-M-R II)	Mixture of three vaccines (rubeola, rubella, mumps) Usually preferred over single immunizing agents	Immunization from age 15 mo to puberty		SC, total volume of reconstituted vial

(continued)

TABLE 43-1	VACCINES AND TOXOIDS FOR ACTIVE IMMUNITY (Continued)

Generic/Trade Name	Characteristics	Clinical Indications	Routes and Dosage Ranges	
			Adults	*Children*
Meningitis vaccine (Menomune-A/C Menomune-A/C/ Y/W-135)	Suspension prepared from groups A and C or A, C, Y, and W-135 of *Neisseria meningitidis*	Immunization of people at risk in epidemic or endemic areas Type A only should be given to infants and children under 2 y of age.	SC 0.5 ml	
Mumps vaccine (Mumpsvax)	Sterile suspension of live, attenuated mumps virus Provides active immunity in about 97% of children and 93% of adults for at least 10 y Most often given in combination with measles and rubella vaccines	Routine immunization of children (1 y and older) and adults	SC 0.5 ml in a single dose of reconstituted vaccine. (Reconstituted vaccine retains potency for 8 h if refrigerated. Discard if not used within 8 h.)	Over 1 y, same as adults (vaccination not indicated in children under 1 y)
Plague vaccine	Sterile suspension of killed plague bacilli	Immunization of high-risk people (*e.g.*, laboratory workers, people in disaster areas)	IM 1.0 ml initially, then 0.2 ml after 1–3 mo and 3–6 mo (total of three doses) Booster doses of 0.1– 0.2 ml every 6 mo during active exposure	Age 5–10 y, ⅔ adult dose Age 1–4 y, ⅖ adult dose Age under 1 y, ⅕ adult dose
Pneumococcal vaccine, polyvalent (Pneumovax 23 Pnu-Imune 23)	Consists of 23 strains of pneumococci, which cause approximately 85%–90% of the serious pneumococcal infections in the United States Protection begins about the third week after vaccination and lasts years. Not recommended for children under 2 y old because they may be unable to produce adequate antibody levels	Adults with chronic cardiovascular or pulmonary diseases Adults with chronic disease associated with increased risk of pneumococcal infection (*e.g.*, splenic dysfunction, Hodgkin's disease, multiple myeloma, cirrhosis, alcohol dependence, renal failure, immunosuppression) Adults 65 y or older who are otherwise healthy Children 2 y or older with chronic disease associated with increased risk of pneumococcal infection (*e.g.*, asplenia, nephrotic syndrome, immunosuppression)	SC IM 0.5 ml as a single dose	Same as adults

TABLE 43-1 VACCINES AND TOXOIDS FOR ACTIVE IMMUNITY (Continued)

Generic/Trade Name	Characteristics	Clinical Indications	Routes and Dosage Ranges	
			Adults	*Children*
Poliomyelitis vaccine, inactivated (IPOL)	A suspension of inactivated poliovirus types I, II, and III	Children not previously immunized Adults not previously immunized and at high risk of exposure (*e.g.*, health care or laboratory workers)	SC 0.5 ml × three doses initially, second dose 1–2 mo after first, third dose 6–12 mo after second dose	SC 0.5 ml × three doses with first at 2 mo of age, second at 4 mo, third at 10–16 mos (6–12 mo after second dose) Booster 0.5 ml × one dose at 4–6 y of age
Poliovirus vaccine, trivalent, oral (Sabin) (Orimune)	A suspension of live, attenuated poliovirus types I, II, and III Effective in >90% of recipients	Routine immunization of all infants and children Immunization of high-risk adults (*e.g.*, health care workers, people who live in or travel to epidemic or endemic areas)	Same as children and adolescents	Infants, PO 0.5 ml at 2, 4, and 6 mo, followed by a fourth dose at approximately 15–18 mo Children and adolescents, PO 0.5 ml for two doses, 6–8 wk apart, followed by a third dose of 0.5 ml 8–12 mo after the second dose. All children who have received the series should be given a single booster dose at 4–6 y of age.
Rabies vaccine (human diploid cell rabies vaccine [HDCV]) (Imovax)	An inactivated virus vaccine Immunity develops in 7–10 d and lasts 1 y or longer	Pre-exposure immunization in people at high risk of exposure (veterinarians, animal handlers, laboratory personnel who work with rabies virus) Postexposure prophylaxis in people who have been bitten by potentially rabid animals or who have skin scratches or abrasions exposed to animal saliva (*e.g.*, animal licking of wound), urine, or blood	Pre-exposure prophylaxis, IM 1.0 ml for three doses. The second dose is given 1 wk after the first: the third dose is given 4 wk after the first. Thereafter, booster doses (1 ml) are given every 2 y in high-risk people. Postexposure, IM 1 ml for five doses. After the initial dose, remaining doses are given 3, 7, 14, and 28 d later. Rabies immunoglobulin is administered at the same time as the initial dose of HDVC vaccine	
Rubella vaccine (Meruvax II)	Sterile suspension of live, attenuated rubella virus Protects about 95% of recipients at least	Routine immunization of children 1 y of age or older Initial or repeat immunization of adoles-	SC 0.5 ml in a single dose	SC same as adults

(continued)

TABLE 43-1 VACCINES AND TOXOIDS FOR ACTIVE IMMUNITY (Continued)

Generic/Trade Name	Characteristics	Clinical Indications	Routes and Dosage Ranges	
			Adults	**Children**
	15 y, probably for lifetime Should not be given for 3 mo after receiving immune serum globulin, plasma, or whole blood Usually given with measles and mumps vaccines. A combination product containing all three antigens is available and preferred.	cent girls or women of childbearing age *if* serum antibody levels are low		
Rubella and mumps vaccine (Biavax II)	A mixture of mumps and rubella virus strains Less frequently used than measles, mumps, and rubella vaccine	Immunization of children		Age 1 y and older, SC, total volume of reconstituted vial
Smallpox vaccine	Preparation of live (cowpox) virus Protection lasts 3–10 y, beginning 8 d after vaccination Not recommended for routine immunization in United States Available from Centers for Disease Control and Prevention	Foreign travel to Africa, Asia, Central America, and South America	Intradermal by multiple puncture technique of one capillary tube	
Tuberculosis vaccine (Bacillus Calmette-Guérin) (TICEBCG)	Suspension of attenuated tubercle bacillus Converts negative tuberculin reactors to positive reactors. Therefore, precludes use of the tuberculin skin test for screening or early diagnosis of tuberculosis. Contraindicated in clients who have not had a (negative) tuberculin skin test within the preceding 2 wk; who are actually ill or suspected of having respiratory tract, skin, or other infection; who have dysgammaglobulinemia; and who have a positive tuberculin skin test	People at high risk for exposure, including newborns of women with tuberculosis	Percutaneous, by multiple puncture disk. 0.2–0.3 ml	Newborns, percutaneous, by multiple puncture disk, 0.1 ml Children >1 mo of age, same as adults

| TABLE 43-1 | VACCINES AND TOXOIDS FOR ACTIVE IMMUNITY (Continued) | | | |

Generic/Trade Name	Characteristics	Clinical Indications	Routes and Dosage Ranges	
			Adults	*Children*
Typhoid vaccine (Vivotif Berna)	Sterile suspension of attenuated or killed typhoid bacilli Protects >70% of recipients	High-risk people (household contacts of typhoid carriers or people whose occupation or travel predisposes to exposure)	SC 0.5 ml for two doses at least 4 wk apart, then a booster dose of 0.5 ml (or 0.1 ml intradermal) at least every 3 y for repeated or continued exposure PO 1 capsule every other day × four doses; repeat every 4 y as a booster dose with repeated or continued exposure	Age over 10 y, SC 0.5 ml for two doses at least 4 wk apart, then a booster dose of 0.5 ml at least every 3 y for repeated or continued exposure Age 6 mo–10 y, SC 0.25 ml for two doses, at least 4 wk apart, then a booster dose of 0.25 ml (or 0.1 ml intradermal) every 3 y if indicated Children >6 y of age, same as adults
Varicella virus vaccine (Varivax)	Vaccine contains live, attenuated varicella virus Contraindicated in people with hematologic or lymphatic malignancy, immunosuppression, febrile illness, or pregnancy	Children 12 mo old or older Adults who have frequent contact with children and have not had chickenpox (*e.g.*, health care personnel, teachers, day care center staff, others)	SC 0.5 ml, followed by a second dose of 0.5 ml 4–8 wk after the first dose	1–12 y of age, SC one dose of 0.5 ml Adolescents, 13 y or older, SC 0.5 ml, followed by a second dose of 0.5 ml 4–8 wk after the first dose
Yellow fever vaccine (YF-Vax)	Suspension of live, attenuated yellow fever virus Protects approximately 95% of recipients for 10 y or longer	Laboratory personnel at risk of exposure Travel to endemic areas (Africa, South America)	SC 0.5 ml; booster dose of 0.5 ml every 10 y if in endemic areas	Age over 6 mo, SC same as adults
Diphtheria and tetanus toxoids and whole-cell pertussis vaccine (DTwP) (Tri-Immunol)	Diphtheria component is a preparation of detoxified growth products of *Corynebacterium diphtheriae* Pertussis component is killed, whole bacterial cells	Routine immunization of infants and children 6 y of age or younger		IM 0.5 ml for three doses at 4- to 6-wk intervals, beginning at 2 mo of age, followed by a reinforcing dose 7–12 mo later and a booster dose when the child is 5–6 y of age
Diphtheria and tetanus toxoids and acellular pertussis vaccine (DTaP) (Acel-Imune, Tripedia)	Differs from Tri-Immunol in that the pertussis component is acellular bacterial particles, formulated to decrease serious adverse reactions associated with the whole-cell vaccine	As fourth or fifth dose, after initial immunization with whole cell vaccine, in children at least 15 mo of age		IM 0.5 ml at approximately 18 mo of age: repeat at 4–6 y of age

(continued)

TABLE 43-1 VACCINES AND TOXOIDS FOR ACTIVE IMMUNITY (Continued)

Generic/Trade Name	Characteristics	Clinical Indications	Routes and Dosage Ranges	
			Adults	*Children*
Diphtheria and tetanus toxoids and whole-cell pertussis and *Haemophilus influenzae* type B conjugate vaccines (DTwP-HibTITER) (Tetramune)	A mixture of DTwP (Tri-Immunol) and Hib vaccine (HibTITER)	Immunization of children 2 mo to 5 y of age when indications for diphtheria, tetanus, pertussis (DTP) and *Haemophilus* b conjugate vaccine coincide (usually at 2, 4, 6, and 15 mo of age)		IM 0.5 ml at age 2, 4, 6, and 15 mo (total of four doses)
Diphtheria and tetanus toxoids adsorbed (pediatric type)	Also called DT Contains a larger amount of diphtheria antigen than tetanus and diphtheria toxoids, adult type (Td)	Routine immunization of infants and children up to 6 y of age in whom pertussis vaccine is contraindicated (*i.e.*, those who have adverse reactions to initial doses of DTP)		Infants and children up to 6 y of age. IM 0.5 ml for two doses at least 4 wk apart, followed by a reinforcing dose 1 y later and at the time the child starts school
Tetanus toxoid, adsorbed	Preparation of detoxified growth products of *Clostridium tetani* Protects approximately 100% of recipients for 10 y or more Usually given in combination with DTP or diphtheria toxoid (DT) for primary immunization of infants and children up to 6 y of age Usually given alone or combined with diphtheria toxoid (Td adult type) for primary immunization of adults	Routine immunization of infants and young children Primary immunization of adults Prevention of tetanus in previously immunized people who sustain a potentially contaminated wound	Primary immunization in adults not previously immunized IM 0.5 ml initially, followed by 0.5 ml in 4–8 wk, followed by 0.5 ml 6–12 mo later (total of three doses). Then, 0.5 ml booster dose every 10 y. Prophylaxis, IM 0.5 ml if wound severely contaminated and no booster dose received for 5 y; 0.5 ml if wound clean and no booster dose received for 10 y	Primary immunization and prophylaxis, same as adults
Tetanus and diphtheria toxoids, adsorbed (adult type)	Also called Td Contains a smaller amount of diphtheria antigen than diphtheria and tetanus toxoids, pediatric type	Primary immunization or booster doses in adults and children over 6 y of age	IM 0.5 ml for two doses, at least 4 wk apart, followed by a reinforcing dose 6–12 mo later and every 10 y thereafter	Age above 6 y, same as adults

Nursing Process

Assessment

Assess the client's immunization status by obtaining the following information:

- Determine the client's previous history of diseases for which immunizing agents are available (*e.g.,* measles, influenza).

- Ask if the client has had previous immunizations.
  - For which diseases were immunizations received?
  - Which immunizing agent was received?
  - Were any adverse effects experienced? If so, what symptoms occurred, and how long did they last?
  - Was tetanus toxoid given for any cuts or wounds?
  - Did any foreign travel require immunizations?

TABLE 43-2 **IMMUNE SERUMS AND ANTITOXINS FOR PASSIVE IMMUNITY**

Generic/Trade Name	Characteristics	Clinical Indications	Routes and Dosage Ranges
Immune Serums			
Cytomegalovirus immune globulin, IV, human (CMV-IGIV) (CytoGam)	Contains antibodies against CMV	Treat CMV infection in renal transplantation patients	IV infusion, 150 mg/kg within 72 h of transplant; 100 mg/kg 2–8 wk after transplantation: 50 mg/kg 12–16 wk after transplantation
Hepatitis B immune globulin, human (H-BIG, Hyper-Hep, Hep-B-Gammagee)	A solution of immunoglobulins that contains antibodies to hepatitis B surface antigen	To prevent hepatitis after exposure	Adults and children: IM 0.06 ml/kg as soon as possible after exposure. Repeat dose in 1 mo.
Immune serum globulin (human) (ISG) (Gammar)	Commonly called gamma globulin Obtained from pooled plasma of normal donors Consists primarily of immunoglobulin G (IgG), which contains concentrated antibodies Produces adequate serum levels of IgG in 2–5 d	To decrease the severity of hepatitis A, measles, and varicella after exposure To treat immunoglobulin deficiency Adjunct to antibiotics in severe bacterial infections and burns To lessen possibility of fetal damage in pregnant women exposed to rubella virus (however, routine use in early pregnancy is not recommended)	Adults and children: Exposure to hepatitis A, IM 0.02–0.04 ml/kg Exposure to measles, IM 0.25 ml/kg given within 6 d of exposure Exposure to varicella, IM 0.6–1.2 ml/kg Exposure to rubella (pregnant women only), IM 0.55 ml/kg Immunoglobulin deficiency, IM 1.3 ml/kg initially, then 0.6 ml/kg every 3–4 wk Bacterial infections, IM 0.5–3.5 ml/kg
Immune serum globulin IV (IGIV) (Gamimune, Sandoglobulin)	Given IV only Provides immediate antibodies Half-life about 3 wk Mechanism of action in idiopathic thrombocytopenic purpura (ITP) unknown	Immunodeficiency syndrome ITP	Gamimune: IV infusion 100–200 mg/kg once a month. May be given more often or increased to 400 mg/kg if clinical response or serum level of IgG is insufficient ITP, IV infusion, 400 mg/kg daily for 5 consecutive days Sandoglobulin: IV infusion, 200 mg/kg once a month. May be given more often or increased to 300 mg/kg if clinical response or level of IgG is inadequate ITP, IV infusion, 400 mg/kg daily for 5 consecutive days
Rabies immune globulin (human) (Hyperab, Imogam)	Gamma globulin obtained from plasma of people hyperimmunized with rabies vaccine Not useful in treatment of clinical rabies infection	Postexposure prevention of rabies, in conjunction with rabies vaccine	Adults and children: IM 20 U/kg (half the dose may be infiltrated around the wound) as soon as possible after possible exposure (e.g., animal bite)
Respiratory syncytial virus immune globulin intravenous (human) (RSV-IGIV) (Hypermune RSV, RespiGam)	Reduces severity of RSV illness and the incidence and duration of hospitalization in high-risk infants	Prevention of serious RSV infections in high-risk children under 2 y old (i.e., those with bronchopulmonary dysplasia or history of premature birth [gestation of 35 wk or less]) Treatment of RSV lower respiratory tract infections in hospitalized infants and young children	Children: IV infusion via infusion pump, 1.5 ml/kg/h for 15 min; then 3 ml/kg/h for 15 min, then 6 ml/kg/h until the infusion is completed, once monthly, if tolerated Maximum monthly dose, 750 mg/kg

(continued)

TABLE 43-2   **IMMUNE SERUMS AND ANTITOXINS FOR PASSIVE IMMUNITY (Continued)**

Generic/Trade Name	Characteristics	Clinical Indications	Routes and Dosage Ranges
Rh$_o$(D) immune globulin (human) (Gamulin Rh, HypRho-D, RhoGAM)	Prepared from fractionated human plasma A sterile concentrated solution of specific immunoglobulin (IgG) containing anti-Rh$_o$(D) For IM use only	To prevent sensitization in a subsequent pregnancy to the Rh$_o$(D) factor in an Rh-negative mother who has given birth to an Rh-positive infant by an Rh-positive father To prevent Rh$_o$(D) sensitization in Rh-negative clients accidently transfused with Rh-positive blood Also available in microdose form (MICRhoGAM) for the prevention of maternal Rh immunization following abortion or miscarriage up to 12 wk gestation	Obstetric use: inject contents of 1 vial IM for every 15 ml fetal packed red cell volume within 72 h following delivery, miscarriage, or abortion Transfusion accidents: inject contents of 1 vial IM for every 15 ml of Rh-positive packed red cell volume Consult package instructions for blood typing and drug administration procedures.
Tetanus immune globulin (human) (Hyper-Tet)	Solution of globulins from plasma of people hyperimmunized with tetanus toxoid Tetanus toxoid should be given at the same time (in a different syringe and injection site) to initiate active immunization.	To prevent tetanus in clients with wounds possibly contaminated with *Clostridium tetani* and whose immunization history is uncertain or included less than two immunizing doses of tetanus toxoid Treatment of tetanus	Adults and children: Prophylaxis, IM 250 units as a single dose Treatment of clinical disease IM 3000–6000 U
Varicella-zoster immune globulin (human) (VZIG) (Varicella-zoster immune globulin)	The globulin fraction of human plasma Antibodies last 1 mo or longer.	To prevent or decrease severity of varicella infections (chickenpox, shingles) in children under 15 y of age who are immunodeficient because of illness (*e.g.,* leukemia, lymphoma) or drug therapy (*e.g.,* corticosteroids, antineoplastics) and who have had significant exposure to chickenpox or herpes zoster (*i.e.,* playmate, household or hospital contact) May be used in other children under 15 and adults on an individualized basis	IM 125 U/10 kg up to a maximum of 625 U as soon as possible after exposure, up to 96 h after exposure. Minimal dose, 125 U
Animal Serums (Antitoxins)			
Antirabies serum, equine	A hyperimmune horse serum used only if human rabies immune globulin is not available	To prevent rabies after severe exposure (*e.g.,* multiple, deep animal bites, especially around the head). Used in conjunction with rabies vaccine.	Adults and children: IM 55 U/kg (half the dose may be infiltrated around the wound) as soon as possible. A test for hypersensitivity to horse serum should precede administration.
Botulism antitoxin	1. Obtained from blood of horses immunized against toxins of *Clostridium botulinum* 2. The only specific agent available for treatment of botulism. Prompt use markedly decreases mortality 3. May be obtained from the Centers for Disease Control and Prevention	For treatment of suspected botulism (a severe form of food poisoning that develops from raw or improperly preserved foods such as home-canned vegetables). Botulism has a 20% to 35% mortality.	Adults and children: Consult the manufacturer's instructions regarding dosages and routes of administration. Testing for hypersensitivity to horse serum should precede administration of the antitoxin.

TABLE 43-2   IMMUNE SERUMS AND ANTITOXINS FOR PASSIVE IMMUNITY (Continued)

Generic/Trade Name	Characteristics	Clinical Indications	Routes and Dosage Ranges
Diphtheria antitoxin	1. Obtained from blood of horses hyperimmunized against diphtheria toxin 2. Used in conjunction with antibiotics (*e.g.*, penicillin, tetracycline, erythromycin), which eliminate bacteria but do not eliminate bacterial toxins	1. To prevent diphtheria in exposed, nonimmunized clients 2. For treatment of diphtheria infection (based on clinical diagnosis, without waiting for bacteriologic confirmation of *Corynebacterium diphtheriae*)	Adults and children: Prophylaxis, IM 10,000 U Treatment, IV 20,000–120,000 U

- Determine whether the client has any conditions that contraindicate administration of immunizing agents (*e.g.*, malignancy, pregnancy, immunosuppressive drug therapy).
- For pregnant women not known to be immunized against rubella, serum antibody titer should be measured to determine resistance or susceptibility to the disease.
- For clients with wounds, assess the type of wound and determine how, when, and where it was sustained. Such information may reveal whether tetanus immunization is needed.
- For clients exposed to infectious diseases, try to determine the extent of exposure (*e.g.*, household or brief, casual contact) and when it occurred.

Nursing Diagnoses

- Knowledge Deficit: Importance of maintaining immunizations for both children and adults
- Knowledge Deficit: Risk of disease development versus risk of immunization
- Risk for Fluid Volume Deficit related to inadequate intake and febrile reactions to immunizing agent
- Noncompliance in obtaining recommended immunizations related to fear of adverse effects
- Risk for Injury related to disease development
- Risk for Injury related to hypersensitivity, fever, and other adverse drug effects

Planning/Goals

The client will:
- Avoid diseases for which immunizations are given
- Obtain recommended immunizations for children and self
- Keep appointments for immunizations

Interventions

Use measures to prevent infectious diseases, and provide information about the availability of immunizing agents. General measures include those to promote health and resistance to disease (*e.g.*, nutrition, rest, and exercise). Additional measures include the following:
- Education of the public, especially parents of young children, regarding the importance of immunizations to personal and public health. Include information about the diseases that can be prevented and where immunizations can be obtained.
- Prevention of disease transmission. The following are helpful measures:
  - Handwashing (probably the most effective method)

- Avoiding contact with people who have known or suspected infectious diseases, when possible
  - Using isolation techniques when appropriate
  - Using medical and surgical aseptic techniques
- For someone exposed to rubeola, administration of measles vaccine within 48 hours to prevent the disease
- For someone with a puncture wound or a dirty wound, administration of tetanus immune globulin to prevent tetanus, a life-threatening disease
- For someone with an animal bite, washing the wound immediately with large amounts of soap and water. Health care should then be sought. Administration of rabies vaccine may be needed to prevent rabies, a life-threatening disease.
- Explaining to the client that contracting rubella or undergoing rubella immunization during pregnancy, especially during the first trimester, may cause severe birth defects in the infant. The goal of immunization is to prevent congenital rubella syndrome. Current recommendations are to immunize children against rubella at 12 to 15 months of age.

It is recommended that previously unimmunized girls ages 11 to 13 years be immunized. Further, nonpregnant women of childbearing age should have rubella antibody tests. If antibody concentrations are low, the women should be immunized. Pregnancy should be avoided for 3 months after immunization.

 Teach clients:

- To maintain immunization records for themselves and their children. This is important because immunizations are often obtained at different places and over a period of years. Written, accurate, up-to-date records help to prevent diseases and unnecessary immunizations.
- That if a physician recommends immunization and it is uncertain whether the client has had a particular immunization or disease, it is probably safer to take the immunization than to risk having the disease. Immunization after a client has been previously immunized or has had the disease is generally not harmful.
- That to avoid rubella-induced abnormalities in fetal development, women of childbearing age who receive a rubella immunization must avoid becoming pregnant (*i.e.*, must use effective contraceptive methods) for 3 months

- That women of childbearing age who receive a varicella immunization must avoid becoming pregnant (*i.e.,* must use effective contraceptive methods) for 3 months

Evaluation

- Interview and observe for symptoms.
- Interview and observe for adverse drug effects.
- Check immunization records when indicated.

Principles of Therapy

SOURCES OF INFORMATION

Recommendations regarding immunizations change periodically as additional information and new immunizing agents become available. Consequently, health care personnel should update their knowledge at least annually. The best sources of information regarding current recommendations are the local health department and the Centers for Disease Control and Prevention, U.S. Public Health Service, Department of Health and Human Services, Atlanta, Georgia. Local health departments can be consulted on routine immunizations and those required for foreign travel.

SELECTION OF PREPARATION

For routine immunizations, combined antigen preparations are preferred (*e.g.,* diphtheria, tetanus, and pertussis [DTP] and measles, mumps, and rubella [MMR]). Single antigens are recommended only when other components are contraindicated.

STORAGE OF VACCINES

To maintain effectiveness of vaccines and other biologic preparations, the products must be stored properly. Most products require refrigeration at 2°C to 8°C (35.6°F to 46.4°F); some (*e.g.,* MMR) require protection from light. Follow the manufacturer's instructions for storage.

USE IN CHILDREN

Routine immunization of children has greatly reduced the prevalence of many common childhood diseases. However, many children are not being immunized appropriately, and diseases for which vaccines are available still occur. Standards of practice, aimed toward increasing immunizations, have been established and are supported by most pediatric provider groups (Box 43-1).

BOX 43-1. STANDARDS FOR PEDIATRIC IMMUNIZATION PRACTICES

The following standards are recommended for use by all health professionals in the public and private sector who administer vaccines to or manage immunization services for infants and children.

Standard 1. . . . Immunization services are *readily* available.

Standard 2. . . . There are no barriers or unnecessary prerequisites to the receipt of vaccines.

Standard 3. . . . Immunization services are available free or for a minimal fee.

Standard 4. . . . Providers use all clinical encounters to screen and, when indicated, immunize children.

Standard 5. . . . Providers educate parents and guardians about pediatric immunizations in general terms.

Standard 6. . . . Providers question parents or guardians about contraindications and, before immunizing a child, inform them in specific terms about the risks and benefits of the immunizations their child is to receive.

Standard 7. . . . Providers follow only true contraindications.

Standard 8. . . . Providers administer simultaneously all vaccine doses for which a child is eligible at the time of each visit.

Standard 9. . . . Providers use accurate and complete recording procedures.

Standard 10. . . . Providers coschedule immunization appointments in conjunction with appointments for other child health services.

Standard 11. . . . Providers report adverse events following immunization promptly, accurately, and completely.

Standard 12. . . . Providers operate a tracking system.

Standard 13. . . . Providers adhere to appropriate procedures for vaccine management.

Standard 14. . . . Providers conduct semiannual audits to assess immunization coverage levels and to review immunization records in the patient population they serve.

Standard 15. . . . Providers maintain up-to-date, easily retrievable medical protocols at all locations where vaccines are administered.

Standard 16. . . . Providers operate with patient-oriented and community-based approaches.

Standard 17. . . . Vaccines are administered by properly trained individuals.

Standard 18. . . . Providers receive ongoing education and training on current immunization recommendations.

Guidelines for children whose immunizations begin in early infancy are listed below. Different schedules are recommended for children ages 1 to 5 years and for those over 6 years of age who are being immunized for the first time.

1. Hepatitis B vaccine to all newborns or infants
2. DTP and trivalent oral poliovirus vaccine (TOPV) at ages 2 months, 4 months, 6 months, 18 months, and 4 to 6 years
3. MMR at 12 to 15 months of age, usually as a combined vaccine. These vaccines are given later than DTP and TOPV because sufficient antibodies may not be produced until passive immunity acquired from the mother dissipates (at 12 to 15 months of age).
4. Tetanus-diphtheria (adult type) at 14 to 16 years of age and every 10 years thereafter
5. For children with acquired immunodeficiency syndrome (AIDS), live viral and bacterial vaccines (MMR, OPV, varicella, Bacillus Calmette-Guérin) are contraindicated because they may cause the disease rather than prevent it. However, immunizations with DTP, inactivated polio vaccine, and *Haemophilus influenzae* type b are recommended even though they may be less effective than in children with competent immune systems. Also recommended are annual administration of inactivated influenza vaccine for children over 6 months old and one-time administration of pneumococcal vaccine for children over 2 years of age.

USE IN HEALTHY ADOLESCENTS, YOUNG ADULTS, AND MIDDLE-AGE ADULTS

Adolescents who completed all primary immunizations as younger children should have hepatitis B vaccine (if not received earlier) and a tetanus-diphtheria (Td) booster. Young adults who are health care workers, are sexually active, or belong to high-risk groups should have hepatitis B vaccine if not previously received; a tetanus diphtheria booster every 10 years; and MMR if not pregnant and rubella titer is inadequate or proof of immunization is unavailable. In addition, young adults who are health care providers should have influenza vaccine annually.

Middle-age adults should maintain immunizations against tetanus; high-risk groups (*e.g.,* those with chronic illness) and health care providers should receive hepatitis B once (if not previously taken) and influenza vaccine annually.

USE IN OLDER ADULTS

Annual influenza vaccine and one-time administration of pneumococcal vaccine are recommended for healthy older adults and those with chronic respiratory, cardiovascular, and other diseases. As with younger adults, immunization for most other diseases is recommended for older adults at high risk of exposure.

USE IN IMMUNOSUPPRESSION

Live, attenuated viral vaccines (MMR, oral polio, varicella) should not be given to people with AIDS, other immune diseases, or impaired immune systems due to leukemia, lymphoma, corticosteroid or anticancer drugs, or radiation therapy. The virus may be able to reproduce and cause infection in these individuals. If one is exposed to measles or varicella, immune globulin or varicella-zoster immune globulin may be given for passive immunization.

NURSING ACTIONS

IMMUNIZING AGENTS

NURSING ACTIONS	*RATIONALE/EXPLANATION*
1. Administer accurately **a.** Read the package insert, and check the expiration date on all biologic products (*e.g.,* vaccines, toxoids, human immune serums, and antitoxins).	Concentration, dosage, and administration of biologic products often vary with the products. Fresh products are preferred; avoid administration of expired products. Also, use reconstituted products within designated time limits because they are usually stable for only a few hours.
b. Give trivalent oral poliovirus vaccine into the side of an infant's mouth with a dropper, by placing on a child's tongue or a sugar cube or by mixing with milk, distilled water, or chlorine-free water.	Several methods of administration are effective and can be varied to meet the needs of individual infants or children. Avoid administering TOPV to a crying child because the dose may be lost or aspirated into the lungs.
c. Check the child's temperature before giving diphtheria, tetanus, pertussis (DTP) vaccine.	If the temperature is elevated, do not give the vaccine.

(continued)

NURSING ACTIONS	*RATIONALE/EXPLANATION*
d. Give DTP in the lateral thigh muscle of the infant.	The vastus lateralis is the largest skeletal muscle mass in the infant and the preferred site for all IM injections.
e. With measles, mumps, rubella (MMR) vaccine, use only the diluent provided by the manufacturer, and administer the vaccine SC, within 8 h after reconstitution.	The reconstituted preparation is stable for approximately 8 h. If not used within 8 h, discard the solution.
f. Give hepatitis B vaccine IM in the anterolateral thigh of infants and young children and in the deltoid of older children and adults. Although the IM route is preferred, the drug can be given SC in people at high risk of bleeding from IM injections (*e.g.*, hemophiliacs).	Higher blood levels of protective antibodies are produced when the vaccine is given in the thigh or deltoid than when it is given in the buttocks, probably because of injection into fatty tissue rather than gluteal muscles.
g. Give IM human immune serum globulin with an 18- to 20-gauge needle, preferably in gluteal muscles. If the dose is 5 ml or more, divide it and inject it into two or more IM sites. Follow manufacturer's instruction for preparation and administration of IV formulations.	To promote absorption and minimize tissue irritation and other adverse reactions
h. Test for sensitivity to horse serum before administering any antitoxin (*e.g.*, botulism, diphtheria). This test is preferably performed by the physician. If done by the nurse, a physician should be in close proximity. Also, a syringe with 1 ml of epinephrine 1:1000 should be prepared *before* testing.	Anaphylactic shock may occur. Epinephrine aqueous solution 1:1000 is used for emergency treatment of anaphylaxis. Epinephrine is injected subcutaneously in a dose of 0.5 ml for adults and 0.01 ml/kg for children.
(1) For the intradermal test, inject 0.1 to 0.2 ml of a 1:1000 dilution of horse serum into the forearm. The test is positive (*i.e.*, indicates allergy to horse serum) if a wheal appears at the injection site within 30 min.	If sensitivity tests are positive and antitoxins are deemed necessary, special desensitization procedures may be performed. Follow the manufacturer's recommendations for desensitization.
(2) For the conjunctival test, 1 drop of a 1:10 dilution of horse serum in isotonic saline solution is instilled in one eye. The test is positive if lacrimation and conjunctivitis appear within 30 min.	
i. Aspirate carefully before IM or SC injection of any immunizing agent.	To avoid inadvertent IV administration and greatly increased risks of severe adverse effects
j. Have aqueous epinephrine 1:1000 readily available before administering any vaccine.	For immediate treatment of allergic reactions
k. After administration of an immunizing agent in a clinic or office setting, have the client stay in the area for at least 30 min.	To be observed for allergic reactions, which usually occur within 30 min
2. Observe for therapeutic effects **a.** Absence of diseases for which immunized **b.** Decreased incidence and severity of symptoms when given to modify disease processes	
3. Observe for adverse effects	Immunizing agents may cause adverse, life-threatening reactions. The risk of serious adverse effects from immunization is usually much smaller than the risk of the disease immunized against. Adverse effects may be caused by the immunizing agent or by foreign protein incorporated with the immunizing agent (*e.g.*, egg protein in viral vaccines grown in chick embryos).

NURSING ACTIONS	RATIONALE/EXPLANATION
a. Pain, tenderness, redness at injection sites	Local tissue irritation may occur with an injected immunizing agent. It is especially likely to occur with adsorbed DTP or tetanus toxoid. With DTP, a nodule or lump may persist for months but eventually resolves.
b. Fever, malaise, myalgia	These adverse effects are relatively common with vaccines and toxoids. They rarely occur with human immune serums given for passive immunity.
c. Severe fever, shock, somnolence, convulsions, encephalopathy	These are rare adverse reactions to DTP. If they occur, they are thought to be caused by the pertussis antigen, and further administration of pertussis vaccine or DTP is contraindicated.
d. Paralysis (Guillain-Barré syndrome)	This is a rare reaction to oral poliovirus vaccine.
e. Anaphylaxis (cardiovascular collapse, shock, laryngeal edema, urticaria, angioneurotic edema, severe respiratory distress)	Anaphylaxis is most likely to occur with injections of antitoxins (horse serum) but may occasionally occur with other immunizing agents. Anaphylaxis is a medical emergency that requires immediate treatment with SC epinephrine (0.5 ml for adults; 0.01 ml/kg for children). Anaphylaxis is most likely to occur within 30 min after immunizing agents are injected.
f. Serum sickness (urticaria, fever, arthralgia, enlarged lymph nodes)	Serum sickness is a delayed hypersensitivity reaction that occurs several days or weeks after an injection of serum. It is most likely to occur with antitoxins (horse serum). Treatment is symptomatic. Symptoms are usually relieved by aspirin, antihistamines, and corticosteroids.
4. Observe for drug interactions **a.** Drugs that alter effects of vaccines: Immunosuppressant agents (*e.g.*, corticosteroids, antineoplastic drugs, phenytoin [Dilantin])	Vaccines may be contraindicated in clients receiving immunosuppressive drugs. These clients cannot produce sufficient amounts of antibodies for immunity and may develop the illness produced by the particular organism contained in the vaccine. The disease is most likely to occur with the live virus vaccines (measles, mumps, rubella). Similar effects occur when the client is receiving irradiation and phenytoin, an anticonvulsant drug that suppresses both cellular and humoral immune responses.
b. With varicella vaccine, salicylates may increase risk of Reye's syndrome.	Aspirin and other salicylates should be avoided for 6 wk after vaccine administration because of potential Reye's syndrome, which has been reported with salicylate use after natural varicella infection.
5. Teach clients **a.** Give acetaminophen (Tylenol) every 4–6 h to children who develop fever 24–48 h after DTP injection.	For symptomatic relief and comfort.
b. Report adverse reactions other than discomfort at the injection site, minor fever, malaise, and muscle aches.	This is especially important when vaccines are given in serial doses or booster doses. Subsequent doses may need to be reduced.
c. With varicella vaccine, avoid close contact with newborns, pregnant women, and anyone whose immune system is impaired. Also, avoid pregnancy for at least 3 mo after immunization.	Vaccinated individuals may potentially transmit the vaccine virus to susceptible close contacts. Effects of the vaccine on the fetus are unknown, but fetal harm has occurred with natural varicella infection during pregnancy.

REVIEW AND APPLICATION EXERCISES

1. What is the difference between active immunity and passive immunity?

2. How do vaccines act to produce active immunity?

3. What are the sources and functions of immune serums?

4. List common childhood diseases for which immunizing agents are available.

5. Which immunizations are recommended for adults?

6. What are advantages of administering a combination of immunizing agents rather than single agents?

7. What are common adverse reactions to immunizing agents, and how may they be prevented or minimized?

8. Why should live vaccines not be given to people whose immune systems are suppressed by drugs or diseases?

SELECTED REFERENCES

Ad hoc working group for the development of standards for pediatric immunization practices (1993). Standards for pediatric immunization practices. *Journal of the American Medical Association, 269,* 1817–1822.

Bertino, J.S. & Casto, D.T. (1997). Vaccines, toxoids, and other immunobiologics. In J.T. DiPiro, R.L. Talbert, G.C. Yee, G.R. Matzke, B.G. Wells & L.M. Posey (Eds.), *Pharmacotherapy: A pathophysiologic approach,* 3rd ed., pp. 2319–2350. Stamford, CT: Appleton & Lange.

Drug facts and comparisons. (Updated monthly). St. Louis: Facts and Comparisons.

Eickhoff, T.C. (1997). Immunizations. In W.N. Kelley (Ed.), *Textbook of internal medicine,* 3rd ed., pp. 151–155. Philadelphia: Lippincott-Raven.

Gardner, P. & Schaffner, W. (1993). Immunization of adults. *The New England Journal of Medicine, 328*(17), 1252–1258.

Porth, C.M. (1994). *Pathophysiology: Concepts of altered health states,* 4th ed. Philadelphia: J.B. Lippincott.

Immunostimulants

Objectives

After studying this chapter, the student will be able to:

1 Describe the goals and methods of enhancing immune functions.

2 Discuss the use of epoetin in the treatment of anemia.

3 Discuss the use of filgrastim in the treatment of neutropenia induced by anticancer chemotherapy.

4 Describe the use of sargramostim in bone marrow transplantation.

5 Describe the adverse effects and nursing process implications of administering filgrastim and sargramostim.

6 Discuss interferons and aldesleukin in terms of clinical uses, adverse effects, and nursing process implications.

Key Terms

Colony-stimulating factors (CSFs)

Immunocompetence

Immunodeficiency

Immunostimulant

Immunotherapy

Myelosuppression

Neutropenia

Description

Activating or enhancing a person's own immune system to fight infection and cancer is an evolving concept. Immunostimulant drug therapy is a type of immunotherapy in which the goal is to restore normal function or increase the ability of the immune system to eliminate potentially harmful invaders. Most immunostimulant drugs are facsimiles of natural endogenous protein substances (see Chap. 42). Techniques of molecular biology are used to delineate the type and sequence of amino acids and to identify the genes responsible for producing the substances. These genes are then inserted into bacteria (usually *Escherichia coli*) or yeasts capable of producing the substances exogenously (called recombinant deoxyribonucleic acid [DNA] biotechnology, genetic engineering, or gene splicing). Laboratory production greatly increased the available amounts of these substances and therefore facilitated their development as drugs for prevention and treatment of disease.

Immunostimulants currently available as pharmaceutical agents include colony-stimulating factors (CSF), interferons, and an interleukin. These drugs are the primary focus of this chapter. Bacillus Calmette-Guérin (BCG) vaccine, used in the treatment of bladder cancer, is also discussed. Other drugs with immunostimulant properties are discussed in other chapters. These include traditional immunizing agents (see Chap. 43); levamisole (Ergamisol), which restores functions of macrophages and T-cells and is used with fluorouracil in the treatment of intestinal cancer (see Chap. 64); lithium, a mood-stabilizing agent used in the treatment of bipolar affective disorder (see Chap. 10), which mobilizes neutrophils and other granulocytes from bone marrow and is sometimes given to patients with neutropenia induced by cancer chemotherapy; and antiviral drugs used in the treatment of acquired immunodeficiency syndrome (AIDS) (see Chap. 39). Levamisole and antiviral drugs are more accurately called immunorestoratives because they help a compromised immune system regain normal function rather than stimulating "supranormal" function. In AIDS, the human immunodeficiency virus (HIV) causes immune system malfunction, so the antiviral drugs indirectly improve immunologic function.

COLONY-STIMULATING FACTORS

Epoetin alfa (Epogen, Procrit) is a recombinant DNA version of erythropoietin, a hormone that stimulates bone marrow production of red blood cells. This drug, classified as a blood modifier rather than an immunostimulant, was the first CSF used clinically. It is used to treat anemia caused by chronic renal failure, cancer chemotherapy, or zidovudine, an anti-AIDS drug. *Filgrastim* and *sargramostim* are the only other Food & Drug Administration (FDA)–approved CSF currently available. These drugs stimulate bone marrow production of white blood cells (WBCs). Although they have similar effects and are considered relatively safe and effective for short-term treatment of patients with bone marrow deficiency associated with cancer chemotherapy or bone marrow transplantation, they are FDA-approved for different uses.

Filgrastim stimulates granulocyte (*e.g.,* neutrophil) production and is used in patients with cancer to prevent infection. These patients are often at risk for infection because of the debilitating disease process and antineoplastic drugs that depress the immune system, including bone marrow production of WBCs. In an immunocompromised patient, infections often result from the normal microbial flora of the patient's body or environmental microorganisms, and they may involve bacteria, fungi, and viruses. The client is most vulnerable to infection when the neutrophil count falls below $500/mm^3$.

Treatment of infections in neutropenic patients consists primarily of antimicrobial therapy, with drugs chosen according to probable organisms, likely effectiveness, the patient's signs and symptoms, and other factors. Antimicrobial drugs are usually given intravenously (IV) and may cause adverse effects, including the emergence of drug-resistant microorganisms. Obviously, it is desirable to prevent infections in neutropenic patients rather than treat them. Filgrastim helps to prevent infection by reducing the incidence, severity, and duration of neutropenia associated with several chemotherapy regimens. Most patients taking filgrastim have fewer days of fever, infection, and antimicrobial drug therapy. In addition, by promoting bone marrow recovery after a course of cytotoxic antineoplastic drugs, filgrastim also may allow higher doses or more timely administration of subsequent antitumor drugs.

Sargramostim stimulates production of granulocytes and macrophages and is used in patients undergoing bone marrow transplantation. Before receiving bone marrow transplantation, the patient's immune system is suppressed by chemotherapeutic drugs or irradiation. After the transplantation, it takes 2 to 4 weeks for the engrafted bone marrow cells to mature and begin producing blood cells. During this time, the patient has virtually no functioning granulocytes and is at high risk for infection. Sargramostim promotes engraftment and function of the transplanted bone marrow, thereby decreasing risks of infection. If the graft is successful, the granulocyte count starts to rise in about 2 weeks. Sargramostim also is used to treat graft failure.

INTERFERONS

Interferons have antiviral, antiproliferative, and immunoregulatory activities. They are designated as alfa, beta, or gamma according to specific characteristics. Interferon-alfa is the most studied and most clinically useful thus far. Interferon-alfa-2a and interferon-alfa-2b, structurally the same except for one amino acid, are both FDA approved to treat hairy cell leukemia and Kaposi's sarcoma associated with AIDS. Interferon-alfa-2b is also approved for the treatment of viral infections, such as chronic hepatitis and condylomata acuminata (genital warts associated with infection by human papillomavirus). Interferon-alfa-n3 is approved only for treatment of refractory or recurring condylomata. Interferon-gamma is approved for the treatment of chronic granulomatous disease; interferon-beta is approved for the treatment of multiple sclerosis.

Interferons are being investigated for additional uses, especially in cancer and viral infections, including AIDS. In cancer, for example, interferon-alfa has demonstrated antitumor effects in non-Hodgkin's lymphoma, chronic myelogenous leukemia, multiple myeloma, malignant melanoma, and renal cell carcinoma. Common solid tumors of the breast, lung, and colon are unresponsive. In chronic hepatitis C, interferon improves liver function in about 50% of patients, but relapse often occurs when drug therapy is stopped. In condylomata, interferons are injected directly into the lesions for several weeks, and a majority of the lesions disappear completely.

Interferons are given only by injection because they are proteins and would be destroyed by digestive enzymes if given orally. Systemic interferons are generally well absorbed, widely distributed, and eliminated primarily by the kidneys.

INTERLEUKIN

Although numerous interleukins have been identified (see Chap. 42), only interleukin-2 (IL-2, aldesleukin) is available for clinical use. Human recombinant aldesleukin is somewhat different from native IL-2, but it has the same biologic activity. Pharmacologic effects include activation of cellular immunity (*e.g.*, produces leukocytosis); production of cytokines, such as tumor-necrosis factor, IL-1, and interferon-gamma; and inhibition of tumor growth. Aldesleukin is approved for treatment of metastatic renal cell carcinoma, and approximately 15% to 25% of patients experience objective therapeutic responses. The best responses occur in patients with prior nephrectomy and low tumor burden. The drug is being investigated for use in malignant melanoma, and other types of cancer.

Various approaches are being researched to elucidate additional clinical uses of aldesleukin. In cancer, for example, cancer-fighting T-cells are found within tumors. These T-cells, called tumor-infiltrating lymphocytes (TILs), can be removed from the tumors, incubated in vitro with aldesleukin, and reinjected into the patient. These reinjected TIL cells return to the tumor and are more active in killing malignant cells than untreated T-cells.

Aldesleukin is a protein that is not absorbed after oral administration. It is given by IV infusion, after which it is rapidly distributed to extravascular, extracellular spaces and eliminated by metabolism in the kidneys.

BACILLUS CALMETTE-GUÉRIN

BCG vaccine is a suspension of attenuated *Mycobacterium bovis,* long used as an immunizing agent against tuberculosis. The drug's immunostimulant properties stem from its ability to stimulate cell-mediated immunity. It is used as a topical agent to treat superficial cancers of the urinary bladder, in which approximately 80% of patients achieve a therapeutic response.

MECHANISMS OF ACTION

Exogenous immunostimulant drugs have the same mechanisms of action as the endogenous products described in Chapter 42. Thus, CSF bind to receptors on the cell surfaces of immature WBCs in the bone marrow and increase the number, maturity, and functional ability of the cells. Interferons also bind to specific cell surface receptors. In viral infections, interferons induce enzymes that inhibit protein synthesis and degrade viral RNA. As a result, viruses are less able to enter uninfected cells, reproduce, and release new viruses.

In cancer, immunostimulant effects enhance activities of immune cells (*i.e.*, natural killer cells, T-cells, B-cells, and macrophages), induce tumor cell antigens (which make tumor cells more easily recognized by immune cells), or alter the expression of oncogenes (genes that can cause a normal cell to change to a cancer cell). Interleukins increase the response of lymphocytes and other WBCs to antigens and other foreign substances. In cancer, interleukins stimulate cytotoxic cells, including lymphokine-activated killer cells, natural killer cells, and TIL. The exact mechanisms by which interferons and interleukins exert antineoplastic effects are unknown. BCG vaccine is thought to act against cancer of the urinary bladder by stimulating the immune system and eliciting a local inflammatory response, but its exact mechanism of action is unknown.

INDICATIONS FOR USE

Immunostimulants are used primarily to prevent or treat infection, neutropenia, and some types of cancer (Table 44-1). In cancer, a major reason for using CSF is to

TABLE 44-1	IMMUNOSTIMULANTS

Generic/Trade Name	Indications for Use	Routes and Dosage Ranges	Comments
Aldesleukin (interleukin-2) (Proleukin)	Metastatic renal cell carcinoma in adults*	IV infusion over 15 min 600,000 IU or 0.037 mg/kg q8h for 14 doses: after 9d, repeat q8h for 14 doses	Adverse reactions are common and may be serious or fatal. Drug administration must be interrupted or stopped for serious toxicity.
Bacillus Calmette-Guérin (TICE BCG, TheraCys)	Bladder cancer	Intravesical instillation by urinary catheter, three vials, reconstituted according to manufacturer's instructions, then diluted further in 50 ml of sterile, preservative-free saline solution (total volume per dose, 53 ml). Repeat once weekly for 6 wk, then give 1 dose monthly for 6–12 mo (TICE BCG) or 1 dose at 3, 6, 12, 18, and 24 mo (TheraCys).	Start 7–14 d after bladder biopsy or transurethral resection
Filgrastim (G-CSF) (Neupogen)	To prevent infection in patients with neutropenia induced by cancer chemotherapy or bone marrow transplantation To mobilize stem cells from bone marrow to peripheral blood, where they can be collected and re-infused after chemotherapy that depresses bone marrow function To treat severe chronic neutropenia	Myelosuppressive chemotherapy, 5 µg/kg/d, up to 2 wk until ANC reaches 10,000/mm³ Bone marrow transplantation, IV or SC infusion, 10 µg/kg/d initially, then titrated according to neutrophil count (5 µg/kg/d if ANC more than 1000/mm³ for 3 consecutive days; stop drug if more than 1000/mm³ for 6 d. If ANC drops below 1000/mm³, restart filgrastim at 5 µg/kg/d). Collection of peripheral stem cells, SC 10 µg/kg/d, by bolus injection or by continuous infusion, for 6–7 d, with collection on the last 3 days of drug administration Severe, chronic neutropenia, SC 5 or 6 µg/kg, once or twice daily, depending on clinical response and ANC	Do not give 24 h before or after a dose of cyto-toxic chemotherapy. Dosage may be increased if indicated by neutrophil count. Stop the drug if the ANC exceeds 10,000/mm³
Interferon-alfa-2a (Roferon-A)	Hairy cell leukemia in adults* AIDS-related Kaposi's sarcoma in adults*	Hairy cell leukemia SC, IM Induction, 3 million IU daily for 16–24 wk Maintenance, 3 million IU three times weekly Kaposi's sarcoma SC, IM Induction, 36 million IU daily for 10–12 wk Maintenance, 36 million IU three times weekly	SC recommended for patients with platelet counts <50,000/mm³ or who are at risk for bleeding Omit single doses or reduce dosage by 50% if severe adverse reactions occur.
Interferon-alfa 2b (Intron A)	Hairy cell leukemia in adults* AIDS-related Kaposi's sarcoma in adults* Condylomata (genital warts) Chronic hepatitis (B and non-A, non-B/C)	Hairy cell leukemia SC, IM Induction and maintenance, 2 million IU/m² three times weekly Kaposi's sarcoma SC, IM Induction and maintenance, 30 million IU/m² three times weekly Chronic hepatitis C SC, IM 3 million IU three times weekly	Omit single doses or reduce dosage by 50% if severe adverse reactions occur.

TABLE 44-1	IMMUNOSTIMULANTS (Continued)		

Generic/Trade Name	Indications for Use	Routes and Dosage Ranges	Comments
	Malignant melanoma, after surgical excision, to delay recurrence and prolong survival	Malignant melanoma induction, IV 20 million IU/m² on 5 consecutive days per week for 4 wk; maintenance, SC 10 million IU/m² three times per week for 48 wk, unless disease progression occurs Chronic hepatitis B SC, IM 5 million IU daily or 10 million IU three times weekly (total of 30–35 million IU per wk) for 16 wk Condylomata intralesionally 1 million IU/lesion (maximum of five lesions) three times weekly for 3 wk.	
Interferon-alfa-n3 (Alferon N)	Condylomata	Intralesionally 250,000 IU/wart, two times weekly up to 8 wk	
Interferon beta-1A (Avonex)	Multiple sclerosis, to reduce frequency of exacerbations	IM, 30 μg once per week	
Interferon beta-1B (Betaseron)	Same as interferon beta-1A, above	SC 0.25 mg every other day	
Interferon-gamma-1b (Actimmune)	Reducing frequency and severity of serious infections associated with chronic granulomatous disease	SC 50 μg/m² if body surface area (BSA) is >0.5 m²; 1.5 μg/kg if BSA <0.5 m² three times weekly (e.g., Mon., Wed., Fri.)	
Sargramostim (GM-CSF) (Leukine, Prokine)	After bone marrow transplantation to promote bone marrow function or to treat graft failure or delayed function Mobilization of stem cells in peripheral blood so they can be collected by leukapheresis	Bone marrow reconstitution, IV infusion over 2 h, 250 μg/m²/d, starting 2–4 h after bone marrow infusion, and continuing for 21 d Graft failure or delay, IV infusion over 2 h, 250 μg/m²/d, for 14 d. Course of treatment may be repeated after 7 d off therapy if engraftment has not occurred. Mobilization of stem cells, SC or IV over 24 h, 250 μg/m²/d	

* = 18 years and older.

stimulate the bone marrow to regenerate normal numbers of WBCs. An increased WBC count increases the ability of patients with cancer to fight infection and to tolerate higher doses or more frequent administration of antineoplastic drugs that depress bone marrow function.

The drugs also are used to treat patients who undergo bone marrow transplantation for Hodgkin's disease, non-Hodgkin's lymphoma, or acute lymphoblastic leukemia. In these patients, CSFs promote engraftment and function of the transplanted bone marrow. They are also effective in treating graft failure. Interferons are used primarily to treat viral infections and some specific cancers. Aldesleukin is used in the treatment of metastatic renal cell carcinoma. These drugs and similar ones

are undergoing intensive investigation for use in other conditions. Thus, the number of immunostimulant drugs and their indications for use are expected to expand during the next few years.

CONTRAINDICATIONS FOR USE

All of the drugs are contraindicated for use in clients who have previously experienced hypersensitivity reactions to any component of the pharmaceutical preparations. In addition, aldesleukin should not be given initially to patients who have had organ transplantation or those with serious cardiovascular disease (e.g., an abnormal thallium stress test, which reflects coronary artery disease) or serious pulmonary disease (*e.g.*, abnormal pulmonary function tests). Also, with aldesleukin, repeated courses of therapy are contraindicated in patients who developed serious toxicity during earlier courses, including the following:

- Cardiac—arrhythmias unresponsive to treatment or ventricular tachycardia lasting for five beats or more, recurrent episodes of chest pain with electrocardiographic evidence of angina or myocardial infarction, pericardial tamponade
- Renal—impairment requiring dialysis for longer than 72 hours
- Gastrointestinal (GI)—bleeding requiring surgery, bowel ischemia or perforation
- Respiratory—intubation required longer than 72 hours
- Central nervous system—coma or toxic psychosis lasting longer than 72 hours, repetitive or hard to control seizures

BCG is contraindicated in immunosuppressed patients, because the live tubercular organisms may cause tuberculosis in this high-risk population.

Individual Immunostimulants

See Table 44-1 for names, uses, and dosages.

Nursing Process

Assessment

- Assess the client's status in relation to infection or cancer.
- Assess nutritional status, including appetite and weight.
- Assess functional abilities in relation to activities of daily living (ADL).
- Assess adequacy of support systems for outpatients (*e.g.*, transportation for clinic visits).
- Assess ability and attitude toward planned drug therapy and associated monitoring and follow-up.
- Assess coping mechanisms of client and significant others in stressful situations.
- Assess client (*e.g.*, skin integrity, invasive devices, cigarette smoking) for factors predisposing to infection.
- Assess environment for factors predisposing to infection (*e.g.*, family or health care providers with infections).
- Assess baseline values of laboratory and other diagnostic test reports to aid monitoring of responses to immunostimulant drug therapy.

Nursing Diagnoses

- Risk for Injury: Infection related to drug-induced neutropenia, immunosuppression, malnutrition, chronic disease
- Risk for Injury: Adverse drug effects
- Altered Nutrition: Less Than Body Requirements related to disease process or drug therapy

- Activity Intolerance related to weakness, fatigue from debilitating disease, or drug therapy
- Anxiety related to the diagnosis of cancer or AIDS, disease progression, and treatment
- Self-Care Deficit related to debilitation from disease process or drug therapy
- Self-Esteem Disturbance related to illness, inability to perform usual ADL
- Knowledge Deficit: Disease process
- Knowledge Deficit: Immunotherapy
- Ineffective Individual Coping related to a medical diagnosis of life-threatening illness
- Ineffective Family Coping related to illness and treatment of a family member

Planning/Goals

The client will:

- Participate in interventions to prevent or decrease infection
- Remain afebrile during immunostimulant therapy
- Experience increased immunocompetence as indicated by increased WBCs (if initially leukopenic) or tumor regression
- Avoid preventable infections
- Experience relief or reduction of disease symptoms
- Maintain independence in ADL when able; be assisted appropriately when unable
- Maintain adequate levels of nutrition and fluids, rest and sleep, and exercise
- Maintain or increase appetite and weight if initially anorexic and underweight
- Be assisted to cope with stresses of the disease process and drug therapy
- Learn to self-administer medications accurately when indicated

Interventions

- Practice and promote good handwashing techniques by patients and all others in contact with the patient.
- Use sterile technique for all injections, IV site care, wound dressing changes, and any other invasive diagnostic or therapeutic measures.
- Allow patients to perform hygienic care when able, or provide assistance when unable.
- Screen staff and visitors for signs and symptoms of infection; if infection is noted, do not allow contact with the patient.
- Allow patients to participate in self-care and decision making when possible and appropriate.
- Use isolation procedures when indicated, usually when the neutrophil count is below 500/mm^3.
- Promote adequate nutrition, with nutritious fluids, supplements, and snacks when indicated.
- Promote adequate rest, sleep, and exercise (*e.g.*, schedule frequent rest periods, avoid interrupting sleep when possible, individualize exercise or activity according to the patient's condition).
- Inform patients about diagnostic test results, planned changes in therapeutic regimens, and evidence of progress.
- Allow family members or significant others to visit patients when feasible.
- Monitor complete blood count (CBC) and other diagnostic test reports for normal or abnormal values.

- Schedule and coordinate drug administration, diagnostic tests, and other elements of care to conserve clients' energy and decrease stress.
- Consult other health care providers (*e.g.,* physician, dietitian, social worker) on the client's behalf when indicated.

Teach clients:

- Ways to prevent or reduce the incidence of infections (*e.g.,* meticulous personal hygiene, avoiding contact with infected people)
- To enhance immune mechanisms and other body defenses by healthy lifestyle habits, such as a nutritious diet, adequate rest and sleep, and avoidance of tobacco and alcohol
- Ways to maintain or improve intake of food and fluids
- Stress management techniques
- The importance of taking the drugs as prescribed
- The importance of keeping appointments for monitoring response to drug therapy and follow-up care
- To inform any other physician, dentist, or health care provider of the disease process and therapeutic plan
- Techniques of preparation, self-administration, and disposal of medications

Evaluation

- Determine the number and type of infections that have occurred in neutropenic patients.
- Compare current CBC reports with baseline values for changes toward normal levels (*e.g.,* WBC 5000 to 10,000/mm³).
- Compare weight and nutritional status to baseline values for maintenance or improvement.
- Observe and interview for decreased numbers or severity of disease symptoms.
- Observe for increased energy and ability to participate in ADL.
- Observe and interview outpatients regarding compliance with follow-up care.
- Observe and interview regarding the mental and emotional status of the client and family members.

Principles of Therapy

INPATIENT VERSUS OUTPATIENT SETTINGS FOR DRUG ADMINISTRATION

Choosing inpatient or outpatient immunostimulant therapy depends on many factors, including the condition of the client, route of drug administration, expected duration of therapy, and potential severity of adverse drug reactions. Most of the immunostimulants are proteins, and anaphylactic or other allergic reactions may occur, especially with parenteral administration. Thus, initial doses should be given when appropriate supplies and personnel are available to treat allergic reactions. Because severe, life-threatening adverse effects may occur with high-dose aldesleukin, this drug should be given only in a hospital with intensive care facilities, under the supervision of health care providers experienced in critical care.

DOSAGE

Optimal dosages for interferons and aldesleukin have not been established. For patients who experience severe adverse reactions with interferon-alfa, dosage should be reduced by 50% or administration stopped until the reaction abates. For patients who experience severe reactions to aldesleukin, dosage reduction is not recommended. Instead, one or more doses should be withheld, or the drug should be discontinued. Withhold the dose for cardiac arrhythmias, hypotension, chest pain, agitation or confusion, sepsis, renal impairment (oliguria, increased serum creatinine), hepatic impairment (encephalopathy, increasing ascites), positive stool guaiac test, or severe dermatitis until the condition is resolved. The drug should be discontinued for the occurrence of any of the conditions listed as contraindications (see the section entitled Contraindications for Use above) for repeat courses of aldesleukin therapy (*e.g.,* sustained ventricular tachycardia, angina, myocardial infarction, pulmonary intubation, renal dialysis, coma, and GI bleeding).

LABORATORY MONITORING

CBC with WBC differential and platelet count should be done before and during immunostimulant drug therapy to monitor response to drug therapy and prevent avoidable adverse drug reactions. With CSF, CBC, WBC differential, and platelet count are recommended twice weekly during drug administration. With aldesleukin, the above tests plus electrolytes and renal and liver function tests are recommended daily during drug administration.

USES IN PATIENTS WITH CANCER

Colony-Stimulating Factors

When filgrastim is given to prevent infection in neutropenic cancer patients, the drug should be started at least 24 hours after the last dose of the antineoplastic agent. It should then be continued during the period of maximum bone marrow suppression and the lowest neutrophil count (nadir) and during bone marrow recovery. CBC and platelet counts should be performed twice weekly during therapy, and the drug should be stopped if the neutrophil count exceeds 10,000/mm³. When sargramostim is given to cancer patients who have had bone marrow transplantation, the drug should be started 2 to 4 hours after the bone marrow infusion and at least 24 hours after the last dose of antineoplastic chemotherapy or 12 hours after the last radiotherapy treatment. CBC should be done twice weekly during therapy, and the neutrophil count should not exceed approximately 20,000/mm³.

Interferons

In hairy cell leukemia, interferons normalize WBC counts in 70% to 90% of patients, with or without prior splenectomy. Drug therapy must be continued indefinitely to avoid relapse, which usually develops rapidly after the drug is discontinued. In AIDS-related Kaposi's sarcoma, larger doses are required than in other clinical uses, with resultant increases in toxicity. Interferon-alfa is recommended for patients with CD4 cell counts higher than 200/ml (CD4 cells are the helper T-cells attacked by the AIDS virus), who have no systemic symptoms, and who have had no opportunistic infections. About 40% of these patients achieve a therapeutic response that lasts an average of 1 to 2 years. In addition to antineoplastic effects, data indicate that viral replication is suppressed in responding patients. Research studies suggest that a combination of interferon-alfa and zidovudine, an antiviral drug used in the treatment of AIDS, may have synergistic antineoplastic and antiviral effects. Lower doses of interferon must be used when the drug is combined with zidovudine, to minimize neutropenia.

Interleukin

Aldesleukin is a highly toxic drug and contraindicated in patients with pre-existing, serious cardiovascular or pulmonary impairment. Therefore, patients must be carefully selected, evaluated, and monitored. One way to decrease toxicity is to give the drug by continuous infusion rather than bolus injection. Another method is to combine aldesleukin with cytotoxic tumor infiltrating lymphocytes harvested from the patient's tumor, which allows lower and therefore less toxic doses of aldesleukin. Although corticosteroids can decrease toxicity, they are not recommended for use because they also decrease the antineoplastic effects of aldesleukin.

In addition, aldesleukin may impair neutrophil function and increase the risk of infections, including septicemia and bacterial endocarditis. Therefore, any pre-existing infection should be treated and resolved before initiating aldesleukin therapy. Patients with indwelling central IV devices should be given prophylactic antibacterials that are effective against *Staphylococcus aureus* (*e.g.,* nafcillin, vancomycin).

Bacillus Calmette-Guérin

BCG, when instilled into the urinary bladder of patients with superficial bladder cancer, causes remission in up to 82% of patients for an average of 4 years. Early and successful treatment of carcinoma-in-situ also prevents development of invasive bladder cancer. A specific protocol has been developed for administration of BCG solution, and it should be followed accurately.

USE IN CHILDREN

There has been limited experience with immunostimulants in children (younger than 18 years), and the drugs' safety and effectiveness have not been established. The CSF (filgrastim, sargramostim) have been used in children with therapeutic and adverse effects similar to those seen in adults. In clinical trials, filgrastim produced a greater incidence of subclinical spleen enlargement in children than in adults, but whether this affects growth and development or has other long-term consequences is unknown. Little information is available about the use of interferons in children. Aldesleukin has been used but has not yet demonstrated effectiveness. Adverse effects were similar to those seen in adults.

USE IN OLDER ADULTS

Generally, immunostimulants have the same uses and responses in older adults as in younger adults. As with many other drugs, older adults may be at greater risk of adverse effects, especially if large doses are used.

IMMUNOSTIMULANTS

NURSING ACTIONS	*RATIONALE/EXPLANATION*
1. Administer accurately	For hospitalized clients, the drugs may be prepared for administration in a pharmacy. When nurses prepare the drugs, they should consult the manufacturer's instructions. Outpatients may be taught self-administration techniques
a. Give filgrastim according to indication for use: (1) With cancer chemotherapy, give by SC bolus injection, IV infusion over 15–30 min, or continuous SC or IV infusion	

NURSING ACTIONS	RATIONALE/EXPLANATION

(2) For BMT, give by IV infusion over 4 h or by continuous IV or SC infusion

(3) For collection of stem cells, give as a bolus or a continuous infusion

(4) For chronic neutropenia, give SC

b. Give sargramostim by IV infusion over 2 h, after reconstitution with 1 ml sterile water for injection and addition to 0.9% sodium chloride.

c. Inject interferon for condylomata intralesionally into the base of each wart with a small-gauge needle. For large warts, inject at several points.

Manufacturer's recommendation

d. With intravesical. *Bacillus Calmette-Guérin (BCG)*.

(1) Reconstitute solution (see Table 44-1).

Reconstituted solution should be used immediately or refrigerated. Discard if not used within 2 h.

(2) Wear gown and gloves.

(3) Insert a sterile urethral catheter and drain bladder.

(4) Instill medication slowly by gravity.

(5) Remove catheter.

(6) Have the patient lie on abdomen, back, and alternate sides for 15 min in each position. Then, allow to ambulate but ask to retain solution for a total of 2 h before urinating, if able.

(7) Dispose of all equipment in contact with BCG solution appropriately.

BCG contains live mycobacterial organisms and is therefore infectious material.

(8) Do not give if catheterization causes trauma (*e.g.*, bleeding), and wait 1 wk before a repeat attempt.

2. Observe for therapeutic effects
a. With aldesleukin, observe for tumor regression (improvement in signs and symptoms).

Tumor regression may occur as early as 4 wk after the first course of therapy and may continue up to 12 mo.

b. With parenteral interferons, observe for improvement in signs and symptoms.

With hairy cell leukemia, hematologic tests may improve within 2 mo, but optimal effects may require 6 mo of drug therapy. With acquired immunodeficiency syndrome (AIDS)–related Kaposi's sarcoma, skin lesions may resolve or stabilize over several weeks. With chronic hepatitis, liver function tests may improve within a few weeks.

c. With intralesional interferons, observe for disappearance of genital warts.

Lesions usually disappear after several weeks of treatment.

3. Observe for adverse effects

Colony-stimulating factors (CSFs) are well tolerated overall. Adverse effects occur more often with sargramostim than filgrastim.

a. With filgrastim, observe for bone pain, erythema at SC injection sites, and increased serum lactate dehydrogenase (LDH), alkaline phosphatase, and uric acid levels.

Bone pain reportedly occurs in 20% to 25% of patients and can be treated with acetaminophen or a nonsteroidal anti-inflammatory drug (NSAID).

b. With sargramostim, observe for bone pain, fever, headache, myalgias, generalized maculopapular skin rash, and fluid retention (peripheral edema, pleural effusion, pericardial effusion).

Pleural and pericardial effusions are more likely at doses greater than 20 μg/kg/d.

(continued)

NURSING ACTIONS	*RATIONALE/EXPLANATION*
c. With interferons, observe for acute flu-like symptoms (*e.g.*, fever, chills, fatigue, muscle aches, headache), chronic fatigue, depression, leukopenia, and increased liver enzymes.	Acute effects occur in most patients, increasing with higher doses and decreasing with continued drug administration. Symptoms can be relieved by acetaminophen. Fatigue and depression occur with long-term administration and are dose-limiting effects.
d. With aldesleukin, observe for capillary leak syndrome (hypotension, shock, angina, myocardial infarction, arrhythmias, edema, respiratory distress, gastrointestinal bleeding, renal insufficiency, mental status changes). Other effects may involve most body systems, such as chills and fever, blood (anemia, thrombocytopenia, eosinophilia), and central nervous system (CNS) (seizures, psychiatric symptoms), skin (erythema, burning, pruritus), hepatic (cholestasis), endocrine (hypothyroidism), and bacterial infections. In addition, drug-induced tumor breakdown may cause hypocalcemia, hyperkalemia, hyperphosphatemia, hyperuricemia, renal failure, and electrocardiogram changes.	Adverse effects are frequent, often serious, and sometimes fatal. Most subside within 2 to 3 d after stopping the drug. Capillary leak syndrome, which may begin soon after treatment starts, is characterized by a loss of plasma proteins and fluids into extravascular space. Signs and symptoms result from decreased organ perfusion, and most patients can be treated with vasopressor drugs, cautious fluid replacement, diuretics, and supplemental oxygen.
e. With intravesical BCG, assess for symptoms of bladder irritation (*e.g.*, frequency, urgency, dysuria, hematuria) and systemic symptoms of fever, chills, and malaise.	These effects occur in more than 50% of patients, usually starting a few hours after administration and lasting 2 to 3 d. They can be decreased by phenazopyridine (Pyridium), an analgesic; propantheline (Pro-Banthine) or oxybutynin (Ditropan), antispasmodics; and acetaminophen (Tylenol) or ibuprofen (Motrin), analgesics, and antipyretics.
4. Observe for drug interactions	
a. Drugs that *increase* effects of sargramostim	
Corticosteroids, lithium	These drugs have myeloproliferative (bone marrow stimulating) effects of their own, which may add to those of sargramostim.
b. Drugs that *alter* effects of interferons	
Other antineoplastic agents	Additive therapeutic and myelosuppressive effects
c. Drugs that *increase* effects of aldesleukin	All of the listed drug groups may potentiate adverse effects of aldesleukin.
(1) Aminoglycoside antibiotics (*e.g.*, gentamicin, others)	Increased nephrotoxicity
(2) Antihypertensives	Increased hypotension
(3) Antineoplastics (*e.g.*, asparaginase, doxorubicin, methotrexate)	Increased toxic effects on bone marrow, heart, and liver. Aldesleukin is usually given as a single antineoplastic agent; its use in combination with other antineoplastic drugs is being evaluated.
(4) Narcotic analgesics	Increased CNS adverse effects
(5) NSAIDs (*e.g.*, ibuprofen)	Increased nephrotoxicity
(6) Sedative-hypnotics	Increased CNS adverse effects
d. Drugs that *decrease* effects of aldesleukin	
Corticosteroids	These drugs should not be given concurrently with aldesleukin. Although they decrease some adverse effects, such as fever, renal impairment, confusion, and others, they also decrease the drug's therapeutic antineoplastic effects.

NURSING ACTIONS	*RATIONALE/EXPLANATION*
5. Teach clients **a.** Report signs of infection, bleeding, weight loss, severe fatigue, and so forth.	These are potential problems that can be managed more effectively if recognized early.
b. Maintain a fluid intake of 2 to 3 quarts daily.	This is adequate for normal metabolic needs; more may be needed with fever or tumor lysis to excrete products of cellular metabolism and maintain kidney function.
c. Drug preparation, administration, and disposal	These drugs are often taken on an outpatient basis, and a client or family member must be taught accurate administration, including injection techniques.

REVIEW AND APPLICATION EXERCISES

1. What are cytokines, and how do they function in normal immunity?

2. What are the clinical uses of interferons and aldesleukin?

3. What are the adverse effects of interferons and aldesleukin, and how can they be prevented or minimized?

4. Describe the origin, functions, and clinical uses of CSF.

5. What are adverse effects of CSF, and how may they be prevented or minimized?

SELECTED REFERENCES

Balmer, C., & Valley, A.W. (1997). Basic principles of cancer treatment and cancer chemotherapy. In J.T. DiPiro, R.L. Talbert, G.C. Yee, G.R. Matzke, B.G. Wells & L. M. Posey (Eds.), *Pharmacotherapy: A pathophysiologic approach*, 3rd ed., pp. 1879–1929. Stamford, CT: Appleton & Lange.

Diasio, R.B. & LoBuglio, A.F. (1996). Immunomodulators: Immunosuppressive agents and immunostimulants. In J.G. Hardman, L.E. Limbird, P.B. Molinoff, & R.W. Ruddon (Eds.), *Goodman & Gilman's The pharmacological basis of therapeutics*, 9th ed., pp. 2403–2465. New York: McGraw-Hill.

Drug facts and comparisons. (Updated monthly). St. Louis: Facts and Comparisons.

Hillman, R.S. (1996). Hematopoietic agents: Growth factors, minerals, and vitamins. In J.G. Hardman, L.E. Limbird, P.B. Molinoff & R.W. Ruddon (Eds.), *Goodman & Gilman's The pharmacological basis of therapeutics*, 9th ed., pp. 1311–1340. New York: McGraw-Hill.

Louie, S.G. & Jung, B. (1993). Clinical effects of biologic response modifiers. *American Journal of Hospital Pharmacy, 50*(Suppl. 3), S10–S18.

Moore, M. (1997). Hematopoietic growth factors. In W.N. Kelley (Ed.), *Textbook of internal medicine*, 3rd ed., pp. 1522–1525. Philadelphia: Lippincott-Raven.

Nemunaitis, J. (1993). Colony-stimulating factors: A new step in clinical practice. Part II. *Annals of Medicine, 25*, 25–29.

Steward, W.P. (1993). Granulocyte and granulocyte-macrophage colony stimulating factors. *The Lancet, 342*, 153–157.

Urba, W.J. & Chabner, B.A. (1997). Principles of biologic therapy. In W.N. Kelley (Ed.), *Textbook of internal medicine*, 3rd ed., pp. 1519–1522. Philadelphia: Lippincott-Raven.

45 Immunosuppressants

Outline

Description

Autoimmune Disorders

Tissue and Organ Transplantation
   rejection reactions with solid organ
      transplantation
   bone marrow transplantation and
      graft-versus-host disease

Corticosteroids

Cytotoxic Agents
   cyclosporine
   mycophenolate
   tacrolimus
   antilymphocyte antibody preparations

Nursing Process
   assessment
   nursing diagnoses
   planning/goals
   interventions
   evaluation

Principles of Therapy
   risk–benefit factors
   drug choices and combinations
   dosage factors
   drug administration schedules
   laboratory monitoring
   use in children
   use in older adults
   home care

Objectives

After studying this chapter, the student will be able to:

1 Describe general characteristics and consequences of immunosuppression.

2 Discuss general characteristics and clinical uses of the major immunosuppressant drugs.

3 Identify adverse effects of immunosuppressant drugs.

4 Discuss nursing interventions to decrease adverse effects of immunosuppressant drugs.

5 Teach clients, family members, and caregivers about safe and effective immunosuppressant drug therapy.

6 Assist clients and family members to identify potential sources of infection in the home care environment.

Key Terms

Autoimmune disorders	**Graft-versus-host disease**
Cytotoxic	**Immunosuppression**
Graft rejection reactions	**Transplantation**

Description

Immunosuppressant drugs interfere with the production or function of immune cells. The drugs are used therapeutically to decrease an inappropriate or undesirable immune response. The immune response is normally a protective mechanism that helps the body defend itself against potentially harmful external (*e.g.*, microorganisms) and internal agents (*e.g.*, cancer cells). However, numerous disease processes are thought to be caused or aggravated when the immune system perceives one's own body tissues as harmful invaders and tries to eliminate them. This inappropriate activation of the immune response is a major factor in a growing list of serious diseases believed to involve autoimmune processes, including rheumatoid arthritis, systemic lupus erythematosus, membranous glomerulonephritis, chronic active hepatitis, inflammatory bowel disease, multiple sclerosis, myasthenia gravis, and others.

An appropriate but undesirable immune response is elicited when foreign tissue is transplanted into the body. If the immune response is not sufficiently suppressed, the body reacts as with other antigens and attempts to destroy (reject) the foreign organ or tissue. Although numerous advances have been made in transplantation technology, the immune response remains a major factor in determining the success or failure of a tissue or organ transplantation.

A major goal of research is to develop pharmacologic agents that suppress the immune response to specific antigens. However, available drugs provide nonspecific inhibition of the immune response. Drugs used therapeutically as immunosuppressants comprise a diverse group, several of which also are used for other purposes. These include corticosteroids (see Chap. 24) and certain cytotoxic antineoplastic drugs (see Chap. 64). These drugs are discussed here primarily in relation to their effects on the immune response. Six drugs (*i.e.*, azathioprine, cyclosporine, antithymocyte globulin, muromonab-CD3, mycophenolate mofetil, and tacrolimus), which are used mainly to prevent or treat transplant rejection reactions, are the main focus of this chapter (Fig. 45-1). These drugs are described below and listed in Table 45-1. To aid understanding of immunosuppressive drug therapy, autoimmune disorders, tissue and organ transplantation, and rejection reactions are briefly discussed.

Autoimmune Disorders

Autoimmune disorders occur when a person's immune system loses its tolerance to its own body tissues (self antigens), perceives body tissues as "nonself" antigens, initiates an immune reponse, and destroys host tissues.

Although much remains to be learned about autoimmunity, disease processes involving virtually every body cell or tissue are associated with autoimmune reactions. The major mechanism of tissue inflammation and destruction is thought to be a cell-mediated immune response in which T-lymphocytes either destroy tissue directly or produce substances that recruit and activate phagocytes, especially macrophages, which then destroy antigen-containing cells.

In most instances, the perceived antigen is thought to be a protein. Thus, in rheumatoid arthritis, the antigen is a protein found in joint tissue; in autoimmune thyroiditis, the antigen is a protein found on thyroid cells; and in insulin-dependent diabetes mellitus, the antigen is a protein on the pancreatic beta cells that normally produce insulin. Systemic lupus erythematosus, a chronic inflammatory disease involving connective tissue of the skin, kidneys, joints, and nervous sytem, is considered the classic autoimmune disease.

Tissue and Organ Transplantation

Tissue and organ transplantation involves replacing diseased host tissue with healthy donor tissue. The goal of such treatment is to save or enhance the quality of the host's life. Skin and renal grafts are commonly and sucessfully performed; heart, liver, lung, pancreas, and bone marrow transplantations are increasing. Although numerous factors affect graft survival, including the degree of matching between donor tissues and recipient tissues, drug-induced immunosuppression is a major part of transplantation technology. The goal is to provide adequate, but not excessive, immunosuppression. If immunosuppression is inadequate, graft rejection reactions occur with solid organ transplantation, and graft-versus-host disease (GVHD) occurs with bone marrow transplantation. If immunosuppression is excessive, the client is likely to develop serious infections and other adverse effects from immunosuppressant drugs.

REJECTION REACTIONS WITH SOLID ORGAN TRANSPLANTATION

A rejection reaction occurs when the host's immune system is stimulated to destroy the transplanted organ. The immune cells (primarily T-lymphocytes) of the recipient react against the antigens of the donor organ. This reaction usually destroys the solid organ graft within 2 weeks unless the recipient's immune system is adequately suppressed by immunosuppressant drugs.

Rejection reactions are designated as hyperacute, acute, or chronic, depending on the time lapse between transplantation and rejection. *Hyperacute* reactions occur as soon as blood from the recipient perfuses the

Figure 45-1
Sites of action of immunosuppressants. Available immunosuppressants provide nonspecific inhibition of the immune response by blocking that response at various sites, as shown here.

grafted organ. This type of reaction is rare and usually occurs in recipients who have previously formed antibodies against antigens in the graft. The antibodies bind to the graft and induce inflammation. *Acute* reactions, which occur about 2 weeks after transplantation, involve an immune response that may be delayed or less intense in clients receiving immunosuppressant drugs. *Chronic* reactions may occur after months or years of normal function and are characterized by progressive organ failure.

Rejection reactions produce general manifestations of inflammation and specific manifestations depending on

the organ involved. With renal transplantation, for example, acute rejection reactions produce fever, flank tenderness over the graft organ site, and symptoms of renal failure (*e.g.*, increased serum creatinine, decreased urine output, edema and weight gain, hypertension).

BONE MARROW TRANSPLANTATION AND GRAFT-VERSUS-HOST DISEASE

With bone marrow transplantation, the donor bone marrow mounts an immune response (mainly by stimulating T-lymphocytes) against antigens on the host's

TABLE 45-1 **IMMUNOSUPPRESSANTS**

Generic/ Trade Name	Indications for Use	Contraindications	Routes and Dosage Ranges
Azathioprine (Imuran)	Prevent renal transplant rejection Severe rheumatoid arthritis unresponsive to other treatment	Pregnancy Allergy to azathioprine	Renal transplant: PO, IV 3–5 mg/kg/d initially, decreased (1–3 mg/kg/d) for maintenance and in presence of renal impairment Rheumatoid arthritis: PO 1 mg/kg/d (50–100 mg), increased by 0.5 mg/kg/d after 8 wk, then every 5 wk to a maximum dose of 2.5 mg/kg/d. Decrease dosage for maintenance.
Cyclosporine (Sandimmune, Neoral)	Prevent rejection of solid organ (*e.g.*, heart, kidney, liver) transplant Prevent and treat graft-versus-host disease (GVHD) in bone marrow transplantation	Allergy to cyclosporine or polyoxyethylated castor oil (in IV preparation only) Cautious use during pregnancy or lactation	Sandimmune, PO 15 mg/kg 4–12 h before transplant surgery, then 15 mg/kg once daily for 1–2 wk, then decrease by 5% per week to a maintenance dose of 5–10 mg/kg/d Neoral, PO, the first dose in patients with new transplants is the same as the first oral dose of Sandimmune; later doses are titrated according to the desired cyclosporine blood level IV 5–6 mg/kg infused over 2–6 h
Lymphocyte immune globulin, antithymocyte globulin (Equine) (Atgam)	Prevent or treat renal rejection Treat aplastic anemia	Allergy to horse serum or prior allergic reaction to ATG	IV 15 mg/kg/d for 14 d, then every other day for 14 d (21 doses)
Methotrexate (MTX) (Rheumatrex)	Severe rheumatoid arthritis unresponsive to other therapy	Allergy to MTX Pregnancy, lactation, liver disease Blood dyscrasias	PO 7.5 mg/wk as single dose, or 2.5 mg q12h for three doses once weekly
Muromonab-CD3 (Orthoclone OKT3)	Treatment of renal transplant rejection	Allergy to muromonab-CD3 Signs of fluid overload (*e.g.*, heart failure, weight gain during week before starting drug therapy) Cautious use during pregnancy	IV 5 mg bolus injection once daily for 10–14 d
Mycophenolate mefetil (CellCept)	Prevention of organ rejection in patients with renal transplants	Hypersensitivity to the drug or any component of the product	PO 1 g q12h (2 g daily), with the first dose within 72 h after transplantation
Tacrolimus (Prograf)	Prevention of organ rejection in patients with liver, kidney, and heart transplants	Hypersensitivity to the drug or the castor oil used in the IV formulation	Adults: IV infusion, 25–50 µg/kg/d, starting no sooner than 6 h after transplantation, until the patient can tolerate oral administration, usually 2–3 d PO 150–200 µg/kg/d, in two divided doses q12h, with the first dose 8–12 h after stopping the IV infusion Children: IV 50–100 µg/kg/d PO 200–300 µg/kg/d

tissues, producing GVHD. Acute GVHD occurs in about 30% to 50% of patients, usually within 6 weeks. Signs and symptoms include delayed recovery of bone marrow production of blood cells, skin rash, liver dysfunction (indicated by increased alkaline phosphatase, transaminase, and bilirubin), and diarrhea. Chronic GVHD occurs more than 100 days after bone marrow transplantation.

Corticosteroids

Corticosteroids have long been used to suppress inflammation and immune reactions. In many disorders, they relieve signs and symptoms by decreasing the accumulation of lymphocytes and macrophages and the production of cell-damaging chemicals at sites of inflammatory reactions. Because inflammation is a common response to chemical mediators or antigens that cause tissue injury, the anti-inflammatory and immunosuppressive actions of corticosteroids often overlap and are indistinguishable. Despite this somewhat arbitrary separation, corticosteroid effects on the immune response are emphasized here. Generally, the drugs suppress growth of all lymphoid tissue and therefore decrease formation and function of antibodies and T-cells. Specific effects include the following:

- Increased numbers of circulating neutrophils (more are released from bone marrow and fewer leave the circulation to enter inflammatory exudates). In terms of neutrophil functions, corticosteroids increase chemotaxis and release of lysosomal enzymes but decrease the release of nonlysosomal proteolytic enzymes, such as collagenase and plasminogen activator.
- Decreased numbers of circulating basophils, eosinophils, and monocytes. The reduced availability of monocytes is thought to be a major factor in the anti-inflammatory activity of corticosteroids. Functions of monocyte–macrophages are also impaired. Corticosteroids suppress phagocytosis and initial antigen processing (necessary to initiate an immune response), impair migration to areas of tissue injury, and block the differentiation of monocytes to macrophages.
- Decreased numbers of circulating lymphocytes (immune cells), resulting from impaired production (i.e., inhibition of deoxyribonucleic acid [DNA], ribonucleic acid [RNA], and protein synthesis), sequestration in lymphoid tissues, or lysis of the cells. T-cells are markedly reduced; B-cells are moderately reduced.
- Impaired function of cellular (mainly T-cells) and humoral (B-cells) immunity. Corticosteroids inhibit the production of immunostimulant cyto-

kines (e.g., interleukins 1 and 2) required for activation and clonal expansion of lymphocytes and cytotoxic cytokines, such as tumor necrosis factor, lymphotoxin, and interferons. When administered for 2 to 3 weeks, the drugs also inhibit immune reactions to antigenic skin tests and reduce serum concentrations of some antibodies (immunoglobulins G and A but not IgM).

Cytotoxic Agents

Cytotoxic drugs damage or kill cells that are able to reproduce, such as immunologically competent lymphocytes. These drugs are used primarily in cancer chemotherapy. However, in small doses, some also exhibit immunosuppressive activities and are used to treat autoimmune disorders (e.g., methotrexate) and to prevent rejection reactions in organ transplantation (azathioprine). These drugs cause generalized suppression of the immune system and can kill lymphocytes and nonlymphoid proliferating cells (e.g., bone marrow blood cells, gastrointestinal mucosal cells, and germ cells in gonads).

Azathioprine is an antimetabolite that interferes with production of DNA and RNA and thus blocks cellular reproduction, growth, and development. Once ingested into the body, azathioprine is metabolized by the liver to 6-mercaptopurine, a purine analog, and incorporated into the DNA of proliferating cells in place of the natural purine bases to produce abnormal DNA. Rapidly proliferating cells are most affected, including lymphocytes, which normally reproduce rapidly in response to stimulation by an antigen. The drug acts especially on T-cells to block cell division, clonal proliferation, and differentiation. Azathioprine is well absorbed following oral administration, with peak serum concentrations occurring in 1 to 2 hours and a half-life of less than 5 hours. The mercaptopurine resulting from initial biotransformation is inactivated mainly by the enzyme xanthine oxidase. Impaired liver function may decrease metabolism of azathioprine to its active metabolite and therefore decrease pharmacologic effects. Azathioprine is used mainly to prevent organ graft rejection and has little effect on established rejection reactions. It is also used to treat severe rheumatoid arthritis not responsive to conventional treatment.

Methotrexate is a folate antagonist. It inhibits dihydrofolate reductase, the enzyme that converts dihydrofolate to the tetrahydrofolate required for biosynthesis of DNA and cell reproduction. The resultant DNA impairment inhibits production and function of immune cells, especially T-cells. Methotrexate has long been used in the treatment of cancer. Other uses have evolved from its immunosuppressive effects, including treatment of autoimmune or inflammatory disorders, such as severe arthritis and psoriasis, that do not respond to other treatment measures. It is also used (with cyclosporine) to prevent GVHD associated with bone marrow transplantation, but it is not FDA approved for this purpose. Much lower doses are given for these conditions than for cancers. Thus, adverse drug effects are minimal.

CYCLOSPORINE

Cyclosporine is a powerful drug used only as an immunosuppressant, primarily in organ transplantation. The drug inhibits cellular and humoral immunity but affects T-lymphocytes more than B-lymphocytes. With T-cells, cyclosporine reduces proliferation of helper and cytotoxic T-cells and synthesis of several lymphokines (*e.g.,* interleukin-2, interferons). Suppressor T-cells seem to be less affected by cyclosporine. With B-cells, cyclosporine reduces production and function to some extent, but considerable activity is retained.

Cyclosporine is used to prevent rejection reactions (destruction of the transplanted tissues by the body's immune system) following solid organ transplantation (*e.g.,* kidney, liver, heart, lung) or to treat chronic rejection in patients previously treated with other immunosuppressive agents. Transplant rejection reactions mainly involve cellular immunity or T-cells. With cyclosporine-induced deprivation of interleukin-2, T-cells stimulated by the graft antigen do not undergo clonal expansion and differentiation, and graft destruction is inhibited. In addition to its use in solid organ transplantation, cyclosporine is used to prevent and treat GVHD, a potential complication of bone marrow transplantation. In GVHD, T-lymphocytes from the transplanted marrow of the donor arouse an immune response against the tissues of the recipient.

Absorption of cyclosporine is slow and incomplete with oral administration. The drug is highly bound to plasma proteins (90%), and about 50% is distributed in erythrocytes, so drug levels in whole blood are significantly higher than those in plasma. Peak plasma levels occur 4 to 5 hours after a dose, and the elimination half-life is about 10 to 27 hours. Cyclosporine is metabolized in the liver and excreted in bile; less than 10% is excreted unchanged in urine. Because the drug is insoluble in water, other solvents are used in commercial formulations. Thus, it is prepared in alcohol and olive oil for oral administration and in alcohol and polyoxyethylated castor oil for intravenous (IV) administration. Anaphylactic reactions, attributed to the castor oil, have occurred with the IV formulation. Neoral is a newer microemulsion formulation of cyclosporine that is better absorbed than oral Sandimmune. The two formulations are not equivalent and cannot be used interchangeably. Neoral is available in capsules and an oral solution; Sandimmune is available in capsules, oral solution, and an IV solution.

MYCOPHENOLATE

Mycophenolate is a newer agent that is similar to azathioprine. It is used mainly for prevention and treatment of rejection reactions with renal transplantation. It inhibits proliferation and function of T- and B-lymphocytes. It has synergistic effects with cyclosporine and prednisone.

After oral administration, the drug is rapidly broken down to mycophenolic acid, the active component. Mycophenolic acid is eliminated in bile and urine. Neutropenia and thrombocytopenia may occur but are less common and less severe than with azathioprine. Infections with mycophenolate occur at about the same rate as with other immunosuppressant drugs. The role of mycophenolate in transplantation is not clearly established.

TACROLIMUS

Tacrolimus, formerly called FK506, is similar to cyclosporine in its mechanisms of action, pharmacokinetic characteristics, and adverse effects. It prevents rejection of transplanted organs by inhibiting growth and proliferation of T-lymphocytes. Although survival of patients and grafts is about the same as with cyclosporine, potential advantages of tacrolimus include less corticosteroid therapy and shorter, less costly hospitalizations. Tacrolimus is not well absorbed orally, so that higher oral doses than IV doses must be given to obtain similar blood levels. It is extensively distributed through the body and reaches higher concentrations in erythrocytes than in plasma. It is metabolized in the liver and intestine to several metabolites. Impaired liver function may slow its metabolism and elimination.

Dosage ranges of tacrolimus vary according to clinical response, adverse effects, and blood concentrations. Serum drug levels are routinely monitored, with therapeutic ranges approximately 10 to 20 ng/ml for 6 months after transplantation, then 5 to 15 ng/ml. Children with transplants metabolize tacrolimus more rapidly than adults with transplants, on a body weight basis. Thus, children require higher doses, based on mg/kg, to maintain similar plasma drug levels. Dosage does not need to be reduced in renal insufficiency because there is little renal elimination of the drug.

There are numerous potential drug interactions that increase or decrease blood levels and effects of tacrolimus. Because tacrolimus is metabolized mainly by the cytochorome P450 enzymes that metabolize cyclosporine, drug interactions known to alter cyclosporine effects are likely to alter tacrolimus effects. In addition, tacrolimus is a macrolide and may have drug interactions similar to those occurring with erythromycin. Erythromycin is known to increase blood levels and risks of toxicity of several drugs, including oral anticoagulants, nonsedating antihistamines (*e.g.*, astemizole), digoxin, and theophylline.

The role of tacrolimus in transplantation immunosuppression is not well defined. Because successful liver and intestinal transplantations have been attributed to the drug, some people suggest that tacrolimus may replace cyclosporine as the immunosuppressant of choice for new patients. It may also be useful for patients who do not respond to cyclosporine. In renal transplantation, its role is less clear because high success rates have been achieved with cyclosporine. However, cyclosporine is given with corticosteroids and tacrolimus may be preferred if clinical trials validate that it may allow corticosteroids to be reduced or stopped, thereby decreasing the adverse effects of long-term corticosteroid therapy. Nephrotoxicity occurs about equally with both drugs.

ANTILYMPHOCYTE ANTIBODY PREPARATIONS

Antilymphocyte antibody preparations are derived from animals injected with human lymphoid tissue to stimulate an immune response. The antibodies may be nonspecific polyclonal or specific monoclonal. Polyclonal preparations are a mixture of antibodies (*e.g.*, IgA, IgD, IgE, IgG, or IgM) produced by several clones of B-lymphocytes. Each clone produces a structurally and functionally different antibody, even though the humoral immune response was induced by a single antigen. Monoclonal antibodies are produced by DNA recombinant techniques that combine B-lymphocytes from animals (usually mice) that have been injected with a specific antigen and B-lymphocytes (plasma cells) from malignant myelomas (plasma cell tumors). The resulting "hybridoma" is a clone of B-lymphocytes that produces antibody against a specific antigen and proliferates indefinitely. Hybridomas are capable of producing relatively large amounts of monoclonal antibodies.

Lymphocyte immune globulin, antithymocyte globulin (ATG) is a nonspecific polyclonal antibody with activity against all blood cells, although it acts mainly against T-lymphocytes. ATG is obtained from the serum of horses immunized with human thymus tissue or T-lymphocytes. It contains antibodies that destroy lymphoid tissues and decrease the number of circulating T-cells, thereby suppressing cellular and humoral immune responses. In addition to its high concentration of antibodies against T-lymphocytes, the preparation contains low concentrations of antibodies against other blood cells. A skin test is recommended before administration to determine whether the patient is allergic to horse serum. Because there is a high risk of anaphylactic reactions in recipients previously sensitized to horse serum, patients with positive skin tests

should be desensitized before drug therapy is begun. ATG is usually given for a few weeks to treat rejection reactions following solid organ transplantation, and it may be used to treat aplastic anemia.

Muromonab-CD3 (OKT3) is a monoclonal antibody that acts specifically against an antigenic receptor called CD3, which is found on the surface membrane of most T-cells in blood and body tissues. CD indicates clusters of differentiation, which are groups of cells with the same antigenic receptors. The CD3 molecule is associated with the antigen recognition structure of T-cells and is essential for T-cell activation. Muromonab-CD3 binds with its antigen (CD3) and therefore blocks all known functions of T-cells containing the CD3 molecule. Because rejection reactions are mainly T-cell mediated immune responses against antigenic (nonself) tissues, the drug's ability to suppress such reactions accounts for its therapeutic effects in treating renal transplant rejection. It is usually given for 10 to 14 days. After treatment, CD3-positive T-cells reappear rapidly and reach pretreatment levels within 1 week. The drug's name is derived from its source (murine or mouse cells) and its action (monoclonal antibody against the CD3 antigen). Because the drug is a protein and induces antibodies in most patients, decreased effectiveness and serious allergic reactions may occur if it is readministered later. Second courses of treatment must be undertaken cautiously.

Nursing Process

Assessment

- Assess clients receiving or anticipating immunosuppressant drug therapy for signs and symptoms of current infection.
- Assess clients receiving or anticipating immunosuppressant drug therapy for factors predisposing them to potential infection (*e.g.*, impaired skin integrity, invasive devices, cigarette smoking).
- Assess the environment for factors predisposing to infection (*e.g.*, family or health care providers with infections, contact with young children, and potential exposure to childhood infectious diseases).
- Assess nutritional status, including appetite and weight.
- Assess response to planned drug therapy and associated monitoring and follow-up.
- Assess coping mechanisms of client and significant others in stressful situations.
- Assess baseline values of laboratory and other diagnostic test reports to aid monitoring of responses to immunosuppressant drug therapy. With pretransplantation patients, this includes assessing for impaired function of the diseased organ and for abnormalities that need treatment before surgery.
- Assess adequacy of support systems for transplantation recipients.
- Assess post-transplantation patients for surgical wound healing, manifestations of organ rejection, and for adverse effects of immunosuppressant drugs.

Nursing Diagnoses

- Risk for Injury: Infection related to immunosuppression and increased susceptibility
- Risk for Injury: Cancer related to immunosuppression and increased susceptibility
- Risk for Injury: Adverse drug effects
- Knowledge Deficit: Disease process or planned treatment
- Knowledge Deficit: Immunosuppressant therapy
- Anxiety related to the diagnosis of serious disease or need for organ transplantation
- Body Image Disturbance: Cushingoid changes with long-term corticosteroid therapy; alopecia with azathioprine
- Ineffective Individual Coping related to chronic illness and long-term treatment
- Ineffective Family Coping related to illness and treatment of a family member
- Fear related to potential transplantation complications, disease progression, or death
- Social Isolation related to activities to reduce exposure to infection

Planning/Goals

The client will:

- Participate in decision making about the treatment plan
- Receive or take immunosuppressant drugs correctly
- Verbalize or demonstrate essential drug information
- Participate in interventions to prevent infection (*e.g.,* avoid known sources of infection) while immunosuppressed
- Experience relief or reduction of disease symptoms
- Maintain adequate levels of nutrition and fluids, rest and sleep, and exercise
- Be assisted to cope with anxiety and fear related to the disease process and drug therapy
- Keep appointments for follow-up care
- Have adverse drug effects prevented or recognized and treated promptly
- Maintain diagnostic test values within acceptable limits
- Maintain family and other emotional or social support systems
- Receive optimal instructions and information about the treatment plan, self-care in activities of daily living, reporting adverse drug effects, and other concerns
- Before and after tissue or organ transplantation, receive appropriate care, including prevention or early recognition and treatment of rejection reactions

Interventions

- Practice and emphasize good personal hygiene and handwashing techniques by patients and all others in contact with the patient.
- Use sterile technique for all injections, IV site care, wound dressing changes, and any other invasive diagnostic or therapeutic measures.
- Screen staff and visitors for signs and symptoms of infection; if infection is noted, do not allow contact with the patient.
- Report fever and other manifestations of infection *immediately*.
- Allow patients to participate in decision making when possible and appropriate.
- Use isolation techniques according to institutional policies, usually after transplantation or when the neutrophil count is below 500/mm^3.

- Assist clients to maintain adequate nutrition, rest and sleep, and exercise.
- Inform patients about diagnostic test results, planned changes in therapeutic regimens, and evidence of progress.
- Allow family members or significant others to visit patients when feasible.
- Monitor complete blood count (CBC) and other diagnostic test reports related to blood, liver, and kidney function throughout drug therapy. Specific tests vary with the client's health or illness status and the immunosuppressant drug(s) being taken.
- Schedule and coordinate drug administration to maximize therapeutic effects and minimize adverse effects.
- Consult other health care providers (*e.g.,* physician, dietitian, social worker) on the client's behalf when indicated. Multidisciplinary consultation is essential for transplantation patients.

Teach clients on long-term immunosuppressant drug therapy:

- Ways to prevent or reduce the incidence of infections (*e.g.,* meticulous personal hygiene, avoiding contact with infected people)
- To report any signs or symptoms of infection to a health care provider immediately
- To enhance immune mechanisms and other body defenses by maintaining healthy lifestyle habits, such as a nutritious diet, adequate rest and sleep, and avoiding tobacco and alcohol
- Stress management techniques
- The importance of taking the drugs as prescribed
- The importance of keeping appointments for monitoring response to drug therapy and other follow-up care
- To carry identification that states the drug(s) being taken; the dosage; the physician's name, address, and telephone number; and instructions for emergency treatment. This information is needed if an accident or emergency situation occurs.
- To inform all health care providers that immunosuppressant drug therapy is being taken and must be considered in any treatment plan
- To maintain regular medical supervision. This is extremely important so the physician can detect adverse reactions, evaluate disease status, and evaluate drug response and indications for dosage change, as well as other responsibilities that can be carried out only with personal contact between the physician and the client. Periodic blood tests and other diagnostic or monitoring studies are needed.
- To take no other drugs, prescription or nonprescription, without notifying the physician who is managing immunosuppressant therapy. Immunosuppressant drugs may influence reactions to other drugs, and other drugs may influence reactions to the immunosuppressants. Thus, taking other drugs may decrease therapeutic effects or increase adverse effects.
- To practice effective contraceptive techniques during immunosuppressive drug therapy if sexually active

Evaluation

- Interview and observe for accurate drug administration.
- Interview and observe for personal hygiene practices and infection-avoiding maneuvers.

- Interview and observe for adverse drug effects with each patient contact.
- Interview regarding knowledge and attitude toward the drug therapy regimen, including follow-up care and symptoms to report to health care providers.
- Determine the number and type of infections that have occurred in the neutropenic patient.
- Compare current CBC and other reports with baseline values for acceptable levels, according to the client's condition.
- Observe and interview outpatients regarding compliance with follow-up care.
- Observe and interview regarding the mental and emotional status of clients and family members or significant others.
- Interview and observe for organ function and absence of rejection reactions in post-transplantation patients.

Principles of Therapy

The use of immunosuppressant drugs in autoimmune disorders and tissue and organ transplantation continues to evolve in drug selection, dosages, routes of administration, scheduling, and other aspects. Specific protocols vary widely among transplantation centers. These drugs are often used in highly technical, complex circumstances to manage life-threatening illness. Consequently, except for corticosteroids, the drugs should be used only by specialist physicians who are adept in their management. In addition, all health care providers need to review research studies and other current literature regularly for ways to maximize safety and effectiveness and minimize adverse effects of immunosuppression.

RISK–BENEFIT FACTORS

Immunosuppression is a serious, life-threatening condition that may result from disease processes or drug therapy. At the same time, most immunosuppressant drugs are used to treat life-threatening illnesses, and their use may therefore be justified. Rational use of immunosuppressant drugs requires thorough assessment of a client's health or illness status, clear-cut indications for use, a lack of more effective and safer alternative treatments, analysis of potential risks versus potential benefits, cautious administration, and vigilant monitoring of the patient's response. If a decision is then made that immunosuppressant drug therapy is indicated and benefits outweigh risks, the therapeutic plan must be discussed with the client (*i.e.,* reasons, expected benefits, consequences for the client's health, behavior, and lifestyle).

In addition to the specific risks or adverse effects of individual immunosuppressant drugs, general risks of immunosuppression include infection and cancer. Infection is a major cause of morbidity and mortality, especially in patients who are neutropenic (neutrophil count less than

1000/mm³) from cytotoxic immunosuppressant drugs or who have had bone marrow or solid organ transplantation. For the latter group who must continue lifelong immunosuppression to avoid graft rejection, serious infection is a constant hazard. Extensive efforts are made to prevent infections; if these efforts are unsuccessful and infections occur, they may be fatal unless recognized promptly and treated vigorously. Common infections are bacterial (gram-positive, such as *Staphylococcus aureus* or *epidermidis,* and gram-negative, such as *Escherichia coli, Klebsiella,* and *Pseudomonas* species), fungal (candidiasis, aspergillosis, pneumocystosis), or viral (cytomegalovirus, herpes simplex or zoster).

Cancer, most commonly lymphoma or skin cancer, may result from immunosuppression. The normal immune system is thought to recognize and destroy malignant cells as they develop, as long as they can be differentiated from normal cells. With immunosuppression, the malignant cells are no longer destroyed and thus are allowed to proliferate.

DRUG CHOICES AND COMBINATIONS

Choices of immunosuppressant drug are limited, and available drugs are relatively toxic. Thus, when feasible, less toxic drugs and nondrug treatment measures should be used to avoid or delay immunosuppressant drug therapy. In many instances, though, there are no acceptable alternatives, and such therapy is required. Moreover, combinations of drugs are often used. For example, most organ transplantation centers use a combination regimen for prevention and treatment of rejection reactions. Generally, once the transplanted tissue is functioning and rejection has been successfully prevented or treated, it is often possible to maintain the graft with fewer drugs or lower drug dosages. Some recommendations to increase safety or effectiveness of drug combinations include the following:

- *Antithymocyte globulin* is usually given concomitantly with azathioprine and a corticosteroid.
- *Azathioprine* may be given alone to treat rheumatoid arthritis but is often combined with other drugs to treat organ transplant rejection reactions. For example, azathioprine, cyclosporine, and prednisone are often coadministered for treatment of liver or pancreatic graft rejection.
- *Corticosteroids* may be given alone or included in multidrug regimens with cyclosporine and muromonab-CD3. A corticosteroid should always accompany cyclosporine administration to enhance immunosuppression. In prophylaxis of organ transplant rejection, the combination seems more effective than azathioprine alone or azathioprine and a corticosteroid. A corticosteroid may not be required, at least long-term, with tacrolimus.

- *Cyclosporine* should be used cautiously with immunosuppressants other than corticosteroids to decrease risks of excessive immunosuppression and its complications.
- *Methotrexate* may be used alone for rheumatoid arthritis and alone or with cyclosporine for prophylaxis of GVHD following bone marrow transplantation.
- *Muromonab-CD3* may be given cautiously with reduced numbers or dosages of other immunosuppressants. When coadministered with prednisone and azathioprine, the maximum daily dose of prednisone is 0.5 mg/kg, and the maximum for azathioprine is 25 mg. When muromonab-CD3 is coadministered with cyclosporine, cyclosporine dosage should be reduced or temporarily discontinued. Cyclosporine is then restarted 3 days before completing the course of muromonab-CD3 therapy to resume a maintenance level of immunosuppression.
- *Mycophenolate* may potentially be used in multidrug regimens instead of azathioprine, and *tacrolimus* may be used instead of cyclosporine. However, these drugs are still undergoing investigation of their efficacy, safety, and comparison to older, similar agents.

DOSAGE FACTORS

Immunosuppressant drugs are relatively toxic, and adverse effects occur more often and are likely to be more severe with higher doses. Thus, the general principle of using the smallest effective dose for the shortest period of time is especially important with immunosuppressant drug therapy. Dosage must be individualized according to the patient's clinical response (*i.e.,* improvement in signs and symptoms or occurrence of adverse effects). Factors to be considered in drug dosage decisions include the following:

- *Azathioprine* dosage should be reduced or the drug discontinued if severe bone marrow depression occurs (*e.g.,* reduced erythrocytes, leukocytes, and platelets on CBC). If necessary to stop the drug, administration may be resumed at a smaller dosage once the bone marrow has recovered. With renal transplant recipients, the dosage required to prevent rejection and minimize toxicity varies. When given long-term for maintenance of immunosuppression, the lowest effective dose is recommended. If given concomitantly with muromonab-CD3, reduce dosage to 25 mg daily.
- *Corticosteroid* dosages vary widely, depending on the disease process and the goal of treatment. For long-term treatment of chronic diseases, the smallest dose that will partially relieve symptoms is

indicated. For short-term use and rapid symptom control in such serious disorders as autoimmune hemolytic anemia, idiopathic thrombocytopenic purpura, or immune-induced glomerulonephritis, large doses are required.

With transplant recipients, doses vary among transplantation centers. The highest doses are usually given immediately after the transplantation and during treatment of acute graft rejection reactions. Doses are usually tapered by 6 months after the transplantation, and long-term maintenance doses of prednisone are usually under 10 mg daily. Doses of corticosteroids may also be reduced when the drugs are given in combination with other immunosuppressants. For some patients, the drugs may be discontinued.

- *Cyclosporine* dosage should be individualized according to blood levels of drug and serum creatinine. When a patient receiving cyclosporine is given muromonab-CD3, cyclosporine is stopped temporarily. If continued, cyclosporine dosage should be reduced. Dosage of cyclosporine also is reduced for long-term maintenance of immunosuppression following solid organ transplantation.
- *Methotrexate* dosages, both initial and maintenance, are much lower for autoimmune disorders than for antineoplastic indications. When given for severe, disabling rheumatoid arthritis, small doses are usually given weekly.
- *Muromonab-CD3* dosage should follow established amounts and protocols.
- Optimal dosage regimens of *mycophenolate* and *tacrolimus* have not been established.

DRUG ADMINISTRATION SCHEDULES

The effectiveness of immunosuppressant drug therapy may be enhanced by appropriate timing of drug administration. For example, corticosteroids are most effective when given just before exposure to the antigen, whereas the cytotoxic agents (*e.g.,* azathioprine, methotrexate) are most effective when given soon after exposure (*i.e.,* during the interval between exposure to the antigen and the production of sensitized T-cells or antibodies).

LABORATORY MONITORING

With *azathioprine,* bone marrow depression (*e.g.,* severe leukopenia or thrombocytopenia) may occur. To monitor bone marrow function, CBC and platelet counts should be checked weekly during the first month, every 2 weeks during the second and third months, then monthly. If dosage is changed or a client's health status worsens at any time during therapy, more frequent blood tests are needed.

With oral *cyclosporine*, monitor blood levels of the drug periodically for low or high values. Subtherapeutic levels may lead to organ transplant rejection, especially with liver transplantation. They are more likely to occur with the Sandimmune formulation than with Neoral because Sandimmune is poorly absorbed. High levels increase adverse effects. The blood levels can be used to regulate dosage. Drug levels are higher in whole blood than in plasma, so the laboratory technique must be known to interpret reported values accurately.

In addition, renal (serum creatinine, blood urea nitrogen) and liver (bilirubin, enzymes) function tests should be performed regularly to monitor for nephrotoxicity and hepatotoxicity.

With *methotrexate*, CBC and platelet counts should be checked periodically to monitor for bone marrow depression.

With *muromonab-CD3*, WBC and differential counts should be performed periodically.

With *mycophenolate*, complete blood counts are recommended weekly during the first month, twice monthly during the second and third months, and monthly during the first year.

With *tacrolimus*, periodic measurements of serum creatinine, potassium, and glucose are recommended to monitor for the adverse effects of nephrotoxicity, hyperkalemia, and hyperglycemia.

USE IN CHILDREN

Corticosteroids and cytotoxic immunosuppressant drugs are used in children, generally for the same disorders as in adults. Cyclosporine has been safely and effectively given to children as young as 6 months old, but extensive studies have not been performed.

Muromonab-CD3 has been used sucessfully in children as young as 2 years old; however, safety and efficacy for use in children have not been established. Mycophenolate has been used in a few children undergoing renal transplantation, but safety and efficacy are not established. Tacrolimus has been used in children under 12 years of age who were undergoing liver transplantation. Children require higher doses to maintain therapeutic blood levels than adults because they metabolize the drug more rapidly. Adverse effects of immunosuppressants in children are similar to those in adults, except that corticosteroids may impair growth in children.

USE IN OLDER ADULTS

Immunosuppressants are generally used for the same purposes and produce similar therapeutic and adverse effects in older adults as in younger adults. Because older adults often have multiple disorders and organ impairments, it is especially important that drug choices, dosages, and monitoring tests are individualized.

 ## HOME CARE

With clients who are taking immunosuppressant drugs, a major role of the home care nurse is to assess the environment for potential sources of infection, assist clients and other members of the household to understand the client's susceptibility to infection, and teach ways to decrease risks of infection. Although infections often develop from the client's own body flora, other potential sources include persons with infections, caregivers, water or soil around live plants, and raw fruits and vegetables. Meticulous environmental cleansing, personal hygiene, and handwashing are required.

 ## IMMUNOSUPPRESSANTS

NURSING ACTIONS	*RATIONALE/EXPLANATION*
1. Administer accurately **a.** Give oral azathioprine in divided doses, after meals; give IV drug by infusion, usually over 30 to 60 min.	To decrease nausea and vomiting with oral drug
b. Measure oral cyclosporine solutions with the dosing syringe provided; add to orange or apple juice that is at room temperature (avoid grapefruit juice); stir well and have the patient drink at once (do not allow diluted solution to stand before drinking). Use a glass container, not plastic. Rinse the glass with more diluent to ensure the total dose is taken. Do not rinse the dosing syringe with water or other cleaning agents. Give on a consistent schedule with regard to time of day and meals.	These are the manufacturer's recommendations. Mixing with orange or apple juice improves taste; grapefruit juice should not be used because it affects metabolism of cyclosporine. The amount of fluid should be large enough to increase palatability, especially for children, but small enough to be consumed quickly. Rinsing ensures the entire dose is taken. Oral administration is preferred. If necessary to give IV temporarily, resume oral use when able. Oral cyclosporine may

NURSING ACTIONS	RATIONALE/EXPLANATION
For IV cyclosporine, dilute just before use in 20–100 ml of 0.9% sodium chloride or 5% dextrose injection; infuse over 2–6 h.	be given to clients who have had anaphylactic reactions to the IV preparation, because the reaction is attributed to the oil diluent rather than the drug.
c. Give muromonab-CD3 in an IV bolus injection once daily. Do not give by IV infusion or mix with other drug solutions.	Manufacturer's recommendations
d. Dilute lymphocyte immune globulin, antithymocyte globulin in 0.9% sodium chloride or 5% dextrose and sodium chloride (0.225% or 0.45%) to a concentration of 1 mg/ml. Using an in-line filter, infuse IV into a large or central vein over at least 4 h. Once diluted, use within 24 h.	Manufacturer's recommendations. Using a high-flow vein decreases phlebitis and thrombosis at the IV site. The filter is used to remove any insoluble particles.
e. Dilute IV tacrolimus with 0.9% sodium chloride or 5% dextrose injection and give as a continuous infusion; give the first dose of oral tacrolimus 8–12 h after stopping the IV infusion.	Oral tacrolimus can usually be substituted for IV drug 2–3 d after transplantation

2. Observe for therapeutic effects

a. When a drug is given to suppress the immune response to organ transplants, therapeutic effect is the absence of signs and symptoms indicating rejection of the transplanted tissue.

b. When azathioprine or methotrexate is given for rheumatoid arthritis, observe for decreased pain.	With azathioprine, therapeutic effects usually occur after 6–8 wk. If no response occurs within 12 wk, other treatment measures are indicated. With methotrexate, therapeutic effects usually occur within 3–6 wk.

3. Observe for adverse effects

a. Observe for infection (fever, sore throat, wound drainage, productive cough, dysuria, and so forth).	Frequency and severity increase with higher drug dosages. Risks are high in immunosuppressed patients. Infections may be caused by almost any microorganism and may affect any part of the body, although respiratory and urinary tract infections may occur more often.
b. With azathioprine, observe for	The incidence of adverse effects is high in renal transplant recipients.
(1) Bone marrow depression (anemia, leukopenia, thrombocytopenia, abnormal bleeding).	
(2) Nausea and vomiting	Can be reduced by dividing the daily dosage and giving after meals
c. With cyclosporine, observe for	
(1) Nephrotoxicity (increased serum creatinine and blood urea nitrogen [BUN], decreased urine output, edema, hyperkalemia)	This is a major adverse effect, and it may produce signs and symptoms that are difficult to distinguish from those caused by renal graft rejection. Rejection usually occurs within the first month after surgery. If it occurs, dosage must be reduced and the patient observed for improved renal function.
	Also, note that graft rejection and drug-induced nephrotoxicity may be present simultaneously. The latter may be decreased by reducing dosage. The reported incidence of nephrotoxicity is 25% in clients with kidney transplants, 38% in those with heart transplants, and 37% in those with liver transplants. It often occurs 2–3 mo after transplantation and results in a stable but decreased level of renal function (BUN of 35–45 mg/dl and serum creatinine of 2.0–2.5 mg/dl).

(continued)

NURSING ACTIONS	RATIONALE/EXPLANATION
(2) Hepatotoxicity (increased serum enzymes and bilirubin)	The reported incidence is less than 8% after kidney, heart, or liver transplantation. It usually occurs during the first month, when high doses are used, and decreases with dosage reduction.
(3) Hypertension	This is especially likely to occur in patients with heart transplant and may require antihypertensive drug therapy. Do not give a potassium-sparing diuretic as part of the antihypertensive regimen because of increased risk of hyperkalemia.
(4) Anaphylaxis (with IV cyclosporine) (urticaria, hypotension or shock, respiratory distress)	This is rare but may occur. The allergen is thought to be the polyoxyethylated castor oil because people who had allergic reactions with the IV drug have later taken oral doses without allergic reactions. During IV administration, observe the patient continuously for the first 30 min and often thereafter. Stop the infusion if a reaction occurs, and give emergency care (*e.g.,* epinephrine 1 : 1000).
(5) Central nervous system toxicity (confusion, depression, hallucinations, seizures, tremor)	These effects are relatively uncommon and may be caused by factors other than cyclosporine (*e.g.,* nephrotoxicity).
(6) Other (gingival hyperplasia, hirsutism)	Gingival hyperplasia can be minimized by thorough oral hygiene.
d. With muromonab-CD3, observe for	
(1) Acute (first dose) reactions—fever, chills, dyspnea, pulmonary edema	These reactions are most likely to occur during the first 6 h, especially chills and fever. Pulmonary edema has occurred only in patients who were already overloaded with fluid. The first two to three doses should be given only in an inpatient setting with resuscitation supplies readily available and when fluid overload has been ruled out (by chest x-ray, assessing weight, fluid intake, and urine output). These effects may be prevented or minimized by premedicating with acetaminophen, an antihistamine, and a corticosteroid (*e.g.,* hydrocortisone or methylprednisolone).
(2) Nausea, vomiting, diarrhea	
e. With lymphocyte immune globulin, antithymocyte globulin, observe for	
(1) Anaphylaxis (chest pain, respiratory distress, hypotension or shock)	An uncommon but serious allergic reaction to the animal protein in the drug that may occur anytime during therapy. If it occurs, stop the drug infusion, inject 0.3 ml epinephrine 1 : 1000, and provide other supportive emergency care as indicated.
(2) Chills and fever	Fever occurs in about 50% of patients; it may be decreased by premedicating with acetaminophen, an antihistamine, or a corticosteroid.
f. With mycophenolate, observe for	
(1) GI effects—nausea, vomiting, diarrhea	GI effects are more likely when mycophenolate is started and may subside if dosage is reduced.
(2) Hematologic effects—anemia, leukopenia	
(3) Sepsis	Sepsis may occur with virtually any immunosuppressant drug.
(4) CNS effects—dizziness, headache, insomnia	
g. With tacrolimus, observe for	
(1) Nephrotoxicity	Nephrotoxicity (increased serum creatinine, decreased urine output) has occurred in one third or more of liver transplant

NURSING ACTIONS	RATIONALE/EXPLANATION
	patients who received tacrolimus. The risk is greater with higher doses.
(2) Neurotoxicity—minor neurologic effects include insomnia, mild tremors, headaches, photophobia, nightmares; major effects include confusion, seizures, coma, expressive aphasia, psychosis and encephalopathy.	Neurologic symptoms are common and occur in about 10%–20% of patients receiving tacrolimus.
(3) Infection—cytomegalovirus (CMV) infection and others	CMV infection commonly occurs.
(4) Hyperglycemia	Glucose intolerance may require insulin therapy.
4. Observe for drug interactions	
a. Drugs that *increase* effects of azathioprine	
(1) Allopurinol	Inhibits hepatic metabolism, thereby increasing pharmacologic effects. If the two drugs are given concomitantly, the dose of azathioprine should be reduced drastically to 25%–35% of the usual dose.
(2) Corticosteroids	Increased immunosuppression and risk of infection
b. Drugs that *increase* effects of cyclosporine	
(1) Aminoglycoside antibiotics (*e.g.,* gentamicin), antifungals (amphotericin B, ketoconazole)	Increased risk of nephrotoxicity. Avoid other nephrotoxic drugs when possible.
(2) Antifungals (fluconazole, itraconazole), calcium channel blockers (diltiazem, nicardipine, verapamil), cimetidine	Decreased hepatic metabolism, increased serum drug levels, and increased risk of toxicity
(3) Erythromycin, metoclopramide	Increased gastrointestinal absorption of cyclosporine
c. Drugs that *decrease* effects of cyclosporine	
Enzyme inducers, including anticonvulsants (carbamazepine, phenobarbital, phenytoin), rifampin, sulfamethoxazole-trimethoprim	Enzyme-inducing drugs stimulate hepatic metabolism of cyclosporine, thereby reducing blood levels. If concurrent administration is necessary, monitor cyclosporine blood levels to avoid subtherapeutic levels and decreased effectiveness.
d. Drugs that *increase* effects of mycophenolate	
(1) Acyclovir, ganciclovir	Increase blood levels of mycophenolate, probably by decreasing renal excretion
(2) Probenecid, salicylates	Increase blood levels
e. Drug that *decrease* effects of mycophenolate	
Cholestyramine	Decreases absorption
f. Drugs that *increase* effects of tacrolimus	
(1) Nephrotoxic drugs (*e.g.,* aminoglycoside antibiotics, amphotericin B, cisplatin, nonsteroidal anti-inflammatory drugs)	Increased risk of nephrotoxicity
(2) Antifungals (clotrimazole, fluconazole, itraconazole, ketoconazole); erythromycin and other macrolides; calcium channel blockers (diltiazem, verapamil), cimetidine, danzaol, methylprednisolone, metoclopramide	These drugs may increase blood levels of tacrolimus, probably by inhibiting or competing for hepatic drug–metabolizing enzymes
(3) Angiotensin-converting enzyme (ACE) inhibitors, potassium supplements	Increased risk of hyperkalemia. Serum potassium levels should be monitored closely.
g. Drugs that *decrease* effects of tacrolimus	

(continued)

NURSING ACTIONS	RATIONALE/EXPLANATION
(1) Antacids	With oral tacrolimus, antacids adsorb the drug or raise the pH of gastric fluids and increase its degradation. If ordered concomitantly, an antacid should be given at least 2 h before or after tacrolimus.
(2) Enzyme inducers—carbamazepine, phenobarbital, phenytoin, rifampin, rifabutin	Induction of drug-metabolizing enzymes in the liver may accelerate metabolism of tacrolimus and decrease its blood levels.
5. Teach clients on long-term immunosuppressant drug therapy **a.** Take drugs as directed.	This is extremely important with these drugs. Missing doses, stopping the drug, changing the amount or time of administration, or taking extra drug or any other alterations may result in the occurrence of the condition the drugs are given to prevent (*e.g.*, rejection of a transplanted organ) or adverse effects of the drugs.
b. Report to the prescribing physician if unable to take a dose orally because of vomiting or some other illness or problem.	
c. Avoid exposure to infection when possible (*e.g.*, avoid crowds and people with infections). Also, wash hands frequently and thoroughly.	These drugs increase the likelihood of infection, so preventive measures are needed.
d. Wear protective clothing, and use sunscreens to decrease exposure of skin to sunlight.	To decrease risks of skin cancers (squamous cell carcinoma, malignant melanoma). In addition, methotrexate may cause photosensitivity reactions.
e. Obtain regular physical examinations and screening tests for cancers of the breast, cervix, colon, and lung.	For early recognition and treatment, especially important in patients who have had solid organ transplants.
f. Report to a health care provider: (1) Sore throat, fever, or other signs of infection (2) Decreased urine output (with cyclosporine) (3) Easy bruising or bleeding (with azathioprine and methotrexate)	These are symptoms of adverse reactions. If they occur, they need to be assessed by a health care provider who can determine whether changes in immunosuppressant therapy are indicated.
g. Use the manufacturer's syringe to measure oral cyclosporine solution.	For accurate dosage
h. Take immunosuppressants about the same time each day.	For more consistent blood levels, possibly improving therapeutic effects and decreasing adverse effects

 REVIEW AND APPLICATION EXERCISES

1. List clinical indications for use of immunosuppressant drug therapy.

2. How do corticosteroids, antineoplastic drugs, azathioprine, cyclosporine, and muromonab-CD3 exert their immunosuppressant effects?

3. What are major adverse effects of immunosuppressant drugs?

4. When assessing a client receiving one or more immunosuppressant drugs, what specific signs and symptoms indicate adverse drug effects?

5. What are the similarities and differences between solid organ and bone marrow transplantations?

6. For a client taking one or more immunosuppressant drugs, prepare a teaching plan related to safe and effective drug therapy.

SELECTED REFERENCES

Burckart, G.J., Venkataramanan, R. & Ptachcinski, R.J. (1997). Overview of transplantation. In J.T. DiPiro, R.L. Talbert, G.C. Yee, G.R. Matzke, B.G. Wells & L.M. Posey (Eds.), *Pharmacotherapy: A pathophysiologic approach,* 3rd ed., pp. 129–147. Stamford, CT: Appleton & Lange.

Diasio, R.B. & LoBuglio, A.F. (1996). Immunomodulators: Immunosuppressive agents and immunostimulants. In J.G. Hardman, L.E. Limbird, P.B. Molinoff, & R.W. Ruddon (Eds.), *Goodman & Gilman's The pharmacological basis of therapeutics,* 9th ed., pp. 1291–1308. New York: McGraw-Hill.

Drug facts and comparisons. (Updated monthly). St. Louis: Facts and Comparisons.

Guyton, A.C. & Hall, J.E. (1996). *Textbook of medical physiology,* 9th ed. Philadelphia: W.B. Saunders.

Kelley, W.N. (Ed.). (1997). *Textbook of internal medicine,* 3rd ed. Philadelphia: Lippincott-Raven.

Munoz, S.J. (1996). Long-term management of the liver transplant recipient. *Medical Clinics of North America, 80*(5), 1103–1119.

Drugs Affecting the Respiratory System

46 Physiology of the Respiratory System

Outline

The Respiratory System

Disorders of the Respiratory System

Drug Therapy

Objectives

After studying this chapter, the student will be able to:

1 Review roles of the main respiratory tract structures in oxygenation of body tissues.

2 Describe the role of carbon dioxide in respiration.

3 List common signs and symptoms affecting respiratory function.

4 Identify general categories of drugs used to treat respiratory disorders.

Key Terms

Anoxia

Hypoxemia

Hypoxia

Oxygenation

Ventilation

The Respiratory System

The respiratory system helps meet the basic human need for oxygen (O_2). Oxygen is necessary for the oxidation of foodstuffs, by which energy for cellular metabolism is produced. When the oxygen supply is inadequate, cell function is impaired; when oxygen is absent, cells die. Permanent brain damage occurs within 4 to 6 minutes of anoxia. In addition to providing oxygen to all body cells, the respiratory system also removes carbon dioxide (CO_2), a major waste product of cell metabolism. Excessive accumulation of CO_2 damages or kills body cells.

The efficiency of the respiratory system depends on the quality and quantity of air inhaled, the patency of air passageways, the ability of the lungs to expand and contract, and the ability of O_2 and CO_2 to cross the alveolar–capillary membrane. In addition to the respiratory system, the circulatory, nervous, and musculoskeletal systems have important functions in respiration.

Some characteristics of the respiratory system and the process of respiration include the following:

1. **Respiration** is the process of gas exchange by which O_2 is obtained and CO_2 is eliminated. This gas exchange occurs between the lung and the blood across the alveolar–capillary membrane and between the blood and body cells. The first phase of respiration depends on the adequacy of air flow to and from alveoli in the lungs (ventilation). The second phase depends on the adequacy of the circulatory system.
2. The **respiratory tract** is a series of branching tubes with progressively smaller diameters. These tubes (nose, pharynx, larynx, trachea, bronchi, and bronchioles) function as air passageways and air "conditioners" that filter, warm, and humidify incoming air. Most of the conditioning is done by the ciliated mucous membrane that lines the entire respiratory tract except the pharynx and alveoli. *Cilia* are tiny, hair-like projections that sweep mucus toward the pharynx to be expectorated or swallowed. The mucous membrane secretes mucus, which forms a protective blanket and traps foreign particles, such as bacteria or dust.
   a. When air is inhaled through the nose, it is conditioned by the nasal mucosa. When the nasal passages are blocked, the mouth serves as an alternate airway. The oral mucosa may warm and humidify air but cannot filter it.
   b. Air passes from the nasal cavities to the *pharynx* (throat). Its walls are composed of skeletal muscle, and its lining is composed of mucous membrane. The pharynx contains the palatine tonsils, which are large masses of lymphatic tissue. The pharynx is a passageway for food,

fluids, and air. Food and fluids go from the pharynx to the esophagus, and air passes from the pharynx into the trachea.
   c. The **larynx** is composed of nine cartilages joined by ligaments and controlled by skeletal muscles. It contains the vocal cords and forms the upper end of the trachea. It closes on swallowing to prevent aspiration of food and fluids into the lungs.
   d. The **trachea** is the passageway between the upper respiratory tract and the lungs. It divides into right and left primary or mainstem *bronchi,* which branch into secondary and smaller bronchi, then into bronchioles. *Bronchioles* are about the size of broom straws. The walls of the bronchioles contain smooth muscle, which is controlled by the autonomic nervous system. Parasympathetic nerves cause constriction; sympathetic nerves cause relaxation or dilation. The bronchioles give rise to the *alveoli,* which are grape-like clusters of air sacs surrounded by capillaries.
   e. Gas exchange occurs across the alveolar-capillary membrane by passive diffusion. O_2 enters the bloodstream to be transported to body cells; CO_2 enters the alveoli to be exhaled from the lungs.
3. Beginning with the bronchi, the respiratory structures are contained in the *lungs.*
   a. Each lung is divided into lobes. The right lung has three lobes, the left has two. Each lobe is supplied by a secondary bronchus. The lobes are further subdivided into bronchopulmonary segments, supplied by smaller bronchi. The bronchopulmonary segments contain lobules, which are the functional units of the lung (the site where gas exchange takes place). Each lobule is supplied by a bronchiole and by an arteriole, a venule, and a lymphatic vessel.
   b. The lungs are encased in a membrane called the *pleura,* which is composed of two layers. The inner layer, which adheres to the surface of the lung, is called the *visceral pleura.* The outer layer, which lines the thoracic cavity, is called the *parietal pleura.* The potential space between the layers is called the pleural cavity. It contains fluid that allows the layers to glide over each other and minimizes friction.
   c. The lungs expand and relax in response to changes in pressure relationships (intrapulmonic and intrapleural pressures). Elastic tissue in the bronchioles and alveoli allows the lungs to stretch or expand to accommodate incoming air. This ability is called *compliance.* The lungs also recoil (like a stretched rubber band) to expel air. Some air remains in the lungs after expiration, which allows gas exchange to continue between respirations.
4. The nervous system regulates the rate and depth of respiration by the respiratory center in the medulla

oblongata, the pneumotaxic center in the pons, and the apneustic center in the reticular formation. The respiratory center is stimulated primarily by increased CO_2 in the fluids of the center. (However, excessive CO_2 will depress the respiratory center.) When the center is stimulated, the rate and depth of breathing are increased, and excessive CO_2 is exhaled. A lesser stimulus to the respiratory center is decreased oxygen in arterial blood.

The nervous system also operates several reflexes important to respiration. The cough reflex is especially important because it helps protect the lungs from foreign particles, air pollutants, bacteria, and other potentially harmful substances. A cough occurs when nerve endings in the respiratory tract mucosa are stimulated by dryness, pressure, cold, irritant fumes, and excessive secretions.

5. The circulatory system transports O_2 and CO_2. After oxygen enters the bloodstream across the alveolar–capillary membrane, it combines with hemoglobin in red blood cells for transport to body cells, where it is released. CO_2 combines with hemoglobin in the cells for return to the lungs and elimination from the body.
6. The musculoskeletal system participates in chest expansion and contraction. Normally, the diaphragm and external intercostal muscles expand the chest cavity and are called muscles of inspiration. The abdominal and internal intercostal muscles are the muscles of expiration.
7. Normal respiration requires:
   a. Atmospheric air containing at least 21% O_2
   b. Adequate ventilation. Ventilation, in turn, requires patent airways, expansion and contraction of the chest, expansion and contraction of the lungs, and maintenance of a normal range of intrapulmonic and intrapleural pressures.
   c. Adequate diffusion of O_2 and CO_2 through the alveolar-capillary membrane. Factors influencing diffusion include the thickness and surface area of the membrane and pressure differences between gases on each side of the membrane.
   d. Adequate perfusion or circulation of blood and sufficient hemoglobin to carry needed O_2
8. Normal breathing occurs 16 to 20 times per minute and is quiet, rhythmic, and effortless. About 500 ml of air is inspired and expired with a normal breath (tidal volume); deep breaths or "sighs" occur six to ten times per hour to ventilate more alveoli. Fever, exercise, pain, and emotions such as anger tend to increase respirations. Sleep or rest and various medications, such as tranquilizers, sedatives, and narcotic analgesics, tend to slow respiration.

Disorders of the Respiratory System

The respiratory system is subject to many disorders that interfere with respiration. Common disorders include respiratory tract infections, allergic disorders, inflammatory disorders, and conditions that obstruct air flow (*e.g.,* excessive respiratory tract secretions, emphysema, and other chronic obstructive pulmonary diseases). Common signs and symptoms of respiratory disorders include cough, increased secretions, mucosal congestion, and bronchospasm.

Drug Therapy

As a general rule, drug therapy is more effective in relieving symptoms than in curing the underlying disorders that cause the symptoms. Major drug groups used to treat respiratory symptoms are bronchodilating and antiasthmatic agents (see Chap. 47), antihistamines (see Chap. 48), and nasal decongestants, antitussives, and cold remedies (see Chap. 49).

 REVIEW AND APPLICATION EXERCISES

1. What is the main function of the respiratory system?
2. Where does the exchange of oxygen and carbon dioxide occur?
3. List factors that stimulate rate and depth of respiration.
4. List factors that depress rate and depth of respiration.
5. What are common signs and symptoms of respiratory disorders for which drug therapy is often used?

SELECTED REFERENCES

Guyton, A.C. & Hall, J.E. (1996). *Textbook of medical physiology,* 9th ed. Philadelphia: W.B. Saunders.
Porth, C.M. (1994). *Pathophysiology: Concepts of altered health states,* 4th ed. Philadelphia: J.B. Lippincott.
Smeltzer, S.C. & Bare, B.G. (1996). *Brunner and Suddarth's Textbook of medical-surgical nursing,* 8th ed. Philadelphia: Lippincott-Raven.

47

Bronchodilating and Antiasthmatic Drugs

Outline

Objectives

After studying this chapter, the student will be able to:

1 Differentiate the types of bronchodilating drugs and their mechanisms of action.

2 Review effects of adrenergic drugs, including consequences of overuse.

3 List advantages of inhaled beta$_2$-adrenergic agonists over systemic, nonselective adrenergic drugs.

4 Differentiate between short-acting and long-acting inhaled beta$_2$-adrenergic agonists in terms of uses and nursing process implications.

5 Describe theophylline preparations in terms of indications for use, routes of administration, adverse effects, and nursing process implications.

6 Compare adrenergic and xanthine bronchodilators in terms of therapeutic and adverse effects and nursing process implications.

7 Discuss the roles of mast cell stabilizers and corticosteroids in the treatment of bronchial asthma.

8 State the rationale for using inhaled corticosteroids in the long-term treatment of bronchoconstrictive respiratory disorders.

9 Discuss principles of therapy and nursing process for a client with an acute asthma attack.

10 Discuss principles of therapy and nursing process for a client with chronic bronchoconstrictive disease.

11 Describe important elements of using antiasthmatic drugs in children and older adults.

Key Terms

Aerosol	Cyanosis
Bronchoconstriction	Nebulization
Bronchodilation	Status asthmaticus
Bronchospasm	Wheezing

Respiratory Disorders

Bronchodilating and antiasthmatic agents are used in the treatment of respiratory disorders characterized by bronchoconstriction or bronchospasm, inflammation, mucosal edema, and excessive mucus production (asthma, bronchitis, and emphysema). Bronchoconstriction involves narrowing of the airways, which is aggravated by the inflammation, mucosal edema, and excessive mucus. Resultant symptoms include dyspnea, wheezing, coughing, and other signs of respiratory distress.

Bronchoconstriction may be precipitated by respiratory infections, odors, smoke, chemical fumes or other air pollutants, cold air, exercise, emotional upsets, tartrazine (a yellow dye found in many foods and drugs), and some drugs (*e.g.,* beta-adrenergic blocking agents, aspirin, and nonsteroidal anti-inflammatory agents). When lung tissues are exposed to these stimuli, mast cells release histamine and other substances that cause bronchoconstriction and inflammation. Mast cells are found throughout the body in connective tissues and are abundant in tissues surrounding capillaries in the lungs.

Bronchoconstrictive substances include acetylcholine, cyclic guanosine monophosphate (GMP), histamine, leukotrienes, prostaglandins, serotonin, and others. These substances are antagonized by adenosine $3':5'$-cyclic monophosphate (cyclic AMP). Cyclic AMP is an intracellular substance that initiates various intracellular activities, depending on the type of cell. In lung cells, cyclic AMP inhibits release of bronchoconstrictive substances and promotes bronchodilation.

ASTHMA

Major characteristics of *asthma* are inflammation, bronchoconstriction, and hyperreactivity of the airways. Bronchoconstriction is usually reversible, either spontaneously or with drug therapy, and clients may be symptom free between periodic attacks. Asthma may occur at any age but is especially common in childhood and early adulthood.

CHRONIC BRONCHITIS AND EMPHYSEMA

In *chronic bronchitis* and *emphysema,* commonly called chronic obstructive pulmonary disease (COPD), bronchoconstriction is more constant and less reversible than with asthma. Anatomic and physiologic changes occur over several years and lead to increasing dyspnea and activity intolerance. These conditions usually affect middle-age or older adults.

Drug Therapy

Drug therapy of these disorders involves dilating the airways, reducing inflammation, and stabilizing mast cells. Several types of drugs are used, including bronchodilators, corticosteroids, and others.

MECHANISMS OF ACTION

Bronchodilators

Adrenergics (see Chap. 18) stimulate beta$_2$-adrenergic receptors in bronchial smooth muscle. The receptors, in turn, stimulate the enzyme adenyl cyclase to increase production of cyclic AMP. The increased cyclic AMP produces bronchodilation. Some beta-adrenergic drugs (*e.g.,* epinephrine) also stimulate beta$_1$-receptors in the heart to increase the rate and force of contraction. Cardiac stimulation is an adverse effect when the drugs are given for bronchodilation. Commonly used and preferred beta-adrenergic bronchodilators (*e.g.,* albuterol) act more selectively on beta$_2$-receptors and cause fewer cardiac effects.

Xanthines (*e.g.,* theophylline) were formerly thought to increase cyclic AMP by inhibiting the enzyme phosphodiesterase, which metabolizes cyclic AMP. However, several other mechanisms (*e.g.,* increasing endogenous catecholamines, inhibiting calcium ion movement into smooth muscle, inhibiting prostaglandin synthesis and release, or inhibiting the release of bronchoconstrictive substances from mast cells and leukocytes) have been proposed. In addition to their bronchodilating effects, xanthines also increase cardiac output, cause peripheral vasodilation, exert a mild diuretic effect, and stimulate the central nervous system (CNS). The cardiovascular and CNS effects are considered adverse effects.

Anticholinergics (see Chap. 21) block the action of acetylcholine in bronchial smooth muscle when given by inhalation. This action reduces intracellular GMP, a bronchoconstrictive substance.

Corticosteroids

In asthma and other bronchoconstrictive disorders, corticosteroids have two major actions. First, the drugs suppress inflammation in the airways by inhibiting the following processes: movement of fluid and protein into tissues; migration and function of neutrophils and eosinophils; synthesis of histamine in mast cells; and production of proinflammatory substances (*e.g.*, prostaglandins, leukotrienes, several interleukins, and others). Beneficial effects of suppressing airway inflammation include decreased mucus secretion, decreased edema of airway mucosa, and perhaps repair of damaged epithelium, with subsequent reduction of airway reactivity. A second action is to increase the number and sensitivity of beta$_2$-adrenergic receptors, which restores or increases the effectiveness of beta$_2$-adrenergic bronchodilators. The number of beta$_2$ receptors increases within about 4 hours, and improved responsiveness to beta$_2$ agonists occurs within about 2 hours.

Leukotriene Inhibitors

Leukotrienes are strong chemical mediators of bronchoconstriction and inflammation, the major pathologic features of asthma. They also increase mucus secretion and mucosal edema in the respiratory tract. They are formed in response to tissue injury, which causes the breakdown of the phospholipid layer of cell membranes and the subsequent release of arachidonic acid. Arachidonic acid is then metabolized to leukotrienes by the lipoxygenase pathway (and prostaglandins by the cyclooxygenase pathway). Leukotrienes are designated by the abbreviation LT, the letter B, C, D, or E, and the number of chemical bonds in their structure (*e.g.*, LTB$_4$, LTC$_4$).

The leukotriene-inhibitor drugs include two agents with different mechanisms of action. Zileuton (Zyflo) inhibits lipoxygenase and thereby reduces formation of leukotrienes. Zafirlukast (Accolate) inhibits leukotriene receptors and is classified as a leukotriene receptor antagonist or LTRA. Both drugs are used for prevention of asthma attacks; they are not effective in relieving acute asthma attacks.

Mast Cell Stabilizers

Cromolyn and nedocromil stabilize mast cells and prevent the release of bronchoconstrictive and inflammatory substances when mast cells are confronted with allergens and other stimuli.

INDICATIONS FOR USE

Bronchodilators are used to prevent and treat bronchoconstriction associated with asthma, acute and chronic bronchitis, and emphysema. Adrenergic bronchodilators, usually beta$_2$ receptor agonists given by inhalation, are used in acute and chronic bronchoconstrictive disorders. Theophylline is now considered a second-line bronchodilator and used less often than formerly. Intravenous (IV) aminophylline may be used for acute bronchoconstriction; oral theophylline preparations may be used for long-term treatment of chronic disor-

ders, especially nocturnal asthma. Inhaled anticholinergic bronchodilators are used primarily for chronic disorders.

Corticosteroids are useful in the treatment of acute and chronic disorders. Leukotriene inhibitors are indicated for the prophylaxis and chronic treatment of asthma in adults and children 12 years and older. Although the drugs are not effective in relieving acute asthma attacks, they may be continued concurrently with other drugs during acute episodes. Cromolyn and nedocromil are indicated only for prophylaxis of asthma attacks.

CONTRAINDICATIONS FOR USE

Adrenergics are contraindicated in clients with cardiac tachyarrhythmias and severe coronary artery disease; they should be used cautiously in clients with hypertension, hyperthyroidism, diabetes mellitus, and seizure disorders. *Xanthines* are contraindicated in clients with acute gastritis and peptic ulcer disease; they should be used cautiously in those with cardiovascular disorders that could be aggravated by drug-induced cardiac stimulation. Inhaled *anticholinergics* should be used with caution in clients with narrow-angle glaucoma and prostatic hypertrophy. *Corticosteroids* should be used with caution in clients with peptic ulcer disease, inflammatory bowel disease, hypertension, congestive heart failure, and thromboembolic disorders. *Leukotriene inhibitors* are contraindicated in clients with hypersensitivity to the drugs and *zileuton* is contraindicated in clients with active liver disease or substantially elevated liver enzymes (three times the upper limit of normal values). *Mast cell stabilizers* are contraindicated in clients who are hypersensitive to the drugs. They should be used with caution in clients with impaired renal or hepatic function. Also, the propellants in the aerosol may aggravate coronary artery disease or arrhythmias.

Individual Bronchodilating and Antiasthmatic Drugs

ADRENERGIC BRONCHODILATORS

Epinephrine (Adrenalin, Bronkaid) may be administered subcutaneously in an acute attack of bronchoconstriction. Therapeutic effects may occur within 5 minutes and last for 4 hours. Epinephrine is available in a pressurized aerosol form without a physician's prescription (*e.g.,* Primatene). When given by inhalation, epinephrine rapidly relieves bronchoconstriction associated with asthma, bronchitis, or emphysema. Almost all over-the-counter aerosol products promoted for use in asthma contain epinephrine. These products are often abused and may delay the client from seeking medical attention. Clients should be cautioned that excessive use may produce tolerance and hazardous adverse effects.

Routes and Dosage Ranges

Adults: Aqueous solution (epinephrine 1:1000), SC 0.2–0.5 ml; dose may be repeated after 20 minutes if necessary

Aqueous suspension (Sus-Phrine 1:200), SC 0.1–0.3 ml; dose may be repeated after 4 h if necessary

Inhalation by inhaler, 1 or 2 inhalations four to six times per day

Inhalation by nebulizer, 0.25–0.5 ml of 2.25% racemic epinephrine in 2.5 ml normal saline

Children: Aqueous solution (epinephrine 1:1000), SC 0.01 ml/kg q4h as needed. A single dose should not exceed 0.5 ml.

Aqueous suspension (Sus-Phrine 1:200), SC 0.005 ml/kg q8–12h if necessary

Inhalation, same as adults for both inhaler and nebulizer

Albuterol (Proventil), **bitolterol** (Tornalate), and **pirbuterol** (Maxair) are short-acting beta$_2$-adrenergic agents used for prevention and treatment of bronchoconstriction. Although they have less effect on the cardiovascular system than epinephrine or isoproterenol, they should be used with caution in clients with cardiac disorders.

Albuterol
Routes and Dosage Ranges

Adults: PO 2–4 mg three or four times per day
Inhalation, 1 or 2 inhalations (90 µg/puff) q4–6h

Children: Safety and effectiveness in children younger than 12 years have not been established.

Bitolterol
Route and Dosage Ranges

Adults and children >12 years: Treatment, 2 inhalations (0.37 mg/puff) at least 1–3 min apart, followed by a third if necessary

Prophylaxis, 2 inhalations q8h; maximum recommended dose, 3 inhalations q6h or 2 inhalations q4h

Pirbuterol
Route and Dosage Range

Adults: Inhalation, 2 puffs (0.4 mg/dose), four to six times per day; maximum dose, 12 inhalations/d

Children over 12 years: Inhalation, same as adults; not recommended for use in children younger than 12 years

Isoetharine (Bronkosol, Bronkometer) is used to treat acute attacks of asthma. Although the drug acts more selectively on beta$_2$-adrenergic receptors than on beta$_1$ receptors, cardiac and CNS stimulation may occur with high doses. Isoetharine is relatively short acting (duration of 1 to 3 hours). It is available as a solution for nebulization or in a pressurized container for inhalation.

Route and Dosage Ranges

Adults and children: Inhalation by nebulizer, 0.25–0.5 ml of 1% isoetharine in 2.5 ml of normal saline

Inhalation by inhaler, 1 or 2 inhalations (0.34 mg/dose) four times per day

Isoproterenol (Isuprel) is a potent bronchodilator and cardiac stimulant. When used for treatment of bronchospasm, isoproterenol is given by inhalation, alone or in combination with other agents. Isoproterenol is a short-acting agent (approximate duration of 1 to 3 hours).

Route and Dosage Ranges

Adults and children: Inhalation by nebulizer, 0.25–0.5 ml of 1:200 Isuprel solution in 2.5 ml saline

Inhalation by inhaler, 1 or 2 inhalations (0.075–0.125 mg/puff) four times per day; maximum dose, 3 inhalations per attack of bronchospasm

Metaproterenol (Alupent) is a relatively selective, intermediate-acting beta$_2$-adrenergic agonist that may be given orally or by metered-dose inhaler. Metaproterenol is used to treat acute bronchospasm and to prevent exercise-induced asthma. In high doses, metaproterenol loses some of its selectivity and may cause cardiac and CNS stimulation.

Routes and Dosage Ranges

Adults: Inhalation, 1–3 puffs (0.65 mg/dose), four times per day; maximum dose, 12 inhalations/d
PO 10–20 mg q6–8h

Children: Inhalation, not recommended for use in children younger than 12 years

9 years or under or weight under 27 kg, PO 10 mg q6–8h

Over 9 years or weight over 27 kg, PO 20 mg q6–8h

Salmeterol (Serevent) is a long-acting beta$_2$-adrenergic agonist used only for prophylaxis of acute bronchoconstriction. Because it has a slow onset of action (about 20 minutes), it should not be used to treat acute bronchospasm. Because effects last 12 hours, it should not be taken more frequently. If additional bronchodilating medication is needed, a short-acting agent (*e.g.*, albuterol) should be used.

Routes and Dosage Ranges

Adults: Oral inhalation, 2 inhalations (42 µg), q12h

Terbutaline (Brethine) is a relatively selective beta$_2$-adrenergic agonist that is a long-acting bronchodilator. When given subcutaneously, terbutaline loses its selectivity and has little advantage over epinephrine. Muscle tremor is the most frequent side effect with this agent.

Routes and Dosage Ranges

Adults: PO 2.5–5 mg q6–8h; maximum dose, 15 mg/d
SC 0.25 mg, repeated in 15–30 min if necessary, q4–6h
Inhalation, 2 inhalations (400 µg/dose) q4–6h
Children: PO 2.5 mg three times per day for children 12 years and older; maximum dose, 7.5 mg/d
SC dosage not established
Inhalation, same as adults for children 12 years and older

ANTICHOLINERGIC BRONCHODILATORS

Atropine (Dey-Dose Atropine Sulfate) is the prototype anticholinergic drug with multiple indications for use. It is occasionally given by inhalation for prevention and treatment of bronchospasm associated with asthma, bronchitis, and emphysema. Systemic absorption is variable and more likely to occur with higher doses.

Route and Dosage Ranges

Adults: Inhalation, 0.025 mg/kg diluted with 3 to 5 ml of saline and given by nebulizer three or four times per day; maximum dose, 2.5 mg/d
Children: Inhalation, 0.05 mg/kg diluted in saline and given by nebulizer three or four times per day

Ipratropium bromide (Atrovent) is similar to atropine in its actions, uses, and effects. It is ineffective in acute bronchospasm when a rapid response is required. It is used in maintenance therapy of bronchoconstriction associated with chronic bronchitis and emphysema. Improved pulmonary function usually occurs within 15 minutes, peaks in 1 to 2 hours, and lasts about 4 hours. The most common adverse effects are cough, nervousness, nausea, gastrointestinal upset, headache, and dizziness. Ipratropium acts synergistically with adrenergic bronchodilators and may be used concomitantly.

Route and Dosage Range

Adults: 2 inhalations (36 µg) from the metered-dose inhaler four times per day
Children: Dosage not established

XANTHINE BRONCHODILATORS

Theophylline may be used in the prevention and treatment of bronchoconstriction associated with asthma, bronchitis, and emphysema. Numerous dosage forms are available. Most formulations contain anhydrous theophylline (100% theophylline) as the active ingredient; some contain theophylline salts. For example, theophylline ethylenediamine (aminophylline) contains about 85% theophylline and is the only formulation that can be given IV. Oral sustained-action tablets (*e.g.,* Theo-Dur, Theobid) are more commonly used than other formulations.

In addition to the single-drug formulations, many combination products are available. These products contain other active ingredients, such as an adrenergic drug (*e.g.,* ephedrine), an expectorant (*e.g.,* guaifenesin), or a sedative (*e.g.,* phenobarbital, hydroxyzine). Although combination products are rarely prescribed by health care providers, several are available over the counter and may be self-prescribed for "asthma." The potential risks of overusing these nonprescription products or combining them with prescribed antiasthmatic drugs are great, and clients should be cautioned against such usage.

Aminophylline
Routes and Dosage Ranges

Adults: PO, 500 mg initially, then 200–300 mg q6–8h; IV infusion, 6 mg/kg over 30 minutes, then 0.1–1.2 mg/kg/h
Children: PO, 7.5 mg/kg initially, then 5–6 mg/kg q6–8h; IV infusion, 6 mg/kg over 30 minutes, then 0.6–0.9 mg/kg/h

Long-Acting Theophylline (e.g., Theo-Dur)
Routes and Dosage Ranges

Adults: PO, 150–300 mg q8–12h; maximal dose 13 mg/kg or 900 mg daily, whichever is less
Children: PO, 100–200 mg q8–12h; maximal dose, 24 mg/kg/d

CORTICOSTEROIDS

Beclomethasone (Beclovent, Vanceril), **flunisolide** (AeroBid), and **triamcinolone** (Azmacort) are topical corticosteroids for inhalation. Topical administration minimizes systemic absorption and adverse effects. These preparations may substitute for or allow reduced dosage of systemic corticosteroids. In persons with asthma who are taking an oral corticosteroid, the oral dosage is reduced slowly (over weeks to months) when an inhaled corticosteroid is added. The goal is to give the lowest oral dose necessary to control symptoms. Beclomethasone and flunisolide also are available in nasal solutions for treatment of allergic rhinitis that does not respond to other treatment.

Beclomethasone
Routes and Dosage Ranges

Adults: Oral inhalation, 2 inhalations (0.84 mg/dose) three or four times daily; maximum dose, 20 inhalations/24 h

Nasal inhalation (Vanceril nasal inhaler), 1 inhalation (0.42 mg) in each nostril two to four times per day

Children 6–12 years: Oral inhalation, 1 or 2 inhalations three or four times per day; maximum dose, 10 inhalations/24 h

Children over 12 years: Nasal inhalation, same as adults

Flunisolide
Routes and Dosage Ranges

Adults: Oral inhalation, 2 inhalations (0.50 mg/dose) twice daily, morning and evening; maximum dose, 4 inhalations twice daily (2 mg)

Nasal inhalation (Nasalide), 2 sprays in each nostril twice daily; maximum dose, 8 sprays in each nostril per day

Children 6–15 years: Oral inhalation, 2 inhalations twice daily

Nasal inhalation, 1 spray in each nostril three times per day, or 2 sprays twice daily; maximum dose, 4 sprays in each nostril per day

Triamcinolone
Route and Dosage Ranges

Adults: Oral inhalation, 2 inhalations three or four times per day; maximum dose, 16 inhalations/24 h

Children 6–12 years: 1 or 2 inhalations three or four times per day; maximum dose, 12 inhalations/24 h

Hydrocortisone, prednisone, and **methylprednisolone** (Solu-Medrol) are given to clients who require systemic corticosteroids. Corticosteroids may be given IV in acute, severe attacks of asthma or bronchospasm; they may be given orally in chronic asthma or bronchospasm.

Hydrocortisone Sodium Phosphate and Sodium Succinate
Route and Dosage Ranges

Adults: IV 100–200 mg q4–6h initially, then decreased or switched to an oral dosage form

Children: IV 1–5 mg/kg q4–6h

Methylprednisolone sodium succinate
Route and Dosage Ranges

Adults: IV 2–60 mg q4–6h

Children: IV 1–4 mg/kg q4–6h

Prednisone
Route and Dosage Ranges

Adults: PO 20–60 mg/d

Children: PO 2 mg/kg/d initially

LEUKOTRIENE INHIBITORS

Zafirlukast and **zileuton** are oral agents used to prevent acute asthma attacks in clients with chronic asthma; they do not relieve bronchospasm in acute asthma attacks. Because of their anti-inflammatory effects, they may be able to reduce the use of corticosteroids. It is important to teach clients to continue drug administration during symptom-free periods.

Zafirlukast is well absorbed when given on an empty stomach. It is extensively metabolized in the liver by the cytochrome P450 enzyme system and may interact with other drugs metabolized by this system. Most metabolites are excreted in the feces. Zafirlukast is excreted in breast milk and should not be taken during lactation. The most common adverse effects reported in clinical trials were headache, nausea, diarrhea, and infection.

Zileuton is well absorbed and may be taken with or without food. It is highly bound to serum albumin (93%), metabolized by the cytochrome P450 liver enzymes, and metabolites are excreted mainly in urine. Hepatic transaminase enzymes should be monitored during zileuton therapy and the drug should be discontinued if enzyme levels reach five times the normal values or if symptoms of liver dysfunction develop. Elevation of liver enzymes was the most serious adverse effect during clinical trials; other adverse effects include headache, pain, and nausea. Zileuton increases serum concentrations of propranolol, theophylline, and warfarin.

Zafirlukast
Route and dosage range

Adults: PO 20 mg twice daily, 1 h before or 2 h after a meal

Children 12 years and older: Same as adults

Zileuton
Route and dosage range

Adults: PO 600 mg four times daily

Children 12 years and older: Same as adults

MAST CELL STABILIZERS

Cromolyn (Intal) and **nedocromil** (Tilade) are used to prevent acute asthma attacks in clients with chronic asthma, including allergic and exercise-induced asthmas. Use of one of these drugs may allow reduced dosage of bronchodilators and corticosteroids. The drugs are used only for prophylaxis; they are not effective in acute bronchospasm or status asthmaticus and should not be used in these conditions.

Cromolyn is available in a capsule and a solution for inhalation. The capsule is placed in a turboinhaler (Spinhaler) that punctures the capsule. When the client places the turboinhaler in the mouth and inhales, the capsule spins and vibrates, causing the micronized powder to be inhaled. The solution is for use with a power-operated nebulizer; hand-operated nebulizers are unsuitable.

Occasionally, the client may experience cough or bronchospasm following cromolyn inhalation. If a significant amount of bronchospasm occurs, the drug should be discontinued. Also, the drug should be discontinued if a therapeutic response is not obtained within 4 weeks of therapy.

A nasal solution (Nasalcrom) is available for prevention and treatment of allergic rhinitis; an ophthalmic solution (Opticrom) is available for prevention and treatment of allergic conjunctivitis and keratitis.

Intal
Route and Dosage Range

Adults: 20 mg (capsule or solution) inhaled four times per day
Children 5 years and older for capsules, 2 years and older for nebulizer solution: Same as adults

Nasalcrom
Route and Dosage Range

Adults and children 6 years and older: 1 spray in each nostril three to six times per day at regular intervals

Opticrom
Route and Dosage Range

Adults and children: 1 or 2 drops (cromolyn 1.6 mg/drop) in each eye four to six times per day at regular intervals

Nedocromil
Route and Dosage Range

Adults and children over 12 years: Inhalation, 4 mg q6–12h

Nursing Process

Assessment

Assess the client's pulmonary function:
- General assessment factors include rate and character of respiration, skin color, arterial blood gas analysis, and pulmonary function tests. Abnormal breathing patterns (*e.g.,* rate below 12 or above 24 per minute, dyspnea, cough, orthopnea, wheezing, "noisy" respirations) may indicate respiratory dis-

tress. Severe respiratory distress is characterized by tachypnea, dyspnea, use of accessory muscles of respiration, and hypoxia. Early signs of hypoxia include mental confusion, restlessness, anxiety, and increased blood pressure and pulse rate. Late signs include cyanosis and decreased blood pressure and pulse. Hypoxemia is confirmed if arterial blood gas analysis shows decreased partial pressure of oxygen (PO_2).
- In acute bronchospasm, a medical emergency, the client is in obvious and severe respiratory distress. A characteristic feature of bronchospasm is forceful expiration or wheezing.
- If the client has chronic asthma, try to determine the frequency and severity of acute attacks, factors that precipitate or relieve acute attacks, antiasthmatic medications taken occasionally or regularly, allergies, and condition between acute attacks, such as restrictions in activities of daily living due to asthma.
- If the client has chronic bronchitis or emphysema, assess for signs of respiratory distress, hypoxia, cough, amount and character of sputum, exercise tolerance (*e.g.,* dyspnea on exertion, dyspnea at rest), medications, and nondrug treatment measures (*e.g.,* breathing exercises, chest physiotherapy).

Nursing Diagnoses
- Impaired Gas Exchange related to bronchoconstriction and excessive mucus production
- Ineffective Breathing Pattern related to bronchoconstriction
- Activity Intolerance related to fatigue
- Self-Care Deficit related to impaired gas exchange
- Altered Nutrition: Less Than Body Requirements related to fatigue
- Risk for Injury: Respiratory infection
- Anxiety related to chronic illness
- Altered Tissue Perfusion related to bronchodilator-induced cardiac stimulation and arrhythmias
- Noncompliance: Overuse of adrenergic bronchodilators
- Sleep Pattern Disturbance: Insomnia with adrenergic and xanthine bronchodilators
- Altered Thought Processes: Confusion and nervousness related to CNS stimulation with adrenergic and xanthine bronchodilators
- Knowledge Deficit: Factors precipitating bronchoconstriction
- Knowledge Deficit: Measures to avoid precipitating factors and respiratory infection
- Knowledge Deficit: Accurate self-administration of drugs, including use of inhalers

Planning/Goals
The client will:
- Self-administer bronchodilating and other drugs accurately
- Experience relief of symptoms
- Avoid preventable adverse drug effects
- Avoid overusing bronchodilating drugs
- Avoid exposure to stimuli that cause bronchospasm when possible
- Avoid respiratory infections when possible

Interventions

Use measures to prevent, relieve, or decrease bronchoconstriction when possible. General measures include those to prevent respiratory disease or promote an adequate airway. Some specific measures include the following:

- Use mechanical measures for removing respiratory tract secretions and preventing their retention. Effective measures include coughing, deep breathing, percussion, and postural drainage.
- Help the client identify and avoid exposure to conditions that precipitate bronchoconstriction. For example, allergens may be removed from the home, school, or work environment. When bronchospasm is precipitated by exercise, prophylaxis by prior inhalation of bronchodilating agents is better than avoiding exercise, especially in children.
- Try to prevent or reduce anxiety, which may cause or aggravate bronchospasm. Stay with the client during an acute asthma attack if feasible. Clients experiencing severe and prolonged bronchospasm (status asthmaticus) should be admitted or transferred to a hospital intensive care unit.

 Teach clients:

- To drink 2000 to 3000 ml of fluids daily to help thin respiratory tract secretions and make them easier to remove.
- To stop smoking and avoid other bronchial irritants (*e.g.,* aerosol hair spray, antiperspirants, and cleaning products) when possible.
- To avoid excessive intake of coffee, tea, and cola drinks. These caffeine-containing beverages may increase bronchodilation but also may increase nervousness and insomnia with bronchodilating drugs.
- To take influenza vaccine annually and pneumococcal vaccine once if they have chronic lung disease.

Evaluation

- Observe for relief of symptoms and improved arterial blood gas values.
- Interview and observe for correct drug administration, including use of inhalers.
- Interview and observe for tachyarrhythmias, nervousness, insomnia, and other adverse drug effects.
- Interview about and observe behaviors to avoid stimuli that cause bronchoconstriction and respiratory infections.

Principles of Therapy

DRUG SELECTION AND ADMINISTRATION

Choice of drug and route of administration are determined largely by the severity of the disease process and the client's response to therapy. Some guidelines include the following:

1. Selective beta$_2$-adrenergic agonists are preferred bronchodilators. An inhaled, short-acting drug (*e.g.,* albuterol) is the initial drug of choice for acute bronchospasm. The long-acting drug salmeterol should *not* be used because its slow onset of action makes it ineffective in acute bronchospasm.
2. Because aerosol products act directly on the lungs, drugs given by inhalation can usually be given in

smaller doses and produce fewer adverse effects than oral or parenteral drugs.
3. Theophylline preparations are used infrequently because of their toxicity and because other effective agents are available. Although IV aminophylline has been used to treat acute asthma attacks, some studies indicate no benefit from its addition to inhaled beta$_2$ agonists and systemic corticosteroids.
4. Anticholinergic bronchodilators are ineffective in relieving acute bronchospasm. They are most useful in the long-term management of COPD.
5. Cromolyn and nedocromil are used prophylactically; they are ineffective in acute bronchospasm.
6. Because inflammation has been established as a major component of asthma and other bronchoconstrictive respiratory disorders, corticosteroids are being used earlier in the disease process, along with bronchodilators or mast cell stabilizers. In acute bronchoconstriction, a corticosteroid is often given orally or IV for several days.

   In chronic bronchoconstriction, inhaled corticosteroids should be given on a regular schedule. These drugs may be effective when used alone or with relatively small doses of an oral corticosteroid. Optimal schedules of administration are not clearly established but more frequent dosing (*e.g.,* q6h) may be more effective than less frequent dosing (*e.g.,* q12h), even if the total amount is the same. As with systemic glucocorticoid therapy, the recommended dose is the lowest amount required to control symptoms. High doses (more than 1500 µg daily in adults and 800 µg daily in children) suppress adrenocortical function but much less than systemic drugs. Small doses (*e.g.,* 600 µg of beclomethasone daily) may impair bone metabolism and predispose adults to osteoporosis by decreasing calcium deposition and increasing calcium resorption from bone. In children, chronic administration of corticosteroids may retard growth. Local adverse effects (oropharyngeal candidiasis, hoarseness) can be decreased by reducing the dose, administering less often, rinsing the mouth after use, or using a spacer device. These measures decrease the amount of drug deposited in the oral cavity. Generally, the inhaled drugs seem to be well tolerated with chronic use.
7. Using a combination of drugs may be more effective than using a single agent. One advantage of a multidrug regimen is that smaller doses of each agent usually can be given. This may decrease adverse effects and allow dosages to be increased when exacerbation of symptoms occurs.
8. A common regimen for treatment of asthma is an inhaled corticosteroid on a regular schedule, two to four times daily, and an inhaled beta$_2$-adrenergic agonist as needed for prevention or treatment of bronchoconstriction. This regimen may change with the

use of leukotrine inhibitors, which reportedly reduce the need for corticosteroids and as-needed inhaled bronchodilators.

DOSAGE FACTORS

Dosage of bronchodilators, corticosteroids, and mast cell stabilizers must be individualized so the smallest effective amounts are given. With theophylline preparations, guidelines include the following:

1. Dosage should be individualized. One way is to start with a low dose and gradually increase the amount according to symptom relief and serum theophylline levels. Serum levels should be monitored because of individual differences in hepatic metabolism; therapeutic range is 5 to 15 μg/ml. Serum levels of 20 μg/ml or above are associated with a high incidence of toxicity. Blood for serum levels should be drawn 1 to 2 hours after immediate-release dosage forms and 4 hours after sustained-release forms.
2. Children and cigarette smokers usually need higher doses to maintain therapeutic blood levels because they metabolize theophylline rapidly.
3. Clients who have liver disease, congestive heart failure, chronic pulmonary disease, or acute viral infections usually need smaller doses because these conditions impair theophylline metabolism.
4. For obese clients, theophylline dosage should be calculated on the basis of lean or ideal body weight, because theophylline is not highly distributed in fatty tissue.

USE OF BETA₂-ADRENERGIC AGONISTS IN ASTHMA

Beta₂-adrenergic bronchodilating drugs have been used in the treatment of asthma for more than 20 years. During that time, the role of inflammation in the pathophysiology of asthma was elucidated and effective methods of treatment continued to evolve. Despite these advances, however, asthma has become more prevalent and has caused an increasing number of deaths. The reasons for these developments are not clear, but some authorities think that regular use of beta₂-adrenergic agonists may play a role because increased use of the drugs occurred concurrently with the increased morbidity and mortality associated with asthma.

As a result of the above difficulties, recommendations for the use of beta₂-adrenergic agonists have changed during the past few years. Although most drug references still list a regular dosing schedule (*e.g.*, every 4 to 6 hours for albuterol inhalations), prevailing opinion is that the drugs should be used when needed and not on a regular schedule.

USE IN CHILDREN

Antiasthmatic medications are used in children for the same indications as for adults. With adrenergic bronchodilators, recommendations for use vary according to route of administration and age of the child. Inhalation of albuterol (Proventil), bitolterol (Tornalate), metaproterenol (Alupent), and terbutaline (Brethine) is not recommended in children under 12 years of age. In addition, extended release tablets of albuterol are not recommended for children under 12 years, and the syrup formulation is not recommended for children under 2 years. Metaproterenol oral tablets are not recommended for children under 6 years, and terbutaline oral tablets are not recommended for children under 12 years of age.

With theophylline, use in children should be closely monitored because dosage needs and rates of metabolism vary widely. In children younger than 6 months, especially premature infants and neonates, drug elimination may be prolonged due to immature liver function. Except for preterm infants with apnea, theophylline preparations are not recommended for use in this age group. Children aged 6 months to 16 years, approximately, metabolize theophylline more rapidly than younger or older clients. Thus, they may need higher doses than adults in proportion to size and weight. If the child is obese, the dosage should be calculated on the basis of lean or ideal body weight because the drug is not highly distributed in fatty tissue. Long-acting dosage forms are not recommended for children younger than 6 years. Children may become hyperactive and disruptive from the CNS-stimulating effects of theophylline. Tolerance to these effects usually develops with continued use of the drug.

With corticosteroids, a major concern in children is potential impairment of bone growth. This should be monitored closely. As with adults, adverse effects of corticosteroids are less likely to occur with inhalation than with oral use. Cromolyn capsules are commonly used for inhalation in children 5 years of age and older, and nebulizer solution is used with children 2 years and older. Nedocromil is not established as safe and effective in children under 12 years of age.

USE IN OLDER ADULTS

Older adults often have pulmonary disorders for which bronchodilators and antiasthmatic medications are used. As with other populations, administering the medications by inhalation and giving the lowest effective dose decrease adverse effects. The main risks with adrenergic bronchodilators are excessive cardiac and CNS stimulation.

Theophylline use must be carefully monitored because drug effects are unpredictable. On one hand, cigarette smoking and drugs that stimulate drug-metabolizing enzymes in the liver (*e.g.,* phenobarbital, phenytoin) increase the rate of metabolism and therefore dosage requirements. On the other hand, impaired liver function, decreased blood flow to the liver, and some drugs (*e.g.,* cimetidine, erythromycin) impair metabolism and therefore decrease dosage requirements.

Adverse effects include cardiac and CNS stimulation. Safety can be increased by measuring serum drug levels and adjusting dosage to maintain therapeutic levels of 5 to 15 µg/ml. If the client is obese, dosage should be based on lean or ideal body weight because theophylline is not highly distributed in fatty tissue.

HOME CARE

All of the drugs discussed in this chapter are used in the home setting. A major role of the home care nurse is to assist clients to use the drugs safely and effectively. Several studies have indicated that many people do not use metered-dose inhalers and other devices correctly. The home care nurse needs to observe a client using an inhalation device when possible. If errors in technique are assessed, teaching or reteaching may be needed. With inhaled medications, a spacer device may be useful, especially for children and older adults, because less muscle coordination is required to administer a dose. Adverse effects may be minimized as well.

For clients with asthma, especially children, assess the environment for potential triggers of acute bronchospasm, such as cigarette smoking. In addition, assist clients to recognize and treat (or get help for) exacerbations before respiratory distress becomes severe.

With theophylline, the home care nurse needs to assess the client and the environment for substances that may affect metabolism of theophylline and decrease therapeutic effects or increase adverse effects. In addition, the nurse needs to reinforce the importance of not exceeding the prescribed dose, not crushing long-acting formulations, reporting adverse effects, and keeping appointments for follow-up care.

NURSING ACTIONS
BRONCHODILATING AND ANTIASTHMATIC DRUGS

NURSING ACTIONS	RATIONALE/EXPLANATION
1. Administer accurately **a.** Be sure clients have adequate supplies of inhaled bronchodilators and corticosteroids available for self-administration. Observe technique of self-administration for accuracy and assist if needed.	
b. Give immediate-release oral theophylline before meals with a full glass of water, at regular intervals around the clock. If GI upset occurs, give with food.	To promote dissolution and absorption. Taking with food may decrease nausea and vomiting.
c. Give sustained-release theophylline q8–12h, with instructions not to chew or crush.	Sustained-release drug formulations should never be chewed or crushed because doing so causes immediate release of potentially toxic doses.
d. Give IV aminophylline no faster than 25 mg/min.	IV aminophylline is usually given as a loading dose for faster effects, followed by a maintenance infusion. Rapid administration may cause toxic effects.
e. Give zafirlukast 1 h before or 2 h after a meal; zileuton may be given with or without food.	The bioavailability of zafirlukast is reduced about 40% if taken with food. Food does not significantly affect the bioavailability of zileuton.
2. Observe for therapeutic effects **a.** Decreased dyspnea and wheezing	Relief of bronchospasm and wheezing should be evident within a few minutes after giving SC epinephrine, IV aminophylline, or aerosolized adrenergic bronchodilators.
b. Reduced rate and improved quality of respirations	

(continued)

c. Reduced anxiety and restlessness

d. Therapeutic serum levels of theophylline (5–15 μg/ml)

e. Improved arterial blood gas levels (normal values: PO_2, 80 to 100 mm Hg; PCO_2, 35 to 45 mm Hg; pH, 7.35 to 7.45)

f. Improved exercise tolerance

g. Decreased incidence and severity of acute attacks of bronchospasm with chronic administration of drugs

3. Observe for adverse effects

a. With adrenergic bronchodilators, observe for tachycardia, arrhythmias, palpitations, restlessness, agitation, insomnia.

These signs and symptoms result from cardiac and central nervous system (CNS) stimulation.

b. With anticholinergic bronchodilators, observe for dry mouth, blurred vision, headache, nervousness, nausea. Ipratropium also may cause cough or exacerbation of symptoms.

When atropine is given by inhalation, a variable amount of systemic absorption occurs. Adverse effects are increased with greater systemic absorption. Ipratropium is not absorbed systemically.

c. With xanthine bronchodilators, observe for tachycardia, arrhythmias, palpitations, restlessness, agitation, insomnia, nausea, vomiting, convulsions.

Theophylline causes cardiac and CNS stimulation. Convulsions occur at toxic serum concentrations (above 20 μg/ml). They may occur without preceding symptoms of toxicity and may result in death. IV diazepam (Valium) may be used to control seizures. Theophylline also stimulates the chemoreceptor trigger zone in the medulla oblongata to cause nausea and vomiting.

d. With inhaled corticosteroids, observe for hoarseness, cough, throat irritation, and fungal infection of mouth and throat.

Inhaled corticosteroids are unlikely to produce the serious adverse effects of long-term systemic therapy (see Chap. 24).

e. With leukotriene inhibitors, observe for headache, infection, nausea, pain, elevated liver enzymes (*e.g.*, ALT), and liver dysfunction.

These drugs are generally well tolerated. A highly elevated ALT and liver dysfunction are more likely to occur with zileuton.

f. With cromolyn, observe for arrhythmias, hypotension, chest pain, restlessness, dizziness, convulsions, CNS depression, anorexia, nausea and vomiting. Sedation and coma may occur with overdosage.

Some of the cardiovascular effects are thought to be caused by the propellants used in the aerosol preparation.

4. Observe for drug interactions

a. Drugs that *increase* effects of bronchodilators:

(1) MAO inhibitors

These drugs inhibit the metabolism of catecholamines. The subsequent administration of bronchodilators may increase blood pressure. Severe hypertensive reactions have been reported with ephedrine.

(2) Erythromycin, clindamycin, cimetidine

These drugs may decrease theophylline clearance and thereby increase plasma levels.

b. Drugs that *decrease* effects of bronchodilators:

(1) Lithium

Lithium may increase excretion of theophylline and therefore decrease therapeutic effectiveness.

(2) Phenobarbital

This drug may increase the metabolism of theophylline by way of enzyme induction.

(3) Propranolol, other nonselective beta-blockers

These drugs may cause bronchoconstriction and oppose effects of bronchodilators.

NURSING ACTIONS	RATIONALE/EXPLANATION
c. Drugs that alter effects of zafirlukast:	
(1) Aspirin	Increases blood levels
(2) Erythromycin, theophylline	Decrease blood levels
5. Teach clients	
a. Take corticosteroids on a regular schedule.	This is necessary for anti-inflammatory effects. The drugs are not effective if taken on an occasional basis.
b. Take bronchodilators only as prescribed. If desired effects are not achieved or if symptoms worsen, inform the prescribing physician. Do not increase dosage or frequency of taking medication.	Tolerance and decreased effectiveness may occur with overuse, especially with the inhalers. Serious cardiac side effects may also occur.
c. To differentiate uses of individual drugs when more than one is prescribed. For example, a short-acting beta$_2$-agonist is the appropriate drug for bronchodilating effects in acute bronchospasm. Corticosteroids or a long-acting beta$_2$-agonist (*e.g.,* salmeterol) are not effective in relieving acute respiratory distress.	Sometimes patients have the misconception that any inhaler should help their breathing. This may lead to life-threatening delays in obtaining appropriate treatment.
d. Use inhalers correctly:	
(1) Shake well immediately before each use.	To disperse medication evenly
(2) Remove the cap from the mouthpiece.	
(3) Exhale fully, expelling as much air from the lungs as possible.	To increase drug effectiveness.
(4) With the inhaler in the upright position, place the mouthpiece just inside the mouth, and use the lips to form a tight seal.	
(5) While inhaling deeply, fully depress the top of the inhaler with the index finger.	
(6) Hold the breath as long as possible. Before exhaling, remove the mouthpiece from the mouth and the finger from the canister.	
(7) Wait 3–5 min before taking a second inhalation of the drug.	
(8) Rinse the mouthpiece and store the inhaler away from heat.	Inhaler contents are pressurized and may explode if heated.

REVIEW AND APPLICATION EXERCISES

1. What are some causes of bronchoconstriction, and how can they be prevented or minimized?

2. How do beta-adrenergic agonists and theophylline act as bronchodilators?

3. Which beta-adrenergic agonists act more selectively on beta$_2$-adrenergic receptors than on beta$_1$ receptors?

4. What adverse effects are associated with bronchodilators, and how can they be prevented or minimized?

5. What is an adverse effect associated with theophylline toxicity?

6. What is the therapeutic range of serum theophylline levels?

7. How do cromolyn and nedocromil act to prevent acute asthma attacks?

8. For what effects are corticosteroids used in the treatment of bronchoconstrictive respiratory disorders?

SELECTED REFERENCES

Busse, W.W. (1996). Long-and short-acting beta$_2$-adrenergic agonists. *Archives of Internal Medicine, 156,* 1514–1520.

Cockcroft, D.W. & Kalra, S. (1996). Outpatient asthma management. *Medical Clinics of North America, 80*(4), 701–718.

Drug facts and comparisons. (Updated monthly). St. Louis: Facts and Comparisons.

Guyton, A.C. & Hall, J.E. (1996). *Textbook of medical physiology,* 9th ed. Philadelphia: W.B. Saunders.

Kelly, H.W. & Kamada, A.K. (1997). Asthma. In J.T. DiPiro, R.L. Talbert, G.C. Yee, G.R. Matzke, B.G. Wells, & L.M. Posey (Eds.), *Pharmacotherapy: A pathophysiologic approach,* 3rd ed., pp. 553–590. Stamford, CT: Appleton & Lange.

Noyes, M.A. & Stratton, M.A. (1997). Chronic obstructive lung disease. In J.T. DiPiro, R.L. Talbert, G.C. Yee, G.R. Matzke, B.G. Wells, & L.M. Posey (Eds.), *Pharmacotherapy: A pathophysiologic approach,* 3rd ed., pp. 591–613. Stamford, CT: Appleton & Lange.

Porth, C.M. (1994). *Pathophysiology: Concepts of altered health states,* 4th ed. Philadelphia: J.B. Lippincott.

Taylor, D.R., Sears, M.R., & Cockcroft, D.W. (1997). The beta-agonist controversy. *Medical Clinics of North America, 80*(4), 719–748.

Antihistamines

Objectives

After studying this chapter, the student will be able to:

1 Delineate effects of histamine on selected body tissues.

2 Identify the effects of histamine that are blocked by histamine₁ receptor antagonist drugs.

3 Describe antihistamines in terms of indications for use, adverse effects, and nursing process implications.

4 Discuss advantages and disadvantages of nonsedating antihistamines.

Key Terms

Allergic reactions	**Pruritus**
Histamine	**Sedation**
Histamine₁ receptor antagonists	

Histamine and Its Receptors

Antihistamines are drugs that antagonize the action of histamine. Thus, to understand the use of these drugs, it is necessary to understand the action of histamine in the body.

Histamine is an important chemical mediator in immune and inflammatory responses. It is found in most body tissues, with high concentrations in tissues exposed to environmental substances (*e.g.,* skin, mucosal surfaces of the lungs and gastrointestinal [GI] tract). It is also found in the central nervous system (CNS), epidermal cells, gastric mucosa, and rapidly growing tissue.

Histamine is synthesized and stored in secretory granules of mast cells and basophils. It is released from these cells during immediate hypersensitivity reactions and cellular injury. Once released, histamine interacts with three types of histamine receptors, called H_1, H_2, and H_3. When H_1 receptors are stimulated, major effects are

> Contraction of bronchial and other smooth muscle
> Stimulation of sensory peripheral nerve endings to cause pain and pruritus
> Stimulation of vagus nerve endings to produce reflex bronchoconstriction and cough
> Increased permeability of capillaries, which allows fluid to flow into subcutaneous tissues and form edema. Mucosal edema produces the nasal congestion characteristic of allergic rhinitis and the common cold.

When H_2 receptors are stimulated, the main effects are increased secretion of gastric acid and pepsin, increased rate and force of mycocardial contraction, and decreased immunologic and proinflammatory reactions (*e.g.,* decreased release of histamine from basophils, decreased movement of neutrophils and basophils into areas of injury, inhibited T- and B-lymphocyte function). Stimulation of both H_1 and H_2 receptors causes peripheral vasodilation (with hypotension, headache, and skin flushing) and increases bronchial, intestinal, and salivary secretion of mucus.

The H_3 receptor was initially described as a presynaptic receptor on histamine-releasing nerve terminals in the CNS that acted to decrease further histamine synthesis and release from the nerve endings. Since then, it has been found to function as a negative feedback mechanism to inhibit histamine synthesis and release in many body tissues. Stimulation of H_3 receptors opposes the effects produced by stimulation of H_1 receptors. In addition, stimulation of H_3 receptors on nerve terminals of the sympathetic nervous system inhibits vasoconstriction and slows heart rate.

Antihistamines

The term *antihistamines* generally indicates classic or traditional drugs. With increased knowledge about histamine receptors, these drugs are often called H_1-receptor antagonists. Many H_1 antagonists or blocking agents are available for clinical use. These drugs are similar in effectiveness as histamine antagonists but differ in potency, dosage, adverse effects, and dosage forms available. These are the antihistamines discussed in this chapter. Cimetidine (Tagamet), ranitidine (Zantac), famotidine (Pepcid), and nizatidine (Axid) are H_2-receptor antagonists or blocking agents used to prevent or treat peptic ulcer disease. These are discussed in Chapter 60. H_3-receptor agonists and antagonists are being developed, but none is available for clinical use. Groups of H_1 antagonists are described below; individual drugs are listed in Table 48-1.

FIRST-GENERATION H_1-Receptor ANTAGONISTS

These drugs cause CNS depression (drowsiness, sedation) with usual therapeutic doses and may cause CNS stimulation (anxiety, agitation) with excessive doses, especially in children. They also have substantial anticholinergic effects. Groups vary in adverse effects. *Alkylamines* are commonly used. They cause relatively little drowsiness and are suitable for daytime use. *Ethanolamines* are strong CNS depressants and cause a high incidence of drowsiness. Incidence of GI distress is low. Diphenhydramine (Benadryl), the prototype, is commonly used. *Ethylenediamines* cause minimal drowsiness but often cause GI distress. *Phenothiazines*, which are related to the phenothiazine antipsychotic drugs discussed in Chapter 9, are strong CNS depressants. They are used mainly for sedative and antiemetic effects. *Piperazines* cause a relatively low incidence of drowsiness except for hydroxyzine, which is often used as an antiemetic, a preoperative sedative, and an antipruritic with allergic skin disorders. A newer drug, cetirizine (Zyrtec), is an active metabolite of hydroxyzine that causes less drowsiness than hydroxyzine. Several first-generation antihistamines are available without prescription, including brompheniramine (Dimetane), chlorpheniramine (Chlor-Trimeton), diphenhydramine (Benadryl), and triprolidine (Actidil).

First-generation antihistamines are well absorbed following oral administration. Immediate-release oral forms act within 15 to 60 minutes and last about 4 to 6 hours. Enteric-coated or sustained-release preparations last 8 to 12 hours. Most drugs are given orally; a few may be given parenterally. These drugs are primarily metabolized by the liver and excreted within 24 hours by the kidneys.

TABLE 48-1 COMMONLY USED ANTIHISTAMINES

| Generic/Trade Name | Routes and Dosage Ranges | |
	Adults	Children
First Generation		
Alkylamines		
Chlorpheniramine (Chlor-Trimeton)	PO 2–4 mg tid–qid Sustained-release preparation, PO 8–12 mg qd–tid IM, IV, SC 5–40 mg	Age 6–12 y, PO, SC 0.35 mg/kg/d in four divided doses Age 7 y and over, sustained-release preparation, PO 8 mg q12h Not recommended for children under 6 y of age
Brompheniramine (Dimetane)	PO 4–8 mg tid–qid Sustained-release preparation, PO 8–12 mg bid IM, IV, SC 10 mg q6–12h; maximal daily dose, 40 mg	Infant 6 y, PO 0.5 mg/kg/d or 15 mg/m²/d in divided doses Age over 6, PO half of adult dose Age under 12, IM, IV, SC 0.5 mg/kg/d or 15 mg/m²/d in divided doses
Dexchlorpheniramine (Polaramine)	PO 2 mg tid or qid Sustained-release preparation, PO 4–6 mg bid	Infants, PO, one fourth of adult dose or 0.15 mg/kg/d in four divided doses. Under 12 years, PO, half of adult dose Do not use sustained-release preparation.
Triprolidine (Actidil)	PO 2.5 mg tid–qid	Age over 6 y, PO 1.25 mg tid–qid Age 4–6 y, PO 0.9 mg tid–qid Age 2–4 y, 0.6 mg tid–qid Age 4 mo–2 y, 0.3 mg tid–qid In children up to 6 y, use syrup only.
Ethanolamines		
Carbinoxamine (Clistin)	PO 12–32 mg daily in divided doses Long-acting preparation, PO 8–12 mg q6–12h	PO 0.2 mg/kg in three or four divided doses or 2–4 mg tid–qid
Clemastine (Tavist)	PO 2.68 mg one to three times daily, not to exceed 8.04 mg/d Long-acting preparation, initially, PO 1.34 mg bid, not to exceed 8.04 mg/d	Safety and efficacy in children under 12 y of age have not been established.
Dimenhydrinate (Dramamine)	PO 50–100 mg q4h Rectal 100 mg qd–bid IM, IV 50 mg	Age 8–12 y, 25–50 mg tid
Diphenhydramine (Benadryl)	PO 25–50 mg tid–qid IM, IV 10–50 mg to a maximal single dose of 100 mg; maximal daily dose, 400 mg	PO 12.5–25 mg tid or 5 mg/kg/d IM, IV 5 mg/kg or 150 mg/m²/d in four divided doses during a 24-h period, to a maximum of 300 mg/d
Ethylenediamines		
Pyrilamine	PO 75–200 mg daily in three or four divided doses	Age 6–12 y, PO 12.5–25 mg qid
Tripelennamine (P8Z)	PO tablets and elixir 25–50 mg q4–6h; maximal daily dose, 600 mg PO sustained-release tablets, 100 mg q12h	PO tablets and elixir 5 mg/kg/d 24 h in four to six divided doses or 150 mg/m²/d in four to six divided doses Do not use sustained-release tablets in children.
Phenothiazines		
Methdilazine (Tacary)	PO 8 mg bid–qid	Infants, PO 2 mg bid Age over 3 y, PO 4 mg bid–qid
Promethazine (Phenergan)	PO 25 mg at bedtime or 12.5 mg qd–bid Rectal 25 mg, may be repeated in 4–6 h IM, IV 12.5–25 mg, may be repeated in 2 h	PO 0.13 mg/kg in AM and, when necessary, 0.5 mg/kg at bedtime: or 25 mg at bedtime and 6.25–12.5 mg tid IM no more than half of adult dose

(continued)

TABLE 48-1	COMMONLY USED ANTIHISTAMINES (Continued)	
	Routes and Dosage Ranges	
Generic/Trade Name	*Adults*	*Children*
Trimeprazine (Temaril)	PO 2.5 mg qid Sustained-release preparation, PO 5 mg q12h	Age under 3 y, PO 1.25 mg tid maximal daily dose, 5 mg Age 3–12 y, PO 2.5 mg qid; maximal daily dose, 10 mg
Piperazines Cetirizine (Zyrtec)	PO 5–10 mg once daily Renal or hepatic impairment, PO 5 mg once daily	Age 12 y and older, PO 5–10 mg once daily
Cyclizine (Marezine)	PO 50 mg ½ h before travel; repeat q4–6h; maximal daily dose, 300 mg IM 50 mg tid–qid or as required	Age 6–10 y, PO, half of adult dose, IM 1 mg/kg tid
Hydroxyzine (Atarax, Vistaril)	PO 75–100 mg daily in three or four divided doses Preoperative and postoperative sedation, prepartum and postpartum sedation, IM 25–100 mg as a single dose Serious psychiatric conditions, IM 50–100 mg q4–6h PRN	PO 2 mg/kg/d in four divided doses Preoperative and postoperative sedation, IM 0.6 mg/kg in a single dose
Meclizine (Antivert)	Motion sickness, PO 25–50 mg qd 1 h before traveling Vertigo, 25–100 mg daily in divided doses	
Second Generation *Nonsedating Antihistamines* Astemizole (Hismanal)	PO 10 mg/d	Age above 12 y, PO 10 mg/d Age below 12 y, safety and efficacy not established
Fexofenadine (Allegra)	PO 60 mg twice daily Renal impairment: PO 60 mg once daily, initially	Children 12 y or older: PO 60 mg twice daily Children <12 y: Dosage not established
Loratadine (Claritin)	PO 10 mg/d Hepatic impairment, PO 10 mg every other day	Dosage not established
Terfenadine (Seldane)	PO 60 mg q12h	Age above 12 y, PO 60 mg twice daily Age 6–12 y, PO 30–60 mg twice daily Age 3–5 y, PO 15 mg twice daily
Miscellaneous Antihistamines Azatadine (Optimine)	PO 1–2 mg bid. Use lower dosage in older adults.	Dosage not established
Cyproheptadine (Periactin)	PO 4 mg tid not to exceed 0.5 mg/kg/d	Age 2–6 y, PO 2 mg bid–tid, not to exceed 12 mg daily Age 6–14 y, 4 mg tid, not to exceed 16 mg daily

SECOND-GENERATION H_1-RECEPTOR ANTAGONISTS

Second-generation H_1 antagonists, also called the nonsedating antihistamines, include astemizole, loratadine, and terfenadine. These prescription drugs are given orally, are highly bound to serum proteins, and are metabolized in the liver to metabolites that are excreted in urine and feces. Astemizole acts slowly and effects last up to 24 hours. Loratadine effects begin within 1 to 3 hours, reach a maximum in 8 to 12 hours, and last 24 hours or longer. Its long duration of action is due, in part, to an active metabolite. Terfenadine effects begin in about 2 hours, reach a maximum in 3 to 4 hours, and last 12 hours or longer. Fexofenadine, a newer drug, is an active metabolite of terfenadine. It is well absorbed and reaches peak serum concentrations in about 2½ hours after oral administration. Most fexofenadine is excreted in bile and urine; only a small portion is metabolized in the liver.

These drugs were developed to produce less sedation than the first-generation antihistamines. They cause less CNS depression because they do not cross the blood-brain barrier. They also do not cause the anticholinergic effects associated with first-generation drugs. A major disadvantage of astemizole and terfenadine, however, is their potential for causing serious cardiac arrhythmias (ventricular fibrillation, ventricular tachycardia, torsades de pointes, cardiac arrest) if taken in overdose, by clients with significant liver dysfunction, or concurrently with erythromycin, itraconazole, or ketoconazole. Astemizole and terfenadine are metabolized by the P450 enzyme system in the liver. The listed drugs, and possibly related drugs, inhibit metabolism of astemizole and terfenadine and increase their blood levels. These drug combinations should be avoided. These interactions have not been reported with loratadine or fexofenadine. (*Note:* Because of its adverse effects, the FDA has recommended that terfenadine be taken off the market.)

MECHANISM OF ACTION

Antihistamines prevent histamine from acting on target tissues and are effective in inhibiting vascular permeability, edema formation, bronchoconstriction, and pruritus associated with histamine release. Because the drugs are structurally related to histamine, they occupy the same receptor sites as histamine and competitively antagonize its actions. They do not prevent histamine release or reduce the amount released. First-generation drugs bind to both CNS and peripheral H_1 receptors; second-generation drugs bind more specifically with H_1 receptors in peripheral tissues than with H_1 receptors in the brain.

INDICATIONS FOR USE

Clinical indications for the use of H_1 antagonist antihistamines include:

1. **Allergic rhinitis and other hypersensitivity reactions.** Of people with hay fever (seasonal allergic rhinitis), 75% to 95% experience some relief of sneezing, rhinorrhea, nasal airway obstruction, and conjunctivitis with the use of antihistamines. People with perennial allergic rhinitis (nonseasonal) usually experience decreased nasal congestion and drying of nasal mucosa. With anaphylaxis and other serious allergic reactions, antihistamines are helpful in treating urticaria and pruritus but are less effective in treating bronchoconstriction and hypotension. Epinephrine, rather than an antihista-

mine, is the drug of choice for treating anaphylaxis and other serious allergic reactions. With pruritus, trimeprazine and cyproheptadine are especially effective. In addition to *treatment* of allergic disorders, antihistamines may be given to *prevent* allergic reactions to blood transfusions and contrast media (*e.g.,* iodine preparations) used for various diagnostic tests.

2. **Dermatologic conditions.** Antihistamines are the drugs of choice for treatment of acute urticaria but are less effective in chronic urticaria. Other indications for use include contact dermatitis, atopic dermatitis, drug-induced allergic skin reactions, pruritus ani, and pruritus vulvae. However, topical preparations containing antihistamines are not recommended because they may induce dermatologic allergic reactions (*e.g.,* skin rashes).

3. **Vascular disorders.** Antihistamines may be useful in treating angioedema, but they are second-choice drugs, after epinephrine.

4. **Miscellaneous.** Some antihistamines are commonly used for nonallergic disorders, such as motion sickness (*e.g.,* dimenhydrinate, meclizine), nausea and vomiting (*e.g.,* promethazine, hydroxyzine), and sleep (*e.g.,* diphenhydramine). The active ingredient in over-the-counter sleep aids (*e.g.,* Compoz, Sominex) is a sedating antihistamine. Antihistamines are also common ingredients in over-the-counter cold remedies (see Chap. 49).

CONTRAINDICATIONS FOR USE

Antihistamines are contraindicated or must be used with caution in clients with hypersensitivity to the drugs, narrow-angle glaucoma, prostatic hypertrophy, stenosing peptic ulcer, and bladder neck obstruction and during pregnancy. Astemizole and terfenadine are contraindicated in clients who are receiving macrolide antibiotics (*e.g.,* erythromycin, clarithromycin) or members of the imidazole group of antifungal agents (*e.g.,* itraconazole, ketoconazole) because life-threatening cardiac arrhythmias may occur.

Nursing Process

Assessment

Assess the client's condition in relation to disorders in which antihistamines are used. For the client with known allergies, try to determine the factors that precipitate or relieve allergic reactions and specific signs and symptoms experienced during a reaction.

Nursing Diagnoses

- Ineffective Airway Clearance related to thick respiratory secretions
- Risk for Injury related to drowsiness and dizziness

- Knowledge Deficit: Safe and accurate drug use
- Knowledge Deficit: Ways of preventing conditions for which antihistamines are used

Planning/Goals

The client will:
- Experience relief of symptoms
- Take antihistamines accurately
- Avoid hazardous activities if sedated from antihistamines
- Avoid preventable adverse drug effects
- Avoid taking sedative-type antihistamines with alcohol or other sedative drugs

Interventions

- Monitor the client closely for excessive drowsiness during the first few days of therapy with antihistamines known to cause sedation.
- Encourage a fluid intake of 2000 to 3000 ml daily, if not contraindicated.

Teach clients:
- With astemizole and terfenadine, do not take more than the prescribed dose and avoid taking erythromycin (an antibacterial drug), itraconazole, or ketoconazole (antifungal drugs) concurrently. Serious cardiac arrhythmias may result.
- Antihistamines are most effective before exposure to the stimulus that causes histamine release.
- Antihistamines may thicken respiratory tract secretions and make them more difficult to remove.
- Avoid using sedating antihistamines with other sedative-type drugs.

Evaluation

- Observe for relief of symptoms.
- Interview and observe for correct drug usage.
- Interview and observe for excessive drowsiness.

Principles of Therapy

PREVENTION OF HISTAMINE-RELEASING REACTIONS

When possible, avoiding exposure to known allergens can prevent allergic reactions. If antihistamine therapy is required, it is more effective if started before exposure to allergens because the drugs can then occupy receptor sites before histamine is released.

DRUG SELECTION AND USAGE

Choosing an antihistamine is based on the desired effect, duration of action, adverse effects, and other characteristics of available drugs. For most people, a nonsedating, second-generation drug is the first drug of choice. For those with conditions contraindicating

astemizole and terfenadine, (*i.e.,* liver disease, taking interacting drugs), loratadine is preferred because it has not been associated with the potentially serious adverse effects of the other two drugs.

A disadvantage of the second-generation drugs is that they are quite expensive. If costs are prohibitive for a client, a first-generation drug may be used with minimal daytime sedation if taken at bedtime. Also, sedation can be reduced by starting a drug at low doses and gradually increasing doses over a week or two. Overall, safety should be the determining factor. Some studies have shown performance impairment with the first-generation drugs even when the person does not feel drowsy or impaired.

For treatment of acute allergic reactions, a rapid-acting agent of short duration is preferred. For chronic allergic symptoms (*e.g.,* allergic rhinitis), long-acting preparations provide more consistent relief. A client may respond better to one antihistamine than to another. Thus, if one does not relieve symptoms or produces excessive sedation, another may be effective.

An antihistamine is often included in prescription and over-the-counter combination products for the common cold. Studies have demonstrated that antihistamines do not relieve cold symptoms and such usage is not recommended.

USE IN CHILDREN

First-generation antihistamines (*e.g.,* diphenhydramine) may cause drowsiness and decreased mental alertness in children as in adults. Young children may experience paradoxical excitement. These reactions may occur with therapeutic dosages. In overdosage, hallucinations, convulsions, and death may occur. Close supervision and appropriate dosages are required for safe drug usage in children.

The three second-generation antihistamines do not cause drowsiness in recommended dosages. With terfenadine, dosages are recommended for children as young as 3 years. Safety and efficacy of astemizole and loratadine have not been established, and dosages are not listed for children under 12 years old.

USE IN OLDER ADULTS

First-generation antihistamines (*e.g.,* diphenhydramine) may cause dizziness, sedation, syncope, confusion, paradoxical CNS stimulation, and hypotension in older adults. Older men with prostatic hypertrophy may have difficulty voiding while taking these drugs. Some of these adverse reactions derive from anticholinergic effects of the drugs and are likely to be more severe if the client is also taking other drugs with anticholinergic effects (*e.g.,* tricyclic antidepressants, antipsychotic drugs, some antiparkinson drugs). Despite the increased risk of adverse effects, however, diphenhydramine is sometimes prescribed as a sleep aid for occasional use in older adults. As with many other drugs, smaller dosages may be indicated in older adults.

HOME CARE

Antihistamines are often taken in the home setting, especially for seasonal and nonseasonal allergic rhinitis and other allergic disorders. Most people are familiar with the use and side effects of first-generation drugs; they may be less familiar with the second-generation, nonsedating drugs. The home care nurse is unlikely to be involved in antihistamine drug therapy unless visiting a client for other care and purposes. If a first-generation drug is being used, the home care nurse needs to assess for drowsiness and safety hazards in the environment (*e.g.*, operating a car or other potentially hazardous machinery). Most people develop tolerance to the sedative effects within a few days if not taking other sedative-type drugs or alcoholic beverages. If a second-generation drug is being taken, the home care nurse needs to assess for conditions that increase risks of adverse effects (*e.g.*, overdosing, liver disease, concurrent use of interacting drugs).

NURSING ACTIONS — ANTIHISTAMINES

NURSING ACTIONS	RATIONALE/EXPLANATION
1. Administer accurately **a.** Give most oral antihistamines with meals; give astemizole 2 h before a meal and instruct to avoid eating for 1 h after taking the medication.	To decrease gastrointestinal (GI) effects of the drugs. Absorption of astemizole is reduced by 60% when taken with meals.
b. Give IM antihistamines deeply into a large muscle mass.	To decrease tissue irritation
c. Inject IV antihistamines slowly, over a few minutes.	Severe hypotension may result from rapid IV injection.
d. When a drug is used to prevent motion sickness, give it 30–60 min before travel.	
2. Observe for therapeutic effects **a.** A verbal statement of therapeutic effect (relief of symptoms)	Therapeutic effects depend on the reason for use.
b. Decreased nausea and vomiting when given for antiemetic effects	
c. Decreased dizziness and nausea when taken for motion sickness	
d. Drowsiness or sleep when given for sedation	
3. Observe for adverse effects **a.** Sedation—ranging from mild drowsiness to deep sleep	Due to central nervous system (CNS) depression, which occurs with most antihistamines. Sedation is the most common adverse effect.
b. Paradoxical excitation—restlessness, insomnia, tremors, nervousness, palpitations	This reaction is more likely to occur in children. It may result from the anticholinergic effects of antihistamines.
c. Convulsive seizures	Antihistamines, particularly the phenothiazines, may lower the seizure threshold.
d. Dryness of mouth, nose, and throat, blurred vision, urinary retention, constipation	Due to antihistamines' anticholinergic effects
e. GI distress—anorexia, nausea, vomiting	These symptoms are especially likely to occur with the ethylenediamine group of antihistamines.

(continued)

NURSING ACTIONS	*RATIONALE/EXPLANATION*
f. Allergic reactions—skin rashes, photosensitivity	These are more likely to occur with topical antihistamine preparations.
g. Teratogenicity	Piperazine antihistamines are teratogenic.
h. Cardiac arrhythmias	Serious ventricular arrhythmias (fibrillation, tachycardia, torsades de pointes) have been reported with higher than recommended doses of astemizole and terfenadine or concurrent administration with erythromycin, itraconazole, or ketoconazole.
4. Observe for drug interactions Drugs that *increase* effects of antihistamines:	
(1) Ethyl alcohol, CNS depressants (*e.g.,* antianxiety and antipsychotic agents, narcotic analgesics, sedative-hypnotics)	Additive CNS depression. Concomitant use may lead to drowsiness, lethargy, stupor, respiratory depression, coma, and death.
(2) MAO inhibitors	Inhibit metabolism of antihistamines, leading to an increased duration of action; increased incidence and severity of anticholinergic adverse effects.
(3) Tricyclic antidepressants	Additive anticholinergic side effects
(4) Erythromycin, itraconazole, and ketoconazole	These antimicrobials increase the risks of serious cardiac arrhythmias with astemizole and terfenadine, probably by interfering with their metabolism and thereby increasing their blood levels.
5. Teach clients **a.** Take antihistamines only as prescribed or as instructed on packages of over-the-counter preparations.	To maximize therapeutic benefit and minimize adverse effects
b. Do not drink alcohol or take other drugs without the physician's knowledge and consent.	To avoid adverse effects and dangerous drug interactions. Alcohol and other drugs with CNS-depressant effects may cause excessive sedation, respiratory depression, and death.
c. Do not smoke, drive a car, or operate machinery until drowsiness has worn off.	To avoid injury. Drowsiness usually decreases after a few days of continuous drug administration.
d. Report adverse effects, such as excessive drowsiness.	The physician may be able to change drugs or dosages to decrease adverse effects.
e. Store antihistamines out of reach of children.	To avoid accidental ingestion
f. Do not exceed prescribed dosage of astemizole or terfenadine.	To avoid potentially serious irregularities of the heart beat
g. Inform any health care provider if taking astemizole or terfenadine.	To increase safety by avoiding possible adverse drug interactions.

 REVIEW AND APPLICATION EXERCISES

1. Describe several factors that cause histamine release from cells.

2. What signs and symptoms are produced by the release of histamine?

3. How do antihistamines act to block the effects of histamine?

4. Differentiate between histamine₁- and histamine₂-receptor antagonists in terms of pharmacologic effects and clinical indications for use.

5. In general, when should an antihistamine be taken to prevent or treat allergic disorders?

6. Describe advantages and disadvantages of the newer, nonsedating antihistamines in comparison with the older antihistamines.

7. In a client taking terfenadine or astemizole, what would you teach about safe usage?

SELECTED REFERENCES

Drug facts and comparisons. (Updated monthly). St. Louis: Facts and Comparisons.

Guyton, A.C. & Hall, J.E. (1996). *Textbook of medical physiology*, 9th ed. Philadelphia: W.B. Saunders.

Hendeles, L. (1993). Efficacy and safety of antihistamines and expectorants in nonprescription cough and cold preparations. *Pharmacotherapy, 13*(2), 154–158.

Lieberman, P. (1996). Antihistamines. In R.R. Rich, T.A. Fleisher, B.D. Schwartz, W.T. Sehearer, & W. Strober (Eds.), *Clinical immunology: Principles and practice*. St. Louis: C.V. Mosby.

May, J.R., Feger, T.A., & Guill, M.F. (1997). Allergic rhinitis. In J.T. DiPiro, R.L. Talbert, G.C. Yee, G.R. Matzke, B.G. Wells, & L.M. Posey (Eds.), *Pharmacotherapy: A pathophysiologic approach,* 3rd ed., pp. 1801–1813. Stamford, CT: Appleton & Lange.

Porth, C.M. (1994). *Pathophysiology: Concepts of altered health states,* 4th ed. Philadelphia: J.B. Lippincott.

Reports of dangerous cardiac arrhythmias prompt new contraindications for the drug Hismanal. (1993). *FDA Medical Bulletin, 23*(1), 2.

Nasal Decongestants, Antitussives, Mucolytics, and Cold Remedies

Outline

Description
nasal decongestants
antitussives
expectorants
mucolytics
cold remedies

Individual Drugs

Nursing Process
assessment
nursing diagnoses
planning/goals
interventions
evaluation

Principles of Therapy
drug selection and administration
use in children
use in older adults
home care

Objectives

After studying this chapter, the student will be able to:

1 Review decongestant effects of adrenergic drugs.

2 Describe general characteristics and effects of antitussive agents.

3 Discuss the rationale for using combination products in treatment of the common cold.

4 Discuss important elements of using antihistamines in children and older adults.

5 Evaluate over-the-counter cough, cold, and allergy remedies for personal or clients' use.

Key Terms

Antitussive	**Expectorant**
Decongestant	**Mucolytic**

Description

Common signs and symptoms of respiratory disorders are nasal congestion, cough, and increased secretions. Characteristics of these signs and symptoms include the following:

1. **Nasal congestion** is manifested by obstructed nasal passages ("stuffy nose") and nasal drainage ("runny nose"). It is a prominent symptom of the common cold and allergic rhinitis. Nasal congestion results from dilation of the blood vessels in the nasal mucosa and engorgement of the mucous membranes with blood. At the same time, nasal membranes are stimulated to increase mucus secretion. Related symptomatic terms are *rhinorrhea* (the discharge of mucus from the nose), *rhinitis* (inflammation of the mucous membrane of the nose), and *coryza* (profuse discharge from the mucous membrane of the nose).

2. **Cough** is a forceful expulsion of air from the lungs. It is normally a protective reflex for removing foreign bodies, environmental irritants, or accumulated secretions from the respiratory tract. The cough reflex involves central and peripheral mechanisms. Centrally, the cough center in the medulla oblongata receives stimuli and initiates the reflex response (deep inspiration, closed glottis, buildup of pressure within the lungs, and forceful exhalation). Peripherally, "cough receptors" in the pharynx, larynx, trachea, or lungs may be stimulated by air, dryness of mucous membranes, or excessive secretions. A cough is described as "productive" when secretions are expectorated; it is "nonproductive" when it is dry and no sputum is expectorated.

    Cough is a prominent symptom of respiratory tract infections (*e.g.,* influenza, bronchitis, pharyngitis) and chronic obstructive pulmonary diseases (*e.g.,* emphysema, chronic bronchitis).

3. **Increased secretions** may result from excessive production or decreased ability to cough or otherwise remove secretions from the respiratory tract. Secretions may seriously impair respiration by obstructing airways and preventing air flow to and from alveoli, where gas exchange occurs. Secretions also may cause atelectasis and cause or aggravate infections by supporting bacterial growth.

    Respiratory disorders characterized by retention of secretions include influenza, pneumonia, upper respiratory infections, acute and chronic bronchitis, emphysema, and acute attacks of bronchial asthma. Nonrespiratory conditions that predispose to secretion retention include immobility, debilitation, cigarette smoking, and postoperative status. Surgical procedures involving the chest or abdomen are most likely to be associated with retention of secretions because pain may decrease the client's ability to cough, breathe deeply, and ambulate.

Numerous drugs are available and widely used to treat these symptoms. Many are nonprescription drugs and can be obtained alone or in combination products. Available products include nasal decongestants, antitussives, and expectorants.

NASAL DECONGESTANTS

Nasal decongestants are used to relieve nasal obstruction and discharge. Adrenergic (sympathomimetic) drugs are most often used for this purpose (see Chap. 18). These agents relieve nasal congestion by constricting arterioles and reducing blood flow to nasal mucosa. Some nasal decongestants are applied topically to the nasal mucosa as nasal sprays or solutions. Some (*e.g.,* ephedrine, phenylephrine) may be used orally or topically; phenylpropanolamine is prepared only for oral use. Nasal decongestants are most often used to relieve rhinitis associated with respiratory infections or allergies. They also may be used to reduce local blood flow before nasal surgery and to aid visualization of the nasal mucosa during diagnostic examinations.

Nasal decongestants are contraindicated in clients with severe hypertension or coronary artery disease because of their cardiac stimulating and vasoconstricting effects. They also are contraindicated for clients with narrow-angle glaucoma and those taking tricyclic or monoamine oxidase inhibitor antidepressants. They must be used with caution in the presence of cardiac arrhythmias, hyperthyroidism, diabetes mellitus, glaucoma, and prostatic hypertrophy.

ANTITUSSIVES

Antitussive agents suppress cough by depressing the cough center in the medulla oblongata or the cough receptors in the throat, trachea, or lungs. Centrally acting antitussives include narcotics (codeine, hydrocodone, hydromorphone, and morphine) and non-narcotics (benzonatate, dextromethorphan). Peripherally acting agents (*e.g.,* glycerin, ammonium chloride) usually contain demulcents or local anesthetics to decrease irritation of pharyngeal mucosa. These agents are used as gargles, lozenges, and syrups. Flavored syrups are often used as vehicles for other drugs. Lozenges and hard candy increase the flow of saliva, which also soothes pharyngeal mucosa and may suppress cough.

The major clinical indication for use of antitussives is a dry, hacking, nonproductive cough that interferes with rest and sleep. It is not desirable to suppress a productive cough.

EXPECTORANTS

Expectorants are agents given orally to liquefy respiratory secretions and allow for their easier removal. Guaifenesin is an ingredient in many combination cough and cold remedies, although many authorities question its effectiveness.

MUCOLYTICS

Mucolytics are administered by inhalation to liquefy mucus in the respiratory tract. Solutions of mucolytic drugs may be nebulized into a face mask or mouthpiece or instilled directly into the respiratory tract through a tracheostomy. Sodium chloride solution and acetylcysteine (Mucomyst) are the only agents currently recommended for use as mucolytics. Acetylcysteine is effective within 1 minute after inhalation, and maximal effects occur within 5 to 10 minutes. It is effective immediately after direct instillation. Oral acetylcysteine is widely used in the treatment of acetaminophen overdosage (see Chap. 7).

COLD REMEDIES

Many combination products are available for treating symptoms of the common cold. Most of the products contain an antihistamine, a nasal decongestant, and an analgesic. Some contain antitussives, expectorants, and other agents as well. Many cold remedies are over-the-counter (OTC) formulations. Commonly used ingredients include chlorpheniramine (antihistamine), pseudoephedrine or phenylpropanolamine (adrenergic nasal decongestants), acetaminophen (analgesic), dextromethorphan (antitussive), and guaifenesin (expectorant). Some products come in several formulations, with different ingredients, and are advertised for different purposes. In addition, components or amounts may change even though trade names remain the same.

Individual Drugs

Individual decongestants, antitussives, expectorants, and mucolytics are listed in Table 49-1; combination cold, cough, and allergy remedies are listed in Table 49-2.

Nursing Process

Assessment

Assess the client's condition in relation to disorders for which the drugs are used.
- With nasal congestion, observe for decreased ability to breathe through the nose. If nasal discharge is present, note the amount, color, and thickness. Question the client about the duration and extent of nasal congestion and factors that precipitate or relieve the symptom.
- With coughing, a major assessment factor is whether the cough is productive of sputum or dry and hacking. If the cough is productive, note the color, odor, viscosity, and amount of sputum. In addition, assess factors that stimulate or relieve cough and the client's ability and willingness to cough effectively.

Nursing Diagnoses
- Risk for Injury related to cardiac arrhythmias, hypertension, and other adverse effects of nasal decongestants
- Noncompliance: Overuse of nasal decongestant and antitussive drugs
- Ineffective Airway Clearance related to suppression of a productive cough
- Constipation with narcotic antitussives
- Knowledge Deficit: Appropriate use of single- and combination-drug formulations

Planning/Goals
The client will:
- Experience relief of symptoms
- Take drugs accurately and safely
- Avoid overuse of nasal decongestants and narcotic antitussives
- Avoid preventable adverse drug effects
- Act to avoid recurrence of symptoms

Interventions
Encourage clients to use measures to prevent or minimize the incidence and severity of symptoms:
- With allergic disorders, avoid exposure to allergens when possible. Common allergens include plant pollens, dust, animal dander, and medications.
- Avoid smoking cigarettes. Cigarette smoke irritates respiratory tract mucosa, and this irritation causes cough, increased secretions, and decreased effectiveness of cilia in cleaning the respiratory tract.
- Avoid exposure to crowds, especially during winter when the incidence of influenza is high.
- Avoid contact with people who have colds or other respiratory infections. This is especially important for clients with chronic lung disease, because upper respiratory infections may precipitate acute attacks of asthma or bronchitis.
- Maintain a fluid intake of 2000 to 3000 ml daily unless contraindicated by cardiovascular or renal disease.
- Maintain nutrition, rest, activity, and other general health measures.
- Practice good handwashing techniques.
- Annual vaccination for influenza is recommended for clients who are elderly or have chronic respiratory, cardiovascular, or renal disorders.

 Teach clients:
- That drugs may relieve symptoms but do not cure the disorder causing the symptoms

TABLE 49-1	NASAL DECONGESTANTS, ANTITUSSIVES, AND EXPECTORANTS	
	Routes and Dosage Ranges	
Generic/Trade Name	*Adults*	*Children*
Nasal Decongestants		
Ephedrine	PO 25–50 mg q3–4h Topically, 1–2 drops of 1%–3% solution as needed	
Naphazoline (Privine)	Topically, 1–2 drops or 2 spray inhalations no more often than q4–6h	Age over 6 y, topically, same as adults Age under 6 y, not recommended
Oxymetazoline (Afrin)	Topically, 2–4 drops or 2–3 spray inhalations in each nostril, morning and bedtime	Age over 6 y, topically, same as adults Age under 6 y, 2–3 drops of 0.025% solution twice daily
Phenylephrine (Neo-Synephrine)	PO 10 mg three times daily Topically, 2–3 drops of 0.25%–1% solution in each nostril as needed	Age over 6 y, PO 5 mg three times daily: topically, same as adults Infants, topically, 1–2 drops of 0.125% solution as needed
Phenylpropanolamine (Propagest)	PO 25 mg q3–4h or 50 mg q6–8h	Age 8–12 y, PO 20–25 mg three times daily
Prophylhexedrine (Benzedrex)	Topically, 2 inhalations (0.6–0.8 mg) in each nostril as needed	
Pseudoephedrine (Sudafed)	PO 60 mg three or four times daily Sustained-release preparations, PO 120 mg twice daily	Age over 6 y, PO 60 mg three or four times daily Age 4 mo–6 y, PO 30 mg three or four times daily
Tetrahydrozoline (Tyzine)	Topically, 2–3 drops or 1–2 sprays of 0.1% solution instilled in each nostril, no more often than q3h	Age 6 y and over, topically, 1–3 drops of 0.05% solution in each nostril q4–6h Age under 6 y, not recommended
Xylometazoline (Otrivin)	Topically, 2–4 drops or inhalations of 0.1% solution in each nostril two or three times daily	Age 6 mo–12 y, topically, 2–3 drops of 0.05% solution in each nostril two or three times daily Age under 6 mo topically, 1 drop of 0.05% solution in each nostril two to three times daily
Narcotic Antitussives		
Codeine	PO 15 mg q4h as needed; maximal dose, 120 mg/24 h	PO 1–1.5 mg/kg/d in six divided doses as necessary
Hydrocodone	PO 5–10 mg three or four times daily	PO 0.6 mg/kg/d in three or four divided doses
Hydromorphone (Dilaudid)	PO 1 mg q3–4h	
Morphine sulfate	PO 2–4 mg three or four times daily	Age over 1 y, PO 0.06 mg/kg three or four times daily
Nonnarcotic Antitussives		
Benzonatate (Tessalon)	PO 100 mg three times daily; maximal dose, 600 mg/d	Age over 10 y, PO same as adults Age under 10 y, PO 8 mg/kg/d in three to six divided doses
Dextromethorphan (Benylin DM, others)	PO 10–30 mg three or four times daily. Maximum dose 120 mg/24 h	Age 2–6 y, PO 2.5–7.5 mg q4–8h. Maximum dose, 30 mg/24/h Age 6–12 y, PO 5–10 mg q4h or 15 mg q6–8h. Maximum dose, 60 mg/24/h
Expectorant		
Guaifenesin (glyceryl guaiacolate) (Robitussin)	PO 200 mg (2 tsp) q4h	Age 12 y or over, PO 200 mg (2 tsp) q4h Age 6–12 y, PO 100 mg (1 tsp) q4h Age 2–6 y, PO 50 mg (½ tsp) q4h

(continued)

TABLE 49-1 NASAL DECONGESTANTS, ANTITUSSIVES, AND EXPECTORANTS (Continued)

Generic/Trade Name	Routes and Dosage Ranges	
	Adults	*Children*
Mucolytic		
Acetylcysteine (Mucomyst)	Nebulization, 1–10 ml of a 20% solution or 2–20 ml of a 10% solution three or four times daily Instillation, 1–2 ml of a 10% or 20% solution q1–4h Acetaminophen overdosage, PO 140 mg/kg initially, then 70 mg/kg q4h for 17 doses; dilute a 10% or 20% solution to a 5% solution with cola, fruit juice, or water	

- That an adequate fluid intake, humidification of the environment, and sucking on hard candy or throat lozenges can help to relieve mouth dryness and cough
- To avoid using OTC cold remedies longer than 1 week
- Not to increase drug dosage if symptoms are not relieved by recommended amounts
- To see a health care provider if symptoms persist longer than 1 week
- To read the labels of OTC allergy and cold remedies for information about indications for use, contraindications, and adverse effects

Evaluation

- Interview and observe for relief of symptoms.
- Interview and observe for tachycardia, hypertension, drowsiness, and other adverse drug effects.
- Interview and observe for compliance with instructions about drug usage.

Principles of Therapy

DRUG SELECTION AND ADMINISTRATION

Choice of drugs and routes of administration are influenced by several client- and drug-related variables. Some guidelines include the following:

1. Single-drug formulations are usually preferred over combination products because they allow flexibility and individualization of dosage. Combination products may contain unneeded or ineffective components and less-than-optimum dosages of individual ingredients.
2. With nasal decongestants, topical preparations (*i.e.*, nasal solutions or sprays) are often preferred for short-term use. They are rapidly effective because they come into direct contact with nasal mucosa. If used longer than 7 days or in excessive amounts, these products may produce rebound nasal congestion. Oral drugs are preferred for long-term use (more than 7 days). Phenylephrine (Neo-Synephrine), phenylpropanolamine, and pseudoephedrine (Sudafed) are commonly used nasal decongestants in prescription and OTC products. For clients with cardiovascular disease, topical nasal decongestants are preferred. Oral agents are generally contraindicated because of cardiovascular effects (*e.g.*, increased force of myocardial contraction, increased heart rate, increased blood pressure).
3. Most antitussives are given orally as tablets or cough syrups. Syrups serve as vehicles for antitussive drugs and may exert antitussive effects of their own by soothing irritated pharyngeal mucosa. Narcotic antitussives are controlled substances. Strong narcotic agents (*e.g.*, morphine, hydromorphone) should be used as antitussives only in severe, painful cough that cannot be controlled by milder narcotics (*e.g.*, codeine, hydrocodone) or non-narcotic antitussives.

   Dextromethorphan is the antitussive drug of choice in most circumstances. Compared with codeine, dextromethorphan is similarly effective without the disadvantages of a narcotic preparation. Dextromethorphan has no analgesic effect, does not produce tolerance or dependence, and does not depress respiration. Further, dextromethorphan is the only non-narcotic antitussive for which efficacy has been demonstrated by extensive research studies. A dose of 15 to 30 mg reportedly equals 8 to 15 mg of codeine in antitussive effectiveness.
4. For treatment of excessive respiratory tract secretions, mechanical measures (*e.g.*, coughing, deep breathing, ambulation, chest physiotherapy, forcing fluids) are more likely to be effective than expectorant drug therapy.

TABLE 49-2	NONPRESCRIPTION COLD, COUGH, AND ALLERGY REMEDIES

Trade Name	Ingredients				
	Antihistamine	Nasal Decongestant	Analgesic	Antitussive	Expectorant
Actifed	Triprolidine 2.5 mg/tab or cap	Pseudoephedrine 60 mg/tab or cap			
Allerest	Chlorpheniramine 2 mg/tab	Phenylpropanol-amine 18.7 mg/tab			
Allerest (children's preparation)	Chlorpheniramine 1 mg/tab	Phenylpropanol-amine 9.4 mg/tab			
Cheracol D Cough Liquid				Dextromethor-phan 10 mg/5 ml	Guaifenesin 100 mg/5 ml
Comtrex	Chlorpheniramine 2 mg/cap	Phenylpropanol-amine 12.5 mg/cap	Acetaminophen 325 mg/cap	Dextromethor-phan 10 mg/cap	
Contac	Chlorpheniramine 8 mg/cap	Phenylpropanol-amine 75 mg/cap			
Coricidin	Chlorpheniramine 2 mg/tab		Acetaminophen 325 mg/tab		
Coricidin D	Chlorpheniramine 2 mg/tab	Phenylpropanol-amine 12.5 mg/tab	Acetaminophen 325 mg/tab		
CoTylenol cold formula	Chlorpheniramine 2 mg/tab or cap	Pseudoephedrine 30 mg/tab or cap	Acetaminophen 325 mg/tab or cap	Dextromethor-phan 15 mg/tab or cap	
CoTylenol liquid (children's preparation)	Chlorpheniramine 1 mg/5 ml	Phenylpropanol-amine 6.25 mg/5 ml	Acetaminophen 160 mg/5 ml		
Dimetapp Elixir	Brompheniramine 2 mg/5 ml	Phenylpropanol-amine 12.5 mg/5 ml			
Dimetapp Tablets	Brompheniramine 4 mg/tab	Phenylpropanol-amine 25 mg/tab			
Dimetapp Extentabs	Brompheniramine 12 mg/tab	Phenylpropanol-amine 75 mg/tab			
Dristan	Chlorpheniramine 2 mg/cap or tab	Phenylephrine 5 mg/cap or tab	Acetaminophen 325 mg/cap or tab		
Drixoral	Dexbromphenir-amine 6 mg/tab	Pseudoephedrine 120 mg/tab			
Novashistine Elixir	Chorpheniramine 2 mg/5 ml	Phenylephrine 5 mg/5 ml			
Novahistine DMX		Pseudoephedrine HCl 30 mg/5 ml		Dextromethor-phan 10 mg/5 ml	Guaifenesin 100 mg/5 ml
Robitussin-CF		Phenylpropanol-amine 12.5 mg/5 ml		Dextromethor-phan 10 mg/5 ml	Guaifenesin 100 mg/5 ml
Robitussin-DM				Dextromethor-phan 15 mg/5 ml	Guaifenesin 100 mg/5 ml
Robitussin-PE		Guaifenesin 100 mg/5 ml			
Sine-Off	Chlorpheniramine 2 mg/tab	Phenylpropanol-amine 12.5 mg/tab	Aspirin 325 mg/tab		
Sinutab	Chlorpheniramine 2 mg/tab	Pseudoephedrine 30 mg/tab	Acetaminophen 325 mg/tab		
Sinutab II		Pseudoephedrine 30 mg/tab or cap	Acetaminophen 500 mg/tab or cap		

USE IN CHILDREN

Upper respiratory infections with nasal congestion, cough, and increased secretions are common in children. The drugs described in this chapter are often used, and general principles apply.

Nasal congestion may interfere with an infant's ability to nurse. Phenylephrine nasal solution, applied just before feeding time, is usually effective.

Excessive amounts or too frequent administration of topical agents may result in rebound nasal congestion and systemic effects of cardiac and central nervous system stimulation. Despite these potential difficulties, topical drugs are less likely to cause systemic effects than oral agents.

USE IN OLDER ADULTS

Older adults are at high risk of adverse effects (*e.g.,* hypertension, arrhythmias, nervousness, insomnia) from oral nasal decongestants. Adverse effects from topical agents are less likely, but rebound nasal congestion and systemic effects may occur with overuse. Older adults with significant cardiovascular disease should generally avoid the drugs.

With codeine and other narcotic antitussives, older adults may experience drowsiness or paradoxical excitement. Serious adverse effects are uncommon with the small doses used to relieve cough but may occur with excessive amounts.

HOME CARE

Clients and others in home settings may ask the home care nurse for advice about OTC cold remedies. Before recommending a particular product, the nurse needs to assess the intended recipient for conditions or other medications that contraindicate the product's use. For example, the nasal decongestant component may cause or aggravate cardiovascular disorders (*e.g.,* hypertension). In addition, any other medications the client is taking need to be evaluated in terms of potential drug interactions with the multi-ingredient cold remedy.

The home care nurse also must emphasize the need to read the label of any OTC medication for administration instructions, precautions, contraindications, and so forth.

| NURSING ACTIONS | NASAL DECONGESTANTS, ANTITUSSIVES, AND COLD REMEDIES |

NURSING ACTIONS	*RATIONALE/EXPLANATION*
1. Administer accurately **a.** With topical nasal decongestants:	
(1) Use only preparations labeled for intranasal use.	Intranasal preparations are usually dilute, aqueous solutions prepared specifically for intranasal use. Some agents (*e.g.,* phenylephrine) are available in ophthalmic solutions as well. The two types of solutions *cannot* be used interchangeably.
(2) Use the drug concentration ordered.	Some drug preparations are available in several concentrations. For example, phenylephrine preparations may contain 0.125%, 0.25%, 0.5% or 1% of drug.
(3) For instillation of nose drops, have the client lie down or sit with the neck hyperextended. Instill medication without touching the dropper to the nares. Rinse the medication dropper after each use.	To avoid contamination of the dropper and medication.
(4) For nasal sprays, have the client sit, squeeze the container once to instill medication, avoid touching the spray tip to the nares, and rinse the spray tip after each use.	Most nasal sprays are designed to deliver one dose when used correctly. If necessary, secretions may be cleared and a second spray used. Correct usage and cleansing prevents contamination and infection.
(5) Give nasal decongestants to infants 20–30 min before feeding.	Nasal congestion interferes with an infant's ability to suck.
b. Administer cough syrups undiluted and instruct the client to avoid eating and drinking for about 30 min.	Part of the therapeutic benefit of cough syrups stems from soothing effects on pharyngeal mucosa. Food or fluid removes the medication from the pharynx.

NURSING ACTIONS	RATIONALE/EXPLANATION
c. Instruct clients to swallow benzonatate perles without chewing.	If perles are chewed, local anesthetic effects numb oral mucosa.
2. Observe for therapeutic effects **a.** When nasal decongestants are given, observe for decreased nasal obstruction and drainage.	Therapeutic effects depend on the reason for use.
b. With antitussives, observe for decreased coughing.	The goal of antitussive therapy is to suppress nonpurposeful coughing, not productive coughing.
c. With cold and allergy remedies, observe for decreased nasal congestion, rhinitis, muscle aches, and other symptoms.	
3. Observe for adverse effects **a.** With nasal decongestants, observe for	
(1) Tachycardia, cardiac arrhythmias, hypertension	These effects may occur with any of the adrenergic drugs (see Chap. 18). When adrenergic drugs are used as nasal decongestants, cardiovascular effects are more likely to occur with oral agents. However, topically applied drugs also may be systemically absorbed through the nasal mucosa or by being swallowed and absorbed through the gastrointestinal tract.
(2) Rebound nasal congestion, chronic rhinitis, and possible ulceration of nasal mucosa	Adverse effects on nasal mucosa are more likely to occur with excessive or long-term (more than 10 d) use.
b. With antitussives, observe for:	
(1) Excessive suppression of the cough reflex (inability to cough effectively when secretions are present)	This is a potentially serious adverse effect because retained secretions may lead to atelectasis, pneumonia, hypoxia, hypercarbia, and respiratory failure.
(2) Nausea, vomiting, constipation, dizziness, drowsiness, pruritus, and drug dependence	These are adverse effects associated with narcotic agents (see Chap. 6). When narcotics are given for antitussive effects, however, they are given in relatively small doses and are unlikely to cause adverse reactions.
(3) Nausea, drowsiness, and dizziness with non-narcotic antitussives	Adverse effects are infrequent and mild with these agents.
c. With combination products (*e.g.*, cold remedies), observe for adverse effects of individual ingredients (*i.e.*, antihistamines, adrenergics, analgesics, and others)	Adverse effects are rarely significant when the products are used as prescribed. There may be subtherapeutic doses of one or more component drugs, especially in over-the-counter formulations. Also, the drowsiness associated with antihistamines may be offset by stimulating effects of adrenergics. Ephedrine, for example, has central nervous system (CNS)–stimulating effects.
4. Observe for drug interactions **a.** Drugs that *increase* effects of nasal decongestants:	These interactions are more likely to occur with oral decongestants than topically applied drugs.
(1) Cocaine, digitalis, general anesthetics, MAO inhibitors, other adrenergic drugs, thyroid preparations, and xanthines	Increased risks of cardiac arrhythmias
(2) Antihistamines, epinephrine, ergot alkaloids, MAO inhibitors, methylphenidate	Increased risks of hypertension due to vasoconstriction

(continued)

NURSING ACTIONS	RATIONALE/EXPLANATION
b. Drugs that *increase* antitussive effects of codeine:	
CNS depressants (alcohol, antianxiety agents, barbiturates, and other sedative-hypnotics)	Additive CNS depression. Codeine is given in small doses for antitussive effects, and risks of significant interactions are minimal.
c. Drugs that alter effects of dextromethorphan:	
MAO inhibitors	This combination is contraindicated. Apnea, muscular rigidity, hyperpyrexia, laryngospasm, and death may occur.
d. Drugs that may alter effects of combination products for coughs, colds, and allergies:	Interactions depend on the individual drug components of each formulation. Risks of clinically significant drug interactions are increased with use of combination products.
(1) Adrenergic (sympathomimetic) agents (see Chap. 18)	
(2) Antihistamines (see Chap. 48)	
(3) CNS depressants (see Chaps. 6, 8, and 13)	
(4) CNS stimulants (see Chap. 16)	
5. Teach clients	
a. Do not use nose drops more often than recommended or for longer than 7 consecutive days.	Excessive or prolonged use may damage nasal mucosa and produce chronic nasal congestion.
b. Blow the nose gently before instilling nasal solutions or sprays.	To clear nasal passages and increase effectiveness of medications.
c. Do not touch the dropper tip to the nostrils when instilling nasal solutions.	To prevent contamination of the solution.
d. Rinse the dropper or spray tip after each use.	To prevent bacterial contamination of the medication.
e. Report palpitations, dizziness, drowsiness, rapid pulse.	These effects may occur with nasal decongestants and cold remedies and may indicate excessive dosage.

REVIEW AND APPLICATION EXERCISES

1. How do adrenergic drugs relieve nasal congestion?

2. Who should generally avoid OTC nasal decongestants and cold remedies?

3. What are advantages and disadvantages of multi-ingredient cold remedies?

4. What is usually the antitussive of choice?

5. When is an antitussive generally contraindicated or undesirable?

6. Given a client with a productive cough, what are nondrug interventions to promote removal of secretions?

SELECTED REFERENCES

Drug facts and comparisons. (Updated monthly). St. Louis: Facts and Comparisons.

Guyton, A.C. & J.E. (1996). *Textbook of medical physiology*, 9th ed. Philadelphia: W.B. Saunders.

Hendeles, L. (1993). Efficacy and safety of antihistamines and expectorants in nonprescription cough and cold preparations. *Pharmacotherapy, 13*(2), 154–158.

Porth, C.M. (1994). *Pathophysiology: Concepts of altered health states*, 4th ed. Philadelphia: J.B. Lippincott.

Drugs Affecting the Cardiovascular System

50 Physiology of the Cardiovascular System

Objectives

After studying this chapter, the student will be able to:

1 Review roles of the heart, blood vessels, and blood in supplying oxygen and nutrients to body tissues.

2 Discuss atherosclerosis as the basic disorder causing many cardiovascular disorders for which drug therapy is required.

3 List cardiovascular disorders for which drug therapy is a major treatment modality.

4 Identify general categories of drugs used to treat cardiovascular disorders.

Key Terms

Arterioles	**Myocardium**
Atria	**Perfusion**
Cardiac conduction system	**Ventricles**
Collateral circulation	

The cardiovascular or circulatory system is composed of the heart, blood vessels, and blood. The general functions of the system are to carry oxygen, nutrients, hormones, antibodies, and other substances to all body cells and to remove waste products of cell metabolism (CO_2 and others). The efficiency of the system depends on the heart's ability to pump blood, the patency of blood vessels, and the quality and quantity of blood.

Heart

The heart is a hollow, muscular organ that functions as a double pump to circulate 5 to 6 liters of blood through the body every minute.

1. The heart has four chambers: two atria and two ventricles. The *atria* are receiving chambers. The right atrium receives deoxygenated blood from the upper part of the body by way of the superior vena cava, from the lower part of the body by way of the inferior vena cava, and from veins and sinuses within the heart itself. The left atrium receives oxygenated blood from the lungs through the pulmonary veins. The *ventricles* are distributing chambers. The right ventricle sends deoxygenated blood through the pulmonary circulation. It is small and thin-walled because it contracts against minimal pressure. The left ventricle pumps oxygenated blood through the systemic circuit. It is much more muscular and thick-walled because it contracts against relatively high pressure. The right atrium and right ventricle form one pump, and the left atrium and left ventricle form another. The right and left sides of the heart are separated by a strip of muscle called the *septum*.

2. The layers of the heart are the endocardium, myocardium, and epicardium. The *endocardium* is the membrane lining the heart chambers. It is continuous with the lining of blood vessels entering and leaving the heart and covers the heart valves. The *myocardium* is the strong muscular layer of the heart that provides the pumping power of the circulation. The *epicardium* is the outer, serous layer of the heart. The heart is enclosed in a fibroserous sac called the *pericardium*.

3. Heart valves function to guide the one-way flow of blood and prevent backflow. The *mitral* valve separates the left atrium and left ventricle. The *tricuspid* valve separates the right atrium and right ventricle. The *pulmonic* valve separates the right ventricle and pulmonary artery. The *aortic* valve separates the left ventricle and aorta.

4. The heart contains special cells that can carry electrical impulses much more rapidly than ordinary muscle fibers. This special conduction system consists of the sinoatrial (SA) node, the atrioventricular node, bundle of His, right and left bundle branches, and Purkinje fibers. The SA node, the normal pacemaker of the heart, can be compared to a battery. It originates a burst of electrical energy about 70 to 80 times each minute under normal circumstances. The electrical current flows over the heart in an orderly way to produce contraction of both atria, then both ventricles.

   A unique characteristic of the heart is that each part can generate its own electrical impulse to contract. For example, the ventricles can beat independently but at a rate of only 30 to 40 beats per minute. In addition, the heart does not require nervous stimulation to contract. However, the autonomic nervous system does influence heart rate. Sympathetic nerves increase heart rate; parasympathetic nerves (by way of the vagus nerve) decrease heart rate.

5. The heart receives its blood supply from the coronary arteries. Coronary arteries branch off the aorta and fill during *diastole*, the resting or filling phase of the cardiac cycle. Coronary arteries branch into "end arteries," which supply certain parts of the myocardium without an overlapping supply from other branches. However, there are many artery-to-artery anastomoses between adjacent vessels. The anastomotic arteries do not supply sufficient blood to the heart if a major artery is suddenly occluded, but they may dilate into arteries of considerable size when disease (usually coronary atherosclerosis) develops slowly. The resultant *collateral circulation* may provide sufficient blood for myocardial function, at least during rest.

Blood Vessels

The three types of blood vessels are arteries, veins, and capillaries. Arteries and veins are similar in that they have three layers. The *intima* is the smooth inner lining of endothelium. The *media* is the middle layer of muscle and elastic tissue. The *adventitia* is the outer layer of connective tissue.

1. **Arteries** and *arterioles* have a thick media and control peripheral vascular resistance. They are sometimes called "resistance" vessels. Their efficiency depends on patency and ability to constrict or dilate in response to various stimuli. The degree of constriction or dilation (vasomotor tone) determines peripheral vascular resistance, which is a major determinant of blood pressure.

2. **Veins** have a thin media and valves that assist blood flow against gravity. They are sometimes called

"capacitance" vessels, because blood may accumulate in various parts of the venous system. Their efficiency depends on patency, competency of valves, and the pumping action of muscles around veins.

3. **Capillaries** are very thin-walled vessels. Exchange of gases, nutrients, and waste products occurs across capillary walls.

4. **Lymphatic vessels** parallel the veins and drain tissue fluids. They carry lymphocytes and large molecules of protein and fat. They empty into the venous system.

Blood

Blood generally functions to nourish and oxygenate all body cells, protect the body from invading microorganisms, and initiate hemostasis when a blood vessel is injured. Specific functions and components include the following:

1. Functions
   a. Transports oxygen to cells and carbon dioxide from cells to lungs for removal from the body
   b. Carries absorbed food products from the gastrointestinal tract to tissues; at the same time, it carries metabolic wastes from tissues to the kidneys, skin, and lungs for excretion
   c. Carries hormones from endocrine glands to other parts of the body
   d. Carries leukocytes and antibodies to sites of injury, infection, and inflammation
   e. Helps regulate body temperature by transferring heat produced by cell metabolism to the skin, where it can be released
   f. Carries platelets to injured areas for hemostasis
2. Components
   a. Plasma comprises about 55% of the total blood volume, and it is more than 90% water. Other ingredients are
      (1) Serum albumin, which helps maintain blood volume by exerting colloid osmotic pressure
      (2) Fibrinogen, which is necessary for hemostasis
      (3) Gamma globulin, which is necessary for defense against microorganisms
      (4) Less than 1% antibodies, nutrients, metabolic wastes, respiratory gases, enzymes, and inorganic salts
   b. Solid particles comprise about 45% of total blood volume. Solid particles are erythrocytes, also called red blood cells (RBCs); leukocytes, also called white blood cells (WBCs); and thrombocytes, also called platelets. The bone marrow produces all RBCs, 60% to 70% of WBCs, and all platelets. Lymphatic tissues (spleen and lymph nodes) produce 20% to 30% of the WBCs, and

reticuloendothelial tissues (spleen, liver, lymph nodes) produce 4% to 8% of WBCs. Characteristics of solid particles include the following:
   (1) Erythrocytes function mainly to transport oxygen. Almost all oxygen (95% to 97%) is transported in combination with hemoglobin; very little is dissolved in blood. The life span of a normal RBC is about 120 days.
   (2) Leukocytes function mainly as a defense mechanism against microorganisms. They leave the bloodstream to enter injured tissues and phagocytize the injurious agent. They also produce antibodies. The life span of a normal WBC is a few hours.
   (3) Platelets are fragments of large cells, called megakaryocytes, found in the red bone marrow. Platelets are essential to blood coagulation.

Drug Therapy in Cardiovascular Disorders

Cardiovascular disorders are leading causes of morbidity and mortality. They may involve any structure or function of the cardiovascular system. Generally, a disorder in one part of the system eventually disturbs the function of all other parts. Cardiovascular disorders usually treated with drug therapy include atherosclerosis, congestive heart failure, cardiac arrhythmias, angina pectoris, hypertension, hypotension, and shock. Peripheral vascular disease and valvular disease are usually treated surgically. Blood disorders that respond to drug therapy include certain types of anemia and coagulation disorders.

Cardiovascular drugs may be given to increase or decrease cardiac output, blood pressure, and heart rate; to alter heart rhythm; increase or decrease blood clotting; alter the quality of blood; and decrease chest pain of cardiac origin. Cardiovascular drugs are often given for palliation of symptoms. For example, in angina pectoris, hypertension, and congestive heart failure, the drugs relieve symptoms but do not alter the underlying disease process.

 REVIEW AND APPLICATION EXERCISES

1. How does the heart muscle differ from skeletal muscle?

2. What is the normal pacemaker of the heart?

3. In what circumstances do other parts of the heart take over as pacemaker?

4. What is the effect of parasympathetic (vagal) stimulation on the heart?

5. What is the effect of sympathetic stimulation on the heart and blood vessels?

6. How does low or high blood volume influence blood pressure?

SELECTED REFERENCES

Guyton, A.C. & Hall, J.E. (1996). *Textbook of medical physiology*, 9th ed. Philadelphia: W.B. Saunders.

Porth, C.M. (1994). *Pathophysiology: Concepts of altered health states*, 4th ed. Philadelphia: J.B. Lippincott.

Smeltzer, S.C. & Bare, B.G. (1996). *Brunner and Suddarth's Textbook of medical-surgical nursing*, 8th ed. Philadelphia: Lippincott-Raven.

Cardiotonic-Inotropic Agents Used in Congestive Heart Failure

51

Outline

Objectives

After studying this chapter, the student will be able to:

1 Describe major manifestations of congestive heart failure (CHF).

2 List characteristics of digoxin in terms of effects on myocardial contractility and cardiac conduction, indications for use, principles of therapy, and nursing process implications.

3 Differentiate therapeutic effects of digoxin in CHF and atrial filbrillation.

4 Differentiate digitalizing and maintenance doses of digoxin.

5 Identify subtherapeutic, therapeutic, and excessive serum digoxin levels.

6 Identify clients at risk of developing digoxin toxicity.

7 Discuss interventions to prevent or minimize digoxin toxicity.

8 Explain the roles of potassium chloride, lidocaine, atropine, and digoxin immune fab in the treatment of digoxin toxicity.

9 Teach clients ways to increase safety and effectiveness of digoxin.

10 Discuss important elements of using digoxin in children and older adults.

Key Terms

Arrhythmia	**Cardiotonic**
Atrial fibrillation	**Compensatory mechanisms**
Bradycardia	
Cardiac output	**Inotropic**

Cardiotonic-inotropic agents increase the force of myocardial contraction and thereby improve the heart's pumping ability. Drugs with cardiotonic-inotropic effects include adrenergics, digitalis preparations (*e.g.*, digoxin), amrinone, and milrinone. Adrenergics (*e.g.*, epinephrine) also increase cardiac workload and oxygen consumption (see Chap. 18). Digitalis preparations, amrinone, and milrinone are the focus of this chapter. A major clinical use of these agents is the treatment of congestive heart failure (CHF); digitalis is also used to treat atrial tachyarrhythmias.

Congestive Heart Failure

CHF is a common condition that occurs when the heart cannot pump enough blood to meet tissue needs for oxygen and nutrients. Most CHF in adults is caused by myocardial ischemia or hypertension. Other causative factors include hyperthyroidism, excessive intravenous (IV) fluids or blood transfusions, and drugs that decrease the force of myocardial contraction (*e.g.*, beta-adrenergic blocking agents) or cause retention of sodium and water (*e.g.*, corticosteroids, estrogens, nonsteroidal anti-inflammatory agents). These factors impair the pumping ability or increase the workload of the heart so an adequate cardiac output cannot be maintained.

When cardiac output falls, compensatory mechanisms help the body maintain blood flow to tissues. One mechanism is increased sympathetic activity, which increases the force of myocardial contraction, increases heart rate, and causes vasoconstriction. Another mechanism involves increased volume of blood and increased pressure within the heart chambers, which stretches muscle fibers and results in ventricular hypertrophy. A third mechanism is activation of the renin-angiotensin-aldosterone system. Renin is an enzyme produced in the kidney in response to impaired blood flow and tissue perfusion. When released into the bloodstream, it stimulates the production of angiotensin II, a powerful vasoconstrictor. The adrenal cortex is also stimulated to increase production of aldosterone, and aldosterone increases reabsorption of sodium and water in renal tubules.

As a result of these compensatory mechanisms, preload (amount of venous blood returning to the heart), workload of the heart, and afterload (amount of resistance in the aorta and peripheral blood vessels that the heart must overcome to pump effectively) are increased. All of these mechanisms act to increase blood pressure. Although initially effective, the compensatory mechanisms increase the workload of the heart, and they are limited in extent and duration of action. Eventually, signs and symptoms of CHF occur when, despite these compensatory mechanisms, an adequate cardiac output can no longer be maintained, and failure or decompensation occurs.

DRUG THERAPY

Drug therapy for CHF is aimed toward improving circulation and altering the compensatory mechanisms. In addition to cardiotonic-inotropic agents, diuretics, vasodilators, and angiotensin-converting enzyme (ACE) inhibitors are used.

1. **Diuretics** are often used in the treatment of CHF. They act to decrease plasma volume (extracellular fluid volume) and increase excretion of sodium and water, thereby decreasing preload. IV furosemide (Lasix) also has a vasodilatory effect that helps relieve vasoconstriction (afterload) in acute CHF (pulmonary edema). With early or mild CHF, a thiazide or related diuretic may be used. With moderate to severe chronic CHF, oral furosemide is usually the diuretic of first choice. Diuretics are discussed in greater detail in Chapter 56.
2. **Angiotensin-converting enzyme (ACE) inhibitors** have become drugs of first choice in treating chronic CHF because they improve cardiac function and decrease mortality. These drugs (*e.g.*, captopril, others) prevent inactive angiotensin I from being converted to angiotensin II. Angiotensin II produces vasoconstriction and retention of sodium and water; inhibition of angiotensin II decreases vasoconstriction and retention of sodium and water. Thus, a major effect of the drugs is dilation of both veins and arteries, decreased preload and afterload, and decreased workload of the heart. In addition, the drugs seem to delay further impairment of myocardial function and progression of CHF.
3. Other **vasodilators** also are frequently used, often with diuretics and digitalis glycosides. Venous dilators (*e.g.*, nitrates) decrease preload; arterial dilators (*e.g.*, hydralazine) decrease afterload. Isosorbide dinitrate and hydralazine may be combined to decrease both preload and afterload. Nitrates are discussed in Chapter 53; hydralazine is discussed in Chapter 55.

Digitalis Preparations

Digoxin (Lanoxin) and **digitoxin** (Crystodigin) are classified as digitalis glycosides and have the same pharmacologic actions (*i.e.*, therapeutic and adverse effects). Digoxin is used much more often and is the one emphasized here. In addition, the terms *digitalis, digitalization,* and *digitalis toxicity* refer mainly to digoxin in the following discussion.

General Characteristics

When digoxin is given orally, absorption varies among available preparations. Lanoxicaps, which are liquid-filled capsules, and the elixir used for children are better absorbed than tablets. With tablets, the most frequently used formulation, differences in bioavailability may become clinically important, because a person who is stabilized on one formulation may be under-dosed or overdosed if another formulation is taken. Differences are attributed to the rate and extent of tablet dissolution rather than amounts of digoxin. In addition to drug dosage forms, other factors that may decrease digoxin absorption include the presence of food in the gastrointestinal (GI) tract, delayed gastric emptying, malabsorption syndromes, and concurrent administration of some drugs (*e.g.,* antacids, cholestyramine, colestipol).

Digoxin is distributed to most body tissues, and high concentrations are found in the myocardium, brain, liver, and skeletal muscle. It also crosses the placenta, and serum levels in newly delivered neonates are similar to those in the mother. It circulates mainly in a free state, with only 20% to 30% bound to serum proteins. Therapeutic serum levels of digoxin are 0.5 to 2 ng/ml; toxic serum levels are above 2 ng/ml. However, toxicity may occur at virtually any serum level.

Most (60% to 70%) of digoxin is excreted unchanged by the kidneys. Dosage must be reduced in the presence of renal failure to prevent drug accumulation and toxicity. The remainder is metabolized or excreted by nonrenal routes.

Mechanisms of Action

In CHF, digoxin exerts a cardiotonic or positive inotropic effect. Increased myocardial contractility allows the ventricles to empty more completely with each heartbeat. With improved cardiac output, heart size, heart rate, end-systolic and end-diastolic pressures, vasoconstriction, sympathetic nerve stimulation, and venous congestion decrease. The mechanism by which digoxin increases the force of myocardial contraction is thought to be inhibition of Na,K-ATPase, an enzyme in cardiac cell membranes that decreases the movement of sodium out of myocardial cells after contraction. As a result, calcium enters the cell in exchange for sodium and causes additional calcium to be released from intracellular binding sites. With the increased intracellular concentration of free calcium ions, more calcium is available to activate the contractile proteins actin and myosin, and increase myocardial contractility.

In atrial arrhythmias, digitalis slows the rate of ventricular contraction (negative chronotropic effect). Negative chronotropic effects are probably caused by several factors. First, digitalis has a direct depressant effect on cardiac conduction tissues, especially the atrioventricular node. This action decreases the number of electrical impulses allowed to reach the ventricles from supraventricular sources. Second, digitalis indirectly stimulates the vagus nerve. Third, increased efficiency of myocardial contraction and vagal stimulation decrease compensatory tachycardia resulting from the sympathetic nervous system response to inadequate circulation.

Indications for Use

The clinical uses of digitalis are treatment of CHF and atrial tachyarrhythmias (atrial fibrillation, atrial flutter, paroxysmal atrial tachycardia). Digoxin may be used in acute or chronic conditions, for digitalization, or for maintenance therapy; digitoxin is used only for maintenance therapy.

Contraindications for Use

Digitalis glycosides are contraindicated in severe myocarditis, ventricular tachycardia, or ventricular fibrillation and must be used cautiously in clients with acute myocardial infarction, heart block, Adams-Stokes syndrome, Wolff-Parkinson-White syndrome (risk of fatal arrhythmias), electrolyte imbalances (hypokalemia, hypomagnesemia, hypercalcemia), and renal impairment.

Administration and Digitalization

Digoxin is usually given orally or IV. Although it can be given intramuscularly, this route is not recommended because pain and muscle necrosis may occur at injection sites. When given orally, onset of action occurs in 30 minutes to 2 hours, and peak effects occur in about 6 hours. When given IV, the onset of action occurs within 10 to 30 minutes, and maximal effects occur in 1 to 5 hours.

In the heart, maximum drug effect occurs when a steady-state tissue concentration has been achieved. This occurs in about 1 week (five half-lives) unless loading doses are given for more rapid effects. Traditionally, a loading dose is called a digitalizing dose. Digitalization (administration of an amount sufficient to produce therapeutic effects) may be accomplished rapidly by giving about 0.75 to 1 mg of digoxin in divided doses 6 to 8 hours apart over a 24-hour period. Because rapid digitalization engenders higher risks of toxicity, it is usually done for atrial tachyarrhythmias rather than for CHF. Slow digitalization may be accomplished by initiating therapy with a maintenance dose of digoxin. When digoxin is discontinued, the drug is eliminated from the body in about 1 week.

Routes and Dosage Ranges

Adults and children >10 years: Digitalizing dose, PO 0.75–1 mg in three or four divided doses over 24 h; IV 0.5–0.75 mg in divided doses over 24 h
Maintenance dose, PO, IV 0.125–0.5 mg/d (average, 0.25)

Children 2–10 years: Digitalizing dose, PO 0.02–0.04 mg/kg in four divided doses q6h; IV 0.015–0.035 mg/kg in four divided doses q6h
Maintenance dose, PO, IV about 20%–35% of the digitalizing dose

Children 1 month–2 years: Digitalizing dose, PO 0.035–0.06 mg/kg in four divided doses q6h; IV 0.035–0.05 mg/kg in four divided doses q6h
Maintenance dose, PO, IV about 20%–35% of the digitalizing dose

Newborns: Digitalizing dose, PO 0.025–0.035 mg/kg in four divided doses q6h; IV 0.02–0.03 mg/kg in four divided doses q6h
Maintenance dose, PO, IV about 20%–35% of the digitalizing dose

DIGOXIN TOXICITY

Digoxin has a low therapeutic index (*i.e.*, a dose adequate for therapeutic effect may be accompanied by signs of toxicity). Digoxin toxicity may result from many contributing factors:

1. Accumulation of larger than necessary maintenance doses
2. Rapid loading or digitalization, whether by one or more large doses or frequent administration of small doses
3. Impaired renal function, which delays excretion of digoxin
4. Age extremes (young or old)
5. Electrolyte imbalance (*e.g.*, hypokalemia, hypomagnesemia, hypercalcemia)
6. Hypoxia, whether resulting from heart or lung disease, which increases myocardial sensitivity to digoxin
7. Hypothyroidism, which slows digoxin metabolism and may cause accumulation
8. Concurrent treatment with other drugs affecting the heart, such as quinidine, verapamil, or nifedipine

Digitoxin (Crystodigin) is rarely used. In comparison to digoxin, digitoxin has a slower onset of action; a longer half-life (about 7 days); and is 90% to 95% protein bound. With the long half-life, it takes about 1 month to reach therapeutic serum levels, unless loading doses are given, and about 1 month for elimination from the body after stopping drug administration. Thus, digitoxin is used for maintenance therapy rather than rapid digitalization.

Digitoxin is metabolized in the liver, excreted in bile, reabsorbed from the GI tract, and eventually excreted in the urine as inactive metabolites. For this reason, digitoxin may be used in clients with renal failure. In most instances, however, digoxin is used in reduced dosages.

Route and Dosage Range

Adults and children >12 years: PO 0.1–0.2 mg daily

AMRINONE AND MILRINONE

Amrinone (Inocor) and **milrinone IV** (Primacor) are cardiotonic-inotropic agents used in short-term management of severe CHF that is not controlled by digoxin, diuretics, and vasodilators. The drugs increase levels of cyclic adenosine monophosphate (cAMP) in myocardial cells by inhibiting phosphodiesterase, the enzyme that normally metabolizes cAMP. They also relax vascular smooth muscle to produce vasodilation and decrease preload and afterload. In CHF, inotropic and vasodilator effects increase cardiac output. Compared to amrinone, milrinone is reportedly more potent as an inotropic agent and causes fewer adverse effects. A high incidence of serious adverse effects was observed with oral preparations of both drugs. Consequently, both drugs are given IV. The dosage of milrinone should be reduced in the presence of renal impairment.

Amrinone
Route and Dosage Ranges

Adults: IV injection (loading dose), 0.75 mg/kg slowly, over 2–3 min
IV infusion (maintenance dose), 5–10 µg/kg/min, diluted in 0.9% or 0.45% NaCl solution to a concentration of 1–3 mg/ml; maximum dosage, 10 mg/kg/d

Milrinone
Route and Dosage Ranges

Adults: IV bolus infusion (loading dose), 50 µg/kg over 10 min
IV continuous infusion (maintenance dose), 0.375–0.75 µg/kg/min, diluted in 0.9% or 0.45% NaCl solution or 5% dextrose injection

Nursing Process

Assessment

Assess clients for current or potential CHF:
● Identify risk factors for CHF:
  ● **Cardiovascular disorders:** atherosclerosis, hypertension, coronary artery disease, myocardial infarction, cardiac arrhythmias, cardiac valvular disease. Myocardial ischemia and hypertension are frequent causes of CHF.
  ● **Noncardiovascular disorders:** severe infections, hyperthyroidism, pulmonary disease (*e.g.*, cor pulmonale—right-sided heart failure resulting from lung disease)

- **Other factors:** excessive amounts of IV fluids, rapid infusion of IV fluids or blood transfusions, advanced age
- A **combination** of any of the above factors
- Interview and observe for signs and symptoms of chronic CHF. Within the clinical syndrome of CHF, clinical manifestations vary from few and mild to many and severe, depending on the heart's pumping ability. Specific signs and symptoms include the following:
  - **Mild CHF.** Common signs and symptoms of mild CHF are ankle edema, dyspnea on exertion, and easy fatigue with exercise. Edema results from increased venous pressure, which allows fluids to leak into tissues; dyspnea and fatigue result from tissue hypoxia.
  - **Moderate or severe CHF.** More extensive edema, dyspnea, and fatigue at rest are likely to occur. Additional signs and symptoms include orthopnea, postnocturnal dyspnea, and cough (from congestion of the respiratory tract with venous blood); mental confusion (from cerebral hypoxia); oliguria and decreased renal function (from decreased blood flow to the kidneys); and anxiety.
- Observe for signs and symptoms of acute heart failure. Acute pulmonary edema indicates acute heart failure and is a medical emergency. Causes include acute myocardial infarction, cardiac arrhythmias, severe hypertension, acute fluid or salt overload, and certain drugs (*e.g.,* quinidine and other cardiac depressants, propranolol and other antiadrenergics, and phenylephrine, norepinephrine, and other alpha-adrenergic stimulants). Pulmonary edema occurs when left ventricular failure causes blood to accumulate in pulmonary veins and tissues. As a result, the person experiences severe dyspnea, hypoxia, hypertension, tachycardia, hemoptysis, frothy respiratory tract secretions, and anxiety.

  Assess clients for signs and symptoms of atrial tachyarrhythmias:
- Record the rate and rhythm of apical and radial pulses. Atrial fibrillation, the most common atrial arrhythmia, is characterized by tachycardia, pulse deficit (faster apical rate than radial rate), and a very irregular rhythm. Fatigue, dizziness, and fainting may occur.
- Check the electrocardiogram (ECG) for abnormal P waves, rapid rate of ventricular contraction, and QRS complexes of normal configuration but irregular intervals.

  Assess baseline vital signs; weight; edema; laboratory reports of potassium, magnesium, and calcium levels; and other tests of cardiovascular function when available.

  Assess a baseline ECG before digoxin therapy when possible. If a client is in normal sinus rhythm, later ECGs may aid recognition of digitalis toxicity (*i.e.,* drug-induced arrhythmias). If a client has an atrial tachyarrhythmia and is receiving digoxin to slow the ventricular rate, later ECGs may aid recognition of therapeutic and adverse effects. For clients who are already receiving digoxin at the initial contact, a baseline ECG can still be valuable because changes in later ECGs may promote earlier recognition and treatment of drug-induced arrhythmias.

Nursing Diagnoses

- Altered Tissue Perfusion related to decreased cardiac output
- Activity Intolerance related to decreased cardiac output
- Self-Care Deficit related to dyspnea and fatigue
- Anxiety related to chronic illness and lifestyle changes

- Impaired Gas Exchange related to venous congestion and fluid accumulation in lungs
- Decreased Cardiac Output related to drug-induced arrhythmias
- Sensory/Perceptual Alterations related to drug-induced changes in vision
- Altered Nutrition: Less Than Body Requirements related to digoxin-induced anorexia, nausea, and vomiting
- Noncompliance related to the need for long-term drug therapy and regular medical supervision
- Knowledge Deficit: Managing drug therapy regimen safely and effectively

Planning/Goals

The client will:
- Take drugs safely and accurately
- Experience improved breathing and less fatigue and edema
- Maintain serum digoxin levels within therapeutic ranges
- Be closely monitored for therapeutic and adverse effects, especially during digitalization, when dosage is being changed, and when other drugs are added to or removed from the treatment regimen
- Keep appointments for follow-up monitoring of vital signs, serum potassium levels, serum digoxin levels, and renal function

Interventions

Use measures to prevent or minimize CHF and atrial arrhythmias. In the broadest sense, preventive measures include sensible eating habits (a balanced diet, avoiding excess saturated fat and salt, weight control), avoiding cigarette smoking, and regular exercise. In the client at risk for developing CHF and arrhythmias, preventive measures include the following:
- Treatment of hypertension
- Avoidance of hypoxia
- Weight control
- Avoidance of excess sodium in the diet
- Avoidance of fluid overload, especially in elderly clients
- Maintenance of treatment programs for CHF, atrial arrhythmias, and other cardiovascular or noncardiovascular disorders

  Monitor vital signs, weight, urine output, and serum potassium regularly, and compare with baseline values.

  Monitor ECG when available, and compare with baseline or previous tracings.

 Teach clients:
- The importance of taking digoxin as prescribed. *Do not* miss a dose. *Do not* take an extra dose. *Do not* take other prescription or nonprescription drugs without consulting the physician who prescribed digoxin. All these precautions are necessary to increase the drug's safety and effectiveness. The drug must be taken regularly to maintain therapeutic blood levels, but overuse may cause serious adverse effects. Also, several drugs interact with digoxin to increase or decrease its effects.
- That when taking a diuretic and a potassium supplement with digoxin, the drugs should not be altered (*i.e.,* in dosage or frequency of administration) or discontinued without con-

sulting the physician. The balance among these drugs must be maintained for safety. If the diuretic is continued and the potassium stopped, hypokalemia may occur and precipitate cardiac arrhythmias. If the diuretic is stopped, edema is likely to recur or worsen. If the diuretic is stopped but the potassium is continued, hyperkalemia may occur.
- That important adverse drug effects should be reported to the physician or nurse, such as undesirable changes in heart rate or rhythm, GI upset, or visual problems.
- *Not* to use salt substitutes without consulting a health care provider. Salt substitutes contain potassium, which may be contraindicated, especially if a potassium supplement is being taken. Excessive potassium is cardiotoxic.

Evaluation

- Interview and observe for relief of symptoms (weight loss, increased urine output, less extremity edema, easier breathing, improved activity tolerance and self-care ability, slower heart rate).
- Observe serum drug levels for normal or abnormal values, when available.
- Interview regarding compliance with instructions for taking the drug.
- Interview and observe for adverse drug effects, especially cardiac arrhythmias.

Principles of Therapy

TREATMENT OF CONGESTIVE HEART FAILURE

The main treatment measures for CHF consist of drug therapy and diet therapy.

1. **Drug therapy** for CHF is controversial in relation to choice of drug and duration of administration. Until recent years, a digitalis preparation and a diuretic were considered the best treatment. Now, however, previous practices are being challenged, and opinions differ about the role of digitalis and other drugs. Factors influencing the viewpoints include the high incidence of adverse drug effects, greater understanding of the basic pathophysiology of CHF, and the development of new drugs or new uses for older drugs. More specifically:
   a. Some authorities recommend monotherapy with either digitalis or a diuretic, or a combination of the two, for initial treatment. Other drugs are added only if signs and symptoms persist or recur despite treatment.
   b. Some authorities suggest that digitalis is indicated when CHF is accompanied by atrial tachyarrhythmias (to slow ventricular response and decrease the workload of the heart), but it may not be needed with normal sinus rhythm. These physicians may use a diuretic as the initial drug of choice, with digitalis as a second or a third choice, after a vasodilator.

   c. For both groups, vasodilators have become the standard of care.
   d. ACE inhibitors are being increasingly used as monotherapy or as part of a multidrug regimen with digitalis, a diuretic, or both. All three types of drugs may be indicated for severe CHF. ACE inhibitors prevent formation of angiotensin II, a strong vasoconstrictor and stimulator of aldosterone release. Beneficial effects of ACE inhibitors stem mainly from the vasodilation and decreased retention of sodium and water that result from decreased formation of angiotensin II. In addition, studies indicate improved survival rates and relief of symptoms in clients with CHF.
   e. Another challenge to traditional therapy is whether digitalis should be continued throughout the client's life or whether it can be safely stopped. Some studies indicate that digitalis can be discontinued in some clients without recurrence of heart failure, but no clear-cut criteria exist for selecting these clients.
   f. Amrinone and milrinone are indicated only for short-term treatment of CHF that does not respond to other measures.
2. **Diet therapy.** Dietary sodium restriction may reduce edema and allow a decrease in dosage of diuretics. For most clients, sodium restriction need not be severe. A common order, "no added salt," may be accomplished by avoiding obviously salty food (*e.g.,* ham, potato chips, snack foods) and by not adding salt during cooking or eating. A major source of sodium intake is table salt: A level teaspoonful contains 2300 mg of sodium.

GUIDELINES FOR DIGITALIS THERAPY

1. **Choice of digitalis preparation** and route of administration depend primarily on the client's condition and the rapidity with which therapeutic effects are desired.
   a. Digoxin is the drug of choice in most situations because it can be used for rapid or slow digitalization, and if toxicity occurs, the drug leaves the body within a few days. It is the most commonly used digitalis preparation for adults and children.
   b. Digitoxin may be used in clients with renal disease, because it is excreted primarily by the liver rather than by the kidneys.
   c. Preferred routes of digitalis administration are oral and IV. The intramuscular route is not recommended because pain and muscle necrosis may occur at intramuscular injection sites.
2. **Dosage of digitalis preparations** must be individualized.
   a. Digitalis dosages are usually stated as the average amounts needed for digitalization and mainte-

nance therapy. These dosages must be interpreted with consideration of specific client characteristics. Digitalizing or loading doses are safe *only* for a short period, usually 24 hours. In addition, loading doses should be used cautiously in clients who have taken a digitalis preparation within the previous 2 or 3 weeks. Maintenance doses, which are much smaller than digitalizing doses, may be safely used to initiate digitalis therapy and are always used for long-term digitalis therapy.

b. Generally, larger doses are needed to slow the heart rate in atrial tachyarrhythmias than to increase myocardial contractility in CHF. Larger doses may also be needed to reach therapeutic serum levels of digoxin in a small group of patients (about 10%) who have digoxin-metabolizing bacteria in their colons. Members of this group are at risk of developing digoxin toxicity if they are given antibacterial drugs that destroy colonic bacteria.

c. Smaller doses (loading and maintenance) should be given to clients who are elderly or who have hypothyroidism. Because metabolism and excretion of digitalis preparations are delayed in such people, the drugs may accumulate and cause toxicity if dosage is not reduced. Dosage also should be reduced in clients with hypokalemia, extensive myocardial damage, or cardiac conduction disorders. These conditions increase risks of digitalis-induced arrhythmias.

d. Dosage can be titrated according to client response. In CHF, severity of symptoms, ECG, and serum drug concentrations are useful. In atrial fibrillation, dosage can be altered to produce the desired decrease in the ventricular rate of contraction. Optimal dosage is the lowest amount that relieves signs and symptoms of heart failure or alters heart rate and rhythm toward normal without producing toxicity.

e. IV dosage of digoxin should be 20% to 30% less than oral dosage.

f. Dosage of digoxin must be reduced by about half in the presence of renal failure or when certain drugs are given concurrently.

(1) With renal failure, digoxin dosage should be based on signs and symptoms of toxicity, creatinine clearance, and serum drug levels. Because most digoxin is excreted renally, failure to reduce dosage in clients with renal failure leads to drug accumulation in the body, with resultant toxicity.

(2) When given concurrently with digoxin, quinidine, nifedipine (Procardia), and verapamil (Calan) slow digoxin excretion and increase serum digoxin levels. As a result, digoxin may accumulate and cause toxicity.

3. **Maintenance therapy in the hospitalized client** must be individualized. Hospitalized clients may be unable to take a daily maintenance dose of digitalis at the scheduled time owing to diagnostic tests, treatment measures, or other reasons. As a general rule, the dose should be given later rather than omitted. If the client is having surgery, the nurse often must ask the physician whether the drug should be given on the day of surgery (*i.e.,* orally with a small amount of water or parenterally) and whether the drug should be reordered postoperatively. Many clients require continued digitalis therapy. However, if a dose is missed, probably no ill effects will occur, because the pharmacologic actions of both digoxin and digitoxin persist longer than 24 hours.

4. **Electrolyte balance** must be monitored and maintained during digitalis therapy, particularly normal serum levels of potassium (3.5 to 5 mEq/L), magnesium (1.5 to 2.5 mg/100 ml), and calcium (8.5 to 10 mg/100 ml). Hypokalemia and hypomagnesemia increase cardiac excitability and ectopic pacemaker activity, leading to arrhythmias; hypercalcemia enhances digitalis effects. These electrolyte abnormalities increase the risk of digitalis toxicity. Hypocalcemia increases excitability of nerve and muscle cell membranes and causes myocardial contraction to be weak (leading to a decrease in digitalis effect).

The most common electrolyte abnormality is hypokalemia because potassium-losing diuretics are often given concurrently with digitalis preparations in the treatment of CHF. Supplemental potassium may be given to maintain normal serum levels.

RECOGNITION AND TREATMENT OF DIGITALIS TOXICITY

Recognition of digitalis toxicity may be difficult because of nonspecific early manifestations (*e.g.,* anorexia, nausea, confusion) and the similarity between the signs and symptoms of heart disease for which digitalis is given and the signs and symptoms of digitalis intoxication. Continued atrial fibrillation with a rapid ventricular response may indicate inadequate dosage. However, other arrhythmias may indicate toxicity. Premature ventricular contractions commonly occur. Serum drug levels and ECG may be helpful in verifying suspected toxicity. Serum digoxin levels should be drawn just before a dose. Drug distribution to tissues requires about 6 hours after a dose is given; if the blood is drawn before 6 hours, the level may be high.

When signs and symptoms of digitalis toxicity occur, treatment may include any or all of the following interventions, depending on the client's condition.

1. Digitalis should be discontinued, not just reduced in dosage. Most clients with mild or early toxicity

recover completely within a few days after the drug is stopped.

2. If serious cardiac arrhythmias are present, several drugs may be used, including

   a. **Potassium chloride,** a myocardial depressant that acts to decrease myocardial excitability. The dose depends on the severity of toxicity, serum potassium level, and client response. Potassium is contraindicated in renal failure and should be used with caution in the presence of cardiac conduction defects.

   b. **Lidocaine,** an antiarrhythmic local anesthetic agent commonly used in the treatment of digitalis-induced arrhythmias. It acts to decrease myocardial irritability.

   c. **Atropine or isoproterenol,** used in the treatment of bradycardia or conduction defects

   d. **Other antiarrhythmic drugs.** These may be used but are generally less effective in digitalis-induced arrhythmias than in arrhythmias due to other causes.

   e. **Digoxin immune fab** (Digibind, Digidote). This is a digoxin-binding antidote derived from anti-digoxin antibodies produced in sheep. It is recommended only for serious toxicity. It combines with digoxin and pulls digoxin out of tissues and into the bloodstream. Note that serum digoxin levels will be high, but the drug is bound to the antibody and therefore inactive. Digoxin immune fab is given IV, as a bolus injection if the patient is in danger of immediate cardiac arrest but preferably over 15 to 30 minutes. Dosage varies and is calculated according to the amount of digoxin ingested (see manufacturers' instructions). The antidote has also been used for digitoxin toxicity.

Use in Children

Digoxin is commonly used in children for the same indications as for adults. The response to a given dose varies with age, size, and renal and hepatic function. There may be little difference between a therapeutic dose and a toxic dose. Very small amounts are often given to children. These factors increase the risks of dosage errors in children, and each dose should be verified with another nurse before it is administered. ECG monitoring is desirable when digoxin therapy is started.

As in adults, dosage of digoxin should be individualized and carefully titrated. Digoxin is primarily excreted by the kidneys, and dosage must be reduced with impaired renal function. Divided daily doses should be given to infants and children under 10 years,

and adult dosages adjusted to their weight should be given to children older than 10. Larger doses are usually needed to slow a too-rapid ventricular rate in children with atrial fibrillation or flutter. Differences in bioavailability of different preparations (parenterals, capsules, elixirs, and tablets) must be considered when switching from one preparation to another.

Neonates vary in tolerance of digoxin, depending on their degree of maturity. Premature infants are especially sensitive to drug effects. Dosage must be reduced, and digitalization should be even more individualized and cautiously approached than in more mature infants and children. Early signs of toxicity in newborns are undue slowing of sinus rate, sinoatrial arrest, and prolongation of the PR interval.

Use in Older Adults

Digoxin is widely used and a frequent cause of adverse effects in older adults. The usual recommended dose is 0.125 to 0.25 mg daily. Reduced dosages are usually required because of decreased liver or kidney function, decreased lean body weight, and advanced cardiac disease. All of these characteristics are common in older adults. Impaired renal function leads to slower drug excretion and increased risk of accumulation, so smaller doses are needed. Dosage must be reduced by about 50% with renal failure or concurrent administration of quinidine, nifedipine, or verapamil. These drugs increase serum digoxin levels and increase risks of toxicity if dosage is not reduced. Antacids decrease absorption of oral digoxin and should not be given at the same time.

A client's need for digoxin should be reevaluated periodically. Dosage needs may change, or the drug may no longer be needed.

Digitoxin, which is excreted by the liver, is rarely used but may be preferred if renal function is impaired.

Home Care

Most digoxin is taken at home and the home care nurse shares responsibility for teaching clients how to use the drug effectively and circumstances to be reported to a health care provider. Accurate dosing is vitally important because underuse may cause recurrence of symptoms and overuse may cause toxicity. Either condition may be life-threatening and require emergency care. The home care nurse also needs to monitor clients' responses to the drug and changes in conditions or drug therapy that increase risks of toxicity.

CARDIOTONIC-INOTROPIC DRUGS

NURSING ACTIONS	*RATIONALE/EXPLANATION*
1. Administer accurately **a.** With digoxin	
(1) Read the drug label and the physician's order carefully when preparing a dose.	For accurate administration
(2) Give only the ordered dosage form (*e.g.*, tablet, Lanoxicap, or elixir).	Digoxin formulations vary in concentration and bioavailability and *cannot* be used interchangeably.
(3) Check the apical pulse before each dose. If the rate is below 60 in adults or 100 in children, omit the dose, and notify the physician.	Bradycardia is an adverse effect.
(4) Have the same nurse give digoxin to the same clients when possible because it is important to detect *changes* in rate and rhythm (see *Observe for therapeutic effects* and *Observe for adverse effects*, below).	
(5) Give oral digoxin with food or after meals.	This may minimize gastric irritation and symptoms of anorexia, nausea, and vomiting. However, these symptoms probably arise from drug stimulation of chemoreceptors in the medulla rather than a direct irritant effect of the drug on the gastrointestinal (GI) tract.
(6) Inject IV digoxin slowly (over at least 5 min).	Digoxin should be given slowly because the diluent, propylene glycol, has toxic effects on the cardiac conduction system if given too rapidly. Digoxin may be given undiluted or diluted with a fourfold or greater volume of sterile water for injection, 0.9% sodium chloride injection, or 5% dextrose injection. If diluted, use the solution immediately.
b. With amrinone:	
(1) Give undiluted or diluted to a concentration of 1 mg/ml to 3 mg/ml.	
(2) Dilute with 0.9% or 0.45% sodium chloride solution, and use the diluted solution within 24 h. Do not dilute with solutions containing dextrose.	Amrinone may be injected into IV tubing containing a dextrose solution because contact is brief. However, a chemical interaction occurs with prolonged contact.
(3) Give bolus injections into the tubing of an IV infusion, over 2 to 3 min.	
(4) Administer maintenance infusions at a rate of 5 to 10 μg/kg/min.	
c. With milrinone	
(1) Dilute with 0.9% or 0.45% sodium chloride or 5% dextrose solution.	Manufacturer's recommendations
(2) Give the loading dose by bolus infusion over 10 min.	
(3) Give maintenance infusions at a standard rate of 0.5 μg/kg/min; this rate may be increased or decreased according to response.	

(continued)

NURSING ACTIONS	RATIONALE/EXPLANATION
2. Observe for therapeutic effects **a.** When the drugs are given in congestive heart failure (CHF), observe for:	
(1) Fewer signs and symptoms of pulmonary congestion (dyspnea, orthopnea, cyanosis, cough, hemoptysis, rales, anxiety, restlessness)	The pulmonary symptoms that develop with CHF are a direct result of events initiated by inadequate cardiac output. The left side of the heart is unable to accommodate incoming blood flow from the lungs. The resulting back pressure in pulmonary veins and capillaries causes leakage of fluid from blood vessels into tissue spaces and alveoli. Fluid accumulation may result in severe respiratory difficulty and pulmonary edema, a life-threatening development. The improved strength of myocardial contraction resulting from cardiotonic-inotropic drugs reverses this potentially fatal chain of events.
(2) Decreased edema—absence of pitting, decreased size of ankles or abdominal girth, decreased weight	Diuresis and decreased edema result from improved circulation and increased renal blood flow.
(3) Increased tolerance of activity	Indicates a more adequate supply of blood to tissues
b. When digoxin is given in atrial arrhythmias, observe for:	
(1) Gradual slowing of the heart rate to 70 to 80 beats/ min	
(2) Elimination of the pulse deficit	In clients with atrial fibrillation, slowing of the pulse rate and elimination of the pulse deficit are rough guides that digitalization has been achieved.
(3) Change in rhythm from irregular to regular	
3. Observe for adverse effects **a.** With digoxin observe for	There is a high incidence of adverse effects with digoxin therapy. Therefore, every client receiving digoxin requires close observation. Severity of adverse effects can be minimized with early detection and treatment.
(1) Cardiac arrhythmias:	Digoxin toxicity may cause any type of cardiac arrhythmia. These are the most serious adverse effects associated with digoxin therapy. They are detected as abnormalities in ECGs and in pulse rate or rhythm.
(a) Premature ventricular contractions (PVCs)	PVCs are among the most common digoxin-induced arrhythmias. They are not specific for digoxin toxicity because there are many possible causes. They are usually perceived as "skipped" heartbeats.
(b) Bradycardia	Excessive slowing of the pulse rate is an extension of the drug's therapeutic action of slowing conduction through the AV node and probably depressing the SA node as well.
(c) Paroxysmal atrial tachycardia with heart block	
(d) AV nodal tachycardia	
(e) AV block (second- or third-degree heart block)	
(2) Anorexia, nausea, vomiting	These GI effects commonly occur with digoxin therapy. Because they are caused at least in part by stimulation of the vomiting center in the brain, they occur with parenteral and oral administration. The presence of these symptoms raises suspicion of digitalis toxicity but they are not specific because many other conditions may cause anorexia, nausea, and vomiting. Also, clients receiving digoxin are often tak-

NURSING ACTIONS	RATIONALE/EXPLANATION
	ing other medications that cause these side effects, such as diuretics and potassium supplements.
(3) Headache, drowsiness, confusion	These CNS effects are most common in older adults.
(4) Visual disturbances (*e.g.*, blurred vision, photophobia, altered perception of colors, flickering dots)	These are due mainly to drug effects on the retina and may indicate acute toxicity.
b. With amrinone, observe for	
(1) Thrombocytopenia	Thrombocytopenia is more likely to occur with prolonged therapy and is usually reversible if dosage is reduced or the drug is discontinued.
(2) Anorexia, nausea, vomiting, abdominal pain	GI symptoms can be decreased by reducing drug dosage.
(3) Hypotension	Hypotension probably results from vasodilatory effects of amrinone.
(4) Hepatotoxicity	If marked changes in liver enzymes occur in conjunction with clinical symptoms, the drug should be discontinued.
c. With milrinone, observe for ventricular arrhythmias, hypotension, and headache	Ventricular arrhythmias reportedly occur in 12% of clients, hypotension and headache in about 3% of clients.
4. Observe for drug interactions	Most significant drug interactions increase risks of toxicity. Some alter absorption or metabolism to produce under-digitalization and decreased therapeutic effect.
a. Drugs that *increase* effects of digoxin	
(1) Adrenergic drugs (*e.g.*, ephedrine, epinephrine, isoproterenol), succinylcholine	Increase risks of cardiac arrthymias
(2) Antiarrhythmics (*e.g.*, amiodarone, propafenone, quinidine)	Decrease clearance of digoxin, thereby increasing serum digoxin levels and risks of toxicity. Dosage of digoxin should be reduced if one of these drugs is given concurrently (about 25% with propafenone and about 50% with amiodarone and quinidine).
(3) Anticholinergics	Increase absorption of oral digoxin by slowing transit time through the GI tract.
(4) Calcium preparations	Increase risks of cardiac arrhythmias. IV calcium salts are contraindicated in digitalized clients.
(5) Calcium channel blockers (*e.g.*, diltiazem, felodipine, nifedipine, verapamil)	Decrease clearance of digoxin, thereby increasing serum digoxin levels and risks of toxicity. Dosage of digoxin should be reduced about 25% if verapamil is given concurrently.
b. Drugs that *decrease* effects of digoxin	
Antacids, cholestyramine, colestipol, laxatives, oral aminoglycosides (*e.g.*, neomycin)	Decrease absorption of oral digoxin
5. Teach clients about digoxin **a.** Name of drug, dose, reason receiving	
b. Teach the client or a family member to check the radial pulse at least once daily. Omit digoxin and report to the physician if the pulse is below 60 or unusually irregular in adults or under approximately 100 in children.	Changes in the pulse may indicate adverse drug effects and a need to discontinue the drug.
c. Take the drug about the same time each day.	To maintain more even blood levels and to assist in remembering to take the drug.

REVIEW AND APPLICATION EXERCISES

1. What signs and symptoms usually occur with CHF? How would you assess for these?

2. What are the physiologic effects of digitalis on the heart?

3. What is digoxin's mechanism of action?

4. How does digoxin produce diuresis?

5. What is digitalization?

6. Differentiate between a digitalizing dose of digoxin and a daily maintenance dose.

7. Why do nurses need to check heart rate and rhythm before giving digoxin?

8. When is it appropriate to withhold a dose of digoxin?

9. What are adverse effects associated with digoxin, and how may they be prevented or minimized?

10. For clients with renal failure who need digoxin, what are the options for safe, effective therapy?

11. Why is it important to maintain a therapeutic serum potassium level during digoxin therapy?

12. Which commonly used cardiovascular drugs increase blood levels of digoxin and risks of toxicity?

13. What is the specific antidote for severe digitalis toxicity?

SELECTED REFERENCES

Brater, D.C. (1997). Clinical pharmacology of cardiovascular drugs. In W.N. Kelley (Ed.), *Textbook of internal medicine*, 3rd ed., pp. 552–569). Philadelphia: Lippincott-Raven.

Brown, K.K. (1993). Boosting the failing heart with inotropic drugs. *Nursing '93, 23,* 34–44.

Cohn, J.N. (1997). Approach to the patient with heart failure. In W.N. Kelley (Ed.), *Textbook of internal medicine*, 3rd ed., pp. 322–328. Philadelphia: Lippincott-Raven.

Drug facts and comparisons. (Updated monthly). St. Louis: Facts and Comparisons.

Guyton, A.C. & Hall, J.E. (1996). *Textbook of medical physiology*, 9th ed. Philadelphia: W.B. Saunders.

Johnson, J.A. & Lalonde, R.L. (1997). Congestive heart failure. In J.T. DiPiro, R.L. Talbert, G.C. Yee, G.R. Matzke, B.G. Wells, & L.M. Posey (Eds.), *Pharmacotherapy: A pathophysiologic approach*, 3rd ed., pp. 219–256. Stamford, CT: Appleton & Lange.

Porth, C.M. (1994). *Pathophysiology: Concepts of altered health states*, 4th ed. Philadelphia: J.B. Lippincott.

Smeltzer, S.C. & Bare, B.G. (1996). *Brunner and Suddarth's Textbook of medical-surgical nursing*, 8th ed. Philadelphia: Lippincott-Raven.

52 Antiarrhythmic Drugs

Outline

Objectives

After studying this chapter, the student will be able to:

1 Differentiate between supraventricular and ventricular dysrhythmias in terms of etiology and hemodynamic effects.

2 Describe nonpharmacologic measures to prevent or minimize tachyarrhythmias.

3 Discuss the roles of beta-adrenergic blocking agents, calcium channel blockers, digoxin, and quinidine in the treatment of supraventricular tachyarrhythmias.

4 Discuss the effects of lidocaine in the treatment of premature ventricular contractions and ventricular tachycardia.

5 Describe adverse effects and nursing process implications related to the use of selected antiarrhythmic drugs.

Key Terms

Automaticity	**Ectopic focus**
Bradyarrhythmia	**Refractory period**
Cardiac depressants	**Tachyarrhythmia**
Dysrhythmia	

Description

Antiarrhythmic agents are diverse drugs used for prevention and treatment of cardiac arrhythmias. Arrhythmias, also called dysrhythmias, are abnormalities in heart rate or rhythm. They become significant when they interfere with cardiac function and ability to perfuse body tissues. To aid in understanding of arrhythmias and antiarrhythmic drug therapy, the physiology of cardiac conduction and contractility is reviewed.

Cardiac Electrophysiology

The heart is an electrical pump. The "electrical" activity resides primarily in the specialized tissues that can generate and conduct an electrical impulse. Although impulses are conducted through muscle cells, the rate is much slower. The mechanical or "pump" activity resides in contractile tissue. Normally, these activities result in effective cardiac contraction and distribution of blood throughout the body. Each heartbeat or cardiac cycle occurs at regular intervals and consists of four events. These are *stimulation* from an electrical impulse, *transmission* of the electrical impulse to adjacent conductive or contractile tissue, *contraction* of atria and ventricles, and *relaxation* of atria and ventricles, during which they refill with blood in preparation for the next contraction.

AUTOMATICITY

Automaticity is the heart's ability to generate an electrical impulse. Any part of the conduction system can spontaneously start an impulse, but the sinoatrial (SA) node normally has the highest degree of automaticity and therefore the highest rate of spontaneous impulse formation. With its faster rate of electrical discharge or depolarization, the SA node serves as pacemaker and controls heart rate and rhythm.

Initiation of an electrical impulse depends on the movement of sodium and calcium ions into a myocardial cell and the movement of potassium ions out of the cell. Normally, the cell membrane becomes more permeable to sodium and opens pores or channels to allow its rapid movement into the cell. Calcium ions follow sodium ions into the cell at a slower rate. As sodium and calcium ions move into cells, potassium moves out of cells. The movement of the ions changes the membrane from its resting state of electrical neutrality to an activated state of electrical energy buildup. When the electrical energy is discharged (depolarization), muscle contraction occurs.

Some cells in the cardiac conduction system depolarize in response to the entry of calcium ions rather than entry of sodium ions. In these calcium-respondent cells, which are found mainly in the SA and AV nodes, the electrical impulse is conducted more slowly and recovery of excitability takes longer than in sodium-respondent cells. Overall, activation of the SA and AV nodes depends on a slow depolarizing current through calcium channels and activation of the atria and ventricles depends on a rapid depolarizing current through sodium channels. These two types of conduction tissues are often called slow and fast channels, respectively, and they differ markedly in their responses to drugs that affect conduction of electrical impulses.

The ability of a cardiac muscle cell to respond to an electrical stimulus is called *excitability* or *irritability*. The stimulus must reach a certain intensity or threshold to cause contraction. Following contraction, there is a period of decreased excitability (called the *refractory period*) during which the cell cannot respond to a new stimulus. During the refractory period, sodium and calcium ions return to the extracellular space, potassium ions return to the intracellular space, muscle relaxation occurs, and the cell prepares for the next electrical stimulus and contraction.

CONDUCTIVITY

Conductivity is the ability of cardiac tissue to transmit electrical impulses. Although the electrophysiology of a single myocardial cell can assist understanding of the process, the orderly, rhythmic transmission of impulses to all cells results in effective myocardial contraction.

Normally, electrical impulses originate in the SA node and are transmitted to atrial muscle, where they cause atrial contraction, and then to the atrioventricular (AV) node, bundle of His, bundle branches, Purkinje fibers, and ventricular muscle, where they cause ventricular contraction. The cardiac conduction system is shown in Figure 52-1.

Cardiac Arrhythmias

Cardiac arrhythmias can originate in any part of the conduction system or from atrial or ventricular muscle. They result from disturbances in electrical impulse formation (automaticity), conduction (conductivity), or both. The characteristic of automaticity allows myocardial cells other than the SA node to depolarize and initiate the electrical impulse that culminates in atrial and ventricular contraction. This may occur when the SA node fails to initiate an impulse or does so too slowly. When the electrical impulse arises anywhere other than the SA node, it is an abnormal or ectopic focus. If the ectopic focus depolarizes at a rate faster than the SA node, the ectopic focus becomes the dominant pacemaker. Ectopic pacemakers may arise in the atria, AV node,

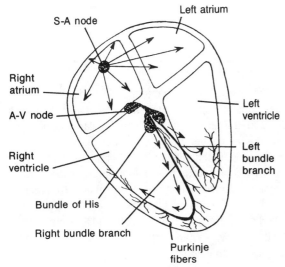

Figure 52-1

The conducting system of the heart. Impulses originating in the SA node are transmitted through the atria, into the AV node to the bundle of His, and by way of Purkinje fibers through the ventricles.

Purkinje fibers, or ventricular muscle. They may be activated by hypoxia, ischemia, or hypokalemia. Ectopic foci indicate myocardial irritability (increased responsiveness to stimuli) and potentially serious impairment of cardiac function.

A common mechanism by which abnormal conduction causes arrhythmias is called *re-entry excitation.* With normal conduction, the electrical impulse moves freely down the conduction system until it reaches recently excited tissue that is refractory to stimulation. This causes the impulse to be extinguished. The SA node then recovers, fires spontaneously, and the conduction process starts over again. Re-entry excitation means that an impulse continues to re-enter an area of the heart rather than becoming extinguished. For this to occur, the impulse must encounter an obstacle in the normal conducting pathway. The obstacle is usually an area of damage, such as myocardial infarction. The damaged area allows conduction in only one direction and causes a circular movement of the impulse (Fig. 52-2).

Arrhythmias may be mild or severe, acute or chronic, episodic or relatively continuous. They are clinically significant if they interfere with cardiac function (*i.e.,* the heart's ability to pump sufficient blood to body tissues). The normal heart can maintain an adequate cardiac output with ventricular rates ranging from 40 to 180 beats per minute. The diseased heart, however, may not be able to maintain an adequate cardiac output with heart rates below 60 or above 120. Arrhythmias are usually categorized by rate, location, or patterns of conduction. Common types of arrhythmias are described in Box 52-1.

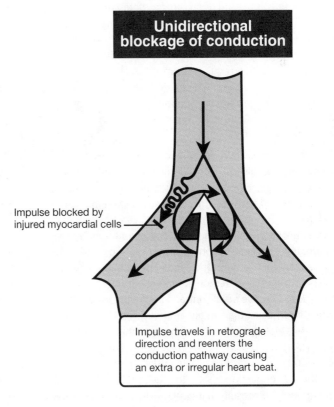

Figure 52-2

Re-entry excitation of arrhythmias.

BOX 52-1. Types of Arrhythmias

Sinus arrhythmias are usually significant only if they are severe or prolonged. Tachycardia increases the workload of the heart and may lead to congestive heart failure or angina pectoris. Sinus tachycardia may cause anginal pain (myocardial ischemia) by two related mechanisms. One mechanism involves increased myocardial oxygen consumption. The other mechanism involves a shortened diastole so that coronary arteries may not have adequate filling time between heartbeats. Thus, additional blood flow to the myocardium is required at the same time that a decreased blood supply is delivered.

Sinus tachycardia may be caused by numerous conditions such as fever, hypotension, congestive heart failure, thyrotoxicosis, stimulation of the sympathetic nervous system (*e.g.*, stress or drugs, including asthma remedies and nasal decongestants), and lifestyle drugs such as alcohol, caffeine, and nicotine. Thus, the initial assessment of a client with sinus tachycardia should include a search for underlying causes. Generally, the rate may be slowed by treating the underlying cause or by stimulating the vagus nerve (*e.g.*, by carotid sinus massage or Valsalva's maneuver).

Sinus bradycardia may occur with excessive vagal stimulation, deficient sympathetic tone, and sinus node dysfunction. It often occurs in healthy young adults, especially in athletes and during sleep. Other conditions associated with sinus bradycardia include hypothyroidism, hypothermia, vasovagal reactions, and drugs such as beta-adrenergic blocking agents, amiodarone, diltiazem, lithium, and verapamil. Thus, as with sinus tachycardia, efforts to identify the underlying cause are needed. Asymptomatic sinus bradycardia does not require treatment. Acute, symptomatic sinus bradycardia can be treated with atropine, epinephrine, or a temporary transvenous pacemaker. Chronic symptomatic sinus bradycardia requires insertion of a permanent pacemaker.

Atrial arrhythmias are most significant in the presence of underlying heart disease. Atrial fibrillation and atrial flutter commonly occur, especially in older adults. Numerous conditions may lead to these arrhythmias, including myocardial ischemia or infarction, hypertension, cardiomyopathy, valvular disorders, pulmonary embolus, pulmonary hypertension, thyrotoxicosis, alcohol withdrawal, sepsis, or excessive physical exertion. One characteristic of atrial fibrillation is disorganized, tremor-like movement of the atria. This lack of effective atrial contraction impairs ventricular filling, decreases cardiac output, and may lead to the formation of atrial thrombi, with a high potential for embolization. Another characteristic is a very rapid atrial rate (400–600 beats/min). Some of the atrial impulses penetrate the AV conduction system to reach the ventricles and some do not. This results in irregular activation of the ventricles and a slower ventricular rate (120–180 beats/min) than atrial rate.

Atrial flutter occurs less often than atrial fibrillation but causes similar symptoms. Atrial flutter is characterized by a rapid (270–330 atrial beats/min) but regular atrial activation and a regular ventricular pulse rate. The main goals of treatment for atrial fibrillation or flutter are restoration of sinus rhythm or slowing the ventricular response rate and prevention of thromboembolic complications. Treatment may include drug therapy (digoxin or a calcium channel blocker) or electrical cardioversion. In addition, antithrombotic therapy with aspirin or warfarin is indicated for all patients with atrial fibrillation.

Nodal arrhythmias may involve tachycardia and increased workload of the heart or bradycardia from heart block. Either tachycardia or bradycardia may decrease cardiac output. Heart block involves impaired conduction of the electrical impulse through the AV node. With first-degree heart block, conduction is slowed but not significantly. With second-degree heart block, every second, third, or fourth atrial impulse is blocked and does not reach the ventricles (2:1, 3:1, or 4:1 block). Thus, atrial and ventricular rates differ. Second-degree heart block may interfere with cardiac output or progress to third-degree block. Third-degree is the most serious type of heart block because no impulses reach the ventricles. As a result, ventricles beat independently at a rate of 30–40/min. This slow ventricular rate severely reduces cardiac output.

Ventricular arrhythmias include premature ventricular contractions (PVCs), ventricular tachycardia, and ventricular fibrillation. PVCs occur in healthy people as well as those with heart disease and may cause no symptoms or only mild palpitations. Serious PVCs often occur with ischemic heart disease, especially after acute myocardial infarction. PVCs are considered serious if they produce significant symptoms (*e.g.*, anginal pain, dyspnea, or syncope), occur more than five times per minute, are coupled or grouped, are multifocal, or occur during the resting phase of the cardiac cycle. Serious PVCs indicate a high degree of myocardial irritability and may lead to life-threatening ventricular tachycardia, ventricular fibrillation, or asystole. The goal of treatment is to decrease myocardial irritability, relieve symptoms, and prevent progression to more serious arrhythmias. With acute, uncomplicated myocardial infarction, some clinicians recommend lidocaine or magnesium sulfate to *prevent* arrhythmias rather than waiting until signs and symptoms of myocardial irritability occur.

Ventricular tachycardia (VT) is characterized by a ventricular rate of 160–250 beats/min. It is diagnosed when three or more PVCs occur in a row at a rate greater than 100 beats/min. VT may be sustained (lasts longer than

BOX 52-1. (Continued)

30 sec or requires termination because of hemodynamic collapse) or nonsustained (stops spontaneously in less than 30 sec). Occasional brief episodes of VT may be asymptomatic; frequent or relatively long episodes may result in hemodynamic collapse, a life-threatening situation. An acute episode most often occurs during an acute myocardial infarction. Other precipitating factors include severe electrolyte imbalances (*e.g.,* hypokalemia), hypoxemia, or digoxin toxicity. Correction of these precipitating factors usually prevents recurrences of VT. Patients with organic heart disease may have a chronic recurrent form of VT. Torsades de pointes is an especially serious type of VT that may deteriorate into ventricular fibrillation. Predisposing factors include severe bradycardia, electrolyte deficiencies (*e.g.,* hypokalemia, hypomagnesemia), and several drug groups (*e.g.,* class IA antiarrhythmics, phenothiazine antipsychotics, tricyclic antidepressants, and the nonsedating antihistamines astemizole and terfe-

nadine). With astemizole and terfenadine, torsades de pointes has been associated with overdose of the drugs or concomitant administration with other drugs (*e.g.,* erythromycin and several antifungal drugs). VT can be treated with lidocaine (a loading dose and continuous infusion), direct current countershock (DCC), or insertion of a transvenous pacing wire for overdrive pacing.

Ventricular fibrillation (VF) produces ineffective myocardial contraction so that there is no cardiac output. Death results unless effective cardiopulmonary resuscitation (CPR) or defibrillation is instituted within about 4–6 min. It most often occurs in patients with ischemic heart disease, especially acute myocardial infarction. Direct current countershock and antiarrhythmic drugs are used to restore a functional heart rhythm. After successful resuscitation, antiarrhythmic drug therapy should be continued until the patient's rhythm and clinical status stabilize. Then, the patient should be monitored closely for recurrence of VT or VF.

Antiarrhythmic Drugs

Antiarrhythmic drugs alter the heart's electrical conduction system. Drugs used for bradyarrhythmias (*e.g.,* atropine and epinephrine) are discussed in Chapters 21 and 18, respectively. Digoxin and its use in treating atrial fibrillation are discussed in Chapter 51. The focus of this chapter is the drugs used for tachyarrhythmias. These drugs are described below and listed in Table 52-1.

INDICATIONS FOR USE

Antiarrhythmic drug therapy is generally indicated in the following conditions:

1. When the ventricular rate is so fast or irregular that cardiac output is impaired. Decreased cardiac output leads to symptoms of decreased systemic, cerebral, and coronary circulation.
2. When premature ventricular contractions (PVCs) may develop into serious episodes of ventricular tachycardia
3. When dangerous arrhythmias have already developed and may be fatal if not quickly terminated. For example, ventricular tachycardia may cause cardiac arrest.

MECHANISMS OF ACTION

Drugs used for rapid arrhythmias mainly *reduce automaticity* (spontaneous depolarization of myocardial cells, including ectopic pacemakers), *slow conduction* of

electrical impulses through the heart, and *prolong the refractory period* of myocardial cells (so they are less likely to be prematurely activated by adjacent cells). Several different groups of drugs perform one or more of these actions. They are classified according to their mechanisms of action and effects on the conduction system, even though they differ in other respects. In addition, some drugs have characteristics of more than one classification.

Classifications and Individual Drugs

CLASS I SODIUM CHANNEL BLOCKERS

Class I drugs block the movement of sodium into cells of the cardiac conducting system. This results in a membrane-stabilizing effect and decreased formation and conduction of electrical impulses.

Class IA

Class IA drugs have a broad spectrum of antiarrhythmic effects and are used for both supraventricular and ventricular arrhythmias. **Quinidine,** the prototype, reduces automaticity, slows conduction, and prolongs the refractory period. It is used for chronic therapy of supraventricular and ventricular tachyarrhythmias. For clients with atrial fibrillation or flutter who have been converted to normal sinus rhythm with digoxin or electrical cardioversion, quinidine may be used to

TABLE 52-1	ANTIARRHYTHMIC DRUGS

Drugs for Tachyarrhythmias	Indications for Use	Routes and Dosage Ranges	
		Adults	**Children**
Class I Sodium Channel Blockers			
Class IA			
Quinidine (Cardioquin, Quinaglute)	Treatment of symptomatic or frequent PVCs, supraventricular tachycardia, and ventricular tachycardia Prevention of ventricular fibrillation	PO 200–600 mg q6h; maximum dose, 3–4 g/d Maintenance dose, PO 200–600 mg q6h, or 1 or 2 extended-action tablets, two or three times per day IM (quinidine gluconate) 600 mg initially, then 400 mg q4–6h IV (quinidine gluconate) 200 mg in 100 ml of solution, given over 20–30 min with continuous ECG and blood pressure monitoring	PO 6 mg/kg q4–6h
Procainamide (Pronestyl, Procanbid)		PO 1 g loading dose initially, then 250–500 mg q3–4h (q6h for sustained-release tablets) IM loading dose, 500–1000 mg, followed by oral maintenance doses IV 25–50 mg/min; maximum dose, 1000 mg	PO 50 mg/kg/d in four to six divided doses
Disopyramide (Norpace)		PO loading dose, 300 mg, followed by 150 mg q6h; usual dose, PO 400–800 mg/d in four divided doses	
Class IB			
Lidocaine (Xylocaine)	Treatment of PVCs, ventricular tachycardia Prevention of ventricular fibrillation	IV 1–2 mg/kg, not to exceed 50–100 mg, as a single bolus injection over 2 min, followed by a continuous infusion (1 g of lidocaine in 500 ml of 5% dextrose in water) at a rate to deliver 1–4 mg/min; maximum dose, 300 mg/h. IM 4–5 mg/kg as a single dose; may repeat in 60–90 min	IV injection 1 mg/kg, followed by IV infusion of 20–50 μg/kg/min
Mexiletine (Mexitil)		PO 200 mg q8h initially, increased by 50–100 mg every 2–3 d if necessary to a maximum of 1200 mg/d	

TABLE 52-1	ANTIARRHYTHMIC DRUGS (Continued)

		Routes and Dosage Ranges	
Drugs for Tachyarrhythmias	**Indications for Use**	*Adults*	*Children*
Tocainide (Tonocard)		PO 400 mg q8h initially, increased up to 1800 mg/d in three divided doses if necessary	
Phenytoin (Dilantin)		PO, loading dose 13 mg/kg (about 1000 mg) first day, 7.5 mg/kg second and third days; maintenance dose, 4–6 mg/kg/d (average 400 mg) in one or two doses starting on the fourth day IV 100 mg every 5 min until the arrhythmia is reversed or toxic effects occur; maximum dose, 1 g/24 h	
Class IC **Flecainide** (Tambocor)	Treatment of life-threatening ventricular tachycardia or fibrillation and supraventricular tachycardia unresponsive to other drugs	PO 100 mg q12h initially, increased by 50 mg q12h every 4 d until effective; maximum dose, 400 mg/d	
Propafenone (Rythmol)		PO 150 mg q8h initially, increased to a maximum dose of 1200 mg/d if necessary; usual maintenance dose 150–300 mg q8h	
Class I Miscellaneous **Moricizine** (Ethmozine)		PO 200–300 mg q8h	
Class II Beta-Blockers **Acebutolol** (Sectral)	Treatment of supraventricular tachycardia	PO 200 mg twice daily, increased gradually until optimal response is obtained (usually 600–1200 mg/d)	
Esmolol (Brevibloc)		IV infusion 500 µg/kg/min initially as a loading dose, followed by a maintenance dose of 50 µg/kg/min over 4 min. Repeat the same loading dose, and increase maintenance doses in 50 µg/kg increments every 5–10 min until therapeutic effects are obtained. Average maintenance dose, 100 µg/kg/min.	

(continued)

TABLE 52-1	ANTIARRHYTHMIC DRUGS (Continued)		
		Routes and Dosage Ranges	
Drugs for Tachyarrhythmias	**Indications for Use**	*Adults*	*Children*
Propranolol (Inderal)		IV injection 1–3 mg at a rate of 1 mg/min PO 10–20 mg three or four times per day	
Class III Potassium Channel Blockers	Treatment of ventricular tachycardia and ventricular fibrillation		
Amiodarone (Cordarone)		Loading dose, PO 800–1600 mg/d for 1–3 wk, with a gradual decrease to 600–800 mg/d for 1 mo Maintenance dose, PO 400 mg/d	
Bretylium (Bretylol)		IM 5 mg/kg, repeated in 1–2 h then q6–8h IV 5–10 mg/kg (diluted in at least 50 ml of IV fluid and infused over 10–20 min). During CPR, IV 5 mg/kg given by direct injection (undiluted); may be repeated q15–30 min to a maximum total dose of 30 mg/kg	
Sotalol (Betapace)		PO 80 mg q12h initially, titrated to response; average dose, 160–320 mg daily. See manufacturer's recommendations for dosing in renal failure.	
Class IV Calcium Channel Blockers	Treatment of supraventricular tachycardia		
Diltiazem (Cardizem)		IV injection 0.25 mg/kg (average dose 20 mg) over 2 min. A second dose of 0.35 mg/kg (average, 25 mg) may be given in 15 min, and an IV infusion of 5–15 mg/h may be given up to 24 h, if necessary.	
Verapamil (Calan, Isoptin)		PO 40–120 mg q6–8h IV 5–10 mg initially, then 10 mg 30 min later, if necessary	*Children up to 1 y*: IV injection 0.1–0.2 mg/kg (usual range, 0.75–2.0 mg for a single dose) over

TABLE 52-1　ANTIARRHYTHMIC DRUGS (Continued)

Drugs for Tachyarrhythmias	Indications for Use	Routes and Dosage Ranges	
		Adults	*Children*
			2 min with continuous ECG monitoring *Children 1–15 y:* IV injection 0.1–0.3 mg/kg (usual range 2–5 mg for a single dose) over 2 min with continuous ECG monitoring; repeat in 30 min if necessary
Unclassified			
Adenosine (Adenocard)	Treatment of supraventricular tachycardia	IV 6 mg given rapidly over 1–2 sec. If first dose does not slow the supraventricular tachycardia within 1–2 min, give 12 mg rapidly, and repeat one time, if necessary.	
Ibutilide (Corvert)	Conversion of recent onset atrial fibrillation or flutter to sinus rhythm	Weight 60 kg or more: IV infusion over 10 min, 1 mg Weight <60 kg: IV infusion over 10 min, 0.01 mg/kg The dose can be repeated once, after 10 min, if necessary.	
Magnesium sulfate	Torsades de pointes	IV 1–2 g (2–4 ml of 50% solution), diluted in 10 ml of 5% dextrose solution	

maintain normal sinus rhythm. However, such usage is being questioned because many patients have recurrent atrial fibrillation despite chronic quinidine therapy. Also, some studies indicate an increased mortality rate with long-term quinidine therapy, usually attributed to proarrhythmic effects. Quinidine is also used to prevent frequent PVCs, paroxysmal tachycardia, and postcountershock arrhythmias.

Quinidine is well absorbed after oral administration. Therapeutic serum levels (2 to 6 µg/ml) are attained within 1 hour and persist for 6 to 8 hours. Quinidine is highly bound to serum albumin and has a half-life of about 6 hours. Quinidine is metabolized by the liver (about 80%) and excreted in the urine (about 20%). In alkaline urine (*i.e.,* pH above 7), renal excretion of quinidine decreases, and serum levels may rise. Serum levels greater than 8 µg/ml are toxic.

Quinidine's low therapeutic ratio and high incidence of adverse effects limit its clinical usefulness. The drug is usually contraindicated in clients with severe, uncompensated congestive heart failure or with heart block because it depresses myocardial contractility and conduction through the AV node.

Quinidine salts used clinically include quinidine gluconate (Quinaglute), quinidine sulfate (Quinora), and quinidine polygalacturonate (Cardioquin). These salts differ in the amount of active drug (quinidine base) they contain and the rate of absorption with oral administration. The sulfate salt contains 83% quinidine base, and peak effects occur in 0.5 to 1.5 hours (4 hours for sustained-release forms). The gluconate salt contains 62% active drug, and peak effects occur in 3 to 4 hours. The polygalacturonate salt contains 60% active drug, and peak effects occur in about 6 hours. Quinidine preparations are usually given orally. The gluconate and polygalacturonate salts reportedly cause less gastrointestinal (GI) irritation than quinidine sulfate; this is probably related to their lower quinidine content. Oral extended-action preparations of quinidine (Quinidex Extentabs, Quinaglute Dura-Tabs) also are available.

Disopyramide is similar to quinidine in pharmacologic actions and is given orally to adults with ventricular tachyarrhythmias. It is well absorbed after oral administration and reaches peak serum levels (2 to 8 µg/ml) within 30 to 60 minutes. Drug half-life is 5 to 8 hours. Disopyramide is excreted by the kidneys and the liver in almost equal proportions. Dosage must be reduced in renal insufficiency.

Procainamide is related to the local anesthetic procaine and is similar to quinidine in actions and uses. Quinidine may be preferred for long-term use because procainamide produces a high incidence of adverse effects, including a syndrome resembling lupus erythematosus. Procainamide has a short duration of action (3 to 4 hours); sustained-release tablets (Procanbid) prolong action to about 6 hours. Therapeutic serum levels are 4 to 8 µg/ml.

Class IB

Lidocaine, a local anesthetic (see Chap. 14), is the prototype of class IB. It is the drug of choice for treating serious ventricular arrhythmias associated with acute myocardial infarction, cardiac surgery, cardiac catheterization, and electrical cardioversion. Lidocaine decreases myocardial irritability (automaticity) in the ventricles. It has little effect on atrial tissue and is not useful in treating atrial arrhythmias. It differs from quinidine in that:

1. It must be given by injection.
2. It does not decrease AV conduction or myocardial contractility with usual therapeutic doses.
3. It has a rapid onset and short duration of action. After intravenous (IV) administration of a bolus dose, therapeutic effects occur within 1 to 2 minutes and last about 20 minutes. This characteristic is advantageous in emergency treatment but limits lidocaine usage to intensive care settings.
4. It is metabolized in the liver. Dosage must be reduced in clients with hepatic insufficiency or congestive heart failure to avoid drug accumulation and toxicity.
5. It is less likely to cause heart block, cardiac asystole, ventricular arrhythmias, and congestive heart failure.

Therapeutic serum levels of lidocaine are 2 to 5 µg/ml. Lidocaine may be given intramuscularly (IM) in emergencies when IV administration is impossible. When given IM, therapeutic effects occur in about 15 minutes and last about 90 minutes. Lidocaine is contraindicated in clients allergic to related local anesthetics (*e.g.,* procaine). Anaphylactic reactions may occur in sensitized people.

Mexiletine and **tocainide** are oral analogs of lidocaine with similar pharmacologic actions. They are used to suppress ventricular arrhythmias, including frequent PVC and ventricular tachycardia. They are

well absorbed from the GI tract, and peak serum levels are obtained within 3 hours. Taking the drug with food delays but does not decrease absorption.

Phenytoin, an anticonvulsant (see Chap. 11), may be used to treat arrhythmias produced by digitalis intoxication. Phenytoin decreases automaticity and improves conduction through the AV node. Decreased automaticity helps control arrhythmias, whereas enhanced conduction may improve cardiac function. Further, because heart block may result from digitalis, quinidine, or procainamide, phenytoin may relieve arrhythmias without intensifying heart block. Phenytoin is not a cardiac depressant. Its only quinidine-like action is to suppress automaticity; otherwise, it counteracts the effects of quinidine and procainamide largely by increasing the rate of conduction. Phenytoin also has a longer half-life (22 to 36 hours) than other antiarrhythmic drugs. Given IV, a therapeutic plasma level (10 to 20 µg/ml) can be obtained rapidly. Given orally, however, the drug may not reach a steady-state concentration for about 1 week unless loading doses are given initially.

Class IC

Flecainide and **propafenone** are oral agents that greatly decrease conduction in the ventricles. They may initiate new arrhythmias or aggravate pre-existing arrhythmias, sometimes causing sustained ventricular tachycardia or ventricular fibrillation. These effects are more likely to occur with high doses and rapid dose increases. The drugs are recommended for use only in life-threatening ventricular arrhythmias.

Miscellaneous Class I Drug

Moricizine is a class I agent with properties of the other subclasses (*i.e.,* IA, IB, and IC). It is indicated for treatment of life-threatening ventricular arrhythmias, such as sustained ventricular tachycardia, and contraindicated in clients with heart block, cardiogenic shock, and hypersensitivity reactions to the drug. Following oral administration, onset of action occurs within 2 hours, and duration of action is 10 to 24 hours. The drug is 95% protein bound, extensively metabolized in the liver, and excreted in the urine. Because moricizine may cause new arrhythmias or aggravate pre-existing arrhythmias, therapy should be initiated in hospitalized clients with continuous electrocardiographic monitoring.

CLASS II BETA-ADRENERGIC BLOCKERS

These agents (see Chap. 19) exert antiarrhythmic effects by blocking sympathetic nervous system stimulation of beta receptors in the heart. Blockage of receptors in the SA node and ectopic pacemakers decreases automaticity, and blockage of receptors in the AV node increases the refractory period. Beta-blockers are most often used to slow the ventricular rate of contraction in supraventricular tachyarrhythmias (*e.g.*, atrial fibrillation, atrial flutter, paroxysmal supraventricular tachycardia). Only four of the beta-blockers marketed in the United States are FDA approved for treatment of arrhythmias. Acebutolol and propranolol may be used for chronic therapy to prevent ventricular arrhythmias, especially those precipitated by exercise. Beta-blockers are contraindicated in the presence of congestive heart failure unless the arrhythmia being treated is the cause of the heart failure.

Acebutolol may be given orally for ventricular arrhythmias. **Esmolol** has a rapid onset and short duration of action. It is given IV for supraventricular tachyarrhythmias, especially during anesthesia, surgery, or other emergency situations when the ventricular rate must be reduced rapidly. It is not used for chronic therapy. **Propranolol** may be given IV for life-threatening arrhythmias or those occurring during anesthesia or orally for chronic therapy. **Sotalol** is a noncardioselective beta-blocker (class II) that also has properties of class III antiarrhythmic drugs. Because its class III characteristics are considered more important in its antiarrhythmic effects, it is a class III drug (see below).

CLASS III POTASSIUM CHANNEL BLOCKERS

These drugs act to slow repolarization and prolong the refractory period in both atria and ventricles. Although the drugs share a common mechanism of action, they are very different drugs. Because of their adverse effects, they have been considered second- or third-line agents and recommended for use only when other drugs are ineffective. More recently, however, use of amiodarone and sotalol seems to be increasing.

Although classified as a potassium channel blocker, **amiodarone** also has electrophysiologic characteristics of sodium channel blockers, beta-blockers, and calcium channel blockers. It may be effective in supraventricular tachycardia, atrial fibrillation and flutter, and ventricular tachycardia. Its main indication for use is chronic oral treatment of recurrent ventricular tachycardia or ventricular fibrillation that does not respond to other drugs. However, studies indicate that low doses (100 to 200 mg/d) may be effective in preventing recurrence of atrial fibrillation with less toxicity than higher doses of amiodarone or usual doses of other agents, including quinidine. If these observations are confirmed in clinical trials, amiodarone may become a first-line agent for treatment of atrial fibrillation.

Amiodarone has a long serum half-life, and therapeutic effects may be delayed 5 to 30 days unless loading doses are given. Effects may persist for several weeks after the drug is discontinued. Adverse effects include hypothyroidism, hyperthyroidism, pulmonary fibrosis, myocardial depression, hypotension, bradycardia,

hepatic dysfunction, central nervous system (CNS) disturbances (depression, insomnia, nightmares, hallucinations), peripheral neuropathy and muscle weakness, bluish discoloration of skin and corneal deposits that may cause photosensitivity, appearance of colored halos around lights, and reduced visual acuity. Most adverse effects are considered dose dependent and reversible.

Bretylium is given parenterally to treat ventricular arrhythmias in intensive care settings. Because it is excreted almost entirely by the kidney, drug half-life is prolonged with renal insufficiency, and dosage must be reduced. Adverse effects include hypotension and arrhythmias.

Sotalol has both beta-blocking and potassium channel blocking activity. It is well absorbed after oral administration, and peak serum level is reached in 2 to 4 hours. It has an elimination half-life of about 12 hours, and 80% to 90% is excreted unchanged by the kidneys. Sotalol is approved for treatment of life-threatening ventricular arrhythmias refractory to other antiarrhythmic drugs. It has also been used, generally in smaller doses, to prevent or treat atrial fibrillation. It is contraindicated in clients with asthma, sinus bradycardia, heart block, cardiogenic shock, heart failure, and previous hypersensitivity to sotalol. Dosage should be individualized, reduced with renal impairment, and increased slowly (*e.g.*, every 2 to 3 days with normal renal function, at longer intervals with impaired renal function). Arrhythmogenic effects are most likely to occur when therapy is started or when dosage is increased. Most adverse effects are attributed to beta-blocking activity.

CLASS IV CALCIUM CHANNEL BLOCKERS

Calcium channel blockers block the movement of calcium into conductile and contractile myocardial cells. As antiarrhythmic agents, these drugs act primarily against tachycardias at SA and AV nodes because the cardiac cells and slow channels that depend on calcium influx are found mainly at these sites. Thus, they reduce automaticity of the SA and AV nodes, slow conduction, and prolong the refractory period in the AV node. They are effective only in supraventricular tachycardias.

Diltiazem and **verapamil** are the only calcium channel blockers approved for treatment of arrhythmias. Both drugs may be given IV to slow the rate of ventricular response and improve cardiovascular function in acute paroxysmal supraventricular tachycardia (PSVT) and in atrial fibrillation and flutter. They are also effective in exercise-related tachycardias. When given IV, the drugs act within 15 minutes and last up to 6 hours. Oral verapamil may be used in the chronic treatment of the above arrhythmias. Diltiazem and verapamil are metabolized by the liver, and metabolites are primarily excreted by the kidneys. The drugs are contraindicated in digitalis toxicity because they may worsen heart block.

If used with propranolol or digitalis, caution must be exercised to avoid further impairment of myocardial contractility. *Do not* use IV verapamil with IV propranolol; potentially fatal bradycardia and hypotension may occur.

UNCLASSIFIED

Adenosine, a naturally occurring component of all body cells, is an antiarrhythmic drug (Adenocard) that differs chemically from other agents. It is used to restore normal sinus rhythm in patients with PSVT; it is ineffective in other arrhythmias. It is thought to act by decreasing calcium movement into cells or increasing vagal tone. The drug has a very short duration of action (serum half-life is less than 10 seconds) and a high degree of effectiveness. It must be given by a rapid bolus injection, preferably through a central venous line. If given slowly, it is eliminated before it can reach cardiac tissues and exert its action.

Ibutilide is a newer drug indicated for treatment of recent onset of atrial fibrillation or atrial flutter, in which the goal is conversion to normal sinus rhythm. The drug is widely distributed and has an elimination half-life of about 6 hours. Most of a dose is metabolized, and the metabolites are excreted in urine and feces. Adverse effects include supraventricular and ventricular arrhythmias and hypotension.

Magnesium sulfate is given IV in the treatment of several arrhythmias, including prevention of recurrent episodes of torsades de pointes and treatment of digitalis-induced arrhythmias. The drug's exact mechanism of antiarrhythmic action is unknown. It is known that hypomagnesemia increases myocardial irritability and is a risk factor for both atrial and ventricular arrhythmias. Thus, it seems clear that serum magnesium levels should be monitored in patients at risk and replacement therapy instituted when indicated. However, in some instances, magnesium sulfate seems to have antiarrhythmic effects even when serum magnesium levels are normal. These effects may derive from the complex interactions among magnesium, potassium and calcium. For example, in the presence of hypomagnesemia, more potassium leaves the cell and treatment of hypokalemia with potassium supplements is less effective. In addition, hypocalcemia often accompanies hypomagnesemia.

Nursing Process

Assessment

Assess the client's condition in relation to cardiac arrhythmias:
- Identify conditions or risk factors that may precipitate arrhythmias. These include the following:
  - Hypoxia
  - Electrolyte imbalances (*e.g.,* hypokalemia, hypomagnesemia)
  - Acid–base imbalances
  - Ischemic heart disease (angina pectoris, myocardial infarction)
  - Cardiac valvular disease
  - Febrile illness
  - Respiratory disorders (*e.g.,* chronic lung disease)
  - Exercise
  - Emotional upset
  - Excessive ingestion of caffeine-containing beverages (*e.g.,* coffee, tea, colas)
  - Cigarette smoking
  - Drug therapy with digoxin, antiarrhythmic drugs, CNS stimulants, anorexiants, and tricyclic antidepressants
  - Hyperthyroidism
- Observe for clinical signs and symptoms of arrhythmias. Mild or infrequent arrhythmias may be perceived by the client as palpitations or skipped heart beats. More severe arrhythmias may produce manifestations that reflect decreased cardiac output and other hemodynamic changes, as follows:
  - Hypotension, bradycardia or tachycardia, and irregular pulse
  - Shortness of breath, dyspnea, and cough from impaired respiration
  - Syncope or mental confusion from reduced cerebral blood flow
  - Chest pain from decreased coronary artery blood flow. Angina pectoris or myocardial infarction may occur.
  - Oliguria from decreased renal blood flow
- When ECGs are available (*e.g.,* 12-lead ECG or continuous ECG monitoring), assess for indications of arrhythmias.

Nursing Diagnoses

- Decreased Cardiac Output related to ineffective pumping action of the heart
- Altered Tissue Perfusion related to decreased cardiac output
- Altered Tissue Perfusion related to drug-induced hypotension
- Activity Intolerance related to weakness and fatigue
- Self-Care Deficit related to decreased tissue perfusion and fatigue
- Impaired Gas Exchange related to decreased tissue perfusion
- Anxiety related to potentially serious illness
- Knowledge Deficit: Pharmacologic and nonpharmacologic management of arrhythmias
- Fluid Volume Excess: Peripheral edema and pulmonary congestion related to decreased cardiac output
- Noncompliance: Underuse of drugs related to adverse drug effects

Planning/Goals

The client will:
- Receive or take antiarrhythmic drugs accurately
- Avoid conditions that precipitate arrhythmias, when feasible
- Experience improved heart rate, circulation, and activity tolerance
- Be closely monitored for therapeutic and adverse drug effects
- Avoid preventable adverse drug effects
- Have adverse drug effects promptly recognized and treated if they occur
- Keep follow-up appointments for monitoring responses to treatment measures

Interventions

Use measures to prevent or minimize arrhythmias:

- Treat underlying disease processes that contribute to arrhythmia development. These include cardiovascular (*e.g.,* acute myocardial infarction) and noncardiovascular (*e.g.,* chronic lung disease) disorders.
- Prevent or treat other conditions that predispose to arrhythmias (*e.g.,* hypoxia, electrolyte imbalance).
- Help the client avoid cigarette smoking, overeating, excessive coffee drinking, and other habits that may cause or aggravate arrhythmias. Long-term supervision and counseling may be needed.
- For the client receiving antiarrhythmic drugs, implement the above measures to minimize the incidence and severity of acute arrhythmias, and help the client comply with drug therapy.
- Monitor heart rate and rhythm and blood pressure every 4 to 6 hours.
- Check laboratory reports of serum electrolytes and serum drug levels when available. Report abnormal values.

Teach clients:

- Ways to prevent or decrease the incidence and severity of fast arrhythmias
- The importance of periodic blood tests, ECGs, and medical supervision
- To avoid over-the-counter cold and asthma remedies, appetite suppressants, and antisleep preparations. These drugs are stimulants that can cause or aggravate irregular heartbeats.

Evaluation

- Check vital signs for improved heart rate and rhythm.
- Interview and observe for relief of symptoms and improved functioning in activities of daily living.
- Interview and observe for hypotension and other adverse drug effects.
- Interview and observe for compliance with instructions for taking antiarrhythmic drugs and other aspects of care.

Principles of Therapy

NONPHARMACOLOGIC TREATMENT OF ARRHYTHMIAS

Nonpharmacologic treatment is preferred, at least initially, for several arrhythmias. For example, sinus tachycardia usually results from such disorders as infection, dehydration, or hypotension, and treatment should be aimed toward relieving the underlying cause. For PSVT with mild or moderate symptoms, Valsalva's maneuver, carotid sinus massage, or other measures to increase vagal tone are preferred. For ventricular fibrillation, immediate defibrillation by electrical countershock is the initial treatment of choice.

In addition to these strategies, others are assuming increased importance. The impetus for nonpharmacologic treatments developed mainly from studies demonstrating that antiarrhythmic drugs could worsen existing arrhythmias, cause new arrhythmias, and cause higher mortality rates in clients receiving the drugs than clients not receiving the drugs. Current technology allows clinicians to insert pacemakers and defibrillators to control bradyarrhythmias or tachyarrhythmias and to use radio waves to deactivate ectopic foci (radio frequency catheter ablation).

PHARMACOLOGIC TREATMENT OF ARRHYTHMIAS

Rational drug therapy for cardiac arrhythmias requires accurate identification of the arrhythmia, understanding of the basic mechanisms causing the arrhythmia, observation of the hemodynamic and ECG effects of the arrhythmia, knowledge of the pharmacologic actions of specific antiarrhythmic drugs, and the expectation that therapeutic effects will outweigh potential adverse effects. Even when these criteria are met, antiarrhythmic drug therapy is somewhat empirical. Although some arrhythmias usually respond to particular drugs, different drugs or combinations of drugs are often required. There is a relative consensus of opinion among clinicians about appropriate treatment for acute, symptomatic arrhythmias, in which the goals are to abolish the abnormal rhythm, restore normal sinus rhythm, and prevent recurrence of the arrhythmia. There is less agreement about long-term use of the drugs, which is probably indicated only for patients who experience recurrent symptomatic episodes. General trends and guidelines include the following:

1. **Verapamil** or **diltiazem** (calcium channel blockers) may be preferred for slowing the ventricular rate in atrial fibrillation or flutter, although digoxin has long been used for this purpose. These drugs are also used to treat PSVT.
2. Although **quinidine** has long been used to prevent recurrence of atrial fibrillation, some clinicians are questioning this approach because up to 50% of the patients taking quinidine have recurrences of atrial fibrillation within a year and their mortality rate may be increased.
3. Use of **amiodarone** and **sotalol** for preventing recurrent atrial fibrillation seems to be increasing. Although approved by the FDA only for treatment of refractory ventricular arrhythmias, the drugs are effective in preventing recurrence of atrial fibrillation. When used for this purpose, the drugs are given in low doses and cause fewer adverse effects than when they are used for severe ventricular arrhythmias.

4. **Lidocaine** is the drug of choice for treating digitalis-induced arrhythmias; phenytoin is a second-line agent for this purpose.
5. **Lidocaine** is the drug of choice for treating PVCs and ventricular tachycardia. Mexiletine and tocainide may be useful because they can be given orally.
6. **Propranolol** and other beta-blockers are not drugs of choice for initial treatment of most arrhythmias but may be useful in treating a variety of arrhythmias, often in combination with other antiarrhythmic drugs.
7. **Amiodarone, bretylium, flecainide, propafenone,** and **sotalol** are used in the treatment of refractory life-threatening ventricular arrhythmias, such as sustained ventricular tachycardia.

USE IN CHILDREN

Antiarrhythmic drugs are less often needed in children than in adults. Supraventricular tachycardias (often occurring with anxiety, fever, or hypovolemia) are the most common arrhythmias in children, and propranolol, quinidine, or verapamil may be used to prevent or treat them. Lidocaine may be used to treat ventricular arrhythmias precipitated by cardiac surgery or digitalis toxicity. As with adults, the drugs should be used only when clearly indicated, and children should be monitored closely because all of the drugs can cause adverse effects, including hypotension and arrhythmias.

USE IN OLDER ADULTS

Cardiac arrhythmias are common in older adults, but generally only those causing symptoms of circulatory impairment should be treated with antiarrhythmic drugs. Compared with younger adults, older adults are more likely to experience serious adverse drug effects, including aggravation of existing arrhythmias, production of new arrhythmias, hypotension, and congestive heart failure. Cautious use is required, and dosage generally needs to be reduced to compensate for heart disease or impaired drug elimination processes.

HOME CARE

Clients receiving chronic antiarrhythmic drug therapy are likely to have significant cardiovascular disease. With each visit, the home care nurse needs to assess the client's physical, mental, and functional status and evaluate pulse and blood pressure. In addition, clients and caregivers should be taught to report symptoms (*e.g.,* dizziness or fainting, chest pain) and avoid over-the-counter drugs unless discussed with a health care provider.

ANTIARRHYTHMIC DRUGS

NURSING ACTIONS	RATIONALE/EXPLANATION
1. Administer accurately	
a. Check apical and radial pulses before each dose. Withhold the dose and report to the physician if marked changes are noted in rate, rhythm, or quality of pulses.	Bradycardia may indicate impending heart block or cardiovascular collapse.
b. Check blood pressure at least once daily in hospitalized clients.	To detect hypotension. Hypotension is most likely to occur when antiarrhythmic drug therapy is being initiated or altered.
c. During IV administration of antiarrhythmic drugs, maintain continuous cardiac monitoring and check blood pressure about every 5 min.	For early detection of hypotension and impending cardiac collapse. These drug side effects are more likely to occur with IV use.
d. Give oral drugs at evenly spaced time intervals.	To maintain adequate blood levels
e. Give mexiletine, quinidine, and tocainide with food.	To decrease gastrointestinal (GI) symptoms
f. Give lidocaine parenterally only, as a bolus injection or a continuous drip. Use only solutions labeled "For cardiac arrhythmias," and do *not* use solutions containing epinephrine. Give an IV bolus over 2 min.	Lidocaine solutions that contain epinephrine are used for local anesthesia only. They should *never* be given intravenously in cardiac arrhythmias because the epinephrine can cause or aggravate arrhythmias. Rapid injection (within about 30 s) produces transient blood levels several times greater than therapeutic range limits. Therefore, there is increased risk of toxicity without a concomitant increase in therapeutic effectiveness.

NURSING ACTIONS	*RATIONALE/EXPLANATION*

g. Give in a peripheral vein (except adenosine).

To allow mixing with blood. Injection into the central circulation (through a central venous pressure line, for example) is hazardous because a high drug concentration develops locally within the heart.

h. Do not add to a blood transfusion assembly.

2. Observe for therapeutic effects

a. Conversion to normal sinus rhythm

b. Improvement in rate, rhythm, and quality of apical and radial pulses and the ECG

c. Signs of increased cardiac output—blood pressure near normal range, urine output more adequate, no complaints of dizziness

After a single oral dose, peak plasma levels are reached in about 1–4 h with quinidine, procainamide, and propranolol and in 6–12 h with phenytoin. A state of equilibrium between plasma and tissue levels is reached in 1 or 2 d with quinidine, procainamide, and propranolol; in about 1 wk with phenytoin; in several weeks with amiodarone (unless loading doses are given); and in just a few minutes with IV lidocaine. Although this information may be helpful in determining when therapeutic effects are most likely to appear, remember that many other factors influence therapeutic effects, such as dose, frequency of administration, presence of conditions that alter drug metabolism, arterial blood gases, serum electrolyte levels, and myocardial status.

d. Serum drug levels within therapeutic ranges:

Serum drug levels must be interpreted in light of the client's clinical status.

Class IA

Quinidine	2–6	µg/ml
Disopyramide	2–8	µg/ml
Procainamide	4–8	µg/ml

Class IB

Lidocaine	1.5–6	µg/ml
Mexiletine	0.5–2	µg/ml
Phenytoin	10–20	µg/ml
Tocainide	4–10	µg/ml

Class IC

Flecainide	0.2–1	µg/ml
Propafenone	0.06–1	µg/ml

Class II

Propranolol	0.05–0.1	µg/ml

Class III

Amiodarone	0.5–2.5	µg/ml
Bretylium	0.5–1.5	µg/ml

Class IV

Verapamil	0.08–0.3	µg/ml

3. Observe for adverse effects

a. Heart block—may be indicated on the ECG by a prolonged P-R interval, prolonged QRS complex, or absence of P waves

Owing to depressant effects on the cardiac conduction system

b. Arrhythmias—aggravation of existing arrhythmia, tachycardia, bradycardia, PVCs, ventricular tachycardia or fibrillation

Because they affect the cardiac conduction system, antiarrhythmic drugs may worsen existing arrhythmias or cause new arrhythmias.

c. Hypotension

Owing to decreased cardiac output

d. Additional adverse effects with specific drugs:

(1) Disopyramide—mouth dryness, blurred vision, urinary retention, other anticholinergic effects

These effects commonly occur.

(continued)

NURSING ACTIONS	RATIONALE/EXPLANATION
(2) Lidocaine—drowsiness, paresthesias, muscle twitching, convulsions, changes in mental status (*e.g.*, confusion), hypersensitivity reactions (*e.g.*, urticaria, edema, anaphylaxis)	Most adverse reactions result from drug effects on the central nervous system (CNS). Convulsions are most likely to occur with high doses. Hypersensitivity reactions may occur in people who are allergic to related local anesthetic agents.
(3) Phenytoin—nystagmus, ataxia, slurring of speech, tremors, drowsiness, confusion, gingival hyperplasia	CNS changes are caused by depressant effects.
(4) Propranolol—weakness or dizziness, especially with activity or exercise	The beta-adrenergic blocking action of propranolol blocks the normal sympathetic nervous system response to activity and exercise. Clients may have symptoms caused by deficient blood supply to body tissues.
(5) Quinidine—hypersensitivity and cinchonism (tinnitus, vomiting, severe diarrhea, vertigo, headache)	
(6) Tocainide—lightheadedness, dizziness, nausea, paresthesia, tremor	These are the most frequent adverse effects. They may be reversed by decreasing dosage, administering with food, or discontinuing the drug.
4. Observe for drug interactions **a.** Drugs that *increase* effects of antiarrhythmics:	These drugs may potentiate therapeutic effects or increase risk of toxicity.
(1) Antiarrhythmic agents	When antiarrhythmic drugs are combined, there are additive cardiac depressant effects.
(2) Antihypertensives, diuretics, phenothiazine antipsychotic agents	Additive hypotension
(3) Cimetidine	Increases effects by inhibiting hepatic metabolism of quinidine, procainamide, lidocaine, tocainide, flecainide, and phenytoin
b. Drugs that *decrease* effects of antiarrhythmic agents:	
(1) Atropine sulfate	Atropine is used to reverse propranolol-induced bradycardia.
(2) Phenytoin, rifampin	Decrease effects by inducing drug-metabolizing enzymes in the liver and accelerating the metabolism of quinidine, disopyramide, and mexiletine
5. Teach clients **a.** Name, dose, and reason for receiving drug	
b. Report ankle edema, fatigue, dyspnea, weight gain.	These symptoms may indicate drug-induced congestive heart failure because these cardiac depressant drugs decrease myocardial contractility.
c. Space activities and rest at intervals.	With these drugs, there is decreased tolerance of activity and exercise.
d. Check pulse at least once daily for irregularity or excessive slowness.	Antiarrhythmic drugs may cause arrhythmias. Bradycardia is a side effect of propranolol.
e. Maintain regular time intervals in taking medication.	To maintain therapeutic blood levels
f. Phenytoin may color urine pink to reddish brown.	This color change is harmless.

REVIEW AND APPLICATION EXERCISES

1. Which tissues in the heart are able to generate an electrical impulse and therefore serve as a pacemaker?

2. What risk factors predispose a client to developing arrhythmias?

3. Name interventions that clients or health care providers can perform to decrease risks of arrhythmias.

4. Differentiate the hemodynamic effects of common arrhythmias.

5. What are the classes of antiarrhythmic drugs?

6. Explain why antiarrhythmic drugs can be called "cardiac depressants."

7. How do quinidine and related drugs and beta-adrenergic blocking agents act on the conduction system to slow heart rate?

8. When is IV lidocaine the drug of choice?

9. What is the main difference between lidocaine and tocainide in treatment of arrhythmias?

10. Why is flecainide reserved for serious ventricular arrhythmias?

11. What are common and potentially serious adverse effects associated with antiarrhythmic drugs?

SELECTED REFERENCES

Bauman, J.L. & Schoen, M.D. (1997). The arrhythmias. In J.T. DiPiro, R.L. Talbert, G.C. Yee, G.R. Matzke, B.G. Wells, & L.M. Posey (Eds.), *Pharmacotherapy: A pathophysiologic approach*, 3rd ed., pp. 323–359. Stamford, CT: Appleton & Lange.

Boisvert, J.T., Reidy, S.J. & Lulu, J. (1995). Overview of pediatric arrhythmias. *Nursing Clinics of North America, 30*(2), 365–379.

Brater, D.C. (1997). Clinical pharmacology of cardiovascular drugs. In W.N. Kelley (Ed.), *Textbook of internal medicine*, 3rd ed., pp. 552–569. Philadelphia: Lippincott-Raven.

Burke, L.J. & Mattson, C.M. (1994). Alterations in cardiac function. In C.M. Porth (Ed.), *Pathophysiology: Concepts of altered health states*, 4th ed., pp. 419–466. Philadelphia: J.B. Lippincott.

Conti, C.R. (1996). Re-examining the clinical safety and roles of calcium antagonists in cardiovascular medicine. *American Journal of Cardiology, 79*(suppl 9A), 13–18.

Drug facts and comparisons. (Updated monthly). St. Louis: Facts and Comparisons.

Fenster, P.E. & Nolan, P.E., Jr. (1993). Antiarrhythmic drugs. In R. Bressler & M.D. Katz (Eds.), *Geriatric pharmacology*, pp. 105–149. New York: McGraw-Hill.

Guyton, A.C. & Hall, J.E. (1996). *Textbook of medical physiology*, 9th ed. Philadelphia: W.B. Saunders.

Nappi, J.M. & McCollam, P.L. (1993). Sotalol: A breakthrough antiarrhythmic? *The Annals of Pharmacotherapy, 27*, 1359–1368.

Porth, C.M. (1994). *Pathophysiology: Concepts of altered health states*, 4th ed., pp. 403–418. Philadelphia: J.B. Lippincott.

Roden, D.M. (1996). Antiarrhythmic drugs. In J.G. Hardman, L.E. Limbird, P.B. Molinoff & R.W. Ruddon (Eds.), *Goodman & Gilman's The pharmacological basis of therapeutics*, 9th ed., pp. 839–874. New York: McGraw-Hill.

Tanel, R.E., Walsh, E.P., Lulu, J.A., & Saul, J.P. (1995). Sotalol for refractory arrhythmias in pediatric and young adult patients: Initial efficacy and long-term outcome. *American Heart Journal, 130*, 791–797.

Antianginal Drugs

Outline

Angina Pectoris
  types of angina
  nonpharmacologic treatment of angina

Antianginal Drugs
  organic nitrates
  beta-adrenergic blocking agents
  calcium channel blocking agents

Individual Antianginal Drugs
  organic nitrates
  beta-adrenergic blocking agents

Nursing Process
  assessment
  nursing diagnoses
  planning/goals
  interventions
  evaluation

Principles of Therapy
  goals of therapy
  choice of drug and dosage form
  titration of dosage
  tolerance to long-acting nitrates
  use in children
  use in older adults
  home care

Objectives

After studying this chapter, the student will be able to:

1 Describe the types, causes, and effects of angina pectoris.

2 Describe general characteristics and types of antianginal drugs.

3 Discuss nitrate antianginals in terms of indications for use, routes of administration, adverse effects, nursing process implications, and drug tolerance.

4 Differentiate between short-acting and long-acting dosage forms of nitrate antianginal drugs.

5 Discuss calcium channel blockers in terms of their effects on body tissues, clinical indications for use, common adverse effects, and nursing process implications.

6 Teach clients ways to prevent, minimize, or treat acute anginal attacks.

Key Terms

Angina pectoris	Myocardial infarction
Coronary atherosclerosis	Myocardial ischemia
Hypoxemia	
Hypoxia	Substernal

Angina Pectoris

Angina pectoris is a clinical syndrome characterized mainly by chest pain or pressure. It occurs when there is a deficit in myocardial oxygen supply (myocardial ischemia) in relation to myocardial oxygen demand. It is most often caused by atherosclerotic plaque formation in the coronary arteries. Atherosclerotic plaque narrows the lumen, decreases elasticity, and impairs dilation of coronary arteries. The result is impaired blood flow to the myocardium, especially with exercise or other factors that increase the cardiac workload and need for oxygen.

Types of Angina

Angina pectoris is generally described as a dull, heavy substernal pain that radiates into the left shoulder and down the left arm. The pain also may radiate to the back, neck, or lower jaw. There are several types of angina pectoris. *Stable angina* is the typical chest pain that is usually precipitated by exercise and relieved by rest or nitroglycerin. It also may be precipitated by stress, anxiety, cigarette smoking, or cold weather. Recurrent episodes of stable angina usually have the same pattern of onset, duration, and intensity of symptoms. *Unstable angina* results from progressive atherosclerosis and produces increased frequency, intensity, and duration of symptoms. Unstable angina is less responsive to rest, nitroglycerin, and other medical therapy. In *vasospastic angina* (also called Prinzmetal's or variant angina), chest pain occurs at rest. It is attributed to spasm in a coronary artery.

Nonpharmacologic Treatment of Angina

Nonpharmacologic measures for prevention and treatment of angina include rest, cessation of smoking, weight control, relaxation or stress-management techniques, and avoidance of circumstances known to precipitate acute attacks.

Antianginal Drugs

Drugs used in angina pectoris are the organic nitrates, the beta-adrenergic blocking agents, and the calcium channel blocking agents. Generally, these drugs relieve anginal pain by decreasing myocardial demand for oxygen or increasing blood supply to the myocardium.

Organic Nitrates

Organic nitrates relax smooth muscle in blood vessel walls. This action produces vasodilation, which relieves anginal pain by several mechanisms. First, dilation of veins reduces venous pressure and venous return to the heart. This decreases blood volume and pressure within the heart (preload), which in turn decreases cardiac workload and oxygen demand. Second, nitrates dilate coronary arteries and can increase blood flow to ischemic areas of the myocardium. Third, nitrates dilate arterioles, which lowers peripheral vascular resistance (afterload). This results in lower systolic blood pressure and, consequently, reduced cardiac workload. The prototype and most widely used nitrate is nitroglycerin.

Clinical indications for nitroglycerin and other nitrates are treatment and prevention of acute chest pain caused by myocardial ischemia. For acute angina and prophylaxis before a situation deemed likely to precipitate acute angina, fast-acting preparations (sublingual or chewable tablets, transmucosal spray or tablet) are used. For management of recurrent angina, long-acting preparations (oral and sustained-release tablets or transdermal ointment and discs) are used. Intravenous (IV) nitroglycerin is used to treat angina that is unresponsive to organic nitrates or beta-adrenergic blocking agents. It also may be used to control blood pressure in perioperative or emergency situations and to reduce preload and afterload in severe congestive heart failure.

Contraindications include hypersensitivity reactions, severe anemia, hypotension, and hypovolemia. The drugs should be used cautiously in the presence of head injury or cerebral hemorrhage because they may increase intracranial pressure.

Beta-Adrenergic Blocking Agents

Beta-adrenergic blocking agents, of which propranolol is the prototype, are often prescribed in a variety of clinical conditions. Their actions, uses, and adverse effects are discussed in Chapter 19. In this chapter, the drugs are discussed only in relation to their use in angina pectoris.

Sympathetic stimulation of beta receptors in the heart increases heart rate and force of myocardial contraction, both of which increase myocardial oxygen demand and may precipitate acute anginal attacks. Beta-blocking drugs prevent or inhibit sympathetic stimulation. Thus, the drugs reduce heart rate and myocardial contractility, particularly when sympathetic output is increased during exercise. Beta-blockers also reduce blood pressure, which in turn decreases myocardial workload and oxygen demand. In angina pectoris, beta-adrenergic blocking agents are used in long-term management to decrease the frequency and severity of anginal attacks, decrease the need for sublingual nitroglycerin, and increase exercise tolerance.

CALCIUM CHANNEL BLOCKING AGENTS

Calcium channel blockers act on contractile and conductive tissues of the heart and on vascular smooth muscle. For these cells to function normally, the concentration of intracellular calcium must be increased. This is usually accomplished by movement of extracellular calcium ions into the cell (through calcium channels or pores in the cell membrane) and release of bound calcium from the sarcoplasmic reticulum in the cell. Thus, calcium plays an important role in maintaining vasomotor tone, myocardial contractility, and conduction. Calcium channel blocking agents prevent the movement of extracellular calcium into the cell. As a result, coronary and peripheral arteries are dilated, myocardial contractility is decreased, and the conduction system is depressed in relation to impulse formation (automaticity) and conduction velocity (Fig. 53-1).

In angina pectoris, the drugs improve the blood supply to the myocardium by dilating coronary arteries and decrease the workload of the heart by dilating peripheral arteries. In atrial fibrillation or flutter and other supraventricular tachyarrhythmias, diltiazem and verapamil slow the rate of ventricular response. In hypertension, the drugs lower blood pressure primarily by dilating peripheral arteries.

Calcium channel blockers are well absorbed after oral administration but undergo extensive first-pass metabolism in the liver. Most of the drugs are more than 90% protein bound and reach peak plasma levels within 1 to 2 hours (6 hours or longer for sustained-release forms). Most also have short elimination half-lives (less than 5 hours), so doses must be given three or four times daily unless sustained-release formulations are used. Amlodipine (30 to 50 hours), bepridil (24 hours), and felodipine (11 to 16 hours) have long elimination half-lives and therefore can be given once daily. The drugs are metabolized in the liver, and dosage should be reduced in clients with severe liver disease. Dosage reductions are not required with renal disease.

The calcium channel blockers approved for use in the United States vary in their chemical structures and effects on body tissues. Seven of these are chemically dihydropyridines, of which nifedipine is the prototype. Bepridil, diltiazem, and verapamil differ chemically from the dihydropyridines and each other. Nifedipine and related drugs act mainly on vascular smooth muscle to produce vasodilation, whereas verapamil and diltiazem have greater effects on the cardiac conduction system.

The drugs also vary in clinical indications for use; most are used for angina or hypertension, and only diltiazem and verapamil are used to treat supraventricular tachyarrhythmias (Table 53-1). In addition,

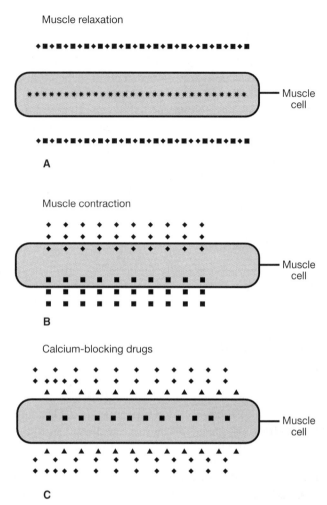

Figure 53-1
Calcium channel blockers: Mechanism of action. (*A*) During muscle relaxation, potassium ions are inside the muscle cell and calcium and sodium ions are outside the muscle cell. (*B*) For muscle contraction to occur, potassium ions leave the cell and sodium and calcium ions enter the cell through open channels in the cell membrane. (*C*) When calcium channels are blocked by drug molecules, muscle contraction is decreased because calcium ions cannot move through the cell membrane into the muscle cell. (Calcium ions = ◆; sodium ions = ■; potassium ions = ✳; calcium channel blocking drugs = ▲.)

nimodipine is approved for use only in subarachnoid hemorrhage to decrease spasm in cerebral blood vessels and thereby limit the extent of brain damage. In animal studies, nimodipine exerted greater effects on cerebral arteries than on other arteries, probably because it is highly lipid soluble and penetrates the blood-brain barrier.

Contraindications include second- or third-degree heart block, cardiogenic shock, and severe bradycardia, congestive heart failure, or hypotension. The drugs should be used cautiously with milder bradycardia, congestive heart failure, or hypotension and with renal or hepatic impairment.

TABLE 53-1 CALCIUM CHANNEL BLOCKERS

Generic/Trade Name	Indications	Routes and Dosage Ranges
Amlodipine (Norvasc)	Angina Hypertension	PO 5–10 mg once daily
Bepridil (Vascor)	Angina	PO 200 mg/d initially, increased to 300 mg daily after 10 d if necessary; maximum dose, 400 mg daily
Diltiazem (Cardizem)	Angina Hypertension Atrial fibrillation and flutter PSVT*	Angina or hypertension, immediate release, PO 60–90 mg four times daily before meals and at bedtime Hypertension, sustained-release only, PO 120–180 mg twice daily Arrhythmias (Cardizem IV only) IV injection 0.25 mg/kg (average dose 20 mg) over 2 min with a second dose of 0.35 mg/kg (average dose 25 mg) in 15 min if necessary, followed by IV infusion of 5–15 mg/h up to 24 h
Felodipine (Plendil)	Hypertension	PO 5–10 mg once daily
Isradipine (DynaCirc)	Hypertension	PO 2.5–5 mg twice daily
Nicardipine (Cardene)	Angina Hypertension	Angina, immediate release only, PO 20–40 mg three times daily Hypertension, immediate release, same as for angina, above; sustained-release, PO 30–60 mg twice daily
Nifedipine (Adalat, Procardia)	Angina Hypertension	Angina, immediate release, PO 10–30 mg three times daily; sustained release, PO 30–60 mg once daily Hypertension, sustained release only, 30–60 mg once daily
Nimodipine (Nimotop)	Subarachnoid hemorrhage	PO 60 mg q4h for 21 consecutive d. If patient unable to swallow, aspirate contents of capsule into a syringe with an 18-gauge needle, administer by nasogastric tube, and follow with 30 ml normal saline.
Nisoldipine (Sular)	Hypertension	PO, initially 20 mg once daily, increased by 10 mg/wk or longer intervals to a maximum of 60 mg daily. Average maintenance dose, 20–40 mg daily. Adults with liver impairment or over 65 y old, PO, initially 10 mg once daily
Verapamil (Calan, Isoptin)	Angina Atrial fibrillation or flutter; PSVT* Hypertension	Angina, PO 80–120 mg three times daily Arrhythmias, PO 80–120 mg three to four times daily; IV injection, 5–10 mg over 2 min or longer, with continuous monitoring of ECG and blood pressure Hypertension, PO 80 mg three times daily or 240 mg (sustained release) once daily

*PSVT = paroxysmal supraventricular tachycardia.

Individual Antianginal Drugs

Specific nitrates and beta-blockers used for angina are described below; calcium channel blockers are listed in Table 53-1.

ORGANIC NITRATES

Nitroglycerin (Nitro-Bid, others), the prototype drug, is used to relieve acute angina pectoris, prevent exercise-induced angina, and decrease the frequency and severity of acute anginal episodes. Oral dosage forms are rapidly metabolized in the liver, and relatively small proportions of doses reach the systemic circulation. In addition, oral doses act slowly and do not help relieve acute chest pain.

For these reasons, several alternative dosage forms have been developed, including transmucosal tablets and sprays administered sublingually or buccally, transdermal ointments and adhesive discs applied to the skin, and an IV preparation. When given sublingually, nitroglycerin is absorbed directly into the systemic circulation. It acts within 1 to 3 minutes and lasts about 30 to 60 minutes. When applied topically to the skin, nitroglycerin is also absorbed directly into the systemic circulation. However, absorption occurs at a slower rate, and topical nitroglycerin has a longer duration of action than other forms. It is available in an ointment, which is effective for 4 to 8 hours, and a transdermal disc, which is effective for about 18 to 24 hours. An IV form of nitroglycerin is used to relieve acute anginal pain that does not respond to other agents.

Routes and Dosage Ranges

Adults: PO 2.5–9 mg two or three times per day; sustained-release tablets or capsules, 2.5 mg three or four times per day
SL 0.15–0.6 mg PRN for chest pain
Translingual spray, one or two metered doses (0.4 mg/dose) sprayed onto oral mucosa at onset of anginal pain, to a maximum of three doses in 15 minutes
Transmucosal tablet, 1 mg q3–5h while awake, placed between lip and gum or cheek and gum
Topical ointment, ½–2 inches q4–8h; do not rub in
Topical transdermal disc, applied once daily
IV 5–10 µg/min initially, increased in 10- to 20-µg/min increments up to 100 µg/min or more if necessary to relieve pain

Amyl nitrite (Vaporole) is dispensed in a container that is crushed to release vapors; the vapors are inhaled. Onset of action and pain relief are rapid, but amyl nitrite is more likely to cause headache and hypotension than other nitrates used in angina pectoris.

Route and Dosage Range

Adults: Inhalation, 0.18–0.3 ml (one container)

Erythrityl tetranitrate (Cardilate) is used for the long-term management or prophylaxis of angina pectoris. The drug is unsuitable for acute episodes of anginal pain, because onset of action occurs after 5 to 10 minutes. Beneficial effects last 3 to 4 hours.

Routes and Dosage Ranges

Adults: SL 10 mg three times per day or before stress
PO 5–15 mg three times per day

Isosorbide dinitrate (Isordil, Sorbitrate) is used to reduce the frequency and severity of acute anginal episodes. When given sublingually or in chewable tablets, isosorbide dinitrate acts in about 2 minutes, and its effects last about 2 to 3 hours. When higher doses are given orally, more drug escapes metabolism in the liver and produces systemic effects in about 30 minutes. Lower doses may be relatively ineffective. Therapeutic effects last about 4 hours after oral administration. The effective oral dose is usually determined by increasing the dose until headache occurs, indicating the maximum tolerable dose. Sustained-release capsules also are available.

Routes and Dosage Ranges

Adults: SL 2.5–10 mg PRN or q2–4h
PO 10–60 mg q4–6h
Sustained-release capsules, PO 40 mg q6–12h

Isosorbide mononitrate (Ismo, Imdur) is the metabolite and active component of isosorbide dinitrate. It is well absorbed after oral administration and about 100% bioavailable. Unlike other oral nitrates, this drug is not subject to first-pass hepatic metabolism. Onset of action occurs within 1 hour, peak effects occur between 1 and 4 hours, and the elimination half-life is about 5 hours. It is used only for prophylaxis of angina; it does not act rapidly enough to relieve acute attacks.

Route and Dosage Range

Adults: PO 20 mg twice daily, with first dose on arising and the second dose 7 hours later
Extended-release tablets (Imdur), PO 30–60 mg once daily in the morning, increased after several days to 120 mg once daily if necessary

Pentaerythritol tetranitrate (Peritrate) is similar to erythrityl tetranitrate in actions and uses. It is used prophylactically in the long-term management of angina pectoris. It is available in short-acting and sustained-release dosage forms.

Route and Dosage Range

Adults: PO 10–40 mg four times daily
Sustained-release PO 30–80 mg q12h

BETA-ADRENERGIC BLOCKING AGENTS

Propranolol (Inderal), the prototype beta-blocker, is used in the treatment of angina pectoris to reduce the frequency and severity of acute attacks. Propranolol is usually added to the antianginal drug regimen when nitrates do not prevent anginal episodes. Propranolol is especially useful in preventing exercise-induced tachycardia, which can precipitate anginal attacks.

Propranolol is well absorbed following oral administration. It is then metabolized extensively in the liver; a relatively small proportion of an oral dose (about 30%) reaches the systemic circulation. For this reason, oral doses of propranolol are much higher than IV doses. Onset of action is 30 minutes after oral administration and 1 to 2 minutes after IV injection. Because of variations in the degree of hepatic metabolism, clients vary widely in the dosages required to maintain a therapeutic response.

Routes and Dosage Ranges

Adults: PO 10–80 mg two to four times per day
IV 0.5–3 mg q4h until desired response is obtained

Atenolol (Tenormin) and **nadolol** (Corgard) have the same actions, uses, and adverse effects as propranolol, but they have long half-lives and can be given once daily. They are excreted by the kidneys, and dosage must be reduced in clients with renal impairment.

Atenolol
Route and Dosage Range

Adults: PO 50 mg once daily, initially, increased to 100 mg/d after 1 week if necessary

Nadolol
Route and Dosage Range

Adults: PO 40–240 mg/d in a single dose

Nursing Process

Assessment

Assess the client's condition in relation to angina pectoris. Specific assessment data vary with each client but usually should include the following:

- During the initial nursing history interview, try to answer the following questions:
  - How long has the client been taking antianginal drugs? For what purpose are they being taken (prophylaxis, treatment of acute attacks, or both)?
  - What is the frequency and duration of acute anginal attacks?
  - Do symptoms other than chest pain occur during acute attacks (*e.g.,* sweating, nausea)?
  - Are there particular activities or circumstances that provoke acute attacks? Do attacks ever occur when the client is at rest?
  - What relieves symptoms of acute angina?
  - If the client takes nitroglycerin, ask how often it is required, how many tablets are needed for relief of pain, how often the supply is replaced, and where the client stores or carries the drug.

- Assess blood pressure and pulse, electrocardiogram reports, presence of symptoms other than chest pain, posture, and facial expression for baseline values.
- During an acute attack, assess the following:
  - Location and quality of the pain. Chest pain is nonspecific. It may be a symptom of numerous disorders, such as pulmonary embolism, esophageal spasm or inflammation (heartburn), costochondritis, or anxiety. Chest pain of cardiac origin is caused by myocardial ischemia and may indicate angina pectoris or myocardial infarction.
  - Precipitating factors. For example, what was the client doing, thinking, or feeling just before the onset of chest pain?

Nursing Diagnoses

- Decreased Cardiac Output related to disease process or drug therapy
- Altered Tissue Perfusion: Cerebral and peripheral, related to drug-induced hypotension
- Pain in chest related to inadequate perfusion of the myocardium
- Pain (headache) related to vasodilating effects of nitrate antianginal drugs
- Activity Intolerance related to chest pain
- Risk for Injury related to hypotension and syncope from antianginal drugs
- Noncompliance related to drug therapy and lifestyle changes
- Impaired Tissue Integrity related to skin irritation from topical nitroglycerin preparations
- Constipation related to drug therapy with calcium channel blockers
- Knowledge Deficit related to management of disease process and drug therapy
- Ineffective Individual Coping related to chronic disease process
- Social Isolation related to activity intolerance
- Body Image Disturbance related to inability to perform usual activities of daily living
- Sexual Dysfunction related to fear of precipitating chest pain

Planning/Goals

The client will:
- Receive or take antianginal drugs accurately
- Experience relief of acute chest pain
- Have fewer episodes of acute chest pain
- Have increased activity tolerance
- Identify and avoid or learn to manage situations that precipitate anginal attacks
- Be closely monitored for therapeutic and adverse effects, especially when drug therapy is started
- Avoid preventable adverse effects
- Verbalize essential information about the disease process, needed dietary and lifestyle changes to improve health status, and drug therapy
- Keep appointments for follow-up care and monitoring

Interventions

Use the following measures to prevent acute anginal attacks:
- Assist in preventing, recognizing, and treating contributory disorders, such as atherosclerosis, hypertension, hyperthyroidism, hypoxia, and anemia.
- Help the client recognize and avoid precipitating factors (*e.g.,* heavy meals, cigarette smoking, strenuous exercise) when

possible. If anxiety is a factor, relaxation techniques or psychological counseling may be helpful.

- Help the client to develop a more healthful lifestyle in terms of diet, adequate rest and sleep, and regular exercise. A supervised exercise program helps to develop collateral circulation.

  During an acute anginal attack in a client known to have angina or coronary artery disease:

- Assume that any chest pain may be of cardiac origin.
- Have the client lie down or sit down to reduce cardiac workload and provide rest.
- Check vital signs and compare them with baseline values.
- Record characteristics of chest pain and the presence of other signs and symptoms.
- Have the client take a fast-acting nitroglycerin preparation (previously prescribed), up to three sublingual tablets or three oral sprays within 15 minutes, if necessary.
- If chest pain is not relieved with rest and nitroglycerin, assume that a myocardial infarction has occurred until proven otherwise. Keep the client at rest and notify the physician immediately.

  Leave sublingual nitroglycerin at the bedside of hospitalized clients. The tablets or spray should be within reach so they can be used immediately. Record the number of tablets used daily, and ensure an adequate supply is available.

Teach clients:

- To seek medical attention immediately if acute chest pain is not relieved by rest and three sublingual tablets or oral sprays 5 minutes apart
- To keep family members or support people informed about the location and use of antianginal medications in case help is needed
- That long-acting forms of nitrates and beta-blocking agents should be tapered and discontinued gradually to avoid rebound angina
- To avoid over-the-counter decongestants, cold remedies, and diet pills, which stimulate the heart and constrict blood vessels and thus may cause angina
- That various dosage forms of nitroglycerin were developed for specific routes of administration and are not interchangeable. Also, that transdermal discs vary in the amount of drug released in a particular time interval.

Evaluation

- Observe and interview for relief of acute chest pain.
- Observe and interview regarding the number of episodes of acute chest pain.
- Interview regarding diet and lifestyle factors that relate to angina.
- Interview regarding compliance with drug therapy.

Principles of Therapy

GOALS OF THERAPY

The goals of drug therapy are to relieve acute anginal pain, reduce the number and severity of acute anginal attacks, and improve exercise tolerance and quality of life.

CHOICE OF DRUG AND DOSAGE FORM

For relief of acute angina and prophylaxis before events that cause acute angina, nitroglycerin (sublingual tablets or translingual spray) is usually the first drug of choice. Sublingual or chewable tablets of isosorbide dinitrate or amyl nitrite also may be used. For long-term prevention or management of recurrent angina, oral or topical nitrates, beta-adrenergic blocking agents, or calcium channel blocking agents are used. Combination drug therapy with a nitrate and one of the other drugs is common. Clients taking one or more long-acting antianginal drugs usually carry a short-acting drug as well to be used for acute attacks.

TITRATION OF DOSAGE

Dosage of all antianginal drugs should be individualized to achieve optimal benefit and minimal adverse effects. This is usually accomplished by starting with relatively small doses and increasing them at appropriate intervals if necessary. Generally, doses may vary widely among individuals.

TOLERANCE TO LONG-ACTING NITRATES

Clients who take long-acting dosage forms of nitrates on a regular schedule develop tolerance to the vasodilating (antianginal) effects of the drug. While this decreases the adverse effects of hypotension, dizziness, and headache, therapeutic effects also may be decreased. As a result, episodes of chest pain may occur more often or be more severe than expected. In addition, short-acting nitrates may be less effective in relieving acute pain.

Opinions seem divided about the best way to prevent or manage nitrate tolerance. Some authorities recommend using short-acting nitrates when needed and avoiding the long-acting forms. Others recommend using the long-acting forms for about 16 hours daily during active periods and omitting them during inactive periods or sleep. Thus, a dose of an oral nitrate or topical ointment would be given every 6 hours for three doses daily, allowing a rest period of 6 hours without a dose. Transdermal discs should be removed at bedtime.

USE IN CHILDREN

The safety and effectiveness of antianginal drugs have not been established for children. Nitroglycerin has been given IV for congestive heart failure and intraoperative control of blood pressure, with the initial dose adjusted for weight and later doses titrated to response. Verapamil (Calan, Isoptin) has been used to treat supraventricular tachycardias in children (see Chap. 52).

USE IN OLDER ADULTS

Antianginal drugs are often used because cardiovascular disease and myocardial ischemia are common problems in older adults. Adverse drug effects, such as hypotension and syncope, are likely to occur, and they may be more severe than in younger adults. Blood pressure and ability to ambulate safely should be closely monitored, especially when drug therapy is started. Ambulatory clients also should be monitored for their ability to take the drugs correctly.

HOME CARE

The role of the home care nurse may vary, depending largely on the severity of the client's illness. Initially, the nurse should assess the frequency and severity of anginal attacks and how the attacks are managed. In addition, the nurse can assess the home setting for lifestyle and environmental factors that may precipitate myocardial ischemia. When causative factors are identified, plans can be developed to avoid or minimize them. Other aspects of home care may include monitoring the client's response to antianginal medications; teaching clients and caregivers how to use, store, and replace medications to ensure a constant supply; and discussing circumstances for which the client should seek emergency care.

ANTIANGINAL DRUGS

NURSING ACTIONS	RATIONALE/EXPLANATION
1. Administer accurately	
a. Check blood pressure and heart rate before each dose of an antianginal drug. Withhold the drug if systolic blood pressure is below 90 mm Hg. If the dose is omitted, record and report to the physician.	Hypotension is an adverse effect of antianginal drugs. Bradycardia is an adverse effect of propranolol and nadolol. Dosage adjustments may be necessary if these effects occur.
b. Give antianginal drugs on a regular schedule, at evenly spaced intervals.	To increase effectiveness in preventing acute attacks of angina
c. If oral nitrates and topical nitroglycerin are being used concurrently, stagger times of administration.	To minimize risks of additive hypotension and headache
d. For sublingual nitroglycerin and isosorbide dinitrate, instruct the client to place the tablets under the tongue until they dissolve.	
e. For oral isosorbide dinitrate, regular and chewable tablets are available. Be sure each type of tablet is taken appropriately.	
f. For sublingual nitroglycerin, check the expiration date on the container.	Sublingual tablets of nitroglycerin are volatile. Once the bottle has been opened, they become ineffective after about 6 mo and should be replaced.
g. To apply nitroglycerin ointment, use the special paper to measure the dose. Place the ointment on a nonhairy part of the body, and apply with the applicator paper. Cover the area with plastic wrap or tape. Rotate application sites.	The measured paper must be used for accurate dosage. The paper is used to apply the ointment because the drug is readily absorbed through the skin. Skin contact should be avoided except on the designated area of the body. Plastic wrap or tape aids absorption and prevents removal of the drug. It also prevents soiling of clothes and linens. Application sites should be rotated because the ointment can irritate the skin.

(continued)

NURSING ACTIONS	RATIONALE/EXPLANATION
h. For nitroglycerin patches, apply at the same time each day to clean, dry, hairless areas on the upper body or arms. Rotate sites. Avoid applying below the knee or elbow or in areas of skin irritation or scar tissue.	To promote effective and consistent drug absorption. The drug is not as well absorbed from distal portions of the extremities because of decreased blood flow. Rotation of sites decreases skin irritation.
i. For IV nitroglycerin, dilute the drug and give by continuous infusion, with frequent monitoring of blood pressure and heart rate. Use only with the special administration set supplied by the manufacturer to avoid drug adsorption onto tubing.	The drug should not be given by direct IV injection. The drug is potent and may cause hypotension. Dosage (flow rate) is adjusted according to response (pain relief or drop in systolic blood pressure of 20 mm Hg).
j. With IV verapamil, inject slowly, over 2–3 min.	To decrease hypotension and other adverse effects
2. Observe for therapeutic effects	
a. Relief of chest pain with acute attacks	Sublingual nitroglycerin usually relieves pain within 5 min. If pain is not relieved, two additional tablets may be given, 5 min apart. If pain is not relieved after 3 tablets, report to the physician.
b. Reduced incidence and severity of acute attacks with prophylactic antianginal drugs	
c. Increased exercise tolerance	
3. Observe for adverse effects	
a. With nitrates, observe for hypotension, dizziness, lightheadedness, tachycardia, palpitations, and headache	Adverse effects are extensions of pharmacologic action. Vasodilation causes hypotension, which in turn causes dizziness from cerebral hypoxia and tachycardia from compensatory sympathetic nervous system stimulation. Hypotension can decrease blood flow to coronary arteries and precipitate angina pectoris or myocardial infarction. Hypotension is most likely to occur within an hour after drug administration. Vasodilation also causes headache, the most common adverse effect of nitrates.
b. With beta-adrenergic blocking agents, observe for hypotension, bradycardia, bronchospasm, and congestive heart failure.	Beta-blockers lower blood pressure by decreasing myocardial contractility and cardiac output. Excessive bradycardia may contribute to hypotension and cardiac arrhythmias. Bronchospasm is more likely to occur in clients with asthma or other chronic respiratory problems.
c. With calcium channel blockers, observe for hypotension, dizziness, lightheadedness, weakness, peripheral edema, headache, congestive heart failure, pulmonary edema, nausea, and constipation. Bradycardia may occur with verapamil and diltiazem; tachycardia may occur with nifedipine and nicardipine.	Adverse effects result primarily from reduced smooth muscle contractility. These effects, except constipation, are much more likely to occur with nifedipine and other dihydropyridines. Nifedipine may cause profound hypotension, which activates the compensatory mechanisms of the sympathetic nervous system and the renin-angiotensin-aldosterone system. Peripheral edema may require the administration of a diuretic. Constipation is more likely to occur with verapamil. Diltiazem reportedly causes few adverse effects.
4. Observe for drug interactions	
a. Drugs that *increase* effects of antianginal drugs.	
(1) Antiarrhythmics, antihypertensive drugs, diuretics, phenothiazine antipsychotic agents	Additive hypotension
(2) Cimetidine	May increase beta-blocking effects of propranolol by slowing its hepatic clearance and elimination. Increases effects of all calcium channel-blockers by inhibiting hepatic metabolism and increasing serum drug levels.
(3) Digoxin	Additive bradycardia when given with beta-blocking agents

NURSING ACTIONS	RATIONALE/EXPLANATION
b. Drugs that *decrease* effects of antianginal drugs:	
(1) Adrenergic drugs (*e.g.*, epinephrine, isoproterenol)	Adrenergic drugs, which stimulate beta receptors, can reverse bradycardia induced by beta-blockers.
(2) Anticholinergic drugs	Drugs with anticholinergic effects can increase heart rate, offsetting slower heart rates produced by beta-blockers.
(3) Calcium salts	May decrease therapeutic effectiveness of calcium channel blockers
(4) Carbamazepine, phenobarbital, phenytoin, rifampin	May decrease effects of calcium channel blockers by inducing hepatic enzymes and thereby increasing their rate of metabolism
5. Teach clients	
a. Take the drugs only as prescribed. Do not increase dosage or discontinue the drugs without specific instructions from the physician.	Dosage of antianginal drugs must be individualized to maximize therapeutic effects and minimize adverse effects. Discontinuing antianginal drugs abruptly has been associated with increased anginal episodes and possibly myocardial infarctions.
b. With sublingual nitroglycerin, keep tablets in the original container, carry them so that they are always within reach but not where they are exposed to body heat, and replace them about every 6 mo.	The tablets lose their potency after about 6 mo, or more rapidly if exposed to light and heat. Tablets should be readily accessible if chest pain occurs.
c. With sublingual or buccal tablets, hold under the tongue or between the cheek and gum until they dissolve. Do not chew the tablets.	Chewing the tablets increases risks of hypotension and headache.
d. Correct application of topical or transdermal preparations (see 1g and 1h). Areas may be shaved.	
e. Record the number and severity of anginal episodes daily, along with the number of nitroglycerin tablets required to relieve the attack and the total number of tablets taken daily.	Antianginal drugs are most often given on an outpatient basis. Information from the client is necessary to monitor therapeutic and adverse effects of drug therapy.
f. Headaches and dizziness may occur when antianginal drugs are started. These effects are usually transient and dissipate with continued therapy. If they persist or prevent normal activities of daily living, report to the physician.	Dosage may need to be reduced.
g. If dizziness occurs, avoid strenuous activity, and assume an upright position slowly for about 1 h after taking the drugs.	Dizziness is caused by a temporary decrease in blood pressure. It is most likely to occur when changing position from lying or sitting to standing and during the first hour after drug administration.

REVIEW AND APPLICATION EXERCISES

1. What is angina pectoris, and what is its cause?

2. How do nitrates relieve angina?

3. Develop a teaching plan for a client who is beginning nitrate therapy.

4. How do beta-blockers relieve angina?

5. Why should beta-blockers be tapered and discontinued slowly in clients with angina?

6. How do calcium channel blockers relieve angina?

7. Develop a teaching plan for a client taking a calcium channel blocker.

SELECTED REFERENCES

Brater, D.C. (1997). Clinical pharmacology of cardiovascular drugs. In W.N. Kelley (Ed.), *Textbook of internal medicine,* 3rd ed., pp. 552–569. Philadelphia: Lippincott-Raven.

Burke, L. & Porth, C.M. (1994). Alterations in cardiac function. In C.M. Porth (Ed.), *Pathophysiology: Concepts of altered health states,* 4th ed., pp. 419–466. Philadelphia: J.B. Lippincott.

Drug facts and comparisons. (Updated monthly). St. Louis: Facts and Comparisons.

Gollub, S.B. (1993). Combination medical therapy in the treatment of angina pectoris. *Hospital Formulary, 28,* 34–44.

Robertson, R.M. & Robertson, D. (1996). Drugs used for the treatment of myocardial ischemia. In J.G. Hardman, L.E. Limbird, P.B. Molinoff, & R.W. Ruddon (Eds.), *Goodman & Gilman's The pharmacological basis of therapeutics,* 9th ed., pp. 759–779. New York: McGraw-Hill.

Talbert, R.L. (1997). Ischemic heart disease. In J.T. DiPiro, R.L. Talbert, G.C. Yee, G.R. Matzke, B.G. Wells, & L.M. Posey (Eds.), *Pharmacotherapy: A pathophysiologic approach,* 3rd ed., pp. 257–294. Stamford, CT: Appleton & Lange.

Drugs Used in Hypotension and Shock

Outline

Hypotension and Shock
  types of shock

Antishock Drugs

Individual Drugs Used in Hypotension and Shock
  dopamine
  dobutamine
  epinephrine
  isoproterenol
  metaraminol
  methoxamine
  norepinephrine
  phenylephrine

Nursing Process
  assessment
  nursing diagnoses
  planning/goals
  interventions
  evaluation

Principles of Therapy
  goal of therapy
  choice of drug
  guidelines for treatment of hypotension
    and shock
  use in children
  use in older adults

Objectives

After studying this chapter, the student will be able to:

1 Identify clients at risk of developing hypovolemia and shock.

2 Identify common causes of hypotension and shock.

3 Discuss assessment of a patient in shock.

4 Describe therapeutic and adverse effects of vasopressor drugs used in the treatment of hypotension and shock.

Key Terms

Alpha-adrenergic effects

Anaphylactic shock

Beta-adrenergic effects

Cardiac output

Cardiogenic shock

Catecholamine

Hypovolemic shock

Perfusion

Vasodilation

Vasopressor

Hypotension and Shock

Shock is a clinical syndrome characterized by decreased blood supply to tissues. Clinical symptoms depend on the degree of impaired perfusion of vital organs (*e.g.,* brain, heart, and kidneys). Common signs and symptoms include oliguria, heart failure, disorientation, clouded sensorium, mental confusion, seizures, cool extremities, and coma. Most, but not all, people in shock are hypotensive. In a previously hypertensive person, shock may be present if a drop in blood pressure of greater than 50 mm Hg has occurred, even if current blood pressure readings are "normal."

TYPES OF SHOCK

Hypovolemic shock is characterized by a decreased circulating blood volume and may occur with acute blood loss, severe burns, or dehydration.

Cardiogenic shock is characterized by decreased cardiac output and may result from myocardial infarction, arrhythmias, or valvular disease.

Septic shock is characterized by profound vasodilation and decreased peripheral vascular resistance. It most often results from gram-negative bacterial infections but may occur with gram-positive infections as well.

Anaphylactic shock is characterized by extensive vasodilation and decreased peripheral vascular resistance. It may result from a hypersensitivity (allergic) reaction to drugs or other substances (see Chap. 18).

Antishock Drugs

Drugs used in the treatment of shock are primarily the adrenergic drugs, which are discussed more extensively in Chapter 18. In this chapter, the drugs are discussed only in relation to their usage in hypotension and shock. In hypotension and shock, drugs with alpha-adrenergic activity (*e.g.,* norepinephrine, phenylephrine, methoxamine) are used to increase peripheral vascular resistance and raise blood pressure. Drugs with beta-adrenergic activity (*e.g.,* dobutamine, isoproterenol) are used to increase myocardial contractility and heart rate, which in turn raises blood pressure. Several drugs have both alpha- and beta-adrenergic activity (*e.g.,* dopamine, epinephrine, metaraminol). In many cases, a combination of drugs is used, depending on the type of shock and the client's response to treatment.

Adrenergic drugs with beta activity may be relatively contraindicated in shock states precipitated or complicated by cardiac arrhythmias. Beta-stimulating drugs also should be used cautiously in cardiogenic shock following myocardial infarction, because increased contractility and heart rate can increase myo-

cardial oxygen consumption and extend the area of infarction.

Individual Drugs Used in Hypotension and Shock

Dopamine (Intropin) is a naturally occurring catecholamine that functions as a neurotransmitter. Dopamine exerts its actions by stimulating alpha, beta, or dopaminergic receptors, depending on the dose being used. In addition, dopamine acts indirectly by releasing norepinephrine from sympathetic nerve endings and the adrenal glands. Peripheral dopamine receptors are located in splanchnic and renal vascular beds. Stimulation of dopamine receptors produces vasodilation in the renal circulation and increases urine output. At low doses (2 to 5 µg/kg/min), dopamine stimulates dopaminergic receptors. At moderate doses (5 to 10 µg/kg/min), dopamine also stimulates beta receptors and increases heart rate, myocardial contractility, and blood pressure. At rates higher than 10 µg/kg/min, beta activity remains, but increasing alpha stimulation (vasoconstriction) may overcome the dopaminergic actions.

Dopamine is useful in hypovolemic and cardiogenic shock. Adequate fluid therapy is necessary for the maximal pressor effect of dopamine. Acidosis decreases the effectiveness of dopamine.

Route and Dosage Range

Adults and children: IV 2 to 5 µg/kg/min initially, gradually increasing to 10 to 15 µg/kg/min if necessary. Prepare by adding 200 mg of dopamine to 250 ml of IV fluid for a final concentration of 800 µg/ml or to 500 ml IV fluid for a final concentration of 400 µg/ml.

Dobutamine (Dobutrex) is a synthetic catecholamine developed to provide an agent with little vascular activity. Dobutamine acts mainly on beta$_1$ receptors in the heart to increase the force of myocardial contraction with minimal increase in heart rate. Dobutamine also may increase blood pressure with large doses. Dobutamine is less likely to induce tachycardia and arrhythmias than dopamine and isoproterenol. It is most useful in cases of shock that require increases in cardiac output without the need for blood pressure support. Dobutamine has a short plasma half-life and therefore must be administered by continuous intravenous (IV) infusion. It is rapidly metabolized to inactive metabolites. It is recommended for short-term use only.

Route and Dosage Range

Adults: IV 2.5 to 10 µg/kg/min, increased to 40 µg/kg/min if necessary. Reconstitute the 250-mg vial with 10 ml of sterile water or 5% dextrose injection.

The resulting solution should be diluted to at least 50 ml with IV solution before administering (5000 µg/ml). Add 250 mg of drug to 500 ml of diluent for a concentration of 500 µg/ml.

Epinephrine (Adrenalin) is a naturally occurring catecholamine produced by the adrenal glands. At low doses, epinephrine stimulates beta receptors, which results in increased cardiac output and bronchodilation. Larger doses act on alpha receptors to increase blood pressure. Epinephrine is the drug of choice for treatment of anaphylactic shock because of its rapid onset of action and its antiallergic effects (it prevents the release of histamine and other mediators that cause symptoms of anaphylaxis). Its use in other types of shock is limited because it may produce excessive cardiac stimulation, ventricular arrhythmias, and reduced renal blood flow. In addition, more potent vasoconstrictors are available (*e.g.*, norepinephrine). Epinephrine is rapidly inactivated to metabolites, which are excreted by the kidneys. It is usually given by continuous IV infusion to treat shock. A single IV dose may be given in emergencies, such as cardiac arrest.

Routes and Dosage Ranges

Adults: IV 1 to 4 µg/min. Prepare the solution by adding 2 mg (2 ml) of epinephrine injection 1:1000 to 250 or 500 ml of IV fluid. The final concentration is 8 or 4 µg/ml, respectively.
  IV direct injection, 100 to 1000 µg of 1:10,000 injection, q5–15 min, injected slowly. Prepare the solution by adding 1 ml epinephrine 1:1000 to 9 ml sodium chloride injection. The final concentration is 100 µg/ml.
Children: IV infusion, 0.025 to 0.3 µg/kg/min
  IV direct injection, 5 to 10 µg/kg, slowly

Isoproterenol (Isuprel) is a synthetic catecholamine that acts exclusively on beta receptors to increase heart rate, myocardial contractility, and systolic blood pressure. However, it also stimulates vascular beta$_2$ receptors, which causes vasodilation and may decrease diastolic blood pressure. For this reason, isoproterenol has limited usefulness as a pressor agent. It also may increase myocardial oxygen consumption and decrease coronary artery blood flow, which in turn causes myocardial ischemia. Cardiac arrhythmias may result from excessive beta stimulation. Because of these limitations, use of isoproterenol is limited to shock associated with slow heart rates and myocardial depression.

Route and Dosage Ranges

Adults: IV infusion, 0.5 to 10 µg/min. Prepare solution by adding 2 mg to 250 ml of IV fluid. Final concentration is 8 µg/ml.
Children: IV infusion, 0.05 to 0.3 µg/kg/min

Metaraminol (Aramine), occasionally used in hypotensive states, acts indirectly by releasing norepinephrine from sympathetic nerve endings. Its actions are similar to those of norepinephrine, except that metaraminol is less potent and has a longer duration of action.

Routes and Dosage Ranges

Adults: IM 2 to 10 mg
  IV injection, 2 to 5 mg
  IV infusion, add 100 to 500 mg of metaraminol to 500 ml of IV fluid. Adjust flow rate (dosage) to maintain the desired blood pressure.
Children: IM 0.1 mg/kg
  IV injection, 0.01 mg/kg
  IV infusion, 1 mg/25 ml of diluent. Adjust flow rate to maintain the desired blood pressure.

Methoxamine (Vasoxyl) acts on alpha-adrenergic receptors to cause vasoconstriction, increase peripheral vascular resistance, and raise blood pressure. The drug acts similarly to phenylephrine and is used occasionally in hypotension.

Routes and Dosage Ranges

Adults: IM 10 to 20 mg
  IV 3 to 5 mg, slowly
Children: IM 0.25 mg/kg
  IV 0.08 mg/kg, slowly

Norepinephrine, also called **levarterenol** (Levophed) is a pharmaceutical preparation of the naturally occurring catecholamine norepinephrine. Norepinephrine increases blood pressure primarily by vasoconstriction. It also increases heart rate and force of myocardial contraction. It is useful in cardiogenic and septic shock, but reduced renal blood flow limits its prolonged use. Norepinephrine is used mainly with clients who are unresponsive to dopamine or dobutamine.

Route and Dosage Ranges

Adults: IV infusion, 2 to 4 µg/min, to a maximum of 20 µg/min. Prepare solution by adding 2 mg to 500 ml of IV fluid. Final concentration is 4 µg/ml.
Children: IV infusion, 0.03 to 0.1 µg/kg/min

Phenylephrine (Neo-Synephrine) is an adrenergic drug that stimulates alpha-adrenergic receptors. As a result, phenylephrine constricts arterioles and raises systolic and diastolic blood pressures. Phenylephrine resembles epinephrine but has fewer cardiac effects and a longer duration of action. Reduction of renal and mesenteric blood flow limits prolonged usage.

Routes and Dosage Ranges

Adults: IV infusion, 100 to 180 µg/min initially, then 40 to 60 µg/min. Prepare solution by adding 10 or

20 mg of phenylephrine to 500 ml of IV fluid. Final concentration is 20 or 40 μg/ml, respectively.
IV injection, 100 to 500 μg
Children: SC, IM 0.1 mg/kg

Nursing Process

Assessment

Assess the client's condition in relation to hypotension and shock.
- Check blood pressure; heart rate; urine output; skin temperature of extremities; level of consciousness; orientation to person, place, and time; and adequacy of respiration. Abnormal values are not specific indicators of hypotension and shock, but they may indicate a need for further evaluation. Generally, report blood pressure below 90/60, heart rate above 100, and urine output below 50 ml/h.
- Check electrocardiogram and other assessment data if available.

Nursing Diagnoses

- Decreased Cardiac Output related to hypotension and vasoconstriction
- Altered Tissue Perfusion: Decreased related to decreased cardiac output
- Fluid Volume Deficit related to fluid loss or vasodilation
- Anxiety related to potentially life-threatening illness
- Risk for Injury: Myocardial infarction, stroke, or renal damage related to decreased blood flow to vital organs

Planning/Goals

The client will:
- Have improved tissue perfusion and relief of symptoms
- Have improved vital signs
- Be guarded against recurrence of hypotension and shock if possible
- Be monitored for therapeutic and adverse effects of adrenergic drugs
- Avoid preventable adverse effects of adrenergic drugs

Interventions

Use measures to prevent or minimize hypotension and shock.
- General measures include those to maintain fluid balance, control hemorrhage, treat infections, prevent hypoxia, and control other causative factors.
- Learn to recognize *impending* shock so treatment can be initiated early. *Do not wait* until symptoms are severe.
  Monitor clients during shock and vasopressor drug therapy.
- Titrate adrenergic drug infusion to maintain blood pressure and tissue perfusion without causing hypertension.
- Check blood pressure and pulse constantly or at least every 5 to 15 minutes during acute shock and vasopressor drug therapy.
- Monitor distal pulses, urine output, and skin temperature closely to assess tissue perfusion.
- Check venipuncture site frequently for infiltration or extravasation.

Teach clients and family:
- Descriptions and purposes of drug therapy and monitoring equipment
- The need for close observation of vital signs, IV infusion site, urine output, and so forth

Evaluation

Observe for improved vital signs, color and temperature of skin, and urine output.

Principles of Therapy

GOAL OF THERAPY

The goal of adrenergic drug therapy in hypotension and shock is to restore and maintain adequate tissue perfusion.

CHOICE OF DRUG

The choice of drug depends primarily on the pathophysiology involved. For cardiogenic shock and decreased cardiac output, dopamine or dobutamine is given. With severe congestive heart failure characterized by decreased cardiac output and high peripheral vascular resistance, vasodilator drugs (*e.g.*, nitroprusside, nitroglycerin) may be given along with the cardiotonic drug. The combination increases cardiac output and decreases the heart's workload by decreasing preload and afterload. However, vasodilators should not be used alone because of the risk of severe hypotension and further compromising tissue perfusion.

For anaphylactic or neurogenic shock characterized by severe vasodilation and decreased peripheral vascular resistance, a vasoconstrictor or vasopressor drug, such as norepinephrine, is the first drug of choice. Drug dosage must be carefully titrated to avoid excessive vasoconstriction and hypertension, which causes impairment rather than improvement in tissue perfusion.

GUIDELINES FOR TREATMENT OF HYPOTENSION AND SHOCK

1. Vasopressor drugs are less effective in the presence of inadequate blood volume, electrolyte abnormalities, and acidosis. These conditions also must be treated if present. Dopamine, dobutamine, or norepinephrine IV infusions may be titrated to maintain a low normal blood pressure.
2. Septic shock requires appropriate antibiotic therapy in addition to other treatment measures. If an abscess is the source of infection, it must be surgically drained.

3. Hypovolemic shock is most effectively treated by IV fluids that replace the type of fluid lost; that is, blood loss should be replaced with whole blood, and gastrointestinal losses should be replaced with solutions containing electrolytes (*e.g.,* Ringer's lactate or sodium chloride solutions with added potassium chloride).

4. Cardiogenic shock may be complicated by pulmonary congestion, for which diuretic drugs are indicated.

5. Anaphylactic shock is often treated by nonadrenergic drugs as well as epinephrine. For example, the histamine-induced cardiovascular symptoms (*e.g.,* vasodilation and increased capillary permeability) are thought to be mediated through both types of histamine receptors. Consequently, treatment may include a histamine₁ receptor blocker (*e.g.,* diphenhydramine 1 mg/kg IV) and a histamine₂ receptor blocker (*e.g.,* cimetidine 4 mg/kg IV), given over at least 5 minutes. In addition, IV corticosteroids are frequently given, such as methylprednisolone (20 to 100 mg) or hydrocortisone (100 to 500 mg). Doses may need to be repeated every 2 to 4 hours. Corticosteroids increase tissue responsiveness to adrenergic drugs in about 2 hours but do not produce anti-inflammatory effects for several hours.

USE IN CHILDREN

Little information is available about adrenergic drugs for the treatment of hypotension and shock in children. Generally, treatment is the same as for adults, with drug dosages adjusted for weight.

USE IN OLDER ADULTS

The use of adrenergic drugs to manage hypotension and shock in the older adult is essentially the same as for younger adults. Older adults often have disorders such as atherosclerosis, peripheral vascular disease, and diabetes mellitus. When adrenergic drugs are given, their vasoconstricting effects may decrease blood flow and increase risks of tissue ischemia and thrombosis. Careful monitoring of pulses and skin color and temperature, especially in the extremities, is required.

DRUGS USED IN HYPOTENSION AND SHOCK

NURSING ACTIONS	RATIONALE/EXPLANATION
1. Administer accurately	
a. Use a large vein for the venipuncture site.	To decrease risks of extravasation
b. Dilute drugs for continuous infusion in 250 or 500 ml of IV fluid. A 5% dextrose injection is compatible with all of the drugs and is most often used. For use of other IV fluids, consult drug manufacturers' literature. Dilute drugs for bolus injections to at least 10 ml with sodium chloride or water for injection.	To avoid adverse effects, which are more likely to occur with concentrated drug solutions
c. Use a separate IV line or a "piggyback" IV setup.	This allows the adrenergic drug solution to be regulated or discontinued without disruption of other IV lines.
d. Use an infusion pump	To administer the drug at a consistent rate. This helps to prevent wide fluctuations in blood pressure and other cardiovascular functions.
e. Discard any solution with a brownish color or precipitate.	Most of the solutions are stable for 24–48 h. Epinephrine and isoproterenol decompose on exposure to light, producing a brownish discoloration.
f. Start the adrenergic drug slowly, and increase as necessary to obtain desired responses in blood pressure and other parameters of cardiovascular function.	Flow rate (dosage) is titrated according to client response.
g. Stop the drug gradually.	Abrupt discontinuance of pressor drugs may cause rebound hypotension.

(continued)

NURSING ACTIONS	RATIONALE/EXPLANATION
2. Observe for therapeutic effects	
a. Systolic blood pressure of 80–100 mm Hg	These levels are adequate for tissue perfusion. Higher levels may increase cardiac workload, resulting in reflex bradycardia and decreased cardiac output. However, higher levels may be necessary to maintain cerebral blood flow in older adults.
b. Heart rate of 60–100, improved quality of peripheral pulses	These indicate improved tissue perfusion and cardiovascular function.
c. Improved urine output	Increased urine output indicates improved blood flow to the kidneys.
d. Improved skin color and temperature	
e. Pulmonary-capillary wedge pressure between 15 and 20 mm Hg in cardiogenic shock	Normal pulmonary-capillary wedge pressure is 6–12 mm Hg. Higher levels are required to maintain cardiac output in cardiogenic shock.
3. Observe for adverse effects	
a. Bradycardia	Reflex bradycardia may occur with levarterenol, metaraminol, methoxamine, and phenylephrine
b. Tachycardia	This is most likely to occur with isoproterenol but may occur with dopamine and epinephrine.
c. Arrhythmias	Fatal arrhythmias due to excessive adrenergic stimulation of the heart may occur with any of the agents used in hypotension and shock.
d. Hypertension	This is most likely to occur with high doses of levarterenol, metaraminol, methoxamine, and phenylephrine.
e. Hypotension	This is most likely to occur with low doses of dopamine and isoproterenol, owing to vasodilation.
f. Angina pectoris—chest pain, dyspnea, palpitations	All pressor agents may increase myocardial oxygen consumption and induce myocardial ischemia.
g. Tissue necrosis if extravasation occurs	This may occur with extravasation of solutions containing dopamine, levarterenol, metaraminol, and phenylephrine, owing to local vasoconstriction and impaired blood supply. Tissue necrosis may be prevented by injecting 5–10 mg of phentolamine (Regitine), subcutaneously, around the area of extravasation. Regitine is most effective if injected within 12 h after extravasation.
4. Observe for drug interactions	
a. Drugs that *increase* effects of pressor agents:	
(1) General anesthetics (*e.g.,* halothane)	Halothane and other halogenated anesthetics increase cardiac sensitivity to sympathomimetic drugs and increase the risks of cardiac arrhythmias.
(2) Anticholinergic drugs (*e.g.,* atropine)	Atropine and other drugs with anticholinergic activity may potentiate the tachycardia that often occurs with pressor agents, especially isoproterenol.
(3) MAO inhibitors (*e.g.,* tranylcypromine)	All effects of exogenously administered adrenergic drugs are magnified in clients taking MAO inhibitors because MAO is the circulating enzyme responsible for metabolism of adrenergic agents.
(4) Oxytocics (*e.g.,* oxytocin)	The risk of severe hypertension is increased.

Nursing Actions	*Rationale/Explanation*
b. Drugs that *decrease* effects of pressor agents: Beta-blocking agents (*e.g.*, propranolol)	Beta-blocking agents antagonize the cardiac stimulation produced by some pressor agents (*e.g.*, dobutamine, isoproterenol). Decreased heart rate, myocardial contractility, and blood pressure may result.
5. Teach clients **a.** To report pain, edema, or cool skin around the venipuncture site	These symptoms may indicate leakage of the drug solution into surrounding tissues. If extravasation occurs, prompt treatment may prevent severe tissue damage.
b. That frequent measurements of blood pressure and pulse and other observations are necessary	Knowing what to expect will decrease the client's anxiety.

REVIEW AND APPLICATION EXERCISES

1. How do adrenergic drugs improve circulation in hypotension and shock?

2. Which adrenergic drug improves renal blood flow?

3. Which adrenergic drug should be readily available for treatment of anaphylactic shock?

4. What are adverse effects of adrenergic drugs?

5. How would you assess the client for therapeutic or adverse effects of an adrenergic drug being given by continuous IV infusion?

6. Why is it important to prevent extravasation of adrenergic drug infusions into tissues surrounding the vein?

7. In hypovolemic shock, should fluid volume be replaced before or after an adrenergic drug is given?

SELECTED REFERENCES

Sypniewski, E., Jr. (1997). Hypovolemic and cardiogenic shock. In J.T. DiPiro, R.L. Talbert, G.C. Yee, G.R. Matzke, B.G. Wells, & L.M. Posey (Eds.), *Pharmacotherapy: A pathophysiologic approach*, 3rd ed., pp. 509–541. Stamford, CT: Appleton & Lange.

Urban, N. (1994). Circulatory shock. In C.M. Porth (Ed.), *Pathophysiology: Concepts of altered health states*, 4th ed., pp. 485–498. Philadelphia: J.B. Lippincott.

Antihypertensive Drugs

Objectives

After studying this chapter, the student will be able to:

1 Describe factors that control blood pressure.

2 Define/describe hypertension.

3 Identify clients at risk of developing hypertension and its sequelae.

4 Discuss nonpharmacologic measures to control hypertension.

5 Review the effects of alpha-adrenergic blockers, beta-adrenergic blockers, and calcium channel blockers in hypertension.

6 Discuss angiotensin-converting enzyme (ACE) inhibitors and angiotensin II receptor antagonists in terms of mechanisms of action, indications for use, adverse effects, and nursing process implications.

7 Describe the rationale for using combination drugs in the treatment of hypertension.

8 Discuss interventions to increase therapeutic effects and minimize adverse effects of antihypertensive drugs.

Key Terms

Angiotensin II	**Peripheral vascular resistance**
Cardiac output	
Hypertension	**Vascular tone**
Hypotension	**Vasoconstriction**
	Vasodilation

ntihypertensive drugs are used to treat hypertension, a common, chronic disorder affecting an estimated 60 million adults and an unknown number of children and adolescents in the United States. Hypertension increases risks of myocardial infarction, congestive heart failure, cerebral infarction and hemorrhage, and renal disease. To understand hypertension and antihypertensive drug therapy, one must first understand the physiologic mechanisms that normally control blood pressure, characteristics of hypertension, and characteristics of antihypertensive drugs.

Regulation of Arterial Blood Pressure

Arterial blood pressure reflects the force exerted on arterial walls by blood flow. Blood pressure normally stays relatively constant because of homeostatic mechanisms that adjust blood flow. The two major determinants of arterial blood pressure are cardiac output (systolic pressure) and peripheral vascular resistance (diastolic pressure). Cardiac output equals the product of the heart rate and stroke volume ($CO = HR \times SV$). Stroke volume is the amount of blood ejected with each heartbeat (about 60 to 90 ml). Thus, cardiac output depends on the force of myocardial contraction, blood volume, and other factors. Peripheral vascular resistance is determined by the degree of constriction or dilation in arterioles (vascular tone). The endothelial cells that line arteries and arterioles synthesize and secrete several vasoactive substances. Vasoconstricting substances, which increase vascular tone and blood pressure, include angiotensin II and endothelin I. Vasodilating substances, which decrease vascular tone and blood pressure, include bradykinin, endothelium-derived relaxing factor (nitric oxide), and prostacyclin. Excessive vasoconstrictors or deficient vasodilators may contribute to the development of atherosclerosis, hypertension, and other diseases.

Thus, regulation of blood pressure involves a complex network of nervous, hormonal, and renal mechanisms and any condition that affects heart rate, stroke volume, or peripheral resistance affects arterial blood pressure. The nervous and hormonal mechanisms act rapidly; renal mechanisms act more slowly.

RESPONSE TO HYPOTENSION

When hypotension (and decreased tissue perfusion) occurs, the sympathetic nervous system (SNS) is stimulated, the hormones epinephrine and norepinephrine are secreted by the adrenal medulla, angiotensin II and aldosterone are formed, and the kidneys retain fluid. These compensatory mechanisms raise the blood pressure. Specific effects include the following:

1. Constriction of arterioles, which increases peripheral vascular resistance
2. Constriction of veins and increased venous tone
3. Stimulation of cardiac beta-adrenergic receptors, which increases heart rate and force of myocardial contraction
4. Activation of the renin-angiotensin-aldosterone mechanism. Renin is an enzyme secreted by the kidneys in response to low renal blood flow and SNS stimulation. It acts on a plasma protein to produce angiotensin I. Then, a converting enzyme acts on angiotensin I to produce angiotensin II. Angiotensin II constricts arterioles, increases peripheral resistance, and increases blood pressure by direct vasoconstriction, stimulation of the SNS, and stimulation of catecholamine release from the adrenal medulla. It also stimulates secretion of aldosterone from the adrenal cortex, which then causes the kidneys to retain sodium and water. Retention of sodium and water increases blood volume, cardiac output, and blood pressure.

RESPONSE TO HYPERTENSION

When arterial blood pressure is elevated, the following sequence of events occurs:

1. Kidneys excrete more fluid (increase urine output).
2. Fluid loss reduces both extracellular fluid volume and blood volume.
3. Decreased blood volume reduces venous blood flow to the heart and therefore decreases cardiac output.
4. Decreased cardiac output reduces arterial blood pressure.
5. The vascular endothelium produces vasodilating substances (*e.g.*, bradykinin, endothelium-derived relaxing factor [nitric oxide], and prostacyclin), which reduce blood pressure.

Hypertension

Hypertension is persistently high blood pressure that results from abnormalities in the regulatory mechanisms described above. It is usually defined as a systolic pressure above 140 mm Hg or a diastolic pressure above 90 mm Hg on multiple blood pressure measurements.

Primary or essential hypertension (that for which no cause can be found) makes up about 90% of known cases. Secondary hypertension may result from renal, endocrine, or central nervous system (CNS) disorders and from drugs that stimulate the SNS or cause retention of sodium and water. Primary hypertension can be controlled with appropriate therapy; secondary hypertension can sometimes be cured by surgical therapy.

The Fifth Report of the Joint National Committee on Detection, Evaluation, and Treatment of High Blood Pressure, published in 1993, classified blood pressures in adults (in mm of Hg), as follows:

- Normal = systolic 130 or below; diastolic 85 or below
- High normal = systolic 130 to 139; diastolic 85 to 89
- Stage 1 hypertension (mild) = systolic 140 to 159; diastolic 90 to 99
- Stage 2 hypertension (moderate) = systolic 160 to 179; diastolic 100 to 109
- Stage 3 hypertension (severe) = systolic 180 to 209; diastolic 110 to 119
- Stage 4 hypertension (very severe) = systolic 210 or above; diastolic 120 or above

A systolic pressure of 140 or above with a diastolic pressure below 90 is usually called isolated systolic hypertension.

Hypertension profoundly alters cardiovascular function by increasing the workload of the heart and causing thickening and sclerosis of arterial walls. As a result of increased cardiac workload, the myocardium hypertrophies as a compensatory mechanism. However, heart failure eventually occurs. As a result of arterial changes, the lumen is narrowed, blood supply to tissues is decreased, and risks of thrombosis are increased. In addition, necrotic areas may develop in arteries, and these may rupture with sustained high blood pressure. The areas of most serious damage are the heart, brain, kidneys, and eyes. These are often called "target organs."

Initially and perhaps for years, primary hypertension may produce no symptoms. If symptoms occur, they are usually vague and nonspecific. Hypertension may go undetected, or it may be incidentally discovered when blood pressure measurements are taken as part of a routine physical examination, screening test, or assessment of other disorders. Eventually, symptoms reflect target organ damage. Not infrequently, hypertension is discovered after a person experiences angina pectoris, myocardial infarction, congestive heart failure, stroke, or renal disease.

Hypertensive emergencies are episodes of severely elevated blood pressure that may be an extension of malignant hypertension or caused by cerebral hemorrhage, dissecting aortic aneurysm, renal disease, pheochromocytoma, or eclampsia. These require immediate treatment, usually intravenous (IV) antihypertensive drugs, to lower blood pressure. Symptoms include severe headache, nausea, vomiting, visual disturbances, neurologic disturbances, disorientation, and decreased level of consciousness (drowsiness, stupor, coma). Hypertensive urgencies are episodes of less severe hyper-tension often managed with oral drugs. The goal of treatment is to lower blood pressure within 24 hours. In most instances, it is better to lower blood pressure gradually (rather than precipitously) and to avoid wide fluctuations in blood pressure.

Antihypertensive Drugs

Drugs used in the treatment of primary hypertension belong to several different groups, including angiotensin-converting enzyme (ACE) inhibitors, angiotensin II receptor antagonists, antiadrenergics, calcium channel blockers, diuretics, and direct vasodilators. These drugs generally act to decrease blood pressure by decreasing cardiac output or peripheral vascular resistance.

ANGIOTENSIN-CONVERTING ENZYME (ACE) INHIBITORS

Angiotensin-converting enzyme (also called kininase) is mainly located in the endothelial lining of blood vessels, and this is where most angiotensin II is produced. This same enzyme also metabolizes bradykinin, an endogenous substance with strong vasodilating properties.

ACE inhibitors block the enzyme that normally converts angiotensin I to the potent vasoconstrictor angiotensin II. By blocking production of angiotensin II, the drugs decrease vasoconstriction (thereby having a vasodilating effect) and decrease aldosterone production (thereby reducing retention of sodium and water). In addition to inhibiting formation of angiotensin II, the drugs also inhibit the breakdown of bradykinin, thereby prolonging its vasodilating effects. Because of their effectiveness in hypertension and beneficial effects on the heart, blood vessels, and kidneys, these drugs are increasing in importance, number, and use.

In clients with normal renal function, ACE inhibitors may be used alone or in combination with other antihypertensive agents, such as thiazide diuretics. In clients with impaired renal function, the drugs are recommended for those who fail to respond or who experience intolerable adverse effects with other antihypertensive agents. Although the drugs can cause or aggravate proteinuria and renal damage in nondiabetics, they decrease proteinuria and slow the development of nephropathy in diabetics.

Most ACE inhibitors (captopril, enalapril, fosinopril, lisinopril, ramipril, and quinapril) also are used in the treatment of congestive heart failure; they decrease vasoconstriction and peripheral vascular resistance, thereby reducing cardiac workload. Captopril is also indicated for the treatment of diabetic nephropathy, in which it slows progression of renal insufficiency. Captopril's "renal protective" effects are thought to be more than its antihypertensive effects, because other antihypertensive agents do not slow nephropathy. Although other ACE inhibitors are not FDA approved for this indication, presumably they would have similar effects.

ACE inhibitors are well absorbed with oral administration, produce effects within 1 hour that last about 24 hours, have prolonged serum half-lives with impaired renal function, and are metabolized to active metabolites, which are excreted in urine and feces. These drugs are generally well tolerated, with a low incidence of serious adverse effects (*e.g.,* neutropenia, agranulocytosis, proteinuria, glomerulonephritis, and angioedema). However, a persistent cough develops in about 10% to 20% of patients and may lead to stopping the drug. Also, acute hypotension may occur when an ACE inhibitor is started, especially in clients with fluid volume deficit. This reaction may be prevented by starting with a low dose, taken at bedtime, or by stopping diuretics and reducing dosage of other antihypertensive drugs temporarily. Hyperkalemia may develop in patients who have diabetes mellitus or renal impairment or who are taking nonsteroidal anti-inflammatory drugs, potassium supplements, or potassium-sparing diuretics. These drugs are contraindicated during pregnancy because serious illnesses, including renal failure, have been identified in neonates whose mothers took an ACE inhibitor during the second and third trimesters.

ANGIOTENSIN II RECEPTOR ANTAGONISTS

Angiotensin II receptor antagonists or inhibitors are a new drug classification. These drugs were developed to block the strong blood pressure–raising effects of angiotensin II. Instead of decreasing production of angiotensin II, as the ACE inhibitors do, these drugs compete with angiotensin II for tissue binding sites and prevent angiotensin II from combining with its receptors in body tissues. Although multiple types of receptors have been identified, the AT_1 receptors located in brain, renal, myocardial, vascular, and adrenal tissue determine most of the effects of angiotensin II on cardiovascular and renal functions. Angiotensin II receptor inhibitors block the angiotensin II AT_1 receptors and decrease arterial blood pressure by decreasing systemic vascular resistance.

Losartan (Cozaar) was the first FDA-approved drug of this class, but several others are being developed. Losartan is similar to ACE inhibitors in its effects on blood pressure and hemodynamics and is considered as effective as an ACE inhibitor in the treatment of hypertension and probably heart failure. Losartan does not cause a cough and is less likely to cause hyperkalemia than ACE inhibitors. Overall, losartan is well tolerated, and the incidence of most adverse effects is similar to that of placebo.

Losartan is readily absorbed and rapidly metabolized by the cytochrome P450 liver enzymes to an active metabolite. Both losartan and the metabolite are highly bound to plasma albumin, and losartan has a shorter duration of action than its metabolite. When losartan therapy is started, maximal effects on blood pressure usually occur within 3 to 6 weeks. If losartan alone does not control blood pressure, a low dose of a diuretic may be added. A combination product (Hyzaar) with 50 mg of losartan and 12.5 mg of hydrochlorothiazide is available.

ANTIADRENERGICS

Antiadrenergic (sympatholytic) drugs inhibit activity of the SNS. When the SNS is stimulated (see Chap. 17), the nerve impulse travels from the brain and spinal cord to the ganglia. From the ganglia, the impulse travels along postganglionic fibers to effector organs (*e.g.,* heart, blood vessels). Although SNS stimulation produces widespread effects in the body, the effects relevant to this discussion are the increases in heart rate, force of myocardial contraction, cardiac output, and blood pressure that occur. When the nerve impulse is inhibited or blocked at any location along its pathway, the result is decreased blood pressure.

Alpha$_1$-receptor blocking agents (*e.g.,* prazosin) dilate blood vessels and decrease peripheral vascular resistance. These drugs can be used alone or in multidrug regimens. One adverse effect, called the first-dose phenomenon, involves orthostatic hypotension with palpitations, dizziness, and perhaps syncope 1 to 3 hours after the first dose or an increased dose. To prevent this effect, first doses and first increased doses are taken at bedtime. Another effect, associated with long-term use or higher doses, leads to sodium and fluid retention and a need for concurrent diuretic therapy. Alpha$_2$-receptor agonists (*e.g.,* clonidine) stimulate presynaptic alpha$_2$ receptors in the brain. As a result, less norepinephrine is released and sympathetic outflow from the vasomotor center is reduced. Stimulation of presynaptic alpha$_2$ receptors peripherally may also contribute to the decreased sympathetic activity. Reduced sympathetic activity leads to decreased cardiac output, heart rate, peripheral vascular resistance, and blood pressure. Chronic use of clonidine and related drugs may result in sodium and fluid retention, especially with higher doses.

Beta-adrenergic blocking agents (*e.g.,* propranolol) decrease heart rate, force of myocardial contraction, cardiac output, and renin release from the kidneys. Other antiadrenergic drugs include guanethidine and related drugs, which act at postganglionic nerve endings; and two other alpha-blockers (phentolamine and phenoxybenzamine), which occasionally are used in hypertension resulting from catecholamine excess. The latter two drugs are discussed in Chapter 19.

CALCIUM CHANNEL BLOCKING AGENTS

Calcium channel blockers (*e.g.*, verapamil) are used for several cardiovascular disorders. Their mechanism of action and use in the treatment of tachyarrhythmias and angina pectoris are discussed in Chapters 52 and 53, respectively. In hypertension, they mainly decrease peripheral vascular resistance. The decrease in peripheral vascular resistance stems largely from their ability to dilate peripheral arteries.

Most of the available drugs are approved for use in hypertension. Nifedipine is often used to treat hypertensive emergencies or urgencies. Because it is available only in a capsule, various methods have been used to obtain rapid drug action; these methods include puncturing the capsule and squeezing the contents under the tongue. Studies indicate that the drug is not absorbed through oral mucosa and that its effects result from the swallowed drug. Thus, clients should bite and swallow the capsule when rapid lowering of blood pressure is the desired effect. Do *not* give a long-acting form of nifedipine by this method; toxicity may result.

DIURETICS

Antihypertensive effects of diuretics are usually attributed to sodium and water depletion. In fact, diuretics generally produce the same effects as severe dietary sodium restriction. In many cases of hypertension, diuretic therapy alone may lower blood pressure. When diuretic therapy is begun, blood volume and cardiac output decrease. With long-term administration of a diuretic, cardiac output returns to normal, but there is a persistent decrease in peripheral vascular resistance. This has been attributed to a persistent small reduction in extracellular water and plasma volume, decreased receptor sensitivity to vasopressor substances such as angiotensin, direct arteriolar vasodilation, and arteriolar vasodilation secondary to electrolyte depletion in the vessel wall.

In moderate or severe hypertension that does not respond to a diuretic alone, the diuretic may be continued and another antihypertensive drug added, or monotherapy with a different type of antihypertensive drug may be tried.

The most commonly used diuretics are the thiazides (*e.g.*, hydrochlorothiazide [HydroDIURIL]). Others are useful in particular circumstances; see Chapter 56 for more information regarding diuretic drugs.

VASODILATORS (DIRECT ACTING)

Vasodilator antihypertensive drugs directly relax smooth muscle in blood vessels to cause dilation and decreased peripheral vascular resistance. They also reduce afterload and may be used in treatment of heart failure. Hydralazine and minoxidil act mainly on arterioles; nitroprusside acts on arterioles and venules. These drugs have a limited effect on hypertension when used alone because the vasodilating action that lowers blood pressure also stimulates the SNS and arouses reflexive compensatory mechanisms (vasoconstriction, tachycardia, and increased cardiac output), which raise blood pressure. This effect can be prevented during long-term therapy by also giving a drug that prevents excessive sympathetic stimulation (*e.g.*, propranolol). These drugs also cause sodium and water retention, which may be minimized by giving a diuretic concomitantly.

Individual Drugs

Diuretics are discussed in Chapter 56 and listed in Table 56-1. Antihypertensive agents are shown in Table 55-1; antihypertensive–diuretic combination products are listed in Table 55-2.

(*text continues on page 712*)

TABLE 55-1	**ANTIHYPERTENSIVE DRUGS**	
	Routes and Dosage Ranges	
Generic/Trade Name	*Adults*	*Children**
Angiotensin II Antagonist		
Losartan (Cozaar)	PO, initial dose 50 mg (25 mg for those who have hepatic impairment or are taking a diuretic). Maintenance dose 25–100 mg daily, in one or two divided doses, adjusted according to blood pressure control.	
Angiotensin-Converting Enzyme (ACE) Inhibitors		
Benazepril (Lotensin)	PO 10 mg once daily initially, increased to 40 mg daily if necessary, in one or two doses	

TABLE 55-1 ANTIHYPERTENSIVE DRUGS (Continued)

Generic/ Trade Name	Routes and Dosage Ranges	
	Adults	*Children*
Captopril (Capoten)	PO 25 mg two to three times daily initially, increased after 1–2 wk if necessary to 50 mg two to three times daily, then to 100 mg two to three times daily, then to 150 mg two to three times daily. Maximal dose, 450 mg/d.	Children PO initially 1.5 mg/kg/d in divided doses, q8h; maximum dose 6 mg/kg/d Neonates PO 0.03–0.15 mg/kg/d, q8–24h. Maximum dose, 2 mg/kg/d PO 0.15 mg q12–24h
Enalapril (Vasotec)	PO 5 mg once daily, increased to 10–40 mg daily, in one or two doses, if necessary	
Fosinopril (Monopril)	Same as benazepril, above	
Lisinopril (Prinivil, Zestril)	PO 10 mg once daily, increased to 40 mg if necessary	
Moexipril (Univasc)	PO, initial dose 7.5 mg (3.75 mg for those who have renal impairment or are taking a diuretic). Maintenance dose 7.5–30 mg daily, in one or two divided doses, adjusted according to blood pressure control.	
Quinapril (Accupril)	PO 10 mg once daily initially, increased to 20, 40, or 80 mg daily if necessary, in one or two doses. Wait at least 2 wk between dose increments	
Ramipril (Altace)	PO 2.5 mg once daily, increased to 20 mg daily if necessary, in one or two doses	
Trandolapril (Mavik)	PO, initial dose 1 mg once daily (0.5 mg for those who have hepatic or renal impairment or are taking a diuretic; 2 mg for African-Americans). Usual maintenance dose 2–4 mg daily, in a single dose, adjusted according to blood pressure control	
Antiadrenergic Agents		
Alpha₁-Blocking Agents		
Doxazosin (Cardura)	PO 1 mg once daily initially, increased to 2 mg, then to 4, 8, and 16 mg if necessary	
Prazosin (Minipress)	PO 1 mg two to three times daily initially, increased if necessary to a total daily dose of 20 mg in divided doses. Average maintenance dose, 6–15 mg/d.	
Terazosin (Hytrin)	PO 1 mg at bedtime initially, increased gradually to maintenance dose, usually 1–5 mg once daily	
Alpha₂-agonists		
Clonidine (Catapres)	PO 0.1 mg two times daily initially, gradually increased if necessary up to 2.4 mg/d. Average maintenance dose, 0.2–0.8 mg/d.	PO 5–25 µg/kg/d, in divided doses, q6h; increase at 5- to 7-d intervals, if needed
Guanabenz (Wytensin)	PO 4 mg twice daily, increased by 4–8 mg daily every 1–2 wk if necessary to a maximal dose of 32 mg twice daily	
Guanfacine (Tenex)	PO 1 mg daily at bedtime, increased to 2 mg after 3–4 wk, then to 3 mg if necessary	
Methyldopa (Aldomet)	PO 250 mg two or three times daily initially, increased gradually at intervals of not less than 2 d until blood pressure is controlled or a daily dose of 3 g is reached	PO 10 mg/kg/d in two to four divided doses initially, increased or decreased according to response. Maximal dose, 65 mg/kg/d or 3 g daily, whichever is less.

(continued)

TABLE 55-1	ANTIHYPERTENSIVE DRUGS (Continued)	

	Routes and Dosage Ranges	
Generic/Trade Name	*Adults*	*Children*
Postganglionic-Active Drugs		
Guanadrel (Hylorel)	PO 10 mg daily initially. Usual dosage range, 20–75 mg daily in divided doses.	
Guanethidine sulfate (Ismelin)	PO 10 mg daily initially, increased every 5–7 d to a maximal daily dose of 300 mg if necessary. Usual daily dose, 25–50 mg. For hospitalized clients, therapy may be initiated with 25–50 mg daily and increased every 1–2 d.	PO 0.2 mg/kg/d initially, increased by the same amount every 7–10 d if necessary to a maximum dose of 3 mg/kg/d
Reserpine (Serpasil)	PO 0.25–0.5 mg daily initially for 1–2 wk, reduced slowly to 0.1–0.25 mg daily for maintenance	
Beta-Adrenergic Blocking Agents		
Acebutolol (Sectral)	PO 400 mg once daily initially, increased to 800 mg daily if necessary	
Atenolol (Tenormin)	PO 50 mg once daily initially, increased in 1–2 wk to 100 mg once daily, if necessary	
Betaxolol (Kerlone)	PO 10–20 mg daily	
Bisoprolol (Zebeta)	PO 5 mg once daily, increased to a maximum dose of 20 mg daily if necessary	
Carteolol (Cartrol)	PO 2.5 mg once daily initially, gradually increased to a maximum daily dose of 10 mg if necessary. Usual maintenance dose, 2.5–5 mg once daily. Extend dosage interval to 48 h for a creatinine clearance of 20–60 ml/min and to 72 h for a creatinine clearance below 20 ml/min.	
Metoprolol (Lopressor)	PO 50 mg twice daily, gradually increased in weekly or longer intervals if necessary, to maximal daily dose of 450 mg	
Nadolol (Corgard)	PO 40 mg daily initially, gradually increased if necessary, by 40–80 mg daily. Average daily dose, 80–320 mg.	
Penbutolol (Levatol)	PO 20 mg once daily	
Pindolol (Visken)	PO 5 mg two or three times daily initially, increased by 10 mg/d at 3- to 4-wk intervals to a maximal daily dose of 60 mg	
Propranolol (Inderal)	PO 40 mg twice daily initially, gradually increased to 160–640 mg daily	PO 1 mg/kg/d initially, gradually increased to a maximum dose of 10 mg/kg/d
Timolol (Blocadren)	PO 10 mg twice daily initially, increased gradually if necessary. Average daily dose, 20–40 mg; maximal daily dose, 60 mg.	
Alpha-Beta-Adrenergic Blocking Agents		
Carvedilol (Coreg)	PO 6.25 mg twice daily for 7–14 d, then increase to 12.5 mg twice daily for 7–14 d, then increase to a maximal dose of 25 mg twice daily if tolerated and needed	
Labetalol (Trandate, Normodyne)	PO 100 mg twice daily, increased by 100 mg twice daily every 2–3 d if necessary. Usual maintenance dose, 200–400 mg twice daily. Severe hypertension may require 1200–2400 mg daily.	

TABLE 55-1   ANTIHYPERTENSIVE DRUGS (Continued)

Generic/Trade Name	Routes and Dosage Ranges	
	Adults	*Children*
	IV injection, 20 mg slowly over 2 min, followed by 40–80 mg every 10 min until the desired blood pressure is achieved or 300 mg has been given. IV infusion, add 200 mg to 250 ml of 5% dextrose or 0.9% sodium chloride solution (concentration 2 mg/3 ml) and infuse at a rate of 3 ml/min. Adjust flow rate according to blood pressure, and substitute oral labetalol when blood pressure is controlled.	
Calcium Channel Blocking Agents		
Amlodipine (Norvasc)	PO 5–10 mg once daily	
Diltiazem (sustained release) (Cardizem SR)	PO 60–120 mg twice daily	
Felodipine (Plendil)	PO 5–10 mg once daily. Extended-release tablets; swallow whole, do not crush or chew.	
Isradipine (DynaCirc)	PO 2.5–5 mg twice daily	
Nicardipine (Cardene, Cardene SR, Cardene IV)	PO 20–40 mg three times daily; sustained release, PO 30–60 mg twice daily; IV infusion 5–15 mg/h.	
Nifedipine (Adalat, Procardia, Procardia XL)	Immediate release, PO 10 mg for hypertensive crisis (have client bite and swallow capsule); sustained release, PO 30–60 mg once daily, increased over 1–2 wk if necessary	
Nisoldipine (Sular)	PO, initially 20 mg once daily, increased by 10 mg/wk or longer intervals to a maximum of 60 mg daily. Average maintenance dose, 20–40 mg daily. Adults with liver impairment or over 65 y old, PO, initially 10 mg once daily	
Verapamil (Calan, Isoptin, Calan SR, Isoptin SR)	Immediate release, PO 80 mg three times daily; sustained release, PO 240 mg once daily	
Vasodilators, Direct Acting		
Hydralazine (Apresoline)	Chronic hypertension, PO 10 mg four times daily for 2–4 d, increased to 25 mg four times daily for 2–4 d if necessary, then increased to 50 mg four times daily if necessary, to a maximal dose of 300 mg/d Hypertensive crisis, IM, IV 10–20 mg, increased to 40 mg if necessary. Repeat dose as needed.	Chronic hypertension, 0.75 mg/kg/d initially in four divided doses. Gradually increased over 3–4 wk to a maximal dose of 7.5 mg/kg/d if necessary Hypertensive crisis, IM, IV 0.1–0.2 mg/kg per dose every 4–6 h as needed
Minoxidil (Loniten)	PO 5 mg once daily initially, increased gradually until blood pressure is controlled. Average daily dose, 10–40 mg; maximal daily dose, 100 mg in single or divided doses	Age under 12 y, PO 0.2 mg/kg/d initially as a single dose, increased gradually until blood pressure is controlled. Average daily dose, 0.25–1.0 mg/kg; maximal dose, 50 mg/d.
Sodium nitroprusside (Nipride)	IV infusion at a flow rate to deliver 0.5–10 µg/kg/min. Average dose is 3 µg/kg/min. Prepare solution by adding 50 mg of sodium nitroprusside to 250–1000 ml of 5% dextrose in water, and wrap promptly in aluminum foil to protect from light.	Same as for adults.

*Children's dosages from *Drug Facts and Comparisons* (1996) and the National High Blood Pressure Education Program Working Group on Hypertension Control in Children and Adolescents (1996).

TABLE 55-2 ORAL ANTIHYPERTENSIVE COMBINATION PRODUCTS*

	Components						
Trade Name	Angiotensin II Antagonist	Angiotensin Converting Enzyme Inhibitor	Beta-blocker	Calcium Blocker	Diuretic	Non-beta-blocker Antiadrenergic	Dosage Ranges
Aldoril					Hydrochlorothiazide (HCTZ) 15, 25, 30, or 50 mg	Methyldopa 250 or 500 mg	1 tablet two to three times daily for 48 h, then adjusted according to response
Capozide		Captopril 25 or 50 mg			HCTZ† 15 or 25 mg		1 tablet two to three times daily
Combipres					Chlorthalidone 15 mg	Clonidine 0.1, 0.2, or 0.3 mg	1 tablet twice daily
Corzide			Nadolol 40 or 80 mg		Bendroflumethiazide 5 mg		1 tablet daily
Hyzaar	Losartan 50 mg				HCTZ† 12.5 mg		1 tablet once daily
Inderide			Propranolol 40 or 80 mg		HCTZ† 25 mg		1–2 tablets twice daily
Inderide LA			Propranolol 80, 120, or 160 mg		HCTZ† 50 mg		1 capsule once daily
Lopressor HCT			Metoprolol 50 or 100 mg		HCTZ† 25 or 50 mg		1–2 tablets daily

Trade Name	Antihypertensive Agent(s)	Diuretic	Dose
Lotensin HCT	Benazepril 5, 10, or 20 mg	HCTZ† 6.25, 12.5, or 25 mg	
Lotrel	Benazepril 10 or 20 mg; Amlodipine 2.5 or 5 mg		
Minizide	Prazosin 1, 2, or 5 mg	Polythiazide 0.5 mg	1 capsule two to three times daily
Prinzide	Lisinopril 10 or 20 mg	HCTZ† 12.5 or 25 mg	
Tarka	Trandolapril 1, 2, or 4 mg; Verapamil 180 or 240 mg		1 tablet daily
Tenoretic	Atenolol 50 or 100 mg	Chlorthalidone 25 mg	1 tablet daily
Timolide	Timolol 10 mg	HCTZ† 25 mg	1–2 tablets one or two times daily
Vaseretic	Enalapril	HCTZ† 25 mg	1–2 tablets daily
Zestoretic	Lisinopril 10 or 20 mg	HCTZ† 12.5 or 25 mg	1 tablet daily
Ziac	Bisoprolol 2.5, 5, or 10 mg	HCTZ† 6.25 mg	1 tablet daily

*Note that one trade name product may be available in multiple formulations, with variable amounts of antihypertensive, diuretic or both components.

†HCTZ = hydrochlorothiazide.

711

Nursing Process

Assessment

Assess the client's condition in relation to hypertension.

- Identify conditions and risk factors that may lead to hypertension. These include
  - Obesity
  - Elevated serum cholesterol and triglycerides
  - Cigarette smoking
  - Sedentary lifestyle
  - Family history of hypertension or other cardiovascular disease
  - African-American race
  - Renal disease (*e.g.*, renal artery stenosis)
  - Adrenal disease (*e.g.*, hypersecretion of aldosterone, pheochromocytoma)
  - Other cardiovascular disorders (*e.g.*, atherosclerosis, left ventricular hypertrophy)
  - Diabetes mellitus
  - Oral contraceptives, corticosteroids, appetite suppressants, nasal decongestants, nonsteroidal anti-inflammatory agents
  - Neurologic disorders (*e.g.*, brain damage)
- Observe for signs and symptoms of hypertension.
  - Check blood pressure accurately and repeatedly. As a rule, multiple measurements in which systolic pressure is above 140 mm Hg, diastolic pressure is above 90 mm Hg, or both are necessary to establish a diagnosis of hypertension.

    The importance of accurate blood pressure measurements cannot be overemphasized because there are many possibilities for errors. Some ways to improve accuracy and validity include using correct equipment (*e.g.*, proper cuff size), having the client in the same position each time blood pressure is measured (*e.g.*, sitting or supine with arm at heart level), using the same arm for repeated measurements, and having the same person do successive recordings on a particular client.
  - In most cases of early hypertension, elevated blood pressure is the only clinical manifestation. If symptoms do occur, they are usually nonspecific (*e.g.*, headache, weakness, fatigue, tachycardia, dizziness, palpitations, epistaxis).
  - Eventually, signs and symptoms occur as target organs are damaged. Heart damage is often reflected as angina pectoris, myocardial infarction, or congestive heart failure. Chest pain, tachycardia, dyspnea, fatigue, and edema may occur. Brain damage may be indicated by transient ischemic attacks or strokes of varying severity with symptoms ranging from syncope to hemiparesis. Renal damage may be reflected by proteinuria, increased blood urea nitrogen, and increased serum creatinine. Ophthalmoscopic examination may reveal hemorrhages, sclerosis of arterioles, and inflammation of the optic nerve (papilledema). Because arterioles can be visualized in the retina of the eye, damage to retinal vessels may indicate damage to arterioles in the heart, brain, and kidneys.

Nursing Diagnoses

- Decreased Cardiac Output related to disease process or drug therapy
- Anxiety related to fear of myocardial infarction or stroke
- Ineffective Individual Coping related to long-term lifestyle changes and drug therapy
- Noncompliance related to lack of knowledge about hypertension and its management, costs and adverse effects of drug therapy, and psychosocial factors
- Body Image Disturbance related to the need for long-term treatment and medical supervision
- Fatigue related to antihypertensive drug therapy
- Knowledge Deficit related to hypertension, antihypertensive drug therapy, and nondrug lifestyle changes
- Sexual Dysfunction related to adverse drug effects
- Risk for Injury related to drug-induced hypotension and dizziness

Planning/Goals

The client will:

- Receive or take antihypertensive drugs correctly
- Be monitored closely for therapeutic and adverse drug effects, especially when drug therapy is started and when changes are made in drugs or dosages
- Use nondrug measures to assist in blood pressure control
- Avoid, manage, or report adverse drug reactions
- Verbalize or demonstrate knowledge of prescribed drugs and recommended lifestyle changes
- Keep follow-up appointments

Interventions

Implement measures to prevent or minimize hypertension. Preventive measures are mainly lifestyle changes to reduce risk factors. These measures should be started in childhood and continued throughout life. Once hypertension is diagnosed, lifetime adherence to a therapeutic regimen may be necessary to control the disease and prevent complications. The nurse's role is important in the prevention, early detection, and treatment of hypertension. Some guidelines for intervention at community, family, and personal levels include the following:

- Participate in programs to promote healthful lifestyles (*e.g.*, improving eating habits, increasing exercise, managing stress more effectively, and decreasing cigarette smoking).
- Participate in community screening programs, and make appropriate referrals when abnormal blood pressures are detected. If hypertension develops in women taking oral contraceptives, the drug is usually discontinued for 3 to 6 months to see whether blood pressure decreases without antihypertensive drugs.
- Help the hypertensive client comply with prescribed therapy. Noncompliance is high among clients with hypertension. Reasons often given for noncompliance include lack of symptoms, lack of motivation and self-discipline to make needed lifestyle changes (*e.g.*, lose weight, stop smoking, restrict salt intake), perhaps experiencing more symptoms from medications than from hypertension, the cost of therapy, and the client's failure to realize the importance of treatment, es-

pecially as related to prevention of major cardiovascular diseases (myocardial infarction, stroke, and death). In addition, several studies have shown that compliance decreases as the number of drugs and number of doses increase.

The nurse can help increase compliance by teaching the client about hypertension, helping the client make necessary lifestyle changes, and maintaining supportive interpersonal relationships. Losing weight, stopping smoking, and other changes are most likely to be effective if attempted one at a time.

Teach clients:

- About the disease process of hypertension, including factors thought to cause or aggravate it
- That hypertension can be controlled by appropriate treatment
- That hypertension rarely causes symptoms unless complications occur
- That uncontrolled hypertension may lead to stroke, myocardial infarction, and kidney failure
- That antihypertensive drug therapy is usually long term, may require more than one drug, and produces side effects. Inform the client that he or she may not feel well when a medication is started or when dosage is increased, that drugs must be taken as prescribed for optimal benefits, and that changes in drugs or dosages may be needed to increase effectiveness or decrease side effects.
- That no antihypertensive drug should be stopped abruptly. If problems develop, they should be discussed with the clinician who is treating the hypertension. If treatment is stopped, blood pressure usually increases gradually as the medication(s) are eliminated from the body. Sometimes, however, blood pressure rapidly increases to pretreatment levels or even higher. With any of these situations, the client is at risk of a heart attack or stroke. In addition, stopping one drug of a multidrug regimen may lead to increased adverse effects as well as decreased antihypertensive effectiveness.

Evaluation

Observe for blood pressure measurements within goal or more nearly normal ranges.

Observe and interview regarding compliance with instructions about drug therapy and lifestyle changes.

Observe and interview regarding adverse drug effects.

Principles of Therapy

THERAPEUTIC REGIMENS

Once the diagnosis of hypertension is established, a therapeutic regimen must be designed and implemented.

The goal of treatment for most clients is to achieve and maintain normal blood pressure range (below 140/90). If this goal cannot be achieved, lowering blood pressure to any extent is still considered beneficial in decreasing the incidence of coronary artery disease and stroke.

The Joint National Committee on Detection, Evaluation, and Treatment of High Blood Pressure recommends a treatment algorithm in which initial interventions are lifestyle modifications (*i.e.,* reduction of weight and sodium intake, regular physical activity, moderate alcohol intake, and no smoking). If these modifications do not produce goal blood pressure or substantial progress toward goal blood pressure within 3 to 6 months, they should be continued along with an antihypertensive drug. Although the Committee recommends monotherapy (use of one antihypertensive drug) with a diuretic or a beta-blocker because research studies demonstrate reduced morbidity and mortality with these agents, a drug from another classification (*e.g.,* ACE inhibitors, angiotensin II receptor antagonists, calcium channel blockers, alpha$_1$-adrenergic blockers) may also be used effectively.

If the initial drug (and dose) does not produce the desired blood pressure, options for further treatment include increasing the drug dose, substituting another drug, or adding a second drug from a different group. If the response is still inadequate, a second or third drug may be added, including a diuretic if not previously prescribed. When current treatment is ineffective, reassess the client's compliance with lifestyle modifications and drug therapy. In addition, review other factors that may be sabotaging the therapeutic regimen, such as over-the-counter appetite suppressants or nasal decongestants, which raise blood pressure.

DRUG SELECTION

Because many effective antihypertensive drugs are available, choices depend primarily on client characteristics and responses. Some general guidelines include the following:

1. **ACE inhibitors** may be effective alone in white hypertensive clients or in combination with a diuretic in African-American hypertensive clients.
2. **Antiadrenergics** may be effective in any hypertensive population. **Alpha agonists and antagonists** are most often used in multidrug regimens for stages 2, 3, or 4, because they may cause postural hypotension and syncope. Clonidine is available in a skin patch that is applied once a week and reportedly reduces adverse effects and increases compliance. An additional advantage of transdermal clonidine is that it can be used by patients who cannot take oral medications. A disadvantage of this system is a delayed

onset of effect (2 to 3 days) so other antihypertensive medications must also be given during the first 2 to 3 days of clonidine transdermal therapy. Other disadvantages include cost, a 20% incidence of local skin rash or irritation, and a 2- to 3-day delay in "offset" of action when transdermal therapy is discontinued. **Beta-blockers** may be the drugs of first choice for clients under 50 years old with high renin hypertension, tachycardia, angina pectoris, or left ventricular hypertrophy. Most beta-blockers are approved for use in hypertension and are probably equally effective. However, the cardioselective drugs (see Chap. 19) are preferred for hypertensive clients who also have asthma, peripheral vascular disease, or diabetes mellitus.

3. **Calcium channel blockers** may be used for monotherapy or in combination with other drugs. They may be especially useful for hypertensive clients who also have angina pectoris or other cardiovascular disorders.

4. **Diuretics** are usually preferred for initial therapy in older clients and African-American hypertensive clients. They are usually included in any multidrug regimen for these and other populations. Thiazide and related diuretics are equally effective. Hydrochlorothiazide is commonly used.

5. **Vasodilators** are usually used in combination with a beta-blocker and a diuretic to prevent hypotension-induced compensatory mechanisms (stimulation of the SNS and fluid retention) that raise blood pressure.

6. **Combination products** usually contain an antiadrenergic drug as the antihypertensive component and a thiazide or related diuretic as the diuretic component. Most are available in various formulations (see Table 55-2). Potential advantages of fixed dose combination products include comparable or improved effectiveness, smaller doses of individual components, fewer adverse effects, improved compliance, and possibly decreased costs.

Historically, combination products were not recommended for initial treatment of hypertension so dosage of each ingredient could be individualized. Then, if individualized dosages of ingredients were comparable to a combination product, the combination product could be used for long-term maintenance therapy. Some authorities are questioning this assumption, citing studies using rational combination products (*i.e.*, two drugs with different mechanisms of action) even in initial therapy.

Dosage Factors

1. Dosage of antihypertensive drugs must be titrated according to individual response. Generally, dosage is started at minimal levels and increased if necessary. Several drugs, including thiazide diuretics, are effective at lower doses than formerly used. Lower doses decrease the incidence and severity of adverse effects.

2. For many clients, it may be more beneficial to add another drug rather than increase dosage. Two or three drugs in small doses may be effective and cause fewer adverse effects than a single drug in large doses. When two or more drugs are given, the dose of each drug may need to be reduced.

Duration of Therapy

Clients who maintain control of their blood pressure for 1 year or so may be candidates for reduced dosages or reduced numbers of drugs. Any such adjustments must be gradual and carefully supervised by a health care provider. Expected benefits include fewer adverse effects and greater compliance.

Sodium Restriction

Any therapeutic regimen for hypertension includes sodium restriction. Severe restrictions are not generally acceptable to clients; however, moderate restrictions (avoiding heavily salted foods, such as cured meats, sandwich meats, pretzels, and potato chips, and not adding salt to food at the table) are beneficial and more easily implemented. These statements are based on research studies that indicate the following:

1. Sodium restriction alone reduces blood pressure.
2. Sodium restriction potentiates the antihypertensive actions of diuretics and other antihypertensive drugs. Conversely, excessive sodium intake decreases the antihypertensive actions of all antihypertensive drugs. Patients with unrestricted salt intake who are taking thiazides may lose excessive potassium and become hypokalemic.
3. Sodium restriction may decrease dosage requirements of antihypertensive drugs, thereby decreasing the incidence and severity of adverse effects.

Genetic/Ethnic Considerations

For most antihypertensive drugs, there have been few research studies comparing their effects in different genetic or ethnic groups. However, several studies indicate that beta-blockers have greater effects in people of Asian heritage, compared with their effects in white people. For hypertension, Asians generally need much smaller doses because they metabolize and excrete beta-blockers slowly. In African-Americans, diuretics are effective and recommended as initial drug therapy; calcium channel blockers, alpha$_1$ receptor blockers, and the alpha–beta-blocker labetalol are reportedly equally effective in African-American and white people. ACE inhibitors and beta-blockers are less effective as mono-therapy in African-Americans. When beta-blockers are used, they are usually one component of a multidrug regimen, and higher doses may be required. Overall, African-Americans are more likely to have severe hypertension and require multiple drugs.

USE IN SURGICAL CLIENTS

The Joint National Committee on Detection, Evaluation, and Treatment of High Blood Pressure recommends that drug therapy be continued until surgery and restarted as soon as possible after surgery. If clients cannot take drugs orally, parenteral diuretics, antiadrenergic agents, ACE inhibitors, calcium blockers, or vasodilators may be given to avoid the rebound hypertension associated with abrupt discontinuance of some antiadrenergic anti-hypertensive agents. Transdermal clonidine also may be used. The anesthesiologist and surgeon must be informed about the client's medication status.

USE IN RENAL IMPAIRMENT

In hypertensive clients with primary renal disease or di-abetic nephropathy, drug therapy may slow progres-sion of renal impairment. Sodium retention may be a causative factor, so diuretics are important in treatment. Thiazides should be used cautiously if at all; metolazone (Zaroxolyn) is the only thiazide or related drug with sig-nificant diuretic activity if serum creatinine is above 2 mg/dl, and relatively large doses may be required. Loop diuretics, such as furosemide (Lasix), are more often used, and relatively large doses may be required. Anti-adrenergics, vasodilators, and ACE inhibitors are usually effective in renal disease. Dosage of ACE inhibitors should be reduced in clients with renal impairment.

USE IN HYPERTENSIVE URGENCIES AND EMERGENCIES

Hypertensive urgencies and emergencies involve dan-gerously high blood pressures, with actual or potential damage to target organs. Although there are risks with severe hypertension, there are also risks associated with lowering blood pressure excessively or too rapidly, including stroke, myocardial infarction, and acute renal failure. Thus, the goal of treatment is usually to lower blood pressure rather gradually, over several minutes to several hours, with careful titration of drug dosage to avoid precipitous drops.

Urgencies can be treated with oral antihypertensive agents such as: **Captopril** 25 to 50 mg q1–2 h; **cloni-dine** 0.2 mg initially, then 0.1 mg hourly until diastolic blood pressure falls below 110 mm Hg or 0.7 mg has been given; **nifedipine** 10 mg (often given sublin-gually, but nifedipine is not absorbed across the mu-cosa and must be swallowed. Rapid effects are ob-tained by perforating the capsule or having the patient bite the capsule).

A hypertensive emergency, defined as a diastolic pressure of 120 mm Hg or higher and target organ dam-age, requires administration of an IV antihypertensive drug. The goal of treatment is usually to lower diastolic pressure to 100 to 110 mm Hg and maintain it there for several days to allow adjustment of the physiologic mechanisms that normally regulate blood pressure. Then, the blood pressure can be lowered to normoten-sive levels.

Any one of several antihypertensive drugs can be given IV to treat a hypertensive emergency. **Nitroprus-side** is often the drug of first choice because it has a rapid onset and short duration of action. It may be given as a continuous infusion at a rate of 0.5 to 8.0 µg/kg/min. Intra-arterial blood pressure should be monitored dur-ing nitroprusside infusion. If nitroprusside must be given longer than 72 hours, serum thiocyanate levels should be measured and the infusion should be stopped if the level is more than 12 mg/dl.

IV **nitroglycerin** is also very effective and especially beneficial in patients with both severe hypertension and myocardial ischemia. The dose is titrated accord-ing to blood pressure response and may range from 5 to 100 µg/min. Tolerance develops to IV nitroglycerin over 24 to 48 hours. Other drugs that may be used include IV **hydralazine, labetalol**, and **nicardipine**; see Table 55-1 for dosages.

USE IN CHILDREN

Most principles of managing adult hypertension apply to managing childhood and adolescent hypertension; some additional elements include the following:

1. Children may have primary or secondary hyperten-sion, but the incidence is unknown, and treatment is not well defined. The National High Blood Pressure Education Program Working Group on Hypertension Control in Children and Adolescents recommends blood pressure measurement as part of routine pedi-atric examinations. This is especially important for children who have a hypertensive parent. Some stud-ies indicate that increased blood pressure in children often correlates with hypertension in young adults.

2. National norms have been established for blood pressure in children and adolescents of comparable age, body size (height and weight), and gender. Nor-mal blood pressure is defined as systolic and dia-stolic values less than the 90th percentile; hyperten-sion is defined as an average of systolic or diastolic pressure that equals or exceeds the 95th percentile on three or more occasions. Blood pressure values obtained with a child or adolescent should be com-

pared with the norms and recorded in permanent health care records. Multiple accurate measurements are especially important in diagnosing hypertension because blood pressure may be more labile in children and adolescents.

3. Children have a greater incidence of secondary hypertension than adults. Generally, the higher the blood pressure and the younger the child, the greater the likelihood of secondary hypertension. Diagnostic tests may be needed to rule out renovascular disease or coarctation of the aorta in those under 18 years of age with blood pressure above 140/90 mm Hg and young children with blood pressures above the 95th percentile for their age group. Oral contraceptives may cause secondary hypertension in adolescents.

4. Treatment of hypertension in children and adolescents should generally be very conservative because long-term effects of drug therapy are unknown. Many antihypertensive drugs are not FDA approved for use in children, and their safety and effectiveness in children are unknown. Therefore, sodium restriction and weight reduction, if needed, may be preferred initially. If this approach is unsuccessful, cautious drug therapy is indicated, especially for those with significantly elevated blood pressures or target organ involvement. The fewest drugs and the lowest doses should be used. Thus, if an initial drug is ineffective, it may be better to give a different single drug than to add a second drug to the regimen.

5. Some guidelines for choosing drugs are as follows:
   a. Beta-blockers are used in children of all ages; they should probably be avoided in children with resting pulse rates under 60.
   b. Thiazide diuretics may be used, and they do not commonly produce hyperglycemia, hyperuricemia, or hypercalcemia in children as they do in adults.
   c. ACE inhibitors may be used to treat hypertension in children of all ages, including secondary hypertension and renal insufficiency. Effects are stronger and last longer in newborns and young infants than in older children. Because of teratogenic effects, these drugs should be used very cautiously, if at all, in adolescent girls who may be sexually active.
   d. Calcium channel blockers are used, most often nifedipine, in treating acute and chronic childhood hypertension. With chronic hypertension, immediate-release forms of nifedipine have a short duration of action and require frequent administration, and long-acting forms contain dosages that are not suitable for young children.
   e. Hydralazine (Apresoline) seems to be less effective in childhood and adolescent hypertension than in adult disease.

6. Although all clients with primary hypertension need regular supervision and assessment of blood pressure, this is especially important with young children and adolescents because of growth and developmental changes.

Use in Older Adults

Most principles of managing hypertension in other populations apply to older adults (over 65 years). In addition, the following factors require consideration:

1. There are basically two types of hypertension in older adults. One is systolic hypertension, in which systolic blood pressure is above 160 mm Hg, but diastolic pressure is below 95 mm Hg or normal. The other type, systolic-diastolic hypertension, involves elevations of both systolic and diastolic pressures.

   Until recently, systolic hypertension was considered a normal aspect of aging that did not require treatment. However, ample evidence indicates that both types of hypertension increase cardiovascular morbidity and mortality, especially congestive heart failure and stroke, and should be treated.

2. Nonpharmacologic treatments should be tried alone or with drug therapy. For example, weight reduction and moderate sodium restriction may be the initial treatment of choice if the client is hypertensive and overweight.

3. If antihypertensive drug therapy is required, drugs used for younger adults may be used alone or in combination. A diuretic is usually the drug of first choice in older adults and may be effective alone. ACE inhibitors and calcium channel blocking agents may also be effective as monotherapy; beta-blockers are usually less effective as monotherapy. Additional guidelines for antihypertensive drug therapy include the following:
   a. The goal of drug therapy may be partial reduction of blood pressure rather than achievement of normal levels.
   b. Older adults may be especially susceptible to the adverse effects of antihypertensive drugs because their homeostatic mechanisms are less efficient. For example, if hypotension occurs, the mechanisms that raise blood pressure are less efficient and syncope may occur. In addition, renal and liver function may be reduced, making accumulation of drugs more likely.
   c. Initial drug doses should be about half of the recommended doses for younger adults, and increases should be smaller and spaced at longer intervals. Lower drug doses (*e.g.*, hydrochlorothiazide 12.5 mg daily) are often effective and reduce risks of adverse effects.

d. Blood pressure should be reduced *slowly* to facilitate adequate blood flow through arteriosclerotic vessels. Rapid lowering of blood pressure may produce cerebral insufficiency (syncope, transient ischemic attacks, stroke).

e. If blood pressure control is achieved and maintained for about 6 months, drug dosage should be gradually reduced, if possible.

HOME CARE

Antihypertensive drugs are very commonly used in the home setting, usually self-administered. The home care nurse is most likely to be involved when making home visits for other reasons. Whether the client or another member of the household is taking antihypertensive medications, the home care nurse may be helpful in teaching about the drugs, monitoring for drug effects, and promoting compliance with the prescribed regimen.

Noncompliance with prescribed antihypertensive drug therapy is a major problem, and consequences may be catastrophic. The home care nurse is well situated to assess for actual or potential barriers to compliance. For example, several antihypertensive medications are quite expensive and clients may not take the drugs at all or they may take fewer-than-needed doses. If the nurse's assessment reveals this sort of situation, he or she may contact the prescribing physician and discuss the possibility of using less expensive drugs. If the physician is unwilling to try alternative drugs, the nurse may be able to identify resources for obtaining the needed medications.

ANTIHYPERTENSIVE DRUGS

NURSING ACTIONS	RATIONALE/EXPLANATION
1. Administer accurately **a.** Check blood pressure before each dose, preferably with the client in supine and standing positions.	To monitor therapeutic and adverse responses to drug therapy. This is especially important when initiating drug therapy, changing medications, or changing dosages.
b. Give oral captopril on an empty stomach.	Food decreases drug absorption.
c. Give other oral antihypertensive agents with or after food intake.	To decrease gastric irritation
d. For IV injection of propranolol or labetalol, the client should be attached to a cardiac monitor. In addition, parenteral atropine and isoproterenol (Isuprel) must be readily available.	For early detection and treatment of excessive myocardial depression and arrhythmias. Atropine may be used to treat excessive bradycardia. Isoproterenol may be used to stimulate myocardial contractility and increase cardiac output.
e. Give the first dose and the first increased dose of prazosin, doxazosin, and terazosin at bedtime	To prevent orthostatic hypotension and syncope
f. For nitroprusside administration, consult the manufacturer's instructions.	Nitroprusside is unstable in solution. It requires special mixing procedures and additional dilution in IV fluids.
2. Observe for therapeutic effects Decreased blood pressure. The usual goal is a normal blood pressure (*i.e.,* below 140/90).	The choice of drugs and drug dosages often requires adjustment to maximize beneficial effects and minimize adverse effects. Thus, optimal therapeutic effects may not occur immediately after drug therapy is begun.
3. Observe for adverse effects	Adverse effects are most likely to occur in clients who are elderly, have impaired renal function, and are receiving multiple antihypertensive drugs or large doses of antihypertensive drugs.
a. Postural hypotension, dizziness, weakness	This is an extension of the expected pharmacologic action. Postural hypotension results from drug blockage of com-

(continued)

NURSING ACTIONS	RATIONALE/EXPLANATION
	pensatory reflexes (vasoconstriction, decreased venous pooling in extremities, and increased venous return to the heart) that normally maintain blood pressure in the upright position. This adverse reaction may be aggravated by other conditions that cause vasodilation (*e.g.*, exercise, heat or hot weather, and alcohol consumption). Postural hypotension is more likely to occur with guanethidine, methyldopa, and reserpine.
b. Sodium and water retention, increased plasma volume, perhaps edema and weight gain	These effects result from decreased renal perfusion. This reaction can be prevented or minimized by concurrent administration of a diuretic.
c. Prolonged atrioventricular conduction, bradycardia	Owing to increased vagal tone and stimulation
d. Gastrointestinal disturbances, including nausea, vomiting, and diarrhea	These effects are more likely to occur with hydralazine, methyldopa, propranolol, and captopril.
e. Mental depression (with reserpine)	Apparently caused by decreased levels of catecholamines and serotonin in the brain
f. Bronchospasm or cardiac failure (with propranolol and other beta-adrenergic blocking agents)	Caused by bronchoconstriction and depression of myocardial contractility. These drugs are contraindicated in asthma, other bronchoconstrictive lung diseases, and congestive heart failure.
g. Hypertensive crisis (with abrupt withdrawal of clonidine or guanabenz).	This may be prevented by tapering the prescribed dosage over a period of at least 2–4 days before discontinuing the drug.
h. Cough and hyperkalemia with ACE inhibitors	A chronic, nonproductive cough is a relatively common adverse effect. Hyperkalemia has been reported with 1%–4% of patients.
4. Observe for drug interactions **a.** Drugs that *increase* effects of antihypertensives:	
(1) Alcohol, phenothiazine antipsychotic agents, peripheral vasodilators	Because these drugs have hypotensive effects when used alone, additive hypotension occurs when they are combined with antihypertensive agents.
(2) Digoxin	Additive bradycardia with beta-blockers
b. Drugs that *decrease* effects of antihypertensives:	
(1) Adrenergics	These drugs stimulate the sympathetic nervous system and raise blood pressure. They include over-the-counter nasal decongestants, cold remedies, bronchodilators, and appetite suppressants.
(2) Amphetamines	When given with guanethidine, amphetamines displace guanethidine from its site of action. When given with methyldopa, amphetamines decrease antihypertensive effects by increasing sympathetic activity.
(3) Tricyclic antidepressants	These drugs inhibit the action of clonidine and guanethidine.
(4) MAO inhibitors	Caused by antagonistic effects, which are apparently most significant with guanethidine
(5) Oral contraceptives	Oral contraceptives tend to increase blood pressure, probably by causing retention of sodium and water. When they are given concurrently with antihypertensive agents, dosage of antihypertensives may need to be increased.

NURSING ACTIONS	RATIONALE/EXPLANATION
(6) Nonsteroidal anti-inflammatory drugs	Aspirin, ibuprofen, and related drugs may cause retention of sodium and water.
5. Teach clients a. Name and purpose of each drug	In few other conditions is client education as important as with hypertension. Every effort must be made to aid understanding and compliance with the treatment regimen.
b. Adverse effects to be reported	Adverse effects can sometimes be prevented or minimized by nondrug measures, by changing drugs, or by reducing drug dosage.
c. Measures to control orthostatic hypotension and dizziness. These include the following: move from supine or sitting positions to a standing position slowly; sleep with the head of the bed elevated; wear elastic stockings; exercise legs; avoid prolonged standing; avoid hot baths.	These measures allow adaptation of normal homeostatic mechanisms, avoid vasodilation, and avoid pooling of blood in the extremities. If symptoms still occur, the person should sit or lie down immediately to avoid a fall and possible injury.
d. Do not stop any antihypertensive drug abruptly or without discussion with the prescribing physician.	Several of the drugs may cause rebound hypertension that may be as severe or worse than the original levels. To avoid this phenomenon, antihypertensive drugs should be tapered in dosage and discontinued gradually.

REVIEW AND APPLICATION EXERCISES

1. Describe the physiologic mechanisms that control blood pressure.

2. What are common factors that raise blood pressure?

3. What signs and symptoms occur with hypertension, and how would you assess for them?

4. Why is it important to measure blood pressure accurately and repeatedly?

5. Does all hypertension require nonpharmacologic or pharmacologic treatment? Justify your answer.

6. What are the potential consequences of untreated or inadequately treated hypertension?

7. How do ACE inhibitors, alpha- and beta-adrenergic blockers, calcium channel blockers, and direct vasodilators lower blood pressure?

8. What are adverse effects of each group of antihypertensive drugs, and how may they be prevented or minimized?

9. For a client newly diagnosed with hypertension, outline a teaching plan for lifestyle and pharmacologic interventions.

10. List interventions by health care providers that may help hypertensive clients adhere to their treatment regimens and maintain quality of life.

11. How would you assess a client being treated for hypertension for compliance with the prescribed lifestyle and drug therapy regimen?

SELECTED REFERENCES

Applegate, W.B. (1997). Approach to the elderly patient with hypertension. In W.N. Kelley (Ed.), *Textbook of internal medicine*, 3rd ed., pp. 2482–2488. Philadelphia: Lippincott-Raven.

Brater, D.C. (1997). Clinical pharmacology of cardiovascular drugs. In W.N. Kelley (Ed.), *Textbook of internal medicine*, 3rd ed., pp. 552–569. Philadelphia: Lippincott-Raven.

Drug facts and comparisons. (Updated monthly). St. Louis: Facts and Comparisons.

Epstein, M. & Bakris, G. (1996). Newer approaches to antihypertensive therapy: Use of fixed-dose combination therapy. *Archives of Internal Medicine 156*, 1969–1978.

Guyton, A.C. & Hall, J.E. (1996). *Textbook of medical physiology*, 9th ed. Philadelphia: W.B. Saunders.

Hawkins, D.W., Bussey, H.I., & Prisant, L.M. (1997). Hypertension. In J.T. DiPiro, R.L. Talbert, G.C. Yee, G.R. Matzke, B.G. Wells, & L.M. Posey (Eds.), *Pharmacotherapy: A pathophysiologic approach*, 3rd ed., pp.195–218. Stamford, CT: Appleton & Lange.

Jackson, E.K. & Garrison, J.C. (1996). Renin and angiotensin. In J.G. Hardman, L.E. Limbird, P.B. Molinoff, & R.W. Ruddon (Eds.), *Goodman & Gilman's The pharmacological basis of therapeutics*, 9th ed., pp. 733–758. New York: McGraw-Hill.

Joint National Committee on Detection, Evaluation, and Treatment of High Blood Pressure (1993). *The Fifth Report: NIH Publication No. 93-1088.* Bethesda, MD: National Institutes of Health.

Jones, W.N. & Fagan, T.C. (1993). Hypertension. In R. Bressler & M.D. Katz (Eds.), *Geriatric pharmacology,* pp. 79–103. New York: McGraw-Hill.

Messerli, F.H., Weber, M.A. & Brunner, H.R. (1996). Angiotensin II receptor inhibition: A new therapeutic principle. *Archives of Internal Medicine 156,* 1957–1978.

National High Blood Pressure Education Program Working Group (1996). Update on the 1987 task force report on high blood pressure in children and adolescents. *Pediatrics 98,* 649–658.

Oates, J.A. (1996). Antihypertensive agents and the drug therapy of hypertension. In J.G. Hardman, L.E. Limbird, P.B. Molinoff, & R.W. Ruddon (Eds.), *Goodman & Gilman's The pharmacological basis of therapeutics,* 9th ed., pp. 780–808. New York: McGraw-Hill.

Porth, C.M. (1994). Alterations in blood pressure: Hypertension and orthostatic hypotension. In C.M. Porth (Ed.), *Pathophysiology: Concepts of altered health states,* 4th ed., pp. 379–402. Philadelphia: J.B. Lippincott.

Weinberger, M.H. (1997). Systemic hypertension. In W.N. Kelley (Ed.), *Textbook of internal medicine,* 3rd ed., pp. 175–183. Philadelphia: Lippincott-Raven.

56 Diuretics

Objectives

After studying this chapter, the student will be able to:

1 List characteristics of diuretics in terms of mechanism of action, indications for use, principles of therapy, and nursing process implications.

2 Discuss major adverse effects of thiazide, loop, and potassium-sparing diuretics.

3 Identify clients at risk of developing adverse reactions to diuretic administration.

4 Recognize commonly used potassium-losing and potassium-sparing diuretics.

5 Discuss the rationale for using combination products containing a potassium-losing and a potassium-sparing diuretic.

6 Teach clients the importance of taking diuretics and potassium supplements as prescribed.

7 Discuss important elements of diuretic therapy in older adults.

Key Terms

Ascites	Hypokalemia
Dehydration	Hyperglycemia
Diuresis	Hyperkalemia
Edema	Hyperuricemia

Description

Diuretics are drugs that increase renal excretion of water, sodium, and other electrolytes, thereby increasing urine formation and output. Diuretics are important therapeutic agents widely used in the treatment of edematous (*e.g.,* congestive heart failure, renal and hepatic disease) and nonedematous (*e.g.,* hypertension, ophthalmic surgery) conditions. To aid understanding of diuretic drug therapy, renal physiology related to drug action and characteristics of edema are reviewed before further discussion of the drugs. Individual diuretics are listed in Table 56-1.

Renal Physiology

The primary function of the kidneys is to regulate the volume, composition, and pH of body fluids. The kidneys receive about 25% of the cardiac output. From this large amount of blood flowing through it, the normally functioning kidney is efficient in retaining substances needed by the body and eliminating those not needed.

THE NEPHRON

The nephron is the functional unit of the kidney; each kidney contains about 1 million nephrons. Each nephron is composed of a glomerulus and a tubule (Fig. 56-1). The glomerulus is a network of capillaries that receives blood from the renal artery. Bowman's capsule is a thin-walled structure that surrounds the glomerulus, then narrows and continues as the tubule. The tubule is a thin-walled structure of epithelial cells surrounded by peritubular capillaries. The tubule is divided into three segments (the proximal tubule, loop of Henle, and distal tubule), which differ in structure and function. The tubules are often called "convoluted" tubules because of their many twists and turns. The convolutions provide a large surface area of close proximity between the blood flowing through the peritubular capillaries and the glomerular filtrate flowing through the tubular lumen. Consequently, substances can be readily exchanged through the walls of the tubules.

The nephron functions by three processes: glomerular filtration, tubular reabsorption, and tubular secretion. These processes normally maintain the fluid volume, electrolyte concentration, and pH of body fluids within a relatively narrow range. They also remove waste products of cellular metabolism. A minimum daily urine output of about 400 ml is required to remove normal amounts of metabolic end-products.

GLOMERULAR FILTRATION

Arterial blood enters the glomerulus by the afferent arteriole at the relatively high pressure of about 70 mm Hg. This pressure "pushes" water, electrolytes, and other solutes out of the capillaries into Bowman's capsule and then to the proximal tubule. This fluid, called *glomerular filtrate,* contains the same components as blood except for blood cells, fats, and proteins.

The glomerular filtration rate is about 180 L/d, or 125 ml/min. Most of this fluid is reabsorbed as the glomerular filtrate travels through the tubules. The end-product is about 2 L of urine daily. Urine flows into collecting tubules, which carry it to the renal pelvis. From the renal pelvis, urine flows through the ureters, bladder, and urethra for elimination from the body.

Blood that does not become part of the glomerular filtrate travels out of the glomerulus through the efferent arteriole. The efferent arteriole branches into the peritubular capillaries, which eventually empty into veins and return the blood to the systemic circulation.

TUBULAR REABSORPTION

The term *reabsorption,* in relation to renal function, indicates movement of substances from the tubule (glomerular filtrate) to the blood in the peritubular capillaries. Most reabsorption occurs in the proximal tubule. Almost all glucose and amino acids are reabsorbed; about 80% of water, sodium, potassium, chloride, and most other substances is reabsorbed. As a result, only some of the glomerular filtrate (about 20%) enters the loop of Henle. In the descending limb of the loop of Henle, water is reabsorbed; in the ascending limb, sodium is reabsorbed. A large fraction of the total amount of sodium (up to 30%) filtered by the glomeruli is reabsorbed in the loop of Henle. Additional sodium is reabsorbed in the distal tubule, primarily by the exchange of sodium ions for potassium ions secreted by epithelial cells of tubular walls. Final reabsorption of water occurs in the distal tubule and small collecting tubules. The remaining water and solutes are now correctly called urine.

Antidiuretic hormone from the posterior pituitary gland promotes reabsorption of water from the distal tubules and the collecting ducts of the kidneys. This conserves water needed by the body and produces a more concentrated urine. Aldosterone, a hormone from the adrenal cortex, promotes sodium–potassium exchange mainly in the distal tubule and collecting ducts. Thus, aldosterone promotes sodium reabsorption and potassium loss.

TUBULAR SECRETION

The term *secretion,* in relation to renal function, indicates movement of substances from blood in the peritubular capillaries to glomerular filtrate flowing through the renal tubules. Secretion occurs in the proximal and distal tubules, across the epithelial cells that line the tubules. In the proximal tubule, uric acid, creatinine, hydrogen ions, and ammonia are secreted; in the distal

TABLE 56-1 DIURETIC AGENTS

Generic/Trade Name	Routes and Dosage Ranges	
	Adults	*Children*
Thiazide and Related Diuretics		
Bendroflumethiazide (Naturetin)	PO 5 mg daily initially. For maintenance, 2.5–20 mg daily or intermittently	PO up to 0.4 mg/kg/d initially, in two divided doses. For maintenance, 0.05–0.1 mg/kg/d in a single dose.
Benzthiazide (Exna)	PO 50–200 mg daily for several days initially, depending on response. For maintenance, dosage is gradually reduced to the minimal effective amount.	PO 1–4 mg/kg/d initially, in three divided doses. For maintenance, dosage is reduced to the minimal effective amount.
Chlorothiazide (Diuril)	PO 500–1000 mg one or two times daily IV 500 mg twice daily	PO 22 mg/kg/d in two divided doses Infants under age 6 mo, up to 33 mg/kg/d in two divided doses IV not recommended
Chlorthalidone (Hygroton)	PO 25–100 mg daily	PO 3 mg/kg three times weekly, adjusted according to response
Hydrochlorothiazide (HydroDIURIL, Esidrix, Oretic)	PO 25–100 mg one or two times daily Elderly adults, 12.5–25 mg daily	PO 2 mg/kg/d in two divided doses Infants under age 6 mo, up to 3.3 mg/kg/d in two divided doses
Hydroflumethiazide (Saluron)	PO 25–200 mg daily	PO 1 mg/kg/d
Indapamide (Lozol)	PO 2.5–5 mg daily	Dosage not established
Methyclothiazide (Enduron)	PO 2.5–10 mg daily	PO 0.05–0.2 mg/kg/d
Metolazone (Zaroxolyn, Mykrox)	PO 5–20 mg daily, depending on severity of condition and response	
Polythiazide (Renese)	PO 1–4 mg daily, depending on severity of condition and response	PO 0.02–0.08 mg/kg/d
Quinethazone (Hydromox)	PO 50–200 mg daily	Dosage not established
Trichlormethiazide (Metahydrin, Naqua)	PO 2–4 mg one or two times daily initially. For maintenance, 1–4 mg once daily	PO 0.07 mg/kg/d in single or divided doses
Loop Diuretics		
Bumetanide (Bumex)	PO 0.5–2 mg daily as a single dose. May be repeated q4–6h to a maximal dose of 10 mg, if necessary. Giving on alternate days or for 3–4 d with rest periods of 1–2 d is recommended for long-term control of edema. IV, IM 0.5–1 mg, repeated in 2–3 h if necessary, to a maximal daily dose of 10 mg. Give IV injections over 1–2 min.	Not recommended for children under age 18 y
Ethacrynic acid (Edecrin)	Edema, PO 50–100 mg daily, increased or decreased according to severity of condition and response, maximal daily dose, 400 mg Rapid mobilization of edema, IV 50 mg or 0.5–1 mg/kg injected slowly to a maximum of 100 mg/dose	PO 25 mg daily No recommended parenteral dose in children
Furosemide (Lasix)	Edema, PO 20–80 mg as a single dose initially. If an adequate diuretic response is not obtained, dosage may be gradually increased by 20- to 40-mg increments at intervals of 6–8 h. For maintenance, dosage range and frequency of administration vary widely and must be individualized. Maximal daily dose, 600 mg.	PO 2 mg/kg one or two times daily initially, gradually increased by increments of 1–2 mg/kg per dose if necessary at intervals of 6–8 h. Maximal daily dose, 6 mg/kg IV 1 mg/kg initially. If diuretic response is not adequate, increase dosage by 1 mg/kg no sooner than 2 h after previous dose. Maximal dose, 6 mg/kg

(continued)

TABLE 56-1   **DIURETIC AGENTS** (Continued)

Generic/Trade Name	Routes and Dosage Ranges	
	Adults	*Children*
Furosemide (cont)	Hypertension, PO 40 mg twice daily, gradually increased if necessary Rapid mobilization of edema, IV 20–40 mg initially, injected slowly. This dose may be repeated in 2 h. With acute pulmonary edema, initial dose is usually 40 mg, which may be repeated in 60–90 min. Acute renal failure, IV 40 mg initially, increased if necessary. Maximum dose, 1–2 g/24 h Hypertensive crisis, IV 40–80 mg injected over 1–2 min. With renal failure, much larger doses may be needed.	
Torsemide (Demadex)	PO, IV 5–20 mg once daily	
Potassium-Sparing Diuretics		
Amiloride (Midamor)	PO 5–20 mg daily	Dosage not established
Spironolactone (Aldactone)	PO 25–200 mg daily	PO 3.3 mg/kg/d in divided doses
Triamterene (Dyrenium)	PO 100–300 mg daily in divided doses	PO 2–4 mg/kg/d in divided doses
Osmotic Agents		
Glycerin (Osmoglyn)	PO 1–1.5 g/kg of body weight, usually given as a 50% or 75% solution, 1–2 h before ocular surgery	Same as adults
Isosorbide (Ismotic)	PO 1.5–3 g/kg, up to four times daily if necessary for glaucoma or ocular surgery	
Mannitol (Osmitrol)	Diuresis, IV infusion 50–200 g over 24 h, flow rate adjusted to maintain a urine output of 30–50 ml/h Oliguria and prevention of renal failure, IV 50–100g Reduction of intracranial or intraocular pressure, IV 1.5–2 g/kg, given as a 20% solution, over 30–60 min	Same as adults
Combination Diuretic Products		
Hydrochlorothiazide 50 mg and **amiloride** 5 mg (Moduretic)	PO 1–2 tablets daily	
Hydrochlorothiazide 25 mg and **spironolactone** 25 mg (Aldactazide 25/25)	PO 1–8 tablets daily	
Hydrochlorothiazide 50 mg and **spironolactone** 50 mg (Aldactazide 50/50)	PO 1–4 tablets daily	
Hydrochlorothiazide 25 mg and **triamterene** 37.5 mg (Dyazide)	Hypertension, PO 1 capsule twice daily initially, then adjusted according to response Edema, 1–2 capsules twice daily	
Hydrochlorothiazide 50 mg and **triamterene** 75 mg (Maxzide)	PO 1 tablet daily	

Figure 56-1
The nephron is the functional unit of the kidney.

tubule, potassium ions, hydrogen ions, and ammonia are secreted. Secretion of hydrogen ions is important in maintaining acid–base balance in body fluids.

Alterations in Renal Function

Many clinical conditions alter renal function. In some conditions, excessive amounts of substances (*e.g.,* sodium and water) are retained; in others, needed substances (*e.g.,* potassium, proteins) are eliminated. These conditions include cardiovascular, renal, hepatic, and other disorders that may be treated with diuretic drugs.

EDEMA

Edema is the excessive accumulation of fluid in body tissues. It is a symptom of many disease processes and may occur in any part of the body. Additional characteristics include the following:

1. Edema formation results from one or more of the following mechanisms that allow fluid to leave the

bloodstream (intravascular compartment) and enter interstitial spaces.

   a. **Increased capillary permeability** occurs as part of the response to tissue injury. Thus, edema may occur with burns and trauma or allergic and inflammatory reactions.

   b. **Increased capillary hydrostatic pressure** results from a sequence of events in which increased blood volume (from fluid overload or sodium and water retention) or obstruction of venous blood flow causes a high venous pressure and a high capillary pressure. This is the primary mechanism for edema formation in congestive heart failure, pulmonary edema, and renal failure.

   c. **Decreased plasma oncotic pressure** may occur with decreased synthesis of plasma proteins (caused by liver disease or malnutrition) or increased loss of plasma proteins (caused by burn injuries or the nephrotic syndrome). Plasma proteins are important in keeping fluids within the bloodstream. When plasma proteins are lacking, fluid leaves the capillaries and accumulates in tissues.

2. Edema interferes with blood flow to tissues. Thus, it interferes with delivery of oxygen and nutrients and removal of metabolic waste products. If severe, edema may distort body features, impair movement, and interfere with activities of daily living.

3. Specific manifestations of edema are determined by its location and extent. A common type of localized edema occurs in the feet and ankles (dependent edema), especially with prolonged sitting or standing. A less common but more severe type of localized edema is pulmonary edema, a life-threatening condition that occurs with circulatory overload (of intravenous [IV] fluids or blood transfusions, for example) or acute heart failure. Generalized massive edema (anasarca) interferes with the functions of many body organs and tissues.

Diuretic Drugs

Diuretic drugs act on the kidneys to decrease reabsorption of sodium, chloride, water, and other substances. Major subclasses are the thiazides and related diuretics, loop diuretics, and potassium-sparing diuretics. These groups differ from each other primarily because they act at different sites in the nephron.

Major clinical indications for diuretics are edema and hypertension. In edematous states, diuretics mobilize tissue fluids by decreasing plasma volume. In hypertension, the exact mechanism by which diuretics lower blood pressure is unknown, but antihypertensive action is usually attributed to sodium depletion. Initially, diuretics decrease blood volume and cardiac output. With chronic use, cardiac output returns to normal, but there is a persistent decrease in plasma volume and peripheral vascular resistance. Sodium depletion may have a vasodilating effect on arterioles.

Use of diuretic agents in the treatment of congestive heart failure and hypertension is discussed further in Chapters 51 and 55, respectively.

THIAZIDE AND RELATED DIURETICS

Thiazide diuretics are synthetic drugs that are chemically related to the sulfonamides. Chlorothiazide (Diuril) is the prototype of thiazide diuretics, but hydrochlorothiazide (HydroDIURIL), a more potent derivative, is more commonly used. Related diuretics are nonthiazides whose pharmacologic actions are essentially the same as those of the thiazides; they include chlorthalidone, metolazone, and quinethazone.

Thiazides and related drugs are frequently prescribed diuretics. They decrease reabsorption of sodium and water in the ascending limb of the loop of Henle and in the distal tubule. They also decrease reabsorption of chloride and bicarbonate.

Thiazides and related drugs are well absorbed with oral administration. They are widely distributed in body fluids but accumulate only in the kidneys. With most of the drugs, diuretic effects occur within 2 hours, peak at 4 to 6 hours, and last 6 to 24 hours. Most of the drugs are excreted unchanged by the kidneys within 3 to 6 hours; some (e.g., polythiazide, chlorthalidone) have longer durations of action (about 48 to 72 hours), attributed to slower excretion.

These drugs are especially useful in long-term treatment of congestive heart failure and hypertension. They are ineffective when immediate diuresis is required and are relatively ineffective with decreased renal function. Because they cross the placenta and may have adverse effects on the fetus, usage during pregnancy must be based on careful consideration of potential benefits versus potential harm. Thiazides and related drugs are contraindicated in clients allergic to sulfonamide drugs.

LOOP DIURETICS

Loop diuretics exert their primary pharmacologic actions in the ascending limb of the loop of Henle. They also are called high-ceiling diuretics because their dosage can be increased to produce greater diuretic effects (in contrast to the thiazides; increasing the dosage of these beyond a certain point does not increase diuretic effects). Loop diuretics are the most effective and versatile diuretics available for clinical use.

Loop diuretics inhibit sodium and chloride reabsorption primarily in the loop of Henle. Their saluretic (sodium-losing) effect is up to 10 times greater than that of thiazide diuretics. These drugs may be given orally or IV. After oral administration, diuretic effects occur within 30 to 60 minutes, peak in 1 to 2 hours, and last 6 to 8 hours. After IV administration, diuretic effects occur within 5 minutes, peak within 30 minutes, and last about 2 hours. Thus, the drugs produce extensive diuresis for short periods of time, after which the kidney tubules regain their ability to reabsorb sodium. Actually, the kidneys reabsorb more sodium than usual during this postdiuretic phase, so a high dietary intake of sodium can cause sodium retention and reduce or cancel the diuretic-induced sodium loss. Thus, dietary sodium restriction is required to achieve optimum therapeutic benefits. The drugs are rapidly excreted by the kidneys, and drug accumulation does not occur even with repeated doses.

The loop diuretics are the diuretics of choice when rapid effects are required (e.g., in pulmonary edema) and when renal function is impaired (creatinine clearance less than 30 ml/min). The drugs are contraindicated during pregnancy unless necessary.

Furosemide is the most commonly used loop diuretic. Bumetanide may be used to produce diuresis in some clients who are allergic to or no longer respond to furosemide. It is more potent than furosemide on a weight basis, and large doses can be given in small volumes. Ethacrynic acid is uncommonly used because it produces more ototoxicity and gastrointestinal symptoms than the other drugs. These drugs differ mainly in potency and produce similar effects at equivalent doses (furosemide 40 mg = bumetanide 1 mg = ethacrynic acid 50 mg).

POTASSIUM-SPARING DIURETICS

Potassium-sparing diuretics include three drugs. One is spironolactone (Aldactone), an aldosterone antagonist. Aldosterone is a hormone secreted by the adrenal cortex. It promotes retention of sodium and water and excretion of potassium by stimulating the sodium-potassium exchange mechanism in the distal tubule and collecting ducts. The other two drugs, amiloride and triamterene, are chemically unrelated to spironolactone but are similar to each other in diuretic activity.

Potassium-sparing diuretics are usually given in combination with potassium-losing diuretics to increase diuretic activity and decrease potassium loss. Amiloride and triamterene act directly on the distal renal tubule to decrease the exchange of sodium for potassium. Spironolactone blocks the sodium-retaining effects of aldosterone, and aldosterone must be present for spironolactone to be effective.

Potassium-sparing diuretics are contraindicated in the presence of renal insufficiency because their use may cause hyperkalemia. Hyperkalemia is the major adverse effect of these drugs; clients receiving potassium-sparing diuretics should *not* be given potassium supplements, encouraged to eat foods high in potassium, or allowed to use salt substitutes. Salt substitutes contain potassium chloride rather than sodium chloride.

OSMOTIC DIURETICS

Osmotic agents produce rapid diuresis by increasing the solute load (osmotic pressure) of the glomerular filtrate. The increased osmotic pressure causes water to be pulled from extravascular sites into the bloodstream, thereby increasing blood volume and decreasing reabsorption of water and electrolytes in the renal tubules. Mannitol (Osmitrol) is useful in treating oliguria or anuria, and it may prevent acute renal failure during prolonged surgery, trauma, or infusion of cisplatin, an antineoplastic agent. Mannitol is effective even when renal circulation and glomerular filtration rate are reduced (*e.g.*, in hypovolemic shock, trauma, or dehydration). Other important clinical uses of hyperosmolar agents include reduction of intracranial pressure before or after neurosurgery, reduction of intraocular pressure before certain types of ophthalmic surgery, and urinary excretion of toxic substances. Other osmotic agents are listed in Table 56-1.

COMBINATION PRODUCTS

Thiazide and related diuretics are available in numerous fixed-dose combinations with nondiuretic antihypertensive agents (see Chap. 55) and with potassium-sparing diuretics (see Table 56-1). A major purpose of the antihypertensive combinations is to increase client convenience and compliance with drug therapy regimens. A major purpose of the diuretic combinations is to prevent potassium imbalances.

Nursing Process

Assessment

Assess the client's status in relation to baseline data and conditions in which diuretic drugs are used.
- Useful baseline data include serum electrolytes, uric acid, blood glucose, creatinine, and urea nitrogen, because diuretics may alter these values. Other data are blood pressure readings, weight, amount and appearance of urine output, and measurement of edematous areas, such as ankles or abdomen.
- Observe for edema. Visible edema often occurs in the feet and legs of ambulatory clients. Rapid weight gain may indicate fluid retention.
  - With congestive heart failure, numerous signs and symptoms result from edema of various organs and tissues. For example, congestion in the gastrointestinal tract may cause nausea and vomiting, liver congestion may cause abdominal pain and tenderness, and congestion in the lungs (pulmonary edema) causes rapid, labored breathing, hypoxemia, frothy sputum, and other manifestations of severe respiratory distress.

- Cerebral edema may be manifested by confusion, headache, dizziness, convulsions, unconsciousness, bradycardia, or failure of the pupils to react to light.
- Ascites, which occurs with hepatic cirrhosis, is an accumulation of fluid in the abdominal cavity. The abdomen appears much enlarged.
- With congestive heart failure, fatigue and dyspnea, in addition to edema, are common symptoms.
- Hypertension (blood pressure above 140/90 mm Hg on several measurements) may be the only clinical manifestation present.

Nursing Diagnoses

- Fluid Volume Excess in edematous clients related to retention of sodium and water
- Fluid Volume Deficit related to increased urine output after a diuretic drug is begun
- Altered Urinary Elimination: Increased frequency
- Altered Nutrition: Less Than Body Requirements related to excessive loss of potassium
- Risk for Injury: Hypotension and dizziness as adverse drug effects
- Knowledge Deficit related to the need for and correct usage of diuretics
- Sexual Dysfunction related to adverse drug effects

Planning/Goals

The client will:
- Take or receive diuretic drugs as prescribed
- Experience reduced edema and improved control of blood pressure
- Reduce dietary intake of sodium and increase dietary intake of potassium
- Avoid preventable adverse drug effects
- Keep appointments for follow-up monitoring of blood pressure, edema, and serum electrolytes

Interventions

Promote measures to prevent or minimize conditions for which diuretic drugs are used.
- With edema, helpful measures include the following:
  - Decreasing dietary sodium intake
  - Losing weight, if obese
  - Elevating legs when sitting
  - Avoiding prolonged standing or sitting
  - Wearing support hose or elastic stockings
  - Treating the condition causing edema
- With congestive heart failure and in older adults, administer IV fluids or blood transfusions carefully to avoid fluid overload and pulmonary edema. Fluid overload may occur with rapid administration or excessive amounts of IV fluids.
- With hypertension, helpful measures include decreasing dietary sodium intake and losing weight, if obese.

 Teach clients:
- That reducing dietary sodium intake will help diuretic drugs be more effective and allow smaller doses to be given. Smaller doses are less likely to cause adverse effects.

- To avoid excessive table salt and obviously salty foods (*e.g.*, ham, packaged sandwich meats, potato chips, dill pickles, most canned soups). These foods may aggravate edema or hypertension by causing sodium and water retention.
- Not to use salt substitutes unless recommended by a health care provider. These preparations contain potassium instead of sodium, and excessive potassium in the blood may have serious adverse effects on the heart.
- To maintain regular medical supervision so drug effects can be monitored and dosages adjusted when indicated

Evaluation

- Observe for reduced edema and body weight.
- Observe for reduced blood pressure.
- Observe for increased urine output.
- Monitor serum electrolytes for normal values.
- Interview regarding compliance with instructions for diet and drug therapy.
- Monitor compliance with follow-up appointments in outpatients.

Principles of Therapy

DRUG SELECTION

The choice of diuretic drug depends primarily on the client's condition.

1. **Thiazides and related diuretics** are the drugs of choice for most clients who require diuretic therapy, especially for long-term treatment of congestive heart failure and hypertension. All the drugs in this group have similar effects and differ mainly in duration of action. For most clients, short-acting (*e.g.*, bendroflumethiazide) or intermediate-acting (*e.g.*, hydrochlorothiazide) agents are preferred. Although long-acting drugs (*e.g.*, several other thiazides and metolazone) may increase client compliance by requiring less frequent administration, they also may cause more hypokalemia. Some of the drugs are also more expensive than others.
2. A **loop diuretic** (*e.g.*, furosemide) is preferred when rapid diuretic effects are required or when renal insufficiency is present.
3. A **potassium-sparing diuretic** may be given concurrently with a potassium-losing diuretic to prevent or treat hypokalemia and to augment the diuretic effect.
4. **Combination products** (see Table 56-1) containing a potassium-losing and a potassium-sparing diuretic are often prescribed because of client convenience and compliance. However, for initial therapy, it is better to titrate the dosage of each drug separately. If titrated doses are similar to the amounts in the combination products, the combination products may then be used.

DOSAGE FACTORS

Dosage of diuretics depends largely on the client's condition and response and should always be individualized to administer the minimal effective amount. With hydrochlorothiazide, for example, research studies indicate that smaller doses (*e.g.*, 25 mg daily) are usually as effective as the larger doses formerly used and are less likely to cause hypokalemia and other adverse effects.

In liver disease, electrolyte imbalances produced by diuretics may precipitate or aggravate hepatic coma. For renal disease, furosemide is often given in large doses to achieve a diuretic response. Bumetanide may be a useful alternative, because it can be given in smaller doses.

USE IN EDEMA

When diuretics are used to treat patients with edema, the underlying cause of the edema should be addressed, not just the edema itself. When treating such patients, it is preferable to aim for a weight loss of about 2 lb (about 1 kg) per day. Rapid and excessive diuresis may cause dehydration and decreased blood volume with circulatory collapse.

USE WITH DIGITALIS

When digitalis preparations and diuretics are given concomitantly, as is common when treating patients with congestive heart failure, the risk of digitalis toxicity is increased. Digitalis toxicity is related to diuretic-induced hypokalemia. Potassium is a myocardial depressant and antiarrhythmic; it has essentially opposite cardiac effects to those of digitalis. In other words, extracellular potassium decreases the excitability of myocardial tissue, but digitalis increases excitability. The higher the serum potassium, the less effective a given dose of digitalis will be. Conversely, decreased serum potassium increases the likelihood of digitalis-induced cardiac arrhythmias, even with "small" doses and therapeutic serum levels of digitalis.

Supplemental potassium chloride, a potassium-sparing diuretic, and other measures to prevent hypokalemia are often used to maintain normal serum potassium levels (3.5 to 5.0 mEq/L).

PREVENTION AND TREATMENT OF POTASSIUM IMBALANCES

Potassium imbalances (see Chap. 32) may occur with diuretic therapy. Hypokalemia and hyperkalemia are cardiotoxic and should be prevented when possible.

1. **Hypokalemia** (serum potassium level under 3.5 mEq/L) may occur with potassium-losing diuretics (*e.g.*, hydrochlorothiazide, furosemide). Mea-

sures to prevent or treat hypokalemia include the following:

a. Giving supplemental potassium, usually potassium chloride, in an average dosage range of 20 to 60 mEq daily

b. Giving a potassium-sparing diuretic along with the potassium-losing drug

c. Increasing food intake of potassium. Many texts advocate this approach as preferable to supplemental potassium or combination diuretic therapy, but the effectiveness of this approach is not clearly established. Although the minimal daily requirement of potassium is unknown, usual recommendations are 40 to 50 mEq daily for the healthy adult. Potassium loss with diuretics may be several times this amount.

Some foods (*e.g.*, bananas) have undeserved reputations for having high potassium content; actually, large amounts must be ingested. To provide 50 mEq of potassium daily, estimated amounts of certain foods include 1000 ml of orange juice, 1600 ml of apple or grape juice, 1200 ml of pineapple juice, four to six bananas, or 30 to 40 prunes. Some of these foods are high in calories and may be contraindicated, at least in large amounts, for obese clients.

d. Using salt substitutes. One teaspoonful of salt substitute contains about 60 to 70 mEq of potassium chloride.

e. Restricting dietary sodium intake. This reduces potassium loss by decreasing the amount of sodium available for exchange with potassium in renal tubules.

2. **Hyperkalemia** (serum potassium level above 5 mEq/L) may occur with potassium-sparing diuretics (spironolactone, triamterene, amiloride). The following measures prevent hyperkalemia:

a. Avoiding use of potassium-sparing diuretics and potassium supplements in clients with renal insufficiency

b. Avoiding excessive amounts of potassium chloride supplements and salt substitutes

c. Maintaining urine output, the major route for eliminating potassium from the body

USE IN CHILDREN

Thiazides are used for treatment of edema in children, and they do not commonly cause hyperglycemia, hyperuricemia, or hypercalcemia in children as they do

in adults. Pediatric doses of hydrochlorothiazide are about 2.2 mg/kg/d.

Furosemide (Lasix) is the loop diuretic that has been used most extensively in children. Oral therapy is preferred when feasible, and doses above 6 mg/kg/d are not recommended. Furosemide stimulates production of prostaglandin E_2 in the kidneys and may therefore increase the incidence of patent ductus arteriosus and neonatal respiratory distress syndrome if given to premature infants. Potassium-sparing diuretics are not usually indicated for use in children.

USE IN OLDER ADULTS

Thiazide diuretics are often prescribed for the treatment of hypertension and congestive heart failure, which are common in older adults. Older adults are especially sensitive to adverse drug effects, such as hypotension and electrolyte imbalance. Thiazides may aggravate renal or hepatic insufficiency. With rapid or excessive diuresis, myocardial infarction, renal impairment, or cerebral thrombosis may occur from fluid volume depletion and hypotension. The smallest effective dose is recommended, usually a daily dose of 12.5 to 25 mg of hydrochlorothiazide or equivalent doses of other thiazides and related drugs. Risks of adverse effects may exceed benefits at doses greater than 25 mg.

With loop diuretics, older adults are at greater risk of excessive diuresis, hypotension, fluid volume deficit, and possibly thrombosis or embolism. Rapid diuresis may cause urinary incontinence. With potassium-sparing diuretics, hyperkalemia is more likely to occur in older adults because of the renal impairment that occurs with aging.

 ## HOME CARE

Diuretics are often taken in the home setting. The home care nurse may need to assist clients and caregivers in using the drugs safely and effectively, monitor client responses (*e.g.*, assess nutritional status, blood pressure, weight, and use of over-the-counter medications that may aggravate edema or hypertension with each home visit), and provide information as indicated. In some cases, the home care nurse may need to assist the client in obtaining medications or blood tests (*e.g.*, serum potassium measurements.)

DIURETICS

NURSING ACTIONS	RATIONALE/EXPLANATION

1. Administer accurately

a. Give in the early morning if ordered daily.

So that peak action will occur during waking hours and not interfere with sleep

b. Take safety precautions. Keep a bedpan or urinal within reach. Keep the call light within reach, and be sure the client knows how to use it. Assist to the bathroom anyone who is elderly, weak, dizzy, or unsteady in walking.

Mainly to avoid falls

2. Observe for therapeutic effects

Decrease or absence of edema, increased urine output, decreased blood pressure

Most oral diuretics start their action within about 2 h; IV diuretics act within minutes. Antihypertensive effects may not be evident for several days.

(1) Weigh the client daily while edema is present and two or three times weekly thereafter. Weigh under standard conditions: early morning before eating or drinking, after urination, with the same amount of clothing, and using the same scales.

Body weight is a very good indicator of fluid gain or loss. A weight change of 2.2 lb (1 kg) may indicate a gain or loss of 1000 ml of fluid. Also, weighing assists in dosage regulation to maintain therapeutic benefit without excessive or too rapid fluid loss.

(2) Record fluid intake and output every shift.

Normally, oral fluid intake approximates urinary output (1500 ml/24 h). With diuretic therapy, urinary output may exceed intake, depending on the amount of edema or fluid retention, renal function, and diuretic dosage. All sources of fluid gain, including IV fluids, must be included; all sources of fluid loss (perspiration, fever, wound drainage, gastrointestinal [GI] tract drainage) are important. Clients with abnormal fluid losses have less urine output with diuretic therapy. Oliguria (decreased excretion of urine) may require stopping the drug. Output greater than 100 ml/h may indicate that side effects are more likely to occur.

(3) Observe and record characteristics of urine.

Excessively dilute urine may indicate excessive fluid intake or greater likelihood of fluid and electrolyte imbalance due to rapid diuresis. Concentrated urine may mean oliguria or decreased fluid intake.

(4) Check daily for edema: ankles for the ambulatory client, sacral area and posterior thighs for clients at bed rest. Also, it is often helpful to measure abdominal girth, ankles, and calves to monitor gain or loss of fluid.

Expect a decrease in visible edema and size of measured areas. If edema reappears or worsens, a thorough reassessment of the client is in order. Questions to be answered include the following:

(1) Is the prescribed diuretic being taken correctly?
(2) What type of diuretic and what dosage is ordered?
(3) Is there worsening of the underlying condition(s) that contributed to edema formation in the first place?
(4) Has other disease developed?

(5) In clients with congestive heart failure or acute pulmonary edema, observe for decreased dyspnea, rales, cyanosis, and cough.

Decreased fluid in the lungs leads to dramatic improvement in respirations as more carbon dioxide and oxygen gas exchange takes place and greater tissue oxygenation occurs.

(6) Record blood pressure two to four times daily when diuretic therapy is initiated.

Although thiazide diuretics apparently do not lower normal blood pressure, other diuretics may, especially with excessive or rapid diuresis.

NURSING ACTIONS	RATIONALE/EXPLANATION
3. Observe for adverse effects **a.** With potassium-losing diuretics (thiazides, bumetanide, furosemide, ethacrynic acid), observe for	Major adverse effects are fluid and electrolyte imbalances.

(1) Hypokalemia
      (a) Serum potassium levels below 3.5 mEq/L
      (b) ECG changes (*e.g.*, low voltage, flattened T wave, depressed ST segment)
      (c) Cardiac arrhythmias; weak, irregular pulse
      (d) Hypotension
      (e) Weak, shallow respirations
      (f) Anorexia, nausea, vomiting
      (g) Decreased peristalsis or paralytic ileus
      (h) Skeletal muscle weakness
      (i) Confusion, disorientation
	Potassium is required for normal muscle function. Thus, potassium depletion causes weakness of cardiovascular, respiratory, digestive, and skeletal muscles. Clients most likely to develop hypokalemia are those who are taking large doses of diuretics, potent diuretics (*e.g.*, furosemide), or adrenal corticosteroids; those who have decreased food and fluid intake; or those who have increased potassium losses through vomiting, diarrhea, chronic laxative or enema use, or GI suction. Clinically significant symptoms are most likely to occur with a serum potassium level below 3 mEq/L.

(2) Hyponatremia, hypomagnesemia, hypochloremic alkalosis, changes in serum and urinary calcium levels	In addition to potassium, sodium chloride, magnesium, and bicarbonate also are lost with diuresis. Thiazides and related diuretics cause hypercalcemia and hypocalciuria. They have been used to prevent calcium nephrolithiasis (kidney stones). Furosemide and other loop diuretics tend to cause hypocalcemia and hypercalciuria.

(3) Dehydration
      (a) Poor skin turgor, dry mucous membranes
      (b) Oliguria, urine of high specific gravity
      (c) Thirst
      (d) Tachycardia; hypotension
      (e) Decreased level of consciousness
      (f) Elevated hematocrit (above 45%)
	Fluid volume depletion occurs with excessive or rapid diuresis. If it is prolonged or severe, hypovolemic shock may occur.

(4) Hyperglycemia—blood glucose above 120 mg/ 100 ml, polyuria, polydipsia, polyphagia, glycosuria	Hyperglycemia is more likely to occur in clients with known or latent diabetes mellitus Larger doses of hypoglycemic agents may be required. The hyperglycemic effect may be reversible when diuretic therapy is discontinued.
(5) Hyperuricemia—serum uric acid above 7.0 mg/100 ml	Hyperuricemia is usually asymptomatic except for clients with gout, a predisposition toward gout, or chronic renal failure. Apparently, decreased renal excretion of uric acid allows its accumulation in the blood.
(6) Pulmonary edema (with osmotic diuretics)	Pulmonary edema is most likely to occur in clients with congestive heart failure who cannot tolerate the increased blood volume produced by the drugs.
(7) Ototoxicity (with furosemide and ethacrynic acid)	Reversible or transient hearing impairment, tinnitus, and dizziness are more common, although irreversible deafness may occur. Ototoxicity is more likely to occur when the drugs are injected rapidly in clients with severe renal impairment, or when other ototoxic drugs (*e.g.*, aminoglycoside antibiotics) are being taken concurrently.

(continued)

NURSING ACTIONS	RATIONALE/EXPLANATION
(8) Hypersensitivity reactions (skin rash, dermatitis) and hematologic reactions (leukopenia, thrombocytopenia)	These effects rarely occur.
b. With potassium-sparing diuretics (spironolactone, triamterene, amiloride), observe for	
(1) Hyperkalemia	
(a) Serum potassium levels above 5 mEq/L	Hyperkalemia is most likely to occur in clients with impaired renal function or those who are ingesting additional potassium (*e.g.*, salt substitutes)
(b) ECG changes (*i.e.*, prolonged P-R interval; wide QRS complex; tall, peaked T wave; depressed ST segment)	
(c) Cardiac arrhythmias, which may progress to ventricular fibrillation and asystole	
4. Observe for drug interactions	
a. Drugs that *increase* effects of diuretics:	
(1) Aminoglycoside antibiotics	Additive ototoxicity with ethacrynic acid
(2) Antihypertensive agents	Additive hypotensive effects
(3) Corticosteriods	Additive hypokalemia
b. Drugs that *decrease* effects of diuretics:	
(1) Nonsteroidal anti-inflammatory drugs (*e.g.*, aspirin, ibuprofen, others)	These drugs cause retention of sodium and water
(2) Oral contraceptives	Retention of sodium and water
(3) Vasopressors (*e.g.*, epinephrine, norepinephrine)	These drugs may antagonize hypotensive effects of diuretics by decreasing responsiveness of arterioles.
5. Teach clients	
a. Take diuretics in the early morning.	To avoid nocturia
b. Expect increased frequency of urination, decreased edema, and weight loss	Polyuria lasts only a few days or weeks in nonedematous clients.
c. Weigh periodically, under standardized conditions	Weighing is most helpful in edematous conditions
d. If the client is taking digoxin, a potassium-losing diuretic, and a potassium supplement, emphasize that these drugs must be taken as prescribed.	This is a frequently ordered combination of drugs for clients with congestive heart failure. To increase therapeutic effectiveness and avoid hypokalemia and digoxin toxicity, the balance among these drugs must be maintained
e. Report adverse effects.	So the treatment regimen can be altered if indicated.

REVIEW AND APPLICATION EXERCISES

1. What are clinical indications for the use of diuretics?

2. What is the general mechanism by which all diuretics act?

3. How can you assess a client for therapeutic effects of a diuretic?

4. Compare and contrast the main groups of diuretics in terms of adverse effects.

5. Why should serum potassium levels be monitored regularly during diuretic therapy?

6. Which prescription and over-the-counter drugs may decrease the effects of a diuretic?

7. For a client who is starting diuretic therapy, what are important points to teach the client about safe and effective drug usage?

8. For a client who is taking a potassium-losing diuretic and a potassium chloride supplement, explain the possible consequences of discontinuing one drug while continuing the other.

SELECTED REFERENCES

Applegate, W.B. (1997). Approach to the elderly patient with hypertension. In W.N. Kelley (Ed.), *Textbook of internal medicine,* 3rd ed., pp. 2482–2488. Philadelphia: Lippincott-Raven.

Brater, D.C. (1997). Clinical pharmacology of cardiovascular drugs. In W.N. Kelley (Ed.), *Textbook of internal medicine,* 3rd ed., pp. 552–569. Philadelphia: Lippincott-Raven.

Drug facts and comparisons. (Updated monthly). St. Louis: Facts and Comparisons.

Guyton, A.C. & Hall, J.E. (1996). *Textbook of medical physiology,* 9th ed. Philadelphia: W.B. Saunders.

Hawkins, D.W., Bussey, H.I. & Prisant, L.M. (1997). Hypertension. In J.T. DiPiro, R.L. Talbert, G.C. Yee, G.R. Matzke, B.G. Wells, & L.M. Posey (Eds.), *Pharmacotherapy: A pathophysiologic approach,* 3rd ed., pp. 195–218. Stamford, CT: Appleton & Lange.

Jackson, E.K. (1996). Diuretics. In J.G. Hardman, L.E. Limbird, P.B. Molinoff & R.W. Ruddon (Eds.), *Goodman & Gilman's The pharmacological basis of therapeutics,* 9th ed., pp. 685–713. New York: McGraw-Hill.

Johnson, J.A. & LaLonde, R.L. (1997). Congestive heart failure. In J.T. DiPiro, R.L. Talbert, G.C. Yee, G.R. Matzke, B.G. Wells, & L.M. Posey (Eds.), *Pharmacotherapy: A pathophysiologic approach,* 3rd ed., pp. 219–256. Stamford, CT: Appleton & Lange.

Joint National Committee on Detection, Evaluation, and Treatment of High Blood Pressure (1993). *The Fifth Report.* NIH Publication No. 93-1088. Bethesda, MD: National Institutes of Health.

Porth, C.M. (1994). *Pathophysiology: Concepts of altered health states,* 4th ed. Philadelphia: J.B. Lippincott.

57 Anticoagulant, Antiplatelet, and Thrombolytic Agents

Objectives

After studying this chapter, the student will be able to:

1 Discuss potential consequences of blood clotting disorders.

2 Compare and contrast heparin and warfarin in terms of indications for use, onset and duration of action, route of administration, blood tests used to monitor effects, and nursing process implications of anticoagulant drug therapy.

3 Discuss nursing process implications of anticoagulant drug therapy.

4 Teach clients on long-term warfarin therapy protective measures to prevent abnormal bleeding.

5 Discuss antiplatelet agents in terms of indications for use and effects on blood coagulation.

6 With aspirin, contrast the dose and frequency of administration for antiplatelet effects with those for analgesic, antipyretic, and anti-inflammatory effects.

7 Describe thrombolytic agents in terms of indications and contraindications for use, routes of administration, and major adverse effects.

Key Terms

Activated partial thromboplastin time (APTT)

Antiplatelet

Coagulation

Embolus

Prothrombin time (PT)

Thromboembolic

Thrombolytic

Thrombus

Description

Anticoagulant, antiplatelet, and thrombolytic drugs are used in the prevention and treatment of thrombotic and thromboembolic disorders. Thrombosis involves the formation (thrombogenesis) or presence of a blood clot (thrombus) within the vascular system. Blood coagulation is a normal body defense mechanism to prevent blood loss. Thus, thrombogenesis may be life saving when it occurs as a response to hemorrhage; however, it may be life threatening when it occurs at other times, because the thrombus can obstruct a blood vessel and impair the blood supply of tissues beyond the clot. When part of a thrombus breaks off and travels to another part of the body, it is called an *embolus*. Ultimate consequences of thrombi and emboli depend primarily on location and size. Thrombi and emboli that lodge in vital organs are major causes of morbidity and mortality from such disorders as myocardial infarction, stroke, and pulmonary embolism.

Under normal circumstances, thrombi are constantly being formed and dissolved (thrombolysis), but the blood stays fluid, and blood flow is not significantly obstructed. If the balance between thrombogenesis and thrombolysis is upset, thrombotic or bleeding disorders result. Thrombotic disorders occur much more often than bleeding disorders. To aid understanding of drug therapy for thrombotic disorders, normal blood coagulation and characteristics of arterial and venous thrombosis are discussed.

Blood Coagulation

Normal blood coagulation is a complex process involving numerous interacting elements. It is initiated by injury to a blood vessel and followed by two successive phases or series of events that result in clot formation.

PLATELET OR VASCULAR PHASE

Platelets, also called thrombocytes, are produced in the bone marrow and released into the bloodstream, where they circulate for about 7 to 10 days before they are removed by the spleen. Platelets are fragments of large cells called *megakaryocytes;* they contain no nuclei and therefore cannot repair or replicate themselves. Their only known function in the body is related to hemostasis (the control of bleeding by blood coagulation).

When injury occurs to a blood vessel wall, platelets elongate and become "sticky" so that they adhere to the vessel wall and to other platelets (platelet aggregation). At the same time, the fragile cell membrane disintegrates and allows leakage of platelet contents (*e.g.,* thromboplastin and other clotting factors, cal-

cium, serotonin, epinephrine, adenosine diphosphate, and thromboxane A_2), which serve various functions to stop bleeding. Thromboplastin activates prothrombin. Serotonin and epinephrine cause vasoconstriction. Thromboxane A_2 (a prostaglandin synthesized by platelets) is a potent stimulus of vasoconstriction and platelet aggregation.

Platelets act within seconds to form a platelet plug and stop bleeding. Platelets usually disappear from a blood clot within 24 hours and are replaced by fibrin.

BLOOD COAGULATION PHASE

Blood coagulation acts more slowly (within 1 to 2 minutes) to cause hemostasis. It involves sequential activation of clotting factors that are normally present in blood and tissues as inactive precursors. Characteristics and functions of coagulation factors are listed in Table 57-1. Major steps in the coagulation process are the following:

1. Release of thromboplastin by disintegrating platelets and damaged tissue
2. Conversion of prothrombin to thrombin, which requires thromboplastin and calcium ions
3. Conversion of fibrinogen to fibrin by thrombin

Thrombotic and Thromboembolic Disorders

Thrombosis may occur in both arteries and veins. Arterial thrombosis is usually associated with atherosclerotic plaque, hypertension, and turbulent blood flow. These conditions damage the inner lining of the artery so platelets adhere, aggregate, and release thromboplastin to initiate the coagulation process. Arterial thrombi cause disease by obstructing blood flow. If the obstruction is incomplete or temporary, local tissue ischemia (deficient blood supply) occurs. If the obstruction is complete or prolonged, local tissue death or infarction occurs.

Venous thrombosis is usually associated with venous stasis. When blood flows very slowly, thrombin and other coagulant substances present in the blood become sufficiently concentrated in local areas to initiate the clotting process. With a normal rate of blood flow, these substances are rapidly removed from the blood, primarily by Kupffer's cells in the liver. A venous thrombus is less cohesive than an arterial thrombus and an embolus can easily become detached and travel to other parts of the body.

Venous thrombi cause disease by two mechanisms. First, thrombosis causes local congestion, edema, and perhaps inflammation by impairing normal outflow of venous blood (*e.g.,* thrombophlebitis, deep vein throm-

TABLE 57-1 **BLOOD COAGULATION FACTORS**

Number	Name	Functions
I	Fibrinogen	Forms fibrin, the insoluble protein strands that compose the supporting framework of a blood clot. Thrombin and calcium are required for the conversion.
II	Prothrombin	Forms thrombin, which catalyzes the conversion of fibrinogen to fibrin
III	Thromboplastin	Converts prothrombin to thrombin
IV	Calcium	Catalyzes the conversion of prothrombin to thrombin
V	Labile factor	Required for formation of active thromboplastin
VII	Proconvertin or stable factor	Accelerates action of tissue thromboplastin
VIII	Antihemophilic factor	Promotes breakdown of platelets and formation of active platelet thromboplastin
IX	Christmas factor	Similar to factor VIII
X	Stuart factor	Promotes action of thromboplastin
XI	Plasma thromboplastin antecedent	Promotes platelet aggregation and breakdown, with subsequent release of platelet thromboplastin
XII	Hageman factor	Similar to factor XI
XIII	Fibrin-stabilizing factor	Converts fibrin meshwork to the dense, tight mass of the completely formed clot

bosis [DVT]). Second, embolization causes obstruction of blood supply when the embolus becomes lodged. The pulmonary arteries are common sites of embolization.

Drugs Used in Thrombotic and Thromboembolic Disorders

Drugs given to prevent or treat thrombosis alter some aspect of the blood coagulation process. Anticoagulants are widely used in thrombotic disorders. They are more effective in preventing venous thrombosis than arterial thrombosis. Antiplatelet drugs are used to prevent arterial thrombosis. Thrombolytic agents are used to dissolve thrombi and limit tissue damage in selected thromboembolic disorders.

ANTICOAGULANTS

Anticoagulant drugs are given to prevent formation of new clots and extension of clots already present. They do not dissolve formed clots, improve blood flow in tissues around the clot, or prevent ischemic damage to tissues beyond the clot. Heparin and warfarin are commonly used anticoagulants. These drugs act by different mechanisms to interfere with certain coagulation factors and prevent thrombus formation (see discussions of the individual drugs).

Clinical indications for anticoagulants include prevention or treatment of thromboembolic disorders, such as thrombophlebitis, DVT, and pulmonary embolism. Heparin is also used for other purposes.

ANTIPLATELET DRUGS

Antiplatelet drugs prevent platelet aggregation and thereby interfere with the initial phase of blood coagulation. Increased platelet aggregation is associated with atherosclerosis and thromboembolic disorders. For example, arterial thrombi, which are composed primarily of platelets, may embolize from abnormal heart valves, mural thrombi, or atherosclerotic plaque.

Drugs used clinically for antiplatelet effects are abciximab, aspirin, dipyridamole, and ticlopidine. Abciximab is used with aspirin and heparin to prevent reclosure of treated coronary arteries after percutaneous transluminal angioplasty or atherectomy (PCTA). The other drugs are used to prevent myocardial infarction, stroke in clients with transient ischemic attacks (TIAs), and thromboembolism in clients with prosthetic heart valves.

THROMBOLYTIC AGENTS

Thrombolytic agents are given to dissolve thrombi. They stimulate conversion of plasminogen to plasmin (also called fibrinolysin). Plasmin is a proteolytic enzyme that breaks down fibrin, the framework of a thrombus. The main use of thrombolytic agents is for treatment of acute, severe thromboembolic disease, such as myocardial infarction, pulmonary embolism, and iliofemoral thrombosis. The goal of thrombolytic therapy is to reestablish blood flow and prevent or limit tissue damage. The drugs also are used to dissolve clots in intravascular catheters. Currently approved thrombolytics are alteplase (Activase), anistreplase (Eminase), streptokinase (Streptase), and urokinase (Abbokinase).

Individual Drugs

ANTICOAGULANTS AND THEIR ANTIDOTES

Heparin is a pharmaceutical preparation of the natural anticoagulant produced primarily by mast cells in pericapillary connective tissue. Endogenous heparin is found in various body tissues, most abundantly in the liver and lungs. Exogenous heparin is obtained from bovine lung or porcine intestinal mucosa and standardized in units of biologic activity.

Heparin combines with antithrombin III to inactivate several clotting factors (IX, X, XI, XII) and thrombin so thrombus formation is prevented. Antithrombin III is an alpha globulin normally present in the blood as a natural anticoagulant substance. Antithrombin III must be present for heparin action.

Heparin acts immediately after intravenous (IV) administration and within 20 to 30 minutes after subcutaneous injection. It is metabolized in the liver and excreted in the urine, primarily as inactive metabolites. Heparin does not cross the placental barrier and is not secreted in breast milk. Disadvantages of heparin are its short duration of action and the subsequent need for frequent administration, the necessity for parenteral injection (because it is not absorbed from the gastrointestinal tract), its relatively high cost, and local tissue reactions at injection sites.

Prophylactically, low doses of heparin are given to prevent DVT and pulmonary embolism in clients at risk of developing these disorders, such as the following:

1. Those having abdominal or thoracic surgery who are over age 40 or have additional risk factors for DVT (*e.g.*, obesity, varicose veins)
2. Those with a history of thrombophlebitis or pulmonary embolism
3. Those having gynecologic surgery, especially if they have been taking estrogens or oral contraceptives or have other risk factors for DVT
4. Those expected to be on bed rest or to have limited activity for longer than 5 days, especially if debilitating conditions are also present (*e.g.*, severe congestive heart failure, stroke, malignant disease)

Low-dose heparin prophylaxis is either ineffective or contraindicated in major orthopedic surgery, abdominal prostatectomy, and brain surgery.

Therapeutically, heparin is used for treatment of acute thromboembolic disorders (*e.g.*, DVT, thrombophlebitis, pulmonary embolism). In these conditions, the aim of therapy is to prevent further thrombus formation and embolization. Heparin is also used in disseminated intravascular coagulation (DIC), a life-threatening condition characterized by widespread clotting, which depletes the blood of coagulation factors. The depletion of coagulation factors then produces widespread bleeding. The goal of heparin therapy in DIC is to prevent blood coagulation long enough for clotting factors to be replenished and thus be able to control hemorrhage.

Although sometimes used in arterial occlusive disease, myocardial infarction, and stroke, heparin therapy has not been proven effective in preventing further thromboembolic problems. However, heparin may be effective in preventing embolization from prosthetic heart valves.

Heparin is also used to prevent clotting during cardiac and vascular surgery, extracorporeal circulation, hemodialysis, and blood transfusions and in blood samples to be used in laboratory tests. It has been used to maintain patency of intermittent IV infusion devices (*e.g.*, catheters and heparin locks). With heparin locks, several studies have indicated that normal saline flushes are effective, and use of heparin for this purpose has declined.

Dalteparin (Fragmin) and **Enoxaparin** (Lovenox) are low-molecular-weight formulations of heparin. Standard heparin is a mixture of high and low molecular weights, but most anticoagulant activity is attributed to the low molecular weight portion. Some studies indicate that subcutaneous dalteparin or enoxaparin may be as effective as IV heparin in treating thrombotic disorders. In addition, these drugs do not require close monitoring of blood coagulation tests. These characteristics may allow outpatient treatment for disorders that have required hospitalization.

Contraindications to heparin therapy include gastrointestinal ulcerations (*e.g.*, peptic ulcer disease, ulcerative colitis), blood dyscrasias, severe kidney or liver disease, severe hypertension, polycythemia vera, and recent surgery of the eye, spinal cord, or brain. It should be used with caution in clients with mild hypertension, renal or hepatic disease, alcoholism, history of gastrointestinal ulcerations, drainage tubes (*e.g.*, nasogastric tubes, indwelling urinary catheters), and any occupation with high risks of traumatic injury.

Heparin
Routes and Dosage Ranges

Adults: IV injection, 5000 units initially, followed by 5000–10,000 units q4–6h, to a maximum dose of 25,000 units/d

DIC, IV injection, 50–100 units/kg q4h

IV infusion, 20,000–40,000 units/d at initial rate of 0.25 units/kg/min, then adjusted according to blood clotting tests (activated partial thromboplastin time [APTT])

SC 10,000–12,000 units q8h, or 14,000–20,000 units q12h

Low-dose prophylaxis, SC 5000 units 2 h before surgery, then q12h until discharged from hospital or fully ambulatory

Children: DIC, IV injection, 25–50 units/kg q4h
IV infusion, 50 units/kg initially, followed by
100 units/kg q4h or 20,000 units/m² over 24 h

Dalteparin
Route and Dosage Range

Adults: SC 2500 IU once daily, with first dose 1–2 h
before surgery, then daily for 5–10 days postoperatively

Enoxaparin
Route and Dosage Range

Adults: SC 30 mg twice daily, with first dose soon
after surgery but not more than 24 h postoperatively. Usual duration, 7–10 d

Protamine sulfate is an antidote or antagonist for
heparin. Heparin is an acid; protamine sulfate is a base.
Thus, protamine neutralizes heparin activity. Protamine dosage depends on the amount of heparin administered during the previous 4 hours. Each milligram of
protamine neutralizes about 100 units of heparin. A single dose should not exceed 50 mg. The drug is given by
slow IV infusion over 10 minutes (to prevent or minimize adverse effects of hypotension, bradycardia, and
dyspnea). Protamine effects occur immediately and
last for about 2 hours. A second dose may be required,
because heparin activity lasts about 4 hours.

Warfarin (Coumadin) is the prototype and most
commonly used coumarin anticoagulant. Warfarin acts
in the liver to prevent synthesis of vitamin K–dependent clotting factors (*i.e.*, factors II, VII, IX, and X). Warfarin is similar to vitamin K in structure and therefore
acts as a competitive antagonist to hepatic use of vitamin K. Anticoagulant effects do not occur for about 3 to
5 days after warfarin is started because clotting factors
already in the blood follow their normal pathway of
elimination. Warfarin has no effect on circulating clotting factors or on platelet function.

Warfarin is well absorbed after oral administration.
Although it can be given parenterally, there is no advantage in therapeutic effect. Warfarin is highly bound
to plasma proteins (about 98%), mainly albumin. It is
metabolized in the liver and primarily excreted as inactive metabolites by the kidneys.

Warfarin is most useful in long-term prevention or
treatment of venous thromboembolic disorders, including deep vein thrombosis, pulmonary embolism, and
embolization associated with atrial fibrillation and prosthetic heart valves. There is also evidence that warfarin
therapy after myocardial infarction decreases reinfarction, stroke, venous thromboembolism, and death. As a
general rule, warfarin is not indicated in arterial thrombosis because arterial thrombi are composed primarily of
platelets, and warfarin has no effect on platelet functions.

Contraindications to warfarin therapy include gastrointestinal ulcerations (*e.g.*, peptic ulcer disease, ulcerative colitis), blood dyscrasias (*e.g.*, hemophilia, thrombocytopenia), severe kidney or liver disease, severe
hypertension, and recent surgery of the eye, spinal
cord, or brain. Warfarin crosses the placenta and is
contraindicated during pregnancy. Warfarin should be
used cautiously with hypertension, renal or hepatic
disease, alcoholism, history of gastrointestinal ulcerations, drainage tubes (*e.g.,* nasogastric tubes, indwelling
urinary catheters), and occupations with high risks of
traumatic injury.

Route and Dosage Range

Adults: PO 10 mg/d for 2–3 d, then adjusted according to the international normalized ratio
(INR); average maintenance dose, 2–10 mg/d

Phytonadione (vitamin K, Mephyton) is the antidote
for warfarin overdosage. An oral dose of 10 to 20 mg
will usually stop minor bleeding and return the INR to
a normal range within 24 hours.

ANTIPLATELET AGENTS

Aspirin is a commonly used analgesic-antipyretic-antiinflammatory drug (see Chap. 7) with potent antiplatelet
effects. Aspirin exerts pharmacologic actions by inhibiting synthesis of prostaglandins. In this instance, aspirin
acetylates the enzyme in platelets that normally synthesizes thromboxane A_2, a prostaglandin that causes
platelet aggregation. Thus, aspirin prevents formation
of thromboxane A_2, thereby preventing platelet aggregation and thrombus formation. Antithrombotic effects
persist for the life of the platelet (about 10 days). Aspirin
may be used as an antiplatelet agent for prevention of
myocardial infarction and in clients with prosthetic heart
valves or TIAs. Adverse effects are uncommon with the
small doses used for antiplatelet effects. However,
there is an increased risk of bleeding.

Route and Dosage Range
Adults: PO 80–325 mg/d

Dipyridamole (Persantine) is an antiplatelet drug
recommended only for prevention of thromboembolism after cardiac valve replacement. It is given with
warfarin.

Route and Dosage Range

Adults: PO 25–75 mg three times per day, 1 h before
meals

Ticlopidine (Ticlid) inhibits platelet aggregation
irreversibly, and effects persist for the life span of the

platelet. The drug is indicated for prevention of thrombosis in people with coronary artery or cerebral vascular disease. Ticlopidine is considered a second-line drug for use in clients who cannot take aspirin, mainly because of adverse effects (*e.g.,* neutropenia, diarrhea) and greater cost. Contraindications include active bleeding disorders (*e.g.,* gastrointestinal bleeding from peptic ulcer or intracranial bleeding), neutropenia, thrombocytopenia, severe liver disease, and hypersensitivity to the drug.

Ticlopidine is rapidly absorbed after oral administration and reaches peak plasma levels about 2 hours after a dose. It is highly protein bound (98%), extensively metabolized in the liver, and excreted in urine and feces. As with other antiplatelet drugs, there is increased risk of bleeding with ticlopidine.

Route and Dosage Range

Adults: PO 250 mg twice daily with food

Abciximab (ReoPro) is a monoclonal antibody that binds with platelets and inhibits platelet aggregation. It is used with PCTA to prevent rethrombosis of treated arteries. It is contraindicated in clients who have recently received an oral anticoagulant or IV dextran. Other contraindications include active bleeding, thrombocytopenia, history of a serious stroke, surgery or major trauma within the previous 6 weeks, uncontrolled hypertension, or hypersensitivity to drug components.

Route and Dosage Range

Adults: IV bolus injection, 0.25 mg/kg 10–60 min before starting PCTA, then a continuous IV infusion of 10 μg/min for 12 h.

THROMBOLYTIC AGENTS AND THEIR ANTIDOTES

Alteplase is a thrombolytic agent produced by recombinant DNA technology. It is a tissue plasminogen activator and is often called tPA. It is used in acute myocardial infarction to dissolve clots obstructing coronary arteries and reestablish perfusion of tissues beyond the thrombotic area. The drug binds to fibrin in a clot and acts locally to dissolve the clot with less systemic effect than streptokinase.

The most common adverse effect is bleeding, which may be internal (*e.g.,*intracranial, gastrointestinal, genitourinary) or external (*e.g.,* venous or arterial puncture sites, surgical incisions). The drug is contraindicated in the presence of bleeding, a history of stroke, central nervous system surgery or trauma within the previous 2 months, and severe hypertension.

Route and Dosage Range

Adults: IV infusion, 100 mg over 3 h (first hour, 60 mg with a bolus of 6–10 mg over 1–2 min initially; second hour, 20 mg; third hour, 20 mg)

Anistreplase is a combination of human plasminogen and streptokinase. Like alteplase, it breaks down fibrin and is used to lyse coronary artery clots in acute myocardial infarction. Adverse effects and contraindications are the same as for other thrombolytic agents. An advantage is that anistreplase can be given in a single IV injection.

Route and Dosage Range

Adults: IV injection, 30 units over 2–5 min

Streptokinase, a protein derived from streptococci, promotes dissolution of blood clots by interacting with a plasminogen proactivator. The resulting substance catalyzes the conversion of plasminogen to plasmin. Plasmin (fibrinolysin) breaks down fibrin. Streptokinase may be used for treatment of acute pulmonary emboli or iliofemoral thrombophlebitis when these conditions are severe and life threatening. Bleeding, fever, and allergic reactions may occur. Heparin and warfarin are given after streptokinase therapy is finished.

Streptokinase also may be injected directly into a coronary artery to dissolve a thrombus if done within 6 hours of onset of symptoms. An additional use is to dissolve clots in arterial or venous cannulas or catheters.

Route and Dosage Range

Adults: IV 250,000 units over 30 min, then 100,000 units/h for 24–72 h

Urokinase is a proteolytic enzyme that catalyzes the conversion of plasminogen to plasmin. Plasmin breaks down fibrin and thereby promotes dissolution of blood clots. Urokinase is recommended for use in clients allergic to streptokinase. Urokinase is contraindicated in children, pregnant women, and clients with wounds, malignancies, and recent strokes. In addition, all other contraindications to heparin and warfarin therapy apply to urokinase. Urokinase causes a high incidence of bleeding and is more expensive than other thrombolytics. Heparin and warfarin are started after urokinase therapy is completed.

Route and Dosage Range

Adults: IV 4400 units/kg over 10 min, followed by continuous infusion of 4400 units/kg/h for 12 h

Aminocaproic acid (Amicar) and **tranexamic acid** (Cyklokapron) are antidotes used to control bleeding induced by overdoses of thrombolytic agents. Aminocaproic acid also may be used in other bleeding disorders caused by hyperfibrinolysis (*e.g.,* cardiac surgery, blood disorders, hepatic cirrhosis, prostatectomy, neoplastic disorders). Tranexamic acid also is used for short periods (2–8 days) in hemophiliacs to prevent or decrease bleeding from tooth extraction. Dosage of tranexamic acid should be reduced in the presence of moderate or severe renal impairment.

Aminocaproic Acid
Route and Dosage Range

Adults: PO, IV infusion, 5 g initially, followed by 1.0 to 1.25 g/h for 8 h or until bleeding is controlled; maximum dose, 30 g/24 h

Tranexamic Acid
Route and Dosage Range

Adults: Hemophiliacs having dental extraction, PO 25 mg/kg three to four times daily, starting 1 d before surgery or IV 10 mg/kg immediately before surgery, followed by 25 mg/kg PO three to four times daily for 2 to 8 d

Nursing Process

Assessment

Assess the client's status in relation to thrombotic and thromboembolic disorders.

- Risk factors for thromboembolism include
  - Immobility (*e.g.,* limited activity or bed rest for more than 5 days)
  - Obesity
  - Cigarette smoking
  - History of varicose veins, thrombophlebitis, or pulmonary emboli
  - Congestive heart failure
  - Pedal edema
  - Lower limb trauma
  - Myocardial infarction
  - Atrial fibrillation
  - Mitral or aortic stenosis
  - Prosthetic heart valves
  - Abdominal, thoracic, pelvic, or major orthopedic surgery
  - Atherosclerotic heart disease or peripheral vascular disease
  - Use of oral contraceptives
- Signs and symptoms of thrombotic and thromboembolic disorders depend on the location and size of the thrombus.
  - DVT and thrombophlebitis usually occur in the legs. The conditions may be manifested by edema (the affected leg is often measurably larger than the other) and pain, especially in the calf when the foot is dorsiflexed (Homans' sign). If thrombophlebitis is superficial, it may be visible as a red, warm, tender area following the path of a vein.
  - Pulmonary embolism, if severe enough to produce symptoms, is manifested by chest pain, cough, hemoptysis,

tachypnea, and tachycardia. Massive emboli cause hypotension, shock, cyanosis, and death.
  - DIC is usually manifested by bleeding, which may range from petechiae or oozing from a venipuncture site to massive internal bleeding or bleeding from all body orifices.

Nursing Diagnoses

- Altered Tissue Perfusion related to thrombus or embolus
- Pain related to tissue ischemia
- Impaired Physical Mobility related to bed rest and pain
- Altered Tissue Perfusion related to drug-induced bleeding
- Decreased Cardiac Output related to hemorrhage and volume depletion
- Anxiety related to fear of myocardial infarction or stroke
- Ineffective Individual Coping related to the need for long-term prophylaxis of thromboembolic disorders or fear of excessive bleeding
- Noncompliance related to anxiety, the need for periodic blood tests, and lack of knowledge about anticoagulant therapy
- Knowledge Deficit related to anticoagulant or antiplatelet drug therapy
- Risk for Injury related to drug-induced impairment of blood coagulation

Planning/Goals

The client will:
- Receive or take anticoagulant and antiplatelet drugs correctly
- Be monitored closely for therapeutic and adverse drug effects, especially when drug therapy is started and when changes are made in drugs or dosages
- Use nondrug measures to decrease venous stasis and prevent thromboembolic disorders
- Act to prevent trauma from falls and other injuries
- Inform any health care provider when taking an anticoagulant
- Avoid or report adverse drug reactions
- Verbalize or demonstrate knowledge of safe management of anticoagulant drug therapy
- Keep follow-up appointments for tests of blood coagulation and drug dosage regulation

Interventions

Use measures to prevent thrombotic and thromboembolic disorders.
- Have the client ambulate and exercise legs regularly, especially postoperatively.
- For clients who cannot ambulate or do leg exercises, do passive range-of-motion and other leg exercises several times daily when changing the client's position or performing other care.
- Have the client wear elastic stockings. Elastic stockings should be removed every 8 hours and replaced after inspecting the skin. Improperly applied elastic stockings can impair circulation rather than aid it.
- Avoid trauma to lower extremities.
- Maintain adequate fluid intake (1500 to 3000 ml/d) to avoid dehydration and hemoconcentration.

For the client receiving anticoagulant therapy, implement safety measures to prevent trauma and bleeding.

- For clients who cannot ambulate safely due to weakness, sedation, or other conditions, keep the call light within reach, keep bedrails elevated, and assist in ambulation.
- Provide an electric razor for shaving.
- Avoid intramuscular injections, venipunctures, and arterial punctures when possible.
- Avoid intubations when possible (*e.g.*, nasogastric tubes, indwelling urinary catheters).

 Teach clients:

- To exercise legs periodically, especially if walking and other activities are limited
- To avoid situations that impair blood circulation, such as wearing tight clothing; crossing the legs at the knees; prolonged sitting, standing, and bed rest; and placing pillows under the knees when in bed
- Risks of thromboembolic disorders
- The importance of continued supervision and monitoring by a health care provider

Evaluation

- Observe for signs and symptoms of thromboembolic disorders or bleeding.
- Check blood coagulation tests for therapeutic ranges.
- Observe and interview regarding compliance with instructions about drug therapy.
- Observe and interview regarding adverse drug effects.

Principles of Therapy

DRUG SELECTION

The choice of anticoagulant or antiplatelet drug depends mainly on the reason for use.

1. Heparin is the drug of choice in acute thromboembolic disorders because the anticoagulant effect begins immediately with IV administration.
2. Warfarin is the drug of choice for long-term maintenance therapy (*i.e.*, several weeks or months) because it can be given orally.
3. Aspirin is the most widely used antiplatelet drug for prevention of myocardial reinfarction and arterial thrombosis in clients with TIAs and prosthetic heart valves.
4. When anticoagulation is required during pregnancy, heparin is used because it does not cross the placenta. Warfarin is contraindicated during pregnancy.

DOSAGE FACTORS

Dosage of anticoagulant drugs must be individualized, primarily according to blood coagulation tests, client characteristics, and concomitant drug therapy.

Heparin

Dosage is regulated by the activated partial thromboplastin time (APTT), which is sensitive to changes in blood clotting factors, except factor VII. Thus, normal or control values indicate normal blood coagulation; therapeutic values indicate low levels of clotting factors and delayed blood coagulation. During heparin therapy, the APTT should be maintained at about 1.5 to 2.5 times the control or baseline value. The normal control value is 25 to 35 seconds; therefore, therapeutic values are 35 to 85 seconds, approximately. With continuous IV infusion, blood for the APTT may be drawn anytime; with intermittent administration, blood for the APTT should be drawn about 1 hour before a dose of heparin is scheduled. APTT is not necessary with low-dose conventional heparin given subcutaneously for prophylaxis of thromboembolism or with enoxaparin or dalteparin.

Warfarin

Dosage is regulated according to the INR, for which therapeutic values are 2.0 to 3.0 in most conditions requiring warfarin therapy. The INR is based on prothrombin time (PT). PT is sensitive to changes in three of the four vitamin K–dependent coagulation factors (*i.e.*, II, VII, IX, and X). Thus, normal or control values indicate normal levels of these blood coagulation factors; therapeutic values indicate low levels of the factors and delayed blood coagulation. A normal baseline or control PT is about 12 seconds; a therapeutic value is about 1.5 times the control, or 18 seconds.

When warfarin is started, PT and INR should be performed daily until a stable daily dose is reached (the dose that maintains PT and INR within therapeutic ranges and does not cause bleeding). Thereafter, PT and INR are performed every 2 to 4 weeks for the duration of oral anticoagulant drug therapy. If the warfarin dose is changed, PT and INR are needed more often until a stable daily dose is again reached.

For many years, the PT test was used to regulate warfarin dosage. PT is performed by adding a mixture of thromboplastin and calcium to citrated plasma and measuring the time (in seconds) it takes for the blood to clot. However, values vary among laboratories according to the type of thromboplastin and the instrument used to measure PT. The INR system standardizes the PT by comparing a particular thromboplastin with a standard thromboplastin designated by the World Health Organization (WHO). Advantages of the INR include consistent values among laboratories, more consistent warfarin dosage with less risk of bleeding or thrombosis, and more consistent reports of clinical trials and other research studies. Some laboratories report both PT and INR.

Warfarin dosage may need to be reduced in clients with biliary tract disorders (*e.g.,* obstructive jaundice), liver disease (*e.g.,* hepatitis, cirrhosis), malabsorption syndromes (*e.g.,* steatorrhea), and hyperthyroidism or fever. These conditions increase anticoagulant drug effects by reducing absorption of vitamin K, decreasing hepatic synthesis of blood-clotting factors, or increasing the rate of degradation of clotting factors. Despite these influencing factors, however, the primary determinant of dosage is the PT and INR.

Warfarin and other coumarin anticoagulants interact with many other drugs to cause increased, decreased, or unpredictable anticoagulant effects. Thus, warfarin dosage may need to be increased or decreased when other drugs are given concomitantly. Most drugs can be given if warfarin dosage is carefully titrated according to the PT or INR and altered appropriately when an interacting drug is added or stopped. INR or PT measurements and vigilant observation are needed whenever a drug is added to or removed from a drug therapy regimen containing warfarin.

THROMBOLYTIC THERAPY

1. Thrombolytic therapy should be performed only by experienced personnel in an intensive care setting with cardiac and other monitoring devices in place.
2. All of the available agents are effective with recommended uses. Thus, the choice of a thrombolytic agent depends mainly on risks of adverse effects and costs. All of the drugs may cause bleeding. Alteplase and anistreplase may act more specifically on the fibrin in a clot and cause less systemic depletion of fibrinogen, but these agents are very expensive. Streptokinase, the least expensive agent, may cause allergic reactions because it is a foreign protein. Combination therapy (*e.g.,* with alteplase and streptokinase) is being investigated for safety, efficacy, and cost.
3. Before a thrombolytic agent is begun, INR, APTT, platelet count, and fibrinogen should be checked to establish baseline values and to determine if a blood coagulation disorder is present. Two or three hours after thrombolytic therapy is started, the fibrinogen level can be measured to determine that fibrinolysis is occurring. Alternatively, INR and/or APTT can be checked for increased values because the breakdown products of fibrin exert anticoagulant effects.
4. Major factors in decreasing risks of bleeding are selecting recipients carefully, avoiding invasive procedures when possible, and omitting anticoagulant or antiplatelet drugs while thrombolytics are being given. If bleeding does occur, it is most likely from a venipuncture or invasive procedure site, and local pressure may control it. If bleeding cannot be controlled or involves a vital organ, the thrombolytic drug should be stopped and fibrinogen replaced with whole blood plasma or cryoprecipitate. Aminocaproic acid or tranexamic acid may also be given.

5. When the drugs are used in acute myocardial infarction, cardiac arrhythmias may occur when blood flow is reestablished. Therefore, antiarrhythmic drugs should be readily available.

USE IN CHILDREN

Little information is available about the use of anticoagulants in children. Heparin solutions containing benzyl alcohol as a preservative should not be given to premature infants because fatal reactions have been reported. When given for systemic anticoagulation, heparin dosage should be based on the child's weight (about 50 units/kg). Safety and effectiveness of enoxaparin and dalteparin have not been established in children.

Warfarin is given to children after cardiac surgery to prevent thromboembolism, but doses and guidelines for safe, effective usage have not been developed. Accurate drug administration, close monitoring of blood coagulation tests, safety measures to prevent trauma and bleeding, avoiding interacting drugs, and informing others in the child's environment (*e.g.,* teachers, babysitters, health care providers) are necessary.

Antiplatelet and thrombolytic drugs have no established indications for use in children.

USE IN OLDER ADULTS

Older adults often develop thromboembolic disorders, especially if mobility is impaired. They are also more likely than younger adults to experience bleeding and other complications of anticoagulant drugs.

With heparin, general principles for safe and effective use apply. With warfarin, dosage should be reduced because impaired liver function and decreased plasma proteins increase the risks of bleeding. Also, many drugs interact with warfarin to increase or decrease its effect, and older adults often take several drugs concurrently. Starting or stopping any drug may require that warfarin dosage be adjusted.

 HOME CARE

Antiplatelet agents and warfarin are used for long-term prevention or treatment of thromboembolism and are often taken at home. Subcutaneous heparin may also be taken at home. The home care nurse needs to assess clients in relation to knowledge about prescribed drugs and ability and willingness to comply with instructions for taking the drugs, obtaining blood tests when indicated, and taking safety precautions. In addition, assess the environment for risk factors for injury. Interventions vary with clients, environments, and assessment data but may include reinforcing instructions for safe usage of the drugs, assisting clients to obtain laboratory tests, and teaching how to observe for signs and symptoms of bleeding.

NURSING ACTIONS

ANTICOAGULANTS

NURSING ACTIONS	RATIONALE/EXPLANATION
1. Administer accurately	
a. With *heparin*:	
(1) When transcribing a physician's order, write out "units" rather than using the abbreviation "U."	This is a safety precaution to avoid erroneous dosage. For example, 1000 U (1000 units) may be misread as 10,000 units.
(2) Check dosage carefully.	Although accurate dosage is important in all drug therapy, it is especially important with anticoagulants because a rather narrow range exists between therapeutic and toxic levels. Therefore, underdosage may cause thromboembolism, and overdosage may cause bleeding. In addition, heparin is available in several concentrations (1000, 2500, 5000, 10,000, 15,000, 20,000, and 40,000 units/ml)
(3) For subcutaneous heparin:	
(a) Use a 26-gauge, 1/2-inch needle.	To minimize trauma and risk of bleeding
(b) Use a tuberculin syringe and a drug volume of 0.5 ml or less.	To measure accurately and minimize trauma
(c) Cleanse injection site gently with an alcohol sponge.	To prevent infection
(d) Grasp a fold of tissue between thumb and fingers of the nondominant hand. Do not pinch tightly.	To give the drug in a deep subcutaneous or fat layer
(e) Insert the needle at a 90-degree angle into the skin fold; inject without aspirating, and withdraw the needle.	To minimize trauma and risk of bleeding
(f) Apply gentle pressure to the site for 30–60 s. Do not rub.	To prevent bleeding
(g) Rotate injection sites (abdomen, upper arms and lateral thighs may be used). Do not inject heparin within 2 inches of the umbilicus.	To minimize tissue irritation and trauma. Avoid the umbilical area to prevent inadvertent injection into umbilical veins.
(4) For intermittent IV administration:	
(a) Give by direct injection into a heparin lock or tubing injection site.	These methods prevent repeated venipunctures
(b) Dilute the dose in 50 to 100 ml of any IV fluid (usually 5% dextrose in water).	
(5) For continuous IV administration:	This is usually the preferred method of administration because it maintains consistent serum drug levels rather than peak levels and trough levels
(a) Use a volume-control device and an infusion-control device.	To regulate dosage and flow rate accurately
(b) Add only enough heparin for a few hours. One effective method is to fill the volume-control set (*e.g.*, Volutrol) with 100 ml of 5% dextrose in water and add 5000 units of heparin to yield a concentration of 50 units/ml. Dosage is regulated by varying the flow rate. For example, administration of 1000 units/h requires a flow rate of 20 ml/h. Another method is to add 25,000 units of heparin to 500 ml of IV solution.	To avoid inadvertent administration of large amounts. Whatever method is used, it is desirable to standardize concentration of heparin solutions within an institution. Standardization is safer, because it reduces risks of errors in dosage.

(continued)

NURSING ACTIONS	RATIONALE/EXPLANATION
b. After the initial dose of warfarin, check the INR before giving a subsequent dose. Do not give the dose if the INR is above 3.0. Notify the physician.	The INR is measured daily until a maintenance dose is established, then periodically throughout warfarin therapy. An elevated INR indicates a high risk of bleeding.
c. With thrombolytic agents, follow manufacturers' instructions for reconstitution and administration.	

2. Observe for therapeutic effects
  a. Absence of signs and symptoms when given prophylactically

  b. Decrease or improvement in signs and symptoms when given therapeutically (*e.g.*, less edema and pain with thrombophlebitis, less chest pain and respiratory difficulty with pulmonary embolism)

  c. INR between 2.0 and 3.0 for warfarin; APTT within 1.5 to 2.5 times the control value for heparin.

3. Observe for adverse effects

a. Bleeding:	Bleeding is the major adverse effect of anticoagulant drugs. It may occur anywhere in the body, spontaneously or in response to minor trauma.
(1) Record vital signs regularly.	Hypotension and tachycardia may indicate internal bleeding.
(2) Check stools for blood (melena).	Gastrointestinal (GI) bleeding is fairly common; risks are increased with intubation. Blood in stools may be bright red, tarry (blood that has been digested by GI secretions), or occult (hidden to the naked eye but present with a guaiac test). Hematemesis also may occur.
(3) Check urine for blood (hematuria).	Genitourinary bleeding also is fairly common; risks are increased with catheterization or instrumentation. Urine may be red (indicating fresh bleeding) or brownish or smokey gray (indicating old blood). Or bleeding may be microscopic (red blood cells are visible only on microscopic examination during urinalysis).
(4) Inspect the skin and mucous membranes daily.	Bleeding may occur in the skin as petechiae, purpura, or ecchymoses. Surgical wounds, skin lesions, parenteral injection sites, the nose, and gums may be bleeding sites.
(5) Assess for excessive menstrual flow.	
b. Other adverse effects:	
(1) With heparin, tissue irritation at injection sites, transient alopecia, reversible thrombocytopenia, paresthesias, hypersensitivity	These effects are uncommon. They are more likely to occur with large doses or prolonged administration.
(2) With warfarin, dermatitis, diarrhea, alopecia	These effects occur only occassionally. Warfarin has been given for prolonged periods without toxicity.
c. With thrombolytic drugs, observe for bleeding with all uses and reperfusion arrhythmias when used for acute myocardial infarction.	Bleeding is most likely to occur at sites of venipuncture or other invasive procedures. Reperfusion arrhythmias may occur when blood supply is restored to previously ischemic myocardium.

4. Observe for drug interactions
  a. Drugs that *increase* effects of heparin:

(1) Aspirin, dipyridamole, ticlopidine	These drugs inhibit platelet function and therefore increase risks of bleeding.
(2) Warfarin (Coumadin)	Additive anticoagulant effects and increased risks of bleeding

NURSING ACTIONS	RATIONALE/EXPLANATION
b. Drugs that *decrease* effects of heparin:	
(1) Antihistamines, digitalis glycosides, tetracyclines	These drugs antagonize the anticoagulant effects of heparin. Mechanisms are not clear.
(2) Protamine sulfate	The antidote for heparin overdose
c. Drugs that *increase* effects of warfarin	
(1) Allopurinol, anabolic steroids (*e.g.*, methandrostenolone), cimetidine, tricyclic antidepressants (*e.g.*, amitriptyline), isoniazid (INH), methylphenidate	These drugs potentiate anticoagulant effects (and increase risks of bleeding) by inhibiting hepatic enzymes and slowing the rate of warfarin metabolism. Other mechanisms also may be involved.
(2) Antibiotics	Potentiate anticoagulant effects by decreasing production of vitamin K by intestinal bacteria. In addition, chloramphenicol and tetracyclines act by other mechanisms to increase risks of bleeding. Alternate antibiotics are preferred.
(3) Antidiabetic agents, oral	Displace anticoagulants from plasma protein binding sites
(4) Antineoplastics	Additive risks of bleeding because antineoplastic drugs depress bone marrow function and platelet counts
(5) Antiplatelet agents (*e.g.*, aspirin)	Decrease platelet aggregation
(6) Aspirin, other salicylates and nonsteroidal anti-inflammatory agents (*e.g.*, indomethacin)	These drugs greatly increase risks of bleeding. They displace warfarin from plasma protein binding sites, decrease platelet aggregation, and are ulcerogenic. None of these drugs should be given concurrently with oral anticoagulants.
(7) Heparin	Additive anticoagulant effects
(8) Thyroid preparations (*e.g.*, Synthroid)	Increase metabolism of clotting factors
d. Drugs that may *increase* or *decrease* effects of oral anticoagulants:	
(1) Alcohol	Alcohol may induce liver enzymes, which *decrease* effects by accelerating the rate of metabolism of the anticoagulant drug. However, with alcohol-induced liver disease (*i.e.*, cirrhosis), effects may be *increased* owing to impaired metabolism of the anticoagulant.
(2) Corticosteroids	These drugs may *decrease* effects by stimulating synthesis of clotting factors or other mechanisms. They may *increase* risks of bleeding by their ulcerogenic effects.
e. Drugs that *decrease* effects of warfarin:	
(1) Antacids and griseofulvin	May decrease GI absorption of oral anticoagulants
(2) Barbiturates and other sedative-hypnotics, carbamazepine, disulfiram, rifampin	These drugs activate liver metabolizing enzymes, which accelerate the rate of metabolism of oral anticoagulant drugs.
(3) Cholestyramine	Decreases absorption
(4) Diuretics	Increase synthesis and concentration of blood clotting factors
(5) Estrogens, including oral contraceptives	Increase synthesis of clotting factors and have thromboembolic effect
(6) Vitamin K	Restores prothrombin and other vitamin K-dependent clotting factors in the blood. Antidote for overdose of oral anticoagulants.

(continued)

NURSING ACTIONS	RATIONALE/EXPLANATION
5. Teach clients receiving long-term therapy	
a. Take the drugs as directed.	This is crucial to avoid underdosage (risks of thromboemboli) and overdosage (risks of bleeding).
b. Do not change from one brand to another.	Different brands may not be equivalent and either increased or decreased anticoagulant effects may occur.
c. Do not take any other drugs without the physician's knowledge and consent, especially over-the-counter cold remedies and analgesics.	Oral anticoagulant drugs interact with many other drugs with subsequent increased or decreased anticoagulant effects, either of which may be harmful to the client. Many nonprescription analgesics and cold remedies contain aspirin. Aspirin and any aspirin-containing products are contraindicated with oral anticoagulants because the risks of bleeding are greatly increased.
d. Do not stop taking any medication without the physician's knowledge and consent.	Dosage of warfarin is carefully regulated or balanced. Stopping a drug may upset the balance and either increase risks of bleeding or increase risks of blood clot formation.
e. Inform any physician, surgeon, or dentist about anticoagulant drug therapy before any treatment measures are begun.	This is mainly a safety measure to prevent bleeding episodes.
f. Keep all appointments for laboratory tests.	These tests are required regularly throughout oral anticoagulant therapy for safety (prevention of bleeding) and titration of dosage.
g. Use safety precautions:	To avoid injury and subsequent bleeding
(1) Avoid walking barefoot.	
(2) Avoid contact sports.	
(3) Use an electric razor.	
(4) Avoid injections when possible.	
h. Carry an identification card, necklace, or bracelet (*e.g.,* MedicAlert) stating the name of the drug and the physician's name and telephone number.	
i. Inspect skin, mucous membranes, urine, and feces for signs of bleeding. Report to the physician if bleeding occurs.	Pinprick hemorrhages, bruising, or frank bleeding may occur in the skin and mucous membranes. Urine may be bright red or smoky gray. Feces may be bright red or black (tarry).
j. Apply direct pressure to superficial bleeding sites for 3 to 5 min or longer if necessary.	To prevent excessive blood loss
k. Do not eat large amounts of green leafy vegetables (*e.g.,* spinach), tomatoes, bananas, or fish.	These foods contain vitamin K, which may decrease anticoagulant effects.

REVIEW AND APPLICATION EXERCISES

1. What are the major factors in blood clotting?

2. What are the indications for use of heparin and warfarin?

3. How do heparin and warfarin differ in mechanism of action, onset and duration of action, and method of administration?

4. List interventions to protect clients from anticoagulant-induced bleeding.

5. Why are clients with low levels of serum albumin at high risk of bleeding with warfarin unless dosage is reduced?

6. When is it appropriate to use protamine sulfate as an antidote for heparin?

7. When is it appropriate to use vitamin K as an antidote for warfarin?

8. How do protamine sulfate and vitamin K act to control bleeding?

9. What is the role of platelets in blood coagulation?

10. List commonly used drugs that inhibit platelet aggregation and function.

11. For what conditions are antiplatelet drugs indicated?

12. How do thrombolytic drugs act to dissolve blood clots?

13. When is it appropriate to use a thrombolytic drug?

14. How do aminocaproic acid and tranexamic acid stop bleeding induced by thrombolytics?

SELECTED REFERENCES

Brater, D.C. (1997). Clinical pharmacology of cardiovascular drugs. In W.N. Kelley (Ed.), *Textbook of internal medicine*, 3rd ed., pp. 552–569. Philadelphia: Lippincott-Raven.

Byers, J.F. (1993). The use of aspirin in cardiovascular disease. *Journal of Cardiovascular Nursing, 8*(1), 1–18.

Drug facts and comparisons. (Updated monthly). St. Louis: Facts and Comparisons.

Erdman, S.M., Rodvold, K.A. & Friedenberg, W.R. (1997). Thromboembolic disorders. In J.T. DiPiro, R.L. Talbert, G.C. Yee, G.R. Matzke, B.G. Wells, & L.M. Posey (Eds.), *Pharmacotherapy: A pathophysiologic approach*, 3rd ed., pp. 399–433. Stamford, CT: Appleton & Lange.

Ezekowitz, M.D. & Hirsh, J. (1997). Use of anticoagulant drugs. In W.N. Kelley (Ed.), *Textbook of internal medicine*, 3rd ed., pp. 569–578. Philadelphia: Lippincott-Raven.

Goodnight, S.H., Coull, B.M., McAnulty, J.H., & Taylor L.M. (1993). Antiplatelet therapy—Part 1. *Western Journal of Medicine, 158,* 385–392.

Guyton, A.C. & Hall, J.E. (1996). *Textbook of medical physiology*, 9th ed. Philadelphia: W.B. Saunders.

Haines, S.T. & Bussey. H.I. (1995). Thrombosis and the pharmacology of antithrombotic agents. *The Annals of Pharmacotherapy, 29*(9), 892–905.

Majerus, P.W., Broze, G.J., Jr., Miletich, J.P. & Tollefsen, D.M. (1996). Anticoagulant, thrombolytic, and antiplatelet drugs. In J.G. Hardman, L.E. Limbird, P.B. Molinoff, & R.W. Ruddon (Eds.). *Goodman & Gilman's The pharmacological basis of therapeutics*, 9th ed., pp. 1341–1359. New York: McGraw-Hill.

Nichols, W.L. & Bowie, E.J.W. (1993). Standardization of the prothrombin time for monitoring orally administered anticoagulant therapy with use of the international normalized ratio system. *Mayo Clinic Proceedings, 68*, 897–898.

Porth, C.M. (1994). *Pathophysiology: Concepts of altered health states*, 4th ed. Philadelphia: J.B. Lippincott.

Smeltzer, S.C. & Bare, B.G. (1996). *Brunner and Suddarth's Textbook of medical-surgical nursing*, 8th ed. Philadelphia: Lippincott-Raven.

58 Antilipemics and Peripheral Vasodilators

Outline

Antilipemic Drugs and Peripheral Vasodilators

Atherosclerosis

Blood Lipids

Hyperlipidemia

Drugs Used to Treat Hyperlipidemia

  types of antilipemic drugs

    bile acid sequestrants

    HMG-CoA reductase inhibitors

    niacin

    gemfibrozil

  hemorrheologic agent

    pentoxifylline

Nursing Process

  assessment

  nursing diagnoses

  planning/goals

  interventions

  evaluation

Principles of Therapy

  initial treatment

  drug selection

  use in children

  use in older adults

  home care

Objectives

After studying this chapter, the student will be able to:

1 Discuss the role of hyperlipidemia in the etiology of atherosclerosis.

2 Identify sources and functions of cholesterol.

3 Describe selected cholesterol-lowering drugs in terms of mechanism of action, indications for use, major adverse effects, and nursing process implications.

4 Teach clients nonpharmacologic measures to prevent or reduce hyperlipidemia.

Key Terms

Antilipemic	**Hyperlipidemia**
Claudication	**Viscosity**
Hypercholesterolemia	

Antilipemic Drugs and Peripheral Vasodilators

Antilipemic drugs are used in the treatment of clients with elevated blood lipids, a major risk factor for atherosclerosis. **Peripheral vasodilator drugs** are occasionally used in the treatment of clients with arterial insufficiency caused by atherosclerosis or vasospasm. However, there is little evidence of efficacy in increasing blood flow to ischemic tissues in the heart, brain, or extremities. These drugs are listed in Table 58-1. Pentoxifylline, a hemorrheologic agent that improves blood flow by decreasing blood viscosity and making erythrocytes more flexible, is also discussed in this chapter.

Although a few other drugs are included here, the main focus is the antilipemic drugs, which have proven efficacy and are being used increasingly to reduce morbidity and mortality from coronary heart disease and total mortality. To understand clinical usage of these drugs, one needs to understand atherosclerosis, characteristics of blood lipids, and types of blood lipid disorders.

Atherosclerosis

Atherosclerosis is a major cause of ischemic heart disease (*e.g.,* angina pectoris, myocardial infarction, heart failure), stroke, peripheral vascular disease, and death. It is characterized by formation of lesions in the endothelial lining of the aorta and its branches, the coronary arteries, and the arteries that supply the brain. These lesions (called fatty plaque or atheromas) result from progressive accumulation of lipids, vascular smooth muscle cells, macrophages, lymphocytes, and connective tissue proteins. Over time, the lesions interfere with nutrition of the blood vessel lining, the normally smooth endothelium becomes roughened, and thrombi, necrosis, scarring, and calcification occur. As the lesions develop and enlarge, they protrude into the lumen of the artery, reduce the size of the lumen, reduce blood flow, and may eventually occlude the artery. Severely impaired blood flow leads to damage or death of tissue supplied by the artery. When an artery is gradually blocked by atheromatous plaque, collateral circulation may develop sufficiently to provide oxygen and nutrients at rest. However, tissue ischemia and infarction are likely to develop with strenuous exercise or other conditions that increase tissue demands for oxygen and nutrients.

Blood Lipids

Blood lipids, which include cholesterol, phospholipids, and triglycerides, are derived from the diet or synthesized by the liver and intestine. Most cholesterol is found in body cells, where it is a component of cell membranes and performs other essential functions. In cells of the adrenal glands, ovaries, and testes, cholesterol is required for the synthesis of steroid hormones (*e.g.,* cortisol, estrogen, progesterone, and testosterone). In liver cells, cholesterol is used to form cholic acid. The cholic acid is then conjugated with other substances to form bile salts, which promote absorption and digestion of fats. In addition, a small amount is found in blood serum. Serum cholesterol is the portion of total body cholesterol involved in the formation of atherosclerotic plaques in arteries throughout the body. Unless a person has a genetic disorder of lipid metabolism, the amount of cholesterol in the blood is strongly related to dietary intake of saturated fat. Phospholipids are essential components of cell membranes, and triglycerides provide energy for cellular metabolism.

Blood lipids are transported in plasma by specific proteins called lipoproteins. Each lipoprotein contains cholesterol, phospholipid, and triglyceride bound to protein. The lipoproteins vary in density and amounts of lipid and protein. Density is determined mainly by the amount of protein, which is more dense than fat. Thus, density increases as the proportion of protein increases. The lipoproteins are differentiated according to these properties, which can be measured in the laboratory. For example, high density lipoprotein (HDL) cho-

TABLE 58-1	PERIPHERAL VASOLIDATORS
Generic/Trade Name	**Routes and Dosage Ranges (Adults)**
Papaverine hydrochloride (Pavabid, others)	PO 100–300 mg three to five times daily. Timed-release capsules, PO 150 mg q12h
Cyclandelate (Cyclospasmol)	PO 1.2–1.6 g daily, in four divided doses, before meals and at bedtime. Decreased to 400–800 mg daily, in two to four divided doses, for maintenance
Isoxsuprine hydrochloride (Vasodilan)	PO 10–20 mg, three or four times daily IM 5–10 mg, two or three times daily

lesterol contains larger amounts of protein and smaller amounts of lipid; low density lipoprotein (LDL) cholesterol contains less protein and larger amounts of lipid. Other plasma lipoproteins are chylomicrons and very low density lipoproteins (VLDL). Additional characteristics of lipoproteins are described in Box 58-1.

The National Cholesterol Education Program Expert Panel on Detection, Evaluation and Treatment of High Blood Cholesterol in Adults, under the auspices of the National Institutes of Health, classifies blood lipid levels as follows:

Total serum cholesterol (mg/dl)
   Normal or desirable = less than 200
   Borderline high = 200–239
   High = 240 or above
LDL cholesterol (mg/dl)
   Normal or desirable = less than 130

BOX 58-1. TYPES OF LIPOPROTEINS

Chylomicrons, the largest lipoprotein molecules, are synthesized in the wall of the small intestine. They carry recently ingested dietary cholesterol and triglycerides that have been absorbed from the gastrointestinal tract. Hyperchylomicronemia normally occurs after a fatty meal, reaches peak levels in 3 to 4 h, and subsides within 12 to 14 h. Chylomicrons carry triglycerides to fat and muscle cells, where the enzyme lipoprotein lipase breaks down the molecule and releases fatty acids to be used for energy or stored as fat. This process leaves a remnant containing cholesterol, which is then transported to the liver. Thus, chylomicrons transport triglycerides to peripheral tissues and cholesterol to the liver.

Low density lipoprotein (LDL) cholesterol, sometimes called "bad cholesterol," transports about 75% of serum cholesterol and carries it to peripheral tissues and the liver. LDL cholesterol is removed from the circulation by receptor and nonreceptor mechanisms. The receptor mechanism involves the binding of LDL cholesterol to receptors on cell surface membranes. The bound LDL molecule is then engulfed into the cell where it is broken down by enzymes and releases free cholesterol into the cytoplasm.

Most LDL cholesterol receptors are located in the liver. However, nonhepatic tissues (e.g., adrenal glands, smooth muscle cells, endothelial cells, and lymphoid cells) also have receptors by which they obtain the cholesterol needed for building cell membranes and synthesizing hormones. These cells can regulate their cholesterol intake by adding or removing LDL receptors.

About two thirds of the LDL cholesterol is removed from the bloodstream by the receptor-dependent mechanism. The number of LDL receptors on cell membranes determines the amount of LDL degradation (i.e., the more receptors on cells, the more LDL is broken down). Conditions that decrease the number or function of receptors (e.g., high dietary intake of cholesterol, saturated fat, or calories), increase blood levels of LDL.

The remaining one third is removed by mechanisms that do not involve receptors. Nonreceptor uptake occurs in various cells, especially when levels of circulating LDL cholesterol are high. For example, macrophage cells in arterial walls can attach LDL, thereby promoting accumulation of cholesterol and the development of atherosclerosis. The amount of LDL cholesterol removed by nonreceptor mechanisms is increased with inadequate numbers of receptors or excessive amounts of LDL cholesterol.

A high serum level of LDL cholesterol is atherogenic and a strong risk factor for coronary heart disease. The body normally attempts to compensate for high serum levels by inhibiting hepatic synthesis of cholesterol and cellular synthesis of new LDL receptors.

Very low density lipoprotein (VLDL) contains about 75% triglycerides and 25% cholesterol. It transports endogenous triglycerides (those synthesized in the liver and intestine, not those derived exogenously, from food) to fat and muscle cells. There, as with chylomicrons, lipoprotein lipase breaks down the molecule and releases fatty acids to be used for energy or stored as fat. The removal of triglycerides from VLDL leaves a cholesterol-rich remnant, which returns to the liver. Then, the cholesterol is secreted into the intestine, mostly as bile acids, or it is used to form more VLDL and recirculated.

High density lipoprotein (HDL) cholesterol, often referred to as "good cholesterol," is a small but very important lipoprotein. It is synthesized in the liver and intestine and some is derived from the enzymatic breakdown of chylomicrons and VLDL. It contains moderate amounts of cholesterol. However, this cholesterol is transported to the liver for catabolism and excretion. This reverse transport of cholesterol is thought to have protective effects against coronary heart disease.

The mechanisms by which HDL cholesterol exerts protective effects are unknown. Possible mechanisms include clearing cholesterol from atheromatous plaque; increasing excretion of cholesterol so less is available for reuse in the formation of LDL cholesterol; and inhibiting cellular uptake of LDL cholesterol. Regular exercise and moderate alcohol consumption are associated with increased levels of HDL cholesterol; obesity, diabetes mellitus, genetic factors, smoking, and some medications (e.g., steroids and beta blockers) are associated with decreased levels. HDL cholesterol levels are not directly affected by diet.

Borderline high = 130–159
    High = 160
HDL cholesterol (mg/dl)
    High = more than 60
    Low = less than 35
Triglycerides (mg/dl)
    Normal or desirable = less than 200
    Borderline high = 200–400
    High = 400–1000
    Very high = more than 1000

Overall, the most effective blood lipid profile for prevention or treatment of atherosclerosis and its sequelae is a high HDL cholesterol, a low LDL cholesterol, and a low total cholesterol. A low triglyceride level is also desirable. For accurate interpretation of a client's lipid profile, blood samples for laboratory testing of triglycerides should be drawn after the client has fasted about 12 hours. Fasting is not required for cholesterol testing.

Hyperlipidemia

Hyperlipidemia is associated with atherosclerosis and its many pathophysiologic effects (*e.g.*, myocardial ischemia and infarction, stroke, peripheral arterial occlusive disease). Ischemic heart disease has a high rate of morbidity and mortality. Elevated total cholesterol and LDL cholesterol and reduced HDL cholesterol are the abnormalities that are major risk factors for coronary heart disease. Elevations in triglyceride levels also play a role in cardiovascular disease. For example, high blood levels reflect excessive caloric intake (excessive dietary fats are stored in adipose tissue; excessive pro-

teins and carbohydrates are converted to triglycerides and also stored in adipose tissue) and obesity. High caloric intake also increases the conversion of VLDL to LDL cholesterol and high dietary intake of triglycerides and saturated fat decrease the activity of LDL receptors and increase synthesis of cholesterol. Very high triglyceride levels are associated with acute pancreatitis.

When blood lipid levels are elevated, there is an accompanying increase in blood levels of lipoproteins (hyperlipoproteinemia). Hyperlipoproteinemia may be primary (*i.e.*, genetic or familial) or secondary to dietary habits or other diseases (*e.g.*, diabetes mellitus, alcoholism, hypothyroidism, obstructive liver disease). Types of hyperlipoproteinemias are described in Box 58-2.

Drugs Used to Treat Hyperlipidemia

Antilipemic drugs are used to decrease blood lipids, especially total and LDL cholesterol, to prevent or delay the development of atheromas, to promote the regression of existing atheromas, and to reduce morbidity and mortality. Antilipemic drugs decrease hyperlipoproteinemias by altering the production, metabolism, or removal of lipoproteins. No drugs currently available are effective in lowering all types of hyperlipoproteinemia. Antilipemic drugs are recommended for use when dietary therapy for 3 to 6 months fails to decrease hyperlipoproteinemia to an acceptable level. They are also recommended for clients with signs and symptoms of coronary heart disease, a strong family history of coronary heart disease or hyperlipoproteinemia, or other risk factors for atherosclerotic vascular disease (*e.g.*, hy-

---

BOX 58-2. TYPES OF HYPERLIPOPROTEINEMIA

Type I is characterized by elevated or normal serum cholesterol, elevated triglycerides, and chylomicronemia. This rare condition may occur in infancy and childhood.

Type IIa (familial hypercholesterolemia) is characterized by a high level of LDL cholesterol, a normal level of VLDL, and a normal or slightly increased level of triglycerides. It occurs in children and is a definite risk factor for development of atherosclerosis and coronary artery disease. **Type IIb** (combined familial hyperlipoproteinemia) is characterized by increased levels of LDL, VLDL, cholesterol, and triglycerides and lipid deposits (xanthomas) in the feet, knees, and elbows. It occurs in adults.

Type III is characterized by elevations of cholesterol and triglycerides plus abnormal levels of LDL and VLDL. This type usually occurs in middle-aged adults (40–60 y) and is

associated with accelerated coronary and peripheral vascular disease.

Type IV is characterized by normal or elevated cholesterol levels, elevated triglycerides, and increased levels of VLDL. This type usually occurs in adults and may be the most common form of hyperlipoproteinemia. Type IV is often secondary to obesity, excessive intake of alcohol, or other diseases. Ischemic heart disease may occur at 40 to 50 y of age.

Type V is characterized by elevated cholesterol and triglyceride levels with an increased level of VLDL and chylomicronemia. This uncommon type usually occurs in adults. Type V is not associated with ischemic heart disease. Instead, it is associated with fat and carbohydrate intolerance, abdominal pain, and pancreatitis, which are relieved by lowering triglyceride levels.

pertension, diabetes mellitus, cigarette smoking). Types of antilipemic drugs are described below; individual drugs are listed in Table 58-2.

TYPES OF ANTILIPEMIC DRUGS

Bile-acid sequestrants (cholestyramine and colestipol) bind bile acids in the intestinal lumen. This causes the bile acids to be excreted in feces and prevents their being recirculated to the liver. Loss of bile acids stimulates hepatic synthesis of more bile acids from cholesterol. As more hepatic cholesterol is used to pro-

duce bile acids, more serum cholesterol moves into the liver to replenish the supply, thereby lowering serum cholesterol (especially LDL). LDL cholesterol levels decrease within a week of starting one of these drugs and reach maximal reductions within a month. When the drugs are stopped, pretreatment LDL cholesterol levels are reached within a month.

The main advantage of these drugs is their safety. They are not absorbed systemically and therefore do not cause serious adverse effects. The main disadvantages are drug interactions. Bile acid sequestrants decrease absorption of many oral medications (*e.g.*, digoxin, glip-

TABLE 58-2	ANTILIPEMIC AGENTS		
Generic/Trade Name	**Clinical Indications (Type of Hyperlipo-proteinemia)**	**Route and Dosage Ranges**	
		Adults	*Children*
Cholestyramine (Questran)	Type IIa	PO tablets 4 g once or twice daily initially, gradually increased at monthly intervals to 8–16 g daily in two divided doses. Maximum daily dose, 24 g. PO powder 4 g one to six times daily	
Colestipol	Type IIa	PO tablets 2 g once or twice daily initially, gradually increased at 1- to 2-mo intervals, up to 16 g daily PO granules 5 g daily initially, gradually increased at 1- to 2-mo intervals, up to 30 g daily in single or divided doses	
Fluvastatin (Lescol)	Types IIa and IIb	PO 20–40 mg once daily at bedtime	
Gemfibrozil (Lopid)	Types IV, V	PO 900–1500 mg daily, usually 1200 mg in two divided doses, 30 min before morning and evening meals	
Lovastatin (Mevacor)	Types IIa and IIb	PO 20 mg daily with a meal, initially, increased up to 80 mg daily if necessary. Dosage increments should be at least 4 wk apart.	
Nicotinic acid (niacin)	Types II, III, IV, V	PO 2–6 g daily, in three or four divided doses, with or just after meals	PO 55–87 mg/kg/d, in three or four divided doses, with or just after meals
Pravastatin (Pravachol)	Types IIa and IIb	PO 10–40 mg once daily at bedtime Elderly, PO 10 mg once daily at bedtime	
Simvastatin (Zocor)	Types IIa and IIb	PO 5–40 mg once daily in the evening Elderly, PO 5–20 mg once daily in the evening	

izide, propranolol, tetracyclines, thiazide diuretics, thyroid hormones, fat-soluble vitamins, and warfarin). When one of these drugs is ordered concomitantly with a bile acid sequestrant, the drug should be given at least 1 hour before or 4 hours after cholestyramine or colestipol administration. In addition, dosage of the interactive drug may need to be changed when a bile acid sequestrant is added or withdrawn.

HMG-CoA reductase inhibitors (also called statins) decrease or block an enzyme (hydroxymethylglutaryl-coenzyme A) required for hepatic synthesis of cholesterol. By decreasing production of cholesterol, these drugs (lovastatin, pravastatin, simvastatin, and fluvastatin) decrease total serum cholesterol, LDL cholesterol, VLDL cholesterol, and triglycerides. They reduce LDL cholesterol within 2 weeks and reach maximal effects in about 4 to 6 weeks. HDL cholesterol levels remain unchanged or increase. Overall, these drugs are the most effective available for lowering cholesterol and are the most widely used antilipemics. They are also well tolerated; the most common adverse effects (nausea, constipation, diarrhea, abdominal cramps or pain, headache, skin rash) are usually mild and transient. More serious reactions include rare occurrences of hepatotoxicity and myopathy. Long-term effects of suppressing cholesterol synthesis are unknown but should be considered because cholesterol is required for cell membranes and several hormones.

Niacin (nicotinin acid) decreases both cholesterol and triglycerides. It decreases hepatic synthesis of VLDL, which leads to decreased production of LDL cholesterol. It also increases HDL cholesterol by reducing its catabolism. Disadvantages of niacin are the high doses required for antilipemic effects and the subsequent adverse effects. Niacin commonly causes flushing and pruritus and may cause hyperglycemia, hyperuricemia, and elevated hepatic transaminase enzymes. Flushing and pruritus can be reduced by starting with small doses, gradually increasing doses, taking doses with meals, and taking aspirin 325 mg about 30 minutes before niacin doses.

Gemfibrozil decreases hepatic production of triglycerides, decreases VLDL cholesterol, and increases HDL cholesterol. Its main adverse effects are gastrointestinal discomfort and diarrhea.

HEMORRHEOLOGIC AGENT

Pentoxifylline (Trental), a methylxanthine derivative, is a hemorrheologic agent that improves blood flow by decreasing blood viscosity rather than by vasodilation. Specific effects include increased flexibility of red blood cells with subsequent decreases in red blood cell aggregation and local hyperviscosity, decreased platelet aggregation, and decreased fibrinogen concentration.

Pentoxifylline is approved for use in intermittent claudication caused by chronic occlusive arterial insufficiency. It is contraindicated in clients who cannot take methylxanthines, such as theophylline or caffeine. It is generally well tolerated, and most adverse reactions (dyspepsia, nausea, vomiting, dizziness, and headache) occur in only 1% to 3% of recipients.

Route and Dosage Range

Adults: PO 400 mg three times per day with meals, reduced to 400 mg twice daily if gastrointestinal and central nervous system side effects occur

Nursing Process

Assessment

Assess the client's status in relation to atherosclerotic vascular disease.
- Identify risk factors:
  - Hypertension
  - Diabetes mellitus
  - High intake of dietary fat and refined sugars
  - Obesity
  - Lack of exercise
  - Cigarette smoking
  - Family history of atherosclerotic disorders
  - Hyperlipidemia
- Signs and symptoms depend on the specific problem:
  - **Hyperlipidemia** is manifested by elevated serum cholesterol (above 240 mg/100 ml) or triglycerides (above 200 mg/100 ml) or both.
  - **Coronary artery atherosclerosis** is manifested by myocardial ischemia (angina pectoris, myocardial infarction).
  - **Cerebrovascular insufficiency** may be manifested by syncope, memory loss, transient ischemic attacks (TIAs) or cerebrovascular accidents (CVAs). Impairment of blood flow to the brain is caused primarily by atherosclerosis in the carotid, vertebral, or cerebral arteries.
  - **Peripheral arterial insufficiency** is manifested by impaired blood flow in the legs (weak or absent pulses; cool, pale extremities; intermittent claudication; leg pain at rest; and development of gangrene, usually in the toes because they are most distal to blood supply). This condition results from atherosclerosis in the distal abdominal aorta, the iliac arteries, and the femoral and smaller arteries in the legs.

Nursing Diagnoses

- Altered Tissue Perfusion related to atherosclerotic plaque in coronary, cerebral, or peripheral arteries
- Altered Nutrition: More Than Body Requirements of fats and calories
- Anxiety related to risks of atherosclerotic cardiovascular disease
- Body Image Disturbance related to the need for lifestyle changes
- Pain related to gastrointestinal distress with drug therapy
- Noncompliance related to dietary restrictions and adverse drug reactions
- Knowledge Deficit related to drug and diet therapy of hyperlipidemia

Planning/Goals

The client will:

- Take lipid-lowering drugs as prescribed
- Decrease dietary intake of saturated fats and cholesterol
- Lose weight if obese and maintain the lower weight
- Have periodic measurements of blood lipids
- Avoid preventable adverse drug effects
- Receive positive reinforcement for efforts to lower blood lipid levels
- Feel less anxious and more in control as risks of atherosclerotic cardiovascular disease are decreased

Interventions

Use measures to prevent, delay, or minimize atherosclerosis.

- Help clients to control risk factors. Ideally, primary prevention begins in childhood with healthful eating habits (*i.e.,* avoiding excessive fats, meat, and dairy products; obtaining adequate amounts of all nutrients, including dietary fiber; avoiding obesity), exercise, and avoiding cigarette smoking. However, changing habits to a more healthful lifestyle is helpful at any time, before or after disease manifestations appear. Weight loss often reduces blood lipids and lipoproteins to a normal range. Changing habits is difficult for most people, even those with severe symptoms.
- Use measures to increase blood flow to tissues:
  - Exercise is helpful in developing collateral circulation in the heart and legs. Collateral circulation involves use of secondary vessels in response to tissue ischemia related to obstruction of the principal vessels. Clients with angina pectoris or previous myocardial infarction require a carefully planned and supervised program of progressive exercise. Those with peripheral arterial insufficiency usually can increase exercise tolerance by walking regularly. Distances should be determined by occurrence of pain and must be individualized.
  - Posture and position may be altered to increase blood flow to the legs in peripheral arterial insufficiency. Elevating the head of the bed and having the legs horizontal or dependent may help. Elevating the feet is usually contraindicated unless edema is present or likely to develop.
- Although drug therapy is being increasingly used to prevent or treat atherosclerotic disorders, a major treatment of occlusive vascular disease is surgical removal of atherosclerotic plaque or revascularization procedures. Thus, severe angina pectoris may be relieved by a coronary artery bypass procedure that detours around occluded vessels. This procedure also may be done after a myocardial infarction. The goal is to prevent infarction or reinfarction. TIAs may be relieved by carotid endarterectomy; the goal is to prevent a stroke. Peripheral arterial insufficiency may be relieved by aortofemoral, femoral-popliteal, or other bypass grafts that detour around occluded vessels. Although these procedures increase blood flow to ischemic tissues, they do not halt progression of atherosclerosis.

The nursing role in relation to these procedures is to provide excellent preoperative and postoperative nursing care to promote healing, prevent infection, maintain patency of grafts, and help the client to achieve optimum function.

- The most effective treatment in hyperlipoproteinemia is diet therapy. Specific diets have been developed for each type.

Any antilipemic drug therapy must be accompani[ed] appropriate diet.

Teach clients:

- That all adults 20 years of age or older should have measurements of total cholesterol and HDL cholesterol at least once every 5 years. People with a personal or family history of hyperlipidemia or other risk factors should be tested more often.
- The most effective measures for preventing hyperlipidemia and atherosclerosis are those related to a healthful lifestyle (diet low in cholesterol and saturated fats, weight control, exercise).
- Drug therapy is relatively ineffective without diet therapy. Overeating or gaining weight may decrease or cancel the lipid-lowering effects of the drugs.
- Dietary restrictions and other lifestyle changes contribute to improved health and decreased risks of heart attack and stroke.

Evaluation

- Observe for decreased blood levels of cholesterol and triglycerides.
- Observe and interview regarding compliance with instructions for drug, diet, and other therapeutic measures.
- Observe and interview regarding adverse drug effects.
- Validate the client's ability to identify foods high and low in cholesterol and saturated fats.

Principles of Therapy

INITIAL TREATMENT

Although several antilipemic drugs are available, none is effective in all types of hyperlipidemia. Although hypercholesterolemia is usually emphasized, hypertriglyceridemia is also associated with most types of hyperlipoproteinemia. Initial treatment for high serum triglycerides includes efforts to achieve desirable body weight, consume low levels of saturated fat and cholesterol, exercise regularly, stop smoking and restrict alcohol, if indicated. In addition, treatment of conditions known to increase blood lipid levels (*e.g.,* diabetes, hypothyroidism, liver disease, corticosteroid drug therapy) may obviate the need for drug therapy. For these reasons, and because all antilipemic drugs may cause adverse effects, diet and exercise are the first-line treatment. Drug therapy is used if there is significant hyperlipidemia and lifestyle changes are ineffective in lowering blood lipids within about 6 months.

DRUG SELECTION

Drug selection is based on the type of hyperlipidemia and its severity. For single drug therapy to lower cholesterol, cholestyramine, colestipol, fluvastatin, lovastatin,

pravastatin, or simvastatin is preferred. To lower both cholesterol and triglycerides, a statin, gemfibrozil, or niacin may be used. To lower triglycerides, gemfibrozil or niacin may be used. Gemfibrozil is preferred for persons with diabetes because niacin increases blood sugar.

When monotherapy is not effective, combination therapy is rational because the drugs act by different mechanisms. In general, an HMG-CoA reductase inhibitor (a statin) and a bile acid sequestrant or niacin and a bile acid sequestrant are the most effective combinations in reducing total and LDL cholesterol. Gemfibrozil or niacin should be included when a goal of therapy is to increase levels of HDL cholesterol. However, giving either of these drugs in combination with lovastatin or a related drug increases the risks of hepatotoxicity.

USE IN CHILDREN

Hyperlipidemia occurs in children and may lead to atherosclerotic cardiovascular disease, including myocardial infarction, in early adulthood. Hyperlipidemia is diagnosed with total serum cholesterol levels of 200 mg/dl or above (desirable level, less than 170) and LDL cholesterol levels of 130 mg/dl or above (desirable level, less than 110). Thus, early identification and treatment are needed. As with adults, initial treatment consists of diet therapy (for 6 to 12 months) and treatment of any secondary causes, especially with younger children. With additional risk factors or primary familial hypercholesterolemia (type IIa), however, these measures are not likely to be effective without drug therapy. Antilipemic drug therapy is not recommended for children younger than 10 years. Although few studies have been done in children, the bile acid sequestrants are considered the drugs of choice, and niacin also may be used. Despite consid-

erable use of bile acid sequestrants, children's dosages have not been established. The HMG-CoA reductase inhibitors (lovastatin and related drugs) are not recommended in children under 18 years of age. The long-term consequences of antilipemic drug therapy in children are unknown.

USE IN OLDER ADULTS

As with younger adults, diet, exercise, and weight control should be tried first. When drug therapy is required, HMG-CoA reductase inhibitors are effective for lowering LDL cholesterol and are generally well tolerated by older adults. However, they are expensive. Niacin and bile acid sequestrants are effective, but older adults do not tolerate their adverse effects very well. In postmenopausal women, estrogen replacement therapy (alone or with a progestin) has beneficial antilipemic effects, lowering LDL cholesterol and raising HDL cholesterol.

Older adults often have diabetes, impaired liver function, or other conditions that raise blood lipid levels. Thus, treatment of secondary causes is especially important. They are also likely to have cardiovascular and other disorders that increase the adverse effects of antilipemic drugs. Overall, use of antilipemic drugs should be cautious, with close monitoring for therapeutic and adverse effects.

HOME CARE

For a client with hyperlipidemia, the home care nurse may teach about the prescribed treatment regimen and the importance of compliance, assist to obtain periodic blood lipid levels and other tests to monitor responses, and consult with a nutritionist.

NURSING ACTIONS

ANTILIPEMICS AND VASODILATORS

NURSING ACTIONS	*RATIONALE/EXPLANATION*
1. Administer accurately	
a. Mix cholestyramine powder and colestipol granules with water or other fluids, soups, cereals, or fruits such as applesauce or crushed pineapple.	These forms should not be taken dry; mixing dissolves or suspends the medication and increases palatability.
b. Do not give cholestyramine or colestipol with other drugs.	These drugs may prevent absorption of other drugs. Give other drugs 1 h before or 4–6 h after cholestyramine or colestipol.
c. Give lovastatin and immediate-release niacin with meals; give fluvastatin, pravastatin, simvastatin, and timed-release niacin without regard to meals.	To decrease gastric irritation associated with lovastatin and niacin.

(continued)

NURSING ACTIONS	*RATIONALE/EXPLANATION*
2. Observe for therapeutic effects **a.** With antilipemic agents, observe for decreased levels of total serum cholesterol, LDL cholesterol, and triglycerides and increased levels of HDL cholesterol.	With cholestyramine and colestipol, effects occur within 1 wk, with maximum effects in about 1 mo. With "statin" drugs, effects occur in 1–2 wk, with maximum effects in 4–6 wk. With gemfibrozil and niacin, effects occur in about 1 mo.
b. With vasodilators, observe for increased warmth and improved color of extremities.	
c. With pentoxifylline, observe for decreased leg pain with exercise.	Improvement in function and symptoms may occur in 2–4 wks.
3. Observe for adverse effects **a.** Gastrointestinal (GI) problems—nausea, vomiting, flatulence, constipation or diarrhea, abdominal discomfort	GI symptoms are the most common adverse effects of antilipemic and vasodilator drugs. Constipation is especially common with cholestyramine and colestipol.
b. With lovastatin and related drugs, observe for GI upset (see 3a), skin rash, pruritus, and myopathy	Adverse effects are usually mild and of short duration. A less common but potentially serious effect is liver dysfunction, usually manifested by increased levels of serum transaminases. Serum transaminases (AST, ALT) should be measured before starting the drug, every 4–6 wk during the first 3 mo, then every 6–12 wk or after dosage increases for 1 y, then every 6 mo.
c. With vasodilator drugs, tachycardia, hypotension, dizziness, and flushing of the face and neck may occur.	These effects result from vasodilation of nonatherosclerotic blood vessels, including the skin capillaries of the face and neck.
d. With nicotinic acid, flushing of the face and neck, pruritus, and skin rash may occur, as well as tachycardia, hypotension, and dizziness.	These symptoms may be prominent when nicotinic acid is used to lower blood lipids because relatively high doses are required. Aspirin 325 mg, given 30 min before nicotinic acid, decreases the flushing reaction.
e. With pentoxifylline, observe for dyspepsia, nausea, vomiting, dizziness, and headache.	These are the more common adverse effects.
4. Observe for drug interactions **a.** Drugs that *increase* effects of lovastatin and related drugs	
Cyclosporine, erythromycin, gemfibrozil, niacin	Increased risk of severe myopathy or rhabdomyolysis
b. Drugs that *increase* effects of nicotinic acid and other vasodilating drugs	
Alcohol and antihypertensive vasodilating drugs, (*e.g.*, hydralazine [Apresoline])	Additive vasodilation with hypotension and dizziness
5. Teach clients **a.** Take cholestyramine and colestipol with ample amounts of fluids, and increase dietary intake of high-fiber.	To prevent constipation, a common adverse effect
b. When taking vasodilator drugs assume an upright position slowly.	To prevent or decrease vertigo, syncope, and weakness

REVIEW AND APPLICATION EXERCISES

1. How would you describe hyperlipidemia to a client?

2. What is the goal of treatment for hyperlipidemia?

3. Differentiate lipid-lowering drugs according to their mechanisms of action.

4. Which groups of lipid-lowering drugs are most effective?

5. What are the limitations and adverse effects of peripheral vasodilating drugs?

6. How does pentoxifylline improve circulation?

SELECTED REFERENCES

Davis, J. & Sherer, K. (1994). *Applied nutrition and diet therapy for nurses,* 2nd ed. Philadelphia: W.B. Saunders.

Drug facts and comparisons. (Updated monthly). St. Louis: Facts and Comparisons.

Ettinger, W.H. & Hazzard, W.R. (1997). Approach to the elderly patient with dyslipidemia. In W.N. Kelley (Ed.), Textbook of internal medicine, 3rd ed., pp. 2494–2497. Philadelphia: Lippincott-Raven.

Guyton, A.C. & Hall, J.E. (1996). *Textbook of medical physiology,* 9th ed. Philadelphia: W.B. Saunders.

Porth, C.M. (1994). *Pathophysiology: Concepts of altered health states,* 4th ed. Philadelphia: J.B. Lippincott.

Talbert, R.L. (1997). Hyperlipidemia. In J.T. DiPiro, R.L. Talbert, G.C. Yee, G.R. Matzke, B.G. Wells & L.M. Posey (Eds.), *Pharmacotherapy: A pathophysiologic approach,* 3rd ed., pp. 459–489. Stamford, CT: Appleton & Lange.

Talbert, R.L. (1997). Peripheral vascular disease. In J.T. DiPiro, R.L. Talbert, G.C. Yee, G.R. Matzke, B.G. Wells & L.M. Posey (Eds.), *Pharmacotherapy: A pathophysiologic approach,* 3rd ed., pp. 491–508. Stamford, CT: Appleton & Lange.

Witztum, J.L. (1996). Drugs used in the treatment of hyperlipoproteinemias. In J.G. Hardman, L.E. Limbird, P.B. Molinoff & R.W. Ruddon (Eds.), *Goodman & Gilman's The pharmacological basis of therapeutics,* 9th ed., pp. 875–897. New York: McGraw-Hill.

Drugs Affecting the Digestive System

59

Physiology of the Digestive System

Outline

- **The Digestive System**
- **Organs of the Digestive System**
- **Secretions of the Digestive System**
- **Effects of Drugs on the Digestive System**

Objectives

After studying this chapter, the student will be able to:

1 Review roles of the main digestive tract structures.

2 List common signs and symptoms affecting gastrointestinal functions.

3 Identify general categories of drugs used to treat gastrointestinal disorders.

4 Discuss the effects of nongastrointestinal drugs on gastrointestinal functioning.

Key Terms

Bile and bile salts	**Gastrin**
Catabolism	**Metabolism**
Enterogastrone	**Peristalsis**

The Digestive System

The digestive system consists of the alimentary canal (a tube extending from the oral cavity to the anus, about 25 to 30 ft [7.5 to 9 m] long) and the accessory organs (salivary glands, gallbladder, liver, and pancreas). The main function of the system is to provide the body with fluids, nutrients, and electrolytes in a form that can be used at the cellular level. The system also disposes of waste products that result from the digestive process.

The alimentary canal has the same basic structure throughout. The layers of the wall are mucosa, connective tissue, and muscle. Peristalsis propels food through the tract and mixes the food bolus with digestive juices. Stimulation of the parasympathetic nervous system (by vagus nerves) increases motility and secretions. The tract has an abundant blood supply, which increases cell regeneration and healing. Blood flow increases during digestion and absorption. Blood flow decreases with strenuous exercise, sympathetic nervous system stimulation (*i.e.,* "fight or flight"), aging (secondary to decreased cardiac output and atherosclerosis), and conditions that shunt blood away from the digestive tract (*e.g.,* congestive heart failure, atherosclerosis).

Organs of the Digestive System

1. In the **oral cavity,** chewing mechanically breaks food into smaller particles, which can be swallowed more easily and provide a larger surface area for enzyme action. Food is also mixed with saliva, which lubricates the food bolus for swallowing and initiates the digestion of starch.
2. The **esophagus** is a musculofibrous tube about 10 inches (25 cm) long; its main function is to convey food from the pharynx to the stomach. It secretes a small amount of mucus and has some peristaltic movement.
3. The **stomach** is a dilated area that serves as a reservoir. It churns and mixes the food with digestive juices, secretes mucus and enzymes, starts protein breakdown, and secretes intrinsic factor, which is necessary for absorption of vitamin B_{12} from the ileum. Although there is much diffusion of water and electrolytes through the gastric mucosa in both directions, there is very little absorption of these substances. Carbohydrates and amino acids are also poorly absorbed. Only a few highly lipid-soluble substances, such as alcohol and some drugs, are absorbed in moderate quantities from the stomach.

 The inlet of the stomach is the end of the esophagus, and the outlet is the pyloric sphincter at the beginning of the duodenum. The stomach normally holds about 1000 ml comfortably and empties in about 4 hours. Numerous factors influence the rate of gastric emptying, including the size of the pylorus, gastric motility, type of food, fluidity of chyme (the material produced by gastric digestion of food), and the state of the duodenum. Generally, factors that cause rapid emptying include carbohydrate foods, increased motility, fluid chyme, and an empty duodenum. The stomach empties more slowly with decreased gastric tone and motility, fatty foods, chyme of excessive acidity, and a duodenum that contains fats, proteins, or chyme of excessive acidity. When fats are present, the duodenal mucosa produces a hormone, enterogastrone, that inhibits gastric secretion and motility. This allows a longer time for the digestion of fats in the small intestine.

4. The **small intestine** consists of the duodenum, jejunum, and ileum and is about 20 ft (6 m) long. The duodenum makes up the first 10 to 12 inches (25 to 30 cm) of the small intestine. The pancreatic and bile ducts empty into the duodenum at the papilla of Vater. The small intestine contains numerous glands that secrete digestive enzymes, hormones, and mucus. For the most part, digestion and absorption occur in the small intestine, including absorption of most orally administered drugs.
5. The **large intestine** consists of the cecum, colon, rectum, and anus. The ileum opens into the cecum. The colon secretes mucus and absorbs water.
6. The **pancreas** secretes enzymes, which are necessary for the digestion of carbohydrates, proteins, and fats. It also secretes insulin and glucagon, hormones that regulate glucose metabolism and blood sugar levels.
7. The **gallbladder** is a small pouch attached to the underside of the liver that stores and concentrates bile. It has a capacity of about 50 to 60 ml. The gallbladder releases bile when fats are present in the duodenum.
8. The **liver** is a vital organ that performs numerous functions. It receives about 1500 ml of blood per minute, or 25% to 30% of the total cardiac output. About three fourths of the blood flow is venous blood from the stomach, intestines, spleen, and pancreas (portal circulation); the remainder is arterial blood through the hepatic artery. The hepatic artery carries blood to the connective tissue of the liver and bile ducts, then empties into the hepatic sinuses. Arterial blood mixes with blood from the portal circulation. Venous blood from the liver flows into the inferior vena cava for return to the systemic circulation. The ample blood flow facilitates specific hepatic functions, which include the following:
   a. **Blood reservoir.** The liver can eject about 500 to 1000 ml of blood into the general circulation in response to stress, decreased blood volume, and sympathetic nervous system stimulation (*e.g.,* hemorrhagic or hypovolemic shock).

b. **Blood filter and detoxifier.** Kupffer's cells in the liver phagocytize bacteria carried from the intestines by the portal vein. They also break down worn-out erythrocytes, saving iron for reuse in hemoglobin synthesis, and form bilirubin, a waste product excreted in bile. The liver metabolizes many body secretions and most drugs to prevent accumulation and harmful effects on body tissues.

Most drugs are active as the parent compound and are metabolized in the liver to an inactive metabolite, which is then excreted by the kidneys. However, some drugs become active only after formation of a metabolite in the liver.

The liver detoxifies or alters substances by oxidation, hydrolysis, or conjugation. Conjugation involves combining a chemical substance with an endogenous substance to produce an inactive or harmless compound. Essentially all steroid hormones, including adrenal corticosteroids and sex hormones, are at least partially conjugated in the liver and secreted into the bile. When the liver is damaged, these hormones may accumulate in body fluids and cause symptoms of hormone excess.

c. **Metabolism of carbohydrate, fat, and protein.** In carbohydrate metabolism, the liver converts glucose to glycogen for storage and reconverts glycogen to glucose when needed to maintain an adequate blood sugar concentration. Excess glucose that cannot be converted to glycogen is converted to fat. The liver also changes fructose and galactose, which cannot be used by body cells, to glucose, which provides energy for cellular metabolism. Fats are synthesized and catabolized by the liver. Amino acids from protein breakdown may be used to form glycogen, plasma proteins, and enzymes.

d. **Storage of nutrients.** In addition to glycogen, the liver also stores fat-soluble vitamins (*i.e.,* vitamins A, D, E, K), vitamin B_{12}, iron, phospholipids, cholesterol, and small amounts of protein and fat.

e. **Synthesis** of bile; serum albumin and globulin; prothrombin; fibrinogen; blood coagulation factors V, VII, VIII, IX, XI, and XII; and urea. Formation of urea removes ammonia from body fluids. Large amounts of ammonia are formed by intestinal bacteria and absorbed into the blood. If the ammonia is not converted to urea by the liver, plasma ammonia concentrations rise to toxic levels and cause hepatic coma and death.

f. **Production of body heat** by continuous cellular metabolism. The liver is the body organ with the highest rate of chemical activity during basal conditions, and it produces about 20% of total body heat.

Secretions of the Digestive System

1. **Mucus** is secreted by mucous glands in every part of the gastrointestinal (GI) tract. The functions of mucus are to protect the lining of the tract from digestive juices, lubricate the food bolus for easier passage, promote adherence of the fecal mass, and neutralize acids and bases.

2. **Saliva** consists of mucus and salivary amylase. It is produced by the salivary glands and totals about 1000 ml daily. Saliva has a slightly acidic to neutral pH (6 to 7); it lubricates the food bolus and starts starch digestion.

3. **Gastric juice** consists of mucus, digestive enzymes, hydrochloric acid, and electrolytes. The gastric glands secrete about 2000 ml of gastric juice daily. The pH is highly acidic (1 to 3). Secretion is stimulated by the parasympathetic nervous system (by the vagus nerve), the hormone gastrin, the presence of food in the mouth, and seeing, smelling, or thinking about food.

The major digestive enzyme in gastric juice is pepsin, a proteolytic enzyme that functions best at a pH of 2 to 3. Hydrochloric acid provides the acid medium to promote pepsin activity. The major function of gastric juice is to begin digestion of proteins. There is also a weak action on fats by gastric lipase and on carbohydrates by gastric amylase. A large amount of mucus is secreted in the stomach to protect the stomach wall from the proteolytic action of pepsin. When mucus is not secreted, gastric ulceration occurs within hours.

4. **Pancreatic juices** are alkaline (pH of 8 or above) secretions that contain amylase for carbohydrate digestion, lipase for fat digestion, and trypsin and chymotrypsin for protein digestion. They also contain large amounts of sodium bicarbonate, a base (alkali) that neutralizes the acid chyme from the stomach by reacting with hydrochloric acid. This protects the mucosa of the small intestine from the digestive properties of gastric juice. The daily amount of pancreatic secretion is about 1200 ml. The hormone cholecystokinin stimulates secretion of pancreatic juices.

5. **Bile** is an alkaline (pH of about 8) secretion that is formed continuously in the liver, carried to the gallbladder by the bile ducts, and stored there. The hormone cholecystokinin causes the gallbladder to contract and release bile into the small intestine when fats are present in intestinal contents. The liver secretes about 600 ml of bile daily. This amount is concentrated to the 50- to 60-ml capacity of the gallbladder. Bile contains bile salts, cholesterol, bilirubin, fatty acids, and electrolytes. Bile salts are required for digestion and absorption of fats, including fat-

soluble vitamins. Most of the bile salts are reabsorbed and reused by the liver (enterohepatic circulation); some are excreted in feces.

Effects of Drugs on the Digestive System

The digestive system and drug therapy have a reciprocal relationship. Many common symptoms (*i.e.,* nausea, vomiting, constipation, diarrhea, abdominal pain) relate to GI dysfunction. These symptoms may result from a disorder in the digestive system, disorders in other body systems, or drug therapy. Many GI symptoms and disorders alter the ingestion, dissolution, absorption, and metabolism of drugs. Drugs may be administered to *relieve* these symptoms and disorders, but drugs administered for conditions unrelated to the digestive system may *cause* such symptoms and disorders. GI conditions may alter responses to drug therapy.

Drugs used in digestive disorders primarily alter GI secretion, absorption, or motility. They may act systemically or locally within the GI tract. The drug groups included in this section are drugs used for peptic ulcer disease, laxatives, antidiarrheals, and antiemetics. Other drug groups used in GI disorders include cholinergics (see Chap. 20), anticholinergics (Chap. 21), corticosteroids (Chap. 24), and anti-infective drugs (Section VI).

REVIEW AND APPLICATION EXERCISES

1. What is the main function of the GI system?
2. What is the role of the parasympathetic nervous system in GI function?
3. List factors affecting GI motility and secretions.
4. Describe important GI secretions and their functions.
5. What factors stimulate or inhibit GI secretions?
6. How does the GI tract affect oral medications?
7. How do oral medications affect the GI tract?

SELECTED REFERENCES

Guyton, A.C. & Hall, J.E. (1996). *Textbook of medical physiology,* 9th ed. Philadelphia: W.B. Saunders.
Porth, C.M. (1994). *Pathophysiology: Concepts of altered health states,* 4th ed., pp. 801–815. Philadelphia: J.B. Lippincott.

60 Drugs Used in Peptic Ulcer Disease

Outline

Objectives

After studying this chapter, the student will be able to:

1 Describe the role of *Helicobacter pylori* and other etiologic factors in peptic ulcer disease.

2 Differentiate the types of antiulcer drugs in terms of their mechanisms of action, indications for use, common adverse effects, and nursing process implications.

3 Describe the similarities and differences of histamine₂ receptor blocking agents.

4 Discuss significant drug–drug interactions with cimetidine (Tagamet).

5 Describe characteristics, uses, and effects of selected antacids.

6 Discuss the rationale for using combination antacid products.

7 Teach clients nonpharmacologic measures to manage gastroesophageal reflux disease and peptic ulcer disease.

Key Terms

Antacid

Autodigestion

Cytoprotective

Gastroesophageal reflux disease

***Helicobacter pylori* organisms**

Histamine₂ receptor blocking agents

Prostaglandin

Proton pump inhibitors

Pyrosis

Ulcerogenic

Peptic Ulcer Disease

Peptic ulcer disease is characterized by ulcer formation in areas of the gastrointestinal (GI) mucosa that are exposed to gastric acid and pepsin (*i.e.*, esophagus, stomach, and duodenum). Although esophageal ulcers are less common than gastric and duodenal ulcers, another esophageal disorder associated with exposure to gastric acid and pepsin is gastroesophageal reflux disease (GERD). This disorder is included here because antiulcer medications are used to prevent and treat GERD. Gastric ulcers (which may be preceded by less severe mucosal defects such as erosions or gastritis) may be acute ulcers associated with stress (*e.g.*, surgery, shock, head injury, severe burn injuries, major medical illness), certain drugs (mainly aspirin and other nonsteroidal anti-inflammatory drugs [NSAIDs]), or *Helicobacter pylori* infection. Duodenal ulcers are usually chronic in nature and are also commonly associated with NSAID ingestion and *H. pylori* infection. Selected acid-peptic disorders for which antiulcer drugs are used are described further in Box 60-1.

CAUSES OF PEPTIC ULCER DISEASE

Peptic ulcer disease is attributed to an imbalance between cell-destructive and cell-protective effects. Cell-destructive effects include those of gastric acid (hydrochloric acid), pepsin and *H. pylori* infection. Gastric acid, a strong acid that can digest the stomach wall, is secreted by the parietal cells in the mucosa of the stomach antrum, near the pylorus. The parietal cells contain receptors for acetylcholine, gastrin, and histamine, substances that stimulate gastric acid production. Acetylcholine is released by vagus nerve endings in response to stimuli, such as thinking about or ingesting food. Gastrin is a hormone released by cells in the stomach and duodenum in response to food ingestion and stretching of the stomach wall. It is secreted into the bloodstream and eventually circulated to the parietal cells. Histamine is released from cells in the gastric mucosa and diffuses into nearby parietal cells. Once produced, gastric acid is released by activation of an enzyme system (hydrogen, potassium adenosine triphosphatase, or H^+,K^+-ATPase) at the surface of parietal cells. This enzyme system acts as a gastric acid (proton) pump to move gastric acid from parietal cells in the mucosal lining of the stomach into the stomach lumen.

Pepsin is a proteolytic enzyme that also can digest the stomach wall. Pepsin is derived from a precursor called pepsinogen, which is secreted by chief cells in the gastric mucosa. Pepsinogen is converted to pepsin only in a highly acidic environment (*i.e.*, when the pH of gastric juices is about 3 or less).

H. pylori is a gram-negative bacterium found in the gastric mucosa of most patients with gastritis, about 75% of patients with gastric ulcers, and more than 90% of patients with duodenal ulcers. The mechanism by which *H. pylori* infection leads to gastritis or ulceration is unknown but may involve impairment of mucosal defense mechanisms. It is known, however, that eradication of the organism accelerates ulcer healing and significantly decreases the rate of ulcer recurrence.

Autodigestion of stomach and duodenal tissues and ulcer formation are normally prevented by the cell-protective effects of mucus, dilution of gastric acid by food and secretions, prevention of diffusion of hydrochloric acid from the stomach lumen back into the gastric mucosal lining, the presence of certain prostaglandins (*e.g.*, PGE), alkalinization of gastric secretions by pancreatic juices and bile, and perhaps other mechanisms. Overall, then, peptic ulcers form when cell-destructive elements exceed cell-protective elements. The main pathophysiologic mechanism may reflect an abnormality in acid and pepsin secretion or impaired mucosal defense mechanisms.

Types of Antiulcer Drugs

Drugs used in the treatment of acid-peptic disorders promote healing of lesions and prevent recurrence of lesions by decreasing cell-destructive effects and/or increasing cell-protective effects. Several types of drugs are used for this purpose, alone or in various combinations. Antacids neutralize gastric acid and decrease pepsin production; antimicrobials and bismuth can eliminate *H. pylori* infection; histamine$_2$ (H$_2$) receptor antagonists and proton pump inhibitors decrease gastric acid secretion; sucralfate provides a barrier between mucosal erosions or ulcers and gastric secretions; and misoprostol restores prostaglandin activity. Types of drugs and individual agents are described further below and listed in Tables 60-1 and 60-2.

ANTACIDS

Antacids are alkaline substances that neutralize acids. They react with hydrochloric acid in the stomach to produce neutral, less acidic, or poorly absorbed salts and to raise the pH (alkalinity) of gastric secretions. Raising the pH to about 3.5 neutralizes more than 90% of gastric acid and inhibits conversion of pepsinogen to pepsin. Commonly used antacids are aluminum, magnesium, and calcium compounds. Small amounts of aluminum, magnesium, and calcium are absorbed from the GI tract. Normally insignificant, these small amounts may cause serious adverse effects in the presence of renal disease.

BOX 60-1. SELECTED UPPER GASTROINTESTINAL DISORDERS

Gastroesophageal Reflux Disease

Gastroesophageal reflux disease (GERD) is a common condition characterized by regurgitation of gastric contents into the esophagus and exposure of esophageal mucosa to gastric acid and pepsin. Depending on the frequency and extent of acid-pepsin reflux, GERD may result in mild to severe esophagitis or esophageal ulceration. The main symptom is heartburn, which most people experience occasionally, without serious consequences. In some people, however, esophageal mucosa becomes damaged and inflamed. The severity of heartburn does not reflect the extent of injury to esophageal mucosa. A hiatal hernia, which allows movement of a portion of the stomach upward into the chest, was once considered the main cause of gastroesophageal reflux. Now, however, the condition is attributed primarily to an incompetent lower esophageal sphincter. GERD occurs in men, women, and children, but is especially common during pregnancy and after 40 y of age.

NSAID Gastropathy

NSAID gastropathy indicates damage to gastroduodenal mucosa by aspirin and other nonsteroidal anti-inflammatory drugs. The damage may range from minor superficial erosions to ulceration and bleeding. NSAID gastropathy is considered one of the most common causes of gastric ulcers, and it may cause duodenal ulcers as well. Many people take NSAIDs daily for pain, arthritis, and other conditions. Chronic ingestion of NSAIDs causes local irritation of gastroduodenal mucosa, inhibits the synthesis of protective prostaglandins, and increases the synthesis of leukotrienes and possibly other inflammatory substances that may contribute to mucosal injury.

Peptic Ulcer Disease

Peptic ulcer disease usually denotes gastric and duodenal ulcers. Although there is considerable overlap in etiology, clinical manifestations, and treatment of gastric and duodenal ulcers, there are some differences as well. Gastric ulcers may be caused by severe physiologic stress, H. pylori infection, and NSAID ingestion. Stress ulcers may occur in any age group and are usually acute in nature. Gastric ulcers associated with H. pylori infection or NSAID ingestion are more likely to occur in older adults, especially in the sixth and seventh decades, and to be chronic in nature. Duodenal ulcers are strongly associated with H. pylori infection,

are more common than gastric ulcers, may occur at any age, and occur more often in men than women.

A gastric or duodenal ulcer may penetrate only the mucosal surface or it may extend into the smooth muscle layers. When superficial lesions heal, no defects remain. When smooth muscle heals, however, scar tissue remains and the mucosa that regenerates to cover the scarred muscle tissue may be defective. These defects contribute to repeated episodes of ulcerations.

Overall, peptic ulcers are thought to result from an imbalance between gastric acid and pepsin production and the ability of the gastroduodenal mucosa to resist the destructive action of these digestive agents. H. pylori organisms colonize the mucus-secreting epithelial cells of the stomach and probably impair mucosal function. H. pylori infection is strongly associated with chronic gastritis and gastric and duodenal ulcers.

Stress Ulcers

Stress ulcers indicate gastric mucosal lesions that develop in patients who are critically ill from trauma, shock, hemorrhage, sepsis, burns or other severe illnesses. They are usually manifested by painless upper GI bleeding. The frequency of occurrence has decreased, possibly because of prophylactic use of antiulcer drugs and improved management of sepsis, hypovolemia and other disorders associated with critical illness.

The exact mechanisms of stress ulcer formation are unknown. However, several factors are thought to play a role, including mucosal ischemia and systemic acidosis. Acidosis increases severity of lesions, and correction of acidosis decreases their formation. In addition, lesions do not form if the pH of gastric fluids is kept above 3.5 to 4.

Zollinger-Ellison Syndrome

Zollinger-Ellison syndrome is a rare condition characterized by excessive secretion of gastric acid and a high incidence of ulcers. It is caused by gastrin-secreting tumors in the pancreas, stomach, or duodenum. About two thirds of the gastrinomas are malignant. Symptoms are those of peptic ulcer disease, and diagnosis is based on high levels of serum gastrin and gastric acid. Treatment may involve long-term use of a proton pump inhibitor or a histamine$_2$ antagonist to diminish gastric acid or surgical excision.

Antacids differ in the amounts needed to neutralize gastric acid (about 50 to 80 mEq of acid are produced hourly), in onset of action, and in adverse effects produced. *Aluminum compounds* have a low neutralizing capacity (*i.e.*, large doses are required) and a slow onset

of action. They can cause constipation. People who ingest large amounts of aluminum-based antacids over a long period may develop hypophosphatemia and osteomalacia because aluminum combines with phosphates

(*text continues on page 771*)

TABLE 60-1 REPRESENTATIVE ANTACID PRODUCTS

Trade Name	Magnesium Oxide or Hydroxide	Aluminum Hydroxide	Calcium Carbonate	Sodium	Other	Route and Dosages Ranges (Adults)
			Components			
Aludrox Amphojel	103 mg/5 ml	307 mg/5 ml 300 or 600 mg/tab, 320 mg/5 ml		1.5 mg/5 ml <7 mg/5 ml		PO 10 ml q4h, or as needed PO 10 ml or 600 mg five or six times daily
Di-Gel	87 mg/5 ml	282 mg/5 ml		8.5 mg/5 ml	Simethicone 20 mg/5 ml	PO 2 tsp liquid q2h, after meals or between meals, and at bedtime. Maximal dose, 20 tsp/24 h. Do not use maximal dose longer than 2 wk.
Gelusil	200 mg/tab	200 mg/tab		< 5 mg/tab	Simethicone 25 mg/tab	PO 10 or more ml or 2 or more tablets after meals and at bedtime or as directed by physician to a maximum of 12 tablets or tsp/24 h
Maalox suspension	200 mg/5 ml	225 mg/5 ml		1.35 mg/5 ml		PO 30 ml four times daily, after meals and at bedtime or as directed by physician; maximal dose, 16 tsp/24 h
Maalox No. 1 tablets	200 mg/tab	200 mg/tab		0.84 mg/tab		PO 2–4 tablets, four times daily, after meals and at bedtime or as directed by physician; maximal dose, 16 tablets/24 h
Maalox No. 2 tablets	400 mg/tab	400 mg/tab		1.84 mg/tab		PO 1–2 tablets, four times daily, after meals and at bedtime, or as directed by physician; maximal dose, 8 tablets/24 h
Maalox Plus	200 mg/tab, 200 mg/5 ml	200 mg/tab, 225 mg/5 ml		1 mg/tab, 1.3 mg/5 ml	Simethicone 25 mg/tab, 20 mg/5 ml	PO 2–4 tsp or tablets, four times daily after meals and at bedtime, or as directed by physician
Mylanta	200 mg/tab, 200 mg/5 ml	200 mg/tab, 200 mg/5 ml		0.77 mg/tab, 0.68 mg/5 ml	Simethicone 25 mg/tab, 20 mg/5ml	PO 5–10 ml or 1–2 tablets q2–4h, between meals and at bedtime or as directed by physician
Mylanta-II	400 mg/tab, 400 mg/5 ml	400 mg/tab, 400 mg/5 ml		1.3 mg/tab, 1.14 mg/5 ml	Simethicone 30 mg/tab, 30 mg/5 ml	Same as Mylanta
Titralac			420 mg/tab, 1 g/5 ml	<0.3 mg/tab, 11 mg/5 ml	Glycine 180 mg/tab, 300 mg/5 ml	PO 1 tsp or 2 tablets, after meals or as directed by physician, to maximal dose of 19 tablets or 8 tsp/24 h

TABLE 60-2 ANTIULCER DRUGS

Generic/Trade Name	Indications for Use	Routes and Dosage Ranges (Adults)
Histamine₂ Receptor Antagonists **Cimetidine** (Tagamet)	Treatment of gastric ulcer, duodenal ulcer, and erosive esophagitis, to promote healing, then maintenance to prevent recurrence Prevention of stress ulcers and GI bleeding; prevention of aspiration pneumonitis Treatment of Zollinger-Ellison syndrome Treatment of heartburn (OTC only)	PO 800 mg once daily at bedtime or 300 mg four times per day *Prophylaxis of recurrent ulcer,* PO 400 mg at bedtime *IV injection,* 300 mg, diluted in 20 ml of 5% dextrose or saline solution and infused over at least 2 min, q6–8h *IV intermittent infusion,* 300 mg diluted in at least 50 ml of dextrose or saline solution and infused over 15–20 min, q6h *IM* 300 mg q6–8h (undiluted) *GERD*,* PO 1600 mg daily in divided doses (800 mg twice daily or 400 mg four times daily) Prevention of upper GI bleeding, IV continuous infusion, 50 mg per hour. *Impaired renal function,* PO, IV 300 mg q8–12h
Famotidine (Pepcid)		*Acute duodenal ulcer,* PO 40 mg once daily at bedtime or 20 mg twice daily for 4–8 wk; maintenance therapy, PO 20 mg once daily at bedtime *Zollinger-Ellison syndrome,* PO 20 mg q6h, increased if necessary *IV injection,* 20 mg q12h, diluted to 5 or 10 ml with 5% dextrose or 0.9% sodium chloride, and injected over at least 2 min *IV infusion,* 20 mg q12h, diluted with 100 ml of 5% dextrose or 0.9% sodium chloride, and infused over 15–30 min *Impaired renal function* (creatinine clearance below 10 ml/min), PO, IV 20 mg q24–48h
Nizatidine (Axid)		*Acute duodenal ulcer,* PO 300 mg once daily at bedtime; maintenance therapy, PO 150 mg once daily at bedtime *Impaired renal function* (creatinine clearance 20–50 ml/min), PO 150 mg daily; (creatinine clearance below 20 ml/min), PO 150 mg q48h
Ranitidine (Zantac)		PO 300 mg once daily at bedtime or 150 mg twice daily *IM* 50 mg q6–8h (undiluted) *IV injection,* 50 mg diluted in 20 ml of 5% dextrose or 0.9% sodium chloride solution and injected over at least 5 min q6–8h *IV intermittent infusion,* 50 mg diluted in 100 ml of 5% dextrose or 0.9% sodium chloride solution and infused over 15–20 min

(continued)

TABLE 60-2	ANTIULCER DRUGS (Continued)

Generic/Trade Name	Indications for Use	Routes and Dosage Ranges (Adults)
Ranitidine (cont)		*Impaired renal function* (creatinine clearance below 50 ml/min), PO 150 mg q24h; IV, IM 50 mg q18–24h
Proton Pump Inhibitors **Lansoprazole** (Prevacid)	Treatment of gastric and duodenal ulcers, for 4–8 wk Treatment of GERD* for 4–8 wk to promote healing, then maintenance to prevent recurrence Treatment of Zollinger-Ellison syndrome	
Omeprazole (Prilosec)		*Duodenal ulcer*, PO 15 mg once daily for 4 wk *GERD**, PO 30 mg once daily for 8 wk, then 15 mg once daily for maintenance *Gastric ulcer*, PO 40 mg once daily for 4–8 wk *Duodenal ulcer*, PO 20 mg once daily for 4–8 wk *GERD**, PO 20 mg once daily *Zollinger-Ellison syndrome*, PO 60 mg once daily initially, increased if necessary
Misoprostol (Cytotec)	Prevention of aspirin and NSAID-induced gastric ulcers in selected clients	PO 100–200 mg four times daily with meals and at bedtime
Sucralfate (Carafate)	Treatment of active duodenal ulcer to promote healing, then maintenance to prevent recurrence	*Treatment of active ulcer*, PO 1 g four times daily before meals and at bedtime *Maintenance therapy*, PO 1 g two times daily
H. pylori Agents		
Antimicrobials **Amoxicillin** **Clarithromycin** **Metronidazole** **Tetracycline**	*H. pylori* infection causing gastric or duodenal ulcers	PO 500 mg four times daily PO 500 mg two to three times daily PO 250 mg four times daily PO 500 mg four times daily
Bismuth subsalicylate	*H. pylori* eradication and GI upset (abdominal cramping, indigestion, nausea, diarrhea)	*Adults:* PO 525 mg (2 tabs or 30 ml) four times daily *Children:* 9–12 y, PO 1 tab or 15 ml; 6–9 y, PO 2/3 tab or 10 ml; 3–6 y, PO 1/3 tab or 5 ml; under 3 y, consult physician. Dosage may be repeated every 30–60 min, if needed, up to eight doses in 24 h.
Combination Regimens **Bismuth subsalicylate, metronidazole, and tetracycline)** (Helidac) **Omeprazole and clarithromycin**		PO Bismuth 525 mg (2 tabs), metronidazole 250 mg (1 tab), tetracycline 500 mg (1 capsule) four times daily for 14 d Omeprazole 40 mg once daily in the morning and clarithromycin 500 mg three times daily for 14 d, then omeprazole 20 mg once daily for 14 more days

*GERD = gastroesophageal reflux disease, including erosive esophagitis.

in the GI tract and prevents phosphate absorption. Aluminum compounds are rarely used alone for acid-peptic disorders. *Magnesium-based antacids* have a high neutralizing capacity and a rapid onset of action. They may cause diarrhea and hypermagnesemia. *Calcium compounds* are effective and have a rapid onset of action but may cause hypersecretion of gastric acid ("acid rebound") and the "milk-alkali syndrome," which includes alkalosis and azotemia. Consequently, calcium compounds are rarely used in peptic ulcer disease.

Commonly used antacids are mixtures of aluminum hydroxide and magnesium hydroxide (*e.g.,* Gelusil, Mylanta, Maalox). Some antacid mixtures contain other ingredients, such as simethicone. Simethicone is an antiflatulent drug available alone as Mylicon. When added to antacids, simethicone does not affect gastric acidity. It reportedly decreases gas bubbles, thereby reducing GI distention and abdominal discomfort.

Antacids act primarily in the stomach and are used to prevent or treat peptic ulcer disease, gastroesophageal reflux disease, esophagitis, pyrosis ("heartburn"), gastritis, GI bleeding, and stress ulcers. Aluminum-based antacids also are given to clients with chronic renal failure and hyperphosphatemia to decrease absorption of phosphates in food.

Magnesium-based antacids are contraindicated in clients with renal failure, and sodium-containing antacids should be used cautiously in clients with hypertension or congestive heart failure.

HELICOBACTER PYLORI AGENTS

Multiple drugs are required to eradicate *H. pylori* organisms. Although the optimal regimen has not been determined, several regimens are effective. A commonly used combination consists of two antimicrobial drugs, a bismuth compound, and a histamine₂ antagonist or a proton pump inhibitor. A single antimicrobial agent is not used because of concern about emergence of drug-resistant *H. pylori* organisms.

For the antimicrobial component, two of the following four drugs (**amoxicillin, clarithromycin, metronidazole, tetracycline**) are used. A common combination is metronida_le and tetracycline. For the bismuth component, **bismuth subsalicylate** is used. Bismuth preparations exert antibacterial effects against *H. pylori* by disrupting the integrity of bacterial cell walls, preventing the organism from adhering to gastric epithelium, and inhibiting bacterial enzymatic and proteolytic activity. They also increase secretion of mucus and bicarbonate, inhibit pepsin activity, and accumulate in ulcer craters. They do not inhibit or neutralize gastric acid.

Patient compliance is a difficulty with all the *H. pylori* eradication regimens. This is usually attributed to the inconvenience of taking several drugs. To promote client convenience and compliance, the components of each dose of a commonly used combination (*i.e.,* two chewable bismuth tablets, one 250-mg tablet of metronidazole, and one 500-mg capsule of tetracycline) are packaged together under the trade name of Helidac.

HISTAMINE₂ RECEPTOR BLOCKING AGENTS

Histamine is a substance found in almost every body tissue and released in response to certain stimuli (*e.g.,* allergic reactions, tissue injury). Once released, histamine causes the following reactions: contraction of smooth muscle in the bronchi, GI tract, and uterus; dilation and increased permeability of capillaries; dilation of cerebral blood vessels; and stimulation of sensory nerve endings to produce pain and itching. Another effect of histamine, and the most important effect in relation to peptic ulcer disease, is strong stimulation of gastric acid secretion. Vagal stimulation causes release of histamine from cells in the gastric mucosa. The histamine then acts on receptors located on the parietal cells to increase production of hydrochloric acid. These receptors are called the H₂ receptors.

Traditional antihistamines or H₁ receptor blocking agents prevent or reduce other effects of histamine but do not block histamine effects on gastric acid production. The H₂ receptor blocking drugs inhibit secretion of gastric acid stimulated by histamine, acetylcholine, and gastrin. They decrease the amount and acidity (hydrogen ion concentration) of gastric juices. They have the same mechanism of action and clinical indications for use.

Clinical indications for use include prevention and treatment of peptic ulcer disease, preventing GI bleeding due to acute stress ulcers, esophagitis resulting from gastroesophageal reflux of gastric acid, and Zollinger-Ellison syndrome. When used therapeutically for gastric or duodenal ulcers, H₂ blockers promote healing within 6 to 8 weeks. Over-the-counter oral preparations are approved for the treatment of heartburn. There are no known contraindications, but the drugs should be used with caution in children, pregnant women, older adults, and clients with impaired renal or hepatic function. Dosage should be reduced in the presence of impaired renal function.

Adverse effects occur infrequently with usual doses and duration of treatment. They are more likely to occur with prolonged use of high doses and in older adults or those with impaired renal or hepatic function.

Cimetidine, ranitidine, famotidine, and **nizatidine** are the four available H₂ blockers. Cimetidine was the first, and it is still widely used. It is well absorbed following oral administration. After a single dose, peak blood level is reached in 1 to 1.5 hours, and an effective concentration is maintained about 4 hours. The drug is distributed in almost all body tissues. Cimetidine should be used with caution during pregnancy because it crosses the placenta, and it should not be taken during lactation because it is excreted in breast milk. Most of an oral dose is excreted unchanged in the urine within 24 hours; some is excreted in bile and eliminated in feces. For acutely ill clients, cimetidine is given intravenously. A major disadvantage of cimetidine is that it inhibits the hepatic metabolism of numerous other drugs, thereby increasing blood levels and risks of toxicity of the inhibited drug.

Ranitidine is more potent than cimetidine, and smaller doses can be given less frequently. In addition, ranitidine causes fewer drug interactions than cimetidine. Oral ranitidine is 50% to 60% bioavailable, reaches peak blood levels 1 to 3 hours after administration, and is metabolized in the liver; about 30% is excreted unchanged in the urine. Parenteral ranitidine is 90% to 100% bioavailable and reaches peak blood levels in approximately 15 minutes; about 65% to 80% is excreted unchanged in the urine. Because of these pharmacokinetic differences, larger doses are required with oral than with parenteral administration. Famotidine and nizatidine are chemically different but pharmacologically similar to cimetidine and ranitidine. They are more potent on a weight basis. The drugs cause similar adverse effects but are less likely to cause mental confusion and gynecomastia (antiandrogenic effects) than cimetidine. In addition, they do not affect the cytochrome P450 drug-metabolizing system in the liver and therefore do not interfere with the metabolism of other drugs, as does cimetidine.

PROTON PUMP INHIBITORS

Proton pump inhibitors are potent gastric acid inhibitors. These drugs bind with H^+,K^+-ATPase to prevent the "pumping" or release of gastric acid into the stomach lumen and therefore block the final step of acid production. Indications for use include treatment of peptic ulcer disease, erosive gastritis, gastroesophageal reflux disease, and Zollinger-Ellison syndrome. The drugs are reportedly more effective than histamine$_2$ receptor antagonists in gastroesophageal reflux disorders and are the treatment of choice for Zollinger-Ellison syndrome. They are generally well tolerated. Nausea, diarrhea, and headache are the most frequently reported adverse effects. However, long-term consequences of profound gastric acid suppression are unknown.

Omeprazole and **lansoprazole** are approved proton pump inhibitors. Omeprazole was the first and is still widely used. It is well absorbed following oral administration, highly bound to plasma proteins (about 95%), metabolized in the liver, and excreted in the urine (about 75%) and bile or feces (about 25%). Acid-inhibiting effects occur within 2 hours and last 72 hours or longer. When the drug is discontinued, effects persist for 3 to 5 days, until the gastric parietal cells can synthesize additional H^+,K^+-ATPase. Lansoprazole is very similar to omeprazole. The drugs are formulated as enteric-coated granules (to prevent destruction by gastric

acid) in an extended-release capsule, which should be swallowed whole.

PROSTAGLANDIN

Naturally occurring prostaglandin E, which is produced in mucosal cells of the stomach and duodenum, inhibits gastric acid secretion and increases mucus and bicarbonate secretion, mucosal blood flow, and perhaps mucosal repair. When synthesis of prostaglandin E is inhibited, erosion and ulceration of gastric mucosa may occur. This is the mechanism by which aspirin and other NSAIDs are thought to cause gastric ulcers (see Chap. 7).

Misoprostol is a synthetic form of prostaglandin E approved for concurrent use with NSAIDs to protect gastric mucosa from NSAID-induced erosion and ulceration. It is indicated for clients at high risk of GI ulceration and bleeding, such as those taking high doses of NSAIDs for arthritis and older adults. It is contraindicated in women of childbearing potential, unless effective contraceptive methods are being used, and during pregnancy because it may induce abortion. The most common adverse effects are diarrhea (occurs in 10% to 40% of recipients) and abdominal cramping. Older adults may be unable to tolerate misoprostol-induced diarrhea and abdominal discomfort.

SUCRALFATE

Sucralfate is a preparation of sulfated sucrose and aluminum hydroxide that binds to normal and ulcerated mucosa. It is used to prevent and treat peptic ulcer disease. When an ulcer is present, the drug combines with ulcer exudate, adheres to the ulcer site, and forms a protective barrier between the mucosa and gastric acid, pepsin, and bile salts. Sucralfate is as effective as other antiulcer agents in healing duodenal ulcers. When an ulcer has healed, sucralfate may be used in small doses as maintenance therapy to prevent ulcer recurrence. Because sucralfate is not absorbed systemically, the incidence and severity of adverse effects are low; constipation and dry mouth are most often reported. However, the drug may bind other drugs and prevent their absorption. As a general rule, sucralfate should be given about 2 hours before or after other drugs.

Nursing Process

Assessment

Assess the client's status in relation to peptic ulcer disease and other conditions in which antiulcer drugs are used.
- Identify risk factors for peptic ulcer disease:
  - Cigarette smoking. Specific effects are thought to include stimulation of gastric acid secretion and decreased blood supply to gastric mucosa. Moreover, patients with peptic ulcers who continue to smoke heal more slowly and have

more recurrent ulcers, despite usually adequate treatment, than those who stop smoking.

- Stress, including physiologic stress (*e.g.,* shock, sepsis, burns, surgery, head injury, severe trauma, or medical illness) and psychological stress. One mechanism may be that stress activates the sympathetic nervous system, which in turn causes vasoconstriction in organs not needed for "fight or flight." Thus, stress may lead to ischemia in gastric mucosa, with ulceration if ischemia is severe or prolonged.
- Genetic influences. Clients with blood type O are more likely to have duodenal ulcers; those with blood type A are more likely to have gastric ulcers. Also, close relatives of clients with peptic ulcer disease have an increased risk of developing ulcers.
- Male sex. Men have a higher incidence of duodenal and gastric ulcers compared with women.
- Drug therapy with aspirin and other NSAIDs, corticosteroids, and antineoplastics.
- Signs and symptoms depend on the type and location of the ulcer:
  - Periodic epigastric pain, which occurs 1 to 4 hours after eating or during the night and is often described as burning or gnawing, is a characteristic symptom of chronic duodenal ulcer.
  - GI bleeding occurs with acute or chronic ulcers when the ulcer erodes into a blood vessel. Clinical manifestations may range from mild (*e.g.,* occult blood in feces and eventual anemia) to severe (*e.g.,* hematemesis, melena, hypotension, and shock).
- Gastroesophageal reflux disease produces heartburn or "indigestion" (a substernal burning sensation), which is caused by the backward flow of gastric acid onto esophageal mucosa. These disorders may occur with obesity and overeating as a result of gastric distention.

Nursing Diagnoses

- Pain related to effects of gastric acid on peptic ulcers
- Ineffective Individual Coping related to acute and chronic manifestations of peptic ulcer disease
- Risk for Injury: GI bleeding, ulcer perforation, bowel obstruction
- Altered Nutrition: Less Than Body Requirements related to anorexia and abdominal discomfort
- Constipation related to aluminum- or calcium-containing antacids and sucralfate
- Diarrhea related to magnesium-containing antacids and misoprostol
- Risk for Injury: Adverse drug effects
- Knowledge Deficit related to the disease process
- Knowledge Deficit related to drug therapy for gastro-esophageal reflux and peptic ulcer disease

Planning/Goals

The client will:
- Take or receive antiulcer drugs accurately
- Experience relief of symptoms
- Avoid situations that cause or exacerbate symptoms, when possible
- Be observed for GI bleeding and other complications of peptic ulcer disease

- Maintain normal patterns of bowel function
- Avoid preventable adverse effects of drug therapy
- Demonstrate use of relaxation techniques

Interventions

Use measures to prevent or minimize peptic ulcer disease and gastric acid–induced esophageal disorders.
- With peptic ulcer disease, helpful interventions may include the following:
  - General health measures such as a well-balanced diet, adequate rest, and regular exercise
  - Avoiding cigarette smoking and gastric irritants (*e.g.,* alcohol, aspirin, caffeine)
  - Reducing psychological stress (*e.g.,* by changing environments) or learning healthful methods of handling it (*e.g.,* relaxation techniques, physical exercise). There is no practical way to avoid psychological stress, because it is part of everyday life.
  - Long-term drug therapy with relatively small doses of H_2 receptor antagonists, antacids, or sucralfate. With "active" peptic ulcer disease, helping the client follow the prescribed therapeutic regimen helps to promote healing and prevent serious complications (*i.e.,* hemorrhage, perforation, obstruction).
  - Diet therapy is of minor importance in prevention or treatment of peptic ulcer disease. Because various studies have failed to demonstrate the effectiveness of ulcer diets, some physicians prescribe no dietary restrictions for clients with peptic ulcer disease, whereas others suggest avoiding highly spiced foods, gas-forming foods, and caffeine-containing beverages.
- With gastric acid-induced esophagitis, helpful measures are those that prevent or decrease gastroesophageal reflux of gastric contents (*e.g.,* elevating the head of the bed, avoiding gastric distention by eating small meals, not lying down for about 1 hour after eating, and avoiding obesity, constipation, or other conditions that increase intra-abdominal pressure).

Teach clients:
- That most conditions for which antiulcer drugs are used are chronic and are usually managed on an outpatient basis. It is important for the client to know about prevention and treatment of the conditions.
- Characteristics of the disease process, nondrug measures to prevent or minimize symptoms, drug therapy, and accurate information related to diet
- To observe for and report signs and symptoms of complications, such as GI bleeding
- Relaxation and stress-management techniques

Evaluation

- Observe and interview regarding drug usage.
- Observe and interview regarding relief of symptoms.
- Observe for signs and symptoms of complications.
- Observe and interview regarding adverse drug effects.
- Observe and interview regarding relaxation techniques.

Principles of Therapy

DRUG SELECTION

All of the antiulcer drugs are effective for indicated uses; the choice of drugs may depend on ulcer etiology, ulcer acuity, cost, and convenience. *H. pylori* infection should be considered in most cases of peptic ulcer disease. If confirmed by appropriate diagnostic tests, agents to eradicate the organisms should be drugs of first choice. Proton pump inhibitors may be drugs of first choice in most situations. They may heal peptic ulcers more rapidly and be more effective in erosive gastritis and Zollinger-Ellison syndrome than H_2 antagonists. However, they are given orally only. If the drug must be injected for a client who is unable to take an oral medication, an H_2 antagonist must be used. When an H_2 antagonist is used, cimetidine may be less expensive but it may cause confusion and antiandrogenic effects. It also increases the risks of toxicity with several commonly used drugs. Compared with cimetidine, famotidine, nizatidine, and ranitidine are more potent on a weight basis and have a longer duration of action, so they can be given in smaller, less frequent doses. In addition, they do not alter the hepatic metabolism of other drugs. Over-the-counter histamine$_2$ antagonists are indicated for the treatment of heartburn. In some cases, clients may depend on self-medication with over-the-counter drugs and delay seeking treatment for peptic ulcer disease or gastroesophageal reflux disease. For prescription or nonprescription uses, cimetidine should probably be used only for clients who are taking no other medications.

Antacids are often used to relieve heartburn and abdominal discomfort. If used to treat peptic ulcer disease, they are more often used with other agents than alone. The frequent administration of relatively large amounts is inconvenient for many clients. Sucralfate must be taken before meals, and this is inconvenient for some clients.

GUIDELINES FOR THERAPY WITH HISTAMINE$_2$ RECEPTOR ANTAGONISTS

1. For an acute ulcer, full dosage may be given for up to 8 weeks. When the ulcer heals, the drug may be discontinued or reduced in dosage for maintenance therapy to prevent recurrence. These drugs are effective and convenient in a single daily dose taken at bedtime to suppress nocturnal secretion of gastric acid. Dosage of all these drugs should be reduced in the presence of impaired renal function.
2. Antacids are often given concurrently with H_2 receptor blocking agents to relieve pain. They should not be given at the same time because the antacid reduces absorption of the other drug. H_2 antagonists relieve pain after about 1 week of administration.

GUIDELINES FOR THERAPY WITH SUCRALFATE

When sucralfate is used to treat an ulcer, it should be administered for 4 to 8 weeks unless healing is confirmed by radiologic or endoscopic examination. When used long-term to prevent ulcer recurrence, dosage should be reduced.

GUIDELINES FOR THERAPY WITH ANTACIDS

1. The choice of antacid depends on characteristics of clients and drug preparations and should be individualized. Combination products containing aluminum hydroxide and magnesium oxide or hydroxide are commonly used. Some guidelines include the following:
   a. **Neutralizing capacity.** Use of an agent with high in vitro neutralizing capacity is probably better. However, the clinical or in vivo capacity may be different, depending on the amount of gastric acid and rate of gastric emptying. In a fasting state, for example, the antacid leaves the stomach in about 30 minutes and thereafter becomes ineffective. After a meal, acid-neutralizing effects last 3 hours or longer.
   b. **Side effects.** Calcium carbonate has a high neutralizing capacity, but doses large and frequent enough to maintain neutralization of gastric acid may cause hypercalcemia and impaired renal function due to systemic absorption. Magnesium hydroxide has a higher buffering capacity than magnesium hydroxide–aluminum hydroxide mixtures, but it may cause diarrhea and hypermagnesemia. Aluminum hydroxide has the least buffering capacity.
   c. **Rapid action.** Magnesium hydroxide, magnesium oxide, and calcium carbonate are effective for rapid action. Sodium bicarbonate is rapidly effective but of short duration. It is contraindicated for long-term use because of systemic absorption and possible metabolic alkalosis. Effervescent antacids have a rapid onset but short duration of action, because they leave the stomach quickly.
   d. **Dosage form.** Antacid liquid suspensions usually act faster than chewable tablets. However, suspensions have not been proven more effective in neutralizing gastric acid. Chewable tablets may be more convenient in some circumstances.
   e. **Antiflatulent.** Simethicone, which is added to several antacid mixtures, has no effect on intragastric pH but may be useful in relieving flatulence or gastroesophageal reflux.
   f. **Ingredients.** Antacids with these ingredients or characteristics are contraindicated as follows:
      (1) Magnesium is contraindicated in renal disease because hypermagnesemia may result.

(2) High sodium content may be contraindicated in edematous states, such as congestive heart failure.

(3) High sugar content may be contraindicated in diabetes mellitus.

g. **Occasional use.** Although sodium bicarbonate (baking soda) and calcium carbonate are generally contraindicated in the large amounts and long-term usage required for treatment of peptic ulcer disease, occasional use is not likely to be harmful.

h. **Palatability.** Efforts should be made to find an antacid preparation that is acceptable to the client in terms of taste, dosage, and convenience of administration.

2. As a general rule, single drugs are preferable to mixtures. However, antacid combinations have several advantages, including the following:

a. Combining an antacid with a laxative effect (*e.g.,* magnesium hydroxide) with one that has a constipating effect (*e.g.,* aluminum hydroxide) tends to prevent or reduce the incidence of both symptoms.

b. Combining fast-acting and slow-acting antacids can prolong gastric acid neutralization.

c. Mixtures allow smaller dosages of individual ingredients, and adverse effects may be prevented or reduced.

d. Client compliance with antacid therapy is usually improved.

3. Antacid dosage, including frequency of administration, depends primarily on the purpose for use, buffering capacity of the antacid, and client response. Some guidelines include the following:

a. To prevent stress ulcers in critically ill clients and to treat acute GI bleeding, nearly continuous neutralization of gastric acid is desirable. Dose and frequency of administration must be sufficient to neutralize about 50 to 80 mEq of gastric acid each hour. This can be accomplished by a continuous intragastric drip through a nasogastric tube or by hourly administration.

b. When a client has a nasogastric tube in place, antacid dosage may be titrated by aspirating stomach contents, determining pH with Nitrazine paper, and then basing the dose on the pH. (Most gastric acid is neutralized and most pepsin activity is eliminated at a pH above 3.5.)

c. For most clients, the standard practice of giving an antacid 1 hour and 3 hours after meals and at bedtime is effective and rational, although gastric acid is buffered intermittently rather than continuously. When an antacid is given on an empty stomach, gastric acid is neutralized for about 30 minutes, depending on gastric emptying time. When an antacid is taken after meals, buffering effects last 3 or more hours.

d. When antacids are used to relieve pain, they may be taken as needed.

e. The usual dose of a liquid antacid is 30 ml (2 tbsp or 6 tsp). This amount is higher than doses recommended by most manufacturers (5 to 20 ml or 1 to 4 tsp).

EFFECTS OF ANTIULCER DRUGS ON OTHER DRUGS

Antacids may prevent absorption of most drugs taken at the same time, including benzodiazepine antianxiety drugs, corticosteroids, digoxin, H_2 blockers (cimetidine, ranitidine), iron supplements, phenothiazine antipsychotic drugs, phenytoin, quinolone antibacterials, salicylates, and tetracyclines. Antacids increase absorption of a few drugs, including levodopa, quinidine, and valproic acid. These interactions can be avoided or minimized by separating administration times by 1 to 2 hours.

Histamine$_2$ receptor blocking drugs may alter the effects of several drugs. Most significant effects occur with cimetidine, which inhibits drug-metabolizing enzymes (cytochrome P450 pathway) in the liver and interferes with the metabolism of several commonly used drugs. Consequently, the affected drugs are eliminated more slowly, their serum levels are increased, and they are more likely to cause adverse effects and toxicity unless dosage is reduced.

Interacting drugs include antiarrhythmics (lidocaine, moricizine, propafenone, quinidine), the anticoagulant warfarin, anticonvulsants (carbamazepine, phenytoin), benzodiazepine antianxiety or hypnotic agents (alprazolam, chlordiazepoxide, diazepam, flurazepam, triazolam), beta-adrenergic blocking agents (labetalol, metoprolol, propranolol), the bronchodilator theophylline, calcium channel blocking agents (*e.g.,* verapamil), tricyclic antidepressants (*e.g.,* amitriptyline), and sulfonylureas (*e.g.,* oral antidiabetic drugs). In addition, cimetidine may increase serum levels (*e.g.,* fluorouracil, procainamide and its active metabolite) and pharmacologic effects of other drugs (*e.g.,* flecainide, respiratory depression with narcotic analgesics or succinylcholine) by unidentified mechanisms. Cimetidine also may decrease effects of several drugs, including drugs that require an acidic environment for absorption (*e.g.,* iron salts, indomethacin, fluconazole, ketoconazole, tetracyclines) and miscellaneous drugs (*e.g.,* digoxin, tocainide), by unknown mechanisms.

Ranitidine, famotidine, and nizatidine do not inhibit the cytochrome P450 metabolizing enzymes. Ranitidine decreases absorption of diazepam if given at the same time and increases hypoglycemic effects of glipizide. Nizatidine increases serum salicylate levels in people taking high doses of aspirin.

Omeprazole increases blood levels of diazepam, phenytoin, and warfarin, probably by inhibiting hepatic metabolism. These interactions have not been reported with lansoprazole.

Sucralfate decreases absorption of ciprofloxacin and other quinolone antibiotics, digoxin, ketoconazole, phenytoin, and warfarin. Apparently, sucralfate binds to these drugs when both are present in the GI tract. This interaction can be avoided or minimized by giving the interacting drug 2 hours before sucralfate.

EFFECTS OF ANTIULCER DRUGS ON NUTRIENTS

Dietary folate, iron, and vitamin B_{12} are better absorbed from an acidic environment. When gastric fluids are made less acidic by antacids, histamine$_2$ antagonists, or proton pump inhibitors, deficiencies of these nutrients may occur. In addition, sucralfate interferes with absorption of fat-soluble vitamins, and magnesium-containing antacids interfere with absorption of vitamin A.

USE IN CHILDREN

Antacids may be given to ambulatory children in doses of 5 to 15 ml every 3 to 6 hours or at 1 and 3 hours after meals and at bedtime, as for adults with acute peptic ulcer disease. For prevention of GI bleeding in critically ill children, 2 to 5 ml may be given to infants and 5 to 15 ml to children every 1 to 2 hours. Safety and effectiveness of other antiulcer drugs have not been established for children.

USE IN OLDER ADULTS

All of the antiulcer drugs may be used in older adults. With antacids, older adults usually secrete less gastric acid than younger adults, and smaller doses may be effective. Further, with decreased renal function, older adults are more likely to have adverse effects. These include neuromuscular effects of magnesium-containing antacids and cardiovascular effects (edema, hypertension, congestive heart failure) of sodium-containing antacids, especially if large or frequent doses are taken. Many physicians recommend calcium carbonate antacids (*e.g.,* TUMS) as a calcium supplement to prevent osteoporosis in older women.

With H$_2$ receptor antagonists, older adults are more likely to experience adverse effects, especially confusion, agitation, and disorientation with cimetidine. In addition, older adults often have decreased renal function, and doses need to be reduced.

Older adults often take large doses of NSAIDs for arthritis and therefore are at risk of developing acute gastric ulcers and GI bleeding. Thus, they may be candidates for treatment with misoprostol. Dosage of misoprostol may need to be reduced to prevent severe diarrhea and abdominal cramping.

Proton pump inhibitors and sucralfate seem to be well tolerated by older adults.

HOME CARE

All of the antiulcer drugs are commonly taken in the home setting, usually by self-administration. The home care nurse can assist clients by providing information about taking the drugs correctly and monitoring responses. If cimetidine is being taken, the home care nurse needs to assess for potential drug-drug interactions. With over-the-counter histamine$_2$ antagonists, clients should be instructed to avoid daily use for longer than 2 weeks. If usage of antacids or over-the-counter histamine$_2$ antagonists seems to be excessive or prolonged, the client should be assessed for peptic ulcer disease or gastroesophageal reflux disease.

ANTIULCER DRUGS

NURSING ACTIONS	*RATIONALE/EXPLANATION*
1. Administer accurately **a.** Give oral cimetidine with meals or at bedtime. Famotidine, nizatidine, and ranitidine may be given without regard to food intake.	When cimetidine is taken with meals, peak serum drug level coincides with gastric emptying, when gastric acidity is usually highest. When taken at bedtime, cimetidine prevents secretion of gastric acid for several hours. Thus, correct timing of drug administration may promote faster healing of the ulcer.

NURSING ACTIONS	RATIONALE/EXPLANATION
b. To give cimetidine or ranitidine intravenously, dilute in 20 ml of 5% dextrose or normal saline solution, and inject over at least 2 min. For intermittent infusion, dilute in at least 50 ml of 5% dextrose or 0.9% sodium chloride solution, and infuse over 15–20 min.	
c. To give famotidine intravenously, dilute with 5–10 ml of 0.9% sodium chloride injection, and inject over at least 2 min. For intermittent infusion, dilute in 100 ml of 5% dextrose or 0.9% sodium chloride, and infuse over 15–30 min.	
d. Do not give antacids within about 1 h of oral H_2 antagonists or sucralfate.	Antacids decrease absorption and therapeutic effectiveness of the other drugs.
e. Shake liquid antacids well before measuring the dose.	These preparations are suspensions. Drug particles settle to the bottom of the container on standing and must be mixed thoroughly to give the correct dose.
f. Instruct clients to chew antacid tablets thoroughly.	To increase the surface area of drug available to neutralize gastric acid
g. Give sucralfate 1 h before meals and at bedtime.	To allow the drug to form its protective coating over the ulcer before high levels of gastric acidity. Sucralfate requires an acidic environment. After it has adhered to the ulcer, antacids and food do not affect drug action.
h. Give omeprazole and lansoprazole before food intake, with instructions to swallow the capsules whole (without crushing or chewing).	The drugs are formulated in an enteric-coated (to prevent destruction by gastric acid), extended-release preparation.
i. Give misoprostol with food.	
2. Observe for therapeutic effects	Therapeutic effects depend on the reason for use.
a. Decreased epigastric pain	Antacids should relieve ulcer pain within a few minutes. H_2 antagonists relieve pain in about 1 wk by healing effects on the ulcer.
b. Decreased gastrointestinal (GI) bleeding (*e.g.,* absence of visible or occult blood in vomitus, gastric secretions, or feces)	
c. Higher pH of gastric contents	The minimum acceptable pH with antacid therapy is 3.5. In acute situations the goal may be a pH of 7 (neutral).
d. Radiologic or endoscopic reports of ulcer healing	
3. Observe for adverse effects **a.** With H_2 antagonists, observe for diarrhea or constipation, headache, dizziness, muscle aches, fatigue, skin rashes, mental confusion, delirium, coma, depression, fever.	Adverse effects are uncommon and usually mild with recommended doses and duration of drug therapy (8 wk). Central nervous system effects have been associated with high doses in elderly clients or those with impaired renal function. With long-term administration of cimetidine, other adverse effects have been observed. These include decreased sperm count and gynecomastia in men and galactorrhea in women.
b. With antacids containing magnesium, observe for diarrhea and hypermagnesemia.	Diarrhea may be prevented by combining these antacids with other antacids containing aluminum or calcium. Hypermagnesemia is unlikely in most clients but may occur in those with impaired renal function. These antacids should not be given to clients with renal failure.

(continued)

Nursing Actions	*Rationale/Explanation*
c. With antacids containing aluminum or calcium, observe for constipation.	Constipation may be prevented by combining these antacids with other antacids containing magnesium. A high-fiber diet and adequate fluid intake (2000–3000 ml daily) also help prevent constipation.
d. With sucralfate, observe for constipation.	Thus far, adverse effects observed with sucralfate have been few and minor. (The drug is not absorbed systemically.) The most common one was constipation (4.7% in 2500 people).
e. With misoprostol, observe for diarrhea, abdominal pain, nausea, and vomiting, headache, uterine cramping, vaginal bleeding.	Diarrhea is the most commonly reported and may be severe enough to indicate dosage reduction or stopping the drug.
f. With omeprazole, observe for headache, diarrhea, abdominal pain, nausea, and vomiting.	These effects occur infrequently and are usually well tolerated.
g. With bismuth, observe for black stools.	This is a harmless discoloration of the stool; it does not indicate GI bleeding.
4. Observe for drug interactions	Most significant drug interactions alter the effect of the other drug rather than that of the antiulcer drug. For example, cimetidine may potentiate anticoagulants; antacids alter the absorption of many oral drugs.
a. Drugs that *decrease* effects of cimetidine and ranitidine: Antacids	Antacids decrease absorption of cimetidine and probably ranitidine. The drugs should not be given at the same time.
b. Drugs that *increase* effects of antacids: Anticholinergic drugs (*e.g.*, atropine)	May increase effects by delaying gastric emptying and by decreasing acid secretion themselves
c. Drugs that *decrease* effects of antacids: Cholinergic drugs (*e.g.*, dexpanthenol [Ilopan])	May decrease effects by increasing GI motility and rate of gastric emptying
d. Drugs that *decrease* effects of sucralfate: Antacids	Antacids should not be given within ½ hour before or after administration of sucralfate.
e. Drug that *increases* effects of omeprazole Clarithromycin	May increase blood levels of omeprazole
f. Drug that *decreases* effects of lansoprazole Sucralfate	Decreases absorption of lansoprazole. Lansoprazole should be given about 30 min before sucralfate if both are being used.
5. Teach clients **a.** Take antiulcer drugs as prescribed.	Underuse decreases therapeutic effectiveness; overuse increases adverse effects. For acute peptic ulcer disease, drugs are given in relatively high doses for 4–8 wk to promote healing. For long-term maintenance therapy, dosage is reduced.
b. Take cimetidine with food; take ranitidine, famotidine, and nizatidine without regard to meals; take sucralfate before meals and at bedtime; take antacids 1 and 3 h after meals and at bedtime; take misoprostol with food and omeprazole before food intake.	For increased therapeutic effects
c. Do not take over-the-counter cimetidine, famotidine, nizatidine or ranitidine continuously for more than 2 wk without the advice and supervision of a physician.	There is a risk of delaying treatment for GERD or peptic ulcer disease.
d. Choose antacids carefully.	Because antacids do not require a prescription, many products are readily available. However, these products are not equally safe or effective in all people.

NURSING ACTIONS	RATIONALE/EXPLANATION
(1) Consult with a physician before choosing an antacid for peptic ulcer disease or when heart or kidney disease is present.	Some antacids are safer and more effective than others in the large doses and long-term usage required for peptic ulcer disease. Some antacids should not be taken with heart disease (because of high sodium content with potential fluid retention and edema) or kidney disease (because of drug accumulation and higher risks of toxicity).
(2) Do not overuse baking soda, Alka-Seltzer effervescent antacid tablets, Titralac, or Tums.	These products may cause serious adverse effects if taken in large amounts or for prolonged periods. Baking soda and Alka-Seltzer effervescent tablets contain large amounts of sodium; the other products contain calcium carbonate.
e. Take antacids at least 1 h before or after other drugs.	Antacids decrease absorption of many other drugs, including cimetidine and other H_2 receptor antagonists and sucralfate.
f. Swallow omeprazole capsules whole. Do not open, chew, or crush the capsules.	To prevent destruction of the drug by stomach acid

REVIEW AND APPLICATION EXERCISES

1. What are risk factors for peptic ulcer disease?

2. How are ulcers thought to develop? What roles do gastric acid, pepsin, *H. pylori* organisms, prostaglandins, and mucus play in ulcer occurrence?

3. How do the various antiulcer drugs heal ulcers or prevent their recurrence?

4. Compare histamine$_2$ antagonists and proton pump inhibitors in indications for use, effectiveness, and convenience of use.

5. List advantages and disadvantages of cimetidine in comparison with other H_2 blockers.

6. What is the rationale for taking H_2 blockers at bedtime?

7. What is the rationale for taking sucralfate before meals?

8. What is the rationale for taking antacids after meals?

9. Why are aluminum and magnesium salts often combined in antacid preparations?

10. For a client who smokes cigarettes and is newly diagnosed with peptic ulcer disease, how would you explain that smoking cessation aids ulcer healing?

11. Is diet therapy important in ulcer occurrence, healing, or recurrence? Why or why not?

SELECTED REFERENCES

Berardi, R.R. (1997). Peptic ulcer disease and Zollinger-Ellison syndrome. In J.T. DiPiro, R.L. Talbert, G.C. Yee, G.R. Matzke, B.G. Wells & L.M. Posey (Eds.), *Pharmacotherapy: A pathophysiologic approach*, 3rd ed., pp. 697–721. Stamford, CT: Appleton & Lange.

Blum, R.A. (1996). Lansoprazole and omeprazole in the treatment of acid peptic disorders. *American Journal of Health-System Pharmacy 53*, 1401–1415.

Brunton, L.L. (1996). Agents for control of gastric acidity and treatment of peptic ulcers. In J.G. Hardman, L.E. Limbird, P.B. Molinoff & R.W. Ruddon (Eds.), *Goodman & Gilman's The pharmacological basis of therapeutics*, 9th ed., pp. 901–915. New York: McGraw-Hill.

Castell, D.O. & Johnston, B.T. (1996). Gastroesophageal reflux disease: Current strategies for patient management. *Archives of Family Medicine 5*, 221–227.

Davis, J. & Sherer, K. (1994). *Applied nutrition and diet therapy for nurses*, 2nd ed. Philadelphia: W.B. Saunders.

Drug facts and comparisons. (Updated monthly). St. Louis: Facts and Comparisons.

Guyton, A.C. & Hall, J.E. (1996). *Textbook of medical physiology*, 9th ed. Philadelphia: W.B. Saunders.

Hentschel, E., Brandstatter, G., Dragosics, B., Hirschl, A.M., Nemec, H., Schutze, K., Taufer, M. & Wurzer, H. (1993). Effect of ranitidine and amoxicillin plus metronidazole on the eradication of *Helicobacter pylori* and the recurrence of duodenal ulcer. *New England Journal of Medicine 328*, 308–312.

Porth, C.M. (1994). *Pathophysiology: Concepts of altered health states*, 4th ed., pp. 817–841. Philadelphia: J.B. Lippincott.

Roth, S.H. (1996). NSAID gastropathy: A new understanding. *Archives of Internal Medicine 156*, 1623–1628.

Walsh, J.H. & Fass, R. (1997). Acid peptic disorders of the gastrointestinal tract. In W.N. Kelley (Ed.), *Textbook of internal medicine*, 3rd ed., pp. 684–702. Philadelphia: J.B. Lippincott.

Williams, D.B. & Welage, L.S. (1997). Gastroesophageal reflux disease. In J.T. DiPiro, R.L. Talbert, G.C. Yee, G.R. Matzke, B.G. Wells & L.M. Posey (Eds.), *Pharmacotherapy: A pathophysiologic approach*, 3rd ed., pp. 675–696. Stamford, CT: Appleton & Lange

61 Laxatives and Cathartics

Outline

Objectives

After studying this chapter, the student will be able to:

1 Differentiate the major types of laxatives according to effects on the gastrointestinal tract.

2 Differentiate the consequences of occasional use from those of chronic use.

3 Discuss rational choices of laxatives for selected client populations or purposes.

4 Discuss bulk-forming laxatives as the most physiologic agents.

5 Discuss possible reasons for and hazards of overuse and abuse of laxatives.

Key Terms

Bowel cleansing	**Laxative dependence**
Laxative abuse	**Propulsive**

Description

Laxatives and cathartics are drugs used to promote bowel elimination (defecation). The term *laxative* implies mild effects and elimination of soft, formed stool. The term *cathartic* implies strong effects and elimination of liquid or semiliquid stool. Because the different effects depend more on the dose than on the particular drug used, the terms often are used interchangeably.

Defecation

Defecation is normally stimulated by movements and reflexes in the gastrointestinal (GI) tract. When the stomach and duodenum are distended with food or fluids, gastrocolic and duodenocolic reflexes cause propulsive movements in the colon, which move feces into the rectum and arouse the urge to defecate. When sensory nerve fibers in the rectum are stimulated by the fecal mass, the defecation reflex causes strong peristalsis, deep breathing, closure of the glottis, contraction of abdominal muscles, contraction of the rectum, relaxation of anal sphincters, and expulsion of the fecal mass.

The cerebral cortex normally controls the defecation reflex so defecation can occur at acceptable times and places. Voluntary control inhibits the external anal sphincter to allow defecation or contracts the sphincter to prevent defecation. When the external sphincter remains contracted, the defecation reflex dissipates, and the urge to defecate usually does not recur until additional feces enter the rectum or several hours later.

People who often inhibit the defecation reflex or fail to respond to the urge to defecate develop constipation as the reflex weakens. *Constipation* is the infrequent and painful expulsion of hard, dry stools. Although there is no "normal" number of stools because of variations in diet and other factors, most people report more than three bowel movements per week. Normal bowel elimination should produce a soft, formed stool without pain.

Laxatives and Cathartics

Laxatives and cathartics are somewhat arbitrarily classified as bulk-forming laxatives, surfactant laxatives or stool softeners, saline cathartics, stimulant cathartics, and lubricant or emollient laxatives. Individual drugs are listed in Table 61-1.

BULK-FORMING LAXATIVES

Bulk-forming laxatives (*e.g.*, methylcellulose, psyllium seed) are substances that are largely unabsorbed from the intestine. When water is added, these substances swell and become gel-like. The added bulk or size of the fecal mass stimulates peristalsis and defecation. The substances also may act by pulling water into the intestinal lumen. Bulk-forming laxatives are the most physiologic laxatives because they act similarly to increased intake of dietary fiber.

SURFACTANT LAXATIVES (STOOL SOFTENERS)

Surfactant laxatives (*e.g.*, docusate sodium) decrease the surface tension of the fecal mass to allow water to penetrate into the stool. They also act as a detergent to facilitate admixing of fat and water in the stool. As a result, stools are softer and easier to expel. These agents have little if any laxative effect. Their main value is to prevent straining while expelling stool.

SALINE CATHARTICS

Saline cathartics (*e.g.*, magnesium citrate, milk of magnesia, sodium phosphate) are not well absorbed from the intestine. Consequently, they increase osmotic pressure in the intestinal lumen and cause water to be retained. Distention of the bowel leads to increased peristalsis and decreased intestinal transit time for the fecal mass. The resultant stool is semifluid.

IRRITANT OR STIMULANT CATHARTICS

The irritant or stimulant cathartics are the strongest and most abused laxative products. These drugs act by irritating the GI mucosa and pulling water into the bowel lumen. As a result, feces are moved through the bowel too rapidly to allow colonic absorption of fecal water, so a watery stool is eliminated. These cathartics are subdivided into three groups, which differ in location and time of action but are similar in mechanism of action, pharmacokinetics, and adverse effects. The groups are castor oil, anthraquinones (senna products, cascara sagrada), and diphenylmethanes (bisacodyl, phenolphthalein). Phenolphthalein is the active ingredient in several over-the-counter laxatives (*e.g.*, Ex-Lax, Feen-a-Mint).

In addition to the oral agents, glycerin is administered as a rectal suppository. Glycerin stimulates bowel evacuation by its irritant effects on rectal mucosa and hyperosmotic effects in the colon. Glycerin is not given orally for laxative effects.

LUBRICANT LAXATIVES

Mineral oil is the only lubricant laxative used clinically. It lubricates the intestine and is thought to soften stool by retarding colonic absorption of fecal water, but the exact mechanism of action is unknown. Mineral oil may cause several adverse effects and is not recommended for long-term use.

TABLE 61-1 LAXATIVES AND CATHARTICS

Generic/Trade Name	Routes and Dosage Ranges	
	Adults	*Children*
Bulk-Forming Laxatives		
Methylcellulose (Citrucel)	PO 1 heaping Tbsp one to three times daily with water (8 oz or more)	PO 1 level Tbsp one to three times daily with water (4 oz)
Polycarbophil (FiberCon, Mitrolan)	PO 1 g four times daily or PRN with 8 oz of fluid; maximum dose, 6 g/24 h	Age 6–12 y, PO 500 mg one to three times daily or PRN; maximum dose, 3 g/24 h Age 2–6 y, PO 500 mg one or two times daily or PRN; maximum dose, 1.5 g/24 h
Psyllium preparations (Metamucil, Effersyllium, Serutan, Perdiem Plain)	PO 4–10 g (1–2 tsp) one to three times daily, stirred in at least 8 oz of water or other liquid	
Surfactant Laxatives (Stool Softeners)		
Docusate sodium (Colace, Doxinate)	PO 50–200 mg daily	Age over 12 y, same dosage as adults Age 3–12 y, 20–120 mg daily Age under 3 y, 10–40 mg daily
Docusate calcium (Surfak)	PO 50–240 mg daily	Age over 12 y, same dosage as adults Age 2–12 y, 50–150 mg daily Age under 2 y, 25 mg daily
Docusate potassium (Dialose)	PO 100–300 mg daily	Age 6–12 y, 100 mg at bedtime
Saline Cathartics		
Magnesium citrate solution	PO 200 ml at bedtime	
Magnesium hydroxide (milk of magnesia, magnesia magma)	Regular liquid, PO 15–60 ml at bedtime. Concentrated liquid, PO 10–20 ml at bedtime	Regular liquid, PO 2.5–5 ml
Polyethylene glycol-electrolyte solution (PEG 3350, sodium sulfate, sodium bicarbonate, sodium chloride, potassium chloride) (Colyte, Colovage, GoLYTELY)	For bowel cleansing before GI examination: PO 240 ml (8 oz) every 10 min until 4 L are consumed	No recommended children's dose
Sodium phosphate and sodium biphosphate (Fleet Phosphosoda, Fleet Enema)	PO 20–40 ml in 8 oz of water Rectal enema, 60–120 ml	Age 10 y and over, PO 10–20 ml in 8 oz of water Age 5–10 y, PO 5–10 ml in 8 oz of water Rectal enema, 60 ml
Irritant or Stimulant Cathartics		
Anthraquinone		
Cascara sagrada (Cas-Evac)	PO, tablets, 325 mg; fluid extract, 0.5–1.5 ml; aromatic fluid extract, 5 ml	
Senna pod preparations (Senokot, Black Draught)	Granules, PO 1 level tsp once or twice daily; geriatric, obstetric, gynecologic clients, PO 0.5 level tsp once or twice daily Syrup, PO 2–3 tsp once or twice daily; geriatric, obstetric, gynecologic clients, 1–1½ tsp once or twice daily	Weight over 27 kg: granules, syrup, tablets, suppositories—½ adult dose

TABLE 61-1	LAXATIVES AND CATHARTICS (Continued)	

	Routes and Dosage Ranges	
Generic/Trade Name	*Adults*	*Children*
	Tablets, PO 2 tablets once or twice daily; geriatric, obstetric, gynecologic clients, 1 tablet once or twice daily Suppositories, 1 suppository at bedtime	
Diphenylmethane Cathartics		
Bisacodyl (Dulcolax)	PO 10–15 mg Rectal suppository, 10 mg	Age 6 y and over, PO 5–10 mg Age under 2 y, rectal suppository 5 mg
Phenolphthalein (Alophen, Feen-a-Mint, Ex-Lax)	PO 30–194 mg daily	
Other Irritant Cathartics		
Castor Oil (Alphamul, Neoloid)	PO 15–60 ml	Age 5–15 y, PO 5–30 ml depending on strength of emulsion Age under 2 y, PO 1.25–7.5 ml depending on strength of emulsion
Glycerin	Rectal suppository, 3 g	Age under 6 y, rectal suppository 1–1.5 g
Lubricant Laxative		
Mineral oil (Agoral Plain, Milkinol, Fleet Mineral Oil Enema)	PO 15–30 ml at bedtime Rectal enema, 30–60 ml	Age over 6 y, PO 5–15 ml at bedtime Rectal enema, 30–60 ml
Miscellaneous Laxatives		
Lactulose (Chronulac, Cephulac)	PO 15–30 ml daily; maximum dose, 60 ml daily Portal systemic encephalopathy, PO 30–45 ml three or four times daily, adjusted to produce two or three soft stools daily Rectally as retention enema, 300 ml with 700 ml water or normal saline, retained 30–60 min, q4–6h	Infants, PO 2.5–10 ml daily in divided doses Older children, PO 40–90 ml daily in divided doses
Sorbitol	PO 30–50 g daily	

MISCELLANEOUS LAXATIVES

Lactulose is a disaccharide that is not absorbed from the GI tract. It exerts laxative effects by pulling water into the intestinal lumen. It is used to treat constipation and hepatic encephalopathy. The latter condition usually results from alcoholic liver disease in which ammonia accumulates and causes stupor or coma. Ammonia is produced by metabolism of dietary protein and intestinal bacteria. Lactulose decreases production of ammonia in the intestine. The goal of treatment is usually to maintain two to three soft stools daily.

Polyethylene glycol-electrolyte solution (Colyte, GoLYTELY) is a nonabsorbable, oral solution that induces diarrhea within 30 to 60 minutes and rapidly evacuates the bowel, usually within 4 hours. It is used

only for bowel cleansing before GI examination (*e.g.*, colonoscopy) and is contraindicated with GI obstruction, gastric retention, colitis, or bowel perforation.

Sorbitol is a monosaccharide that pulls water into the intestinal lumen and has laxative effects. It is often given with sodium polystyrene sulfonate (Kayexalate), a potassium-removing resin used to treat hyperkalemia, to prevent constipation and aid expulsion of the potassium-resin complex.

INDICATIONS FOR USE

Laxatives and cathartics are widely available on a non-prescription basis. They are among the most frequently used and abused drugs. One reason for overuse is the common misconception that a daily bowel movement is necessary for health and well-being. This notion may lead to a vicious cycle of events in which a person fails to have a bowel movement, takes a strong laxative, again fails to have a bowel movement, and takes another laxative before the fecal column has had time to become reestablished (2 to 3 days). Thus, a pattern of laxative dependence and abuse is established. Despite widespread abuse of laxatives and cathartics, there are several rational indications for use:

1. To **relieve constipation** in pregnant women, elderly clients whose abdominal and perineal muscles have become weak and atrophied, children with megacolon, and clients receiving drugs that decrease intestinal motility (*e.g.*, narcotic analgesics, anticholinergics, tricyclic antidepressants)
2. To **prevent straining** at stool in clients with coronary artery disease (*e.g.*, postmyocardial infarction), hypertension, cerebrovascular disease, and hemorrhoids and other rectal conditions
3. To **empty the bowel** in preparation for bowel surgery or diagnostic procedures (*e.g.*, proctoscopy, colonoscopy, barium enema)
4. To **accelerate elimination** of potentially toxic substances from the GI tract (*e.g.*, orally ingested drugs or toxic compounds)
5. To **prevent absorption** of intestinal ammonia in clients with hepatic encephalopathy
6. To **obtain a stool specimen** for parasitologic examination
7. To **accelerate excretion of parasites** after anthelmintic drugs have been administered

CONTRAINDICATIONS FOR USE

Laxatives and cathartics should not be used in the presence of undiagnosed abdominal pain. The danger is that the drugs may cause an inflamed organ (*e.g.*, the appendix) to rupture and spill GI contents into the abdominal cavity with subsequent peritonitis, a life-threatening situation. The drugs also are contraindicated with intestinal obstruction and fecal impaction.

Nursing Process

Assessment

Assess clients for current or potential constipation.
- Identify risk factors:
  - Diet with minimal fiber (*i.e.*, small amounts of fruits, vegetables, and whole-grain products)
  - Low fluid intake (*e.g.*, less than 2000 ml daily)
  - Immobility or limited activity
  - Drug therapy with central nervous system depressant drugs (*e.g.*, narcotic analgesics), anticholinergics, and others that reduce intestinal motility. Overuse of antidiarrheal agents also may cause constipation.

- Hemorrhoids, anal fissures, or other conditions characterized by painful bowel elimination
- Elderly or debilitated clients
- Signs and symptoms include the following:
  - Decreased number and frequency of stools
  - Passage of dry, hard stools
  - Abdominal distention and discomfort
  - Flatulence

Nursing Diagnoses

- Constipation related to decreased activity, inadequate dietary fiber, inadequate fluid intake, drugs, or disease processes
- Pain (abdominal cramping and distention) related to constipation or use of laxatives
- Impaired Tissue Integrity: Loss of normal bowel function related to overuse of laxatives
- Noncompliance with recommendations for nondrug measures to prevent or treat constipation
- Noncompliance with instructions for appropriate use of laxatives
- Risk for Fluid Volume Deficit related to diarrhea from frequent or large doses of laxatives
- Altered Nutrition: Poor absorption of nutrients during laxative-induced diarrhea
- Risk for Injury: Falls from weakness induced by vigorous bowel cleansing before GI surgery or diagnostic tests
- Knowledge Deficit: Nondrug measures to prevent constipation
- Knowledge Deficit: Appropriate use of laxatives

Planning/Goals

The client will:
- Take laxative drugs appropriately
- Use nondrug measures to promote normal bowel function and prevent constipation
- Regain normal patterns of bowel elimination
- Avoid excessive losses of fluids and electrolytes from laxative use
- Be protected from excessive fluid loss, hypotension, and other adverse drug effects, when possible
- Be assisted to avoid constipation when at risk (*i.e.*, has illness or injury that prevents activity, food and fluid intake; has medically prescribed drugs that decrease GI function)
- Be assisted as needed to prevent falls and other injuries when weak from vigorous bowel cleansing before surgery or diagnostic tests

Interventions

When not contraindicated by the client's condition, assist clients with constipation to
- Increase activity and exercise
- Increase intake of dietary fiber (vegetables, fruits, cereal grains)
- Drink at least 2000 ml of fluid daily
- Establish and maintain a routine for bowel elimination (*e.g.*, going to the bathroom immediately after breakfast)
Monitor client responses:
- Record number, amount, and type of bowel movements.
- For clients who become weak from laxatives and enemas, assist in ambulation or other activities.
- Record vital signs. Hypotension and weak pulse may indicate fluid volume deficit.

Teach clients:

- That diet, exercise, and fluid intake influence the frequency and type of bowel movements
- Nondrug measures to promote normal bowel function and prevent constipation:
  - Eat foods high in dietary fiber daily. Fiber is the portion of plant food that is not digested. It is contained in fruits, vegetables, and whole-grain cereals and breads. Bran, the outer coating of cereal grains, such as wheat or oats, is an excellent source of dietary fiber and is available in numerous cereal products.
  - Drink at least 6 to 10 glasses (8 oz each) of fluid daily if not contraindicated.
  - Exercise regularly. Walking and other activities aid movement of feces through the bowel.
  - Establish regular bowel habits. The defecation urge is usually strongest after eating or drinking. This knowledge may help to establish a regular time for defecation. The defecation reflex is weakened or lost if repeatedly ignored. The place chosen for defecation should allow adequate privacy.
- To avoid regular use of self-prescribed laxatives because it may prevent normal bowel function, cause adverse drug reactions, and delay treatment for conditions that cause constipation
- *Never* to take laxatives when acute abdominal pain is present. Doing so may cause a ruptured appendix or other serious complication.
- That 2 to 3 days of normal eating are required to reestablish the fecal column after a strong oral laxative has been taken
- That frequent use of strong oral laxatives promotes laxative dependence
- That bulk-forming laxatives act the same way as increasing fiber in the diet and are usually best for long-term use. When taken daily, these drugs are effective in preventing constipation, but they are not effective in relieving acute constipation.

Evaluation

- Observe and interview for improved patterns of bowel elimination.
- Observe for use of nondrug measures to promote bowel function.
- Observe for appropriate use of laxatives.
- Observe and interview regarding adverse effects of laxatives.

Principles of Therapy

DRUG SELECTION

Choice of a laxative or cathartic depends on the reason for use and the client's condition.

1. For long-term use of laxatives or cathartics in clients who are elderly, unable or unwilling to eat an adequate diet, or debilitated, bulk-forming laxatives (*e.g.,* Metamucil, Effersyllium) usually are preferred. However, because obstruction may occur, these agents should not be given to clients with dysphagia,

adhesions or strictures in the GI tract, or to those who are unable or unwilling to drink adequate fluids.

2. For clients in whom straining is potentially harmful or painful, stool softeners (*e.g.,* docusate sodium) are agents of choice.

3. For occasional use to cleanse the bowel for endoscopic or radiologic examinations, saline or stimulant cathartics are acceptable (*e.g.,* magnesium citrate, polyethylene glycol-electrolyte solution, castor oil, bisacodyl). These drugs should not be used more than once per week. Frequent use is likely to produce laxative abuse.

4. Oral use of mineral oil may cause potentially serious adverse effects (decreased absorption of fat-soluble vitamins and some drugs, lipid pneumonia if aspirated into the lungs). Thus, mineral oil is not an oral laxative of choice in any condition, although occasional use in the alert client is unlikely to be harmful. Mineral oil is probably most useful as a retention enema to soften hard, dry feces and aid in their expulsion. Mineral oil should not be used regularly.

5. In fecal impaction, a rectal suppository (*e.g.,* bisacodyl) or an enema (*e.g.,* oil retention or Fleet enema) is preferred. Oral laxatives are contraindicated when fecal impaction is present but may be given after the rectal mass is removed. Once the impaction is relieved, measures should be taken to prevent recurrence. If dietary and other nonpharmacologic measures are ineffective or contraindicated, use of a bulk-forming agent daily or another laxative once or twice weekly may be necessary.

6. Saline cathartics containing magnesium, phosphate, or potassium salts are contraindicated in clients with renal failure because hypermagnesemia, hyperphosphatemia, or hyperkalemia may occur.

7. Saline cathartics containing sodium salts are contraindicated in clients with edema or congestive heart failure because enough sodium may be absorbed to cause further fluid retention and edema. They also should not be used in clients with impaired renal function or those following a sodium-restricted diet for hypertension.

8. Polyethylene glycol-electrolyte solution is formulated for rapid and effective bowel cleansing without significant changes in water or electrolyte balance.

USE IN CHILDREN

As in adults, increasing fluids, high-fiber foods, and exercise is preferred when possible. For acute constipation, glycerin suppositories are often effective in infants and small children. Stool softeners may be given to older children. Children generally should not use strong, stimulant laxatives. Parents should be advised not to use any laxative more than once a week without consulting a health care provider.

USE IN OLDER ADULTS

Constipation is a common problem in older adults, and laxatives are often used or overused. Nondrug measures to prevent constipation (*e.g.,* increasing fluids, high-fiber foods, and exercise) are much preferred to laxatives. If a laxative is required on a regular basis, a psyllium compound (*e.g.,* Metamucil) is best because it is most physiologic in its action. If taken, it should be accompanied by a full glass of fluid. There have been reports of obstruction in the GI tract when taken with insufficient fluid. Strong stimulant laxatives should generally be avoided.

HOME CARE

Laxatives are commonly self-prescribed and self-administered in the home setting. The home care nurse may become involved when visiting a client for other purposes. The role of the home care nurse may include assessing usual patterns of bowel elimination, identifying clients at risk of developing constipation, promoting lifestyle interventions to prevent constipation, and obtaining laxatives when indicated.

NURSING ACTIONS — LAXATIVES AND CATHARTICS

NURSING ACTIONS	*RATIONALE/EXPLANATION*
1. Administer accurately **a.** Give bulk-forming laxatives with at least 8 oz of water or other fluid. Mix with fluid immediately before administration.	To prevent thickening and expansion in the GI tract with possible obstruction. These substances absorb water rapidly and solidify into a gelatinous mass.
b. With bisacodyl tablets, instruct the client to swallow the tablets without chewing and not to take them within an hour after ingesting milk or gastric antacids or while receiving cimetidine therapy.	The tablets have an enteric coating to delay dissolution until they reach the alkaline environment of the small intestine. Chewing or giving the tablets close to antacid substances or to cimetidine-treated clients causes premature dissolution and gastric irritation and results in abdominal cramping and vomiting.
c. Give saline cathartics on an empty stomach with 240 ml of fluid.	To increase effectiveness
d. Refrigerate magnesium citrate and polyethylene glycol-electrolyte solution before giving.	To increase palatability and retain potency
e. Castor oil may be chilled and followed by fruit juice or other beverage.	To increase palatability
f. Insert rectal suppositories to the length of the index finger, next to rectal mucosa.	These drugs are not effective unless they are in contact with intestinal mucosa.
2. Observe for therapeutic effects **a.** Soft to semiliquid stool	Therapeutic effects occur in approximately 1 to 3 d with bulk-forming laxatives and stool softeners; 6 to 8 h with bisacodyl tablets, cascara sagrada, phenolphthalein, and senna products; 15 to 60 min with bisacodyl and glycerin suppositories.
b. Liquid to semiliquid stool	Effects occur in approximately 1 to 3 h with saline cathartics and castor oil
c. Decreased abdominal pain when used in irritable bowel syndrome or diverticulosis	
d. Decreased rectal pain when used in clients with hemorrhoids or anal fissures	Pain results from straining to expel hard, dry feces.
3. Observe for adverse effects **a.** Diarrhea—several liquid stools, abdominal cramping. Severe, prolonged diarrhea may cause hyponatremia, hypokalemia, dehydration, and other problems.	Diarrhea is most likely to result from strong, stimulant cathartics (*e.g.,* castor oil, bisacodyl, phenolphthalein, senna preparations) or large doses of saline cathartics (*e.g.,* milk of magnesia).

NURSING ACTIONS	*RATIONALE/EXPLANATION*
b. With bulk-forming agents, impaction or obstruction	Impaction or obstruction of the gastrointestinal (GI) tract can be prevented by giving ample fluids with these agents and not giving the drugs to clients with known dysphagia or strictures anywhere in the alimentary canal.
c. With saline cathartics, hypermagnesemia, hyperkalemia, fluid retention, and edema	Hypermagnesemia and hyperkalemia are more likely to occur in clients with renal insufficiency because of impaired ability to excrete magnesium and potassium. Fluid retention and edema are more likely to occur in clients with congestive heart failure or other conditions characterized by edema. Polyethylene glycol-electrolyte solution produces the least change in water and electrolyte balance.
d. With mineral oil, lipid pneumonia and decreased absorption of vitamins A, D, E, and K	Lipid pneumonia can be prevented by not giving mineral oil to clients with dysphagia or impaired consciousness. Decreased absorption of fat-soluble vitamins can be prevented by not giving mineral oil with or shortly after meals or for longer than 2 wk.

4. Observe for drug interactions
  a. Drugs that *increase* effects of laxatives and cathartics:
 	
    Cholinergics (*e.g.*, dexpanthenol [Ilopan])
	Additive stimulation of intestinal motility. There is probably no reason to use such a combination.

b. Drugs that *decrease* effects of laxatives and cathartics: (1) Anticholinergic drugs (*e.g.*, atropine) and other drugs with anticholinergic properties (*e.g.*, phenothiazine antipsychotic drugs, tricyclic antidepressants, some antihistamines, and antiparkinsonism drugs)	These drugs slow intestinal motility. Clients receiving these agents are at risk for developing constipation and requiring laxatives, perhaps on a long-term basis.
(2) Central nervous system depressants (*e.g.*, narcotic analgesics)	Narcotic analgesics commonly cause constipation.
5. Teach clients **a.** With bulk-forming laxatives, mix in 8 oz of fluid immediately before taking and follow with additional fluid, if able. *Never* take the drug dry.	Adequate fluid intake is essential with these drugs. GI obstruction has been reported in clients taking the drug dry or with inadequate fluid.
b. With bisacodyl tablets, swallow whole (do not crush or chew), and do not take with antacids.	The drug is a strong gastric irritant formulated to dissolve in the alkaline fluids of the small intestine. Crushing, chewing, or taking with antacids allows it to dissolve in the stomach.
c. Do not exceed recommended doses of laxatives.	To avoid adverse effects
d. Discoloration of the urine may occur with cascara sagrada, phenolphthalein, or senna preparations.	Color of the urine may be pink-red, red-violet, red-brown, or yellow-brown, depending on the acidity or alkalinity of the urine.

REVIEW AND APPLICATION EXERCISES

1. What are risk factors for developing constipation?

2. Describe nonpharmacologic strategies to prevent constipation.

3. Which type of laxative is generally the most desirable for long-term use? Which is the least desirable?

4. What are the most significant adverse effects of strong laxatives?

5. If an adult client asked you to recommend an over-the-counter laxative, what information about the client's condition would you need, and what would you recommend? Why?

SELECTED REFERENCES

Barnett, J.L. (1997). Approach to the patient with constipation and fecal incontinence. In W.N. Kelley (Ed.), *Textbook of internal medicine*, 3rd ed., pp. 632–637. Philadelphia: Lippincott-Raven.

Brunton, L.L. (1996). Agents affecting gastrointestinal water flux and motility; emesis and antiemetics; bile acids and pancreatic enzymes. In J.G. Hardman, L.E. Limbird, P.B. Molinoff, & R.W. Ruddon (Eds.), *Goodman & Gilman's The pharmacological basis of therapeutics*, 9th ed., pp. 917–936. New York: McGraw-Hill.

Drug facts and comparisons. (Updated monthly). St. Louis: Facts and Comparisons.

Longe, R.L., & DiPiro, J.T. (1997). Diarrhea and constipation. In J.T. DiPiro, R.L. Talbert, G.C. Yee, G.R. Matzke, B.G. Wells, & L.M. Posey (Eds.), *Pharmacotherapy: A pathophysiologic approach*, 3rd ed., pp. 767–783. Stamford, CT: Appleton & Lange.

Porth, C.M. (1994). *Pathophysiology: Concepts of altered health states*, 4th ed., pp. 817–841. Philadelphia: J.B. Lippincott.

Smeltzer, S.C., & Bare, B.G. (1996). *Brunner and Suddarth's Textbook of medical-surgical nursing*, 8th ed. Philadelphia: Lippincott-Raven.

62 Antidiarrheals

Objectives

After studying this chapter, the student will be able to:

1 Identify clients at risk of developing diarrhea.

2 Discuss guidelines for assessing diarrhea.

3 Describe types of diarrhea in which antidiarrheal drug therapy may be indicated.

4 Differentiate the major types of antidiarrheal drugs.

5 Discuss characteristics, effects, and nursing process implications of opiate-related antidiarrheal agents.

Key Terms

Infectious diarrhea

Pseudomembranous colitis

Inflammatory bowel diseases

Description

Antidiarrheal drugs are used to treat diarrhea, defined as the frequent expulsion of liquid or semiliquid stools. Diarrhea is a symptom of numerous conditions that increase bowel motility, cause secretion or retention of fluids in the intestinal lumen, and cause inflammation or irritation of the gastrointestinal (GI) tract. As a result, bowel contents are rapidly propelled toward the rectum, and absorption of fluids and electrolytes is limited. Some causes of diarrhea include the following:

1. Excessive use of laxatives
2. Intestinal infections with viruses, bacteria, or protozoa. A common source of infection is ingestion of food or fluid contaminated by *Salmonella*, *Shigella*, or *Staphylococcus* microorganisms. So-called travelers' diarrhea is usually caused by an enteropathogenic strain of *Escherichia coli*.
3. Undigested, coarse, or highly spiced food in the GI tract. The food acts as an irritant and attracts fluids in a defensive attempt to dilute the irritating agent. This may result from inadequate chewing of food or lack of digestive enzymes.
4. Lack of digestive enzymes. Deficiency of pancreatic enzymes inhibits digestion and absorption of carbohydrates, proteins, and fats. Deficiency of lactase, a sugar-splitting intestinal enzyme, inhibits digestion of milk and milk products.
5. Inflammatory bowel disorders, such as gastroenteritis, diverticulitis, ulcerative colitis, and regional enteritis (Crohn's disease). In these disorders, the inflamed mucous membrane secretes large amounts of fluids into the intestinal lumen. In addition, when the ileum is diseased or a portion is surgically excised, large amounts of bile salts reach the colon, where they act as cathartics and cause diarrhea. Bile salts are normally reabsorbed from the ileum.
6. Drug therapy. Many oral drugs may irritate the GI tract and cause diarrhea. Antibacterial drugs often do so. Antibacterial drugs also may cause diarrhea by altering the normal bacterial flora in the intestine.

   Pseudomembranous colitis (also called antibiotic-associated colitis and *Clostridium difficile* colitis) is a serious condition that results from oral or parenteral antibiotic therapy. By suppressing normal flora, antibiotics allow gram-positive, anaerobic *Clostridium difficile* organisms to proliferate. The organisms produce a toxin that causes fever, abdominal pain, inflammatory lesions of the colon, and severe diarrhea with stools containing mucus, pus, and sometimes blood. Symptoms may develop within a few days or several weeks after the causative antibiotic is discontinued. Pseudomembranous colitis is more often associated with ampicillin, cephalosporins, and clindamycin but may occur with any antibacterial drug that alters intestinal microbial flora.

7. Intestinal neoplasms. Tumors may increase intestinal motility by occupying space and stretching the intestinal wall. Diarrhea sometimes alternates with constipation in colon cancer.
8. Functional disorders. Diarrhea may be a symptom of stress or anxiety in some clients. No organic disease process can be found in such circumstances.
9. Hyperthyroidism. This condition increases bowel motility.
10. Surgical excision or bypass of portions of the intestine, especially the small intestine. Such procedures decrease the absorptive area and increase fluidity of stools.
11. HIV/AIDS. Diarrhea occurs in most clients with HIV infection, often as a chronic condition that contributes to malnutrition and weight loss. It may be caused by drug therapy, infection with a variety of microorganisms, or other factors.

Diarrhea may be acute or chronic and mild or severe. Most episodes of acute diarrhea are defensive mechanisms by which the body tries to rid itself of irritants, toxins, and infectious agents. These are usually self-limiting and subside within 24 to 48 hours without serious consequences. If severe or prolonged, acute diarrhea may lead to serious fluid and electrolyte depletion, especially in young children and elderly adults. Chronic diarrhea may cause malnutrition and anemia and is often characterized by remissions and exacerbations.

ANTIDIARRHEAL DRUGS

Antidiarrheal drugs include a variety of agents, most of which are discussed in other chapters. When used for treatment of diarrhea, the drugs may be given to relieve the symptom (nonspecific therapy) or the underlying cause of the symptom (specific therapy). Individual drugs are listed in Table 62-1.

Nonspecific Therapy

For symptomatic treatment of diarrhea, opiates and opiate derivatives (see Chap. 6) are the most effective. These drugs decrease diarrhea by slowing propulsive movements in the small and large intestines. Morphine, codeine, and related drugs are effective in relieving diarrhea but are rarely used for this purpose because of their potentially serious adverse effects. Although paregoric is occasionally useful, other opiates have largely been replaced by the synthetic drugs diphenoxylate, loperamide, and difenoxin, which are used only for treatment of diarrhea and do not cause morphine-like adverse effects in recommended doses.

(*text continues on page 795*)

TABLE 62-1	ANTIDIARRHEAL DRUGS

Generic/ Trade Name	Characteristics	Clinical Indications	Routes and Dosage Ranges	
			Adults	*Children*
Opiates and Related Drugs				
Camphorated tincture of opium (paregoric)	1. Contains 0.04% morphine, alcohol, camphor, anise oil, and benzoic acid 2. Antidiarrheal activity is caused by morphine content. Morphine slows propulsive movements in small and large intestines. 3. Under Controlled Substances Act, a Schedule III drug when used alone and a Schedule V drug in the small amounts combined with other drugs. 4. Recommended doses and short-term duration of administration do not produce euphoria, analgesia, or dependence.	Symptomatic treatment of acute diarrhea	PO 5–10 ml one to four times daily (maximum of four doses) until diarrhea is controlled	PO 0.25–0.5 ml/kg one to four times daily (maximum of four doses) until diarrhea is controlled
Difenoxin with atropine sulfate (Motofen)	1. It is the main active metabolite of diphenoxylate. 2. It slows intestinal motility by a local effect on the GI wall. 3. Overdose may cause severe respiratory depression and coma. 4. Each tablet contains 1 mg of difenoxin and 0.025 mg of atropine. The subtherapeutic dose of atropine is added to discourage overdose and abuse for opiate-like effects 5. Contraindicated in children under age 2 y, clients allergic to the ingredients, and clients with hepatic impairment. 6. A Schedule IV drug under the Controlled Substances Act	Symptomatic treatment of acute or chronic diarrhea	PO 2 mg initially, then 1 mg after each loose stool or 1 mg q3–4h as needed; maximum dose, 8 mg (8 tablets)/24 h	Safety and effectiveness not established for children under 12 y
Diphenoxylate with atropine sulfate (Lomotil)	1. A derivative of meperidine (Demerol) used only for treatment of diarrhea 2. Most commonly prescribed antidiarrheal drug. Decreases intestinal motility. 3. As effective as paregoric and more convenient to administer 4. In recommended doses, does not produce euphoria,	Symptomatic treatment of acute or chronic diarrhea	PO 5 mg (2 tablets or 10 ml of liquid) three or four times daily; maximal daily dose, 20 mg	Liquid preparation recommended Ages 8–12 y, PO 10 mg daily in five divided doses Ages 5–8 y, PO 8 mg daily in four divided doses Ages 2–5 y, PO 6 mg daily in three divided doses

(continued)

| TABLE 62-1 | ANTIDIARRHEAL DRUGS (Continued) | | | |

| Generic/ Trade Name | Characteristics | Clinical Indications | Routes and Dosage Ranges | |
			Adults	**Children**
	analgesia or dependence. In high doses, produces morphine-like effects including euphoria, dependence, and respiratory depression. Antidote for overdose is the narcotic antagonist naloxone (Narcan). 5. Each tablet or 5 ml of liquid contains 2.5 mg of diphenoxylate and 0.025 mg of atropine. The subtherapeutic dose of atropine is added to discourage drug abuse by producing unpleasant anticholinergic side effects. 6. Contraindicated in severe liver disease, glaucoma, and children under 2 y. Safety during pregnancy and lactation has not been established. The drug is excreted in breast milk. 7. A Schedule V drug under the Controlled Substances Act			Under age 2 y contraindicated
Loperamide (Imodium)	1. A derivative of meperidine (Demerol) used only for treatment of diarrhea 2. Decreases intestinal motility 3. Compared to diphenoxylate, loperamide is equally effective and may cause fewer adverse reactions in recommended doses. High doses may produce morphine-like effects. 4. Safety has not been established for use in pregnancy, lactation, and in children under age 2 y. 5. Antidote for overdose is the narcotic antagonist naloxone. 6. Each capsule or 10 ml of liquid contains 2 mg of loperamide.	Symptomatic treatment of acute or chronic diarrhea	PO 4 mg initially, then 2 mg after each loose stool to a maximal daily dose of 16 mg. For chronic diarrhea, dosage should be reduced to the lowest effective amount (average 4–8 mg daily).	Ages 8–12 y, PO 6 mg daily in three divided doses (as liquid or capsule) Ages 5–8 y, PO 4 mg daily in two divided doses (as liquid or capsule) Ages 2–5 y, PO 3 mg daily in three divided doses (as liquid) Under age 2 y, contraindicated

Antibacterial Agents

Ampicillin (Omnipen, Penbriten, others)	A broad-spectrum penicillin	1. Bacillary dysentery caused by sensitive strains of *Shigella* 2. Typhoid fever resistant to chloramphenicol	PO, IM, 2–4 g/d, in divided doses, q6h	PO, IM, IV 50–100 mg/kg/d, in divided doses, q6h

TABLE 62-1	ANTIDIARRHEAL DRUGS (Continued)

Generic/ Trade Name	Characteristics	Clinical Indications	Routes and Dosage Ranges	
			Adults	*Children*
		3. Typhoid fever to eliminate the postinfective carrier state		
Chloramphenicol (Chloromycetin)		Typhoid fever (gastroenteritis caused by *Salmonella typhi*)	PO, IV 50 mg/kg/d, in divided doses, q6h	PO 50 mg/kg/d, in divided doses, q6h
Neomycin		Bacillary dysentery caused by strains of *Shigella* that are resistant to other antibiotics but sensitive to neomycin	PO 4 g/d in divided doses, q6h	PO 50–100 mg/ kg/d, in divided doses, q6h
Tetracycline		1. Cholera 2. Bacillary dysentery caused by sensitive strains of *Shigella*	PO 2 g/d in divided doses, q6h	PO 40 mg/kg/d in divided doses, q6h
Trimethoprim-sulfamethoxazole (TMP-SMX) (Bactrim, Septra)		1. Bacillary dysentery caused by susceptible strains of *Shigella* 2. Typhoid fever resistant to chloramphenicol and ampicillin 3. Enteritis caused by susceptible strains of *E. coli*	PO 160 mg of trimethoprim and 800 mg of sulfamethoxazole daily, in divided doses, q12h IV 8–10 mg/kg of trimethoprim and 50 mg/kg sulfamethoxazole daily, in two to four divided doses	PO 8 mg/kg of trimethoprim and 40 mg/kg of sulfamethoxazole daily, in divided doses, q12h IV 8–10 mg/kg of trimethoprim and 50 mg/kg sulfamethoxazole daily, in two to four divided doses
Vancomycin (Vancocin)		1. Pseudomembranous colitis due to suppression of normal bacterial flora by antibiotics and overgrowth of *Clostridium* organisms 2. Staphylococcal colitis due to broad-spectrum antibiotic therapy, combined with parenteral nafcillin (Unipen)	PO 2 g/d in divided doses, q6h	PO 44 mg/kg/d in divided doses, q6h
Miscellaneous Drugs				
Bismuth subsalicylate (Pepto-Bismol)	Has antimicrobial, antisecretory, and possibly anti-inflammatory effects	Control of diarrhea, including travelers' diarrhea, and relief of abdominal cramping	PO 2 tablets or 30 ml, every 30–60 min, if needed, up to 8 doses in 24 h	9–12 y: PO 1 tablet or 15 ml; 6–9 y: PO 2/3 tablet or 10 ml; 3–6 y: PO 1/3 tablet or 5 ml; under 3 y, consult pediatrician

(continued)

| TABLE 62-1 | ANTIDIARRHEAL DRUGS (Continued) | | | |

Generic/ Trade Name	Characteristics	Clinical Indications	Routes and Dosage Ranges	
			Adults	*Children*
Cholestyramine (Questran)	Binds and inactivates bile salts in the intestine	Diarrhea due to bile salts reaching the colon and causing a cathartic effect. "Bile salt diarrhea" is associated with Crohn's disease or surgical excision of the ileum.	PO 16–32 g/d in 120–180 ml of water, in two to four divided doses before or during meals and at bedtime	
Colestipol (Colestid)	Same as cholestyramine, above	Same as cholestyra-mine	PO 15–30 g/d in 120–180 ml of water, in two to four divided doses before or during meals and at bedtime	
Kaolin, pectin, and paregoric (Parepectolin)	1. Effectiveness, if any, attributed to paregoric (3.7 ml paregoric/30 ml of preparation) 2. Schedule V drug under Controlled Substances Act 3. Not recommended for use	Possibly effective for symptomatic treatment of mild, acute diarrhea	PO 15–30 ml after each loose stool to a maximum of 8 doses/24 h	PO 2.5–10 ml after each loose stool to a maximum of 8 doses/24 h
Octreotide (Sandostatin)	In GI tract, decreases secretions and motility	Control diarrhea associated with carcinoid tumors, vasoactive intestinal peptide tumors, AIDS, cancer chemotherapy or radiation or diarrhea that does not respond to other antidiarrheal agents	SC, IV 50 µg two to three times daily initially, then adjusted according to response	Dosage not established
Pancreatin or pancrelipase (Viokase, Pancrease, Cotazym)	Pancreatic enzymes used only for replacement	Diarrhea and mal-absorption due to deficiency of pancreatic enzymes	PO 1–3 tablets or capsules or 1–2 packets of powder with meals and snacks	PO 1–3 tablets or capsules or 1–2 packets of powder with each meal
Psyllium preparations (Metamucil, Effersyllium)	Absorbs water and decreases fluidity of stools	Possibly effective for symptomatic treatment of diarrhea	PO 6–10 g (1–2 tsp), two or three times daily, in a full glass of water or other fluid, mixed immediately before ingestion	
Sulfasalazine (Azulfidine)	A poorly absorbed sulfon-amide	Ulcerative colitis	PO 2 g/d in four divided doses	Over age 2 mo, PO 40–60 mg/kg/d in three to six divided doses initially. Maintenance, PO 30 mg/kg/d day in four divided doses

Bismuth salts have antibacterial and antiviral activity; bismuth subsalicylate (Pepto-Bismol, a commonly used over-the-counter drug) also has antisecretory and possibly anti-inflammatory effects attributed to the salicylate component.

Octreotide acetate is a synthetic form of somatostatin, a hormone produced in the anterior pituitary gland and in the pancreas. The drug may be effective in diarrhea because it decreases GI secretion and motility. It is used for diarrhea associated with carcinoid syndrome, intestinal tumors, HIV/AIDS, and diarrhea that does not respond to other antidiarrheal drugs.

Other nonspecific agents sometimes used in diarrhea are anticholinergics (see Chap. 21), and polycarbophil and psyllium preparations (see Chap. 61). Anticholinergic drugs, of which atropine is the prototype, are infrequently used because doses large enough to decrease intestinal motility and secretions cause intolerable adverse effects. The drugs are occasionally used to decrease abdominal cramping and pain (antispasmodic effects) associated with acute nonspecific diarrhea and chronic diarrhea associated with inflammatory bowel disease.

Psyllium preparations (*e.g.*, Metamucil) are most often used as bulk-forming laxatives. They are occasionally used in diarrhea to decrease fluidity of stools. The preparations absorb large amounts of water and produce stools of gelatin-like consistency.

Specific Therapy

Specific drug therapy for diarrhea depends on the cause of the symptom and may include the use of antibacterial, enzymatic, and bile salt-binding drugs. Antibacterial drugs are recommended for use only in carefully selected cases of bacterial enteritis. Although effective in preventing travelers' diarrhea, antibiotics are generally not recommended because their use may promote the emergence of drug-resistant microorganisms. Although effective in reducing diarrhea due to *Salmonella* and *Escherichia coli* intestinal infections, antibiotics may induce a prolonged carrier state during which the infection can be transmitted to other people.

Indications for Use

Despite the limitations of drug therapy in prevention and treatment of diarrhea, antidiarrheal drugs are generally indicated in the following circumstances:

1. Severe or prolonged diarrhea (more than 2 to 3 days), to prevent severe fluid and electrolyte loss
2. Relatively severe diarrhea in young children and elderly adults. These groups are less able to adapt to fluid and electrolyte losses.
3. In chronic inflammatory diseases of the bowel (ulcerative colitis and Crohn's disease), to allow a more nearly normal lifestyle. Ulcerative colitis also is

treated with adrenal corticosteroids and poorly absorbed sulfonamides.
4. In ileostomies or surgical excision of portions of the ileum, to decrease fluidity and volume of stool
5. HIV/AIDS-associated diarrhea
6. When specific causes of diarrhea have been determined

Contraindications for Use

Contraindications for the use of antidiarrheal agents include diarrhea caused by toxic materials, microorganisms that penetrate intestinal mucosa (*e.g.*, pathogenic *Escherichia coli*, *Salmonella*, *Shigella*), or pseudomembranous colitis caused by broad-spectrum antibiotic therapy. In these circumstances, antidiarrheal agents that slow peristalsis may aggravate and prolong diarrhea. Opiates (morphine, codeine, paregoric) usually are contraindicated in chronic diarrhea because of possible opiate dependence. Difenoxin, diphenoxylate, and loperamide are contraindicated in children under 2 years of age.

Nursing Process

Assessment

Assess for acute or chronic diarrhea.

- Try to determine the duration of diarrhea; number of stools per day; amount, consistency, color, odor, and presence of abnormal components (*e.g.*, undigested food, blood, pus, mucus) in each stool; precipitating factors; accompanying signs and symptoms (*i.e.*, nausea, vomiting, fever, abdominal pain or cramping); and measures used to relieve diarrhea. When possible, observe stool specimens.
- Try to determine the *cause* of the diarrhea. This includes questioning about causes such as chronic inflammatory diseases of the bowel, food intake, possible exposure to contaminated food, living or traveling in areas of poor sanitation, and use of laxatives or other drugs that may cause diarrhea. When available, check laboratory reports on stool specimens (*e.g.*, culture reports).
- With severe or prolonged diarrhea, especially in young children and elderly adults, assess for dehydration, hypokalemia, and other fluid and electrolyte disorders.

Nursing Diagnoses

- Diarrhea related to GI infection or inflammatory disorders, other disease processes, dietary irritants, or overuse of laxatives
- Altered Nutrition: Less Than Body Requirements related to impaired absorption of nutrients with diarrhea
- Anxiety related to availability of bathroom facilities
- Body Image Disturbance with chronic diarrhea related to loss of control and possible incontinence of stool
- Social Isolation with chronic diarrhea related to frequent bowel movements
- Fluid Volume Deficit related to excessive losses in liquid stools
- Pain (abdominal cramping) related to intestinal hypermotility and spasm
- Impaired Tissue Integrity: Perianal skin excoriation related to irritants in liquid stools

- Self-Care Deficit related to weakness
- Constipation related to use of antidiarrheal drugs
- Knowledge Deficit: Factors that cause or aggravate diarrhea
- Knowledge Deficit: Appropriate use of antidiarrheal drugs

Planning/Goals

The client will:
- Take antidiarrheal drugs appropriately
- Obtain relief from acute diarrhea (reduced number of liquid stools, reduced abdominal discomfort)
- Maintain fluid and electrolyte balance
- Maintain adequate nutritional intake
- Be assisted when weak from diarrhea
- Avoid adverse effects of antidiarrheal medications
- Reestablish normal bowel patterns after an episode of acute diarrhea
- Have fewer liquid stools with chronic diarrhea

Interventions

Use measures to prevent diarrhea:
- Prepare and store food properly and avoid improperly stored foods and those prepared under unsanitary conditions. Dairy products, cream pies, and other foods may cause diarrhea ("food poisoning") if not refrigerated.
- Wash hands before handling any foods, after handling raw poultry or meat, and always before eating.
- Chew food well.
- Do not overuse laxatives (*i.e.,* amount per dose or frequency of use). Many commonly used over-the-counter products contain phenolphthalein, a strong stimulant laxative.

Whether or not antidiarrheal drugs are used, supportive therapy is required for the treatment of diarrhea. Elements of supportive care include the following:
- Replacement of fluids and electrolytes. If diarrhea is not severe, fluids such as weak tea, water, bouillon, clear soup, and gelatin may be sufficient. If diarrhea is severe or prolonged, intravenous fluids may be needed (*i.e.,* solutions containing dextrose, sodium chloride, and potassium chloride). Also, oral intake may be restricted to decrease bowel stimulation.
- Avoid foods and fluids that may further irritate GI mucosa (*e.g.,* highly spiced foods or "laxative" foods, such as raw fruits and vegetables).
- Increase frequency and length of rest periods, and decrease activity. Exercise and activity stimulate peristalsis.
- If perianal irritation occurs because of frequent liquid stools, cleanse the area with mild soap and water after each bowel movement, then apply an emollient, such as white petrolatum (Vaseline).

Teach clients:
- To maintain a fluid intake of 2 to 3 quarts daily. This will help prevent dehydration from fluid loss in stools. Clear broths and noncarbonated, caffeine-free beverages are recommended because they are unlikely to cause further diarrhea.
- To avoid highly spiced or "laxative" foods, such as fresh fruits and vegetables, until diarrhea is controlled and peristaltic movements have returned to normal
- Measures to prevent diarrhea (*e.g.,* frequent and thorough handwashing, careful food storage and preparation)

- To consult a health care provider if diarrhea is accompanied by severe abdominal pain or fever

Evaluation

- Observe and interview for decreased number of liquid or loose stools.
- Observe for signs of adequate food and fluid intake (*e.g.,* good skin turgor and urine output, stable weight).
- Observe for appropriate use of antidiarrheal drugs.
- Observe and interview for return of prediarrheal patterns of bowel elimination.
- Interview regarding knowledge and use of measures to prevent or minimize diarrhea.

Principles of Therapy

DRUG SELECTION

Choice of antidiarrheal agent depends largely on the cause, severity, and duration of diarrhea.

1. For symptomatic treatment of diarrhea, difenoxin with atropine (Motofen), diphenoxylate with atropine (Lomotil), or loperamide (Imodium) is probably the drug of choice for most people.
2. In bacterial gastroenteritis or diarrhea, choice of antibacterial drug depends on the causative microorganism and susceptibility tests.
3. In ulcerative colitis, sulfonamides and adrenal corticosteroids are the drugs of choice.
4. In pseudomembranous colitis, stopping the causative drug is the initial treatment. If symptoms do not improve within 3 or 4 days, oral metronidazole or vancomycin is given for 7 to 10 days. Both are effective against *Clostridium difficile,* but metronidazole is the first drug of choice and is much less expensive. Vancomycin may be given for severe disease. For about 6 weeks following recovery, relapse often occurs and requires retreatment. Because relapse is not due to emergence of drug-resistant strains, the same drug used for the initial bout may be used to treat the relapse.
5. In diarrhea caused by enzyme deficiency, pancreatic enzymes are given rather than antidiarrheal drugs.
6. In bile salt diarrhea, cholestyramine is the drug of choice. Colestipol, a similar drug, may be effective also.
7. Although morphine and codeine are contraindicated in chronic diarrhea, they may occasionally be used in the treatment of acute, severe diarrhea. Dosages required for antidiarrheal effects are smaller than those required for analgesia. The following oral drugs and dosages are approximately equivalent in antidiarrheal effectiveness: 4 mg morphine, 30 mg codeine, 10 ml paregoric, 5 mg diphenoxylate, and 2 mg loperamide.

USE IN CHILDREN

Antidiarrheal drugs, including antibiotics, are often used in children to prevent excessive losses of fluids and electrolytes. Small children especially may rapidly develop fluid volume deficit with diarrhea. Drug therapy should be accompanied by appropriate fluid replacement and efforts to decrease further stimuli.

Difenoxin and **diphenoxylate** contain atropine, and signs of atropine overdose may occur with usual doses. Difenoxin, diphenoxylate, and **loperamide** are contraindicated in children younger than 2 years. Loperamide is a nonprescription drug. See Table 62-1 for doses.

USE IN OLDER ADULTS

Diarrhea is less common than constipation in older adults, but it may occur from laxative abuse and bowel cleansing procedures before GI surgery or diag-nostic tests. With diarrhea, older adults may rapidly develop fluid volume deficits. General principles of fluid and electrolyte replacement, measures to decrease GI irritants, and drug therapy apply as for younger adults. Most antidiarrheal drugs may be given to older adults, but cautious use is indicated to avoid inducing constipation.

HOME CARE

Prescription and over-the-counter antidiarrheal aids are often taken in the home setting. The role of the home care nurse may include advising clients and caregivers about appropriate use of the drugs, trying to identify the cause and severity of the diarrhea (*i.e.*, risk of fluid and electrolyte deficit), and teaching strategies to manage the present episode and prevent future episodes. If octreotide is taken at home, the home care nurse may need to teach the client and a caregiver how to administer subcutaneous injections.

ANTIDIARRHEALS

NURSING ACTIONS	*RATIONALE/EXPLANATION*
1. Administer accurately **a.** With liquid diphenoxylate, use only the calibrated dropper furnished by the manufacturer for measuring dosage.	For accurate measurement
b. Add at least 30 ml of water to each dose of paregoric. The mixture appears milky.	To add sufficient volume for the drug to reach the stomach
c. Do not exceed maximal daily doses of diphenoxylate, loperamide, difenoxin, and paregoric. Also, stop the drugs when diarrhea is controlled.	To decrease risks of adverse reactions, including drug dependence
d. Give cholestyramine and colestipol with at least 120 ml of water. Also, do not give within approximately 4 h of other drugs.	The drugs may cause obstruction of the gastrointestinal (GI) tract if swallowed in a dry state. They may combine with and inactivate other drugs.
2. Observe for therapeutic effects **a.** Decreased number, frequency, and fluidity of stools	Therapeutic effects are usually evident within 24 to 48 h.
b. Decreased or absent abdominal cramping pains	
c. Signs of normal fluid and electrolyte balance (adequate hydration, urine output, and skin turgor)	
d. Resumption of usual activities of daily living	
3. Observe for adverse effects **a.** Constipation	Constipation is the most common adverse effect. It can be prevented by using antidiarrheal drugs only as prescribed and stopping the drugs when diarrhea is controlled.

(continued)

NURSING ACTIONS	RATIONALE/EXPLANATION
b. Drug dependence	Dependence is unlikely with recommended doses but may occur with long-term use of large doses of paregoric, diphenoxylate, and probably loperamide.
c. With diphenoxylate, anorexia, nausea, vomiting, dizziness, abdominal discomfort, paralytic ileus, toxic megacolon, hypersensitivity (pruritus, urticaria, angioneurotic edema), headache, tachycardia	Although numerous adverse reactions have been reported, their incidence and severity are low when diphenoxylate is used appropriately.
With overdoses of a diphenoxylate-atropine or difenoxin-atropine combination, respiratory depression and coma may result from diphenoxylate or difenoxin content and anticholinergic effects (e.g., dry mouth, blurred vision, urinary retention) from atropine content	Deliberate overdose and abuse are unlikely because of unpleasant anticholinergic effects. Overdose can be prevented by using the drug in recommended doses and only when required. Overdose can be treated with naloxone (Narcan) and supportive therapy.
d. With loperamide, abdominal cramps, dry mouth, dizziness, nausea and vomiting	Abdominal cramps are the most common adverse effect. No serious adverse effects have been reported with recommended doses of loperamide. Overdose may be treated with naloxone, gastric lavage, and administration of activated charcoal.
e. With cholestyramine and colestipol, constipation, nausea, abdominal distention	Adverse effects are usually minor and transient because these drugs are not absorbed from the GI tract.
f. With octreotide, diarrhea, headache, cardiac dysrhythmias, injection site pain	These are commonly reported adverse effects.
4. Observe for drug interactions	Few clinically significant drug interactions have been reported with commonly used antidiarrheal agents.
Drugs that increase effects of antidiarrheal agents:	
(1) Central nervous system (CNS) depressants (alcohol, sedative-hypnotics, narcotic analgesics, antianxiety agents, antipsychotic agents)	Additive CNS depression with opiate and related antidiarrheals. Narcotic analgesics have additive constipating effects.
(2) Anticholinergic agents (atropine and synthetic anticholinergic antispasmodics; antihistamines and antidepressants with anticholinergic effects)	Additive anticholinergic adverse effects (dry mouth, blurred vision, urinary retention) with diphenoxylate-atropine (Lomotil) and difenoxin-atropine (Motofen)
5. Teach clients **a.** Take antidiarrheal drugs only as prescribed, and stop them when diarrhea is controlled.	To avoid adverse effects
b. Report to the physician if diarrhea persists longer than 3 d, if stools contain blood or mucus, and if fever or abdominal pain develops.	These signs and symptoms may indicate more serious disorders for which other treatment measures are needed.

REVIEW AND APPLICATION EXERCISES

1. What are some common causes of diarrhea?

2. In which patient populations is diarrhea most likely to cause serious problems?

3. Which types of diarrhea do not require antidiarrheal drug therapy and why?

4. How do antidiarrheal drugs decrease frequency or fluidity of stools?

5. What are adverse effects of commonly used antidiarrheal drugs?

6. If a client asked you to recommend an over-the-counter antidiarrheal agent, which would you recommend and why?

7. Would your recommendation differ if the proposed recipient were a child? Why or why not?

SELECTED REFERENCES

Bonis, P.A., & Plaut, A.G. (1997). Gastrointestinal infections. In W.N. Kelley (Ed.), *Textbook of internal medicine,* 3rd ed., pp. 752–761. Philadelphia: Lippincott-Raven.

Brunton, L.L. (1996). Agents affecting gastrointestinal water flux and motility; emesis and antiemetics; bile acids and pancreatic enzymes. In J.G. Hardman, L.E. Limbird, P.B. Molinoff, & R.W. Ruddon (Eds.), *Goodman & Gilman's The pharmacological basis of therapeutics,* 9th ed., pp. 917–936. New York: McGraw-Hill.

Drug facts and comparisons. (Updated monthly). St. Louis: Facts and Comparisons.

George, W.L., & Finegold, S.M. (1997). Clostridial infections. In W.N. Kelley (Ed.), *Textbook of internal medicine,* 3rd ed., pp. 1673–1678. Philadelphia: Lippincott-Raven.

Longe, R.L., & DiPiro, J.T. (1997). Diarrhea and constipation. In J.T. DiPiro, R.L. Talbert, G.C. Yee, G.R. Matzke, B.G. Wells, & L.M. Posey (Eds.), *Pharmacotherapy: A pathophysiologic approach,* 3rd ed., pp. 767–783. Stamford, CT: Appleton & Lange.

Porth, C.M. (1994). *Pathophysiology: Concepts of altered health states,* 4th ed., pp. 817–841. Philadelphia: J.B. Lippincott.

Powell, D.W. (1997). Approach to the patient with diarrhea. In W.N. Kelley (Ed.). *Textbook of internal medicine,* 3rd ed., pp. 617–632. Philadelphia: Lippincott-Raven.

Smeltzer, S.C., & Bare, B.G. (1996). *Brunner and Suddarth's Textbook of medical-surgical nursing,* 8th ed. Philadelphia: Lippincott-Raven.

63 Antiemetics

Outline

Nausea and Vomiting

Antiemetic Drugs
phenothiazines
antihistamines
corticosteroids
benzodiazepine antianxiety drugs
selective serotonin antagonists
prokinetic agents
miscellaneous antiemetics
indications for use
contraindications for use

Nursing Process
assessment
nursing diagnoses
planning/goals
interventions
evaluation

Principles of Therapy
drug selection
dosage and administration factors
timing of drug administration
chemotherapy-induced nausea and vomiting
use in children
use in older adults
home care

Objectives

After studying this chapter, the student will be able to:

1 Identify clients at risk of developing nausea and vomiting.

2 Discuss guidelines for preventing, minimizing, or treating nausea and vomiting.

3 Differentiate the major types of antiemetic drugs.

4 Discuss the advantages and adverse effects of serotonin receptor antagonists.

5 Discuss characteristics, effects, and nursing process implications of selected antiemetic drugs.

Key Terms

Chemoreceptor trigger zone
Emetogenic
Prokinetic

Nausea and Vomiting

Antiemetic drugs are used to prevent or treat nausea and vomiting. *Nausea* is an unpleasant sensation of abdominal discomfort accompanied by a desire to vomit. *Vomiting* is the expulsion of stomach contents through the mouth. Nausea may occur without vomiting, and vomiting may occur without prior nausea, but the two symptoms most often occur together.

Nausea and vomiting are common symptoms experienced by virtually everyone. These symptoms may accompany almost any illness or stress situation. Causes of nausea and vomiting include the following:

1. Systemic illness or infection
2. Gastrointestinal (GI) infection or inflammation (*e.g.*, any portion of the GI tract, liver, gallbladder, or pancreas)
3. Impaired GI motility and muscle tone (*e.g.*, gastroparesis)
4. Overeating or ingestion of foods or fluids that irritate the GI mucosa
5. Drug therapy. Nausea and vomiting are the most common adverse reactions to drug therapy. Although the symptoms may occur with most drugs, they are especially associated with alcohol, aspirin, digoxin, anticancer drugs, antimicrobials, estrogen preparations, and narcotic analgesics.
6. Pain and other noxious stimuli, such as unpleasant sights and odors
7. Emotional disturbances, physical or mental stress
8. Radiation therapy
9. Motion sickness
10. Postoperative status, which may include pain, impaired GI motility, and receiving various medications

Vomiting occurs when the vomiting center in the medulla oblongata is stimulated. Stimuli may be relayed to the vomiting center from peripheral (*e.g.*, gastric mucosa, peritoneum, intestines, joints) and central (*e.g.*, cerebral cortex, vestibular apparatus of the ear, and neurons in the fourth ventricle, called the *chemoreceptor trigger zone* or CTZ) sites. The vomiting center, CTZ, and GI tract contain benzodiazepine, cholinergic, dopamine, histamine, opiate, and serotonin receptors, which are stimulated by emetogenic drugs and toxins circulating in blood and cerebrospinal fluid. In motion sickness, rapid changes in body motion stimulate receptors in the inner ear (vestibular branch of the auditory nerve, which is concerned with equilibrium), and nerve impulses are transmitted to the CTZ and the vomiting center.

When stimulated, the vomiting center initiates efferent impulses that cause closure of the glottis, contraction of abdominal muscles and the diaphragm, relaxation of the gastroesophageal sphincter, and reverse peristalsis, which moves stomach contents toward the mouth for ejection.

Antiemetic Drugs

Drugs used in nausea and vomiting belong to several different therapeutic classifications, and most have anticholinergic, antidopaminergic, antihistaminic, or antiserotonergic effects. The drugs are generally more effective in prophylaxis than treatment. Most antiemetics prevent or relieve nausea and vomiting by acting on the vomiting center, CTZ, cerebral cortex, vestibular apparatus, or a combination of these. Major drugs are described below and in Table 63-1.

PHENOTHIAZINES

Phenothiazines, of which chlorpromazine (Thorazine) is the prototype, are central nervous system depressants used in the treatment of psychosis and psychotic symptoms in other disorders (see Chap. 9). These drugs have widespread effects on the body. Their therapeutic effects in psychosis and vomiting are attributed to their ability to block dopamine from receptor sites in the brain (antidopaminergic effects). When used as antiemetics, phenothiazines act on the CTZ and the vomiting center. Not all phenothiazines are effective antiemetics.

Phenothiazines are usually effective in preventing or treating nausea and vomiting induced by drugs, radiation therapy, surgery, and most other stimuli but are generally ineffective in motion sickness. Drowsiness usually occurs with these drugs.

ANTIHISTAMINES

Antihistamines (*e.g.*, hydroxyzine) are used primarily to prevent histamine from exerting its widespread effects on body tissues (see Chap. 48). Antihistamines used as antiemetic agents are the "classic" antihistamines or H_1 receptor blocking agents (as differentiated from cimetidine and related drugs, which are H_2 receptor blocking agents). The drugs are thought to relieve nausea and vomiting by blocking the action of acetylcholine in the brain (anticholinergic effects). Antihistamines are especially effective in preventing and treating motion sickness. Not all antihistamines are effective as antiemetic agents.

CORTICOSTEROIDS

Although corticosteroids are used mainly as antiallergic, anti-inflammatory, and antistress agents (see Chap. 24), they have antiemetic effects as well. The mechanism by which the drugs exert antiemetic effects is unknown. Dexamethasone and methylprednisolone are commonly

(*text continues on page 804*)

| TABLE 63-1 | ANTIEMETIC DRUGS | |

Generic/ Trade Name	Routes and Dosage Ranges	
	Adults	**Children**
Phenothiazines		
Chlorpromazine (Thorazine)	PO 10–25 mg q4–6h IM 25 mg q3–4h until vomiting stops, followed by oral administration if necessary Rectal suppository 25–100 mg q6–8h	PO 0.5 mg/kg q4–6h IM 0.5 mg/kg q6–8h. Maximal daily dose: up to age 5 y or weight 50 lb, 40 mg: age 5–12 y or weight 50–100 lb, 75 mg Rectal suppository 1 mg/kg q6–8h Not recommended for children under age 6 mo
Perphenazine (Trilafon)	PO 8–16 mg daily in divided doses IM 5 mg as a single dose	
Prochlor- perazine (Compazine)	PO 5–10 mg three or four times daily (sustained-release capsule, 10 mg twice daily) IM 5–10 mg q3–4h to a maximum of 40 mg daily Rectal suppository 25 mg twice daily	Weight over 10 kg: PO 0.4 mg/kg/d, in three or four divided doses IM 0.2 mg/kg as a single dose Rectal suppository 0.4 mg/kg/d, in three or four divided doses
Promethazine (Phenergan)	PO, IM, rectal suppository 12.5–25 mg q4–6h	Age over 3 mo: PO, IM, rectal suppository 0.25–0.5 mg/kg q4–6h
Thiethylper- azine (Torecan)	PO, IM, rectal suppository 10–30 mg/d	
Triflupromazine (Vesprin)	PO 20–30 mg/d IM 5–15 mg q4–6h; maximal dose, 60 mg/d IV 1–3 mg as a single dose	Age over 2 y: PO, IM 0.2 mg/kg/d in three divided doses; maximal daily dose, 10 mg
Antihistamines		
Buclizine (Bucladin-S)	Motion sickness, PO 50 mg 30 min before departure and 4–6 h later, if needed; maintenance dose, 50 mg twice daily	
Cyclizine (Marezine)	Motion sickness, PO 50 mg 30 min before departure, then q4–6h as needed, to a maximal daily dose of 300 mg, IM 50 mg three or four times daily as needed, rectal suppository 100 mg three or four times daily as needed Postoperative vomiting, IM 50 mg preoperatively, 20–30 min before surgery is completed or q4–6h as needed	Age 6–10 y: Motion sickness, PO, IM 3 mg/kg/d in three divided doses; rectal suppository 6 mg/kg/d, in three divided doses Maximal daily dose, 75 mg
Dimenhydrinate (Dramamine)	PO 50–100 mg q4h IM 50 mg as needed Rectal suppository 100 mg once or twice daily	PO, IM 5 mg/kg/d in four divided doses; maximal daily dose, 150 mg
Diphenhy- dramine (Benadryl)	Motion sickness, PO 50 mg 30 min before departure and 50 mg before each meal; IM, IV 20–50 mg q2–3h to a maximal daily dose of 400 mg	PO, IM 5 mg/kg/d, in four divided doses; maximal daily dose, 300 mg
Hydroxyzine (Vistaril, Atarax)	PO, IM 25–100 mg, three or four times daily	Age over 6 y, PO 50–100 mg daily in four divided doses Age under 6 y, PO 50 mg daily in four divided doses
Meclizine (Antivert, Bonine)	PO 25–100 mg daily	Dosage not established
Prokinetic Agents		
Cisapride (Propulsid)	PO 10–20 mg 15 min before meals and at bedtime (four doses daily)	Dosage not established

TABLE 63-1	ANTIEMETIC DRUGS (Continued)	

| Generic/ Trade Name | Routes and Dosage Ranges | |
	Adults	*Children*
Metoclopramide (Reglan)	PO 10 mg 30 min before meals and at bedtime for 2–8 wk IV 2 mg/kg 30 min before injection of cisplatin and 2 h after injection of cisplatin, then 1–2 mg/kg q2-3h if needed, up to four doses	Dosage not established
Granisetron (Kytril)	Cancer chemotherapy, PO 1 mg twice daily, first dose about 1 h before emetogenic drug, second dose 12 h later, only on days receiving chemotherapy; IV 10 µg/kg infused over 5 min, 30 min before emetogenic drug, only on days receiving chemotherapy	2–16 y of age, IV 10 µg/kg
Ondansetron (Zofran)	Cancer chemotherapy, PO 8 mg 30 min before emetogenic drug, repeat in 8 h, then 8 mg q12h for 1–2 d IV 0.15 mg/kg for three doses (first 30 min before emetogenic drug, then at 4 and 8 h after the first dose) or a single dose of 32 mg 30 min before emetogenic drug Postoperative nausea and vomiting, PO 16 mg 1 h before anesthesia or IV 4 mg just before anesthesia or postoperatively	Cancer chemotherapy, 12 y or older PO 8 mg; 4–11 y of age PO 4 mg 30 min before emetogenic drug, repeat in 4 and 8 h, then q8h for 1–2 d 4–18 y of age, IV 0.15 mg/kg for three doses as for adults Dosage not established

Miscellaneous Agents

Benzquinamide (Emete-con)	IM 0.5–1.0 mg/kg at least 15 min before administering antineoplastic drugs or emergence from anesthesia, then q3–4h as needed IV 0.2–0.4 mg/kg as a single dose, injected over 1–3 min	
Diphenidol (Vontrol)	PO 25–50 mg four times daily IM 20–40 mg four times daily IV 20 mg, repeated in 1 h if necessary. Subsequent doses should be given PO or IM	Age over 6 mo or weight over 12 kg, PO 5 mg/kg/d in four divided doses; IM 3 mg/kg/d in four divided doses
Dronabinol (Marinol)	PO 5 mg/m² (square meter of body surface area) 1–3 h before chemotherapy, then q2–4h for a total of four to six doses daily. Dosage can be increased by 2.5 mg/m² increments to a maximal dose of 15 mg/m² if necessary.	
Droperidol (Inapsine)	Preoperatively, IM 2.5–10 mg 30–60 min before procedure	Age 2–12 y, preoperatively, IM 1–1.5 mg/ 20–25 lb 30–60 min before procedure
Phosphorated carbohydrate solution (Emetrol)	PO 15–30 ml repeated at 15-min intervals until vomiting ceases	PO 5–10 ml repeated at 15-min intervals until vomiting ceases
Trimethobenza-mine (Tigan)	PO 250 mg three to four times daily IM, rectal suppository 200 mg three or four times daily	PO, rectal suppository 15 mg/kg/d in three or four divided doses; IM not recommended
Scopolamine (Transderm Scop)	Motion sickness, PO, SC, 0.6–1 mg/kg as a single dose Transdermal disc (1.5 mg scopolamine) placed behind the ear every 3 d if needed	Motion sickness, PO, SC 0.006 mg as a single dose

used in the management of chemotherapy-induced emesis, usually in combination with one or more other antiemetic agents. Regimens vary from a single dose before chemotherapy to doses every 4 to 6 hours for 24 to 48 hours. With this short-term usage, adverse effects are mild (*e.g.*, euphoria, insomnia, mild fluid retention).

BENZODIAZEPINE ANTIANXIETY DRUGS

These drugs (see Chap. 8) are not antiemetics, but they are often used in multidrug regimens to prevent nausea and vomiting associated with cancer chemotherapy. They produce sedation and relaxation, especially in clients who experience anticipatory nausea and vomiting before administration of anticancer drugs. Lorazepam (Ativan) is commonly used.

SELECTIVE SEROTONIN ANTAGONISTS

Ondansetron and **granisetron** are used to prevent or treat postoperative and chemotherapy-induced nausea and vomiting. Some anticancer drugs apparently cause nausea and vomiting by combining with a subset of serotonin (5-hydroxytryptamine or 5HT) receptors located centrally in the CTZ and peripherally on vagal nerve endings. The drugs antagonize 5-HT$_3$ receptors and prevent their activation by emetogenic anticancer drugs. It is unknown whether the drugs' antiemetic effects are central, peripheral, or both. The drugs may be given intravenously or orally, and are metabolized in the liver. Adverse effects are usually mild to moderate, and the most common ones reported in clinical trials were diarrhea, headache, constipation, and transient elevation of liver enzymes.

PROKINETIC AGENTS

Cisapride and **metoclopramide** are structurally related, prokinetic drugs. Prokinetic agents increase GI motility and the rate of gastric emptying by increasing the release of acetylcholine from nerve endings in the GI tract (peripheral cholinergic effects). As a result, they can decrease nausea and vomiting associated with gastroparesis and other nonobstructive disorders characterized by gastric retention of food and fluids. Metoclopramide also has central antiemetic effects; it antagonizes the action of dopamine, a catecholamine neurotransmitter. Metoclopramide is given orally in diabetic gastroparesis and esophageal reflux. Large doses of the drug are given intravenously during chemotherapy with cisplatin (Platinol) and other emetogenic antineoplastic drugs. Cisapride lacks the antidopaminergic activity of metoclopramide and therefore does not have direct antiemetic effects in the brain. Cisapride is well absorbed following oral administration, and the presence of food increases the rate and extent of absorption. Extensive first-pass hepatic metabolism occurs. Peak plasma levels occur in 1 to 2 hours. The drug is 98% protein bound and widely distributed in body tissues. It is eliminated about 50% in urine and 50% in feces. Cisapride reportedly causes fewer adverse effects than metoclopramide but may cause diarrhea.

MISCELLANEOUS ANTIEMETICS

Miscellaneous antiemetics include several drugs with varied mechanisms of action, as listed below.

Benzquinamide apparently acts on the CTZ.

Diphenidol is thought to act on the vestibular apparatus of the inner ear. Because of adverse effects of confusion and hallucinations, it is recommended for use only in hospital or closely supervised settings.

Dronabinol is a cannabinoid (derivative of marijuana) used in the management of nausea and vomiting associated with anticancer drugs and unrelieved by other drugs. Dronabinol may cause the same adverse effects as marijuana, including psychiatric symptoms, and has a high potential for abuse. As a result, it is a Schedule II drug under federal narcotic laws.

Droperidol is a butyrophenone related to the antipsychotic drug haloperidol. It is often used in combination with fentanyl, a narcotic analgesic, for neuroleptanalgesia. The combination product (Innovar) is usually administered by anesthesiologists, but droperidol may be used alone to prevent nausea and vomiting during surgical or diagnostic procedures. Droperidol may be given preoperatively or during surgery for induction and maintenance of anesthesia.

Phosphorated carbohydrate solutions (Emetrol, Nausetrol) are hyperosmolar carbohydrate solutions with phosphoric acid. They are thought to exert a direct local action on the wall of the GI tract, reducing smooth muscle contraction. These preparations are available over the counter.

Scopolamine, an anticholinergic drug (see Chap. 21), is effective in relieving nausea and vomiting associated with motion sickness. A transdermal patch is often used to prevent seasickness.

Trimethobenzamide may act on the CTZ but is considered minimally effective.

INDICATIONS FOR USE

Antiemetic drugs are indicated to prevent and treat nausea and vomiting associated with surgery, pain, motion sickness, cancer chemotherapy, radiation therapy, and other causes. Phenothiazines, because of their relatively high incidence and severity of adverse effects, are indicated only when other antiemetic drugs are ineffective or when only a few doses are expected to be required.

CONTRAINDICATIONS FOR USE

Antiemetic drugs are generally contraindicated when their use may prevent or delay diagnosis, when signs and symptoms of drug toxicity may be masked, and for routine use to prevent postoperative vomiting.

Nursing Process

Assessment

Assess for nausea and vomiting.

- Identify risk factors (*e.g.,* digestive or other disorders in which nausea and vomiting are symptoms; drugs associated with nausea and vomiting).
- Interview regarding frequency, duration, and precipitating causes of nausea and vomiting. Also, question the client about accompanying signs and symptoms, characteristics of vomitus (amount, color, odor, presence of abnormal components, such as blood), and any measures that relieve nausea and vomiting. When possible, observe and measure the vomitus.

Nursing Diagnoses

- Fluid Volume Deficit related to uncontrolled vomiting
- Altered Nutrition: Less Than Body Requirements related to impaired ability to ingest and digest food
- Altered Tissue Perfusion: Hypotension related to fluid volume depletion or antiemetic drug effect
- Risk for Injury related to adverse drug effects
- Knowledge Deficit related to nondrug measures to reduce nausea and vomiting
- Knowledge Deficit related to appropriate use of antiemetic drugs

Planning/Goals

The client will:

- Have antiemetic drugs administered at appropriate times by indicated routes
- Take antiemetic drugs as prescribed for outpatient use
- Obtain relief of nausea and vomiting
- Eat and retain food and fluids
- Have increased comfort
- Maintain body weight
- Maintain normal bowel elimination patterns
- Have fewer vomiting episodes and less discomfort with cancer chemotherapy

Interventions

Use measures to prevent or minimize nausea and vomiting:

- Avoid exposure to stimuli when feasible (*e.g.,* unpleasant sights and odors; excessive ingestion of food, alcohol, or aspirin).
- Because pain may cause nausea and vomiting, administration of analgesics before painful diagnostic tests and dressing changes or other therapeutic measures may be helpful.
- Administer antiemetic drugs before radiation therapy, cancer chemotherapy, or travel.
- Many oral drugs cause less gastric irritation, nausea, and vomiting if taken with or just after food. Thus, scheduling and administering drugs may be an important measure in pre-

venting nausea and vomiting. However, food delays or prevents absorption of many drugs and may decrease therapeutic effectiveness. For any drug likely to cause nausea and vomiting, check reference sources to determine whether it can be given with food without altering beneficial effects.

- When nausea and vomiting occur, assess the client's condition and report to the physician. In some instances, a drug (*e.g.,* digoxin, an antibiotic) may need to be discontinued or reduced in dosage. In other instances (*e.g.,* paralytic ileus, GI obstruction), preferred treatment is restriction of oral intake and nasogastric intubation.
- Eating dry crackers before rising in the morning may help prevent nausea and vomiting associated with pregnancy.
- Avoid oral intake of food, fluids, and drugs during acute episodes of nausea and vomiting. Oral intake may increase vomiting and risks of fluid and electrolyte imbalances.
- Avoid activity during acute episodes of nausea and vomiting. Lying down and resting quietly are often helpful.

Give supportive care during vomiting episodes:

- Give replacement fluids and electrolytes. Offer small amounts of food and fluids orally when tolerated and according to client preference.
- Record vital signs, intake and output, and body weight at regular intervals if nausea or vomiting occurs frequently.
- Decrease environmental stimuli when possible (*e.g.,* noise, odors). Allow the client to lie quietly in bed when nauseated. Decreasing motion may decrease stimulation of the vomiting center in the brain.
- Help the client rinse his or her mouth after vomiting. This decreases the bad taste and corrosion of tooth enamel by gastric acid.
- Provide requested home remedies when possible (*e.g.,* a cool wet washcloth to the face and neck).

Teach clients:

- To avoid situations that cause or aggravate nausea and vomiting, when possible
- To avoid intake of food, fluids, and medications during acute vomiting episodes
- To avoid or decrease activity during episodes of nausea
- To take an antiemetic drug about 30 to 60 minutes before a nausea-producing event, when possible

Evaluation

- Observe and interview for decreased nausea and vomiting.
- Observe and interview regarding ability to maintain adequate intake of food and fluids.
- Compare current weight with baseline weight.
- Observe and interview regarding appropriate use of antiemetic drugs.

Principles of Therapy

DRUG SELECTION

Choice of an antiemetic drug depends largely on the cause of nausea and vomiting and the client's condition.

1. For ambulatory clients, drugs causing minimal sedation are preferred. However, most antiemetic drugs cause some sedation in usual therapeutic doses.
2. Promethazine, a phenothiazine, is often used clinically for its antihistaminic, antiemetic, and sedative effects.
3. Drugs with anticholinergic and antihistaminic properties are preferred for motion sickness.
4. Prokinetic drugs are preferred when nausea and vomiting are associated with nonobstructive gastric retention.
5. Although phenothiazines are effective antiemetic agents, they may cause serious adverse effects (*e.g.,* hypotension, sedation, anticholinergic effects, extrapyramidal reactions that simulate signs and symptoms of Parkinson's disease). Consequently, phenothiazines other than promethazine generally should not be used, especially for pregnant, young, elderly, and postoperative clients, unless vomiting is severe and cannot be controlled by other measures.
6. The serotonin antagonists, ondansetron and granisetron are often used for chemotherapy-induced nausea.

DOSAGE AND ADMINISTRATION FACTORS

Dosage and route of administration depend primarily on the reason for use.

1. Doses of phenothiazines are much smaller for antiemetic effects than for antipsychotic effects.
2. Most antiemetic agents are available in oral, parenteral, and rectal dosage forms. As a general rule, oral dosage forms are preferred for prophylactic use, and rectal or parenteral forms are preferred for therapeutic use.
3. Antiemetic drugs are often ordered PRN (as needed). As for any PRN drug, the client's condition should be assessed before drug administration.

TIMING OF DRUG ADMINISTRATION

When nausea and vomiting are likely to occur because of travel, administration of emetogenic anticancer drugs, diagnostic tests, or therapeutic procedures, an antiemetic drug should be given before the emetogenic event. Pretreatment usually increases patient comfort and allows use of lower drug doses. It also may prevent aspiration and other potentially serious complications of vomiting.

CHEMOTHERAPY-INDUCED NAUSEA AND VOMITING

Several anticancer drugs may cause severe nausea and vomiting and much discomfort for clients. Cisplatin is one of the most emetogenic drugs. For this reason, new antiemetics are usually compared with older drugs in the treatment of cisplatin-induced nausea and vomiting. Some general guidelines for managing this difficult problem include the following:

1. Chemotherapy may be given during sleeping hours.
2. Some clients may experience less nausea and vomiting if they avoid or decrease food intake for a few hours before scheduled chemotherapy.
3. Antiemetic drugs should be given before the emetogenic drug to *prevent* nausea and vomiting when possible. Most often, they are given intravenously for rapid effects.
4. Metoclopramide, given intravenously in high doses, may be used alone or in combination with various other drugs. Diphenhydramine (Benadryl) or another drug with anticholinergic effects may be given at the same time or PRN because high doses of metoclopramide often cause extrapyramidal effects (see Chap. 9).
5. Numerous combinations have been tried, with varying degrees of success. Most of them include two to five antiemetic and sedative-type drugs, usually in moderate to high doses. The client should be closely observed for excessive sedation.

USE IN CHILDREN

The use of antiemetics in children is not clearly defined. Phenothiazines (*e.g.,* chlorpromazine) are more likely to cause dystonias and other neuromuscular reactions in children than in adults. Promethazine is probably preferred because its action is more like the antihistamines than the phenothiazines. Several other antiemetics are not recommended for use in children younger than 12 years of age. These include benzquinamide, buclizine (Bucladin-S), cyclizine (Marezine), and scopolamine. Thus, antiemetic drug therapy should generally be cautious and limited to prolonged vomiting of known etiology.

USE IN OLDER ADULTS

Most antiemetic drugs cause drowsiness, especially in older adults, and therefore should be used cautiously. Efforts should be made to prevent nausea and vomiting when possible. Older adults are at risk of fluid volume depletion and electrolyte imbalances with vomiting.

 ## HOME CARE

Antiemetics are usually given orally or by rectal suppository in the home setting. The home care nurse may need to assist clients and caregivers with appropriate use of the drugs and other interventions to prevent fluid and electrolyte depletion. Teaching safety precautions with sedating drugs may also be needed.

NURSING ACTIONS	RATIONALE/EXPLANATION

1. Administer accurately

a. For prevention of motion sickness, give antiemetics about 30 min before travel and q3–4h, if necessary.

To allow time for drug dissolution and absorption

b. For prevention of vomiting with cancer chemotherapy and radiation therapy, give antiemetic drugs 30–60 min before treatment.

Drugs are more effective in preventing than in aborting nausea and vomiting.

c. Inject intramuscular antiemetics deeply into a large muscle mass (*e.g.*, gluteal area).

To decrease tissue irritation.

d. As a general rule, do not mix parenteral antiemetics in a syringe with other drugs. An exception is promethazine (Phenergan), which is often mixed with meperidine (Demerol) and atropine sulfate for preanesthetic medication.

To avoid physical incompatibilities

e. Omit antiemetic agents and report to the physician if the client appears excessively drowsy or is hypotensive.

To avoid potentiating adverse effects and central nervous system (CNS) depression

f. Mix IV ondansetron in 50 ml of 5% dextrose or 0.9% sodium chloride injection and infuse over 15 min

g. Mix granisetron in 20–50 ml of 5% dextrose or 0.9% sodium chloride injection and infuse over 5 min

2. Observe for therapeutic effects

a. Verbal reports of decreased nausea

b. Decreased frequency or absence of vomiting

3. Observe for adverse effects

a. Excessive sedation and drowsiness

Excessive sedation may occur with usual therapeutic doses of antiemetics and is more likely to occur with high doses. This may be minimized by avoiding high doses and assessing the client for responsiveness before each dose.

b. Anticholinergic effects—dry mouth, urinary retention

These effects are common to many antiemetic agents and are more likely to occur with large doses.

c. Hypotension, including orthostatic hypotension

Most likely to occur with phenothiazines and droperidol

d. Extrapyramidal reactions—dyskinesia, dystonia, akathisia, parkinsonism

These disorders may occur with phenothiazines and metoclopramide. They are more likely to occur when phenothiazines are used as antipsychotics rather than as antiemetics.

e. With dronabinol, observe for alterations in mood, cognition, and perception of reality, depersonalization, dysphoria, drowsiness, dizziness, anxiety, tachycardia, and conjunctivitis.

According to the manufacturer, these adverse effects are well tolerated. Tachycardia may be prevented with a beta-adrenergic blocking drug, such as propranolol (Inderal).

4. Observe for drug interactions

Drugs that *increase* effects of antiemetic agents:

(1) CNS depressants (alcohol, sedative-hypnotics, anti-anxiety agents, other antihistamines or antipsychotic agents)

Additive CNS depression

(continued)

NURSING ACTIONS	RATIONALE/EXPLANATION
(2) Anticholinergics (*e.g.*, atropine)	Additive anticholinergic effects. Some phenothiazines and antiemetic antihistamines have strong anticholinergic properties.
(3) Antihypertensive agents	Additive hypotension
5. Teach clients **a.** Take the drugs as prescribed.	To avoid adverse effects
b. Do not drive an automobile or operate dangerous machinery if drowsy from antiemetic drugs.	To avoid injury
c. If taking antiemetic drugs regularly, do not take other drugs without the physician's knowledge and consent.	Several drugs interact with antiemetic agents to increase incidence and severity of adverse effects.
d. Report excessive drowsiness or other adverse reactions.	The drug may need to be discontinued or reduced in dose or frequency of administration. Also, a change in drugs may reduce adverse effects in a particular individual.
e. With dronabinol, teach clients to take the drug only when they can be supervised by a responsible adult.	To increase safety, owing to the mind-altering effects of the drug.

REVIEW AND APPLICATION EXERCISES

1. List common causes of nausea and vomiting or circumstances in which nausea and vomiting often occur.

2. How do antiemetic drugs prevent or relieve nausea and vomiting?

3. What are adverse effects of commonly used antiemetics?

4. Are antiemetics more effective if given before, during, or after nausea and vomiting?

5. Which antiemetics are often given to control nausea and vomiting that occur with certain antineoplastic drugs?

SELECTED REFERENCES

Brunton, L.L. (1996). Agents affecting gastrointestinal water flux and motility; emesis and antiemetics; bile acids and pancreatic enzymes. In J.G. Hardman, L.E. Limbird, P.B. Molinoff, & R.W. Ruddon (Eds.), *Goodman & Gilman's The pharmacological basis of therapeutics*, 9th ed., pp. 917–936. New York: McGraw-Hill.

Drug facts and comparisons. (Updated monthly). St. Louis: Facts and Comparisons.

Hasler, W.L. (1997). Approach to the patient with nausea and vomiting. In W.N. Kelley (Ed.), *Textbook of internal medicine*, 3rd ed., pp. 608–617. Philadelphia: Lippincott-Raven.

Porth, C.M. (1994). *Pathophysiology: Concepts of altered health states*, 4th ed., pp. 817–841. Philadelphia: J.B. Lippincott.

Taylor, A.T., & Holland, E.G. (1997). Nausea and vomiting. In J.T. DiPiro, R.L. Talbert, G.C. Yee, G.R. Matzke, B.G. Wells, & L.M. Posey (Eds.), *Pharmacotherapy: A pathophysiologic approach*, 3rd ed., pp. 751–765. Stamford, CT: Appleton & Lange.

Drugs Used in Special Conditions

64 Antineoplastic Drugs

Outline

Objectives

After studying this chapter, the student will be able to:

1 Contrast normal and malignant cells.

2 Describe major types of antineoplastic drugs in terms of mechanism of action, indications for use, administration, and nursing process implications.

3 Discuss common and serious adverse drug effects.

4 Describe pharmacologic interventions to prevent or minimize adverse drug effects.

5 Describe nonpharmacologic interventions to prevent or minimize adverse drug effects.

6 Teach clients about their chemotherapy regimens.

Key Terms

Alopecia	**Malignant**
Anaplastic	**Metastasis**
Anemia	**Nephropathy**
Cell cycle	**Neuropathy**
Cell differentiation	**Neutropenia**
Cytotoxic	**Oncogenes and antioncogenes**
Extravasation	
Hyperuricemia	**Stomatitis**
Leukopenia	**Thrombocytopenia**

Antineoplastic drugs are used in the treatment of cancer. Cancer chemotherapy is a major treatment modality, alone or in conjunction with surgery and radiation therapy. It may cure some malignant tumors and is important in the treatment of many others. To participate effectively in cancer chemotherapy, nurses must know the characteristics of normal and malignant cells and of the drugs used to arrest tumor growth.

Characteristics of Normal Cells

Normal cells undergo an orderly process of replication and differentiation into specialized cells that perform specialized functions. Some specific characteristics of normal cells include the following:

1. They reproduce according to a predetermined sequence of events. The normal cell cycle (the interval between the "birth" of a cell and its division into two daughter cells) involves several phases. During the resting phase (G_0), cells perform all usual functions except replication. That is, they are not dividing but are capable of doing so when stimulated. Different types of cells spend different lengths of time in this phase, after which they either reenter the cell cycle and differentiate or die. During the first active phase (G_1), ribonucleic acid (RNA) and enzymes required for production of deoxyribonucleic acid (DNA) are developed. During the next phase (S), DNA is synthesized for chromosomes. During G_2, RNA is synthesized, and the mitotic spindle is formed. Mitosis occurs in the final phase (M). The resulting two daughter cells may then enter the resting phase (G_0) or proceed through the reproductive cycle.
2. Normal cells reproduce in response to a need (*e.g.,* growth or tissue repair) and stop reproduction when the need has been met.
3. They are well differentiated in appearance and function. Thus, they can be examined under a microscope and the tissue of origin can be determined.

Characteristics of Malignant Neoplasms

Malignant neoplasms, malignant tumors, and *cancer* are terms used to describe more than 100 disease processes. A cancer develops from a single normal cell that is transformed into a malignant cell. The transformation probably begins with a random mutation (abnormal structural changes within the genetic material of a cell). A mutated cell may be destroyed by body defenses (*e.g.,* an immune response), or it may replicate. During succeeding cell divisions, additional changes and mu-

tations may produce cells with progressively fewer normal and more malignant characteristics. Malignant cells differ from normal cells in several ways, including the following:

1. Malignant cells reproduce with the same sequence of events as normal cells, but they grow in an uncontrolled fashion. They do not differentiate, mature, or function like normal cells, and they can proliferate indefinitely. Generally, it takes years for malignant cells to produce a clinically detectable mass or tumor. Factors influencing the rate of tumor growth include blood and nutrient supply, the immunocompetence of the host, and hormonal stimulation of some types of cancer.
2. Malignant cells serve no useful purpose in the body. Instead, they occupy space and act as parasites by taking blood and nutrients away from normal tissues.
3. Malignant cells are anaplastic or undifferentiated. This means they have lost the structural and functional characteristics of the cells from which they originated. In comparison to normal cells of the same type, malignant cells are usually larger, more immature or primitive, and differ in appearance from normal cells and other malignant cells. Generally, cells that are more anaplastic or undifferentiated are more malignant. These cells grow into masses that are disorganized and irregular.
4. Malignant cells can invade normal tissues to cause widespread tissue destruction and eventual death unless treatment measures intervene. Owing to a lack of cohesiveness, increased motility, and production of proteolytic enzymes that break down normal tissues, malignant cells are able to break away from the primary tumor and spread to other body parts. Malignant cells invade normal tissues primarily by extending into tissues adjacent to the tumor and by traveling through blood and lymph vessels into tissues distant from the tumor site.

ETIOLOGIC AND RISK FACTORS

Despite extensive study, the cause of cancer is not clear. Because "cancer" is actually many diseases, many etiologic factors are probably involved. Most (about 80%) cancers are thought to be environmental in origin. Carcinogens (cancer-causing agents) and risk factors that predispose people to develop cancer include chemical, physical, and biologic agents. Chemical carcinogens (Table 64-1) include substances used to manufacture various products, tobacco products, and therapeutic drugs. Physical carcinogens include radiation from radioisotopes, ultraviolet light, and sunlight. Biologic carcinogens include viruses, which have been linked to the development of leukemia and cancers of the lymph

TABLE 64-1   **CHEMICAL CARCINOGENS**

Chemical	Source of Exposure	Location of Associated Cancer
Aflatoxins	Foods contaminated with aspergillus fungus, such as peanuts, soybeans, corn, wheat, and rice. Contamination is most likely with warm, moist storage conditions.	Liver
Alcohol	Ingestion of alcoholic beverages, such as whiskey, beer, or wine	Mouth, pharynx, larynx, esophagus, liver
Alkylating agents (*e.g.*, melphalan [Alkeran], others)	Cytotoxic, immunosuppressive drugs used in the treatment of several types of cancer	Lymphoid tissue (lymphoma, leukemia), bladder (cyclophosphamide [Cytoxan])
Alpha-naphthyline (1 NA) and beta-naphthylamine (2 NA)	Manufacturing, handling, or storing substances containing this chemical. It is used in a wide variety of products, including herbicides, dyes, food colors, color film, paint, plastics, rubber, and petroleum products.	Bladder
Anabolic steroids (androgens)	Large doses used by athletes to gain weight and muscle strength	Liver
Arsenic	Drinking contaminated water; spraying insecticides and herbicides; working in oil refineries	Lung, skin
Asbestos	Working in shipyards, reconstructing or demolishing buildings containing asbestos	Lung
Azathioprine, cyclosporine	Immunosuppressant drugs used mainly to prevent rejection of transplanted organs	Lymphoma, skin
Benzene	Working with paints, petrochemicals, dyes, glues, rubber, furniture varnishes	Myelogenous leukemia
Benzidine	Working in chemical plants where benzidine is used in the production of aniline dyes, rubber, plastics, printing inks, fireproofing of textiles, various laboratory chemicals. Living in neighborhoods where such plants are located also may result in significant exposure over the years.	Bladder
Bis (chloromethyl) ether (BCME)	Working in chemical plants where BCME is used for water-softening products, to remove impurities such as salt from water or to decolorize or clarify food beverages. BCME is not present in the finished product.	Lung
Dichlorbenzidine (DCB)	Working in chemical plants where DCB is used in the production of pigments for printing inks, textile dyes, plastics, and crayons. DCB is destroyed during the manufacturing process and is not contained in the final products.	Liver, bladder, breasts, skin
Diesel fumes	Working with buses, trucks, and other diesel-powered machines	Lung
Estrogens	Drugs prescribed for menopausal symptoms and menstrual problems. Estrogen is a component of oral contraceptives.	Uterine endometrium, possibly breasts
Etoposide, teniposide	Antineoplastic drugs used to treat acute leukemias, lymphomas, and other cancers	Leukemia
Hair dyes	Working as barbers or hairdressers	Bladder
Hydrocarbons	Cigarette smoke; soot (chimney sweeps may develop cancer of the scrotum); air pollution from industrial wastes, automobile exhausts; coal tar ointments used in treating some skin disorders; gases and particles produced by burning of coal, wood, and oil; foods such as smoked meats, foods burned by charcoal grilling, some vegetables and cereals; food packaging materials; many groups of industrial workers	Lungs, skin
Metallic ores (specific agent unknown)	Workers exposed to chromium in production of chromates and nickel refiners	Lungs

(continued)

TABLE 64-1	CHEMICAL CARCINOGENS (Continued)	
Chemical	**Source of Exposure**	**Location of Associated Cancer**
Polyvinyl chloride (PVC)	Workers in chemical plants that use PVC in the production of floor tiles, shoes, phonograph records, automobile upholstery, blood bags, and many other widely used products	Liver
Tamoxifen	An antiestrogen drug used in the treatment of advanced breast cancer in postmenopausal women	Endometrium
Tobacco	Cigarette smoking, pipe smoking, chewing tobacco	Lungs, mouth, pharynx, larynx, esophagus, bladder

nodes, liver, pharynx, and cervix and other genitalia. Risk factors cannot predict whether cancer will occur in a person, but they can help identify people who are more likely to develop cancer. Some common risk factors are listed below.

Geographic and racial factors are considered more environmental than hereditary or racial in nature. Studies of immigrants from various geographic areas and ethnic origins indicate that adoption of dietary and lifestyle habits of people in industrialized countries leads to a similar incidence of particular cancers. In addition, people who live in cities are more likely to develop cancer because of greater exposure to air pollutants and other carcinogens. In the United States, African-Americans have higher rates of multiple myeloma and cancers of the lung, prostate, esophagus, and pancreas than white people.

Age and gender may also be risk factors. The incidence of cancer increases with age and reaches a peak as a cause of death in the sixth and seventh decades. A smaller peak in cancer mortality occurs during the first 4 years of life. Lung cancer and colon cancer occur about equally in both sexes, but men are more likely to have leukemia and cancer of the urinary bladder, stomach, and pancreas, whereas women are at risk of developing cancer of the breast, cervix, and endometrium.

Use of tobacco is a major lifestyle risk factor. The incidence of lung cancer is greatly increased among people who smoke cigarettes and increased to a lesser extent among nonsmokers who are exposed to other people's smoke. Cancers of the mouth, throat, and esophagus are associated with smoking cigarettes or a pipe, chewing tobacco, and using "smokeless tobacco." In addition, ingesting alcohol probably increases the cancer-producing effects of cigarette smoking.

Dietary factors also influence the occurrence of cancer. Cancers of the colon, breast, prostate gland, ovary, and endometrium are associated with a high intake of carbohydrate, fat, and animal protein and a low intake of fiber. These eating patterns are more prevalent in affluent, industrialized parts of the world.

Hereditary factors are less important than environmental factors in cancer development. Most relatives of people with cancer are generally no more likely to develop cancer than the general population. However, some specific types of cancer are related to heredity. For example, close relatives of premenopausal women with breast cancer are more likely to develop breast cancer.

Therapeutic drugs may be associated with an increased risk of cancer. These include anticancer drugs (especially the alkylating group), female sex hormones, and immunosuppressants. With alkylating anticancer drugs used to treat Hodgkin's and non-Hodgkin's lymphoma, multiple myeloma, and ovarian, gastric, or colorectal cancer, surviving clients have a relatively high risk of developing acute nonlymphocytic leukemia for about 15 to 20 years. With female sex hormones, risks are increased for endometrial cancer and possibly for breast cancer, especially with long-term use. With immunosuppressants used for solid organ or bone marrow transplant, clients have an increased risk for non-Hodgkin's lymphoma within a few months after transplant and later risks of skin (*e.g.*, squamous cell carcinoma and malignant melanoma) and soft-tissue sarcoma (Kaposi's sarcoma).

ONCOGENES AND ANTIONCOGENES

Oncogenes (cancer-causing genes) are mutations of normal growth-regulating genes called proto-oncogenes, which are present in all body cells. Normally, proto-oncogenes are active for a brief period in the cell reproductive cycle. When exposed to carcinogens and genetically altered to oncogenes, however, they may operate continuously, causing abnormal, disordered, and unregulated cell growth. Unregulated cell growth and proliferation increases the probability of neoplastic transformation of the cell. Tumors of the breast, colon, lung, and bone have been linked to activation of oncogenes.

Antioncogenes, also called tumor suppressor genes, normally inhibit growth and proliferation of cells.

Absent, damaged or inactivated tumor suppressor genes may be inherited or result from exposure to carcinogens. When tumor suppressing genes are inactivated, a block to cellular proliferation is removed and the cells begin unregulated growth. Breast cancer has been associated with the absence of an antioncogene.

Thus, activation of oncogenes and inactivation of antioncogenes probably both play roles in cancer development. Multiple genetic abnormalities are usually characteristic of cancer cells and may occur concurrently or sequentially.

CLASSIFICATION OF MALIGNANT NEOPLASMS

Malignant neoplasms are classified in several different ways according to the type of tissue involved, the rate of growth, and other characteristics. With the exception of the acute leukemias, they are considered chronic diseases. These diseases can be broadly categorized as hematologic or solid neoplasms.

Hematologic Malignancies

Hematologic malignancies involve the bone marrow and lymphoid tissues; they include leukemias, lymphomas, and multiple myeloma.

Leukemias are cancers of the bone marrow characterized mainly by overproduction of abnormal white blood cells. These cells range from very primitive and immature to nearly normal in morphology. They cannot function normally as a body defense mechanism against microorganisms and tissue injuries. They also prevent or decrease production of normal red blood cells, white blood cells, and platelets. They eventually infiltrate other organs (liver, spleen, kidneys) and interfere with organ function.

Leukemias are more specifically classified according to the type of abnormal white blood cell. Acute leukemias involve more immature and less functional cells; chronic leukemias involve cells that are more nearly normal and somewhat functional. Granulocytic leukemia indicates abnormal granulocytes, most often neutrophils; myelogenous leukemia indicates that the abnormal cells originate in the bone marrow. Lymphocytic, lymphatic, or lymphogenous leukemia is characterized by abnormal lymphoid tissue.

The four main types of leukemia are acute lymphocytic leukemia, which is more common in children; acute myelogenous leukemia, which occurs in all ages but more often in young adults; chronic lymphocytic leukemia, which is more common in elderly people; and chronic myelogenous leukemia, which is more common in middle age.

Lymphomas are malignant tumors of lymphoid tissue that are characterized by abnormal proliferation of the white blood cells normally found in lymphoid tissue.

Lymphomas usually develop within lymph nodes and may occur anywhere in the body, because virtually all body tissues contain lymphoid structures. They develop as a solid tumor mass without involving peripheral blood. They impair immunity and increase susceptibility to infection. As the disease progresses, the liver, spleen, bone marrow, and other organs become functionally impaired. The two main types of malignant lymphomas are Hodgkin's disease and non-Hodgkin's lymphoma.

Multiple myeloma is a malignant tumor of the bone marrow in which abnormal plasma cells proliferate. Because normal plasma cells produce antibodies or immunoglobulins and abnormal plasma cells cannot fulfill this function, the body's immune system is impaired. As the tumor grows, it crowds out normal cells and interferes with other bone marrow functions. Although multiple myeloma is a slow-growing tumor, the abnormal plasma cells eventually infiltrate bone and cause extensive destruction. Metastasis eventually occurs in tissues outside bone, such as the spleen, liver, and lymph nodes.

Solid Neoplasms

Solid tumors are composed of a mass of malignant cells (parenchyma) and a supporting structure of connective tissue, blood vessels, and lymphatics (stroma). The growing tumor develops its own blood supply as new blood vessels grow from preexisting blood vessels of the host. Apparently, neoplastic cells secrete a substance that acts on capillaries to stimulate their growth into the tumor. The two major classifications of solid malignant neoplasms are carcinomas and sarcomas. Each is then subclassified according to the particular kind of body cell involved.

Carcinomas are derived from epithelial tissues (skin, mucous membrane, linings and coverings of viscera) and are the most common type of malignant tumors. They are further classified by cell type, such as adenocarcinoma or basal cell carcinoma.

Sarcomas are derived from connective tissue (muscle, bone, cartilage, fibrous tissue, fat, blood vessels). They are subclassified by cell type (*e.g.,* osteogenic sarcoma, angiosarcoma).

EFFECTS OF CANCER ON THE BODY

Effects of cancer on the host vary according to the extent and location of the disease process. There are few effects initially. As the neoplasm grows, effects occur when the tumor becomes large enough to cause pressure, distortion, or deficient blood supply in surrounding tissues; interfere with organ function; obstruct ducts and organs; and cause malnutrition of normal tissues. More specific effects include anemia, malnutrition, pain, infection, hemorrhagic tendencies, thromboembolic problems, hypercalcemia, cachexia, and occurrence of symptoms related to impaired function of affected organs and tissues.

Characteristics of Antineoplastic Drugs

1. Many antineoplastic drugs damage body cells (*i.e.,* they are cytotoxic). They kill malignant cells by interfering with cell replication. Nutrients and genetic materials are necessary for cell replication. To be effective, the drugs must interfere with the supply and use of nutrients (amino acids, purines, pyrimidines) or with the genetic materials in the cell nucleus (DNA or RNA).
2. Some antineoplastic drugs act during specific phases of the cell cycle, such as DNA synthesis or formation of the mitotic spindle. These cell cycle-specific (CCS) agents include the antimetabolites, the plant alkaloids, and some miscellaneous agents (*e.g.,* asparaginase, hydroxyurea). These drugs are more effective when administered continuously because this method prolongs exposure of malignant cells to drug action. Other drugs act during any phase of the cell cycle and are called cell cycle-nonspecific (CCNS) agents. This group includes the alkylating agents, the antibiotic antineoplastics, the nitrosoureas, and some miscellaneous agents (*e.g.,* cisplatin, dacarbazine). CCNS agents are more effective when administered intermittently.
3. Cytotoxic antineoplastic drugs are generally most active against rapidly dividing and proliferating cells. Because the drugs do not act specifically against malignant cells, normal cells are damaged as well. The normal cells especially endangered are the rapidly proliferating cells of the bone marrow, the lining of the gastrointestinal tract, and the hair follicles. The cytotoxic effects of antineoplastic drugs account for therapeutic and adverse effects.
4. Each dose of antineoplastic drugs kills some but not all malignant cells. The cell kill effect follows "first-order kinetics," meaning that a drug dose kills a specific percentage of cells. If the drug destroys 99% of cells, it reduces 1 million cells to 10,000. Succeeding doses would destroy 99% of remaining cells but not all of them. This is important because all malignant cells must be killed to effect a cure.
5. Antineoplastic drugs are given mainly by oral and intravenous (IV) routes of administration. In some circumstances, they may be given topically, intraarterially, intrathecally, or by instillation into a body cavity.
6. Antineoplastic drugs may induce drug-resistant malignant cells. Mechanisms may involve the ability of malignant cells to act on the drug (*e.g.,* by inhibiting drug uptake or activation, increasing the rate of drug inactivation, or pumping the drug out of the cell before it can act) or to act on themselves (*e.g.,* increase cellular repair of DNA damaged by the drugs or alter metabolic pathways and target enzymes of the drugs). Mutant cells also may emerge.
7. Most cytotoxic antineoplastic drugs are potential teratogens.

CLASSIFICATION OF ANTINEOPLASTIC DRUGS

Antineoplastic drugs are classified in several different ways. Some are described in terms of their mechanisms of action (alkylating agents and antimetabolites), others according to their sources (plant alkaloids, antibiotics, enzymes). Other drugs used in cancer chemotherapy are immunostimulants (see Chap. 44), hormones, antihormones, and miscellaneous agents.

Alkylating Agents

Alkylating agents include nitrogen mustard and its derivatives (busulfan, chlorambucil, cyclophosphamide, and melphalan), nitrosoureas (carmustine, lomustine, and streptozocin) and platinum compounds (carboplatin and cisplatin). Nitrogen mustard derivatives interfere with cell division and structure of DNA during dividing and resting stages of the malignant cell cycle. Consequently, their spectrum of activity is relatively broad compared with other antineoplastic drugs. They are most effective in hematologic malignancies but also are used to treat breast, lung, and ovarian tumors. All of these drugs cause significant bone marrow depression (also called myelosuppression). All except nitrogen mustard may be given orally.

Nitrosoureas are classified as alkylating agents, although they also may inhibit essential enzymatic reactions of cancer cells. They have been used in clients with gastrointestinal, lung, and brain tumors. One unique feature of the nitrosoureas is their high lipid solubility, which allows them to enter the brain and cerebrospinal fluid more effectively than most antineoplastic drugs. A second unique characteristic is that they cause delayed bone marrow depression, with maximum leukopenia and thrombocytopenia occurring about 5 to 6 weeks after drug administration.

The platinum compounds inhibit DNA synthesis. Cisplatin is widely used to treat cancers of the bladder, cervix, esophagus, head and neck, lung, prostate, and testes. It is also used to treat lymphomas, multiple myeloma, osteosarcoma, and other sarcomas. Adverse effects are mainly renal, neurologic, and otologic damage. Carboplatin is structurally similar to cisplatin but differs in other aspects. For example, it is most often used to treat endometrial and ovarian carcinomas, and it produces bone marrow depression as a major adverse effect.

Antimetabolites

Antimetabolites include a folic acid antagonist (methotrexate), purine antagonists (mercaptopurine and thioguanine), pyrimidine antagonists (fluorouracil and floxuridine), and an inhibitor of DNA polymerase (cytarabine). The drugs are similar to nutrients needed by the cells for reproduction and are allowed to enter the cells. Once inside the cell, the drugs deprive the cell of necessary substances or cause formation of abnormal DNA. Either action kills the cell.

The antimetabolites have been used to treat the entire spectrum of cancers. Effectiveness of individual drugs varies with different kinds of cancer. Toxic effects mainly involve the bone marrow, epithelial lining of the gastrointestinal tract, and hair follicles.

Some antimetabolites can be given orally and parenterally; others are given only by one route. The effectiveness of these drugs depends greatly on the schedule of administration. They exert their cytotoxic effects during only one phase of the reproductive cycle of the cell (*i.e.,* when DNA is being synthesized). Although there is no way a chemotherapist can determine exactly when a drug is likely to be most effective (*i.e.,* kill the largest number of malignant cells), information has been accumulated empirically through extensive clinical trials. Thus, recommendations regarding dosage schedules should be followed as precisely as possible.

Plant Alkaloids

Plant alkaloids include the podophyllotoxin derivatives (etoposide, teniposide) and the vinca derivatives (vinblastine, vincristine, vinorelbine). These drugs exert their cytotoxic effects by inhibiting cell division (antimitotic effects). Etoposide is used mainly in a multidrug regimen to treat small-cell lung cancer and to treat testicular cancer that does not respond adequately to surgery, radiation, and other chemotherapy. Teniposide is used mainly in a multidrug regimen to treat childhood acute lymphocytic leukemia. Common adverse effects are bone marrow depression, nausea and vomiting, and peripheral neuropathy.

Vinblastine and vincristine have similar structures but different ranges of antineoplastic activity and adverse effects. Either may be effective in treating Hodgkin's disease and choriocarcinoma. Vinblastine also is useful in testicular carcinoma, and vincristine is used in acute lymphoblastic leukemia, non-Hodgkin's lymphomas, oat-cell carcinoma of the lung, and Wilms' tumor. Vinorelbine, a semisynthetic agent, is used to treat non-small cell lung cancer. In terms of adverse effects, vinblastine and vinorelbine are more likely to cause bone marrow depression, and vincristine is more likely to cause peripheral nerve toxicity.

Antineoplastic Antibiotics

Antibiotics with antineoplastic activity include bleomycin, dactinomycin, daunorubicin, doxorubicin, idarubicin, mitomycin, mitoxantrone, pentastatin, and plicamycin. These drugs differ in activity and toxicity. They have some anti-infective activity, but they are too toxic for this use. The major toxicity is bone marrow depression. The anthracycline drugs, daunorubicin, doxorubicin, and idarubicin, also cause cardiotoxicity. Bleomycin may cause significant pulmonary toxicity. All of these drugs except bleomycin must be given IV because they are extremely irritating to tissues and cause tissue necrosis if extravasation occurs.

Hormones and Hormone Inhibitors

Hormones used in cancer chemotherapy exert beneficial effects by altering the hormonal environment that promotes cancer growth. The sex hormones (estrogens, progestins, androgens) are useful in cancers of the sex organs, including the breast and prostate gland. The adrenal corticosteroids suppress formation and function of lymphocytes and are therefore most useful in the treatment of acute leukemia in children and of malignant lymphoma. They also may be used in treating complications of cancer, such as intracranial metastases and hypercalcemia. Hormone inhibitors include tamoxifen, an antiestrogen that competes with estrogen for binding sites in breast tissue; aminoglutethimide, an adrenocorticosteroid-inhibiting agent that produces a "medical adrenalectomy"; and goserelin and leuprolide, which inhibit testosterone secretion in advanced prostatic cancer.

Radioactive Iodine

Radioactive iodine (^{131}I) is used only for treatment of thyroid cancer.

Miscellaneous Agents

Miscellaneous antineoplastic agents vary greatly in their sources, mechanisms of action, indications for use, and toxic effects.

INDICATIONS FOR USE

Cytotoxic antineoplastic drugs are used in the treatment of malignant neoplasms. Goals of chemotherapy vary according to the clinical situation. In some cases, chemotherapy is curative; in others, it is palliative. In still others, it induces or maintains remissions (symptom-free periods that last for varying lengths of time).

Chemotherapy is the primary treatment of choice for a few types of cancer, including Burkitt's lymphoma, choriocarcinoma, Hodgkin's disease, acute leukemia, carcinoma of the testes, Wilms' tumor, Ewing's sarcoma, and retinoblastoma. Most of these malignant tumors are relatively rare. Chemotherapy is less effective in cancers of the lung, rectum, pancreas, colon, and prostate gland.

In hematologic neoplasms, drug therapy is the primary treatment of choice because the systemic distribution of the disease precludes use of the other two treatments for cancer (surgery and radiation). In solid tumors, drug therapy is often used to kill malignant cells remaining after surgery or radiation therapy. Chemotherapy is more effective when the tumor mass has been removed or reduced. Chemotherapy used in conjunction with surgery or irradiation is called *adjuvant chemotherapy*, which is used to destroy malignant cells in breast and other cancers. Drug therapy also is used in advanced malignant disease for palliation of symptoms. Once metastasized, solid tumors become systemic diseases and are no longer readily accessible to surgical excision or radiation therapy.

Antineoplastic drugs are sometimes used in the treatment of nonmalignant conditions. One of these is polycythemia vera, an uncommon condition characterized by abnormal proliferation of blood cells. Methotrexate may be used, in smaller doses than those used for malignant diseases, to treat rheumatoid arthritis and psoriasis.

Individual Drugs

Cytotoxic antineoplastic drugs are listed in Table 64-2; hormones and hormone inhibitors are listed in Table 64-3.

(*text continues on page 823*)

TABLE 64-2 CYTOTOXIC ANTINEOPLASTIC DRUGS

Generic/Trade Name	Routes and Dosage Ranges*	Clinical Uses	Common or Potentially Severe Adverse Reactions
Alkylating Drugs			
Nitrogen Mustard Derivatives			
Busulfan (Myleran)	PO 4–8 mg daily until white blood cell count decreases by half, then maintenance doses up to 4 mg daily	Chronic granulocytic leukemia	Bone marrow depression (leukopenia, thrombocytopenia, anemia), pulmonary toxicity
Chlorambucil (Leukeran)	PO 0.1–0.2 mg/kg/d for 3–6 wk. If maintenance therapy is required, 0.03–0.1 mg/kg/d	Chronic lymphocytic leukemia, non-Hodgkin's lymphomas, carcinomas of breast and ovary	Bone marrow depression, hyperuricemia
Cyclophos-phamide (Cytoxan)	Induction of therapy, PO 1–5 mg/kg/d; IV 35–40 mg/kg over several days (20–30 mg/kg for clients with prior chemotherapy or radiation) Oral maintenance therapy, 1.5–2 mg/kg daily	Hodgkin's disease, non-Hodgkin's lymphomas, neuroblastoma. Often combined with other drugs for acute lymphoblastic leukemia in children, carcinomas of breast, ovary, and lung; multiple myeloma and other malignancies	Bone marrow depression, anorexia, nausea, vomiting, alopecia, hemorrhagic cystitis
Ifosfamide (Ifex)	IV 1.2 g/m²/d for 5 consecutive days. Repeat every 3 wk or after WBC and platelet counts return to normal after a dose.	Germ cell testicular cancer	Bone marrow depression, hemorrhagic cystitis, nausea and vomiting
Mechloretha-mine (nitrogen mustard) (Mustargen)	IV 0.4 mg/kg in one or two doses. Repeat in 3–6 wk. Intracavitary 0.4 mg/kg instilled into pleural or peritoneal cavities	Hodgkin's disease and non-Hodgkin's lymphomas, lung cancer, pleural and peritoneal malignant effusions	Bone marrow depression, nausea, vomiting. Extravasation may lead to tissue necrosis.
Melphalan (Alkeran)	PO 0.25 mg/kg/d for 7 d, followed by 21 drug-free days, then maintenance dose of 2 mg daily	Multiple myeloma	Bone marrow depression, nausea and vomiting

TABLE 64-2   CYTOTOXIC ANTINEOPLASTIC DRUGS (Continued)

Generic/Trade Name	Routes and Dosage Ranges*	Clinical Uses	Common or Potentially Severe Adverse Reactions
Nitrosoureas			
Carmustine (BCNU)	IV 200 mg/m² every 6 wk	Hodgkin's disease, malignant melanoma, multiple myeloma, brain tumors	Bone marrow depression, nausea, vomiting. Extravasation may lead to tissue necrosis.
Lomustine (CCNU)	PO 130 mg/m² every 6 wk	Hodgkin's disease, brain tumors	Bone marrow depression, nausea and vomiting
Streptozocin (Zanosar)	IV 500 mg/m² for 5 consecutive days every 6 wk	Metastatic islet cell carcinoma of pancreas	Nephrotoxicity, nausea, vomiting
Others			
Carboplatin (Paraplatin)	IV infusion 360 mg/m² over at least 15 min on day 1 every 4 wk	Palliation of ovarian cancer	Bone marrow depression, nausea and vomiting
Cisplatin (Platinol)	IV 100 mg/m² once every 4 wk	Carcinomas of testes, bladder, ovary, head and neck, and endometrium	Renal toxicity and ototoxicity
Antimetabolites			
Cytarabine (ARA-C, cytosine arabinoside) (Cytosar-U)	IV 2 mg/kg/d for 10 d	Leukemias of adults and children	Bone marrow depression, nausea, vomiting, stomatitis, diarrhea
Floxuridine (FUDR)	Intra-arterial infusion, 0.1–0.6 mg/kg/d until toxicity occurs	Head and neck tumors, carcinomas of the GI tract, liver, pancreas, and biliary tract	Same as cytarabine, above
Fludarabine (Fludara)	IV 25 mg/m² daily for 5 consecutive days	Chronic lymphocytic leukemia	Bone marrow depression, fever, nausea, vomiting
Fluorouracil (5-FU) (Adrucil) (Efudex, Fluoroplex)	IV 12 mg/kg/d for 5 d	Carcinomas of the breast, colon, rectum, stomach, and pancreas	Same as cytarabine, above
	Topical, apply to skin cancer lesion twice daily for several weeks	Solar keratoses, basal cell carcinoma	Pain, pruritus, burning at site of application
Mercaptopurine (Purinethol)	PO 2.5 mg/kg/d	Acute and chronic leukemias	Bone marrow depression, nausea, hyperuricemia
Methotrexate (MTX, Amethopterin) (Mexate)	Induction of remission of acute leukemia in children PO, IV 3 mg/m²/d. Maintenance of remission, PO 30 mg/m² two times per week (combined with prednisone for induction and maintenance of remission) Choriocarcinoma, PO, IM 15 mg/m² daily for 5 d	Acute lymphoblastic leukemia in children, lymphocytic lymphoma, choriocarcinoma of the testes, osteogenic carcinoma, others	Bone marrow depression, nausea, diarrhea, stomatitis
Thioguanine	PO 2 mg/kg/d	Acute and chronic leukemias	Bone marrow depression, nausea
Antibiotics			
Bleomycin (Blenoxane)	IV, IM 0.25–0.5 units/kg once or twice weekly	Squamous cell carcinoma, lymphomas, testicular carcinoma, Hodgkin's disease	Pulmonary toxicity, stomatitis, alopecia, hyperpigmentation and ulceration of skin

(continued)

TABLE 64-2 **CYTOTOXIC ANTINEOPLASTIC DRUGS** (Continued)

Generic/ Trade Name	Routes and Dosage Ranges*	Clinical Uses	Common or Potentially Severe Adverse Reactions
Dactinomycin (**Actinomycin D**) (Cosmegen)	IV 15 μg/kg/d for 5 d and repeated every 2–4 wk	Rhabdomyosarcoma, Wilms' tumor	Bone marrow depression, anorexia, nausea, vomiting. Extravasation may lead to tissue necrosis.
Daunorubicin (Cerubidin)	IV 60 mg/m^2 daily for 3 d every 3–4 wk	Acute granulocytic and acute lymphocytic leukemias, lymphomas	Same as doxorubicin, below
Daunorubicin (liposomal formulation) (DaunoXome)	IV infusion, 40 mg/m^2 over 1 h, every 2 wk, until disease progression or complications occur	AIDS-related Kaposi's sarcoma	Bone marrow depression, pain, nausea, vomiting, diarrhea, cough, fever, dyspnea, fatigue, headache
Doxorubicin (Adriamycin)	Adults, IV 60–75 mg/m^2 every 21 d Children, IV 30 mg/m^2 daily for 3 d, repeated every 4 wk	Acute leukemias, lymphomas, carcinomas of breast, lung, and ovary	Bone marrow depression, alopecia, stomatitis, GI upset, cardiomyopathy. Extravasation may lead to tissue necrosis.
Doxorubicin (liposomal formulation) (Doxil)	IV infusion, 20 mg/m^2 over 30 min, once every 3 wk, as long as patient responds and tolerates	AIDS-related Kaposi's sarcoma	Bone marrow depression, nausea, vomiting, fever, alopecia, chest pain, weakness, skin eruptions of hands and feet
Idarubicin (Idamycin)	IV injection 12 mg/m^2 daily for 3 d, with concomitant cytarabine	Acute myelogenous leukemia in adults, with other antileukemic drugs	Same as doxorubicin, above
Mitomycin (Mutamycin)	IV 2 mg/m^2/d or 50 μg/kg/d for 5 d, repeated after 2 d. This course of therapy may be repeated after recovery of the bone marrow.	Carcinomas of stomach, colon, rectum, pancreas, bladder, breast, lung, head and neck, and malignant melanoma	Bone marrow depression, nausea, vomiting, diarrhea, stomatitis. Extravasation may lead to tissue necrosis.
Mitoxantrone (Novantrone)	IV infusion 12 mg/m^2 on days 1–3, for induction	Acute nonlymphocytic leukemia	Fever, cough, dyspnea, congestive heart failure, cardiac arrhythmias, nausea, vomiting, diarrhea
Pentastatin (Nipent)	IV 4 mg/m^2 every other week	Hairy cell leukemia unresponsive to alpha-interferon	Bone marrow depression, hepatotoxicity, nausea, vomiting, fever, skin rash
Plicamycin (Mithracin)	IV 25–30 μg/kg/d or every other day for eight to ten doses or until toxicity occurs	Testicular tumors, severe hypercalcemia	Toxicity affecting the bone marrow, liver, and kidneys. Extravasation can cause local tissue inflammation.
Plant Alkaloids			
Etoposide (VePesid)	IV 50–100 mg/m^2/d on days 1–5, or 100 mg/m^2/d on days 1, 3, and 5, every 3–4 wk	Testicular cancer, acute leukemias, lymphomas, small-cell lung cancer	Bone marrow depression, anaphylaxis, nausea, vomiting, alopecia
Teniposide (Vumon)	IV infusion 165 mg/m^2 twice weekly (with cytarabine)	Acute lymphocytic leukemia in children	Same as etoposide, above
Vinblastine (Velban)	IV 0.1 mg/kg weekly, increased gradually by 0.05 mg/kg increments	Metastatic testicular carcinoma, Hodgkin's disease, carcinoma of breast	Bone marrow depression, especially leukopenia, neurotoxicity. Extravasation may lead to tissue necrosis.
Vincristine (Oncovin)	Adults, IV 0.01–0.03 mg/kg weekly Children, IV 0.4–1.4 mg/m^2 weekly	Hodgkin's disease and other lymphomas, acute leukemia	Neurotoxicity with possible foot drop from muscle weakness, paresthesias, constipation, and other manifestations. Extravasation may lead to tissue necrosis.

TABLE 64-2 **CYTOTOXIC ANTINEOPLASTIC DRUGS** (Continued)

Generic/ Trade Name	Routes and Dosage Ranges*	Clinical Uses	Common or Potentially Severe Adverse Reactions
Vinorelbine (Navelbine)	IV injection 30 mg/m² once weekly, over 6–10 min, until disease progression or dose-limiting toxicity occurs	Non-small cell lung cancer	Bone marrow depression, peripheral neuropathy, chest pain, fatigue, nausea, alopecia
Miscellaneous Antineoplastic Agents			
Altretamine (Hexalen)	PO 260 mg/m²/d for 14 or 21 d in four doses, after meals and at bedtime	Advanced ovarian cancer	Nausea, vomiting, bone marrow depression, peripheral neuropathy
Asparaginase (Elspar)	IV 1000 IU/kg/d for 10 d	Acute lymphocytic leukemia refractory to other drugs. Usually used in conjunction with other agents.	Abnormal functioning of the liver, kidneys, pancreas, central nervous system, and the blood-clotting mechanism; hypersensitivity reactions
Cladribine (Leustatin)	IV infusion 0.09 mg/kg/d for 7 consecutive d	Hairy cell leukemia	Bone marrow depression, nausea, vomiting, fever
Dacarbazine (DTIC-Dome)	IV 3.5 mg/kg/d for 7 consecutive d	Malignant melanoma, Hodgkin's disease, sarcoma	Bone marrow depression, nausea and vomiting; increased blood urea nitrogen, aspartate aminotransferase and alanine aminotransferase. Extravasation may cause severe pain and tissue damage.
Docetaxol (Taxotere)	IV 60–100 mg/m², infused over 1 h, every 3 wk	Advanced breast cancer	Bone marrow depression, nausea, vomiting, diarrhea, edema, hypotension, oral mucositis, changes in liver enzymes, skin rash, alopecia
Gemcitabine (Gemzar)	IV 1000 mg/m² over 30 min once weekly. First cycle, up to 7 wk or toxicity occurs, then withhold for 1 wk. Later cycles, once weekly for 3 wk, then off for 1 wk	Pancreatic cancer	Bone marrow depression, nausea, vomiting, fever, influenza-like symptoms, edema, skin rash, alopecia
Hydroxyurea (Hydrea)	PO 80 mg/kg as single dose every third day or 20–30 mg/kg as a single dose daily	Chronic granulocytic leukemia, malignant melanoma	Bone marrow depression, GI upset
Irinotecan (Camptosar)	IV infusion over 90 min, 125 mg/m² once weekly for 4 wk, followed by a 2-wk rest period	Advanced colorectal cancer that has relapsed or progressed with 5-fluorouracil therapy	Bone marrow depression, nausea, vomiting, diarrhea, abdominal cramping
Levamisole (Ergamisol)	PO 50 mg every 8 h for 3 d every 2 wk for 1 y	Colon cancer, with fluorouracil	Nausea, vomiting, diarrhea, dermatitis
Mitotane (Lysodren)	PO 8–10 g daily in three to four divided doses. Maximal daily dose, 19 g	Inoperable carcinoma of the adrenal cortex	Anorexia, nausea, damage to adrenal cortex
Paclitaxel (Taxol)	IV 135 mg/m² every 3 wk	Advanced ovarian cancer	Bone marrow depression, allergic reactions, hypotension, bradycardia, peripheral neuropathy, nausea, vomiting, muscle and joint pain, alopecia
Procarbazine (Matulane)	PO 100–200 mg/d for 1 wk, then 300 mg/d until maximal response or toxicity occurs	Hodgkin's disease	Bone marrow depression, nausea, vomiting

(continued)

TABLE 64-2 CYTOTOXIC ANTINEOPLASTIC DRUGS (Continued)

Generic/Trade Name	Routes and Dosage Ranges*	Clinical Uses	Common or Potentially Severe Adverse Reactions
Topetecan (Hycamtin)	IV infusion 1.5 mg/m² over 30 min daily for 5 consecutive days	Advanced ovarian cancer	Bone marrow depression, nausea, vomiting, diarrhea, constipation, abdominal pain, alopecia, fatigue, fever
Tretinoin (Vesanoid)	PO 45 mg/m²/d in two divided doses until complete remission occurs, then for 30 additional days or a total of 90 d	Acute promyelocytic leukemia that has relapsed after other therapy	Fever, headache, bone pain, nausea, vomiting, diarrhea, constipation, dyspnea, mucositis, weakness, hypotension, cardiac arrhythmias

*Dosages change frequently according to use in different types of cancer and in combination with other antineoplastic drugs.

TABLE 64-3 ANTINEOPLASTIC HORMONES AND HORMONE INHIBITORS

Generic/Trade Name	Routes and Dosage Ranges	Clinical Uses	Common or Potentially Severe Adverse Reactions
Hormones			
Adrenocorticosteroid			
Prednisone (Meticorten, others)	PO 60–100 mg/m²/d for first few days, then gradual reduction to 20–40 mg/d	Used as adjunct for palliation of symptoms in acute leukemia, Hodgkin's disease, lymphomas, complications of cancer, such as thrombocytopenia, hypercalcemia, intracranial metastases	Potentially toxic to almost all body systems. See Chapter 24.
Androgens			
Fluoxymesterone (Halotestin)	PO 10 mg three times daily (30 mg/d)	Advanced breast cancer in premenopausal women	Masculinizing effects, hypercalcemia
Testolactone (Teslac)	PO 250 mg four times daily	Advanced breast cancer	Anorexia, nausea, vomiting, alopecia, paresthesias
Estrogens			
Diethylstilbestrol (DES) (Stilbestrol)	Breast cancer, PO 1–5 mg three times daily Prostate cancer, PO 1–3 mg daily	Carcinoma of prostate gland, carcinoma of breast in postmenopausal women	Feminizing effects in men, anorexia, nausea, vomiting, edema, hypercalcemia, and others. See Chapter 28.
Ethinyl estradiol (Estinyl, others)	Breast cancer, PO 0.5 mg/d initially, gradually increased to 3 mg/d in three divided doses Prostate cancer, PO 0.15–2 mg daily	Carcinoma of prostate, advanced carcinoma of breast in postmenopausal women	Feminizing effects in men, anorexia, nausea, vomiting, edema, hypercalcemia, and others. See Chapter 28.
Progestins			
Medroxyprogesterone (Provera, Depo-Provera)	IM 400–800 mg twice weekly PO 200–300 mg/d	Advanced endometrial carcinoma	Usually well tolerated. May cause edema and irritation at injection sites.
Megestrol (Megace)	PO 40–320 mg/d in divided doses	Advanced endometrial carcinoma, breast carcinoma	Usually produces minimal adverse reactions

TABLE 64-3 ANTINEOPLASTIC HORMONES AND HORMONE INHIBITORS

Generic/ Trade Name	Routes and Dosage Ranges	Clinical Uses	Common or Potentially Severe Adverse Reactions
Hormone Inhibitors			
Adrenocorticosteroid Inhibitor			
Amino- glutethimide (Cytadren)	PO 250 mg four times daily	Advanced prostatic cancer	Adrenal insufficiency
Antiandrogens			
Bicalutamide (Casodex)	PO 500 mg once daily (with goserelin or leuprolide)	Advanced prostatic cancer	Nausea, vomiting, diarrhea, constipation, hot flashes, gynecomastia, pain, weakness
Flutamide (Eulexin)	PO 250 mg every 8 h	Advanced prostatic cancer	Hot flashes, decreased libido, impotence, nausea, vomiting, diarrhea, gynecomastia
Nilutamide (Nilandron)	PO 300 mg daily for 30 d, then 150 mg daily	Advanced breast cancer in postmenopausal women with disease progression after tamoxifen therapy	Diarrhea, GI bleeding, heart failure, cough, hyperglycemia
Antiestrogens			
Anastrazole (Arimidex)	PO 1 mg once daily	Advanced breast cancer in postmenopausal women with disease progression after tamoxifen therapy	Nausea, vomiting, diarrhea, constipation, hot flashes, gynecomastia, pain, weakness
Tamoxifen (Nolvadex)	PO 20–40 mg/d in two divided doses	Advanced breast cancer in postmenopausal women	Hot flashes, nausea and vomiting, ocular toxicity
Gonadotropin-Releasing Hormone Analogues (Antitestosterone Effects)			
Goserelin (Zoladex)	SC 3.6 mg every 28 d	Advanced prostatic cancer, advanced breast cancer, endometriosis	Worsening of symptoms during first few weeks, especially bone pain
Leuprolide (Lupron)	SC 1 mg/d	Advanced prostatic cancer	Same as for goserelin, above

Drugs That Reduce Toxicity of Antineoplastic Drugs

Because cytotoxic antineoplastic drugs damage normal cells as well as malignant cells, adverse drug effects may be severe, debilitating, and even life-threatening to patients. Severe adverse effects may also limit drug dosage or frequency of administration, thereby limiting the potential effectiveness of chemotherapy. To reduce the toxic effects of chemotherapeutic agents, several drugs have been developed. These "antidotes" may protect certain body cells from one or more adverse effects and allow a more optimal dose and schedule of cytotoxic agents. It is important to note that:

A cytoprotective agent does not prevent or treat all adverse effects of a particular cytotoxic agent.

The cytoprotective agent may have adverse effects of its own.

Administration and scheduling must be precise in relation to administration of the cytotoxic agent.

Amifostine produces a metabolite that combines with cisplatin and ameliorates cisplatin-induced renal damage. **Dexrazoxane** decreases cardiac toxicity of doxorubicin. **Erythropoietin, filgrastim,** and **sargramostim** are colony-stimulating factors (see Chap. 44) that stimulate the bone marrow to produce blood cells. Erythropoetin is used for anemia; filgrastim and sargramostim are used to shorten neutropenia and the accompanying risk of severe infection. **Leucovorin** is used with high-dose methotrexate. **Mesna** is used with ifosfamide. Ifosfamide produces a metabolite that causes hemorrhagic cystitis. Mesna combines with and inactivates the metabolite and thereby decreases cystitis. Dosages and routes of administration for these medications are listed in Table 64-4.

TABLE 64-4 CYTOPROTECTIVE AGENTS

Generic/ Trade Name	Clinical Uses	Routes and Dosage Ranges
Amifostine (Ethyol)	Reduction of cisplatin-induced renal toxicity	IV infusion 910 mg/m^2 once daily, over 15 min, within 30 min of starting chemotherapy
Dexrazoxane (Zinecard)	Reduction of doxorubicin-induced cardiomyopathy in women with metastatic breast cancer who have received a cumulative dose of 300 mg/m^2 and would benefit from additional doxorubicin	IV 10 times the amount of doxorubicin (*e.g.,* dexrazoxane 500 mg/m^2 per doxorubicin 50 mg/m^2), then administer the doxorubicin dose within 30 min of completing administration of dexrazoxane
Erythropoietin (Epogen, Procrit)	Treatment of chemotherapy-induced anemia	SC 150 units/kg three times weekly, increased to 300 units/kg if necessary, adjusted to maintain desired hematocrit
Filgrastrim (Neupogen)	Treatment of chemotherapy-induced neutropenia	SC, IV 5 μ/kg/d, at least 24 h after a dose of cytotoxic chemotherapy, up to 2 wk or an absolute neutrophil count of 10000/mm^3
Leucovorin (Wellcovorin)	"Rescue" after high dose methotrexate (MTX) for osteosarcoma Advanced colorectal cancer, with 5-Fluorouracil (5-FU)	"Rescue," PO, IV, IM 15 mg q6h for 10 doses, starting 24 h after MTX begun Colorectal cancer, IV injection, 20 mg/m^2 or 200 mg/m^2, followed by 5-FU injection, daily for 5 d, then repeated every 28 d
Mesna (Mesnex)	Prevention of ifosfamide-induced hemorrhagic cystitis	IV injection, 20% of ifosfamide dose for three doses; first dose at time of ifosfamide administration; repeat at 4 h and 8 h after ifosfamide dose. (Total dose, 60% of ifosfamide dose).
Sargramostim (Leukine)	To decrease neutropenia associated with induction chemotherapy for acute myelogenous leukemia in patients older than 55 y	IV 250 μ/m^2/d, over 4 h, starting 4 d after completing induction chemotherapy

Nursing Process

Assessment

Assess the client's condition before drug therapy is started and frequently throughout the course of treatment. Knowledge about the type of malignancy the client has is necessary for adequate assessment. Useful information includes the main organs affected, whether the tumor grows slowly or rapidly, and usual patterns of metastasis. Specific assessment data include the following:

- Grade of the malignancy. Tumor grading describes the degree of malignancy. It is done by biopsy and histologic examination. Grade 1 and 2 tumors show cellular differentiation and are similar to the normal tissue of origin. Grade 3 and 4 tumors are less differentiated, bear little resemblance to the normal tissue of origin, and are more malignant. Generally, the higher the tumor grade, the poorer the prognosis. Criteria for each grade vary with the type of cancer.
- Stage of the malignancy. Staging describes the extent of the malignant process (*i.e.,* whether the tumor is localized or has spread). It also determines which organs are involved in the malignant process. One system of staging is the TNM system. *T* stands for the primary tumor; subcategories (T_1, T_2, T_3) indicate increasing size. *N* indicates involvement of regional lymph nodes; N_0 means no involvement, and N_1 and N_2 indicate increasing nodal disease. *M* stands for metastasis; M_0 indicates absence of metastasis, and M_1 indicates metastatic spread.

Staging is done by the physician on the basis of a medical history, physical examination, and diagnostic tests, such as x-ray studies, radioisotope scans, tissue biopsies, cytologic examination of various body secretions, endoscopies, liver and other organ function studies, and sometimes exploratory laparotomy or thoracotomy.

- Laboratory test results. Several laboratory tests are useful in cancer chemotherapy. These are usually done before the beginning of drug therapy to establish baseline data for later comparison and during drug therapy to monitor drug effects.
  - **Blood tests for "tumor markers."** Alpha-fetoprotein is a fetal antigen normally present during intrauterine and early postnatal life but absent in adulthood. Increased amounts may indicate hepatic or testicular cancer. Carcinoembryonic antigen (CEA) is secreted by several types of malignant cells, especially by cells originating in the gastrointestinal tract. It is not a good screening test because false-positive and false-negative results occur. It can be useful in selected circumstances, however. For example, a rising CEA level may indicate progression of malignant disease and a need for evaluation or treatment. If CEA levels are elevated before surgery and disappear after surgery, this is a good indication of adequate tumor excision. If CEA levels rise later, it proba-

bly indicates recurrence of the tumor. In chemotherapy, falling CEA levels indicate drug effectiveness. Other tumor markers are immunoglobulins (elevated levels may indicate multiple myeloma), prostatic acid phosphatase (elevated levels may indicate prostatic cancer), and prostate-specific antigen (elevated levels may indicate prostatic cancer).

- **Complete blood count (CBC)** to check for anemia and other abnormalities. Of special interest are the leukocyte and platelet counts, because most antineoplastic drugs cause bone marrow depression manifested mainly by leukopenia and thrombocytopenia. A CBC and white blood cell differential are done before each cycle of chemotherapy. The tests are used to determine dosage and frequency of drug administration, to monitor bone marrow function so fatal bone marrow depression does not occur, and to assist the nurse in planning care. For example, the client is very susceptible to infection when the leukocyte count is low, and bleeding is likely when the platelet count is low. Nursing measures can be taken to prevent or minimize both of these complications of chemotherapy.
  - **Other tests.** These include serum calcium, uric acid, and others, depending on the particular organs affected by the malignant disease.
- Clinical manifestations of the malignancy. Common signs and symptoms include anemia, malnutrition, weight loss, pain, and infection; other symptoms depend on the particular organs affected.
- Other disease conditions. Determine whether other diseases are present and, if the client has had previous cancer treatment, the response obtained.
- Emotional and mental status. Anxiety and depression are common features at any point in cancer diagnosis and treatment. Other aspects of nursing assessment include the client's coping mechanisms, family relationships, and financial resources.

Nursing Diagnoses

- Pain, nausea and vomiting, and weakness related to disease process or drug therapy
- Altered Nutrition: Less Than Body Requirements related to disease process or drug therapy
- Activity Intolerance related to anemia and weakness from disease process or drug therapy
- Self-Care Deficit related to debilitation from disease process or drug therapy
- Anxiety related to the disease, its possible progression, and its treatment
- Ineffective Individual Coping related to medical diagnosis of cancer
- Ineffective Family Coping related to illness and treatment of a family member
- Altered Tissue Perfusion related to anemia
- Fluid Volume Deficit related to chemotherapy-induced nausea, vomiting, and diarrhea
- Body Image Disturbance related to drug-induced alopecia
- Risk for Injury: Infection related to drug-induced neutropenia
- Risk for Injury: Bleeding related to drug-induced thrombocytopenia
- Risk for Injury: Stomatitis (mucositis) related to damage of oral mucosal cells

- Sexual Dysfunction related to adverse drug effects
- Knowledge Deficit about cancer
- Knowledge Deficit about cancer chemotherapy

Planning/Goals

The client will:
- Receive assistance in coping with the diagnosis of cancer
- Experience reduced anxiety and fear
- Receive chemotherapy accurately
- Experience reduction of tumor size, change of laboratory values toward normal, or other therapeutic effects of chemotherapy
- Experience minimal bleeding, infection, nausea and vomiting, and other consequences of adverse drug effects
- Maintain adequate intake of food and fluid
- Maintain body weight
- Receive assistance in activities of daily living when needed
- Be informed about community resources for cancer care (*e.g.,* hospice, Reach to Recovery, other support groups)

Interventions

Because all antineoplastic drugs may cause adverse reactions ranging from relatively minor to life-threatening, measures are needed to prevent or minimize the incidence and intensity of adverse reactions. If they cannot be prevented, they must be detected as early as possible so treatment may be started and damaging effects may be decreased.

- **Nausea and vomiting** are common with most antineoplastic drugs. They usually occur within 1 or 2 hours of drug administration and may last for several hours. Various measures to prevent or treat nausea and vomiting have met with varying amounts of success.
  - Giving antineoplastic drugs at bedtime, often with a sedative, may allow the client to sleep through the hours when nausea and vomiting are likely to be most severe.
  - Antiemetic drugs (see Chap. 63) are probably most effective when started before administration of antineoplastic drugs and given on a regular schedule up to 48 hours afterward. The serotonin receptor antagonists, ondansetron and granisetron, are among the most effective antiemetics, especially when accompanied by a corticosteroid such as dexamethasone (usually a single dose of 10 to 20 mg). A benzodiazepine such as lorazepam is often included for anticipatory nausea and vomiting. Several other agents and regimens may also be used.
  - Oral intake after drug administration is probably best determined by the client through trial and error. Some clients feel better if they avoid oral intake for a few hours; others tolerate small amounts of liquid and dry carbohydrates, such as crackers. As soon as nausea and vomiting are relieved, a normal diet can be resumed.
- **Anorexia** and altered taste perception are related problems that interfere with nutrition. Well-balanced meals, consisting of foods the client is able and willing to eat, are very important. Also, nutritional supplements can be used to increase intake of protein and calories.
- **Alopecia** occurs with several of the more frequently used antineoplastic drugs, such as cyclophosphamide, doxorubicin, methotrexate, and vincristine. Complete hair loss can be psychologically devastating, especially for women. Mea-

sures to help decrease the impact of alopecia include the following:

- Warn clients before drug therapy is started. Reassure them that alopecia is usually temporary and reversible when drug therapy is stopped. Sometimes hair growth returns even while drug therapy continues. Hair may grow back a different color and texture.
- Suggest the purchase of wigs, hats, and scarves. This should be done before hair loss is expected to occur.
- Suggest that clients avoid permanent waves, hair coloring, or other hair treatments that damage the hair and may affect the degree of hair loss.
- Allow clients to express feelings about altered body image.
- **Mucositis** (stomatitis) occurs often with the antimetabolites, antibiotics, and plant alkaloids used in cancer chemotherapy. It is likely to interfere with nutrition, lead to oral infections and bleeding, and cause considerable discomfort. Some guidelines for minimizing or treating stomatitis follow; most of these can be done by the client after the nurse has explained their purpose, whereas others must be done by or with the assistance of the nurse:
  - Brush the teeth at least twice daily with a soft-bristled toothbrush. Stop brushing the teeth if the platelet count drops below 20,000/mm^3 because gingival bleeding is likely. Teeth may then be cleaned with toothettes (soft sponge-tipped devices) or cotton-tipped applicators dipped in a dilute hydrogen peroxide solution.
  - Floss teeth daily with unwaxed floss. Stop if the platelet count drops below 20,000/mm^3 to prevent gingival bleeding.
  - Rinse the mouth several times daily, especially before meals (to decrease unpleasant taste and increase appetite) and after meals (to remove food particles that promote growth of microorganisms). One suggested solution is 1 tsp of table salt and 1 tsp of baking soda in 1 quart of water. Commercial mouthwashes are irritating and drying to oral mucosa and are not recommended for use.
  - Encourage the client to drink fluids. Systemic dehydration and local dryness of the oral mucosa contribute to the development and progression of mucositis. Pain and soreness contribute to dehydration. Fluids usually tolerated include tea, carbonated beverages, and ices, such as popsicles. Gelatin desserts also are usually well tolerated and add to fluid intake. Fruit juices are not usually recommended, especially citrus juices, such as orange and grapefruit, because they may produce pain, burning, and further tissue irritation. They may be tolerated if diluted with water or carbonated beverages, such as Sprite or 7-Up. Drinking fluids through a straw may be more comfortable, because this decreases contact of fluids with painful ulcerations.
  - Encourage the client to eat soft, bland, cold, nonacidic foods. Although individual tolerances vary, it is usually better to avoid highly spiced or rough foods.
  - Remove dentures entirely or for at least 8 hours daily, because they may irritate oral mucosa.
  - Inspect the mouth daily for signs of inflammation and lesions.
  - Give medications for pain. Local anesthetic solutions, such as viscous lidocaine, can be used about 15 minutes before meals to make eating more comfortable. Because the mouth and throat are anesthetized, swallowing and detecting the temperature of hot foods may be difficult, and aspiration or burns may occur. Doses should not exceed 15 ml every 3 hours or 120 ml in 24 hours. If systemic analgesics are used, they should be given about 30 to 60 minutes before eating.
  - In oral infections resulting from stomatitis, local or systemic anti-infective drugs are used. Fungal infections with *Candida albicans,* which are common, can be treated with antifungal tablets, suspensions, or lozenges. Severe infections may require systemic antibiotics, depending on the causative organism as identified by cultures of mouth lesions.
- **Infection** is common because the disease and its treatment lower host resistance to infection. Measures to prevent infection are aimed toward increasing host resistance and decreasing exposure to pathogenic microorganisms. Measures to minimize infection are aimed toward early detection and treatment.
  - Help the client maintain a well-balanced diet. Oral hygiene before meals and analgesics when appropriate may increase food intake. High-protein, high-calorie foods and fluids can be given between meals. Several types of nutritional supplements are available commercially and can be taken with or between meals. Provide fluids with high nutritional value (*e.g.,* milkshakes or nutritional supplements) rather than coffee, tea, or carbonated beverages if the client can tolerate them and has an adequate intake of water and other fluids.
  - Instruct and assist the client to avoid exposure to infection by avoiding crowds, anyone with a known infection, and contact with fresh flowers, soil, animals, or animal excrement.
  - Frequent and thorough handwashing by the client and everyone involved in his or her care is probably the best way to reduce exposure to pathogenic microorganisms.
  - The client should take a bath daily and put on clean clothes. In addition, the perineal area should be washed with soap and water after each urination or defecation.
  - When venous access devices are used, take particular care to prevent them from becoming sources of infection. For implanted catheters, for example, inspect and cleanse around exit sites according to agency policies and procedures. Use strict sterile technique when changing dressings or flushing the catheters. For peripheral venous lines, the same principles of care apply, except that sites should be changed about every 3 days or if signs of phlebitis occur.
  - Avoid indwelling urinary catheters when possible. If they are necessary, cleanse the perineal area with soap and water at least once daily and provide sufficient fluids to ensure an adequate urine output.
  - Signs and symptoms of infection may not be obvious in the person whose defenses against infection are compromised. Fever is probably the most consistent symptom. If it occurs, assume it is caused by infection, and try to determine the source. Rectal temperature measurements are usually avoided because of the risk of mucosal trauma and subsequent infection.
  - When infection is suspected, possible sources are cultured and antibiotics initiated without waiting for culture reports.

- Severe leukopenia can be prevented or its extent and duration minimized by administering colony-stimulating factors (*e.g.,* filgrastim or sargramostim) that stimulate the bone marrow to produce leukocytes (see Chap. 44). If severe leukopenia develops, a protective environment is indicated to decrease exposure to pathogens. Recommendations, resources, and policies vary regarding protective environments, at least partly because most infections are caused by microorganisms from the client's own body rather than exogenous sources. Transfusions of white blood cells may be given in some circumstances.
- **Bleeding** may be caused by thrombocytopenia, and precautions should be instituted if the platelet count drops to 50,000/mm³ or below. Bleeding may occur spontaneously or with seemingly minor trauma. Measures to avoid bleeding include
  - Avoid trauma, including venipuncture, injections, and rectal temperatures when possible.
  - Use an electric razor for shaving.
  - Check skin, urine, and stool for blood.
  - For platelet counts less than 20,000/mm³, stop brushing the teeth. Platelet transfusions may be given.
- **Extravasation** is the leakage of drug into subcutaneous tissues around an IV injection site. Many of the cytotoxic antineoplastic drugs cause severe inflammation, pain, and even tissue necrosis if extravasation occurs. Thus, efforts are needed to prevent extravasation if possible or to minimize tissue damage if it occurs.
  - Start an IV infusion. Avoid veins that are small, located in an edematous extremity, or located near a joint.
  - With the IV infusion running rapidly, inject the drug into the IV tubing with a small-gauge needle. This provides for relatively slow administration and rapid dilution of the drug. In addition, if extravasation should occur, it can be detected quickly and stopped when only small amounts of drug have been injected into subcutaneous tissues.
  - After the drug has been injected, continue the rapid flow rate of the IV fluid for 2 to 5 minutes to thoroughly flush the vein.
  - If extravasation occurs, various techniques have been suggested to decrease tissue damage. These include aspiration of the drug or injection of hydrocortisone through the IV line before it is removed, subcutaneous infiltration of hydrocortisone around the extravasated area, and application of ice bags or cold compresses. Nurses involved in cancer chemotherapy must know the procedure to be followed if extravasation occurs so it can be instituted immediately.
- **Hyperuricemia** results from rapid breakdown or destruction of malignant cells, whether it occurs spontaneously or as a result of antineoplastic drugs. Uric acid crystals can cause kidney damage. Uric acid nephropathy is the main danger to the client. The following measures minimize these effects:
  - Maintain a high fluid intake, with IV fluids if necessary, and a high urine output.
  - Alkalinize the urine with sodium bicarbonate or other agents.
  - Administer allopurinol to inhibit uric acid formation.
  Provide supportive care to clients and families.

- Physiologic care includes pain management, comfort measures, and assistance with nutrition, hygiene, ambulation, and other activities of daily living when needed.
- Psychological care includes allowing family members or significant others to be with the client and participate in care when desired and keeping clients and families informed. In addition, mental health professionals may be consulted to assist in coping with the distress that often accompanies cancer and its treatment.

 Teach clients:

- To practice meticulous personal hygiene, including frequent and thorough handwashing, and to avoid potential sources of infection when possible
- Ways to maintain or improve intake of food and fluids
- To use wigs, scarves, and hats to minimize the impact of alopecia, if expected with chemotherapy. These should be purchased before starting chemotherapy if possible.
- To decrease risks of bleeding by shaving with an electric razor, avoiding aspirin and other nonsteroidal anti-inflammatory drugs (*e.g.,* ibuprofen), and avoiding injections when possible
- To report fever, mouth soreness or ulcerations, or any sign of bleeding (*e.g.,* bruising, bleeding from gums, nose, seeing blood in urine or feces). If these occur, drug therapy may need to be changed or stopped.
- To inform any other physician, dentist, or health care provider that chemotherapy is being taken before any diagnostic test or treatment is begun. Some procedures may be contraindicated or require special precautions.
- To keep all appointments for drug therapy and blood tests for maximal benefits and minimal adverse effects

Evaluation

- Monitor drug administration for accuracy.
- Observe and interview for therapeutic effects of chemotherapy.
- Compare current laboratory reports with baseline values for changes toward normal values.
- Compare weight and nutritional status with baseline values for maintenance or improvement.
- Observe and interview for adverse drug reactions and interventions to prevent or control them.
- Observe and interview for adequate pain management and other symptom control.
- Observe and interview regarding mental and emotional status of the client and family members.
- Interview for knowledge of resources (*e.g.,* family, health care providers, hospice, others).

Principles of Therapy

PLANNING WITH CLIENT AND FAMILY

Once the diagnosis of cancer is made, the tumor is graded and staged, the client's physical and mental status is assessed, and the physician decides that chemotherapy is indicated, additional factors must be discussed with the client and family.

1. **What is the goal of chemotherapy?** It may be to cure the malignant disease, decrease tumor size, relieve symptoms, kill metastatic cells left after surgery or radiation therapy, or prolong life. When the goal is cure or induction of remission, adverse reactions and other disadvantages of chemotherapy may be acceptable. When expected benefit is minimal, even moderate morbidity due to drug therapy may be unacceptable.

2. **What adverse reactions are likely to occur?** Which reactions should be reported to the physician? How will they be managed if they occur? Even if the realities of chemotherapy are unpleasant, it is usually better for the client to know what they are than to fear the unknown. Some specific effects that should be discussed, depending on the drugs to be used, include alopecia, amenorrhea, oligospermia, and possibly permanent sterility. Because most of these drugs are teratogenic, clients in the reproductive years are advised to avoid pregnancy during treatment.

3. **Who will administer the drugs; where and for how long will they be administered?** Cancer chemotherapy is highly specialized. Because the drugs are highly toxic to both normal and malignant body cells and require meticulous techniques of administration, they are preferably given at a cancer treatment center. Some clients undergo chemotherapy at a cancer center far from home; others undergo treatment at a nearby hospital, clinic, physician's office, or even at home. The duration of treatment may be short or long, depending largely on the type of tumor and response to drug therapy. Thus, estimates of weeks, months, or years of drug therapy must be discussed. The time required for one drug treatment should be described as well so the client can schedule other activities.

    Usual practice requires that blood be drawn for a CBC and perhaps other tests. The results of these tests must be reported before antineoplastic drugs are given. If excessive leukopenia or thrombocytopenia is reported, drug therapy may be discontinued or postponed. Clients should be informed about the frequent venipunctures required for blood tests and drug administration.

4. **How can the client help to maximize therapeutic benefits of chemotherapy and minimize adverse effects?** One self-help measure is to eat a well-balanced diet. This may require great effort in the presence of anorexia, nausea, vomiting, diarrhea, or stomatitis. Another self-help measure is frequent and thorough oral hygiene. A third measure is to

keep all appointments for drug administration and blood tests.

DRUG SELECTION

Choice of drug or combination of drugs depends largely on which drugs have been effective in similar types of cancer. Other factors to be considered include primary tumor sites, presence and extent of metastases, physical status of the client, and other disease conditions that affect chemotherapy, such as liver or kidney disease.

COMBINATION DRUG THERAPY

Combinations of several drugs are often used in the continuing effort to increase therapeutic effects without increasing toxic effects. The effectiveness of various combinations is determined by clinical testing and is usually expressed as a percentage of the clients who respond favorably. Combinations also may prevent or delay the development of drug resistance. Combinations are based on knowledge of tumor cell kinetics and drug actions. Some general characteristics of effective drug combinations include the following:

1. Each drug should exert antineoplastic activity when used alone.
2. Each drug should act by a different mechanism. Drugs can be combined to produce either sequential inhibition or concurrent inhibition. For example, one drug can be chosen to damage the DNA, RNA, or proteins of the malignant cell, and another drug can be chosen to prevent their repair or synthesis.
3. Drugs should act at different times in the reproductive cycle of the malignant cell. For example, more malignant cells are likely to be destroyed by combining CCS and CCNS drugs. The first group kills only dividing cells; the second group kills cells during any part of the life cycle, including the resting or nondividing phase.
4. Consecutive doses kill a percentage of the tumor cells remaining after earlier doses and further decrease the tumor burden.
5. Toxic reactions of the various drugs should not overlap so maximal tolerated doses may be given. It is preferable to use drugs that are not toxic to the same organ system (*e.g.*, bone marrow, kidney) and to use drugs that do not exert their toxic effects at the same time. However, adverse reactions to drug combinations may differ considerably from those of each drug when given alone.
6. Combinations may require different dosages and schedules than single-agent drug therapy.

7. Recommendations about combination chemotherapy change as new drugs are developed or different combinations and schedules of older drugs are tried. Numerous combinations have been developed for use in specific types of cancer. For information about specific combinations and their clinical uses, see a current reference on cancer chemotherapy.

DOSAGE AND ADMINISTRATION FACTORS

Antineoplastic drugs are usually given in relatively high doses, on an intermittent or cyclic schedule. This regimen seems to be more effective than low doses given continuously or massive doses given once. It also produces less immunosuppression and provides drug-free periods during which normal tissues can repair themselves from damage inflicted by the drugs. Fortunately, normal cells repair themselves faster than malignant cells. Succeeding doses are given as soon as tissue repair becomes evident, usually when leukocyte and platelet counts return to acceptable levels.

Each antineoplastic drug must be used in the schedule, route, and dose judged to be most effective for a particular type of cancer. With combinations of drugs, the recommended schedule should be followed precisely because safety and effectiveness may be schedule dependent. When chemotherapy is used as an adjuvant to surgery, it usually should be started as soon as possible after surgery, given in maximal tolerated doses just as if advanced disease were present, and continued for several months (usually 1 year for breast cancer).

Dosage of antineoplastic drugs must be calculated and regulated carefully to avoid unnecessary toxicity. The age, nutritional status, blood count, kidney and liver function, and previous chemotherapy or radiation therapy must all be considered when determining dosage for a client. Additional factors that influence dosage are as follows:

1. Dosage is usually based on the recipient's body weight (mg/kg) or surface area (mg/m^2).
2. The usual dosages listed for individual drugs apply only when the drug is used as a single agent. In drug combinations, the amount of each agent must be determined by clinical investigations.
3. Dosage may be reduced on the basis of bone marrow depression (as indicated by leukopenia or thrombocytopenia), liver disease, or kidney disease.
4. Sex hormones used in cancer chemotherapy must be given in larger amounts (pharmacologic doses) than when they are used in hormone replacement therapy (physiologic doses). Consequently, adverse reactions are likely to be increased in incidence and severity.

GUIDELINES FOR HANDLING ANTINEOPLASTIC DRUGS

Antineoplastic drugs may exert adverse effects on nurses and other people who prepare and administer them. These effects include contact dermatitis and mutagenic cells in the urine. The extent and long-term consequences of the mutagenic cells are not yet known. Guidelines for handling the drugs to avoid adverse effects include the following:

1. Avoid contact with solutions for injection by wearing disposable gloves, eye protectors, and protective clothing (*e.g.*, long-sleeved garments).
2. If handling a powder form of a drug, wear a mask to avoid inhaling the powder.
3. Prepare the drugs on disposable trays or towels so spills can be contained.
4. Dispose of contaminated materials in specific chemotherapy waste containers. The containers should be incinerated at temperatures of 1800°F to 2000°F.

USE IN CHILDREN

Safety and effectiveness of most antineoplastic drugs have not been established, and few controlled studies have been done in children. However, children are at risk for a wide range of malignant diseases, including acute leukemias, lymphomas, brain tumors (neuroblastomas and others), Wilms' tumor (nephroblastoma), and sarcomas of muscle (*e.g.*, rhabdomyosarcoma) and bone (*e.g.*, osteosarcoma, Ewing's sarcoma).

Cancer chemotherapy is often used in conjunction with surgical excision or irradiation. Basic principles of therapy apply to children (*e.g.*, preventing or minimizing adverse effects and others). Long-term effects on growth and development of survivors are not clearly defined. Special efforts are needed to maintain nutrition, organ function, psychological support, and other aspects of growth and development.

USE IN OLDER ADULTS

Older adults are at risk of developing a wide range of malignant diseases. Although they also are likely to have renal impairment, chronic cardiovascular disorders, and other diseases that increase their risks of serious adverse effects, they should not be denied the potential benefits of chemotherapy on the basis of age alone. Instead, greater vigilance is needed to maximize benefits and minimize hazards of chemotherapy.

With impaired renal function, dosages of cyclophosphamide and methotrexate may need to be reduced. Creatinine clearance should be monitored; serum creatinine level is not a reliable indicator of renal function in older adults because of their decreased muscle mass.

With cardiovascular disorders, careful assessment and monitoring of cardiovascular status are required with the use of doxorubicin and other cardiotoxic drugs.

Older adults are especially sensitive to the neurotoxic effects of vincristine.

HOME CARE

Clients may receive injected cytotoxic drugs as outpatients at hospitals or physicians' offices and return home or the drugs may be administered in the home setting by the client or a caregiver. The home care nurse may be involved in a wide range of patient-care activities associated with cancer chemotherapy, including administering the antineoplastic drugs, administering drugs to prevent or manage adverse effects, and assessing client and family responses to therapy. In addition, a major role involves teaching about the disease process, management of pain and other symptoms, the anticancer drugs, prevention or management of adverse drug effects, preventing infection, maintaining food and fluid intake, and other aspects of care. If a client is receiving erythropoietin subcutaneously, the client or a caregiver may need to be taught injection technique.

NURSING ACTIONS

ANTINEOPLASTIC DRUGS

NURSING ACTIONS	*RATIONALE/EXPLANATION*
1. Administer accurately **a.** If not accustomed to giving cytotoxic antineoplastic drugs regularly, read package inserts, research protocols, or other recent drug references for specific instructions on administration of individual drugs.	Cancer chemotherapy has evolved into a highly specialized area of nursing practice with most agencies requiring training and demonstration of competency. Obtaining current information is necessary because of the large number and varied characteristics of the drugs; differences in administration according to the type of neoplasm being treated and other client characteristics; and continuing development of new drugs, dosages, routes, schedules of administration, and combinations of drugs.
b. For cytotoxic drugs to be given intravenously:	
(1) Compare labels on pre-prepared solutions to medication orders in terms of the drug, concentration, expiration date, and instructions for administration.	Many of the drugs must be reconstituted from a powder form and further diluted in an IV solution. Drug solutions should generally be prepared in the pharmacy to maintain sterility and avoid dispersing drug particles into the environment.
(2) A commonly used method is to inject the drug into the tubing of a rapidly flowing IV infusion.	To decrease tissue irritation and allow rapid detection of extravasation
(3) For clients with a long-term venous access device (*e.g.*, Hickman or Groshong catheter), follow agency protocols for drug administration and catheter care.	Long-term venous access devices are often desirable, to decrease the number of venipunctures a patient must undergo. These devices require special care to maintain patency and prevent infection of the patient's bloodstream.
(4) Follow agency protocols for skin exposure or spills of cytotoxic drug solutions.	These solutions are considered hazardous materials that require special handling.
c. For drugs to be given orally, the total dose of most drugs can be given at one time. An exception is mitotane, which is given in three or four divided doses.	
2. Observe for therapeutic effects **a.** Increased appetite **b.** Increased sense of well-being **c.** Improved mobility	Therapeutic effects depend to a large extent on the type of malignancy being treated. They may not become evident for several weeks after chemotherapy is begun. Some clients experience anorexia, nausea, and vomiting for 2 to 3 wk after each cycle of drug therapy.

NURSING ACTIONS	RATIONALE/EXPLANATION

d. Decreased pain

e. With busulfan, given for chronic myelogenous leukemia, also observe for decreased white blood cell count and decreased size of the spleen.

Decreased white blood cell count and splenomegaly usually become evident about the second or third week of drug therapy.

f. With melphalan, given for multiple myeloma, also observe for decreased amounts of abnormal proteins in urine and blood, decreased levels of serum calcium, and increased hemoglobin.

3. Observe for adverse effects

Because they are toxic to both normal and malignant cells, cytotoxic antineoplastic drugs may have adverse effects on almost any body tissue. These adverse effects range from common to rare, from relatively mild to life threatening. Some are expected, such as bone marrow depression, and this is used to guide drug therapy. Most of the adverse effects occur with usual dosage ranges and are likely to be increased in incidence and severity with larger doses.

a. Hematologic effects:

(1) Bone marrow depression with leukopenia (decreased white blood cell count), thrombocytopenia (decreased platelets), and anemia (decreased red blood cell count, hemoglobin, and hematocrit)

For most of these drugs, white blood cell count and platelet counts reach their lowest points about 7 to 14 d after drug administration and return toward normal after about 21 d. Normal leukocyte and platelet counts signify recovery of bone marrow function. Anemia may occur later because the red blood cell lives longer than white cells and platelets.

(2) Decreased antibodies and lymphocytes

Most of these drugs have immunosuppressant effects, which impair body defenses against infection.

b. Gastrointestinal (GI) effects—anorexia, nausea, vomiting, diarrhea, constipation, stomatitis and other mucosal ulcerations, oral candidiasis

Anorexia, nausea, and vomiting are very common. They usually occur within a few hours of drug administration. Nausea and vomiting often subside within approximately 12 to 24 h, but anorexia may persist. Constipation is most likely to occur with vincristine. Mucosal ulcerations may occur anywhere in the GI tract and can lead to serious complications (infection, hemorrhage, perforation). Their occurrence is usually an indication to stop drug therapy, at least temporarily. Fungal and bacterial infections may interfere with nutrition. They may be relatively mild or severe.

c. Integumentary effects—alopecia, dermatitis, tissue irritation at injection sites.

Complete hair loss may take several weeks to occur. Alopecia is most significant in terms of altered body image, possible mental depression, and other psychological effects. Several drugs may cause phlebitis and sclerosis of veins used for injections, as well as pain and tissue necrosis if allowed to leak into subcutaneous tissues around the injection site.

d. Renal effects:

(1) Hyperuricemia and uric acid nephropathy

When malignant cells are destroyed by drug therapy, they release uric acid into the bloodstream. Uric acid crystals may precipitate in the kidneys and cause impaired function or even renal failure. Adverse effects on the kidneys are especially associated with methotrexate and cisplatin. Hyperuricemia can be decreased by an ample fluid intake or by administration of allopurinol.

(2) With cyclophosphamide, hemorrhagic cystitis (blood in urine, dysuria, burning on urination)

Hemorrhagic cystitis is thought to occur in about 10% of the clients who receive cyclophosphamide and to result from ir-

(continued)

Nursing Actions	*Rationale/Explanation*
	ritating effects of drug metabolites on the bladder mucosa. The drug is stopped if this occurs. Cystitis can be decreased by an ample fluid intake.
e. Pulmonary effects—cough, dyspnea, chest x-ray changes	Adverse reactions affecting the lungs are associated mainly with bleomycin, busulfan, and methotrexate. With bleomycin particularly, pulmonary toxicity may be severe and progress to pulmonary fibrosis.
f. Cardiovascular effects—congestive heart failure (dyspnea, edema, fatigue), arrhythmias, ECG changes	Cardiomyopathy is associated primarily with daunorubicin and doxorubicin. This is a life-threatening adverse reaction. The heart failure may be unresponsive to digitalis preparations.
g. CNS effects—peripheral neuropathy with vincristine, manifested by muscle weakness, numbness and tingling of extremities, foot drop, and decreased ability to walk	This fairly common effect of vincristine may worsen for several weeks after drug administration. There is usually some recovery of function eventually.
h. Endocrine effects—menstrual irregularities, sterility in males and females	
4. Observe for drug interactions	
a. Drugs that *increase* effects of cytotoxic antineoplastic drugs:	
(1) Allopurinol	Allopurinol is usually given to prevent or treat hyperuricemia, which may occur with cancer chemotherapy. When given with mercaptopurine, allopurinol facilitates the formation of the active metabolite. Consequently, doses of mercaptopurine must be reduced to one third to one fourth the usual dose.
(2) Anticoagulants, oral	Increased risk of bleeding
(3) Bone marrow depressants	Increased bone marrow depression
(4) Other antineoplastic drugs	Additive cytotoxic effects, both therapeutic and adverse
b. Drugs that *increase* effects of cyclophosphamide:	
(1) Anesthetics, inhalation	Lethal combination. Discontinue cyclophosphamide at least 12 h before general inhalation anesthesia is to be given.
(2) Barbiturates	Potentiate cyclophosphamide by induction of liver enzymes, which accelerate transformation of the drug into its active metabolites
(3) Other alkylating antineoplastic drugs	Increased bone marrow depression
c. Drugs that *increase* effects of methotrexate:	
(1) Alcohol	Additive liver toxicity. Avoid concomitant use.
(2) Aspirin; analgesics and antipyretics containing aspirin or other salicylates; barbiturates; phenytoin; sulfonamides	Potentiate methotrexate by displacing it from protein-binding sites in plasma. Salicylates also block renal excretion of methotrexate. This may cause pancytopenia and liver toxicity. Salicylates are present in many prescription and nonprescription drugs, such as headache remedies, pain relievers, and cold remedies.
(3) Other hepatotoxic drugs	Additive liver toxicity
(4) Other antineoplastic drugs	Additive cytotoxic effects, both therapeutic and adverse. Methotrexate is one component of several drug combinations used to treat breast cancer.

NURSING ACTIONS	*RATIONALE/EXPLANATION*
d. Drugs that *decrease* effects of methotrexate: Leucovorin (citrovorum factor, folinic acid)	Leucovorin antagonizes the toxic effects of methotrexate and is used as an antidote for high-dose methotrexate regimens or for overdose. It must be given exactly at the specified time, before affected cells become too damaged to respond.
5. Teach clients **a.** With vincristine, eat high-fiber foods, such as raw fruits and vegetables and whole cereal grains, if able. Also try to maintain a high fluid intake. A stool softener or bulk laxative may be prescribed on a daily basis.	To prevent the constipation that may occur during vincristine therapy
b. With cyclophosphamide, drink 2 or 3 quarts of fluid daily, if possible, and urinate often, especially at bedtime. If blood is seen in the urine or signs of cystitis occur despite precautions, report this immediately.	Products of cyclophosphamide breakdown are irritating to the bladder lining and may cause bleeding, burning on urination, and other signs of cystitis. High fluid intake and frequent emptying of the bladder help to decrease bladder damage. If blood appears in the urine or if cystitis occurs, the drug should be discontinued.
c. With doxorubicin, the urine may turn red for 1 to 2 d after drug administration.	To decrease the anxiety that may occur if the client thinks the red urine is from bleeding. The discoloration is harmless.
d. Also with doxorubicin, the client should report edema, shortness of breath, and excessive fatigue.	These are signs of heart failure and require that drug therapy be stopped.

✔ REVIEW AND APPLICATION EXERCISES

1. Compare and contrast normal cells and malignant cells.

2. Which common or major cancers are attributed mainly to environmental factors? Which are attributed to genetic factors?

3. How do cytotoxic antineoplastic drugs destroy malignant cells?

4. Which cytotoxic antineoplastic drugs are associated with bone marrow suppression?

5. Which antineoplastic drugs are cardiotoxic? Which are nephrotoxic? Which are neurotoxic?

6. Which drugs are associated with second malignancies?

7. What is the basis for the anticancer effects of hormones and antihormones?

8. What is the rationale for combination chemotherapy in cancer?

9. Why are antiemetics, drugs for hypercalcemia, and allopurinol often used with clients who are taking antineoplastic drugs?

SELECTED REFERENCES

Abrahn, J.L. (1997). Cancer pain management. In W.N. Kelley (Ed.), *Textbook of internal medicine,* 3rd ed., pp. 1538–1543. Philadelphia: Lippincott-Raven.

Balmer, C. & Valley, A.W. (1997). Basic principles of cancer treatment and cancer chemotherapy. In J.T. DiPiro, R.L. Talbert, G.C. Yee, G.R. Matzke, B.G. Wells, & L.M. Posey (Eds.), *Pharmacotherapy: A pathophysiologic approach,* 3rd ed., pp. 2403–2465. Stamford, CT: Appleton & Lange.

Calabresi, P. & Chabner, B.A. (1996). Chemotherapy of neoplastic diseases: Introduction. In J.G. Hardman, L.E. Limbird, P.B. Molinoff, & R.W. Ruddon (Eds.), *Goodman & Gilman's The pharmacological basis of therapeutics,* 9th ed., pp. 1225–1232.

Chabner, B.A., Allegra, C.J., Curt, G.A., & Calabresi, P. (1996). Antineoplastic agents. In J.G. Hardman, L.E. Limbird, P.B. Molinoff, & R.W. Ruddon (Eds.), *Goodman & Gilman's The pharmacological basis of therapeutics,* 9th ed., pp. 1233–1287.

Dorr, R.T., & Dalton, W.S. (1993). Cancer chemotherapy. In R. Bressler & M.D. Katz (Eds.), *Geriatric pharmacology,* pp. 535–583. New York: McGraw-Hill.

Drug facts and comparisons. (Updated monthly). St. Louis: Facts and Comparisons.

Fessele, K.S. (1996). Managing the multiple causes of nausea and vomiting in the patient with cancer. *Oncology Nursing Forum* 23(9), 1409–1415.

Furlong, T.G. (1993). Neurologic complications of immunosuppressive cancer therapy. *Oncology Nursing Forum,* 20, 1337–1354.

Graham, K.M., Pecoraro, D.A., Ventura, M., & Meyer, C.C. (1993). Reducing the incidence of stomatitis using a quality assessment and improvement approach. *Cancer Nursing,* 16(2), 117–122.

McEnroe, L.E. (1996). Role of the oncology nurse in home care: Family-centered practice. *Seminars in Oncology Nursing, 12*(3), 188–192.

Porth, C.M. (1994). *Pathophysiology: Concepts of altered health states,* 4th ed., pp. 71–99. Philadelphia: J.B. Lippincott.

Rokita, S. (1996). Oncology: Nursing the patient with cancer. In Smeltzer, S.C. & Bare, B.G. *Brunner and Suddarth's Textbook of medical-surgical nursing,* 8th ed., pp. 265–316. Philadelphia: Lippincott-Raven.

Seiden, M., Urba, W., & Chabner, B.A. (1997). Principles of chemotherapy and hormonal therapy. In W.N. Kelley (Ed.), *Textbook of internal medicine,* 3rd ed., pp. 1508–1518. Philadelphia: Lippincott-Raven.

Urba, W.J. & Chabner, B.A. (1997). Principles of biologic therapy. In W.N. Kelley (Ed.), *Textbook of internal medicine,* 3rd ed., pp. 1518–1522. Philadelphia: Lippincott-Raven.

Weinberg, R.A. (September 1996). How cancer arises. *Scientific American,* 62–70.

65

Drugs Used in Ophthalmic Conditions

Outline

Objectives

After studying this chapter, the student will be able to:

1 Review characteristics of ocular structures that influence drug therapy of eye disorders.

2 Discuss autonomic nervous system (ANS), antimicrobial, anti-inflammatory, and selected miscellaneous drugs in relation to their use in ocular disorders.

3 Use correct techniques to administer ophthalmic medications.

4 Assess for ocular effects of systemic drugs and systemic effects of ophthalmic drugs.

5 Teach clients, family members, or caretakers correct administration of eye medications.

6 For a client with an eye disorder, teach about the importance of taking medications as prescribed to protect and preserve eyesight.

Key Terms

Conjunctiva	**Mydriasis**
Glaucoma	**Refraction**
Miosis	**Tonometry**

Structures of the Eye

The eye is the major sensory organ through which the person receives information about the external environment. An in-depth discussion of vision and ocular anatomy is beyond the scope of this chapter, but some characteristics and functions are described to facilitate understanding of ocular drug therapy. These include the following:

1. The eyelids and lacrimal system function to protect the eye. The *eyelid* is a covering that acts as a barrier to the entry of foreign bodies, strong light, dust, and other potential irritants. The *conjunctiva* is the mucous membrane lining of the eyelids. The *canthi* (singular, canthus) are the angles where upper and lower eyelids meet. The *lacrimal system* produces a fluid that constantly moistens and cleanses the anterior surface of the eyeball. The fluid drains through two small openings in the inner canthus and flows through the nasolacrimal duct into the nasal cavity. When the conjunctiva is irritated or certain emotions are experienced (*e.g.,* sadness), the lacrimal gland produces more fluid than the drainage system can accommodate. The excess fluid overflows the eyelids and becomes *tears.*

2. The eyeball is a spherical structure composed of the sclera, cornea, choroid, and retina, plus special refractory tissues. The *sclera* is a white, opaque fibrous tissue that covers the posterior five sixths of the eyeball. The *cornea* is a transparent, special connective tissue that covers the anterior sixth of the eyeball. The cornea contains no blood vessels. The *choroid,* composed of blood vessels and connective tissue, continues forward to form the iris. The *iris* is composed of pigmented cells, the opening called the *pupil,* and muscles that control the size of the pupil by contracting or dilating in response to stimuli. The *retina* is the innermost layer of the eyeball.

   For vision to occur, light rays must enter the eye through the cornea; travel through the pupil, lens, and vitreous body (see below); and be focused on the retina. Light rays do not travel directly to the retina. Instead, they are deflected in various directions according to the density of the ocular structures through which they pass. This process, called *refraction,* is controlled by the aqueous humor, lens, and vitreous body. The *optic disk* is the area of the retina where ophthalmic blood vessels and the optic nerve enter the eyeball.

3. The structure and function of the eyeball are further influenced by the lens, aqueous humor, and vitreous body. The *lens* is an elastic, transparent structure; its function is to focus light rays to form images on the retina. It is located behind the iris and held in place by suspensory ligaments attached to the ciliary body. The *aqueous humor* is a clear fluid produced by capillaries in the ciliary body. Most of the fluid flows through the pupil into the anterior chamber (between the cornea and the lens and anterior to the iris). A small amount flows into a passage called Schlemm's canal, from which it enters the venous circulation. Under normal circumstances, production and drainage of aqueous humor are approximately equal, and normal intraocular pressure (about 10 to 20 mm Hg) is maintained. Impaired drainage of aqueous humor causes increased intraocular pressure. The *vitreous body* is a transparent, jelly-like mass located in the posterior portion of the eyeball. It functions to refract light rays and maintain the normal shape of the eyeball.

Disorders of the Eye

The eye is subject to the development of many disorders that threaten its structure, function, or both. Some disorders in which ophthalmic drugs play a prominent role include the following.

REFRACTIVE ERRORS

Refractive errors include myopia (nearsightedness), hyperopia (farsightedness), presbyopia, and astigmatism. These conditions impair vision by interfering with the eye's ability to focus light rays on the retina. Ophthalmic drugs are used only in the diagnosis of the conditions; treatment involves prescription of eyeglasses or contact lenses.

GLAUCOMA

Glaucoma, a common preventable cause of blindness, was formerly defined as increased intraocular pressure. The definition has changed because glaucoma may occur with normal intraocular pressure and because some people have increased intraocular pressure without having glaucoma. Thus, glaucoma is now described as a group of diseases characterized by optic nerve damage and changes in visual fields. Diagnostic tests for glaucoma include ophthalmoscopic examination of the optic disk, measurement of intraocular pressure (tonometry), and testing of visual fields.

The most common type of glaucoma is called primary open-angle glaucoma. It is a chronic disorder of unknown cause. A less common but more dramatic type is called narrow-angle glaucoma. Acute narrow-angle glaucoma, which occurs with a sudden, severe increase in intraocular pressure, causes progressive ocular damage and loss of vision unless promptly and effectively treated. Acute increases in intraocular pressure occur in people with narrow-angle glaucoma when pupils are dilated and the outflow of aqueous humor is blocked. Darkness and numerous drugs (*e.g.,* anticholinergics, antihistamines, antipsychotics, and tricyclic antidepressants) may precipitate acute glaucoma. Secondary glaucoma may follow traumatic or inflammatory conditions of the eye.

INFLAMMATORY OR INFECTIOUS CONDITIONS

Inflammation may be caused by bacteria, viruses, allergic reactions, or irritating chemicals. Infections may result from foreign bodies, contaminated hands, contaminated equipment or solutions used in treatment, or infections in contiguous structures (*e.g.,* nose, face, sinuses). Common inflammatory and infectious disorders include the following:

1. **Conjunctivitis** is often caused by allergic reactions that are characterized by a watery discharge and pruritus. A highly contagious form of conjunctivitis ("pink eye") commonly occurs in children. Chronic conjunctivitis is usually caused by *Staphylococcus aureus, Streptococcus viridans,* or *Diplococcus pneumoniae* and is characterized by mucoid or mucopurulent discharge and red, edematous conjunctiva. Conjunctivitis with a purulent discharge is most often caused by the gonococcus; corneal ulcers and scarring may result.
2. **Blepharitis** is a chronic infection of glands and lash follicles on the margins of the eyelids. A hordeolum (commonly called a sty) is often associated with blepharitis. The most common causes are seborrhea and staphylococcal infections.
3. **Keratitis** (inflammation of the cornea) may be caused by microorganisms, trauma, allergy, ischemia, and drying of the cornea (*e.g.,* from inadequate lacrimation or inability to close the eyelid). The major symptom is pain, which ranges from mild to severe. Vision may not be affected initially. However, if not treated effectively, corneal ulceration, scarring, and impaired vision may result.
4. Bacterial **corneal ulcers** are most often caused by pneumococci and staphylococci. Pseudomonal ulcers are less common but may rapidly progress to perforation. Fungal ulcers may follow topical corticosteroid therapy or injury with vegetable matter, such as a tree branch. Viral ulcers are usually caused by the herpesvirus.

Ophthalmic Drugs

Drugs used to diagnose or treat ophthalmic disorders represent numerous therapeutic classifications, most of which are discussed in other chapters. Some drugs are used primarily by ophthalmologists. Major classes of drugs used in ophthalmology include the following:

1. Anti-infective drugs are used to treat bacterial, viral, and fungal infections (see Chaps. 33 through 41). They are usually applied topically but may be injected subconjunctivally or intravenously in severe infections.
2. Autonomic drugs are used extensively in ophthalmology for diagnostic and therapeutic purposes (see Chaps. 17 through 21). Some are used to dilate the pupil before ophthalmologic examinations or surgical procedures; some are used to decrease intraocular pressure in glaucoma. Ophthalmic beta-adrenergic blocking agents are the most commonly used drugs for treatment of glaucoma, in which they decrease intraocular pressure by decreasing formation of aqueous humor.

    Autonomic drugs indicated in one disorder may be contraindicated in another (*e.g.,* anticholinergic drugs are usually contraindicated in glaucoma). In addition, adrenergic mydriatics (*e.g.,* epinephrine, phenylephrine) should be used cautiously in clients with hypertension, cardiac arrhythmias, arteriosclerotic heart disease, and hyperthyroidism. Ophthalmic beta-blockers generally have the same contraindications and precautions as oral or injected drugs (*e.g.,* bradycardia, heart block, congestive heart failure, bronchospastic disorders).
3. Corticosteroids (see Chap. 24) are often used to treat inflammatory conditions of the eye, thereby reducing scarring and preventing loss of vision. Corticosteroids are generally more effective in acute than chronic inflammatory conditions. Because these drugs are potentially toxic, they should not be used to treat minor disorders or disorders that can be effectively treated with safer drugs. When used, corticosteroids should be administered in the lowest effective dose and for the shortest effective time. Long-term use should be avoided when possible. When used in ophthalmologic conditions, corticosteroids may be administered topically, systemically, or both. Corticosteroids are contraindicated in eye infections caused by the herpes virus because the drugs increase the severity of the infection.
4. Ophthalmic preparations of some nonsteroidal anti-inflammatory drugs (NSAIDs) (see Table 65-3 and Chap. 7) may be used in eye disorders.
5. Carbonic anhydrase inhibitors and osmotic diuretics are given to decrease intraocular pressure in glaucoma and before certain surgical procedures. Carbonic anhydrase inhibitors lower intraocular pressure by decreasing production of aqueous humor.
6. Fluorescein (Ful-Glo) is a dye used in diagnosing lesions or foreign bodies in the cornea, fitting contact lenses, and studying the lacrimal system and

flow of aqueous humor. Rose bengal is another dye that may be used.

Drug therapy of ophthalmic conditions is unique because of the location, structure, and function of the eye. Many systemic drugs are unable to cross the blood-eye barrier and achieve therapeutic concentrations in ocular structures. Some drugs penetrate the eye better than others, however, depending on the serum drug concentration, size of drug molecules, solubility of the drug in fat, extent of drug protein binding, and whether inflammation is present in the eye. Generally, penetration is greater if the drug achieves a high concentration in the blood, has small molecules, is fat soluble, is poorly bound to serum proteins, and if inflammation is present.

METHODS OF ADMINISTRATION

Because of the difficulties associated with systemic therapy, various methods of administering drugs locally have been developed. The most common method of drug administration in ocular therapeutics is topical application of ophthalmic solutions (eye drops) to the conjunctiva. Drugs are distributed through the tear film covering the eye and may be used for superficial disorders (*e.g.,* conjunctivitis) or for relatively deep ocular disorders (*e.g.,* when epinephrine is given for glaucoma, the drug must penetrate the cornea, anterior chamber, and ciliary processes to exert therapeutic effects). Other topical dosage forms include ophthalmic ointments and a specialized method of administering pilocarpine so the drug is slowly released over a 1-week period (Ocusert). Ocusert is a small plastic device inserted into the conjunctival area and replaced weekly by the client. It may be used for long-term management of glaucoma.

Other methods of local administration of drugs involve special injection techniques used by ophthalmologists. These include injections through the conjunctiva to subconjunctival tissues or under the fibrous capsule beneath the conjunctiva (sub-Tenon's injection). These injections are painful, and topical anesthetic solutions should be applied before the procedure. Antibiotics and corticosteroids are the drugs most likely to be administered by subconjunctival or sub-Tenon's injection. A third type of injection, called retrobulbar injection, involves injecting a drug behind the globe of the eyeball. Corticosteroids and preoperative local anesthetics may be administered this way.

Individual Drugs

See Tables 65-1, 65-2, and 65-3.

(*text continues on page 844*)

TABLE 65-1   DRUGS USED IN OCULAR DISORDERS*

Ocular Effects	Clinical Indications	Generic/ Trade Name	Routes and Dosage Ranges Adults	Children
Autonomic Drugs				
Adrenergics				
1. Decreased production of aqueous humor	1. Glaucoma	**Dipivefrin (0.1% solution) (Propine)**	Topically, 1 drop in affected eye(s) twice daily q12h	
2. Mydriasis	2. Ophthalmoscopic examination			
3. Decreased intraocular pressure	3. Reduction of adhesion formation with uveitis	**Epinephrine hydrochloride (0.25%, 0.5%, 1%, and 2% solutions) (Epifrin, Glaucon)**	Topically 1 drop in each eye once or twice daily	Same as adults
4. Vasoconstriction	4. Preoperative and postoperative mydriasis	**Hydroxyamphetamine (1% solution) (Paredrine)**	Before ophthalmoscopy, topically, 1 drop in each eye	
5. Photophobia	5. Local hemostasis	**Phenylephrine (2.5% and 10% solutions) (Neo-Synephrine)**	Before ophthalmoscopy or refraction, topically, 1 drop of 2.5% or 10% solution	Refraction, topically, 1 drop of 2.5% solution
			Preoperatively, topically, 1 drop of 2.5% or 10% solution 30–60 min before surgery	

TABLE 65-1	DRUGS USED IN OCULAR DISORDERS* (Continued)

Ocular Effects	Clinical Indications	Generic/Trade Trade Name	Routes and Dosage Ranges	
			Adults	**Children**
			Postoperatively, topically, 1 drop of 10% solution once or twice daily	
Antiadrenergic (Beta-Blocking) Drugs 1. Decreased production of aqueous humor 2. Reduced intraocular pressure	Glaucoma	**Betaxolol (Betoptic)**	Topically to each eye, 1 drop q12h	
		Carteolol (Ocupress)	Topically to affected eye(s), 1 drop q12h	
		Levobunolol (Betagan)	Topically to the affected eye, 1 drop once or twice daily	
		Metipranolol (OptiPranolol)	Topically to affected eye(s), 1 drop q12h	
		Timolol maleate (Timoptic)	Topically, 1 drop of 0.25% or 0.5% solution in each eye twice daily q12h	
Cholinergics 1. Increased outflow of aqueous humor 2. Miosis	Glaucoma	**Pilocarpine (0.25%–10% solutions) (Almocarpine, Isopto Carpine, Pilocar, Pilocel, Pilomiotin)**	Chronic glaucoma, topically, 1 drop of 1% or 2% solution instilled in each eye q6–8h initially. Then, drug concentration and frequency of administration are adjusted to maintain intraocular pressure in the desired range. Drops are usually instilled four times daily.	
		Pilocarpine ocular therapeutic system (Ocusert Pilo-20, Ocusert Pilo-40)	One system placed into conjunctival sac per week, according to package directions. Each system releases 20 or 40 µg pilocarpine per hour for 1 wk.	
		Carbachol (Carbacel, Isopto Carbachol)	Topically, 1 drop of 0.75%–3% solution instilled in each eye initially. Then drug concentration and frequency of administration are adjusted to maintain intraocular pressure in the desired range.	
Anticholinesterase Agents 1. Increased outflow of aqueous humor 2. Miosis	Glaucoma	**Demecarium bromide (Humorsol)**	Topically, 1 drop of 0.125%–0.25% solution in each eye twice a day to twice a week, depending on condition	

(continued)

TABLE 65-1 **DRUGS USED IN OCULAR DISORDERS*** (Continued)

Ocular Effects	Clinical Indications	Generic/ Trade Name	Routes and Dosage Ranges	
			Adults	**Children**
		Echothiopate iodide (Phospholine Iodide)	Topically, 1 drop of solution (0.03%, 0.06%, 0.125%, or 0.25%) in each eye q12–48h	
		Isoflurophate (Floropryl)	Topically, ¼-inch strip of ointment in the lower conjunctival sac of each eye q12–72h	
		Physostigmine sulfate (Eserine Sulfate)	Topically, 0.25% ointment three or four times daily	
		Physostigmine salicylate (Isopto Eserine)	Topically, 1–2 drops of 0.25%–0.5% solution in each eye up to four times daily	
Anticholinergics 1. Mydriasis 2. Cycloplegia 3. Photophobia	1. Mydriasis for refraction and other diagnostic purposes 2. Pre- and postoperatively in intraocular surgery 3. Treatment of uveitis 4. Treatment of some secondary glaucoma	**Atropine sulfate** (0.5%–3% solutions)	Before intraocular surgery, topically, 1 drop of solution Following intraocular surgery, topically, 1 drop of solution once daily	
		Cyclopentolate hydrochloride (Cyclogyl)	For refraction, topically, 1 drop of 0.5% or 2% solution instilled once Before ophthalmoscopy, 1 drop of 0.5% solution	For refraction, topically, 1 drop of 0.5%, 1%, or 2% solution, repeated in 10 min
		Homatropine hydrobromide (2% and 5% solutions)	Refraction, topically, 1 drop of 5% solution every 5 min for two or three doses or 1–2 drops of 2% solution every 10–15 min for five doses Uveitis, topically, 1 drop of 2% or 5% solution two or three times daily	
		Scopolamine hydrobromide (0.25% solution) (Isopto Hyoscine)	Refraction, topically, 1–2 drops in affected eye(s) 1 h before examination	
		Tropicamide (0.5% and 1% solutions) (Mydriacyl)	Before refraction or ophthalmoscopy, topically, 1 drop of 0.5% or 1% solution, repeated in 5 min, then every 20–30 min as needed to maintain mydriasis	
Diuretics *Carbonic Anhydrase Inhibitors* 1. Decreased production of aqueous humor 2. Decreased intraocular pressure	1. Glaucoma 2. Preoperatively in intraocular surgery	**Acetazolamide** (Diamox)	PO 250 mg q6h Sustained-release capsules (Diamox Sequels), PO 500 mg q12h IV, IM 5–10 mg/kg/d in divided doses, q6h	PO 10–15 mg/kg/d in divided doses IV, IM 5–10 mg/kg/d in divided doses, q6h

			Routes and Dosage Ranges	
Ocular Effects	**Clinical Indications**	**Generic/ Trade Name**	*Adults*	*Children*
		Dichlorphenamide (Daranide)	PO 50–200 mg q6–8h. Maintenance dosage, 25–50 mg one to three times daily	
		Dorzolamide (Trusopt)	Topically, 1 drop in affected eye(s) three times daily	
		Methazolamide (Neptazane)	PO 50–100 mg q8h	
Osmotic Agents 1. Reduced volume of vitreous humor 2. Decreased intraocular pressure	1. Preoperatively in intraocular surgery 2. Treatment of acute glaucoma	**Glycerin** (Osmoglyn)	PO 1–1.5 g/kg, usually given as a 50% or 75% solution 1–1 ½ h before surgery	Same as adults
		Isosorbide (Ismotic)	Emergency reduction of intraocular pressure (*e.g.*, acute angle-closure glaucoma), PO 1.5 g/kg up to four times daily if necessary	
		Mannitol (Osmitrol)	IV 1.5–2 g/kg given as a 20% solution over 30–60 min	Same as adults

Miscellaneous Agents

Alpha$_2$-Adrenergic Agonist

	1. Glaucoma 2. Prevention of increased intraocular pressure after ocular surgery	**Apraclonidine** (Iopidine)	1–2 drops in affected eye(s) three times daily	
Anesthetics, Local Surface anesthesia of conjunctiva and cornea	1. Tonometry 2. Subconjunctival injections 3. Removal of foreign bodies 4. Removal of sutures	**Proparacaine hydrochloride** (Alcaine, Ophthaine)	Minor procedures, topically, 1–2 drops of 0.5% solution; instillation may be repeated for deeper anesthesia	
		Tetracaine hydrochloride (Pontocaine)	Minor procedures, topically, 1–2 drops of 0.5% solution; two to four instillations are required for deeper anesthesia	
Antiseptic	Prophylaxis of gonorrheal ophthalmia neonatorum	**Silver nitrate ophthalmic**		Newborns, topically, 2 drops of 1% solution in each eye
Lubricants Serve as "artificial tears"	1. Prevent damage to the cornea in clients with keratitis	**Methylcellulose** (Methulose, Visculose, others)	Topically, 1–2 drops as needed	

(continued)

TABLE 65-1 **DRUGS USED IN OCULAR DISORDERS*** (Continued)

Ocular Effects	Clinical Indications	Generic/ Trade Name	Routes and Dosage Ranges	
			Adults	**Children**
Lubricants *(cont)*	2. Protect the cornea during gonioscopy and other procedures 3. Moisten contact lenses 4. Lubricate artificial eyes	**Polyvinyl alcohol** (Liquifilm, others)	Topically, 1–2 drops as needed	
Prostaglandin	Glaucoma	**Latanoprost** (Xalatan)	Topically, 1 drop in affected eye(s) once daily in the evening	

*Anti-infective agents are listed in Table 65-2; anti-allergic and anti-inflammatory agents are listed in Table 65-3.

TABLE 65-2 **OPHTHALMIC ANTI-INFECTIVE AGENTS**

Generic/Trade Name	Routes and Dosage Ranges	
	Adults	**Children**
Antibacterial Agents		
Bacitracin (Baciguent)	Ophthalmic ointment, topically, instill in infected eye one to three times daily	
Chloramphenicol (Chloromycetin)	Mild conjunctivitis: topically, 1 drop of 0.5% ophthalmic solution q1–2h or ointment instilled three or four times daily	Topically, same as adults
(Chloroptic [0.5% solution, 1% ointment])	Severe conjunctivitis, corneal ulcers: topically, 1 drop of 0.5% solution every 30 min	
Ciprofloxacin ophthalmic solution (Ciloxan)	Corneal ulcers, topically to affected eye. Day 1, 2 drops q15min for 6 h, then q30min for rest of day; day 2, 2 drops q1h; days 3–14, 2 drops q4h. Conjunctivitis, 1–2 drops q2h while awake for 2 d, then 1–2 drops q4h while awake for 5 d	Safety and effectiveness not established for children younger than 12 y
Erythromycin (Ilotycin ophthalmic [0.5% ointment])		Prevention of neonatal gonococcal or chlamydial conjunctivitis, topically, 0.5–1 cm in each eye
Gentamicin sulfate (Garamycin)	Topically, ophthalmic solution (0.3%) 1 drop q1–4h; ophthalmic ointment (0.3%), instill two or three times daily	Topically, same as adults
Norfloxacin ophthalmic solution (Chibroxin)	Topically to affected eye(s), 1–2 drops four times daily, up to 7 d	Same as adults for children 1 y and older; safety not established for children younger than 1 y
Ofloxacin (Ocuflox)	Bacterial conjunctivitis: topically, 1–2 drops of 0.3% solution q2–4h while awake for 2 d, then 1–2 drops four times daily for up to 5 more days	Same as adults for children 1 y and older
Polymyxin B sulfate	Corneal ulcers due to *Pseudomonas aeruginosa*: topically, 1 drop of a freshly prepared solution (20,000 units/mL), instilled two to ten times hourly	

TABLE 65-2 OPTHALMIC ANTI-INFECTIVE AGENTS (Continued)

Generic/Trade Name	Routes and Dosage Range	
	Adults	**Children**
Sulfacetamide sodium (Bleph-10 Liquifilm [10% solution or ointment] Isopto Cetamide [15% solution]) (Cetamide [10% oitment]) Sodium Sulamyd (10% and 30% solution, 10% ointment]) (Also available generically as 10% and 30% solutions)	Acute catarrhal conjunctivitis caused by *Staphylococcus aureus, Diplococcus pneumoniae, Haemophilus influenzae, Neisseria catarrhalis*: topically, 1 drop of 10% or 15% solution every 10–30 min Chronic conjunctivitis due to *Proteus* organisms: topically, 10% ointment instilled three of four times daily Chronic blepharoconjunctivitis due to *S. aureus*: topically, 1 drop of 30% solution three of four times daily Corneal ulcers due to *Escherichia coli* or *Klebsiella pneumoniae*: 1 drop of 10% solution every 30 min or 10% ointment instilled three or four times daily	
Sulfisoxazole diolamine (Gantrisin [4% solution])	Topically, 2–3 drops in affected eye three or more times daily	
Tetracycline (Achromycin)	Inclusion conjunctivitis: topically, 1% solution or ointment instilled three or four times daily for 30 d	Conjunctivitis, same as adults Prevention of neonatal gonococcal or chlamydial conjunctivitis, 0.5–1 cm of ointment into each eye
Tobramycin (Tobrex [0.3% solution and ointment])	Topically, 1–2 drops two to six times daily or ointment two or three times daily	
Antiviral Agents		
Idoxuridine (Herplex)	Herpes simplex infection of eyelids, conjunctiva, and cornea: topically, 1 drop of 0.1% solution q1h during daytime hours and q2h at night, or 0.5% ointment instilled four or five times daily. Treatment should be continued for at least 2 wk.	
Trifluridine (Viroptic)	Keratoconjunctivitis or corneal ulcers caused by herpes simplex virus: topically, 1 drop of 1% solution q2h while awake (maximal daily dose, 9 drops) until corneal ulcer heals, then 1 drop q4h (minimal dose, 5 drops daily for 7 d)	
Vidarabine (Vira-A)	Keratoconjunctivitis caused by herpes simplex virus: topically, 3% ointment instilled q3h	
Antifungal Agent		
Natamycin (Natacyn)	Topically, 1 drop of 5% suspension q1–2h	

TABLE 65-3 TOPICAL OPHTHALMIC ANTI-ALLERGIC AND ANTI-INFLAMMATORY AGENTS

Generic/Trade Name	Indications for Use	Dosage Ranges
Anti-allergic Agents		
Cromolyn (Crolom, Opticrom)	Treatment of seasonal allergic conjunctivitis, keratitis, and keratoconjunctivitis	1–2 drops in each eye four to six times daily at regular intervals
Levocabastine (Livostin)	Treatment of seasonal allergic conjunctivitis	1 drop in affected eyes four times daily, for up to 2 wk

(continued)

TABLE 65-3 TOPICAL OPHTHALMIC ANTI-ALLERGIC AND ANTI-INFLAMMATORY AGENTS

Generic/Trade Name	Indications for Use	Dosage Ranges
Corticosteroids		
Dexamethasone (Decadron, Maxidex)	Inflammatory disorders of the conjunctiva, cornea, eyelid, and anterior eyeball (e.g., conjunctivitis, keratitis) Corneal injury from chemical, radiation or thermal burns or penetration of foreign bodies Prevention of graft rejection after corneal transplant	Solution or suspension 1–2 drops q1h daytime, q2h nighttime until response; then 1 drop q4h Postoperative inflammation, 1–2 drops four times daily, starting 24 h after surgery, for 2 wk Ointment thin strip three to four times daily until response, then once or twice daily
Fluorometholone (FML)		Solution 1 drop q1–2h until response, then less often Ointment thin strip three to four times daily until response, then once or twice daily
Medrysone (HMS)		1 drop q1–2h until response obtained, then less frequently
Prednisolone (Econopred, others)		Solution or suspension 1–2 drops q1–2h until response, then 1 drop q4h, then less frequently Ointment thin strip three to four times daily until response, then once or twice daily
Nonsteroidal Anti-inflammatory Drugs (NSAIDs)		
Diclofenac (Voltaren)	Treatment of inflammation after cataract surgery	1 drop to affected eye four times daily, starting 24 h postoperatively, for 2 wk
Flurbiprofen (Ocufen)	Inhibition of pupil constriction during eye surgery	1 drop every 30 min for four doses, starting 2 h before surgery
Ketorolac (Acular)	Treatment of ocular itching due to seasonal allergic conjunctivitis	1 drop four times daily for about 1 wk
Suprofen (Profenal)	Inhibition of pupil constriction during eye surgery	2 drops at 3, 2, and 1 h before surgery or q4h while awake the day before surgery

Nursing Process

Assessment

Assess the client's condition in relation to ophthalmic disorders.

- Determine whether the client has impaired vision and, if so, the extent or severity of the impairment. Minimal assessment includes the vision-impaired client's ability to participate in activities of daily living, including safe ambulation. Maximal assessment depends on the nurse's ability and working situation. Some nurses do complete vision testing and ophthalmoscopic examinations.
- Identify risk factors for eye disorders. These include trauma, allergies, infection in one eye (a risk factor for infection in the other eye), use of contact lenses, infections of facial structures or skin, and occupational exposure to chemical irritants or foreign bodies.

- Signs and symptoms vary with particular disorders:
  - Pain is usually associated with corneal abrasions or inflammation. Sudden, severe pain may indicate acute angle-closure glaucoma. Acute glaucoma requires immediate treatment to lower intraocular pressure and minimize damage to the optic nerve.
  - Signs of inflammation (redness, edema, heat, tenderness) are especially evident with infection or inflammation of external ocular structures, such as the eyelids and conjunctiva. A mucoid or purulent discharge also often occurs.
  - Pruritus is most often associated with allergic conjunctivitis.
  - Photosensitivity commonly occurs with keratitis.

Nursing Diagnoses

- Sensory-Perceptual Alteration: Impaired vision
- Pain in eyes related to infection, inflammation, or increased intraocular pressure (glaucoma)

- Risk for Injury: Blindness related to inadequately treated glaucoma or ophthalmic infections
- Risk for Injury: Trauma related to blurred vision from disease process or drug therapy
- Impaired Physical Mobility related to impaired vision
- Body Image Disturbance related to impaired vision and chronic illness
- Anxiety related to acute and chronic disturbances in vision
- Knowledge Deficit related to prevention and treatment of ocular disorders

Planning/Goals

The client will:
- Take ophthalmic medications as prescribed
- Follow safety precautions to protect eyes from trauma and disease
- Experience improvement in signs and symptoms (*e.g.,* decreased drainage with infections, decreased eye pain with glaucoma)
- Avoid injury from impaired vision (*e.g.,* falls)
- Avoid systemic effects of ophthalmic drugs
- Have regular eye examinations to monitor effects of anti-glaucoma drugs

Interventions

Use measures to minimize ocular disorders.
- Promote regular eye examinations. This is especially important among middle-age and older adults, who are more likely to develop several ocular disorders. They are also more likely to develop ocular disorders as adverse effects of drugs taken for nonocular disorders.
- Treat eye injuries appropriately:
  - For chemical burns, irrigate the eyes with copious amounts of water as soon as possible (*i.e.,* near the area where the injury occurred). Do not wait for transport to a first-aid station, hospital, or other health care facility. Damage continues as long as the chemical is in contact with the eye.
  - For thermal burns, apply cold compresses to the area.
  - Superficial foreign bodies may be removed by irrigation with water. Foreign bodies embedded in ocular structures must be removed by a physician.
- Warm wet compresses are often useful in ophthalmic inflammation or infections. They relieve pain and promote healing by increasing the blood supply to the affected area.

Teach clients:
- Wear safety goggles when working in high-risk areas. These are often provided by employers.
- Follow instructions for care of contact lenses (*e.g.,* cleaning, inserting or removing, and duration of wear). Improper or infrequent cleaning may lead to infection. Overwearing is a common cause of corneal abrasion and may cause corneal ulceration. The lens wearer should consult a physician when eye pain occurs. Antibiotics are often prescribed for corneal abrasions to prevent development of ulcers.

- Avoid regular use of nonprescription eye drops (*e.g.,* Murine, Visine). Persistent eye irritation and redness should be reported to a physician.
- Avoid eyestrain by using appropriate lighting for reading and handwork. Also, limit periods of reading, watching television, and other visual activities.
- Minimize exposure to dust, smog, cigarette smoke, and other eye irritants when possible.
- Have regular eye examinations and testing for glaucoma after 40 years of age.
- Avoid straining at stool (use laxatives or stool softeners if necessary), heavy lifting, bending over, coughing, and vomiting when possible. These activities increase intraocular pressure, which may cause ocular damage in glaucoma and after intraocular surgery.

Evaluation

- Observe and interview for compliance with instructions regarding drug therapy and follow-up care.
- Observe and interview for relief of symptoms.
- Observe for systemic adverse effects of ophthalmic drugs (*e.g.,* tachycardia and arrhythmias with adrenergics; bradycardia and congestive heart failure with beta-blockers).

Principles of Therapy

OCULAR INFECTIONS

Guidelines for drug therapy of ocular infections include the following:

1. Drug therapy is usually initiated as soon as culture material (eye secretions) has been obtained, often with a broad-spectrum antibacterial agent or a combination of two or more antibiotics.
2. Topical administration is used most often, and recommended drugs include bacitracin, colistimethate, chloramphenicol, polymyxin B, and sulfacetamide. These agents are rarely given systemically. They do not cause sensitization to commonly used systemic antibiotics and do not promote growth of drug-resistant microorganisms.
3. In severe infections, antibacterial drugs may be given both topically and systemically. Because systemic antibiotics penetrate the eye poorly, large doses are required to attain therapeutic drug concentrations in ocular structures. Drugs that reach therapeutic levels in the eye when given in proper dosage include ampicillin and dicloxacillin. Gentamicin and other antibiotics penetrate the eye when inflammation is present.
4. Combination products containing two or more antibacterials are available for topical treatment of external ocular infections. These products are most

useful when therapy must be initiated before the infecting microorganism is identified. Mixtures provide a broader spectrum of antibacterial activity than a single drug. Some of the available combination products contain polymyxin B and bacitracin.

5. Fixed-dose combinations of an antibacterial agent and corticosteroid are available for topical use in selected conditions (*e.g.,* staphylococcal keratitis, blepharoconjunctivitis, allergic conjunctivitis, and some postoperative inflammatory reactions). Chloramphenicol and corticosteroid mixtures include Chloromycetin-Hydrocortisone and Chloroptic. Neomycin and corticosteroid mixtures include Neo-Cortef and NeoDecadron. Neomycin, polymyxin B, and corticosteroid mixtures include Poly-Pred and Maxitrol. Neomycin, polymyxin B, bacitracin, and corticosteroid mixtures include Cortisporin. Sulfacetamide and corticosteroid mixtures include Blephamide, Cetapred, Metimyd, and Vasocidin.

6. Trifluridine (Viroptic) is the drug of choice in eye infections caused by the herpes simplex virus.

7. In fungal infections, natamycin (Natacyn) may be preferred because it has a broad spectrum of antifungal activity and is nonirritating and nontoxic.

Glaucoma

For drug therapy of chronic, primary open-angle glaucoma, beta-adrenergic blocking agents are the most commonly used drugs. Several beta-blockers are now available for ophthalmic use. Most adverse effects occurring with systemic beta-blockers also have been reported with ophthalmic preparations.

Use of Ophthalmic Ointments

Many ophthalmic drugs are available as eye drops (solutions or suspensions) and ointments. Ointments do not need to be administered as frequently and often produce higher concentrations of drug in target tissues. However, ointments also cause blurred vision, which limits their daytime use, at least for ambulatory clients. In some situations, drops may be used during waking hours and ointments at bedtime. However, the two formulations are *not* interchangeable.

Use in Children

Topical ophthalmic drug therapy in children differs little from that in adults. Few studies of ophthalmic drug therapy in children have been reported, and many conditions for which adults need therapy (*e.g.,* cataract, glaucoma) rarely occur in children. A major use of topical ophthalmic drugs in children is to dilate the pupil and paralyze accommodation for ophthalmoscopic examination. As a general rule, the short-acting mydriatics and cycloplegics (*e.g.,* cyclopentolate, tropicamide) are preferred because they cause fewer systemic adverse effects than atropine and scopolamine. In addition, lower drug concentrations are usually given empirically because of the smaller size of children and the potential risk of systemic adverse effects.

Use in Older Adults

Older adults are at risk for developing ocular disorders, especially glaucoma and cataracts. General principles of ophthalmic drug therapy are the same as for younger adults. In addition, older adults are likely to have cardiovascular disorders, which may be aggravated by systemic absorption of topical eye medication. Thus, accurate dosage and occlusion of the nasolacrimal duct in the inner canthus of the eye are needed to prevent adverse drug effects (*e.g.,* hypertension, tachycardia, or arrhythmias with adrenergic drugs and bradycardia or congestive heart failure with beta-blockers).

 Home Care

The home care nurse may be involved in the care of clients with acute or chronic eye disorders. As with other drug therapy, the nurse may need to teach clients and caregivers reasons for use, accurate administration, and assessment of therapeutic and adverse responses to eye medications. The nurse may also need to encourage periodic eye examinations to promote optimal vision and prevent blindness.

NURSING ACTIONS   OPHTHALMIC DRUGS

NURSING ACTIONS	*RATIONALE/EXPLANATION*
1. Administer accurately **a.** Read labels of ophthalmic medications carefully.	To avoid error. For example, many drugs are available in several concentrations. The correct concentration and the correct drug must be given.
b. Read medication orders carefully and accurately.	To avoid error. Abbreviations (*e.g.*, O.S., O.D., O.U.) are often used in physicians' orders and must be interpreted accurately.
c. For hospitalized clients, keep eye medications at the bedside when possible.	Eye medications should be ordered for and used by one person only. They are dispensed in small amounts for this purpose. This minimizes cross-contamination and risk of infection.
d. Wash hands before approaching the client for instillation of eye medications.	To reduce risks of infection
e. To administer eye drops, have the client lie down or tilt the head backward and look upward. Then, pull down the lower lid to expose the conjunctival sac, and drop the medication into the sac. Alternate method: gently grasp the lower lid and pull it outward to form a pouch into which medication is instilled. After instillation, have the client close the eyes gently, and apply pressure to the inner canthus briefly (nurse or client).	Absorption of the drug and its concentration in ocular tissues depend partly on the length of time the medication is in contact with ocular tissues. Contact time is increased by the "pouch" method of administration, closing the eyes (delays outflow into the nasolacrimal) duct), and pressure on the inner canthus (delays outflow and decreases side effects resulting from systemic absorption).
f. When instilling ophthalmic ointments, position the client as above, and apply a ¼-inch to ½-inch strip of ointment to the conjunctiva.	
g. Do not touch the dropper tip or ointment top to the eye or anything else.	To avoid contamination of the medication and infection
h. When crusts or secretions are present, cleanse the eye before administering medication.	If the eye is not cleansed, the drug may not be absorbed.
i. When two or more eye drops are scheduled for the same time, they should be instilled about 5 min apart.	To avoid drug loss by dilution and outflow into the nasolacrimal duct
2. Observe for therapeutic effects **a.** With beta-blocking agents, observe for decreased intra-ocular pressure.	Therapeutic effects depend on the reason for use. Lowering of intraocular pressure usually occurs within a month; periodic measurements should be done.
b. With mydriatics, observe for dilation of the pupil.	Mydriasis begins within 5 to 15 min after instillation.
c. With miotics, observe for constriction of the pupil.	
d. With anti-infective drugs, observe for decreased redness, edema, and drainage.	
e. With osmotic agents, observe for decreased intraocular pressure.	With oral glycerin, maximal decrease in intraocular pressure occurs approximately 1 h after administration, and effects persist for about 5 h. With IV mannitol, maximal decrease in intraocular pressure occurs within 30 to 60 min, and effects last 6 to 8 h.

(continued)

Nursing Actions	*Rationale/Explanation*
3. Observe for adverse effects **a.** Local effects	
(1) Irritation, burning, stinging, blurred vision, discomfort, redness, itching, tearing, conjunctivitis, keratitis, allergic reactions	These effects may occur with any topical ophthalmic agents. Burning and stinging discomfort occur with instillation and are usually transient. Allergic reactions may occur with the active ingredient, preservatives, or other components.
(2) With antibacterial agents—superinfection or sensitization	Superinfection caused by drug-resistant organisms may occur. Sensitization means that topical application induces antibody formation. Therefore, if the same or a related drug is subsequently administered systemically, an allergic reaction may occur. The allergic reaction most often involves dermatitis; occasionally urticaria or anaphylaxis occurs. Penicillin is the most frequently involved drug. Other drugs include streptomycin, neomycin, gentamicin, and sulfonamides (with the exception of sulfacetamide sodium). Sensitization can be prevented or minimized by avoiding topical administration of antibacterial agents that are commonly given systemically.
(3) With anticholinergics, adrenergics, topical corticosteroids—glaucoma	Mydriatic drugs (anticholinergics and adrenergics) may cause an acute attack of angle-closure glaucoma in clients with narrow angles by blocking outflow of aqueous humor. Topical corticosteroids raise intraocular pressure in some clients. The "glaucomatous" response occurs most often in clients with chronic, primary open-angle glaucoma and their relatives. It also may occur in clients with myopia or diabetes mellitus. The magnitude of increased intraocular pressure depends on the concentration, frequency of administration, duration of therapy, and anti-inflammatory potency of the corticosteroid. Increased intraocular pressure has been reported most often with 0.1% dexamethasone (Decadron). This adverse effect can be minimized by checking intraocular pressure every 2 mo in clients receiving long-term therapy with topical corticosteroids.
(4) Cataract formation	This is most likely to occur with long-term use of anticholinesterase agents.
(5) With miotic drugs—decreased vision in dim light	These agents prevent pupil dilation, which normally occurs in dim light or darkness.
b. Systemic effects:	Systemic absorption and adverse effects of eye drops can be prevented or minimized by applying pressure to the inner canthus during and after instillation of the medications. Pressure may be applied by the nurse or the client.
(1) With beta-blocking agents—bradycardia, congestive heart failure, bronchospasm, and others (see Chap. 19)	These agents may be absorbed systemically and cause all the adverse effects associated with oral or injected drugs.
(2) With miotics—sweating, nausea, vomiting, diarrhea, abdominal pain, bradycardia, hypotension, bronchoconstriction. Toxic doses produce ataxia, confusion, convulsions, coma, respiratory failure, and death	These cholinergic or parasympathomimetic effects occur rarely with pilocarpine or carbachol. They are more likely to occur with the long-acting anticholinesterase agents, especially echothiophate (Phospholine Iodide). Acute toxicity may be reversed by an anticholinergic agent, atropine, given IV.
(3) With anticholinergic mydriatics—dryness of the mouth and skin, fever, rash, tachycardia, confusion, hallucinations, delirium	These effects are most likely to occur with atropine and in children and older adults. Tropicamide (Mydriacyl) rarely causes systemic reactions.
(4) With adrenergic mydriatics—tachycardia, hypertension, premature ventricular contractions, tremors, headache	Systemic effects are uncommon. They are more likely to occur with repeated instillations of high drug concentrations (*e.g.*, epinephrine 2%, phenylephrine [Neo-Synephrine] 10%).

NURSING ACTIONS	RATIONALE/EXPLANATION
(5) With carbonic anhydrase inhibitors—anorexia, nausea, vomiting, diarrhea, paresthesias, weakness, lethargy	Nausea, malaise, and paresthesias (numbness and tingling of extremities) commonly occur.
(6) With osmotic diuretics—dehydration, nausea, vomiting, headache, hyperglycemia and glycosuria with glycerin (Osmoglyn)	These agents may produce profound diuresis and dehydration. Oral agents (*e.g.*, glycerin) are less likely to cause severe systemic effects than IV agents (*e.g.*, mannitol). These agents are usually given in a single dose, which decreases the risks of serious adverse reactions unless large doses are given.
(7) With corticosteroids, see Chapter 24.	Serious adverse effects may occur with long-term use of corticosteroids.
(8) With antibacterial agents, see Chapter 33 and the chapter on the individual drug group.	Adverse effects may occur with all antibacterial agents.
(9) With apraclonidine—bradycardia, orthostatic hypotension, headache, insomnia	This drug is related to clonidine, an alpha$_2$-adrenergic agonist antihypertensive agent (see Chaps. 19 and 55).
(10) With latanoprost—common cold or flu-like upper respiratory infection, muscle and joint pain, angina pectoris, skin rash	These were the most commonly reported systemic adverse effects in clinical trials.
(11) With ophthalmic NSAIDs—potential for increased bleeding	Systemic absorption may interfere with platelet function and increase risks of bleeding with surgery or anticoagulant therapy.

4. Observe for drug interactions
a. Drugs that *increase* effects of adrenergic (sympathomimetic) ophthalmic drugs.

(1) Anticholinergic ophthalmic drugs	The combination (*e.g.*, atropine and phenylephrine) produces additive mydriasis
(2) Systemic adrenergic drugs	Additive risks of adverse effects (*e.g.*, tachycardia, cardiac arrhythmias, hypertension)

b. Drugs that *decrease* effects of adrenergic ophthalmic preparations.

(1) Cholinergic and anticholinesterase ophthalmic drugs	Antagonize mydriatic effects of adrenergic drugs

c. Drugs that *increase* effects of antiadrenergic ophthalmic preparations.

(1) Systemic antiadrenergics (*e.g.*, propranolol, atenolol, metoprolol, nadolol, timolol)	When the client is receiving a topical beta-blocker in ocular disorders, administration of systemic beta-blocking agents in cardiovascular disorders may cause additive systemic toxicity.

d. Drugs that *increase* effects of anticholinergic ophthalmic drugs:

(1) Adrenergic ophthalmic agents	Additive mydriasis
(2) Systemic anticholinergic drugs (*e.g.*, atropine) and other drugs with anticholinergic effects (*e.g.*, some antihistamines, antipsychotic agents, and tricyclic antidepressants)	Additive anticholinergic effects (mydriasis, blurred vision, tachycardia). These drugs are hazardous in glaucoma.

e. Drugs that *decrease* effects of cholinergic and anticholinesterase ophthalmic drugs:

(1) Anticholinergics and drugs with anticholinergic effects (*e.g.*, atropine, antipsychotic agents, tricyclic antidepressants, some antihistamines)	Antagonize antiglaucoma (miotic) effects of cholinergic and anticholinesterase drugs
(2) Corticosteroids	Long-term use of corticosteroids, topically or systemically, raises intraocular pressure and may cause glaucoma. There-

(continued)

NURSING ACTIONS	RATIONALE/EXPLANATION
	fore, corticosteroids decrease effects of all drugs used for glaucoma.
(3) Sympathomimetic drugs	Antagonize miotic (antiglaucoma) effects
5. Teach clients **a.** The correct procedure for administering eye medications (including maintenance of sterility)	If the client cannot administer the drugs, a family member may be taught the procedure. Written instructions are preferred to verbal ones.
b. To discard cloudy or discolored solutions	These changes indicate deterioration. Phenylephrine (Neo-Synephrine) solutions become cloudy, epinephrine solutions turn brown, and physostigmine becomes pink or red.
c. With glaucoma: (1) Do not take any drugs without the physician's knowledge and consent.	Many drugs given for purposes other than eye disorders may cause or aggravate glaucoma.
(2) Wear a MedicAlert bracelet or carry identification that states that the person has glaucoma.	To avoid administration of drugs that aggravate glaucoma or to maintain treatment of glaucoma, in emergencies
d. With eye infections: (1) Avoid touching the unaffected eye. (2) Wash hands before and after contact with the infected eye. (3) Use a separate towel.	These measures are indicated to avoid spreading the infection to the unaffected eye or to other people.

REVIEW AND APPLICATION EXERCISES

1. What is the main function of the eye?

2. List common disorders of the eye for which drug therapy is indicated.

3. Do ophthalmic medications need to be sterile? Why or why not?

4. What are important principles and techniques related to the nurse's administration of ophthalmic drugs?

5. For a client with newly prescribed eye drops, how would you teach self-administration principles and techniques?

SELECTED REFERENCES

Cioffi, G.A., & VanBuskirk, E.M. (1997). Glaucoma therapy. In K.W. Wright (Ed.), *Textbook of ophthalmology*, pp. 627–645. Baltimore: Williams & Wilkins.

Curtis, S.M., & Carroll, E.M. (1994). Alterations in vision. In C.M. Porth (Ed.), *Pathophysiology: Concepts of altered health states*, 4th ed., pp. 1113–1153. Philadelphia: J.B. Lippincott.

Drug facts and comparisons. (Updated monthly). St. Louis: Facts and Comparisons.

Ellis, P.P. (1995). Commonly used eye medications. In D.G. Vaughan, T. Asbury, & P. Riordan-Eva (Eds.), *General ophthalmology*, 14th ed., pp. 62–77. Norwalk, CT: Appleton & Lange.

Johns, M.D., & Ponte, C.D. (1995). Acute pulmonary edema associated with ocular metipranolol use. *The Annals of Pharmacotherapy* 29(4), 370–373.

Lesar, T.S. (1997). Glaucoma. In J.T. DiPiro, R.L. Talbert, G.C. Yee, G.R. Matzke, B.G. Wells, & L.M. Posey (Eds.), *Pharmacotherapy: A pathophysiologic approach*, 3rd ed., pp. 1783–1799. Stamford, CT: Appleton & Lange.

Liesegang, T.J. (1996). Glaucoma: Changing concepts and future directions. *Mayo Clinic Proceedings, 71,* 689–694.

Moroi, S.E., & Lichter, P.R. (1996). Ocular pharmacology. In J.G. Hardman, L.E. Limbird, P.B. Molinoff, & R.W. Ruddon (Eds.), *Goodman & Gilman's The pharmacological basis of therapeutics*, 9th ed., pp. 1619–1645. New York: McGraw-Hill.

66 Drugs Used in Dermatologic Conditions

Outline

Functions of the Skin

Disorders of the Skin
inflammatory disorders
dermatologic infections
trauma
ulcerations
acne
external otitis
anorectal disorders

Types of Dermatologic Drugs
antiseptics
anti-infective agents
anti-inflammatory agents
retinoids
astringents
emollients
enzymes
keratolytic agents
sunscreens
melanizing agents
demelanizing agents
application of dermatologic drugs

Individual Drugs

Nursing Process
assessment
nursing diagnoses
planning/goals
interventions
evaluation

Principles of Therapy
drug selection in various skin conditions
dosage forms

use in children
use in older adults
home care

Objectives

After studying this chapter, the student will be able to:

1 Review characteristics of skin structures that influence drug therapy of dermatologic disorders.

2 Discuss antimicrobial, anti-inflammatory, and selected miscellaneous drugs in relation to their use in dermatologic disorders.

3 Use correct techniques to administer dermatologic medications.

4 Teach clients, family members, or caretakers correct administration of dermatologic medications.

5 For clients with "open lesion" skin disorders, teach about the importance and techniques of preventing infection.

6 Practice and teach measures to protect the skin from the damaging effects of sun exposure.

Key Terms

Acne	**Pruritus**
Candidiasis	**Psoriasis**
Dermatitis	**Tinea pedis**
Dermatophytosis	**Urticaria**

Functions of the Skin

The skin, the largest organ of the body, is the interface between the body's internal and external environments. The skin is composed of the epidermis and dermis. Epidermal or epithelial cells begin in the basal layer of the epidermis and migrate outward, undergoing degenerative changes in each layer. The outer layer, called the *stratum corneum,* is composed of dead cells and keratin. The dead cells are constantly being shed (desquamated) and replaced by newer cells. Normally, about 1 month is required for cell formation, migration, and desquamation. When dead cells are discarded, keratin remains on the skin. Keratin is a tough protein substance that is insoluble in water, weak acids, and weak bases. Hair and nails, which are composed of keratin, are referred to as appendages of the skin.

Melanocytes are pigment-producing cells located at the junction of the epidermis and the dermis. These cells produce yellow, brown, or black skin coloring in response to genetic influences, melanocyte-stimulating hormone released from the anterior pituitary gland, and exposure to ultraviolet (UV) light (*e.g.,* sunlight).

The dermis is composed of elastic and fibrous connective tissue. Dermal structures include blood vessels, lymphatic channels, nerves and nerve endings, sweat glands, sebaceous glands, and hair follicles. The dermis is supported underneath by subcutaneous tissue, which is composed primarily of fat cells.

The skin has numerous functions, most of which are protective. Functions include the following:

1. Serves as a physical barrier against loss of fluids and electrolytes and against entry of potentially harmful substances (*e.g.,* microorganisms and other foreign bodies)
2. Detects sensations of pain, pressure, touch, and temperature through sensory nerve endings
3. Assists in regulating body temperature through production and elimination of sweat
4. Serves as a source of vitamin D when exposed to sunlight or other sources of UV light. Skin contains a precursor for vitamin D.
5. Serves as an excretory organ. Water, sodium, chloride, lactate, and urea are excreted in sweat.
6. Inhibits growth of many microorganisms by its acidic pH (about 4.5 to 6.5)

Mucous membrane is composed of a surface layer of epithelial cells, a basement membrane, and a layer of connective tissue. Mucous membranes line body cavities that communicate with the external environment (*i.e.,* mouth, vagina, anus). They receive an abundant blood supply. Capillaries lie just beneath the epithelial cells.

Dermatologic disorders may be primary (*i.e.,* originate in the skin or mucous membranes) or secondary (*i.e.,* result from a systemic condition, such as measles, lupus erythematosus, or adverse drug reactions). This chapter focuses on primary skin disorders and the topical medications used to prevent or treat them.

Disorders of the Skin

Because the skin is constantly exposed to the external environment, it is susceptible to numerous disorders. Dermatologic disorders include the following.

INFLAMMATORY DISORDERS

Dermatitis

Dermatitis is a general term denoting an inflammatory response of the skin to various injuries from irritants, allergens, or trauma. *Eczema* is often used as a synonym for dermatitis. Whatever the cause, dermatitis is usually characterized by erythema, pruritus, and skin lesions. Dermatitis may be acute or chronic.

1. **Atopic dermatitis** is a chronic disorder characterized primarily by pruritus. Its cause is uncertain but may involve allergic, hereditary, or psychological elements.
2. **Contact dermatitis** results from irritants (*e.g.,* strong soaps, detergents, acids, alkalis) or allergens (*e.g.,* clothing materials or dyes, jewelry, cosmetics, hair dyes). Irritants cause dermatitis in anyone with sufficient contact or exposure. Allergens cause dermatitis only in sensitized or hypersensitive people. The location of the dermatitis may indicate the cause (*e.g.,* facial dermatitis may indicate an allergy to cosmetics).
3. **Seborrheic dermatitis** is a disease of the sebaceous glands characterized by excessive production of sebum. A simple form of seborrheic dermatitis involving the scalp is dandruff, which is characterized by flaking and itching of the skin. More severe forms of seborrheic dermatitis are characterized by greasy, yellow scales or crusts with variable amounts of erythema and itching. Seborrheic dermatitis may occur on the scalp, face, or trunk.
4. **Urticaria** ("hives") is an allergic reaction to external agents (*e.g.,* insect bites) or to internal allergens that reach the skin through the bloodstream (*e.g.,* from foods or drugs). The characteristic skin lesion of urticaria is the wheal, a raised edematous area with a pallid center and erythematous border, which itches severely. Topical medications may be applied to relieve itching, but systemic drug therapy with antihistamines and perhaps epinephrine is the major element of drug therapy.

Psoriasis

Psoriasis is a chronic skin disorder characterized by erythematous, dry, scaling lesions. The lesions may occur anywhere on the body but commonly involve the skin covering bony prominences, such as the elbows and knees. The disease is characterized by remissions and exacerbations. It is not contagious.

The cause of psoriasis is unknown. The pathophysiology involves excessively rapid turnover of epidermal cells. Instead of approximately 30 days from formation to elimination of normal epidermal cells, epidermal cells involved in psoriasis are abnormal in structure and have a life span of about 4 days.

Skin lesions may be tender, but they do not usually cause severe pain or itching. However, the lesions are unsightly and usually cause embarrassment and mental distress.

Dermatologic Infections

Bacterial Infections

Bacterial infections of the skin are common; they are most often caused by streptococci or staphylococci.

1. **Cellulitis** is characterized by erythema, tenderness, and edema, which may spread to subcutaneous tissue. Erysipelas is a form of cellulitis. Generalized malaise, chills, and fever may occur.
2. **Folliculitis** is an infection of the hair follicles that most often occurs on the scalp or bearded areas of the face.
3. **Furuncles** and **carbuncles** are infections usually caused by staphylococci. Furuncles (boils) may result from folliculitis. They usually occur in the neck, face, axillae, buttocks, thighs, and perineum. Furuncles tend to recur. Carbuncles involve many hair follicles and include multiple pustules. Carbuncles may cause fever, malaise, leukocytosis, and bacteremia. Healing of carbuncles often produces scar tissue.
4. **Impetigo** is a superficial skin infection caused by streptococci or staphylococci. An especially contagious form is caused by group A beta-hemolytic streptococci. This form occurs most often in children.

Fungal Infections

Fungal infections of the skin and mucous membranes are most often caused by *Candida albicans*.

1. **Oral candidiasis** (thrush) involves mucous membranes of the mouth. It often occurs as a superinfection following the use of broad-spectrum systemic antibiotics.
2. **Candidiasis of the vagina and vulva** occurs with systemic antibiotic therapy and in women with diabetes mellitus.

3. **Intertrigo** involves skin folds or areas where two skin surfaces are in contact (*e.g.*, groin, pendulous breasts).
4. **Tinea** infections (ringworm) are caused by fungi (dermatophytes). These infections may involve the scalp (tinea capitis), the body (tinea corporis), the foot (tinea pedis), and other areas of the body. Tinea pedis, commonly called "athlete's foot," is the most common type of ringworm infection.

Viral Infections

Viral infections of the skin include veruccal (warts) and herpes infections. There are two types of herpes simplex infections. Type 1 infections usually involve the face or neck (*e.g.*, fever blisters or cold sores on the lips), and type 2 infections involve the genital organs. Other herpes infections include herpes zoster (shingles) and varicella (chickenpox).

Trauma

Trauma refers to a physical injury that disrupts the skin. When the skin is broken, it may not be able to function properly. The major problem associated with skin wounds is infection. Common wounds include lacerations (cuts or tears), abrasions (shearing or scraping of the skin), and puncture wounds; surgical incisions; and burn wounds.

Ulcerations

Cutaneous ulcerations are usually caused by trauma and impaired circulation. They may become inflamed or infected.

1. **Pressure ulcers** may occur anywhere on the body where external pressure decreases blood flow. Common sites include the sacrum, trochanters, ankles, and heels. Cutaneous ulcers also may result from improper moving and lifting techniques. For example, when a person is pulled across bed linens rather than lifted, friction and shearing force may cause skin abrasions. Abraded skin is susceptible to infection and ulcer formation.

    Pressure ulcers are most likely to develop in clients who are immobilized, incontinent, malnourished, and debilitated.
2. **Venous stasis ulcers** are commonly located on the lower extremities.

Acne

Acne is a common disorder characterized by excessive production of sebum and obstruction of hair follicles, which normally carry sebum to the skin surface. As a result, hair follicles expand and form comedones (blackheads and whiteheads). The most severe form of acne is acne vulgaris, in which follicles become infected and irritating secretions leak into surrounding tissues to form pustules, cysts, and abscesses.

Acne occurs most often on the face, upper back, and chest because large numbers of sebaceous glands are located in these areas. Etiologic factors include increased secretion of male hormones (which occurs at puberty in males and females); bacteria, which cause sebum to break down into irritating fatty acids; oil-based cosmetics, which plug hair follicles; and certain medications (*e.g.,* phenytoin, corticosteroids, and iodides). There is no evidence that certain foods and emotional stress cause acne.

EXTERNAL OTITIS

External otitis is an infection of the external ear characterized by pain, itching, and drainage. The external ear, including the meatus, canal, and tympanic membrane (eardrum), is lined with epidermal tissue. The epidermal tissue is susceptible to the same skin disorders that affect other parts of the body. External otitis is most often caused by *Pseudomonas aeruginosa* and *Staphylococcus aureus* organisms and may be treated with antimicrobial ear drops for about 7 to 10 days.

ANORECTAL DISORDERS

Hemorrhoids and anal fissures are common anorectal disorders characterized by pruritus, bleeding, and pain. Inflammation and infection may occur.

Types of Dermatologic Drugs

Many different agents are used to prevent or treat dermatologic disorders. Most agents fit into one or more of the following categories:

1. **Antiseptics** kill or inhibit the growth of bacteria, viruses, or fungi. They are used primarily to prevent infection. They are occasionally used to treat dermatologic infections. Soaps and detergents are not antiseptics because they do not kill or inhibit growth of microorganisms. However, soaps and detergents facilitate mechanical cleansing of the skin, especially when applied with friction. Skin surfaces should generally be clean before application of antiseptics. Antiseptics are sometimes called "skin disinfectants," but generally the term *disinfectant* refers to agents used for sterilizing inanimate objects (*e.g.,* instruments). Disinfectants are usually too strong for application to the skin and mucous membranes.

2. **Anti-infective agents** are used to treat infections caused by bacteria, fungi, and viruses (see Chaps. 33 through 41). When used in dermatologic infections, anti-infective drugs may be administered locally (topically) or systemically (orally or parenterally). In many bacterial infections (*e.g.,* furuncles), systemic antibiotics are preferred. Generally, topical antibiotics have limited use in bacterial infections. However, topical therapy of fungal infections is effective. Topical antiviral therapy is available for treatment of ophthalmic viral infections (see Chap. 65); herpes genitalis, an infectious viral disease transmitted primarily by sexual contact; and herpes labialis ("fever blisters") in immunosuppressed clients (see Chap. 39).

3. **Anti-inflammatory agents** are used to treat the inflammation present in many dermatologic conditions. The major anti-inflammatory agents are the adrenal corticosteroids (see Chap. 24). When used in dermatologic conditions, corticosteroids are most often applied topically. However, they also may be administered orally and parenterally in severe dermatologic disorders.

4. **Retinoids** are vitamin A derivatives that are active in proliferation and differentiation of skin cells. These agents are being increasingly used to treat dermatologic disorders. Although tretinoin and isotretinoin are approved for treatment of acne and etretinate is approved for treatment of severe psoriasis, the drugs are being used in many other disorders as well (*e.g.,* aging and wrinkling of skin from sunlight exposure, skin cancers). Etretinate and isotretinoin are contraindicated in women of childbearing potential unless the women have negative pregnancy tests; agree to use effective contraception before, during, and after drug therapy; and agree to take the drugs as prescribed. These oral drugs have been associated with severe fetal abnormalities.

5. **Astringents** (*e.g.,* dilute solutions of aluminum salts) are used for their drying effects on exudative lesions.

6. **Emollients** or lubricants (*e.g.,* mineral oil, lanolin, petrolatum) are used to relieve pruritus and dryness of the skin.

7. **Enzymes** are used to débride burn wounds, decubitus ulcers, and venous stasis ulcers. They promote healing by removing necrotic tissue.

8. **Keratolytic agents** (*e.g.,* salicylic acid) are used to remove warts, corns, calluses, and other keratin-containing skin lesions.

9. **Sunscreens** are used to protect the skin from the damaging effects of UV radiation, thereby decreasing skin cancer and signs of aging, including wrinkles. Dermatologists recommend sunscreen preparations that block both UVA and UVB and have a "sun protection factor" (SPF) value of 30 or higher.

These highly protective sunscreens are especially needed by people who are fair skinned, allergic to sunlight, or using medications that increase skin sensitivity to sunlight (*e.g.*, estrogens, tetracycline).

10. Agents affecting skin pigmentation may be used with variable degrees of effectiveness to increase or decrease pigmentation. **Melanizing agents** (*e.g.*, trioxsalen, methoxsalen) may be used to increase skin pigmentation in vitiligo, a disorder characterized by white patches of skin surrounded by normally pigmented skin. **Demelanizing agents** (*e.g.*, hydroquinone, monobenzone) are occasionally used for hyperpigmented areas of the skin, such as freckles or chronic inflammatory lesions.

APPLICATION OF DERMATOLOGIC DRUGS

Most dermatologic medications are applied topically. To be effective, topical agents must be in contact with the underlying skin or mucous membrane. Numerous dosage forms have been developed for topical application of drugs to various parts of the body and for various therapeutic purposes. Basic components of topical agents are one or more active ingredients and a usually inactive vehicle. The vehicle is a major determinant of the drug's ability to reach affected skin and mucous membranes. Many topical preparations contain other additives (*e.g.*, preservatives, emulsifiers, emollients, dispersing agents) that further facilitate application to skin and mucous membranes. Commonly used vehicles and dosage forms include ointments, creams, lotions, powders, sprays, aerosols, gels, otic solutions, and vaginal and rectal suppositories. Many topical drug preparations are available in several dosage forms.

Topical medications are used primarily for local effects when systemic absorption is undesirable. Factors that influence percutaneous absorption of topical agents include the following:

1. **Degree of skin hydration.** Drug penetration and percutaneous absorption are increased when keratin in the outermost layer of the epidermis is well hydrated.
2. **Drug concentration.** Because percutaneous absorption occurs by passive diffusion, higher concentrations increase the amount of drug absorbed.
3. **Skin condition.** Absorption from abraded or damaged skin is much greater than from intact skin.
4. **Length of contact time.** Absorption is increased when drugs are left in place for prolonged periods.
5. **Size of area.** Absorption is increased when topical medications are applied to large areas of the body.
6. **Location of area.** Absorption from mucous membranes and facial skin is comparatively rapid. Absorption from thick-skinned areas (*e.g.*, palms of hands and soles of feet) is comparatively slow.

Individual Drugs

See Tables 66-1 to 66-3.

(*text continues on page 862*)

TABLE 66-1	ANTISEPTICS	
Generic/ Trade Name	Characteristics	Clinical Indications
Alcohols		
Ethanol (ethyl alcohol) Isopropyl alcohol (Rubbing Alcohol U.S.P. [70% ethanol]), (Isopropyl Alcohol [99% solution], Isopropyl Rubbing Alcohol [70% solution])	1. Bactericidal to common bacteria. When applied to skin, kills approximately 90% of bacteria within 2 min if the area is kept moist for that period. When applied in a single wipe and left to evaporate (*e.g.*, before injections), approximately 75% of bacteria are killed. 2. Erratic against viruses and fungi; ineffective against spores 3. Irritating to intact skin with prolonged contact. Irritating to denuded skin areas or open wounds; causes burning type of pain, increases tissue injury, and coagulates protein to form a mass under which bacteria may proliferate 4. Isopropyl alcohol is slightly more antiseptic than ethyl alcohol. It has the same indications for use.	Cleansing of intact skin before injections or surgical incisions

(continued)

TABLE 66-1 | **ANTISEPTICS** (Continued)

Generic/ Trade Name	Characteristics	Clinical Indications
Biguanide		
Chlorhexidine gluconate (Hibiclens [4% Aqueous Emulsion])	1. Effective against gram-positive and gram-negative bacteria 2. Some studies indicate that chlorhexidine (4%) is more effective than 3% hexachlorophene (pHiso-Hex) or povidone-iodine (Betadine) for handwashing and surgical scrubs 3. Little, if any, absorption occurs through the skin of adults. Absorption from the skin of neonates is unknown but probably slight. 4. Some gram-negative organisms are resistant to the drug, and infection may occur.	1. Handwashing 2. Preoperative skin cleansing for client and health care personnel (surgical scrub) 3. Treatment of superficial cutaneous infections 4. Wound cleansing 5. Neonatal skin cleansing to reduce incidence of staphylococcal and streptococcal infections 6. Treatment of oral ulcers (as an ingredient in mouthwashes) 7. Prevention of dental caries
Iodine Preparations		
Iodine tincture, U.S.P. (2% iodine and 2.4% sodium iodide diluted in 50% ethanol) **Iodine topical solution U.S.P.** (2% iodine and 2.4% sodium iodide in water) **Povidone-iodine** (a 10% solution contains 1% available iodine) (Betadine, Isodine, others)	1. Iodine preparations kill most microorganisms (bacteria, fungi, viruses). When applied to the skin, a 1% solution kills approximately 90% of bacteria within 90 sec. 2. Antiseptic activity depends on the concentration of iodine. Sodium iodide increases solubility; polyvinyl-pyrrolidone (povidone) is a carrier substance that increases solubility of iodine and releases iodine slowly for a sustained action. 3. Betadine, a commonly used iodine preparation, is available in numerous concentrations and dosage forms. These include the following (concentrations expressed in terms of available iodine): aerosol spray 0.5%; ointment 1%; shampoo 0.75%; skin cleanser 0.75%; solution 1%; surgical scrub 0.75%; vaginal douche solution and vaginal gel 1%. 4. Iodine topical solution should not be confused with strong iodine solution (Lugol's solution) used for the treatment of hyperthyroidism.	1. Prevention or treatment of infections of the skin, scalp, and mucous membranes of the mouth and vagina 2. Preoperative cleansing of the skin 3. Treatment of wounds and abrasions
Chlorine Preparations		
Sodium hypochlorite solution, diluted (Modified Dakin's solution)	1. Exerts bactericidal action by releasing hypochlorous acid 2. Irritating to tissues 3. Dissolves necrotic materials 4. Dissolves blood clots and delays clotting 5. Undiluted solutions are too strong for use as antiseptics.	Infected wounds when other methods or agents are not available
Sodium oxychlorosene (Clorpactin sodium)	A mixture of sodium hypochlorite solution and alkylbenzene sulfonates. The alkylbenzene sulfonates have surfactant properties that increase penetration and antibacterial effects.	Treatment of infected wounds
Metallic Antiseptics		
Silver nitrate	Silver nitrate is available in solid form (Toughened silver nitrate U.S.P.) for use as a caustic in removing warts and cauterizing wounds; an ophthalmic solution for use in newborn infants; and a solution (0.5%)	1. Cauterizing warts or wounds 2. Prophylaxis of ophthalmia neonatorum in newborns

TABLE 66-1   **ANTISEPTICS** (Continued)

Generic/ Trade Name	Characteristics	Clinical Indications
	for use in treating burn wounds. It is infrequently used in burn treatment because it stains the skin black and causes hypochloremia.	3. Treatment of burn wounds
Silver sulfadiazine (Silvadene)	1. Silver sulfadiazine is widely used in treatment of burn wounds. 2. Exerts antibacterial action against *Pseudomonas* and many other organisms that infect burn wounds. The drug penetrates eschar. 3. Does not stain the skin or cause pain at application sites.	Prevention of infection in burn wounds
Zinc oxide (Zinc Oxide Ointment [20% zinc oxide]) (Calamine Lotion U.S.P. [8% calamine and 8% zinc oxide])	1. Available in many preparations and dosage forms (powders, ointments, pastes, lotions) 2. Also has astringent properties	1. Eczema 2. Impetigo 3. Tinea infections (ringworm) 4. Venous stasis ulcers 5. Pruritus 6. Psoriasis
Zinc pyrithione (Zincon, others)	1. Used in concentrations of 0.1%–2% 2. A common ingredient in over-the-counter dandruff shampoos	1. Seborrhea 2. Dandruff
Oxidizing Agents		
Hydrogen peroxide topical solution U.S.P. (3% hydrogen peroxide in water)	1. Hydrogen peroxide is more effective as a débriding and cleansing agent than as an antiseptic. It is of doubtful value on intact skin. However, when it comes in contact with wounds or blood, it rapidly decomposes into oxygen and water. The liberated oxygen exerts a brief antibacterial effect and loosens infected material. 2. Prolonged use of hydrogen peroxide as a mouthwash, even at half strength, may cause hypertrophy of filiform papillae of the tongue ("hairy tongue"). This condition is reversible when hydrogen peroxide is discontinued.	1. Wound cleansing 2. Mouthwash (diluted in equal parts with water or normal saline and a commercial mouthwash such as Cepacol) 3. To remove cerumen from the external ear 4. Cleansing of tracheostomy tubes (inner cannulae)
Benzoyl peroxide (Benzoyl peroxide lotion U.S.P. [5% or 10% hydrous benzoyl peroxide])	1. Benzoyl peroxide slowly releases oxygen and is bactericidal for anaerobic bacteria (*e.g.*, *Corynebacterium*). 2. This agent also has irritant, keratolytic, and antiseborrheic properties	Acne
Phenol Derivatives		
Hexachlorophene and entsufon sodium emulsion (pHisoHex)	1. pHisoHex is a commonly used preparation of hexachlorophene. It contains 3% hexachlorophene and entsufon sodium, a detergent. 2. Bacteriostatic against gram-positive bacteria, including staphylococci. Relatively ineffective against gram-negative organisms and fungi. Gram-negative bacterial and fungal infections may increase in incidence during chronic use of hexachlorophene preparations. 3. A single washing with a hexachlorophene substance is no more effective than soap in reducing the number of microorganisms on the skin. Repeated washings leave a residual film on the skin	1. Handwashing, especially for health care personnel and food handlers 2. Preoperative skin cleansing

(continued)

TABLE 66-1	ANTISEPTICS (Continued)

Generic/ Trade Name	Characteristics	Clinical Indications
Hexachlorophene, entsufon (cont)	that produces a steady reduction in bacterial flora. Cleansing with alcohol or washing with soap removes the antibacterial residual film. 4. Hexachlorophene is absorbed systemically from intact skin, especially after repeated applications. Systemic absorption is increased if the skin is broken; thus, hexachlorophene should *not* be applied to open wounds. 5. Use should be followed by thorough rinsing.	
Resorcinol	1. Bactericidal and fungicidal 2. Also has mild irritant and keratolytic characteristics 3. Usually applied as a 10% ointment or lotion	1. Acne 2. Ringworm (tinea) infections 3. Dermatitis 4. Psoriasis 5. Other cutaneous lesions
Miscellaneous Antiseptics		
Acetic acid	1. Bactericidal to many microorganisms, including *Pseudomonas aeruginosa*, in a 5% concentration 2. Bacteriostatic in concentrations lower than 5%	1. Irrigations and dressings of surgical wounds (1% solution), bladder irrigations (0.25% solution) 2. Vaginal infections due to *Trichomonas, Candida*, or *Haemophilus* organisms. Administered as a vaginal douche. 3. External otitis (2% solution, instilled in the auditory canal)
Sulfur	1. Has fungicidal and keratolytic properties 2. May be used alone or in combination with other keratolytic agents (*e.g.*, coal tar, resorcinol, 2% salicylic acid). 3. Widely used in dermatology	1. Psoriasis 2. Seborrhea 3. Dermatitis

TABLE 66-2	DERMATOLOGIC ANTI-INFECTIVE AND ANTI-INFLAMMATORY AGENTS

Generic/ Trade Name	Routes and Dosage Ranges (Adults and Children)
Antibacterial Agents	
Bacitracin (Baciguent ointment)	Topically to skin lesions once or twice daily
Mupirocin (Bactroban)	Impetigo: topically to skin, three times daily
Neomycin sulfate (Myciguent ointment)	Topically to skin once or twice daily
Nitrofurazone (Furacin)	Topically to burn wounds once daily or every few days when dressings are changed
Combination Agents	
Bacitracin and polymyxin B (Polysporin ointment)	Topically to skin two to five times daily

TABLE 66-2   DERMATOLOGIC ANTI-INFECTIVE AND ANTI-INFLAMMATORY AGENTS

Generic/Trade Name	Routes and Dosage Ranges (Adults and Children)
Polymyxin B sulfate, neomycin sulfate, and bacitracin (Neosporin ointment)	Topically to skin two to five times daily
Antifungal Agents	
Amphotericin B (Fungizone)	Cutaneous candidiasis: topically to skin two to four times daily
Clioquinol (Vioform)	Localized dermatophytosis: topically to skin several times daily
Clotrimazole (Lotrimin, Mycelex)	Cutaneous dermatophytosis, cutaneous and vaginal candidiasis: topically to skin or vaginal mucosa once daily
Ciclopirox (Loprox)	Same as econazole
Econazole (Spectazole)	Tinea infections, cutaneous candidiasis: topically to skin twice daily for 2–4 wk
Haloprogin (Halotex)	Tinea pedis (athlete's foot), cutaneous candidiasis: topically to skin twice daily for 2–4 wk
Miconazole (Micatin)	Dermatophytosis, cutaneous candidiasis: topically to skin once or twice daily for 4 wk
Naftifine (Naftin)	Tinea infections: topically to skin once daily (cream) or twice daily (gel)
Nystatin (Mycostatin)	Candidiasis of skin and oral mucous membranes: topically to lesions two or three times daily. Vaginal candidiasis: topically to vaginal mucosa once or twice daily for 14 d
Oxiconazole (Oxistat)	Tinea infections: topically to skin twice daily for 2–4 wk
Sulconazole (Exelderm)	Tinea infections: topically to skin once or twice daily
Terbinafine (Lamisil)	Tinea infections: topically to skin twice daily for at least 1 wk and no longer than 4 wk
Tolnaftate (Tinactin)	Dermatophytosis: topically to skin twice daily
Undecylenic acid (Desenex, others)	Dermatophytosis, especially tinea pedis (athlete's foot): topically to skin or mucous membranes. Dosage recommendations vary among manufacturers.
Antiviral Agent	
Acyclovir (Zovirax)	Herpes genitalis (initial lesions) and herpes labialis in immunosuppressed clients: topically to lesions q3h or at least six times daily for 7 d
Corticosteroids	
Alclometasone (Aclovate)	Topically to skin two to four times daily
Amcinonide (Cyclocort)	Topically to skin two to three times daily
Betamethasone (Benisone, Valisone)	Topically to skin one to four times daily
Clobetasol (Temovate)	Topically to skin two to four times daily
Clocortolone (Cloderm)	Topically to skin one to three times daily
Desonide (Tridesilon)	Topically to skin two or three times daily
Desoximetasone (Topicort)	Topically to skin one or two times daily
Dexamethasone (Decaderm, Decadron)	Topically to skin two or three times daily
Diflorasone (Florone, Maxiflor)	Topically to skin two or three times daily
Fluocinonide (Lidex, Synalar)	Topically to skin three or four times daily
Flurandrenolide (Cordran)	Topically to skin two or three times daily
Halcinonide (Halog)	Topically to skin two or three times daily
Hydrocortisone (Cortril, Hydrocortone)	Topically to skin three or four times daily
Methylprednisolone acetate (Medrol acetate)	Topically to skin one to four times daily, then reduced when disease process is controlled
Triamcinolone acetonide (Aristocort, Kenalog, other	Topically to skin three or four times daily

TABLE 66-3	MISCELLANEOUS DERMATOLOGIC AGENTS

Generic / Trade Name	Dermatologic Effects	Clinical Indications	Method of Administration
Demelanizing Agents			
Hydroquinone (Eldoquin)	Decreases skin pigmentation	1. Freckles 2. Melasma	Topically to hyperpigmented areas of the skin one or two times daily
Monobenzone (Benoquin)	Decreases skin pigmentation	Vitiligo—for permanent depigmentation of areas containing normal pigmentation (*i.e.*, to relieve "spotted" appearance)	Topically, to pigmented areas only, two or three times daily
Melanizing Agents			
Methoxsalen (Oxsoralen-ultra)	Increases skin pigmentation	1. Vitiligo 2. Psoriasis	Topically to small lesions, followed by sunlight or ultraviolet light Psoriasis, PO 10–40 mg daily, followed in 2 h by sunlight or ultraviolet light
Trioxsalen (Trisoralen)	Increases skin pigmentation	1. Vitiligo 2. Increase tolerance to sunlight	Vitiligo: PO 10 mg daily, followed in 2 h by exposure to sunlight To increase tolerance to sunlight: PO 10 mg daily for no longer than 14 d
Enzymes			
Collagenase (Santyl)	Débriding effects	Enzymatic débridement of infected wounds (*e.g.*, burn wounds, decubitus ulcers)	Topically once daily until the wound is cleansed of necrotic material
Fibrinolysin-deoxyribonuclease (Elase)	See collagenase, above	See collagenase, above	See collagenase, above
Papain (Panafil)	Débriding effects	Débridement of surface lesions	Topically one or two times daily
Sutilains (Travase)	Débriding effects	Débridement of wounds	Topically to wound three or four times daily
Trypsin (Granulex)	Débriding effects	Débridement of infected wounds (*e.g.*, decubitus and varicose ulcers)	Topically by spray twice daily
Retinoids			
Adalapene (Differin)	Reportedly causes less burning, itching, redness, and dryness than tretinoin	Acne vulgaris	Topically to skin lesions once daily
Etretinate (Tegison)	Anti-inflammatory and anti-keratinizing effects	Severe psoriasis	PO 0.75–1 mg/kg/d in divided doses
Isotretinoin (Accutane)	Inhibits sebum production and keratinization	1. Severe cystic acne 2. Disorders characterized by excessive keratinization (*e.g.*, pityriasis, ichthyosis) 3. *Mycosis fungoides*	PO 1–2 mg/kg/d, in two divided doses, for 15–20 wk

TABLE 66-3 **MISCELLANEOUS DERMATOLOGIC AGENTS** (Continued)

Generic / Trade Name	Dermatologic Effects	Clinical Indications	Method of Administration
Tretinoin (Retin-A)	Irritant	Acne vulgaris	Topically to skin lesions once daily
Other Agents			
Aluminum acetate solution (Burow's solution)	Astringent, antipruritic, anti-inflammatory	1. Weeping or "wet" skin lesions due to infection or inflammation 2. External otitis	Topically to skin, as wet dressings Topically to external ear, as irrigating solution to remove debris
Anthralin (Anthra-Derm, others)	Slows the rate of skin cell growth and replication	Psoriasis	Topically to lesions once daily or as directed
Azelaic acid (Azelex)	Decreases skin bacteria and comedone formation	Acne	Topically to lesions twice daily
Calcipotriene (Dovonex)	Synthetic analogue of vitamin D that helps to regulate skin cell production and development	Psoriasis	Topically to lesions twice daily
Capsaicin (Zostrix)	Depletes substance P (which transmits pain impulses) in sensory nerves of the skin	Relief of pain associated with rheumatoid arthritis, osteoarthritis, and neuralgias	Topically to affected area, up to three to four times daily
Coal tar (Balnetar, Zetar, others)	Irritant	1. Psoriasis 2. Dermatitis	Topically to skin, in various concentrations and preparations (*e.g.*, creams, lotions, shampoos, bath emulsion). Also available in combination with hydrocortisone and other substances
Colloidal oatmeal (Aveeno)	Antipruritic	Pruritus	Topically as a bath solution (1 cup in bathtub of water)
Dextranomer (Debrisan)	Absorbs exudates from wound surfaces	Cleansing of ulcers (*e.g.*, venous stasis, decubitus) and wounds (*e.g.*, burn, surgical, traumatic)	Apply to a clean, moist wound surface q12h initially, then less often as exudate decreases
Fluorouracil (Efudex)	Antineoplastic	1. Actinic keratoses 2. Superficial basal cell carcinomas	Topically to skin lesions twice daily for 2–6 wk
Masoprocol (Actinex)	Inhibits proliferation of keratin-containing cells	Actinic keratoses	Topically to skin lesions morning and evening for 28 d
Salicylic acid	Keratolytic, antifungal	1. Removal of warts, corns, calluses 2. Superficial fungal infections 3. Seborrheic dermatitis 4. Acne 5. Psoriasis	Topically to lesions
Selenium sulfide (Selsun)	Antifungal, antidandruff	1. Dandruff 2. Tinea versicolor	Topically to scalp as shampoo once or twice weekly

Nursing Process

Assessment

Assess the client's skin for characteristics or lesions that may indicate current or potential dermatologic disorders.

- When a skin rash is present, interview the client and inspect the area to determine the following:
  - **Appearance of individual lesions.** Lesions should be described as specifically as possible so changes can be identified. Terms commonly used in dermatology include *macule* (flat spot), *papule* (raised spot), *nodule* (small solid swelling), *vesicle* (blister), *pustule* (pus-containing lesion), *petechia* (flat, round, purplish-red spot the size of a pinpoint, caused by intradermal or submucosal bleeding), and *erythema* (redness). Lesions also may be described as weeping or dry and scaly or crusty.
  - **Location or distribution.** Some skin rashes occur exclusively or primarily on certain parts of the body (*e.g.*, face, extremities, trunk), and distribution may indicate the cause.
  - **Accompanying symptoms.** Pruritus occurs with most dermatologic conditions. Fever, malaise, and other symptoms may occur as well.
  - **Historic development.** Appropriate questions include
    - When and where did the skin rash appear?
    - How long has it been present?
    - Has it changed in appearance or location?
    - Has it occurred previously?
  - **Etiologic factors.** In many instances, appropriate treatment is determined by the cause. Some etiologic factors include the following:
    - **Drug therapy.** Many commonly used drugs may cause skin lesions, including antibiotics (*e.g.*, penicillins, sulfonamides, tetracyclines), narcotic analgesics, phenothiazine antipsychotic agents (*e.g.*, chlorpromazine), and thiazide diuretics. Skin rashes due to drug therapy are usually generalized and appear abruptly.
    - **Irritants or allergens** may cause contact dermatitis. For example, dermatitis involving the hands may be caused by soaps, detergents, or various other cleansing agents. Dermatitis involving the trunk may result from allergic reactions to clothing.
    - **Communicable diseases** (*i.e.*, measles, scarlatina, chickenpox) cause characteristic skin rashes and systemic signs and symptoms.
- When skin lesions other than rashes are present, assess appearance, size or extent, amount and character of any drainage, and whether the lesion appears infected or contains necrotic material. Bleeding into the skin is usually described as *petechiae* (pinpoint hemorrhages) or *ecchymoses* (bruises). Burn wounds are usually described in terms of depth (partial or full thickness of skin) and percentage of body surface area. Burn wounds with extensive skin damage are rapidly colonized with potentially pathogenic microorganisms. Venous stasis, pressure, and other cutaneous ulcers are usually described in terms of diameter and depth.
- When assessing the skin, consider the age of the client. Infants are likely to have "diaper" dermatitis, miliaria (heat rash), and tinea capitis (ringworm infection of the scalp). School-age children have a relatively high incidence of measles, chickenpox, and tinea infections. Adolescents often have acne. Older adults are more likely to have dry skin, actinic keratoses, and skin neoplasms.
- Assess for skin neoplasms. *Basal cell carcinoma* is the most common type of skin cancer. It may initially appear as a pale nodule, most often on the head and neck. *Squamous cell carcinomas* may appear as ulcerated areas. These lesions may occur anywhere on the body but are more common on sun-exposed parts, such as the face and hands. *Malignant melanoma* is the most serious skin cancer. It involves melanocytes, the pigment-producing cells of the skin. Malignant melanoma may occur in pigmented nevi (moles) or previously normal skin. In nevi, malignant melanoma may be manifested by enlargement and ulceration. In previously normal skin, lesions appear as irregularly shaped pigmented areas. Although it can occur in almost any area, malignant melanoma is most likely to be located on the back in white people and in toe webs and soles of the feet in African-American or Asian people.
- When assessing dark-skinned clients, color changes and skin rashes are more difficult to detect. Some guidelines include the following:
  - Adequate lighting is required. Nonglare daylight is best. The illumination provided by overbed lights or flashlights is inadequate for most purposes.
  - Some skin rashes may be visible on oral mucous membranes.
  - Petechiae are not visible on dark-brown or black skin, but they may be visible on oral mucous membranes or the conjunctiva.
- When skin disorders are present, assess the client's psychological response to the condition. Many clients, especially those with chronic disorders, feel self-conscious and depressed.

Nursing Diagnoses

- Body Image Disturbance related to visible skin lesions
- Anxiety related to potential for permanent scarring or disfigurement
- Pain related to skin lesions and pruritus
- Risk for Injury: Infection related to entry of microbes through damaged skin
- Knowledge Deficit related to prevention and treatment of skin disorders

Planning/Goals

The client will:
- Apply topical drugs correctly
- Experience relief of symptoms
- Use techniques to prevent or minimize skin damage and disorders
- Avoid scarring and disfigurement when possible
- Be encouraged to express concerns about acute and chronic body image changes

Interventions

Use measures to prevent or minimize skin disorders.
- Use general measures to promote health and increase resistance to disease (*i.e.*, maintain nutrition, rest, and exercise).
- Practice good personal hygiene, with at least once daily cleansing of skin areas with high bacterial counts, such as underarms and perineum.

- Practice safety measures to avoid injury to the skin. Any injury, especially one that disrupts the integrity of the skin (*e.g.*, lacerations, puncture wounds, scratching of skin lesions), increases the likelihood of skin infections.
- Avoid known irritants or allergens. Have the client substitute nonirritating soaps or cleaning supplies for irritating ones; use hypoallergenic jewelry and cosmetics if indicated; wear cotton clothing if indicated.
- Use measures to relieve dry skin and pruritus. Dry skin causes itching, and itching promotes scratching. Scratching relieves itching only if it is strong enough to damage the skin and serve as a counterirritant. Skin damaged or disrupted by scratching is susceptible to invasion by pathogenic microorganisms. Thus, dry skin may lead to serious skin disorders. Older adults are especially likely to have dry, flaky skin. Measures to decrease skin dryness include the following:
  - Alternating complete and partial baths. For example, the client may alternate a shower or tub bath with a sponge bath (of face, hands, underarms, and perineal areas). Warm water, mild soaps, and patting dry are recommended because hot water, harsh soaps, and rubbing with a towel have drying effects on the skin.
  - Liberal use of lubricating creams, lotions, and oils. Bath oils, which usually contain mineral oil or lanolin oil and a perfume, are widely available. If bath oils are used, precautions against falls are necessary, because the oils make bathtubs and shower floors slippery. Creams and lotions may be applied several times daily.
- Prevent pressure ulcers by avoiding trauma to the skin and prolonged pressure on any part of the body. In clients at high risk for developing pressure ulcers, major preventive measures include frequent changes of position and correct lifting techniques. Various pressure-relieving devices also are useful. These include special beds and mattresses. Daily inspection of the skin is needed for early detection and treatment of beginning pressure ulcers.
- Avoid excessive exposure to sunlight and other sources of UV light. Although controlled amounts of UV light are beneficial in some dermatologic disorders (*i.e.*, acne, psoriasis), excessive amounts cause wrinkling, dryness, and malignancies. If prolonged exposure is necessary, protective clothing and sunscreening lotions decrease skin damage.
- When skin rashes are present, cool, wet compresses or baths are often effective in relieving pruritus. Water or normal saline may be used alone or with additives, such as aluminum acetate solution (Burow's solution), colloidal oatmeal (Aveeno), or baking soda. A cool environment also tends to decrease pruritus. The client's fingernails should be cut short and kept clean to avoid skin damage and infection from scratching.

  For severe itching, a systemic antihistamine may be needed. Topical antihistamines are not recommended because they may sensitize the skin and cause allergic reactions with later exposures.

Teach clients:

- To promote healthy skin by a balanced diet, personal hygiene measures, avoiding excessive exposure to sunlight, avoiding skin injuries, and lubricating dry skin. Healthy skin is less sus-

ceptible to inflammation, infections, and other disorders. It also heals more rapidly when disorders or injuries occur.
- To avoid scratching, squeezing, or rubbing skin lesions. These behaviors cause additional skin damage.
- Ways to mask unavoidable lesions or scars (*e.g.*, with makeup or clothing)

Evaluation

- Observe and interview regarding use of dermatologic drugs.
- Observe for improvement in skin lesions and symptoms.
- Interview regarding use of measures to promote healthy skin and prevent skin disorders.

Principles of Therapy

DRUG SELECTION IN VARIOUS SKIN CONDITIONS

The choice of dermatologic agents depends primarily on the reason for use and client response. Some guidelines include the following:

1. For routine handwashing of health care personnel and preoperative skin cleansing of surgical staff and clients, chlorhexidine (Hibiclens) and povidone-iodine (Betadine) are the antiseptics of first choice. Alcohol is effective but too drying for routine use. pHisoHex is not effective against gram-negative bacteria and is absorbed systemically from intact skin.
2. Topical medications for inflammatory and noninflammatory skin disorders vary greatly. Generally, though, astringents and lotions are used as drying agents for "wet," oozing lesions, and ointments and creams are used as "wetting" agents for dry, scaling lesions. Topical corticosteroids are available in several dosage forms for use in acute and chronic inflammatory disorders. Hydrocortisone is the topical corticosteroid of choice for use on the face or other cosmetically important areas. It is available over the counter in a 0.5% concentration. The fluorinated corticosteroids may cause skin eruptions, dermatitis, and acne; therefore, these compounds are generally used on areas other than the face.
3. For topical antibiotic therapy, bacitracin, neomycin, and polymyxin are usually preferred. These drugs are often used in combination, and various preparations are available (*e.g.*, Neosporin). Although other antibiotics are available in dosage forms for topical use (*e.g.*, gentamicin, chloramphenicol, tetracyclines), they generally should not be used. These drugs may cause sensitization when used topically. If a sensitized client receives the drug systemically at a later time, serious allergic reactions may occur.
4. In acne, benzoyl peroxide, 5% or 10%, is one of the most effective topical agents. Systemic tetracycline in

low doses may be used for long-term treatment of acne. Because of potentially serious adverse effects, isotretinoin and tretinoin are recommended for use only in severe acne. Because of teratogenic effects, these drugs are contraindicated during pregnancy. Women of childbearing potential should use an effective method of contraception during and for at least 1 month after treatment with isotretinoin or tretinoin.

5. In external otitis, otic preparations of various dermatologic medications are used. Polymyxin B (Cortisporin Otic Solution) and neomycin (Otobiotic Otic Solution) are the most commonly used antibiotics, although others (*e.g.*, tetracyclines, sulfonamides, gentamicin) are available. Acetic acid solution 2% also may be administered as an otic anti-infective agent. Acetic acid is effective against *Pseudomonas* and many other organisms that cause external ear disease. It establishes an acidic environment, which prevents growth of the organisms, and does not produce resistant organisms. Hydrocortisone is the corticosteroid most often included in topical otic preparations. It relieves pruritus and inflammation in chronic external otitis. Local anesthetics, usually benzocaine, are included in some otic formulations. However, local anesthetics are not well absorbed from the ear and are generally ineffective in relieving the severe pain associated with acute external otitis or otitis media. Systemic analgesics are usually required.

6. In pressure ulcers, the only clear-cut guideline for treatment is avoiding further pressure on the affected area. Many topical agents are used, most often with specific procedures for dressing changes, skin cleansing, and so on. No one agent or procedure is clearly superior. Consistent implementation of a protocol (*i.e.*, position changes, inspection of current or potential pressure areas, dressing changes, use of alternating, pressure-relieving mattresses) may be more effective than drug therapy.

7. In anorectal disorders, most preparations contain a local anesthetic, emollients, and perhaps a corticosteroid. These preparations relieve pruritus and pain but do not cure the underlying condition. Some preparations contain ingredients of questionable value, such as vasoconstrictors, astringents, and weak antiseptics. No particular mixture is clearly superior.

DOSAGE FORMS

The choice of dosage form for topical drug therapy depends largely on the reason for use. Guidelines include the following:

1. **Ointments** are oil-based substances that usually contain a medication in an emollient vehicle, such as petrolatum or lanolin. Ointments occlude the skin and promote retention of moisture. Thus, they are especially useful in chronic skin disorders characterized by dry lesions. Ointments should generally be avoided in hairy, moist, and intertriginous areas of the body because of potential maceration, irritation, and secondary infection.

2. **Creams** (emulsions of oil in water, which may be greasy or nongreasy) and *gels* (transparent colloids, which dry and leave a film over the area) retain moisture in the skin but are less occlusive than ointments. These preparations are cosmetically acceptable for use on the face and other visible areas of the body. They also may be used in hairy, moist, intertriginous areas. Creams and gels are especially useful in subacute dermatologic disorders.

3. **Lotions** are suspensions of insoluble substances in water. They cool, dry, and protect the skin. They are most useful in subacute dermatologic disorders. *Sprays* and *aerosols* are similar to lotions.

4. **Powders** have absorbent, cooling, and protective effects. Generally, powders should not be applied in acute, exudative disorders or on denuded areas because they tend to cake, occlude the lesions, and retard healing. Also, some powders (*e.g.*, cornstarch) may lead to secondary infections by promoting growth of bacteria and fungi.

5. **Pastes** are semisolid preparations composed primarily of powder. Pastes adhere strongly to the area of application and are difficult to remove. They are generally less macerating, penetrating, and occlusive than ointments. Pastes should not be used on hairy areas of the body.

6. Topical otic medications are usually delivered in a liquid vehicle. However, creams or ointments may be used for dry, crusted lesions, and powders may be used for drying effects.

7. Topical vaginal medications may be applied as douche solutions, vaginal tablets, or vaginal creams used with an applicator.

8. Dosage of corticosteroids applied topically to skin depends on the potency of the preparation (percentage of drug contained in the ointment, lotion, or other vehicle), the area of application, and the method of application. The skin covering the face, scalp, scrotum, and axillae is more permeable to corticosteroids than other skin surfaces, and these areas can usually be treated with less potent formulations, smaller amounts, or less frequent applications. In addition, drug absorption is increased by applying an occlusive dressing over the affected area. Systemic toxicity may occur. For this reason, drug application is usually done less frequently when occlusive dressings are used.

9. Anorectal medications may be applied as ointments, creams, foams, and rectal suppositories.

USE IN CHILDREN

Children are at risk of developing a wide range of dermatologic disorders, including dermatitis and skin rashes in younger children and acne in adolescents. Few guidelines have been developed for drug therapy of these disorders. Infants, and perhaps older children, have more permeable skin and are more likely to absorb topical drugs than adults. In addition, absorption is increased in the presence of broken or damaged skin. Therefore, cautious use of topical agents is advised.

With topical corticosteroids, suppression of the hypothalamic-pituitary-adrenal axis (see Chap. 24), Cushing's disease, and intracranial hypertension have been reported. Signs of impaired adrenal function may include delayed growth in height and weight and low plasma cortisol levels. Signs of intracranial hypertension may include headaches, bulging fontanelles, and swelling of the optic nerve (papilledema) on ophthalmoscopic examination. The latter may lead to blindness if pressure on the optic nerve is not re-lieved. These drugs should be used only if clearly indicated, in the least effective dose, and for the shortest effective time.

USE IN OLDER ADULTS

Older adults often have dry skin and are at risk of pressure ulcers if mobility, nutrition, or elimination is impaired. Principles of topical drug therapy are the same as for younger adults.

HOME CARE

Skin disorders are commonly treated at home by clients or caregivers. When a home care nurse is involved, responsibilities may include assessing clients, other members of the household, and the home environment for risks of skin disorders; teaching preventive or treatment measures; assisting with treatment; and assessing response to treatment.

NURSING ACTIONS

DERMATOLOGIC DRUGS

NURSING ACTIONS	RATIONALE/EXPLANATION
1. Administer accurately **a.** Use the correct preparation for the intended use (*i.e.,* dermatologic, otic, vaginal, anorectal)	Preparations may differ in drug contents and concentrations.
b. For topical application to skin lesions: (1) Wash the skin, and pat it dry.	To cleanse the skin and remove previously applied medication. This facilitates drug contact with the affected area of the skin.
(2) Apply a small amount of the drug preparation, and rub it in well.	A thin layer of medication is effective and decreases the incidence and severity of adverse effects.
(3) For burn wounds, broken skin, or open lesions, apply the drug with sterile gloves or sterile cotton-tipped applicators.	To prevent infection
(4) Use the drug only for the individual client (*i.e.,* do not use the same tube for more than one client).	To avoid bacterial cross-contamination between clients
(5) Wash hands before and after application.	Wash hands before to avoid exposing the client to infection; wash hands afterward to avoid transferring the drug to your own face or eyes and causing adverse reactions.
2. Observe for therapeutic effects **a.** With dermatologic conditions, observe for healing of skin lesions.	Therapeutic effects depend on the medication being used and the disorder being treated.
b. With external otitis, observe for decreased pain and pruritus.	

(continued)

NURSING ACTIONS	RATIONALE/EXPLANATION
c. With vaginal disorders, observe for decreased vaginal discharge and pruritus.	
d. With anorectal disorders, observe for decreased pain and pruritus.	
3. Observe for adverse effects **a.** Local irritation or inflammation—burning on application, erythema, skin rash, pruritus	Incidence of adverse effects is low with topical agents. Local adverse effects may occur with most topical agents but may be more likely with antiseptics, local anesthetics, and antimicrobials.
b. With topical corticosteroids, observe for acneiform facial lesions and other skin changes (atrophy, thinning, development of striae).	Facial lesions occur with chronic use of fluorinated corticosteroids. They can be avoided by using hydrocortisone on facial lesions. Other skin changes occur with prolonged use of topical corticosteroids.
c. With topical antibiotics, superinfection and sensitization may occur.	Superinfection with drug-resistant organisms may occur with any antibacterial agent. It is less likely to occur with mixtures that have a broad spectrum of antibacterial activity. Sensitization may cause serious allergic reactions if the same drug is given systemically at a later time.
d. With isotretinoin and etretinate, observe for hypervitaminosis A (nausea, vomiting, headache, blurred vision, eye irritation, conjunctivitis, skin disorders, abnormal liver function, musculoskeletal pain, increased plasma triglycerides, others).	Adverse effects commonly occur with usual doses but are more severe with higher doses.
4. Observe for drug interactions	Clinically significant drug interactions rarely occur with topical agents.
5. Teach clients **a.** Use topical medications only as prescribed or according to the manufacturer's instructions (for over-the-counter products).	Most topical agents are safe if used properly but may cause adverse effects if used improperly.
b. For minor wounds and abrasions, cleansing with soap and water is usually adequate. If an antiseptic is used, an iodine preparation (*e.g.*, aqueous iodine solution 1%) is preferred.	Iodine preparations are effective in preventing infection. Alcohol should not be applied to open wounds. Hydrogen peroxide may facilitate mechanical cleansing, but it is a weak antiseptic. Common household agents, for instance, merbromin (Mercurochrome) and thimerosal (Merthiolate), are weak antiseptics. These mercury compounds are generally not recommended for use.
c. With isotretinoin and etretinate, avoid vitamin supplements containing vitamin A and excessive exposure to sunlight.	To decrease risks of excessive vitamin A intake and photosensitivity

REVIEW AND APPLICATION EXERCISES

1. What are the main functions of the skin?

2. Describe interventions to promote skin health and integrity.

3. During initial assessment of a client, what signs and symptoms may indicate common skin disorders?

4. Which client groups are at risk of developing common skin disorders (*e.g.*, skin infections, pressure ulcers)?

5. Compare topical and systemic corticosteroids in terms of adverse effects.

6. If an adolescent client with acne asks your advice about over-the-counter topical drugs, which would you recommend and why?

7. List general principles of using topical agents for common skin disorders.

SELECTED REFERENCES

Allman, R.M. (1997). Approach to the elderly patient with pressure ulcers. In W.N. Kelley (Ed.), *Textbook of internal medicine,* 3rd ed., pp. 2530–2532. Philadelphia: Lippincott-Raven.

Arndt, K.A., LeBoit, P.E., Robinson, J.K., & Wintroub, B.U. (1996). *Cutaneous medicine and surgery.* Philadelphia: W.B. Saunders.

Barnard, C.M., Kim, Y.H., & Bauer, E.A. (1997). Approach to the patient with skin lesions. In W.N. Kelley (Ed.), *Textbook of internal medicine,* 3rd ed., pp. 1215–1222. Philadelphia: Lippincott-Raven.

Deters, G.E. (1996). Management of patients with dermatologic problems. In S.C. Smeltzer & B.G. Bare (Eds.), *Brunner and Suddarth's Textbook of medical-surgical nursing,* 8th ed., pp. 1493–1543. Philadelphia: Lippincott-Raven.

Diehl, K.B. (1996). Topical antifungal agents: An update. *American Family Physician, 54*(5), 1687–1692.

Drug facts and comparisons. (Updated monthly). St. Louis: Facts and Comparisons.

Guzzo, C.A., Lazarus, G.S., & Werth, V.P. (1996). Dermatological pharmacology. In J.G. Hardman, L.E. Limbird, P.B. Molinoff, & R.W. Ruddon (Eds.), *Goodman & Gilman's The pharmacological basis of therapeutics,* 9th ed., pp. 1593–1616. New York: McGraw-Hill.

Nowakowski, P.A., Rumsfield, J.A., & West, D.P. (1997). Common skin disorders: Acne and psoriasis. In J.T. DiPiro, R.L. Talbert, G.C. Yee, G.R. Matzke, B.G. Wells, & L.M. Posey (Eds.), *Pharmacotherapy: A pathophysiologic approach,* 3rd ed., pp. 1815–1833. Stamford, CT: Appleton & Lange.

Simandl, G. (1994). Alterations in skin function and integrity. In C.M. Porth (Ed.), *Pathophysiology: Concepts of altered health states,* 4th ed., pp. 187–220. Philadelphia: J.B. Lippincott.

Drug Use During Pregnancy and Lactation

Objectives

After studying this chapter, the student will be able to:

1 Discuss reasons for avoiding or minimizing drug therapy during pregnancy and lactation.

2 Describe selected teratogenic drugs.

3 Discuss guidelines for drug therapy of pregnancy-induced signs and symptoms.

4 Discuss guidelines for drug therapy of chronic disorders during pregnancy and lactation.

5 Teach adolescent and young adult women to avoid prescribed and over-the-counter drugs when possible and to inform physicians and dentists if there is a possibility of pregnancy.

6 Discuss drugs used during labor and delivery in terms of their effects on the mother and newborn infant.

7 Describe abortifacients in terms of characteristics and nursing process implications.

Key Terms

Abortifacient	**Prostaglandins**
Oxytocic	**Tocolytic**

rug use during pregnancy and lactation requires special consideration because both the mother and the fetus or nursing infant are affected. Few drugs are considered safe, and drug use is generally contraindicated. However, many pregnant or lactating women take drugs for various reasons, including acute disorders that may or may not be associated with pregnancy, chronic disorders that require continued treatment during pregnancy or lactation, and habitual use of nontherapeutic drugs (*e.g.*, alcohol, tobacco, others). The major purpose of this chapter is to describe potential drug effects on the fetus and maternal drug therapy to protect the fetus while providing therapeutic effects to the pregnant woman.

Pregnancy and Lactation

Pregnancy is a dynamic state: mother and fetus undergo physiologic changes that influence drug effects. In the pregnant woman, physiologic changes alter drug pharmacokinetics (Table 67-1), and drug effects are less predictable than in the nonpregnant state. Most of the drugs in this chapter are described more fully elsewhere; they are discussed here in relation to pregnancy and lactation. Other drugs are used mainly to influence some aspect of pregnancy. These drugs are discussed in greater detail and include those used to induce abortion (abortifacients), drugs used to stop preterm labor (tocolytics), and drugs used during labor and delivery.

Maternal-Placental-Fetal Circulation

Drugs ingested by the pregnant woman reach the fetus through the maternal-placental-fetal circulation, which is completed about the third week after conception. On the maternal side, arterial blood pressure carries blood and drugs to the placenta. In the placenta, maternal and fetal blood are separated by a few thin layers of tissue over a large surface area. Drugs readily cross the placenta, mainly by passive diffusion. This process, called placental transfer, begins about the fifth week after conception. When drugs are given on a regular schedule, serum levels reach equilibrium, with fetal blood containing 50% to 100% of the amount in maternal blood.

After drugs enter the fetal circulation, relatively large amounts are pharmacologically active because the fetus has low levels of serum albumin and thus low levels of drug binding. Drug molecules are distributed in two ways. Most are transported to the liver, where they are metabolized. Metabolism occurs slowly because the fetal liver is immature in quantity and quality of drug-metabolizing enzymes. Drugs metabolized by the fetal liver are excreted by fetal kidneys into amniotic fluid. Excretion also is slow and inefficient owing to immature development of fetal kidneys. In addition, the fetus swallows some amniotic fluid, and some drug molecules are recirculated.

TABLE 67-1	PREGNANCY: PHYSIOLOGIC AND PHARMACOKINETIC CHANGES
Physiologic Change	**Pharmacokinetic Change**
Increased plasma volume and body water, approximately 50% in a normal pregnancy	Once absorbed into the bloodstream, a drug (especially if water soluble) is distributed and "diluted" more than in the nonpregnant state. Drug dosage requirements may increase. However, this effect may be offset by other pharmacokinetic changes of pregnancy.
Increased weight (average 25 lb) and body fat	Drugs (especially fat-soluble ones) are distributed more widely. Drugs that are distributed to fatty tissues tend to linger in the body because they are slowly released from storage sites into the bloodstream.
Decreased serum albumin. The rate of albumin production is increased. However, serum levels fall because of plasma volume expansion. Also, many plasma protein-binding sites are occupied by hormones and other endogenous substances that increase during pregnancy.	The decreased capacity for drug binding leaves more free or unbound drug available for therapeutic or adverse effects on the mother and for placental transfer to the fetus. Thus, a given dose of a drug is likely to produce greater effects than it would in the nonpregnant state. Some commonly used drugs with higher unbound amounts during pregnancy include dexamethasone (Decadron), diazepam (Valium), lidocaine (Xylocaine), meperidine (Demerol), phenobarbital, phenytoin (Dilantin), propranolol (Inderal), and sulfisoxazole (Gantrisin).
Increased renal blood flow and glomerular filtration rate secondary to increased cardiac output	Increased excretion of drugs by the kidneys, especially those excreted primarily unchanged in the urine. These include penicillins, digoxin (Lanoxin), and lithium. In late pregnancy, the increased size and weight of the uterus may decrease renal blood flow when the woman assumes a supine position. This may result in decreased excretion and prolonged effects of renally excreted drugs.

Other drug molecules are transported directly to the heart, which then distributes them to the brain and coronary arteries. Drugs enter the brain easily because the blood-brain barrier is poorly developed in the fetus. About half of the drug-containing blood is then transported through the umbilical arteries to the placenta, where it reenters the maternal circulation. Thus, the mother can metabolize and excrete some drug molecules for the fetus.

Drug Effects on the Fetus

The fetus, which is exposed to any drugs circulating in maternal blood, is very sensitive to drug effects because it is small, it has few plasma proteins that can bind drug molecules, and it has a weak capacity for metabolizing and excreting drugs. Once drug molecules reach the fetus, they may cause teratogenicity (anatomic malformations) or other adverse effects. The teratogenicity of many drugs is unknown. However, since 1984, the US Food & Drug Administration (FDA) has required that new drugs be assigned a risk category (Table 67-2).

Drug teratogenicity is most likely to occur when drugs are taken during the first trimester of pregnancy, when fetal organs are formed. For drugs taken during the second and third trimesters, adverse effects are usually manifested in the neonate (birth to 1 month) or infant (1 month to 1 year) as growth retardation, respiratory problems, infection, or bleeding. Overall, effects are determined mainly by the type and amount of drugs, the duration of exposure, and the level of fetal growth and development when exposed to the drugs.

Therapeutic and nontherapeutic drugs may affect the fetus. Effects of commonly used therapeutic drugs are listed in Table 67-3. Nontherapeutic drugs include alcohol, caffeine, tobacco, cocaine, marijuana, and heroin.

Alcohol is contraindicated during pregnancy; no amount is considered safe. Heavy intake may cause fetal alcohol syndrome, a condition characterized by multiple congenital defects and mental retardation. High caffeine intake is associated with an increased incidence of spontaneous abortion, preterm labor, and small (for gestational age) infants. Caffeine is present in coffee, tea and cola drinks, over-the-counter analgesics, and antisleep preparations.

Cigarette smoking (nicotine and carbon monoxide ingestion) also is contraindicated. It interferes with fetal growth (decreases infant birth weight and size) and increases the incidence of preterm delivery. Nicotine causes vasoconstriction and decreases blood flow to the fetus; carbon monoxide decreases the oxygen available to the fetus. Chronic fetal hypoxia from heavy smoking has been associated with mental retardation.

Cocaine, marijuana, and heroin are illegal drugs of abuse. Use of these drugs during pregnancy is particu-

larly serious. Cocaine may cause maternal vasoconstriction, tachycardia, hypertension, cardiac arrhythmias, and seizures. These effects increase the risk of spontaneous abortion during the first and second trimesters. During the third trimester, cocaine causes increased uterine contractility, vasoconstriction and decreased blood flow in the placenta, fetal tachycardia, and increased risk of fetal distress and abruptio placentae. These life-threatening effects on mother and fetus are even more likely to occur with "crack" cocaine, a highly purified and potent form.

Marijuana impairs formation of deoxyribonucleic acid (DNA) and ribonucleic acid (RNA), the basic genetic material of body cells. It also may decrease the oxygen supply of mother and fetus. Heroin ingestion increases the risks of pregnancy-induced hypertension, malpresentation, third-trimester bleeding, complications of labor and delivery, and postpartum morbidity.

Fetal Therapeutics

Although the major concern about drugs ingested during pregnancy is adverse effects on the fetus, a few drugs are given to the mother specifically for their therapeutic effects on the fetus. These include digoxin (Lanoxin) for fetal tachycardia or congestive heart failure, levothyroxine (Synthroid) for hypothyroidism, penicillin for exposure to maternal syphilis, and corticosteroids to promote lung function and decrease respiratory distress syndrome in preterm infants.

Maternal Therapeutics

Thus far, the main emphasis on drug use during pregnancy has related to actual or potential adverse effects on the fetus. Despite the general principle that drug use should be avoided when possible, pregnant women may require drug therapy for increased nutritional needs, pregnancy-induced problems, chronic disease processes, treatment of preterm labor, induction of labor, and pain management during labor.

PREGNANCY-INDUCED SYMPTOMS AND THEIR MANAGEMENT

Anemias

Three types of anemia are common during pregnancy. One is physiologic anemia, which results from expanded blood volume. A second is iron-deficiency anemia, which is often related to long-term nutritional deficiencies. Iron supplements are usually given for prophylaxis (*e.g.*, ferrous sulfate 300 mg or ferrous gluconate 600 mg three times daily). Iron preparations should be given with food to decrease gastric irritation. A third type is megaloblastic anemia, caused by folic acid

TABLE 67-2   FDA DRUG CATEGORIES REGARDING PREGNANCY

Category	Drugs
A. Adequate studies in pregnant women demonstrate no risk to the fetus	Digitalis preparation: digoxin Thyroid hormones: levothyroxine, others
B. Animal studies indicate no risk to the fetus, but there are no adequate studies in pregnant women; or animal studies show adverse effects, but adequate studies in pregnant women have not demonstrated a risk.	Angiotensin-converting enzyme (ACE) inhibitors (first trimester): captopril, enalapril, others Antiarrhythmics: lidocaine Antibiotics: penicillins, cephalosporins, erythromycin, cinoxacin, aztreonam Antidepressants: fluoxetine, imipramine, maprotiline, paroxetine, sertraline Antihypertensives: guanadrel, guanfacine Beta-adrenergic blocking agents: acebutolol, metoprolol, pindolol Histamine$_1$ antagonists: azatadine, chlorpheniramine, clemastine, cyproheptadine, dexchlorpheniramine, diphenhydramine, loratidine, triprolidine Histamine$_2$ antagonists: famotidine, ranitidine Thiazide diuretics: hydrochlorothiazide, others Miscellaneous drugs: cromolyn, ketoprofen, naproxen, terbutaline
C. A potential risk, usually because animal studies have either not been performed or indicated adverse effects, and there are no data from human studies. These drugs may be used when potential benefits outweigh the potential risks.	Adrenergics: albuterol, epinephrine, ephedrine, bitolterol, isoetharine, metaproterenol Angiotensin-converting enzyme (ACE) inhibitors (second and third trimesters): captopril, enalapril, others Antianxiety drugs: diazepam, others Antiarrhythmics: flecainide, mexilitene, procainamide, quinidine, tocainide Antibiotics: aminoglycosides, imipenem/cilastatin, norfloxacin, vancomycin Anticholinergics: atropine, scopolamine Anticonvulsants: carbamazepine, gabapentin, lamotrigine Antidepressants: amitriptyline and other tricyclics, trazodone, venlafaxine Antihypertensives: guanabenz, minoxidil, nitroprusside Antiulcer drug: omeprazole Beta-adrenergic blocking agents: atenolol, labetalol, nadolol, propranolol, timolol Calcium channel blocking agents: diltiazem, felodipine, nifedipine, verapamil Histamine$_1$ antagonists: astemizole, brompheniramine, carbinoxamine, terfenadine Narcotic analgesics Nitrate antianginals: nitroglycerin
D. There is evidence of human fetal risk, but the potential benefits to the mother may be acceptable despite the potential risk.	Anticonvulsants: phenytoin, valproic acid Antimanic agent: lithium Salicylate: aspirin
X. Studies in animals or humans or adverse reaction reports or both have demonstrated fetal abnormalities; the risk of use in a pregnant woman clearly outweighs any possible benefit.	Antiviral: ribavirin Retinoids (oral): etretinate, isotretinoin

deficiency. A folic acid supplement (0.8 mg daily) is often prescribed for prophylaxis.

Constipation

Constipation often occurs during pregnancy, probably from decreased peristalsis. Preferred treatment, if effective, is to increase intake of fluids and high-fiber foods. If a laxative is required, a bulk-producing agent (*e.g.*, Metamucil) is the most physiologic for the mother and safest for the fetus because it is not absorbed systemi-

cally. A stool softener, such as docusate (Colace), may be used occasionally. Mineral oil should be avoided because it interferes with absorption of fat-soluble vitamins. Strong laxatives or any laxative used in excess may initiate uterine contractions and labor.

Heartburn

Heartburn (pyrosis) often occurs in the later months of pregnancy, when increased abdominal pressure and a

(*text continues on page 876*)

TABLE 67-3	DRUG EFFECTS IN PREGNANCY
Adrenergics	These drugs stimulate the heart to increase rate and force of contractions. They also may increase blood pressure. Several are teratogenic and embryocidal in animal studies, but no adequate studies have been done in pregnant women. These drugs are common ingredients in over-the-counter decongestants, cold remedies, and appetite suppressants. Oral and parenteral adrenergics may inhibit uterine contractions during labor; cause hypokalemia, hypoglycemia, and pulmonary edema in the mother; and cause hypoglycemia in the neonate. These effects are unlikely with inhaled adrenergics. Oral albuterol (Proventil, Ventolin) and oral or intravenous terbutaline (Brethine) relax uterine muscle and inhibit preterm labor. Terbutaline is used therapeutically for this purpose.
Analgesics, Narcotic	Safety is not established. The drugs rapidly cross the placenta and reach the fetus. Maternal addiction and neonatal withdrawal symptoms result from regular use. Use of *codeine* during the first trimester has been associated with congenital defects. *Alfentanil* (Alfenta) and *sufentanil* (Sufenta) had embryocidal effects in animal studies. When given to women in labor, narcotic analgesics may decrease uterine contractility and slow progress toward delivery. They also may cause respiratory depression in the neonate. *Meperidine* (Demerol) reportedly causes less neonatal respiratory depression than other narcotics and is usually preferred for obstetric analgesia. If respiratory depression occurs, it can be reversed by administration of *naloxone* (Narcan), a narcotic antagonist.
Angiotensin-Converting Enzyme (ACE) Inhibitors	In animal studies, captopril (Capoten) was embryocidal, and enalapril (Vasotec) produced conflicting data. There are no adequate studies in pregnant women.
Antianginal Agents (Nitrates)	Animal studies have not been conducted, and safety for use has not been established. Because the drugs lower blood pressure, a potential effect is decreased blood supply to the fetus.
Antianxiety and Sedative-Hypnotic Agents (Benzodiazepines)	These drugs should generally be avoided. The benzodiazepines and their metabolites cross the placenta freely and accumulate in fetal blood. If taken during the first trimester, they may cause physical malformations. If taken during labor, they may cause sedation, respiratory depression, hypotonia, lethargy, and sucking difficulties in the neonate. Neonatal tremors and irritability also have been attributed to maternal use of the drugs.
Antiarrhythmics	*Quinidine* (Quinaglute) crosses the placenta and reaches fetal serum levels similar to maternal levels. However, there are no reports of congenital defects. Neonatal thrombocytopenia has been reported. *Procainamide* (Pronestyl, Procan) crosses the placenta. Although adverse effects on the fetus have not been identified, quinidine is preferred because of more clinical experience in its use. *Disopyramide* (Norpace) has been found in human fetal blood, and it may stimulate contraction of the pregnant uterus. Adequate studies have not been done, and experience in its use is limited. *Lidocaine* (Xylocaine) has not been established as safe. In animal studies with large doses, *tocainide* (Tonocard) was not teratogenic but apparently increased the incidence of abortions and stillbirths. *Mexilitene* (Mexitil) has not been studied adequately. *Flecainide* (Tambocor) had teratogenic and embryotoxic effects in animal studies.
Antibiotics	
Beta Lactams	*Penicillins* cross the placenta but apparently produce no adverse effects on the fetus. They are considered safer than other antibiotics. *Cephalosporins* cross the placenta and seem to be safe, although they have not been studied extensively in pregnancy. They apparently have shorter half-lives, lower serum concentrations, and a faster rate of elimination during pregnancy. *Aztreonam* (Azactam) crosses the placenta and enters fetal blood, but fetal effects are unknown. *Imipenem/cilastatin* (Primaxin) showed no teratogenicity in animal studies but has not been studied in pregnant women.
Aminoglycosides	*Aminoglycosides* cross the placenta, and fetal serum levels may reach 15% to 50% of maternal levels. Deafness has been reported in children whose mothers received streptomycin during pregnancy. Serious adverse effects on the fetus or neonate have not been reported with other aminoglycosides, but there is potential for harm because the drugs are nephrotoxic and ototoxic.
Tetracyclines	*Tetracyclines* are contraindicated during pregnancy. They cross the placenta, and fetal serum levels reach 60% to 70% of maternal levels. They interfere with development of teeth and bone in the fetus. Animal studies indicate embryotoxicity.

TABLE 67-3	**DRUG EFFECTS IN PREGNANCY** (Continued)
Sulfonamides	*Sulfonamides* should not be used during the last 2 wk of pregnancy because they displace bilirubin from binding sites on serum albumin and may cause kernicterus in the neonate.
Erythromycin	*Erythromycin* (E-Mycin, others) crosses the placenta to reach fetal serum levels up to 20% of maternal level, but no fetal abnormalities have been reported.
Nitrofurantoin	*Nitrofurantoin* (Macrodantin) should not be used during late pregnancy because of possible hemolytic anemia in the neonate.
Clindamycin	*Clindamycin* (Cleocin) should be used only when infection with *Bacteroides fragilis* is suspected.
Antitubercular Drugs	*Isoniazid* (INH) was embryocidal in some animal studies and should be used only if necessary. *Ethambutol* (Myambutol) was teratogenic in animal studies, but administration to pregnant women produced no detectable effects on the fetus. The effects of combination with other antitubercular drugs are unknown. *Rifampin* (Rifadin) was teratogenic in animal studies.
Antiviral Agents	*Acyclovir* (Zovirax), *amantadine* (Symmetrel), *vidarabine* (Vira-A), and *zidovudine* (Retrovir) were teratogenic in animal studies. None of these drugs should be given unless clearly necessary, and *ribavarin* (Virazole) is contraindicated.
Miscellaneous	*Trimethoprim* (Proloprim), often given in combination with *sulfamethoxazole* (Bactrim, Septra), was teratogenic in small animals. It crosses the placenta to reach levels in fetal serum and amniotic fluid that are similar to those in maternal serum. It may interfere with folic acid metabolism in the fetus. A few studies in pregnant women have not indicated teratogenic effects.
Anticholinergics	*Atropine* crosses the placenta rapidly with IV injection; effects on the fetus depend on the maturity of its parasympathetic nervous system. *Scopolamine* may cause respiratory depression in the neonate and may contribute to neonatal hemorrhage by reducing vitamin K-dependent clotting factors in the neonate.
Anticoagulants	*Heparin* does not cross the placenta and has not been associated with congenital defects. However, its use during pregnancy has been associated with 13% to 22% unfavorable outcomes, including stillbirths and prematurity. *Warfarin* (Coumadin) crosses the placenta, and fetal hemorrhage, spontaneous abortion, prematurity, stillbirth, and congenital anomalies may occur. About 31% of fetuses exposed to warfarin may experience a problem related to the anticoagulant. If a woman becomes pregnant during warfarin therapy, inform her of the potential risks to the fetus, and discuss the possibility of terminating the pregnancy.
Anticonvulsants	Although a large majority of women receiving anticonvulsant drugs deliver normal infants, reports suggest an increased incidence of birth defects. Data are more extensive with *phenytoin* (Dilantin) and *phenobarbital*. The drugs may be discontinued before and during pregnancy when the type, frequency, and severity of seizures do not seriously threaten the client's well-being. They should not be discontinued when given for major seizures because of the risk of precipitating status epilepticus with resultant hypoxia and risk to mother and fetus. It is not known whether minor seizures cause fetal risk. Maternal ingestion of these drugs, especially barbiturates, may cause neonatal bleeding during the first 24 h after birth. This neonatal coagulation defect is characterized by decreased levels of vitamin K-dependent clotting factors and prolongation of either the prothrombin time or partial thromboplastin time or both. This may be prevented by giving vitamin K to the mother 1 mo before delivery and during delivery and to the infant immediately after birth.
Antidepressants	Tricyclic antidepressants such as *amitriptyline* (Elavil) have been associated with teratogenicity and embryotoxicity when given in large doses, and there have been reports of congenital malformations and neonatal withdrawal syndrome. *Trazodone* (Desyrel), in animal studies with large doses, caused increased fetal resorption and congenital anomalies. Monoamine oxidase inhibitors, such as *phenelzine* (Nardil), were associated with fewer viable offspring and growth retardation in animal studies with large doses. Overall, clinical experience with these drugs in pregnant women is limited.
Antidiabetic Drugs	*Insulin* is the only acceptable hypoglycemic drug during pregnancy. Dosage requirements usually change, generally increasing during the second and third trimesters. Blood sugar must be monitored closely. Oral antidiabetic drugs are contraindicated. They cross the placenta and may cause hypoglycemia and death in the fetus. They also may be teratogenic.

(continued)

TABLE 67-3	DRUG EFFECTS IN PREGNANCY (Continued)
Antidiarrheals	*Diphenoxylate* (Lomotil) has been used without reported teratogenic or other adverse effects. *Loperamide* (Imodium) has not been studied in relation to pregnancy.
Antiemetics	None of the available antiemetic drugs has been proven safe for use. Nondrug measures are preferred for controlling nausea and vomiting because of possible drug effects on the fetus.
Antihistamines	Histamine$_1$ receptor blocking agents, such as *diphenhydramine* (Benadryl), have been associated with teratogenic effects, but the extent and significance are unknown. Safety has not been established. The drugs should not be used during the third trimester because of possible convulsions and other adverse effects in the neonate. Histamine$_2$ receptor blocking agents, such as *cimetidine* (Tagamet), have not been established as safe. Animal studies indicated no harmful effects on the fetus, but studies in pregnant women have not been done.
Antihypertensives	Beta-blocking agents, such as *propranolol* (Inderal) and others, apparently improve fetal survival. *Methyldopa* (Aldomet) crosses the placenta and reaches fetal concentrations similar to those of maternal serum However, no teratogenic effects have been reported despite widespread use during pregnancy. Neonates of mothers receiving methyldopa may have decreased blood pressure for about 48 h. *Hydralazine* (Apresoline) is often used and is generally considered safe. *Captopril* (Capoten), *clonidine* (Catapres), *guanabenz* (Wytensin), and *guanfacine* (Tenex) are not recommended because effects in pregnant women are unknown.
Antimanic Agent	*Lithium* crosses the placenta. About 11% of infants exposed to lithium during the first trimester had major congenital defects, 72% of which were cardiovascular. In the neonate, lithium has a prolonged half-life due to slow elimination and has caused bradycardia, cyanosis, diabetes insipidus, hypotonia, hypothyroidism, and ECG abnormalities. Most of these effects resolve within 1 to 2 wk.
Antipsychotic Drugs	Phenothiazines, such as *chlorpromazine* (Thorazine) and related drugs, readily cross the placenta. Several studies indicate that the drugs are not teratogenic, but animal studies indicate potential embryotoxicity, increased neonatal mortality, and decreased performance. The possibility of permanent neurologic damage cannot be excluded. Use near term may cause abnormal movements, abnormal reflexes, and jaundice in the neonate and hypotension in the mother.
Antithyroid Drugs	The drugs readily cross the placenta and can cause fetal goiter and cretinism. If given, dosage must be carefully regulated so sufficient but not excessive amounts are given. In some women, thyroid function decreases as pregnancy progresses, and dosage must be reduced. Propylthiouracil is the preferred antithyroid drug. Neonatal goiter occurs in about 10% of cases.
Aspirin	*Aspirin* is generally contraindicated because of potential adverse effects on the mother and fetus. Maternal effects include prolonged gestation, prolonged labor, and antepartal and postpartal hemorrhage. Fetal effects include constriction of the ductus arteriosus, low birth weight, and increased incidence of stillbirth and neonatal death. However, for the pregnant client with rheumatoid arthritis, aspirin is considered the nonsteroidal anti-inflammatory of choice. The lowest possible doses should be given. For analgesic and antipyretic effects during pregnancy, acetaminophen (Tylenol) is preferred.
Beta-Adrenergic Blocking Agents	Safety for use of propranolol (Inderal) and related drugs has not been established. Animal studies with large doses indicated embryotoxicity. Teratogenicity has not been reported in humans. However, problems have been reported during delivery. These include maternal bradycardia and neonatal bradycardia, hypoglycemia, apnea, low Apgar scores, and low birth weight. Neonatal effects may last up to 72 h.
Bronchodilators (Xanthine)	*Theophylline* (Theo-Dur, Aminophylline) has not been associated with teratogenic effects, but adequate studies have not been done in animals or humans. Thus, drug effects during pregnancy are unknown. Theophylline crosses the placenta, and therapeutic serum levels have been found in neonates. There have been reports of tachycardia and irritability in neonates whose mothers took the drug until labor and delivery.

TABLE 67-3 DRUG EFFECTS IN PREGNANCY (Continued)

Calcium Channel Blocking Agents	Teratogenic and embryotoxic effects occurred in small animals given large doses. Diltiazem (Cardizem) caused fetal death, skeletal abnormalities, and increased incidence of stillbirths. Verapamil (Calan) crosses the placenta, but effects are unknown. Adequate studies have not been done in pregnant women. Because the drugs decrease blood pressure, there is a potential risk of inadequate blood flow to the placenta and the fetus.
Corticosteroids	These drugs cross the placenta. Animal studies indicate that large doses of cortisol early in pregnancy may produce cleft palate, stillborn fetuses, and decreased fetal size. Chronic maternal ingestion during the first trimester has shown a 1% incidence of cleft palate in humans. Adequate human reproduction studies have not been done. Infants of mothers who received substantial amounts of corticosteroids during pregnancy should be closely observed for signs of adrenal insufficiency.
Digitalis Preparations	*Digoxin* (Lanoxin) is apparently safe for use during pregnancy. It crosses the placenta to reach fetal serum levels that are 50% to 80% those of maternal serum. Fetal toxicity and neonatal death have occurred with maternal overdose. Dosage requirements may be less predictable during pregnancy, and serum drug levels and other assessment parameters must be closely monitored. Digoxin also has been administered to the mother for treatment of fetal tachycardia and congestive heart failure. *Digitoxin* (Crystodigin) also crosses the placenta and reaches fetal serum levels similar to those of digoxin.
Diuretics	Thiazide diuretics such as *hydrochlorothiazide* (HydroDIURIL) cross the placenta. They are not associated with teratogenesis, but they may cause other adverse effects. Because the drugs decrease plasma volume, decreased blood flow to the uterus and placenta may occur with resultant impairment of fetal nutrition and growth. Other adverse effects may include fetal or neonatal jaundice, thrombocytopenia, hyperbilirubinemia, hemolytic jaundice, fluid and electrolyte imbalances, and impaired carbohydrate metabolism. These drugs are not indicated for treatment of dependent edema caused by uterine enlargement and restriction of venous blood flow. They also are not effective in prevention or treatment of pregnancy-induced hypertension (preeclampsia). They may be used for treatment of pathologic edema from cardiovascular and other conditions. Loop diuretics such as *furosemide* (Lasix) have not been studied adequately in pregnant women. Teratogenesis has not been reported, but animal studies indicated fetal toxicity and death. Like the thiazides, loop diuretics may decrease plasma volume and blood flow to the placenta and fetus. Potassium-conserving diuretics, such as *triamterene* (an ingredient in Dyazide and Maxide), cross the placenta in animal studies, but effects on the human fetus are unknown.
Laxatives	If a laxative is required, a bulk-forming agent, such as Metamucil, is preferred. It is more physiologic than other laxatives and is not absorbed systemically. It is unlikely to harm the fetus. Mineral oil should be avoided because it interferes with absorption of fat-soluble vitamins. Strong laxatives such as castor oil or bisacodyl (Dulcolax) or excessive use of any laxative may cause fluid and electrolyte imbalances or initiate labor.
Nonsteroidal Anti-Inflammatory Drugs (NSAIDs)	Use of *ibuprofen* (Motrin, Advil, others) and other NSAIDs has not been established as safe during pregnancy and should be avoided. There are no adequate studies in pregnant women. In animal studies, delayed delivery occurred. Because the drugs inhibit prostaglandin synthesis, they may cause premature closure of the ductus arteriosus and other adverse effects on the fetus. If taken during the third trimester, they may delay onset of labor and delivery. If taken within 1 wk of labor and delivery, they increase risks of excessive bleeding.
Thyroid Hormones	These drugs do not readily cross the placenta. No adverse effects have been reported in human fetuses, and the drugs are apparently safe to use in appropriate dosages. When given as replacement therapy in hypothyroid women, the drugs should be continued through pregnancy. *Levothyroxine* (Synthroid) also has been given to the mother to treat hypothyroidism in the fetus.

relaxed cardiac sphincter allow gastric acid to reflux into the esophagus and cause irritation and discomfort. Interventions to decrease abdominal pressure (*e.g.,* eating small meals, sitting in an upright position, avoiding gas-producing foods and constipation) may be helpful. Antacids may be used if necessary. Because little systemic absorption occurs, the drugs are unlikely to harm the fetus if used in recommended doses.

Nausea and Vomiting

Nausea and vomiting often occur, especially during early pregnancy. Dietary management (*e.g.,* eating a few crackers when awakening and waiting a few minutes before arising) and maintaining fluid and electrolyte balance are recommended. Antiemetic drugs should be given only if nausea and vomiting are severe enough to threaten the mother's nutritional or metabolic status. Meclizine (Antivert), 25 to 50 mg daily, and dimenhydrinate (Dramamine), 50 mg q3–4h, are thought to have low teratogenic risks. However, possible teratogenesis cannot be ruled out.

Pregnancy-Induced Hypertension

Pregnancy-induced hypertension includes preeclampsia and eclampsia. These serious complications endanger the lives of mother and fetus. Preeclampsia is most likely to occur during the last 10 weeks of pregnancy or during labor. It is characterized by edema, hypertension, and proteinuria. Nonpharmacologic management includes bed rest, in a left lateral position, and a high-protein, high-carbohydrate, low-salt, low-fat diet. The left lateral position increases blood flow to the kidneys and placenta, promotes diuresis, and lowers blood pressure. Drug therapy includes intravenous hydralazine (Apresoline), which does not cause adverse fetal effects.

Eclampsia, characterized by severe symptoms and convulsions, occurs if preeclampsia is not treated effectively. Intravenous magnesium sulfate is the drug of choice to prevent or treat convulsive seizures. Delivery of the fetus is the only known cure for preeclampsia or eclampsia.

MANAGEMENT OF CHRONIC DISEASES DURING PREGNANCY

Asthma

Pharmacologic treatment of pregnant women with asthma is similar to treatment of nonpregnant women. For mild symptoms or infrequent attacks, inhaled adrenergic bronchodilators, such as albuterol (Proventil, Ventolin) or metaproterenol (Alupent), are the drugs of choice. For more severe or more frequent attacks, oral theophylline, oral terbutaline, or an inhaled corticosteroid, such as beclomethasone (Vanceril), may be

required. Severe episodes or status asthmaticus are managed as in nonpregnant women. Although large doses of corticosteroids in early pregnancy are teratogenic, cautious use of smaller amounts may benefit the mother sufficiently to risk adverse effects on the fetus. Cromolyn and nedocromil, which are prophylactic agents, are not recommended during pregnancy because their safety and fetal effects are unknown.

Diabetes Mellitus

For diabetic women who become pregnant, maintaining normal or near-normal blood sugar levels is required for successful outcomes because poor glycemic control increases the risks of birth defects. Pregnancy causes significant metabolic changes, and insulin is the only hypoglycemic drug acceptable for use during pregnancy. Because insulin requirements vary according to the stage of pregnancy, the diabetic client's condition must be monitored very closely and insulin therapy individualized. At the same time, careful dietary control and other treatment measures are necessary. Some guidelines for insulin therapy during antepartal, intrapartal, and postpartal periods are as follows.

Antepartal period. Pregnancy has a diabetogenic effect because of several hormonal changes. First, human placental lactogen (HPL) exerts an increasing diabetogenic effect throughout pregnancy. This hormone increases mobilization of free fatty acids and decreases effects of maternal insulin. Second, estrogen levels increase as pregnancy advances; estrogen is thought to be an insulin antagonist. Third, progesterone may decrease insulin effectiveness. Fourth, cortisol from the adrenal cortex is thought to increase gluconeogenesis and thus cause maternal hyperglycemia.

Some women first show signs of diabetes during pregnancy. This is called *gestational diabetes.* These women may revert to a nondiabetic state when pregnancy ends, but they are at increased risk of developing diabetes at a later time. Other women, who were previously able to control diabetes with diet alone, may become insulin dependent during pregnancy. Still other women, already insulin dependent, are likely to need larger doses as pregnancy advances.

More specifically, insulin requirements usually decrease during the first trimester and increase during the second and third trimesters. During the first trimester, decreased need for insulin is attributed to fetal use of maternal glucose for growth and development. This lowers maternal blood glucose levels and may cause hypoglycemia. During the second trimester, insulin requirements increase along with increasing blood levels of HPL, estrogen, progesterone, and cortisol. It is recommended that women be screened for diabetes between 24 and 28 weeks (by measuring blood sugar after an oral glucose dose of 50 or 100 g). During the third trimester, insulin requirements increase still further, and the largest amounts are likely to be needed near term.

It is especially important that sufficient insulin is given to prevent maternal acidosis. Uncontrolled acidosis is likely to interfere with neurologic development of the fetus.

Intrapartal period. Women with diabetes usually deliver at 37 to 38 weeks of gestation because of increased incidence of fetal death closer to full term. Early delivery is usually induced by oxytocin (Pitocin) or accomplished by cesarean section. Either method precipitates a high-risk situation. During labor, for example, strenuous muscular contractions increase cellular use of glucose and deplete glycogen stores. Thus, less insulin is needed, and hypoglycemia may occur. If a cesarean section is done, the stress of surgery may increase insulin requirements. Regular, short-acting insulin and frequent blood sugar tests are used to control diabetes during labor and delivery as during other acute situations.

Postpartal period. Insulin requirements continue to fluctuate during the immediate postpartal period because stress, trauma, infection, surgery, or other factors associated with delivery tend to increase blood glucose levels and insulin requirements. At the same time, termination of the pregnancy reverses the diabetogenic hormonal changes and decreases insulin requirements. Usually, women are at higher risk of hypoglycemia during the first 24 to 48 hours after delivery, and some may require no insulin during this time. As during the intrapartal period, regular, short-acting insulin is given, and dosage is based on frequent measurements of blood sugar. Once the insulin requirement is stabilized, the client can return to the prepregnancy treatment regimen unless she is breast-feeding. Insulin does not enter breast milk; however, breast-feeding may decrease insulin requirements. Gestational diabetes usually subsides within 6 weeks after delivery.

Oral antidiabetic drugs are contraindicated in pregnancy and lactation. In pregnancy, they cross the placenta, stimulate the fetal pancreas, and may cause fetal hypoglycemia or death. They also increase the risk of congenital anomalies and may cause overt diabetes in women with gestational diabetes because they stimulate an already overstimulated pancreas. If these drugs are taken by a woman of childbearing potential, they should be discontinued before conception if possible or as soon as pregnancy is suspected. In lactation, chlorpropamide (Diabinese) and tolbutamide (Orinase) are excreted in breast milk. The status of other oral agents is unknown. However, they are not recommended for use during lactation because there is a risk of hypoglycemia in the nursing infant. If an oral agent is given to the mother, she should not breast-feed.

Seizure Disorders

Women with seizure disorders, whether receiving anticonvulsant drugs or not, are more likely to have children with congenital defects and mental retardation than women who do not have epilepsy. Thus, the disease and anticonvulsant drugs have potential teratogenic effects, and none of the drugs has been proven safe for use. Despite this, however, women on medication have a 90% chance of having a normal child. Because seizures adversely affect the fetus, the goal of drug therapy is to prevent seizures with the fewest possible effects on the fetus.

If a client has been seizure free for several years, it may be possible to discontinue drug therapy before pregnancy. If drug therapy is required, phenobarbital or phenytoin (Dilantin) may be preferred. Because dosage requirements may be altered during pregnancy, serum drug levels should be measured monthly and the dosage adjusted accordingly.

The effects of gabapentin (Neurontin) and lamotrigine (Lamictal) during pregnancy and lactation are largely unknown. They are assigned to FDA risk category C and are not recommended for use during pregnancy or lactation. Valproic acid (Depakene) is considered the most teratogenic and should not be given to women of childbearing potential.

Hypertension

Chronic hypertension (hypertension beginning before conception or up to 20 weeks of pregnancy) is associated with increased maternal and fetal risks. Thus, appropriate management is mandatory. Nonpharmacologic interventions (avoiding excessive weight gain, sodium restriction, increased rest) should be emphasized. If drug therapy is required, methyldopa (Aldomet) is the first drug of choice because it has not been associated with adverse effects on the fetus or neonate.

Although diuretics are commonly used in the treatment of hypertension, they should not be given during pregnancy. They decrease blood volume, cardiac output, and blood pressure and may cause fluid and electrolyte imbalances, all of which may have adverse effects on the fetus.

Abortifacients

Abortion is the termination of pregnancy before 20 weeks. It may occur spontaneously or be intentionally induced. Medical abortion may be induced by prostaglandins and an antiprogestin (Table 67-4). Prostaglandins may be used to terminate pregnancy during the second trimester. In the female reproductive system, prostaglandins E and F are found in the ovaries, myometrium, and menstrual fluid. They stimulate uterine

TABLE 67-4	ABORTIFACIENTS, TOCOLYTICS, AND OXYTOCICS
Generic/ Trade Name	**Routes and Dosage Ranges**
Abortifacients	
Progesterone Antagonist Mifepristone (RU-486)	PO 600 mg as a single dose or smaller amounts for 4–7 d
Prostaglandins	
Carboprost tromethamine (Hemabate)	IM 250 µg q1.5–3.5h, depending on uterine response, increased to 500 µg per dose if uterine contractility is inadequate after several 250-µg doses
Dinoprostone (Prostin E$_2$)	Intravaginally 20 mg, repeated q3–5h until abortion occurs
Tocolytics	
Ritodrine (Yutopar)	IV infusion 0.1 mg/min initially, increased by 50 µg/min every 10 min to a maximal dose of 350 µg/min if necessary to stop labor. The infusion should be continued for 12 h after uterine contractions cease. PO 10 mg 30 min before discontinuing the IV infusion, then 10 mg q2h for 24 h, then 10–20 mg q4–6h as long as necessary to maintain the pregnancy. Maximal oral dose, 120 mg daily.
Terbutaline (Brethine)	IV infusion 10 µg/min, titrated up to a maximum dose of 80 µg/min until contractions cease PO 2.5 mg q4–6h as maintenance therapy until term
Magnesium sulfate	IV infusion, loading dose 3–4 g mixed in 5% dextrose injection and administered over 15–20 min. Maintenance dose 1–2 g/h, according to serum magnesium levels and deep tendon reflexes. PO 250–450 mg q3h, to maintain a serum level of 2.0–2.5 mEq/L.
Oxytocics	
Oxytocin (Pitocin)	During labor and delivery, IV 2 milliunits/min, gradually increased to 20 milliunits/min, if necessary, to produce three or four contractions within 10-min periods. Prepare solution by adding 10 units (1 ml) of oxytocin to 1000 ml of 0.9% sodium chloride or 5% dextrose in 0.45% sodium chloride. To control postpartal hemorrhage, IV 10–40 units added to 1000 ml of 0.9% sodium chloride, infused at a rate to control bleeding To prevent postpartal bleeding, IM 3–10 units (0.3–1 ml) as a single dose To promote milk ejection, topically, 1 spray of nasal solution to one or both nostrils 2–3 min before nursing
Ergonovine maleate (Ergotrate)	After delivery of the placenta, IM 0.2 mg, repeated in 2–4 h if bleeding is severe Severe uterine bleeding, IV 0.2 mg To prevent excessive postpartal bleeding, PO 0.2 mg two to four times daily for 2–7 d if necessary
Methylergonovine maleate (Methergine)	Same as ergonovine maleate, above

contraction and are probably important in initiating and maintaining the normal birth process. Drug preparations of prostaglandins are capable of inducing labor at any time during pregnancy.

A newer drug, mifepristone, is a progesterone antagonist that may be used to terminate pregnancy during the first trimester. The optimal regimen for clinical use is still being investigated. Both single dose and multidose (over several days) regimens are effective. After a single dose, uterine bleeding usually occurs in about 5 days. Major adverse effects occur infrequently but

may include heavy uterine bleeding and abdominal pain. A prostaglandin is usually given about 48 hours after the mifepristone to augment uterine contractions and ensure expulsion of the conceptus.

Tocolytics

Drugs given to inhibit labor and maintain the pregnancy are called tocolytics. Uterine contractions between about 20 and 37 weeks of gestation are considered premature labor. Nonpharmacologic treatment includes bed rest, hydration, and sedation. Drug therapy is most effective when the cervix is dilated less than 4 cm and membranes are intact.

Ritodrine (Yutopar), terbutaline (Brethine), and magnesium sulfate are used as tocolytics (see Table 67-4). Ritodrine and terbutaline are beta-adrenergic agents that relax uterine smooth muscle and thereby slow or stop uterine contractions. Magnesium sulfate is most often used as an anticonvulsant in the treatment of pregnancy-induced hypertension (preeclampsia), but it also inhibits preterm labor. Hypermagnesemia may occur because tocolytic serum levels (about 4 to 7 mEq/L) are higher than normal levels (1.5 to 2.5 mEq/L). Close monitoring of serum levels and signs of hypermagnesemia is required.

Drugs Used During Labor and Delivery at Term

At the end of gestation, labor usually begins spontaneously and proceeds through delivery of the neonate. Drugs often used during labor, delivery, and the immediate postpartal period include oxytocics, analgesics, and anesthetics.

OXYTOCICS

Oxytocic drugs include oxytocin and ergot alkaloids (see Table 67-4). Oxytocin is a hormone produced in the hypothalamus and released by the posterior pituitary gland (see Chap. 23). Oxytocin functions in childbirth by stimulating uterine contractions and in lactation by promoting movement of breast milk to the nipples. Pitocin is a synthetic form used to induce labor at or near full-term gestation and to stimulate labor when uterine contractions are weak and ineffective. It also is used to prevent or control uterine bleeding after delivery, to complete an incomplete abortion, and to promote milk ejection during lactation. It is contraindicated for antepartal use in the presence of fetal distress, cephalopelvic disproportion, preterm labor, placenta previa, previous uterine surgery, and severe preeclampsia. Ergot alkaloids markedly increase the force and frequency of uterine contractions. They are used after delivery of the infant and placenta to prevent postpartum uterine atony and hemorrhage.

ANALGESICS

Parenteral narcotic analgesics are used to control discomfort and pain during labor and delivery. They may prolong labor and cause sedation and respiratory depression in the mother and neonate. Meperidine (Demerol) is usually the drug of choice because it may cause less neonatal depression than other narcotic analgesics. If neonatal respiratory depression does occur, it can be reversed by the narcotic antagonist naloxone (Narcan).

ANESTHETICS

Local anesthetics also are used to control discomfort and pain. They are injected by physicians for regional anesthesia in the pelvic area. Paracervical blocks involve injection of the anesthetic agent around the cervix; epidural blocks involve injection into the epidural space of the spinal cord. With regional anesthesia, the mother is usually conscious and comfortable, and the neonate is rarely depressed.

Neonatal Therapeutics

In the neonate, any drug must be used cautiously. Drugs are usually given less often because they are metabolized and excreted slowly. Immature liver and kidney function prolong drug action and increase risks of toxicity. Also, drug therapy should be initiated with low doses, especially with drugs that are highly bound to plasma proteins. Neonates have few binding proteins, which leads to increased amounts of free, active drug and increased risk of toxicity. When assessing the neonate, drugs received by the mother during pregnancy, labor and delivery, and lactation must be considered.

At birth, some drugs are routinely administered to prevent hemorrhagic disease of the newborn and ophthalmia neonatorum. Hemorrhagic disease of the newborn occurs because the intestinal tract lacks the bacteria that normally synthesize vitamin K. Vitamin K is required for liver production of several clotting factors, including prothrombin. Thus, the neonate is at increased risk of bleeding during approximately the first week of life. One dose of phytonadione (AquaMEPHYTON) 0.5 to 0.1 mg is given intramuscularly in the thigh at delivery or on admission to the nursery.

Ophthalmia neonatorum, an eye infection that may cause ulceration and blindness, is usually caused by exposure to *Neisseria gonorrhoeae* during passage through the birth canal. It is a sexually transmitted disease for which prophylaxis is legally required. Another serious eye infection is caused by *Chlamydia trachomatis,* also a sexually transmitted microorganism. Erythromycin 0.5% or tetracycline 1% is applied to each eye at delivery. The drugs are effective against gonorrheal and chlamydial infections. Silver nitrate 1% is rarely used because it is effective only against the gonococcus.

Nursing Process

Assessment

Assess each female client of reproductive age for possible pregnancy. If the client is known to be pregnant, assess status in relation to pregnancy, as follows:

- Length of gestation
- Use of prescription, over-the-counter, nontherapeutic, and illegal drugs
- Acute and chronic health problems that may influence the pregnancy or require drug therapy
- With premature labor, length of gestation, the frequency and quality of uterine contractions, the amount of vaginal bleeding or discharge, and the length of labor. Also determine whether any tissue has been expelled from the vagina. When abortion is inevitable, oxytocics may be given. When stopping labor is possible or desired, a tocolytic may be given.
- When spontaneous labor occurs in normal, full-term pregnancy, frequency and quality of uterine contractions, amount of cervical dilatation, fetal heart rate and quality, and maternal blood pressure
- Assess antepartal women for intention to breast-feed.

Nursing Diagnoses

- Risk for Injury: Damage to fetus or neonate from maternal ingestion of drugs
- Risk for Injury: Damage to the pregnant client from acute and chronic health problems
- Altered Nutrition: Less Than Body Requirements related to pregnancy-induced anemia and nausea and vomiting
- Altered Nutrition: More Than Body Requirements related to excessive weight gain with pregnancy
- Anxiety about outcome of pregnancy
- Noncompliance related to ingestion of nonessential drugs during actual or potential pregnancy
- Pain related to uterine contractions
- Risk for Injury related to possible damage to mother or infant during the birth process
- Knowledge Deficit: Drug effects during pregnancy and lactation

Planning/Goals

The client will:

- Avoid unnecessary drug ingestion when pregnant or likely to become pregnant
- Use nondrug measures to relieve symptoms associated with pregnancy or other health problems when possible
- Maintain nutritional status and appropriate weight gain to support maternal health and fetal growth and development
- Obtain optimal care during pregnancy, labor and delivery, and the postpartal period
- Avoid complications of pregnancy and labor and delivery
- Breast-feed safely and successfully if desired

Interventions

- Use nondrug measures to prevent the need for drug therapy during actual or potential pregnancy.
- Provide optimal prenatal care and counseling to promote a healthy pregnancy (*e.g.,* regular monitoring of blood pres-

sure, weight, blood sugar, urine protein, and counseling about nutrition and other health-promotion activities).

- Help clients and families cope with complications of pregnancy, including therapeutic abortion.
- Counsel candidates for therapeutic abortion about methods and expected outcomes; counsel postabortion clients about contraceptive techniques.

Teach clients:

- That any drug taken by a pregnant woman reaches the fetus and may interfere with fetal growth and development. For most drugs, safety during pregnancy has not been established, and all drugs are relatively contraindicated. Therefore, any drug usage (including prescription drugs) must be cautious and minimal to avoid potential damage to the fetus.
- To avoid drugs when possible and use them very cautiously when necessary. If women who are sexually active and not using contraception take *any* drugs, there is a high risk that potentially harmful agents may be ingested before pregnancy is suspected or confirmed.
- Measures to prevent the need for drug therapy, such as a healthful lifestyle (adequate nutrition, exercise, rest and sleep; avoiding alcohol and cigarette smoking) and avoiding infection (personal hygiene, avoiding contact with people known to have infections, maintaining indicated immunizations)
- Nondrug measures to relieve common health problems (positioning, adequate food and fluid intake, deep breathing)
- To see a health care provider as soon as pregnancy is suspected
- To inform any health care provider from whom treatment is sought if there is a possibility of pregnancy
- That many drugs are excreted in breast milk to some extent and reach the nursing infant

Evaluation

- Interview regarding actions taken to promote reproductive and general health.
- Observe and interview regarding compliance with instructions for promoting and maintaining a healthy pregnancy.
- Interview regarding ingestion of therapeutic and nontherapeutic drugs during prepregnant, pregnant, and lactating states.
- Observe and interview regarding the health status of the mother and neonate.

Principles of Therapy

GENERAL GUIDELINES: PREGNANCY

1. Give medications only when clearly indicated, weighing anticipated benefits to the mother against the risk of harm to the fetus.
2. When drug therapy is required, the choice of drug should be based on the stage of pregnancy and available drug information (see Tables 67-2 and 67-3). During the

first trimester, for example, an older drug that has not been associated with teratogenic effects is usually preferred over a newer drug of unknown teratogenicity.

3. Any drugs used during pregnancy should be given in the lowest effective doses and for the shortest effective time.

2. Give medications only when clearly indicated, weighing potential benefit to the mother against possible harm to the nursing infant.

3. Any drugs used during lactation should be given in the lowest effective dose for the shortest effective time.

GENERAL GUIDELINES: LACTATION

1. Many drugs given to the mother reach the infant in breast milk. For some, the amount of drug is too small to cause significant effects; for others, effects on the nursing infant are unknown or potentially adverse. For the latter drugs, it is usually recommended that the mother stop the drug or stop breast-feeding. Effects of commonly used therapeutic drugs are listed in Table 67-5.

USE OF OXYTOCIN

Oxytocin is the drug of choice for induction or augmentation of labor because physiologic doses produce a rhythmic uterine contraction–relaxation pattern that approximates the normal labor process. It is also the drug of choice for prevention or control of postpartal uterine bleeding because it is less likely to cause hypertension than the ergot alkaloids.

(*text continues on page 886*)

TABLE 67-5	DRUG EFFECTS IN LACTATION
Adrenergics	Parenteral *epinephrine* (Adrenalin) is excreted in breast milk; the status of other adrenergic bronchodilators is not known. *Albuterol* (Proventil, Ventolin) had tumorigenic effects in animals; if considered necessary, breast-feeding should be discontinued. Oral drugs used as nasal decongestants (*e.g., pseudoephedrine* [Sudafed], others) are contraindicated in nursing mothers because of higher than usual risks to infants from sympathomimetic drugs.
Analgesics	*Acetaminophen* (Tylenol) is excreted in breast milk in low concentrations. No adverse effects have been reported, and it is probably the analgesic-antipyretic drug of choice for nursing mothers. Salicylates (*e.g., aspirin*) are excreted in breast milk in small amounts. Adverse effects on nursing infants have not been reported but are a potential risk. Narcotic analgesics such as *meperidine* (Demerol) are excreted in breast milk, but amounts may not be enough to cause adverse effects in the nursing infant. Some authorities recommend waiting 4 to 6 h after a dose before nursing. *Alfentanil* (Alfenta) should probably not be given. Significant amounts were found in breast milk 4 h after a dose.
Angiotensin-Converting Enzyme (ACE) Inhibitors	*Captopril* (Capoten) is excreted in breast milk, but effects on the infant are unknown. It is not known whether *enalapril* (Vasotec) or *lisinopril* (Prinivil, Zestril) is excreted in breast milk. In general, nursing is not recommended while taking these drugs.
Antianginal Agents (Nitrates)	Safety for use in the nursing mother has not been established.
Antianxiety and Sedative-Hypnotic Agents (Benzodiazepines)	*Diazepam* (Valium) and other benzodiazepines should generally be avoided. They are excreted in breast milk and may cause lethargy and weight loss in the infant. The drugs and their metabolites may accumulate to toxic levels in neonates because of slow drug metabolism.
Antiarrhythmics	When these agents are required for a nursing mother, breast-feeding should generally be discontinued. *Quinidine* (Quinaglute), *disopyramide* (Norpace), and *mexiletine* (Mexitil) are excreted in breast milk; it is unknown whether *procainamide* (Pronestyl, Procan), *lidocaine* (Xylocaine), and *flecainide* (Tambocor) are excreted. There is a potential for serious adverse effects on infants.
Antibiotics	*Penicillins* are excreted in breast milk in low concentrations and may cause diarrhea, candidiasis, or allergic responses in nursing infants. *Cephalosporins* are excreted in small amounts and may alter bowel flora, cause pharmacologic effects, and interfere

(continued)

TABLE 67-5	DRUG EFFECTS IN LACTATION (Continued)
Antibiotics (cont)	with interpretation of culture reports with fever or infection. *Aztreonam* (Azactam) is excreted in small amounts; discontinuing breast-feeding temporarily is probably indicated. It is unknown whether *imipenem/cilastatin* (Primaxin) is excreted. The aminoglycosides *netilmicin* (Netromycin) and *streptomycin* are excreted in small amounts. Because these drugs are nephrotoxic and ototoxic, the immature kidney function of neonates and infants should be considered. *Tetracyclines* are excreted in breast milk and should be avoided. *Sulfonamides* are excreted and generally contraindicated. They may cause kernicterus in the neonate and diarrhea and skin rash in the nursing infant. *Erythromycin* is excreted and may become concentrated in breast milk. No adverse effects on nursing infants have been reported. However, the potential exists for alteration in bowel flora, pharmacologic effects, and interference with fever workup. *Nitrofurantoin* (Macrodantin) is excreted in very small amounts. However, safety for use in nursing mothers has not been established, and infants with glucose-6-phosphate dehydrogenase (G-6-PD) deficiency may be adversely affected. *Clindamycin* (Cleocin) is excreted. Breast-feeding is probably best discontinued if the drug is necessary, to avoid potential problems in the infant. *Cinoxacin* (Cinobac) and *norfloxacin* (Noroxin) are probably excreted, and there is a potential for severe adverse effects in nursing infants. Depending on the mother's need for the drug, either the drug or breast-feeding should be discontinued. *Isoniazid* (INH) and *rifampin* (Rifadin) are excreted in breast milk, and nursing infants should be observed for adverse drug effects. *Trimethoprim* (Proloprim, Bactrim) is excreted and may interfere with folic acid metabolism in the infant.
Anticholinergics	*Atropine* and others are excreted and may cause infant toxicity or decreased breast milk production. Safety for use is not established.
Anticoagulants	*Heparin* is not excreted in breast milk; *warfarin* (Coumadin) is excreted, but some evidence suggests no harm to the nursing infant. More data are needed, and heparin is preferred if anticoagulant therapy is required.
Anticonvulsants	*Phenytoin* (Dilantin) and other hydantoins are excreted and may cause serious adverse effects in nursing infants. The drug or breast-feeding should be discontinued. *Phenobarbital* is excreted in small amounts and may cause drowsiness in the infant.
Antidepressants	Tricyclic antidepressants such as *amitriptyline* (Elavil) and others are excreted in small amounts; effects on nursing infants are not known. Other antidepressants have not been established as safe for use.
Antidiabetic Drugs	*Insulin* does not enter breast milk and is not known to affect the nursing infant. However, insulin requirements of the mother may be decreased while breast-feeding. Oral agents *chlorpropamide* (Diabinese) and *tolbutamide* (Orinase) are excreted in breast milk; the status of other sulfonylureas is unknown. There is a potential for hypoglycemia in nursing infants.
Antidiarrheals	*Diphenoxylate* (Lomotil) and *loperamide* (Imodium) should be used cautiously during lactation; effects on the nursing infant are unknown.
Antiemetics	Although information is limited, most of the drugs (*e.g.*, phenothiazines such as *promethazine* [Phenergan] and antihistamines such as *dimenhydrinate* [Dramamine]) are apparently excreted in breast milk and may cause drowsiness and possibly other effects in nursing infants. Antihistamines used for antiemetic effects also may inhibit lactation. *Metoclopramide* (Reglan) is excreted and concentrated in breast milk; it should be used cautiously, if at all.
Antihistamines	Histamine$_1$ receptor antagonists such as *diphenhydramine* (Benadryl) may inhibit lactation by their drying effects and may cause drowsiness in nursing infants. For most of the commonly used drugs, including over-the-counter allergy and cold remedies, little information is available about excretion in breast milk or effects on nursing infants. Histamine$_2$ receptor antagonists such as *cimetidine* (Tagamet) and *ranitidine*

TABLE 67-5	DRUG EFFECTS IN LACTATION (Continued)

(Zantac) are excreted in breast milk. *Famotidine* (Pepcid) was excreted in animals, but it is not known whether it is excreted in human breast milk. It is generally recommended that either the drug or nursing be discontinued.

Antihypertensives
Beta-adrenergic blocking agents should generally be avoided by nursing mothers. *Propranolol* (Inderal) and *metoprolol* (Lopressor) are excreted in low concentrations; *acebutolol* (Sectral) and its major metabolite are excreted; it is unknown whether *nadolol* (Corgard) and *timolol* (Blocadren) are excreted. *Methyldopa* (Aldomet) is excreted; effects on nursing infants are unknown. It is unknown whether *hydralazine* (Apresoline) is excreted; safety for use is not established. *Captopril* (Capoten), *clonidine* (Catapres), *guanabenz* (Wytensin), and *guanfacine* (Tenex) are not generally recommended because information about effects on nursing infants is limited. Calcium channel blocking drugs should not be given to nursing mothers. *Verapamil* (Calan) and *diltiazem* (Cardizem) are excreted in breast milk.

Antimanic Agent
Lithium is excreted in breast milk and reaches about 40% of the mother's serum level. Infant serum and milk levels are about equal. If the drug is required, nursing should be discontinued.

Antipsychotic Drugs
Little information is available considering the extensive use of these drugs. *Chlorpromazine* (Thorazine) and *haloperidol* (Haldol) have been detected in breast milk in small amounts. Safety has not been established.

Antithyroid Drugs
Nursing is contraindicated for clients on the antithyroid drugs *propylthiouracil* and *methimazole* (Tapazole).

Beta-Adrenergic Blocking Agents
See **Antihypertensives**.

Bronchodilators (Xanthine)
Theophyline (Theo-Dur) enters breast milk readily; use in caution.

Calcium Channel Blocking Agents
See **Antihypertensives**.

Corticosteroids
Prednisone (Deltasone), *dexamethasone* (Decadron), and others appear in breast milk and could suppress growth, interfere with endogenous corticosteroid production, or cause other adverse effects in nursing infants. Advise mothers taking pharmacologic doses not to breast-feed.

Digitalis
Digoxin (Lanoxin) is excreted. However, infants receive very small amounts, and no adverse effects have been reported.

Diuretics
If diuretic drug therapy is required, nursing mothers should discontinue breast-feeding. Thiazide diuretics such as *hydrochlorothiazide* (HydroDIURIL) and the loop diuretic *furosemide* (Lasix) are excreted in breast milk. It is unknown whether *bumetanide* (Bumex) and *ethacrynic acid* (Edecrin) are excreted. Little information is available about potassium-sparing diuretics, such as *amiloride* (Midamor), *triamterene* (Dyrenium, Dyazide, Maxide), and *spironolactone* (Aldactone). They are not recommended for use.

Laxatives
Cascara sagrada is excreted in breast milk and may cause diarrhea in the nursing infant. It is not known whether *docusate* (Colace) is excreted.

Nonsteroidal Anti-Inflammatory Drugs
Most of the drugs, such as *ibuprofen* (Motrin, Advil), are excreted in breast milk, and nursing is not recommended. However, occasional use of therapeutic doses is probably acceptable.

Thyroid Hormones
Small amounts are excreted in breast milk. The drugs are not associated with adverse effects on nursing infants but should be used with caution in nursing mothers.

ABORTIFACIENTS, TOCOLYTICS, AND OXYTOCICS

NURSING ACTIONS	RATIONALE/EXPLANATION
1. Administer accurately	
a. Give abortifacients PO, IM, or intravaginally.	Physicians administer intra-amniotic agents.
b. Give tocolytics IV initially, then PO. With IV ritodrine, have the client lie in the left lateral position.	The side-lying position decreases risks of hypotension.
c. For IV oxytocin, dilute the drug in an IV sodium chloride solution, and piggyback the solution into a primary IV line. Use an infusion pump to administer.	Oxytocin has an antidiuretic effect and may cause water intoxication. This is less likely to occur if the drug is given in a saline solution rather than a water solution, such as 5% dextrose in water. Piggybacking allows regulation of the oxytocin drip without interrupting the main IV line. Infusion pumps deliver more accurate doses and minimize the possibility of overdosage.
d. Give IM oxytocin immediately after delivery of the placenta.	To prevent excessive postpartal bleeding
2. Observe for therapeutic effects	
a. When an abortifacient is given, observe for the onset of uterine bleeding and the expulsion of the fetus and placenta.	Abortion usually occurs within 24 h after a prostaglandin is given and about 5 d after mifepristone administration. Uterine contractions may be perceived by the client as abdominal cramping or low back pain.
b. When a tocolytic drug is given in threatened abortion or premature labor, observe for absent or decreased uterine contractions.	The goal of drug therapy is to stop the labor process.
c. When oxytocin is given to induce or augment labor, observe for firm uterine contractions at a rate of three to four per 10 min. Each contraction should be followed by a palpable relaxation period. Examine periodically for cervical dilatation and effacement.	Oxytocin is given to stimulate the normal labor process. Contractions should become regular and increase in duration and intensity.
d. When oxytocin or an ergot alkaloid is given to prevent or control postpartal bleeding, observe for a small, firm uterus and minimal vaginal bleeding.	These agents control bleeding by causing strong uterine contractions. The uterus can be palpated in the lower abdomen.
3. Observe for adverse effects	
a. With mifepristone, observe for excessive uterine bleeding and abdominal pain	These effects are uncommon but may occur.
b. With prostaglandins, observe for	
(1) Nausea, vomiting, diarrhea	These are the most common adverse effects. They occur with all routes of prostaglandin administration and result from drug-induced stimulation of gastrointestinal smooth muscle.
(2) Fever, cardiac arrhythmias, bronchospasm, convulsive seizures, chest pain, muscle aches	These effects occur less frequently and are not clearly related to prostaglandin administration. Bronchospasm is more likely to occur in clients with asthma; seizures are more likely in clients with known epilepsy.
c. With ritodrine, observe for	
(1) Change in fetal heart rate	This is a common adverse effect and may be significant if changes are extreme or prolonged.

NURSING ACTIONS	RATIONALE/EXPLANATION
(2) Maternal effects, such as changes in heart rate, arrhythmias, palpitations, nausea and vomiting, tremors, hypokalemia, hyperglycemia, dyspnea, chest pain and anaphylactic shock.	
d. With oxytocin, observe for	
(1) Excessive stimulation of uterine contractility (hypertonicity, tetany, rupture, cervical and perineal lacerations, fetal hypoxia, arrhythmias, death or damage from rapid, forceful propulsion through the birth canal)	Most likely to occur when excessive doses are given to initiate or augment labor
(2) Hypotension or hypertension	Usual obstetric doses do not cause significant change in blood pressure. Large doses may cause an initial drop in blood pressure, followed by a sustained elevation.
(3) Water intoxication (convulsions, coma)	Unlikely with usual doses but may occur with prolonged administration of large doses (more than 20 milliunits/min)
(4) Allergic reactions, including anaphylactic shock	
(5) Nausea and vomiting	
e. With ergot preparations, observe for	
(1) Nausea, vomiting, diarrhea	These drugs have a direct effect on the vomiting center of the brain and stimulate contraction of gastrointestinal smooth muscle.
(2) Symptoms of ergot poisoning—coolness, numbness and tingling of extremities, headache, vomiting, dizziness, thirst, convulsions, weak pulse, confusion, chest pain, tachycardia or bradycardia, muscle weakness and pain, cyanosis, gangrene of the extremities	The ergot alkaloids are highly toxic; poisoning may be acute or chronic. Acute poisoning is rare; chronic poisoning usually results from overdosage. Circulatory impairments may result from vasoconstriction and vascular insufficiency. Large doses also damage capillary endothelium and may cause thrombosis and occlusion. Gangrene of extremities rarely occurs with usual doses unless peripheral vascular disease or other contraindications also are present.
(3) Hypertension	Blood pressure may rise as a result of generalized vasoconstriction induced by the ergot preparation. Hypertension is most likely to occur when ergonovine or methylergonovine is given to postpartal women with previous hypertension or to those who have had regional anesthesia with vasoconstrictive agents (*e.g.*, epinephrine).
(4) Allergic reactions—local edema, pruritus, anaphylactic shock	Allergic reactions are relatively uncommon.
4. Observe for drug interactions	
a. Drugs that alter effects of prostaglandins:	
(1) Aspirin and other nonsteroidal anti-inflammatory agents, such as ibuprofen (Motrin)	These drugs inhibit effects of prostaglandins. When given concurrently with abortifacient prostaglandins, the abortive process is prolonged.
b. Drugs that alter effects of ritodrine:	
(1) Beta-adrenergic blocking agents, such as propranolol (Inderal)	Decreased effectiveness of ritodrine, which is a beta-adrenergic stimulating (agonist) agent
(2) Corticosteroids	Increased risk of pulmonary edema
c. Drugs that alter effects of oxytocin:	

(continued)

NURSING ACTIONS	RATIONALE/EXPLANATION
Vasoconstrictors, such as epinephrine (Adrenalin) and other adrenergic drugs	Additive vasoconstriction with risks of severe, persistent hypertension and intracranial hemorrhage
d. Drugs that alter effects of ergot alkaloids:	
(1) Propranolol (Inderal)	Additive vasoconstriction
(2) Vasoconstrictors	See oxytocin, above.
5. Teach clients Purpose and expected effects of drugs	The drugs are indicated for short-term use, with close supervision by a health care provider.

REVIEW AND APPLICATION EXERCISES

1. Why should drugs be avoided during pregnancy and lactation when possible?

2. How does insulin therapy for diabetes mellitus differ during pregnancy?

3. What is the rationale for using methyldopa and hydralazine to treat hypertension during pregnancy?

4. Which anticonvulsant agents are generally preferred during pregnancy? Which should not be given during pregnancy?

5. In a client receiving ritodrine or terbutaline to inhibit uterine contractions, how and when would you assess the client for adverse drug effects?

6. In a client receiving an oxytocin infusion to induce or augment labor, what interventions are needed to increase safety and decrease adverse drug effects?

7. Which drugs may be used to increase uterine muscle tone and decrease postpartum hemorrhage?

SELECTED REFERENCES

Drug facts and comparisons. (Updated monthly). St. Louis: Facts and Comparisons.

Graves, C.R. (1996). Agents that cause contraction or relaxation of the uterus. In J.G. Hardman, L.E. Limbird, P.B. Molinoff, & R.W. Ruddon (Eds.), *Goodman & Gilman's The pharmacological basis of therapeutics,* 9th ed., pp. 939–949. New York: McGraw-Hill.

Jones, D.P., & Collins, B.A. (1996). The nursing management of women experiencing preterm labor; Clinical guidelines and why they are needed. *Journal of Obstetrics, Gynecology & Neonatal Nursing, 25,* 569–592.

McCombs, J. (1995). Update on tocolytic therapy. *The Annals of Pharmacotherapy, 29,* 515–522.

McCombs, J. (1997). Therapeutic considerations in pregnancy and lactation. In J.T. DiPiro, R.L. Talbert, G.C. Yee, G.R. Matzke, B.G. Wells, & L.M. Posey (Eds.), *Pharmacotherapy: a pathophysiologic approach,* 3rd ed., pp. 1565–1583. Stamford, CT: Appleton & Lange.

Miscellaneous Drugs

Generic/Trade Name	Clinical Use	Characteristics	Routes and Dosage Ranges
Alprostadil (Caverject, Muse)	Treatment of impotence	A form of prostaglandin E-1 Induces erection within 5–20 min	Injection into penis (Caverject) or insertion into urethra with applicator (Muse). Dosage individualized to lowest dose effective for sexual intercourse
Brimonidine (Alphagan)	Glaucoma, increased intra-ocular pressure	Alpha$_2$ adrenergic agonist Contains benzalkonium chloride, which may be absorbed by soft contact lenses. Teach clients to wait at least 15 min after instilling medication before inserting soft contact lenses.	Topically to eye 1 drop q8h
Epoprostenol (Flolan)	Pulmonary hypertension	Adverse effects include hypotension, headache, nausea, vomiting, diarrhea, anxiety, influenza-like symptoms	Continuous IV infusion via central venous catheter. Dosage individually titrated (see manufacturer's instructions.)
Fosfomycin (Monuril)	Urinary tract infection	Broad-spectrum, structurally unique, long-acting anti-bacterial Most common adverse effects were diarrhea and headache	PO 3 g in a single dose. Teach client to mix powder with one-half cup water and drink immediately. May be taken with or without food.
Lidocaine 2.5%/prilo-caine 2.5% (EMLA)	Topical anesthesia for proce-dures involving skin and subcutaneous tissue (e.g., venipuncture)	Contraindicated for use on mucous membranes or abraded skin	Apply on intact skin and cover with an occlusive dressing for at least 1 h.
Midodrine (ProAmatine)	Severe orthostatic hypotension	An alpha$_1$ adrenergic agonist May cause hypertension Recommended only when orthostatic hypotension seri-ously interferes with activities of daily living	PO 10 mg three times daily
Pentosan polysulfate sodium (Elmiron)	Relieves bladder pain asso-ciated with interstitial cystitis	Mechanism of action un-known; it may adhere to bladder mucosa and prevent mucosal irritation by urine.	PO 100 mg three times daily

(continued)

Generic/Trade Name	Clinical Use	Characteristics	Routes and Dosage Range
Remifentanil (Ultiva)	Opioid analgesic for induction and maintenance of general anesthesia	Has a rapid onset and short duration of action	IV, dosage individualized
Riluzole (Rilutek)	Amyotrophic lateral sclerosis (ALS)	Mechanism of action unknown. Adverse effects include drowsiness, nausea, increased liver enzymes.	PO 50 mg q12 h
Ropivacaine (Naropin)	Local anesthetic	Used for obstetric or postoperative analgesia and local or regional surgical anesthesia.	Injection or epidural infusion, dosage variable
Tizanidine (Zanaflex)	Treatment of increased muscle tone and spasm associated with neuromuscular disorders, such as multiple sclerosis and spinal cord injury	Effects peak in 1 to 2 hours and last about 6 hours Adverse effects include dizziness and sedation	PO 4 mg q6–8h initially, increased gradually if needed. Maximum of 3 doses and 36 mg in 24 h

The International System of Units

The International System of Units (Systeme International d'Unites or SI units), which is based on the metric system, has been adopted by many countries in an attempt to standardize reports of clinical laboratory data among nations and disciplines. A major reason for using SI units is that biologic substances react in the human body on a molar basis.

The international system, like the conventional system, uses the kilogram for measurement of mass or weight and the meter for measurement of length. The major difference is that the international system uses the mole for measurement of amounts per volume of a substance. A mole is the amount of a chemical compound of which its weight in grams equals its molecular weight. Thus, the concentration of solutions is expressed in moles, millimoles, or micromoles per liter (mol/L, mmol/L, μmol/L)

rather than the conventional measurement of mass per volume, such as grams or milligrams per 100 ml or dl. A few laboratory values are the same in conventional and SI units, but many differ dramatically. Moreover, "normal values" in both systems often vary, depending on laboratory methodologies and reference sources. Thus, laboratory data should be interpreted in light of the client's clinical status and with knowledge of the "normal values" of the laboratory performing the test.

In addition to other laboratory tests, measuring the amount of a drug in blood plasma or serum is often useful in the clinical management of various disorders. For example, serum drug levels may be used to guide drug dosage (eg, aminoglycoside antibiotics such as gentamicin), to evaluate an inadequate therapeutic response, and to diagnose drug toxicity.

Therapeutic Serum Drug Concentrations for Selected Drugs

Listed below are generally accepted therapeutic serum drug concentrations, in conventional and SI units, for several commonly used drugs. In addition, toxic concentrations are listed for selected drugs. SI units have not been established for some drugs.

Drug	Conventional Units	SI units
Acetaminophen	0.2–0.6 mg/dL	13–40 µmol/L
	Toxic >5 mg/dL	>300 µmol/L
Amikacin	(peak) 16–32 µg/mL	
	(trough) 8 µg/mL or less	20–30 mg/L
Amitriptyline	110–250 ng/mL	375–900 nmol/L
Carbamazepine	4–12 µg/mL	17–50 µmol/L
Desipramine	125–300 ng/mL	470–825 nmol/L
Digoxin	0.5–2.2 ng/mL	1–2.6 nmol/L
Disopyramide	2–8 µg/mL	6–18 µmol/L
Ethosuximide	40–110 µg/mL	280–780 µmol/L
Gentamicin	(peak) 4–8 µg/mL	
	(trough) 2 µg/mL or less	5–10 mg/L
Imipramine	200–350 ng/ml	530–950 nmol/L
Lidocaine	1.5–6 µg/mL	6–21 µmol/L
Lithium	0.5–1.5 mEq/L	0.5–1.5 mmol/L
Maprotiline	50–200 ng/mL	180–270 nmol/L
Netilmicin	(peak) 6–10 µg/mL	5–10 mg/L
	(trough) 2 µg/mL or less	
Nortriptyline	50–150 ng/mL	190–570 nmol/L
Phenobarbital	15–50 µg/mL	65–170 µmol/L
Phenytoin	10–20 µg/mL	40–80 µmol/L
Primidone	5–12 µg/mL	25–45 µmol/L
Procainamide	4–8 µg/mL	17–40 µmol/L
Propranolol	50–200 ng/mL	190–770 nmol/L
Protriptyline	100–300 ng/mL	380–1140 nmol/L
Quinidine	2–6 µg/mL	4.6–9.2 µmol/L
Salicylate	100–200 mg/L	724–1448 µmol/L
	Toxic >200 mg/L	>1450 µmol/L
Theophylline	10–20 µg/mL	55–110 µmol/L
Tobramycin	(peak) 4–8 µg/mL	5–10 mg/L
	(trough) 2 µg/mL or less	
Valproic acid	50–100 µg/mL	350–700 µmol/L
Vancomycin	(peak) 30–40 mg/mL	(peak) 20–40 mg/L
	(trough) 5–10 mg/mL	(trough) 5–10 mg/L

µg = microgram, ng = nanogram, µmol = micromole.

Canadian Drug Laws and Standards

Two national laws, with their amendments, regulate drug-related standards and practices. The Health Protection Branch of the Department of National Health and Welfare is responsible for administering and enforcing the laws, which are described below.

The Food and Drugs Act, initially passed in 1953 and amended periodically since then, regulates the manufacture, distribution, advertising, labeling, and use of drugs. Specific provisions:

- Empower the government to control the marketing of drugs according to proof of safety and effectiveness
- Require that drugs comply with the standards under which the drugs are approved for sale or the standards listed in "specific pharmacopeiae"
- Direct the government to supervise the manufacturing processes of some drugs
- Classify drugs (e.g., antihypertensives, antimicrobials, hormones) that require a prescription and specify that refills must be designated on the original prescription and obtained within 6 months (Schedule F)
- Specify symbols to be placed on containers of the different classifications of drugs
- Require proof of appropriate drug release from oral dosage formulations
- Prohibit advertising of prescription and controlled drugs to the public
- Prohibit the sale of contaminated, adulterated, or unsafe drugs
- Establish requirements for labeling
- Prohibit false, misleading, or deceptive labeling of drug products

The Narcotic Control Act, originally passed in 1961 and amended periodically since then, restricts the sale, possession, and use of opiates, cocaine, marijuana, and methadone. Additional provisions:

- Restrict possession of the above drugs to authorized people
- Require people possessing the drugs to keep them in a secure place, maintain strict dispensing records, and promptly report any thefts or other losses
- Require prescriptions for dispensing narcotics
- Require that containers with prescribed narcotics be labeled with the symbol N
- Specify four levels of controlled drugs. The first level, narcotics, includes single drugs and preparations containing camphorated tincture of opium (paregoric), cocaine, codeine, heroin, hydrocodone, hydromorphone, methadone, morphine, oxycodone, and pentazocine. The second level, controlled drugs or Schedule G, includes non-narcotic prescription drugs, the use of which is restricted to treatment of certain disorders (e.g., amphetamines, methylphenidate, pentobarbital, and secobarbital). The third level restricts anabolic steroids, amobarbital, phenobarbital, diethylpropion, and nalbuphine. The fourth level (Schedule H), includes substances with no recognized medicinal uses (e.g., hallucinogens such as LSD).

Nurses in Canada are governed by these national laws; there also may be local and provincial laws. Legal possession of a narcotic by a nurse is restricted to the following circumstances:

- When administering to a client according to a physician's order
- When performing custodial care of narcotics as an agent of a health-care facility
- When receiving a prescribed narcotic for medical treatment.

Canadian Drug Names

Many drugs are distributed by international pharmaceutical companies, and most names (generic and trade) are the same in the United States and Canada. To assist the Canadian reader in identifying the drugs discussed in this book, generic names and Canadian trade names are listed below. Generic names used in Canada but not in the United States are designated by an asterisk. The chapter number is listed in parentheses. Canadian trade names that include Apo, Novo, or Nu are drugs manufactured by Apotex, Novo-Pharm and Nu-Pharm companies, respectively.

Generic/Canadian Trade Names

Acebutolol (19)
Monitan, Rhotral, Sectral
Acetaminophen (7), Paracetamol*
APAP, Abenol, Atasol, Panadol,
Tantaphen, Tempra, Tylenol
Acetazolamide (65)
Diamox
Acetohexamide (27)
Dimelor
Acetylcysteine (49)
Mucomyst
Acyclovir (39, 66)
Zovirax
Albuterol (18, 47), Salbutamol*
Novo-Salmol, Ventodisc,
Ventolin, Volmax
Alfentanil (6)
Alfenta
Allopurinol (7)
Purinol, Zyloprim
Alprazolam (8)
Apo-Alpraz, Novo-Alprazol,
Nu-Alpraz, Xanax
Alteplase (57)
Activase rt-PA
Aluminum hydroxide (60)
Amphojel
**Aluminum hydroxide gel/
magnesium hydroxide (60)**
Diovol Ex, Maalox, Mylanta,
Neutralca-S

Amantadine (12, 39)
Symmetrel
Amcinonide (66)
Cyclocort
Amikacin (35)
Amikin
Amiloride (56)
Apo-Amilzide, Moduret,
Novamilor, Nu-Amilzide
Aminocaproic acid (57)
Amicar
Aminoglutethimide (64)
Cytadren
Aminophylline (16, 47)
Phyllocontin
Amiodarone (52)
Cordarone
Amitriptyline (10)
Elavil
Amlodipine (53)
Norvasc
Amobarbital (8), Amylobarbitone*
Amytal, Novamobarb
Amoxapine (10)
Asendin
Amoxicillin (34)
Amoxil, Apo-Amoxi, Novamoxin,
Nu-Amoxi
**Amoxicillin/potassium
clavulanate (34)**
Clavulin

Amphotericin B (40)
Fungizone
Ampicillin (34)
Ampicin, Apo-Ampi, Nu-Ampi,
Penbriten
Amrinone (51)
Inocor
Antithymocyte globulin (45)
Atgam
Ascorbic acid (31)
Apo-C, Ce-Vi-Sol
Asparaginase, Colaspase*
Kidrolase
Aspirin (7)
Entrophen, Novasen
Astemizole (48)
Hismanal
Atenolol (19, 53, 55)
Apo-Atenol, Novo-Atenol,
Nu-Atenol, Tenormin
Atracurium (14)
Tracium
Atropine sulfate (21, 65)
Atropisol, Isopto Atropine,
R.O.-Atropine
Azatadine (48)
Optimine
Azathioprine (45)
Imuran
Bacampicillin (34)
Penglobe

Generic/Canadian Trade Names

Bacitracin (65, 66)
Baciguent, Bacitin
Baclofen (13)
Lioresal
Beclomethasone (24, 47)
Beclodisk, Becloforte, Beclovent,
Beconase, Propaderm,
Vancenase, Vanceril
Bendroflumethiazide (56)
Bendrofluazide*
Naturetin
Benzocaine (14)
Topicaine
Benzoyl peroxide (66)
Acetoxyl, Acnomel, Benoxyl, Ben-
zac, Benzagel, Dermoxyl, Desquam-
X, Loroxide, Panoxyl, Solugel
Benztropine (12, 21)
Cogentin
Betamethasone (24, 66)
Beben, Betacort, Betaderm,
Betnesol, Betnovate, Celestoderm,
Celestone, Diprosone, Occlucort,
Rhoprosone, Tara-Sone, Valisone
Betaxolol (19, 65)
Betoptic
Bethanechol (20)
Duvoid, Myotonachol, Urecholine
Biperiden (12, 21)
Akineton
Bisacodyl (61)
Dulcolax
Bleomycin (64)
Blenoxane
Bretylium (52)
Bretylate
Bromocriptine (12)
Parlodel
Brompheniramine (48)
Parabromdylamine*
Dimetane
Bupivacaine (14)
Marcaine
Busulfan (64)
Myleran
Calcitonin-salmon (26)
Calcimar
Calcitriol (26)
Calcijex, Rocaltrol
Calcium carbonate (26)
Apo-Cal, Calsan, Caltrate, Nu-Cal,
Os-Cal, Tums
Captopril (55)
Apo-Capto, Capoten, Novo-
Captoril, Nu-Capto
Carbachol (65)
Isopto Carbachol, Miostat

Carbamazepine (11)
Novo-Carbamaz, Tegretol
Carbenicillin (34)
Geopen, Pyopen
Carboplatin (64)
Paraplatin
Carisoprodol (13), **Isomeprobamate***
Soma
Carmustine (64)
BiCNU
Cefaclor (34)
Ceclor
Cefadroxil (34)
Duricef
Cefamandole (34)
Mandol
Cefazolin (34)
Ancef, Kefzol
Cefoperazone (34)
Cefobid
Cefotaxime (34)
Claforan
Cefotetan (34)
Cefotan
Cefoxitin (34)
Mefoxin
Ceftazidime (34)
Ceptaz, Tazidime
Ceftizoxime (34)
Cefizox
Ceftriaxone (34)
Rocephin
Cefuroxime (34)
Ceftin, Kefurox, Zinacef
Cephalexin (34)
Apo-Cephalex, Keflex, Novo-Lexin,
Nu-Cephalex
Cephalothin (34)
Keflin
Cephradine (34)
Velosef
Chlorambucil (64)
Leukeran
Chloramphenicol (37, 65)
Chloromycetin, Diochloram,
Ophtho-Chloram, Sopamycetin
Chlordiazepoxide (8)
Librium, Solium
Chlorhexidine (66)
Hexifoam, Hibidil, Hibitane
Chlorpheniramine (48)
Chlorphenamine*
Chlor-Tripolon
Chloroprocaine (14)
Nesacaine
Chloroquine (41)
Aralen

Chlorpromazine (9, 63)
Largactil
Chlorpropamide (27)
Diabinese
Chlorthalidone (56)
Hygroton
Cholestyramine resin (58)
Questran
Ciclopirox (66)
Loprox
Cimetidine (60)
Novo-Cimetine, Nu-Cimet, Peptol,
Tagamet
Ciprofloxacin (35, 65)
Ciloxin, Cipro
Cisapride (63)
Prepulsid
Cisplatin, _cis_-platinum (64)
Platinol AQ
Clarithromycin (37)
Biaxin
Clemastine (48)
Tavist
Clindamycin (37)
Dalacin
Clofibrate (58)
Atromid-S
Clomipramine (8)
Anafranil
Clonazepam (8)
Rivotril
Clonidine (55)
Catapres, Dixarit
Clorazepate (8)
Novo-Clopate, Tranxene
Clotrimazole (40)
Canesten, Clotrimaderm, Myclo
Cloxacillin (34)
Apo-Cloxi, Novo-Cloxin, Nu-Cloxi,
Orbenin, Tegopen
Clozapine (9)
Clozaril
Coal tar (66)
Balnetar, Estar, Ionil T Plus,
Tersa-Tar, Zetar
Colestipol (58)
Colestid
Cortisone (24)
Cortone
Cromolyn (47)
Sodium cromoglycate*
Intal, Opticrom, Rynacrom
Crotamiton (41)
Eurax
Cyanocobalamin (31)
Rubion, Rubramin

(continued)

Generic/Canadian Trade Names

Cyclandelate (58)
Cyclospasmol
Cyclizine (48)
Marezine
Cyclobenzaprine (13)
Flexeril
Cyclopentolate (65)
Cyclogyl, Diopentolate
Cyclophosphamide (64)
Cytoxan, Procytox
Cyclosporine (45)
Sandimmune
Cyproheptadine (48)
Periactin
Cytarabine, cytosine arabinoside (64)
Cytosar
Dacarbazine (64)
DTIC
Dactinomycin (Actinomycin D) (64)
Cosmegen
Danazol (29)
Dantrolene (13)
Dantrium
Daunorubicin (daunomycin) (64)
Cerubidine
Deferoxamine (32)
Desferal
Demeclocycline (36)
Declomycin
Desipramine (10)
Norpramin, Pertofrane
Desonide (66)
Tridesilon
Desoximetasone (66)
Topicort
Dexamethasone (24, 65, 66)
Decadron, Dexasone, Diodex,
Hexadrol, Maxidex, Oradexon,
Spersadex
Dexchlorpheniramine (48)
Polaramine
Dextroamphetamine (16)
 Dexamphetamine*
Dexedrine
Dextromethorphan (49)
Balminil DM, Benylin DM,
Formula 44, Koffex DM, Robidex
Diazepam (8)
Diazemuls, Valium, Vivol
Dibucaine (14)
Nupercainal
Diclofenac (7)
Apo-Diclo, Novo-Difenac,
Nu-Diclo, Voltaren
Dicyclomine (21)
Bentylol

Didanosine (39)
Videx
Dienestrol (28)
 Dienoestrol*
Ortho Dienestrol Creme
Diethylpropion (30)
Tenuate
Diflorasone (66)
Florone
Diflunisal (7)
Dolobid
Digoxin (51)
Lanoxin
Digoxin immune Fab (51)
 **Digoxin-specific antibody
fragments***
Digibind
Dihydrotachysterol (26)
Hytakerol
Diltiazem (52, 53, 55)
Apo-Diltiaz, Cardizem, Novo-
Diltazem, Nu-Diltiaz
Dimenhydrinate (48, 63)
Gravol, Nauseatol, Travel Aid,
Travel-Eze
Dinoprostone (prostaglandin E_2)
(67)
Prepidil, Prostin E_2
Diphenhydramine (12, 48, 63)
Allerdryl, Benadryl, Nytol, Sleep-Eze
Diphenoxylate (62)
Lomotil
Dipivefrin (65)
Propine
Dipyridamole (57)
Novo-Dipiradol, Persantine
Disopyramide (52)
Norpace, Rythmodan
Dobutamine (18, 54)
Dobutrex
Docusate calcium (61)
Calax, Colax-C, Doxate-C, Surfak
Docusate sodium (61)
Colace, Colax-S, Doxate-S, Selax,
Silace
Dopamine (18, 54)
Intropin, Revimine
Doxacurium (14)
Nuromax
Doxazosin (19, 55)
Cardura
Doxepin (9)
Sinequan, Triadapin
Doxorubicin (64)
Adriamycin

Doxycycline (36)
Apo-Doxy, Doryx, Doxycin, Novo
Doxylin, Vibramycin, Vibra-Tabs
Droperidol (14, 63)
Inapsine
Echothiophate (65)
Phospholine
Econazole (40)
Ecostatin
Edrophonium (20)
Enlon, Tensilon
Enalapril (55)
Vasotec
Enflurane (14)
Ethrane
Epinephrine (18, 47, 54)
Adrenalin, Bronkaid Mistometer,
EpiPen, Vaponefrin
Ergocalciferol (26)
Calciferol, Drisdol, Ostoforte,
Radiostol
Ergonovine (67)
 Ergometrine*
Ergotrate
Ergotamine (7)
Ergomar, Gynergen
Ergotamine/caffeine (7)
Cafergot
Erythromycin (37, 65)
Apo-Erythro, Diomycin, EES, E-Mycin,
Erybid, Eryc, Eryped, Erythrocin,
Erythromid, Ilosone, Ilotycin,
Novo-Rythro
Esmolol (52)
Brevibloc
Estradiol (28)
Delestrogen, Estraderm, Estrase
Estrogens, conjugated (28)
Congest, Premarin
Estrogens, esterified (28)
Neo-Estrone
Estrone (28)
Neo-Estrone, Oestrilin
Estropipate (28)
 Piperazine estrone sulfate*
Ogen
Ethacrynic acid (56)
Edecrin
Ethambutol (38)
Myambutol
Ethinyl estradiol (28)
Estinyl
Ethinyl estradiol/ethynodiol (28)
Demulen
Ethinyl estradiol/levonorgestrel (28)
Min-Ovral, Triphasil, Triquilar

Generic/Canadian Trade Names

Ethinyl estradiol/norethindrone (28)
Brevicon, Loestrin, Minestrin, Nor-lestrin, Ortho 0.5/35, Ortho 1/35, Ortho 7/7/7, Ortho 10/11, Synphasic

Ethinyl estradiol/norgestrel (28)
Ovral

Ethopropazine (12)
Parsitan

Ethosuximide (11)
Zarontin

Etidronate (26)
Didronel

Etoposide (64)
VePesid

Famotidine (60)
Pepcid

Felodipine (53)
Plendil

Fenfluramine (30)
Ponderal, Pondimin

Fenoprofen (7)
Nalfon

Fentanyl (6)
Duragesic, Sublimaze

Ferrous sulfate (32)
Fer-In-Sol, Fero-Grad, Slow-Fe

Fibrinolysin/desoxyribonuclease (66)
Elase

Filgrastim (44)
Neupogen

Flavoxate (21)
Urispas

Flecainide (52)
Tambocor

Fluconazole (40)
Diflucan

Flucytosine (40)
Ancotil

Fludarabine (64)
Fludara

Fludrocortisone (24)
Florinef

Flumazenil (8)
Anexate

Flunisolide (24, 47)
Bronalide, Rhinalar

Fluocinolone (66)
Lidemol, Lidex, Lyderm, Topsyn Gel

Fluocinolone acetonide (66)
Dermalar, Fluoderm, Fluonide, Synalar, Synamol

Fluorometholone (65)
Flarex

Fluorouracil, 5-FU (64)
Adrucil, Efudex, Fluoroplex

Fluoxetine (10)
Prozac

Fluoxymesterone (29)
Halostestin

Fluphenazine (9)
Moditen

Flurazepam (8)
Dalmane, Somnol

Flurbiprofen (7, 65)
Froben, Ocufen

Flutamide (64)
Euflex

Folic acid (31)
Folvite

Fosinopril (55)
Monopril

Furosemide (26, 56)
Frusemide*
Lasix, Uritol

Gallamine (14)
Flaxedil

Ganciclovir (39)
Cytovene

Gemfibrozil (58)
Lopid

Gentamicin (35, 65)
Alcomicin, Cidomycin, Diogent, Garamycin, Gentacidin, R.O.-Gentycin

Glyburide (27)
Glibenclamide*
DiaBeta, Euglucon, Gen-Glybe

Glycopyrrolate (21)
Glycopyrronium*
Robinul

Goserelin (64)
Zoladex

Guaifenesin (49)
Glyceryl guaiacolate*
Balminil Expectorant, Benylin-D, Resyl, Robitussin

Griseofulvin (40)
Fulvicin, Grisovin

Haemophilus B conjugate vaccine (43)
HibTITER, Pedvax HIB

Halcinonide (66)
Halog

Haloperidol (9)
Haldol

Halothane (14)
Fluothane

Heparin sodium (57)
Hepalean

Hepatitis B immune globulin, human (43)
Hyperhep

Hepatitis B vaccine, recombinant (43)
Engerix-B, Recombivax-HB

Hexachlorophene (66)
pHisoHex

Hydralazine (55)
Apresoline, Novo-Hylazin, Nu-Hydral

Hydrochlorothiazide (56)
Apo-Hydro, HydroDIURIL

Hydrocodone (6, 49)
Hycodan, Robidone

Hydrocortisone (24, 47, 66)
A-Hydrocort, Cortacet, Cortate, Cortef, Cortenema, Corticreme, Cortiment, Cortifoam, Cortoderm, Hyderm, Solu-Cortef

Hydromorphone (6, 49)
Dilaudid

Hydroquinone (66)
Eldopaque, Eldoquin, NeoStrata HQ, Solaquin

Hydroxychloroquine (41)
Plaquenil

Hydroxyurea (64)
Hydrea

Hydroxyzine (8, 48, 63)
Multipax

Ibuprofen (7)
Actiprofen, Advil, Medipren, Motrin, Novo-Profen

Idarubicin (64)
Idamycin

Ifosfamide (64)
Ifex

Imipramine (10)
Tofranil

Imipenem/cilastatin (34)
Primaxin

Immune serum globulin (human) (ISG-IM) (43)
Gammabulin

Immune serum globulin (IV) (43)
Gamimune N, Iveegam

Indapamide (56)
Lozide

Indomethacin (7)
Indocid, Novo-methacin, Nu-Indo

Influenza vaccines (43)
Fluviral, Fluzone

Insulins, animal (27)
Regular
Iletin Regular, Insulin-Toronto, Velosulin

Isophane (NPH)
Iletin NPH, Insulatard, NPH Insulin

Zinc suspension
Iletin Semilente, Iletin Lente, Iletin Ultralente, Insulin Semilente, Insulin Lente, Insulin Ultralente

Mixtures
Mixtard 30/70 (30% regular, 70% isophane), Initard 50/50 (50% regular, 50% isophane)

(continued)

Generic/Canadian Trade Names

Insulins, human (27)
  Regular
    Humulin-R, Novolin-Toronto,
    Velosulin Human (Regular)
  Isophane (NPH)
    Humulin-N, Insulatard Human
    NPH, Novolin-NPH
  Zinc suspension
    Humulin-L, Humulin-U, Novolin-
    Lente, Novolin-Ultralente
  Mixtures
    Humulin 30/70 (30% regular,
    70% isophane), Mixtard 15/85
    human, Novolin 30/70
Interferon alfa-2a (44)
  Roferon A
Interferon alfa-2b (44)
  Intron A
Iodochlorhydroxyquin (66)
  Clioquinol*
    Vioform
Ipratropium (47)
  Atrovent
Isoflurane (14)
  Forane
Isoproterenol (18, 47)
  Isoprenaline*
    Isuprel
Isosorbide dinitrate (53)
  Sorbide nitrate*
    Apo-ISDN, Cedocard-SR, Coradur,
    Coronex, Isordil
Isotretinoin (66)
  Accutane, Isotrex
Ketamine (14)
  Ketalar
Ketoconazole (40)
  Nizoral
Ketoprofen (7)
  Apo-Keto, Novo-Keto, Orudis,
  Oruvail, Rhodis
Ketorolac (7)
  Acular, Toradol
Labetalol (19, 55)
  Trandate
Lactulose (61)
  Cephulac, Chronulac, Comalose-
  R, Gel-Ose, Lactulax, Rhodialax,
  Rhodialose
Leuprolide (64)
  Lupron
Levobunolol (19, 65)
  Betagan
Levodopa (12)
  Larodopa
Levorphanol (6)
  Levo-Dromoran

Levothyroxine (25)
  Eltroxin, Synthroid
Lidocaine (14, 52)
  Lignocaine*
    Xylocaine, Xylocard
Liothyronine (25)
  Cytomel
Lisinopril (55)
  Prinivil, Zestril
Lithium (10)
  Carbolith, Duralith, Lithane
Lomustine (64)
  CCNU, CeeNu
Loperamide (62)
  Imodium
Loratadine (48)
  Claritin
Lorazepam (8)
  Ativan, Novo-Lorazem, Nu-Loraz
Lovastatin (58)
  Mevacor
Loxapine (9)
  Oxilapine*
    Loxapac
Magnesium citrate (61)
  Citro-Mag
Mannitol (56, 65)
  Osmitrol
Maprotiline (10)
  Ludiomil
Mazindol (30)
  Sanorex
Measles, mumps, and rupella
vaccine (43)
  M-M-R II
Mebendazole (41)
  Vermox
Meclizine (48, 63)
  Histamethizine*
    Bonamine
Mechlorethamine (nitrogen
mustard), chlormethine (64)
  Mustargen
Medroxyprogesterone (28)
  Depo-Provera, Provera
Megastrol (28)
  Megace
Melphalan (64)
  Alkeran
Meperidine (6)
  Pethidine*
    Demerol
Mepivacaine (14)
  Carbocaine, Polocaine
Mercaptopurine (64)
  Purinethol

Mesoridazine (9)
  Serentil
Mestranol/norethindrone (28)
  Norinyl, Ortho 1/50
Methoxsalen (66)
  Oxsoralen, UltraMOP
Metoclopramide (63)
  Apo-Metoclop, Maxeran, Reglan
Metolazone (56)
  Zaroxolyn
Metaproterenol (18, 47)
  Orciprenaline*
    Alupent
Methazolamide (65)
  Neptazane
Methenamine (36)
  Dehydral, Hip-Rex, Mandelamine
Methimazole (25)
  Thiamazole*
    Tapazole
Methocarbamol (13)
  Robaxin
Methohexital (14)
  Brietal
Methotrexate (45, 64)
  Amethopterin*
    Rheumatrex
Methyclothiazide (56)
  Duretic
Methylcellulose (61)
  Citrucel, Murocel
Methyldopa (55)
  Aldomet, Novo-Medopa,
  Nu-Medopa
Methylphenidate (16)
  Ritalin
Methylprednisolone (24, 47, 66)
  Depo-Medrol, Medrol, Solu-Medrol
Methyltestosterone (29)
  Metandren
Methysergide (7)
  Sansert
Metocurine (14)
  Metubine
Metoprolol (19, 55)
  Betaloc, Lopressor, Novo-Metoprol,
  Nu-Metop
Metronidazole (37, 41)
  Flagyl, Metrogel, Novo-Nidazol,
  Trikacide
Mexiletine (52)
  Mexitil
Miconazole (40, 66)
  Micatin, Monistat
Midazolam (8)
  Versed

Generic/Canadian Trade Names

Minocycline (36)
Minocin
Minoxidil (55)
Apo-gain, Loniten, Rogaine
Misoprostol (7, 60)
Cytotec
Mitomycin (64)
Mutamycin
Mitotane (64)
Lysodren
Mitoxantrone (64)
Novantrone
Morphine (6)
MOS, MS Contin, MSIR, Oramorph,
Statex
Mumps vaccine (43)
Mumpsvax
Muromonab-CD3 (45)
Orthoclone OKT 3
Nadolol (19, 53, 55)
Apo-Nadol, Corgard
Nafcillin (34)
Unipen
Nalbuphine (6)
Nubain
Nalidixic acid (36)
NegGram
Naloxone (6)
Narcan
Nandrolone (29)
Deca-Durabolin, Durabolin
Naphazoline (18, 49)
Diopticon, Privine, Naphcon,
R.O.-Naphz, Vasocon
Naproxen (7)
Anaprox, Naprosyn, Naxen,
Novo-Naprox, Nu-Naprox,
Synflex
Nedocromil (47)
Tilade
Neomycin (35)
Mycifradin, Myciguent
Neostigmine (20)
Prostigmin
Netilmicin (35)
Netromycin
Nicardipine (53)
Cardene
Nifedipine (53)
Adalat, Apo-Nifed, Novo-Nifedin,
Nu-Nifed
Nimodipine (53)
Nimotop
Nitrofurantoin (36)
Macrodantin
Nitroprusside (55)
Nipride

Nitroglycerin (53)
Glyceryl trinitrate*
Nitro-Bid, Nitro-Dur, Nitrogard-SR,
Nitrol, Nitrolingual, Nitrong, Nitrostat,
Transderm-Nitro, Tridil
Nizatidine (60)
Axid
Norepinephrine (18, 54)
Levarterenol
Noradrenaline*
Levophed
Norethindrone (28)
Norlutate
Norfloxacin (35, 65)
Noroxin
Nortriptyline (10)
Aventyl
Nystatin (40, 66)
Mycostatin, Nadostine, Nilstat,
Nyaderm
Ofloxacin (35)
Floxin
Omeprazole (60)
Prilosec
Ondansetron (63)
Zofran
Orphenadrine (12, 13)
Disipal, Norflex
Oxazepam (8)
Serax
Oxycodone (6)
Supeudol
Oxymetazoline (18, 65)
Ocuclear
Oxymetholone (29)
Anapolon
Oxymorphone (6)
Numorphan
Oxytocin (23, 67)
Syntocinon, Toesen
Pamidronate (26)
Aredia
Pancreatin (30)
Entozyme
Pancrelipase (30)
Cotazym, Creon, Pancrease, Viokase
Pancuronium (14)
Pavulon
Penicillamine (32)
Cuprimine, Depen
Penicillin G benzathine (34)
Bicillin, Megacillin
Penicillin G potassium (34)
Benzylpenicillin potassium*
Megacillin
Penicillin G procaine (34)
Ayercillin, Wycillin

Penicillin V (34)
Phenoxymethyl penicillin*
Apo-Pen VK, Ledercillin VK,
Nadopen-V, Novo-Pen-VK,
Nu-Pen-VK, Pen-Vee, V-Cillin K
Pentaerythritol (53)
Peritrate
Pentamidine (41)
Pentacarinat, Pneumopent
Pentazocine (6)
Talwin
Pentobarbital (8)
Nembutal
Pentoxifylline (58)
Trental
Pergolide (12)
Permax
Perphenazine (9)
Trilafon
Phenazopyridine (36)
Pyridium
Phenelzine (10)
Nardil
Phenobarbital (8, 11)
Phenobarbitone*
Phentermine (30)
Fastin, Ionamin
Phenylephrine (18, 49)
Dionephrine, Mydfrin, Neo-
Synephrine, Novahistine
decongestant
Phenytoin (11)
Dilantin
Phytonadione (vitamin K) (57)
Phytomenadione*
Konakion
Pilocarpine (65)
Diocarpine, Isopto Carpine,
Miocarpine, Pilopine, R.O.-Carpine,
Spersacarpine
Pindolol (19, 55)
Apo-Pindol, Novo-Pindol, Nu-Pindol,
Visken
Piperacillin (34)
Pipracil
Piperazine (41)
Entacyl
Piroxicam (7)
Feldene, Novo-Pirocam, Nu-Pirox
Pneumococcal vaccine (43)
Pneumovax 23
Polycarbophil (61)
Mitrolan
Polyvinyl alcohol (65)
Hypotears, PMS-Artificial Tears,
R.O.-Dry Eyes

(continued)

Generic/Canadian Trade Names

Thiamine (31)
Betaxin, Bewon
Thiabendazole (41)
Mintezol
Thiethylperazine (63)
Torecan
Thioguanine (64)
Lanvis
Thiopental (14)
Pentothal
Thioridazine (9)
Mellaril
Thiothixene (9)
Navane
Ticarcillin (34)
Ticar
Ticarcillin/potassium clavulanate (34)
Timentin
Ticlopidine (57)
Ticlid
Timolol (19, 55, 65)
Apo-Timol, Apo-Timop,
Blocadren, Novo-Timol, Timoptic
Tioconazole (40)
Gyno-Trosyd, Trosyd
Tobramycin (35, 65)
Nebcin, Tobrex
Tocainide (52)
Tonocard
Tolbutamide (27)
Orinase
Tolmetin (7)
Tolectin
Tolnaftate (40, 66)
Pitrex, Tinactin
Tranexamic acid (57)
Cyklokapron
Tranylcypromine (10)
Parnate
Trazodon e (10)
Desyrel

Tretinoin (retinoic acid) (66)
Retin-A, StieVAA, Vitamin A Acid
Triamterene (56)
Dyrenium
Triazolam (8)
Apo-Triazo, Halcion, Novo-Triolam,
Nu-Triazo
Triamcinolone (24, 47, 66)
Aristocort, Aristospan, Azmacort,
Kenalog, Nasacort, Oracort, Triaderm,
Trimacort
Trifluoperazine (9)
Stelazine
Trifluridine (39, 65)
Viroptic
Trihexyphenidyl (12)
Benzhexol*
Apo-Trihex, Artane
Trimeprazine (48)
Alimemazine*
Panectyl
Trimethoprim (36)
Proloprim
Trimipramine (10)
Apo-Trimip, Novo-Tripramine,
Rhotrimine, Surmontil
Trioxsalen (66)
Trisoralen
Tripelennamine (48)
Pyribenzamine
Tropicamide (65)
Diotrope, Mydriacyl, R.O.-Tropamide
Tubocurarine (14)
Tubarine
Urokinase (57)
Abbokinase
Valproic acid (11)
Depakene
Vancomycin (37)
Vancocin
Vecuronium (14)
Norcuron

Verapamil (52, 53, 55)
Apo-Verap, Isoptin, Novo-Veramil,
Nu-Verap
Vidarabine (39, 65)
Vira-A
Vinblastine (64)
Velbe
Vincristine (64)
Oncovin
Vitamin A (31)
Retinol*
Aquasol A
Vitamin B$_1$ (31)
Betaxin, Bewon
Vitamin B$_2$ (31)
Hexa-Betalin
Vitamin B$_{12}$ (31)
Rubion, Rubramin
Vitamin C (31)
Apo-C, Ce-Vi-Sol
Vitamin D (26)
Calcijex, Rocaltrol
Vitamin E (31)
Tocofersolan, alpha-tocopheryl*
Aquasol E
Vitamin K (31, 57)
Phytomenadione*
Konakion
Warfarin (57)
Coumadin, Warfilone
Xylometazoline (18, 49)
Otrivin
Zalcitabine (39)
Hivid
Zidovudine (39)
Azidothymidine, AZT
Novo-AZT, Retrovir
Zinc oxide (66)
Prevex, Zincofax
Zinc sulfate (66)
Anusol, PMS-Egozin

Index

Page numbers followed by f indicate figures; those followed by t indicate tables; those followed by b indicate boxes.

carbohydrates
  description of, 376, 377t
  imbalances of, 381t
  metabolism of, 276–277
    glucocorticoids and, 276–277
    glucocorticoids in, 276–277
    insulin effect on, 324b
    liver and, 763
    vitamins in, 393
Carbolith (lithium), as Canadian trade name, 896
carbonic anhydrase inhibitors
  in ocular disorders, 840t–841t
carbon monoxide, pregnancy and, 870
carboplatin (Paraplatin), 819t
  Canadian trade name for, 893
carboprost tromethamine (Hemabate), 878t
carbuncles, 853
carcinogenicity, 21
carcinogens, chemical, 813t–814t
carcinoma, 815. See also cancer
Cardene IV (nicardipine), 709t
Cardene (nicardipine), 687t, 709t
  as Canadian trade name, 897
Cardene SR (nicardipine [sustained release]), 709t
cardiac arrhythmias. See arrhythmias
Cardilate (erythrityl tetranitrate), 688
cardiogenic shock
  defined, 696
  drugs in, 698, 699
cardiopulmonary resuscitation, adrenergic drugs in, 220
Cardioquin (quinidine), 672t, 675, 679, 681, 682
  as Canadian trade name, 896
Cardioquin (quinidine polygalacturonate), 675
cardioselective blocking drugs, 19
cardiotonic-inotropic drugs, 658
  administration of, 657–658, 663
  amrinone, 658, 660, 663, 665
  client teaching with, 659–660, 665
  in congestive heart failure, 655–666
  contraindications to, 657
  digitalis glycosides, 656–658, 660–662
  in geriatrics, 661, 662
  indications for, 657
  mechanism of action of, 657
  milrinone, 658, 660, 663, 665
  nursing actions for, 663–665
  nursing process for, 658–660
  in pediatrics, 662
  principles of therapy with, 660–662
cardiovascular system
  alcohol abuse and, 188b
  disorders of, 653
    diabetes and, 327b
    drug therapy in, 653
Cardizem (diltiazem), 674t, 677–678, 679, 687t, 883t, 885t, 894
Cardizem SR (diltiazem [sustained release]), 709t
Cardura (doxazosin), 229, 230t, 707t
  as Canadian trade name, 894
carisoprodol (Rela, Soma), 165t
  Canadian trade name for, 893
carmustine (BCNU), 819t
  Canadian trade name for, 893
carteolol (Cartrol, Ocupress), 229, 231t, 708t
  ophthalmic, 839t
Cartrol (carteolol), 229, 231t, 708t
carvedilol (Coreg), 229, 232t, 708t
cascara sagrada (Cas-Evac), 782t
  lactation and, 883t
Casec, 381
Cas-Evac (cascara sagrada), 782t
Casodex (bicalutamide), 823t
castor oil (Alphamul, Neoloid), 783t
  pregnancy and, 875t
Catapres (clonidine), 229, 230t, 707t, 715
  as Canadian trade name, 893
  lactation and, 883t
  pregnancy and, 874t
cathartics, 781, 782t–783t, 783–787. See also laxatives
  administration of, 786
  adverse effects of, 786–787

client teaching with, 785
contraindications to, 784, 785
definition of, 781
diphenylmethane, 783t
drug interactions with, 787
in geriatrics, 786
indications for, 783–784
irritant, stimulant, 781, 782t–783t
nursing actions for, 786–787
nursing process for, 784–785
in pediatrics, 785
principles of therapy with, 785–786
rational use of, 784
saline, 781, 782t, 785
  in congestive heart failure, 785
selection of, 785
therapeutic effects of, 786
cation exchange resin (Kayexalate), 413
caudal anesthesia, 171
Caverject (alprostadil), 887
CCNU (lomustine), 819t
  as Canadian trade name, 896
Ceclor (cefaclor), 458t
  as Canadian trade name, 893
Cedax (ceftibuten), 458t
Cedocard-SR (isosorbide dinitrate), as Canadian trade name, 896
CeeNU (lomustine), as Canadian trade name, 896
cefaclor (Ceclor), 458t
  Canadian trade name for, 893
cefadroxil (Duricef, Ultracef), 458t
  Canadian trade name for, 893
Cefadyl (cephapirin), 459t
cefamandole (Mandol), 459t
  Canadian trade name for, 893
cefazolin (Ancef, Kefzol), 459t
  Canadian trade name for, 893
cefepime (Maxipime), 462t, 463
cefixime (Suprax), 458t
Cefizox (ceftizoxime), 461t
  as Canadian trade name, 893
cefmetazole (Zefazone), 459t
Cefobid (cefoperazone), 460t–461t
  as Canadian trade name, 893
cefonicid (Monocid), 459t
cefoperazone (Cefobid), 460t
  Canadian trade name for, 893
ceforanide (Precef), 460t
Cefotan (cefotetan), 460t
  as Canadian trade name, 893
cefotaxime (Claforan), 461t
  Canadian trade name for, 893
cefotetan (Cefotan), 460t
  Canadian trade name for, 893
cefoxitin (Mefoxin), 460t
  Canadian trade name for, 893
cefpodoxime (Vantin), 458t
cefprozil (Cefzil), 458t
ceftazidime (Fortaz, Tazicef, Tazidime), 461t
  Canadian trade name for, 893
ceftibuten (Cedax), 458t
Ceftin (cefuroxime), 458t, 460t
  as Canadian trade name, 893
ceftizoxime (Cefizox), 461t
  Canadian trade name for, 893
ceftriaxone (Rocephin), 461t
  Canadian trade name for, 893
cefuroxime (Ceftin, Kefurox, Zinacef), 460t
  Canadian trade name for, 893
cefuroxime (Ceftin, Kefurox, Zincef), 458t
Cefzil (cefprozil), 458t
Celestoderm (betamethasone)
  as Canadian trade name, 893
Celestone (betamethasone), 280t
  as Canadian trade name, 893
Celestone Soluspan (betamethasone acetate and sodium phosphate), 280t
CellCept (mycophenolate mefetil), 599t, 601
cells
  immune, 559–564, 560f
  injury to, 7
    inflammatory and immune responses to, 7–10
  malignant, 812

melanocytes, 852
  normal, 6, 7f, 9–10, 812
  skin, 852
cellulitis, 853
central nervous system. See also narcotic analgesics
  abnormalities of
    psychiatric symptoms and, 57
  adverse effects in, 20
  alcohol effect on, 187–188, 188b
  anabolic steroids and, 367
  androgens and, 367
  drug distribution in, 13
  drugs affecting, 60
  drug therapy for. See also narcotic analgesics
  neurotransmitters affecting, classification of, 54–57
  pain and, 62
  physiology of, 54–60
central nervous system stimulants, 192–194, 201–205
  of abuse and dependence, 192–194
  administration of, 204
  adverse effects of, 204
  amphetamines as, 192, 201
  analeptics as, 201, 202, 203
  in attention-deficit-hyperactivity disorder, 201, 203
  client teaching with, 206
  contraindications to, 201
  drug interactions with, 204–205
  in geriatrics, 203
  indications for, 201
  individual, 201–202
  in narcolepsy, 102
  nursing actions for, 204–205
  nursing process for, 202–203
  in pediatrics, 203
  principles of therapy for, 203
  therapeutic effects of, 204
  types of, 192–194
  xanthines as, 201, 202
Centrax (prazepam), 98t
cephalexin (Keflex), 458t
  Canadian trade name for, 893
cephalosporins, 458t, 459t–462t, 463–464
  administration of, 466, 468
  client teaching with, 470
  contraindications to, 464
  description of, 463
  dosage of, 466
  drug interactions with, 470
  first-generation, 458t, 459t, 463
  fourth-generation, 462t, 463
  in geriatrics, 449, 467
  indications for, 464
  lactation and, 881t–882t
  mechanism of action with, 464
  nursing process for, 465
  oral, 458t
  parenteral, 459t–462t
  in pediatrics, 448, 467
  perioperative use of, 467
  pregnancy and, 872t
  principles of therapy with, 465–466
  in renal failure or impairment, 466, 467
  second-generation, 459t–460t, 463
  selection of, 465–466
  third-generation, 460t–462t, 463
cephalothin (Keflin), 459t
  Canadian trade name for, 893
cephapirin (Cefadyl), 459t
cephradine (Anspor, Velosef), 458t, 459t
  Canadian trade name for, 893
Cephulac (lactulose), as Canadian trade name, 896
Ceptaz (ceftazidime), as Canadian trade name, 893
cerebellum, structure and function of, 59
cerebral cortex, structure and function of, 58
Cerebyx (fosphenytoin), 143
  administration of, 149–150
Cerubidin (daunorubicin [daunomycin]), 820t
Cerubidine (daunorubicin [daunomycin])
  as Canadian trade name, 894

cytoprotective agents, 823, 824t
Cytosar (cytarabine, cytosine arabinoside), as Canadian trade name, 894
Cytosar-U (cytarabine ARA-C, cytosine arabinoside), 819t
Cytotec (misoprostol), 770t, 772
    as Canadian trade name, 897
cytotoxic drugs. *See also* antineoplastic drugs, immunosuppressants
    as antineoplastics, 818t–822t
    in immunosuppression, 600–602
Cytotoxin (cyclophosphamide), 818t
Cytovene (ganciclovir), 522t, 524, 530, 531
    as Canadian trade name, 895
Cytoxan (cyclophosphamide), as Canadian trade name, 894

D

dacarbazine (DTIC-Dome), 821t
    Canadian trade name for, 894
dactinomycin (actinomycin D [Cosmegen]), 820t
    Canadian trade name for, 894
Dakin's solution, modified (sodium hypochlorite solution, diluted), 856t
Dalacin (clindamycin), as Canadian trade name, 893
Dalgan (dezocine), 67
Dalmane (flurazepam), 98t
    as Canadian trade name, 895
dalteparin (Fragmin), 737, 738
danazol (Danocrine), 368t
    Canadian trade name for, 894
Danocrine (danazol), 368t, 894
dantrium (Dantrolene), 165t
    Canadian trade name for, 894
Dantrolene (dantrium), 165t
    Canadian trade name for, 894
Daranide (dichlorphenamide), 841t
Daraprim (pyrimethamine), 548
    as Canadian trade name, 898
Darbid (isopropamide chloride), 250t
Daricon (oxyphencyclimine bromide), 250t
daunorubicin (daunomycin [Cerubidin]), 820t
    Canadian trade name for, 894
daunorubicin (liposomal formulation [DaunoXone]), 820t
DaunoXome (daunorubicin [liposomal formulation]), 820t
Daypro (oxaprozin), 81t, 82, 83
DCB (dichlorbenzidene), 813t
DDAVP (desmopressin acetate [DDAVP]), 270
ddi (didanosine [Videx]), 523t, 525
D-Dur (potassium chloride), as Canadian trade name, 898
debridement, enzymes in, 860t
Debrisan (dextranomer), 861t
Decaderm (dexamethasone), 858t
Decadron (dexamethasone), 281t, 286, 858t
    as Canadian trade name, 894
    lactation and, 883t
    in ophthalmology, 844t
Decadron Respihaler (dexamethasone sodium phosphate), 281t
Decadron Turbinaire (dexamethasone sodium phosphate), 281t
Decadron with Xylocaine (dexamethasone lidocaine), 281t
Deca-Durabolin (nandrolone), as Canadian trade name, 897
Deca-Durabolin (nandrolone decanoate), 368t
Declomycin (demeclocycline), 484t
    as Canadian trade name, 894
defecation, 781
deferoxamine (Desferal), Canadian trade name for, 894
deferoxamine mesylate (Desferal), 413–414
Dehydral (methenamine), as Canadian trade name, 896
Delatestryl (testosterone), as Canadian trade name, 898
Delatestryl (testosterone enanthate), 368t
Delestrogen (estradiol valerate), 356t

Delgestrogen (estradiol), as Canadian trade name, 894
delirium, etiology of, 111
delivery
    analgesics in, 879
    anesthetics in, 178, 1778
    ergot alkaloids following, 878t
    oxytocin and, 878t
Delta-Cortef (prednisolone), 282t
delta cortisone, Canadian trade name for, 898
Delta-D (cholecalciferol), 312t
delta hydrocortisone, Canadian trade name for, 8998
Deltasone (prednisone)
    as Canadian trade name, 898
    lactation and, 883t
delusions, 111
Demadex (torsemide), 724t
demecarium bromide (Humorsol), 839t
demeclocycline (Declomycin), 484t, 487
    Canadian trade name for, 894
demelanizing agents, 855, 860t
Demerol (meperidine), 66
    as Canadian trade name, 896
    lactation and, 881t
    pregnancy and, 872t
Demulen (ethinyl estradiol and ethynodiol), as Canadian trade name, 894
Demulen (ethinyl estradiol and ethynodiol diacetate), 358t
Depakene (valproic acid), 145
    as Canadian trade name, 899
    pregnancy and, 877
Depen (penicillamine), 88
    as Canadian trade name, 897
Depo-Estradiol (estradiol cypionate), 356t
Depo-Medrol (methylprenisolone), as Canadian trade name, 896
Depo-Provera (medroxyprogesterone), 357t, 359t, 822t
    as Canadian trade name, 896
Depo-Testosterone (testosterone cypionate), 368t
depression. *See also* antidepressants
    description of, 127
    dysthymic, 127
    etiology of, 127
    major, 127
    pharmacologic management of, 128–136
    types of, 127
    unipolar, 127
Dermalar (fluocinolone acetonide), as Canadian trade name, 895
dermatitis, types of, 852
dermatologic disorders, 852–854
dermatologic drugs
    absorption of, 12
    administration of, 34, 865
    adverse effects of, 866
    antifungals as, 536t–537t, 859t
    anti-infectives as, 854, 858t–859t
    anti-inflammatory drugs as, 854, 859t
    antiseptics as, 854, 855t–858t
    antivirals as, 859t
    application of, 855
    astringents as, 854
    client teaching with, 863, 866
    corticosteroids as, 280
    demelanizing agents as, 855, 860t
    dosage forms of, 864
    emollients as, 854
    enzymes as, 854, 860t
    in geriatrics, 865
    individual, 855t–858t, 858t–859t, 860t–861t
    keratolytics, 854
    melanizing agents as, 855, 860t
    nursing actions for, 865–866
    nursing process for, 862–863
    in pediatrics, 865
    principles of therapy with, 863–865
    retinoids as, 854, 860t–861t
    selection of, 863–864
    sunscreens, 854–855
    therapeutic effects of, 866=867
    types of, 854–855

dermatophytosis, 535, 537, 859t
dermis, 852
Dermoxyl (benzoyl peroxide), as Canadian trade name, 893
DES. *See* diethylstilbestrol (DES [Stilbestrol])
Desenex (undecylenic acid, zinc undecylenate), 537t
Desenex (undecylenic acid, zinc undecylenate), 858t
Desferal (deferoxamine), as Canadian trade name, 894
Desferal (deferoxamine mesylate), 413–414
desflurane (Suprane), 172t
desipramine (Norpramin, Pertofrane), 131t
    Canadian trade name for, 894
    therapeutic serum concentrations of, 890
desmopressin acetate (DDAVP [Stimate]), 270
Desogen (ethinyl estradiol and desogestrel), 358t
desonide (Tridesilon), 858t
    Canadian trade name for, 894
desoximetasone (Topicort), 858t
    Canadian trade name for, 894
Desoxyn (methamphetamine), 202
Desquam-X (benzoyl peroxide), as Canadian trade name, 893
Desyrel (trazodone), 130, 132t
    as Canadian trade name, 899
    pregnancy and, 873t
dexamethasone acetate, 281t, 286
dexamethasone (Decaderm, Decadron, Maxidex), 281t, 286
    as antiemetic, 801, 804
    Canadian trade name for, 894
    dermatologic, 858t
    lactation and, 883t
    ophthalmologic, 844t
dexamethasone lidocaine (Decadron with Xylocaine), 281t
dexamethasone sodium phosphate (Decadron Respihaler, Decadron Turbinaire), 281t
dexamphetamine, Canadian trade name for, 894
Dexasone (dexamethasone), as Canadian trade name, 894
Dexatrim (phenylpropanolamine), 215t, 218–219
dexchlorpheniramine maleate (Polaramine), 633t
    Canadian trade name for, 894
Dexedrine (dextroamphetamine), 201–202
    as Canadian trade name, 894
dexfenfluramine (Redux), 382t
dexrazone (Zinecard), in cytotoxicity, 823, 824t
dexrazoxane, in doxorubicin toxicity, 823
dextranomer (Debrisan), 861t
dextroamphetamine (Dexedrine), 201–202
    Canadian trade name for, 894
dextromethorphan (Benylin DM), 643t, 644
    Canadian trade name for, 894
dextrose and sodium chloride injection, 383
dextrose injection, 382–383
Dey-Dose (atropine), 622
dezocine (Dalgan), 67
DHE 45 (dihydroergotamine mesylate), 85
DiaBeta (glyburide), 331t, 332
    as Canadian trade name, 895
diabetes, gestational, 329
diabetes mellitus. *See also* hypoglycemic drugs, oral; insulin
    biguanide for, 333
    characteristics of, 325
    classification of, 325
    client teaching in, 335–336
    combination therapy in, 339–340
    complications of, 326, 327b–328b
    drug therapy for, 328–333, 329t–330t, 331t–332t
    etiology of, 326
    home care in, 342–343
    hormone-induced, 326
    hypoglycemic drugs for, oral, 331t–332t, 332–333
    insulin-dependent, 325
    insulin therapy for, 328, 329t–330t, 332

M

Maalox (aluminum hydroxide-magnesium hydroxide), 771
Maalox No 1 and No 2 tablets, 768t
Maalox Plus, 768t
Maalox suspension, 768t
MAC. See also *mycobacterium avium* complex (MAC) disease
Macrodantin (nitrofurantoin), 488t
  as Canadian trade name, 897
  lactation and, 882t
  pregnancy and, 873t
macrolides, 495–504. See also anti-infective drugs; anti-infective drugs, erythromycin
  administration of, 502
  adverse effects of, 502–503
  client teaching with, 504
  contraindications to, 497
  culture and susceptibility studies with, 500
  drug interactions with, 503–504
  erythromycin as prototype, 496
  in geriatrics, 449, 501
  indications for, 496–497
  in liver disease, 501
  mechanism of action of, 496
  in *Mycobacterium avium* complex disease, 496
  nursing process for, 500
  in pediatrics, 501
  principles of therapy with, 500–501
  in renal failure, 501
  therapeutic effects with, 502
macronutrients, 409, 409t–410t, 411. See also minerals
mafenide (Sulfamylon), 487t
magnesia magma (magnesium hydroxide), 782t
magnesium
  description of, 410t
  imbalances of, 413t
    treatment of, 425
  preparation of, 421
magnesium citrate, Canadian trade name for, 896
magnesium citrate solution, 782t
magnesium hydroxide (milk of magnesia, magnesia magma), 421, 782t
magnesium oxide, 421
magnesium sulfate, 421, 428, 429
  administration of, 428
  in arrhythmia, 675t, 678
  in pregnancy, 878t, 879
malaria, 543–544, 550
malathion (Ovide), 550
malignancies. See neoplasms, malignant
Mandelamine (methenamine mandelate), 488t
  as Canadian trade name, 896
Mandol (cefamandole), 459t
  as Canadian trade name, 893
mannitol (Osmitrol), 724t
  Canadian trade name for, 896
  in ocular disorders, 841t
Maolate (chlorphenesin), 165t
maprotiline (Ludiomil), 129, 132t
  Canadian trade name for, 896
  therapeutic serum concentrations of, 890
Marcaine (bupivacaine), 176t
  as Canadian trade name, 893
Marezine (cyclizine), 634t, 802t
  as Canadian trade name, 894
marijuana, 194–195. See also drug abuse
  abuse of, 194–195
  dependence on, 195
  pregnancy and, 870
Marinol (dronabinol), 194–195, 803t, 804
masoprocol (Actinex), 861t
mast cell stabilizers, 623–624
  in bronchoconstrictive disorders, 623–624
  contraindications to, 620
  mechanism of action with, 620
Matulane (procarbazine), 822t
Mavik (trandolapril), 707t
Maxair (pirbuterol), 215t, 621, 626
Maxenal (pseudoephedrine), as Canadian trade name, 898

Maxeran (metoclopramide), as Canadian trade name, 896
Maxidex (dexamethasone)
  as Canadian trade name, 894
  in ophthalmology, 844t
Maxiflor (diflorasone), 858t
Maxipime (cefepime), 462t, 463
Maxzide (hydrochlorothiazide and triamterene), 724t
  lactation and, 883t
mazindol (Sanorex), 382t
  Canadian trade name for, 896
MCT Oil, 382
MDR-TB. See multidrug-resistant tuberculosis (MDR-TB)
measles, mumps, rubella vaccine (M-M-R-II), 571t, 581
  Canadian trade name for, 896
measles and rubella vaccine (M-R-Vax II), 571t
measles vaccine (Attenuvax), 571t
Mebaral (mephobarbital), 96t
mebendazole (Vermox), 549
  Canadian trade name for, 896
mechlorethamine (nitrogen mustard [Mustargen]), 818t
meclizine (Antivert, Bonine), 634t
  as antiemetic, 802t
  Canadian trade name for, 896
meclofenamate (Meclomen), 84
Meclomen (meclofenamate), 84
mechlorethamine (nitrogen mustard), chlormethine, Canadian trade name for, 896
medication. See drugs, drug therapy
medication errors, prevention of, 23
medication history, 40b
medication orders, 24
medication system, 24
Medipren (ibuprofen), as Canadian trade name, 895
Medrol acetate (methylprednisolone acetate), 858t
Medrol (methylprednisolone), 282t
Medrol (methylprenisolone), as Canadian trade name, 896
medroxyprogesterone (Depo-Provera, Provera), 359t
  as antineoplastic agent, 822t
  Canadian trade name for, 896
  indications, routes, dosages for, 357t
medrysone (HMS Liquifilm), in ocular disorders, 844t
medulla oblongata, structure and function of, 58
mefenamic acid, 84
mefloquine (Lariam), 547
Mefoxin (cefoxitin), 460t
  as Canadian trade name, 893
Megace (megestrol), 357t
  as Canadian trade name, 896
Megacillin (penicillin G benzathine)
  as Canadian trade name, 897
megestrol (Megace), 822t
  Canadian trade name for, 896
melanizing agents, 855t, 860t
melanocyte-stimulating hormone, 268
melanocyte-stimulating hormone-inhibiting factor, 267
melanocyte-stimulating hormone-releasing factor, 267
Mellaril (thioridazine), 115t
  as Canadian trade name, 899
melphalan (Alkeran), 818t
  Canadian trade name for, 896
menadione sodium diphosphate (Synkayvite), 401t
meningitis vaccine (Menomune A/C, Menomune A/C/Y/W/-135), 572t
Menomune A/C (meningitis vaccine), 572t
Menomune A/C/Y/W/-135 (meningitis vaccine), 572t
menopause, estrogen replacement in, 354, 355t–356t, 360
menotropins (Pergonal), 269
menstrual cycle, estrogens during, 352
mepenzolate bromide (Cantil), 250t

meperidine (Demerol), 66
  Canadian trade name for, 896
  in delivery, 879
  lactation and, 881t
  pregnancy and, 872t
mephobarbital (Mebaral), 96t
Mephyton (phytonadione)
  routes and dosage ranges for, 401t
mepivacaine (Carbocaine), 176t
  Canadian trade name for, 896
Mepron (atovaquone), 548
mercaptopurine (Purinethol), 819t
  Canadian trade name for, 896
meropenem (Merrem), 464
Merrem (meropenem), 464
Meruvax II (rubella vaccine), 573t–574t
mescaline, 195
mesgestrol acetate (Megace)
  indications, routes, dosages for, 357t
mesna (Mesnex), 823, 824t
  in ifosfamide toxicity, 823
Mesnex (mesna), 823, 824t
mesoridazine (Serentil), 114t
  Canadian trade name for, 896
Mestinon (pyridostigmine), 242
  as Canadian trade name, 898
mestranol and norethindrone
  Canadian trade name for, 896
metabolism
  brain, 59
  defined, 13
  enzyme induction in, 13–14
  enzyme inhibition in, 14
  estrogens and, 352
  in geriatrics, 45t
  glucocorticoids and, 276–277
  liver in, 762
  in pediatric patient, 43t
  vitamins in, 393
metacortandracin, Canadian trade name for, 898
metacortandrolone, Canadian trade name for, 898
Metahydrin (trichlormethiazide), 723t
metal chelating agents, 413–414, 419
metallic antiseptics, 856t
metallic ores, as carcinogens, 813t
Metamucil (psyllium hydrophilic muciloid), 782t, 794t, 795
  as Canadian trade name, 898
Metandren (methylestosterone), as Canadian trade name, 896
metaproterenol (Alupent), 215t, 621, 626
  Canadian trade name for, 896
  in pediatrics, 626
  in pregnancy, 876
metaraminol (Aramine), 215t, 697
metaxalone (Skelaxin), 165t
metformin (Glucophage), 332t, 333, 346
  contraindications to, 333–334
methadone, 187t
  in opiate dependence, 191–192
methadone (Dolophine), 66
methamphetamine (Desoxyn), 202
methamphetamine (ice), 192
methantheline bromide (Banthine), 250t
methazolamide (Neptazane)
  Canadian trade name for, 896
  in ocular disorders, 841t
methdilazine (Tacaryl), 633t
methenamine, Canadian trade name for, 896
methenamine hippurate (Hiprex), 488t
methenamine mandelate (Mandelamine), 488t
  urine pH and, 491
Methergine (methylergonovine maleate), postpartum, 878t, 879
methicillin (Staphcillin), 456t, 457
  resistance to, *Staphylococcus aureus*, 442b
methimazole (Tapazole), 300
  adverse effects of, 305
  Canadian trade name for, 896
  in geriatrics, 303
  lactation and, 883t
  in pediatrics, 303

O

beta-adrenergic, 214, 215
in drug action, 14–16
of narcotic analgesics, 63, 64t
neurotransmitter, 128
opiate, 63, 64t
receptor theory of drug action, 14–15
Recombivax HB (hepatitis B vaccine [recombinant]), 570t
rectal suppositories
in fecal impaction, 785
insertion of, 35
Redux (dexfenfluramine), 382t
refractive errors, diagnostic ophthalmic drugs in, 838
Regitine (phentolamine), 229, 230t
Reglan (metoclopramide), 803t, 804
as Canadian trade name, 896
lactation and, 882t
Regonol (pyridostigmine), as Canadian trade name, 898
Rela (carisoprodol), 165t
Relafen (nabumetone), 81t, 83
Remeron (mirtazapine), 129–130, 132t
remifentanil (Ultiva), 888
renal colic, anticholinergics in, 250
renal disorders, corticosteroids in, 284
renal failure
antacids and, 771
beta-blockers and, 234
macrolides in, 501
tetracyclines in, 487, 489
renal function, alterations in, 725
renal impairment
antihypertensive drugs in, 714
vancomycin in, 501
renal insufficiency
anti-infective drugs and, 448
hypoglycemic drugs in, oral, 342
renal physiology, 722, 725
Renese (polythiazide), 723t
Renoquid (sulfacytine), 485t
ReoPro (abciximab), 739
reserpine (Serpasil), 708t
resorcinol, 858t
RespiGam (respiratory syncytial virus immune globulin intravenous) (human [RSV-IGIV]), 577t
respiration
defined, 616
requirements for, 617
respiratory disorders
theophylline in, 202
respiratory syncytial virus immune globulin intravenous (human [RSV-IGIV]) (Hypermune RSV, RespiGam), 577t
respiratory syncytial virus (RSV) respiratory infections, antiviral drugs in, 524t, 526–527
respiratory system
disorders of, 617
anticholinergics in, 250
asthma, 619
bronchitis, chronic, 619
corticosteroids in, 284, 286
drug therapy for, 417
emphysema, 619
glucocorticoids and, 277
infections of, macrolides in, 496–497
physiology of, 615–617
signs and symptoms of, 641
Restoril (temazepam), 98t
Restorit (temazepam), as Canadian trade name, 898
Resyl (guaifenesin), as Canadian trade name, 895
reticular activating system, structure and function of, 59
Retin-A (tretinoin [retinoic acid]), 861t
as Canadian trade name, 899
retinoids, 854, 860t–861t
in dermatology, 854, 860t–861t
retinol (vitamin A), 393t
retinopathy, diabetic, 327b–328b

Retrovir (zidovudine), 523t–524t, 525, 530, 531
as Canadian trade name, 899
pregnancy and, 873t
Revex (nalmefene), 68
ReVia (naltrexone), 68, 187t, 192
Revimine (dopamine), as Canadian trade name, 894
Rezulin (troglitazone), 332t, 333
rheumatoid arthritis, 81t, 88
Rheumatrex (methotrexate [MXT]), 88
as Canadian trade name, 896
in immunosuppression, 599t, 600–601
Rhinalar (flunisolide), as Canadian trade name, 895
rhinitis, 641
Rhinocort (budesonide), 280t
rhinorrhea, 641
Rhodialax (lactulose)
as Canadian trade name, 896
Rhodialose (lactulose), as Canadian trade name, 896
Rho (D) immune globulin, human, Canadian trade name for, 898
Rho (D) immune globulin (human) (Gamulin Rh, HypRho-D, Rho-GAM), 577t
Rhodis (ketoprofen), as Canadian trade name, 896
Rho-GAM (Rho (D) immune globulin [human]), 577t
Rhoprosone (betamethasone), as Canadian trade name, 893
Rhotrimine (trimipramine), as Canadian trade name, 899
Rhythmol (propafenone), 673t, 676, 680, 681
ribavirin (Virazole), 524t, 526–527
Canadian trade name for, 898
pregnancy and, 871t, 873t
Ribodex (dextromethorphan), as Canadian trade name, 894
riboflavin (vitamin B$_2$)
imbalance of, 395t–396t
as nutrient, 395t–396t
routes and dosage ranges for, 401t
RID (pyrethrin), 550
rifabutin (Mycobutin), 511–512
Rifadin (rifampin)
as Canadian trade name, 898
lactation and, 882t
pregnancy and, 873t
rifamate, in multidrug-resistant tuberculosis, 511
rifampin (Rifadin), 509–510
Canadian trade name for, 898
in combination therapy, 510
lactation and, 882t
in liver disease, 513
pregnancy and, 873t
Rifater, in multidrug-resistant tuberculosis, 511
Rilutek (riluzole), 888
riluzole (Rilutek), 888
Rimactane (rifampin), as Canadian trade name, 898
rimantadine (Flumadine), 524t, 526, 531
Ringer's solution, 422
ringworm (tinea), 853
Risperdal (risperidone), 117
risperidone (Risperdal), 117
Ritalin (methylphenidate), 203
ritodrine (Yutopar)
Canadian trade name for, 898
in pregnancy, 878t, 879
ritonavir (Norvir), 523t, 525, 530, 531
Rivotril (clonazepam), as Canadian trade name, 893
R.O.-Atropine (atropine sulfate), as Canadian trade name, 892
R.O.-Carpine (pilocarpine), as Canadian trade name, 897
R.O.-Dry Eyes (polyvinyl alcohol), as Canadian trade name, 897
R.O.-Eye Drops (tetrahydrozoline), as Canadian trade name, 898
R.O.-Gentycin (gentamicin), as Canadian trade name, 895
R.O.-Naphz (naphazoline), as Canadian trade name, 897

R.O.-Predphate (prednisolone), as Canadian trade name, 898
R.O.-Tropamide (tropicamide), as Canadian trade name, 899
Robaxin (methocarbamol), 165t
as Canadian trade name, 896
Robidone (hydrocodone), as Canadian trade name, 895
Robidrine (pseudoephedrine), as Canadian trade name, 898
Robinul (glycopyrrolate), 250t, 255
as Canadian trade name, 895
Robitussin-CF (guaifenesin), 645t
Robitussin-DM (guaifenesin), 645t
Robitussin (guaifenesin), 643t
as Canadian trade name, 895
Robitussin-PE (guaifenesin), 645t
Rocaltrol (calcitriol), 312t
as Canadian trade name, 893, 899
Rocephin (ceftriaxone), 461t
as Canadian trade name, 893
rocuronium (Zemuron), 175t
Rofact (rifampin), as Canadian trade name, 898
Roferon-A (interferon-alfa-2a), 588t
Roferon A (interferon alfa-2a), as Canadian trade name, 896
Rogaine (minoxidil), as Canadian trade name, 897
Romazicon (flumazenil), 186t
ropivacaine (Naropin), 888
Rose bengal, ophthalmic dye, 838
Roubac (trimethoprim-sulfamethoxazole [TMP-SMX]), as Canadian drug name, 898
roundworm infections (ascariasis), 544. See also anthelmintics
route, drug administration
abbreviations for, 24t
drug action and, 16
intramuscular, 28, 28f, 29f
intravenous, 28
nasogastric, 27, 32
nursing process and, 48
oral, 27
parenteral, 27–29
subcutaneous, 27–28, 28f
topical, 29
nursing actions in, 34
Roxicodone (oxycodone), 66
Roychlor (potassium chloride), as Canadian trade name, 898
Rubbing Alcohol U.S.P. (isopropyl alcohol), dermatologic, 855t
rubella and mumps vaccine (Biavax-II), 574t
rubella vaccine (Meruvax II), 573t–574t
Rubion (cyanocobalamin, vitamin B$_{12}$), as Canadian trade name, 893, 899
Rubramin (cyanocobalamin, vitamin B$_{12}$)
Canadian trade name for, 893, 899
routes and dosage ranges for, 401t
RU-486 (mifepristone), 878t
Rynacrom (cromolyn), as Canadian trade name, 893
Rythmodan (disopyramide), as Canadian trade name, 894
Rythmol (propafenone), as Canadian trade name, 898

S

Sabin poliovirus vaccine, 573t
Sabin vaccine (poliovirus vaccine trivalent [Onmune]), 573t
Salazopyrin (sulfazalazine), as Canadian trade name, 898
salbutamol. See albuterol
salicylate
lactation and, 881t
therapeutic serum concentrations of, 890
salicylic acid, 854, 861t
salicylism, 87
saline cathartics, 781, 782t, 785
edema and congestive heart failure and, 785
renal failure and, 785